*Swearingen's*

# All-in-One

## NURSING CARE PLANNING RESOURCE

*Medical-Surgical, Pediatric, Maternity, and Psychiatric–Mental Health*

EDITION 6

# *Swearingen's*
# All-in-One
## NURSING CARE PLANNING RESOURCE

*Medical-Surgical, Pediatric, Maternity, and Psychiatric–Mental Health*

## Julie S. Snyder, MSN, RN-BC
Adjunct Faculty
School of Nursing
Old Dominion University
Virginia Beach, Virginia

## Christine A. Sump, DNP, RN, CNE
Clinical Assistant Professor
School of Nursing
Old Dominion University
Virginia Beach, Virginia

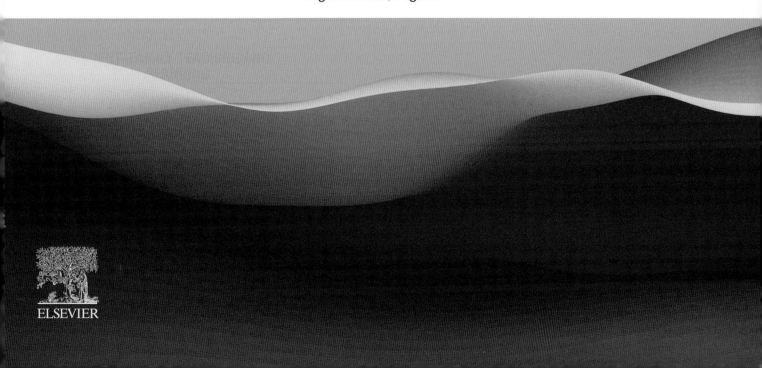

ELSEVIER

Elsevier
3251 Riverport Lane
St. Louis, Missouri 63043

**SWEARINGEN'S ALL-IN-ONE NURSING CARE PLANNING RESOURCE, SIXTH EDITION**     ISBN: 978-0-323-82536-8

*Senior Content Strategist:* Sandra Clark
*Content Development Specialist:* Rebecca Corradetti
*Publishing Services Manager:* Deepthi Unni
*Project Manager:* Thoufiq Mohammed
*Design Direction:* Amy Buxton

Printed in India

Last digit is the print number:  9  8  7  6  5  4  3  2  1

Working together
to grow libraries in
developing countries

www.elsevier.com • www.bookaid.org

# Preface

*Swearingen's All-in-One Nursing Care Planning Resource* is a unique textbook that features nursing care plans for the four core clinical areas: medical-surgical, pediatric, maternity, and psychiatric–mental health nursing, which enables students to use one book throughout the entire nursing curriculum. The distinctive design of this textbook, including its evidence-based content, open and accessible format, and clinically relevant features, makes this a must-have care plan book for nursing students.

In this sixth edition, we continued to shift toward a standard terminology of health care—*patient problems*—and away from NANDA, which tends to be more nursing focused. In this way we hope to better coordinate our language with all clinical practice for optimal interprofessional collaboration. The majority of our patient problems use the format developed by the International Council of Nurses, known as the International Classification for Nursing Practice (ICNP). This system helps to standardize the language used to describe patient problems, using clear, simple, and easier-to-understand terminology. In this way we hope to better coordinate our language with all clinical practice for optimal interprofessional collaboration (see https://www.icn.ch).

## ORGANIZATION

This book is divided into four separate sections for medical-surgical, pediatric, maternal, and psychiatric–mental health care plans. Within each section, care plans are listed alphabetically by disorder or condition (the medical-surgical nursing care plans are organized alphabetically within each body system). General information that applies to more than one disorder can be found in the *General Care Plans* section, where patient problems and interventions for immobility, perioperative care, pain, cancer care, psychosocial support for patients, psychosocial support for the patient's family and significant others, older adult care, palliative and end-of-life care, and support for lesbian, gay, bisexual, transgender, queer/questioning, or intersex patient are discussed.

Each disorder uses the following consistent format:
- Overview/Pathophysiology
- Health Care Setting
- Assessment

- Diagnostic Tests
- Patient Problems/Analyze Cues/Prioritize Hypotheses
- Desired Outcomes/Generate Solutions
- Assessment-Recognize Cues and Interventions-Take Action, With Rationales in a Clear, Two-Column Format
- Patient–Family Teaching and Discharge Planning

This book is organized to provide the most important information related to various disorders. By providing a consistent format for each disorder, key information that a nurse needs to know is fully covered. For example, the rationales given for the interventions are supported by supplemental information provided in the "Overview/Pathophysiology" and "Assessment" sections.

## FEATURES

The care plans in this book were written by clinical experts in each subject area to ensure the most current and accurate information. In addition to reliable content, the book offers the following special features:
- Consistent, easy-to-use format
- Health care setting identification aligned with each patient problem
- Patient problems that include etiology, assessment, outcome criteria, interventions, and intervention rationales
- "Patient–Family Teaching and Discharge Planning" section that highlights key patient education topics as well as resources for further information
- Safety alert icons alert nurses to interventions that necessitate special attention and care
- Complementary and Alternative Therapies icons alert nurses to supplements that patients may be using and how they can interact with conventional medication

**New to this edition are:**
- **Patient problems** using the ICNP terminology for the majority of the plans
- **Next Generation NCLEX (NGN)® headings** added to each care plan to tie the nursing process to the NGN critical decision-making process
- **New care plans** added include infection, delirium, and breastfeeding

# Acknowledgments

We would like to express our appreciation to the editorial staff, especially Rebecca Corradetti, Umarani Natarajan, Thoufiq Mohammed, Lee Henderson, and Sandra Clark, for their professional support and contributions in guiding this text to publication. We acknowledge and appreciate the work on the first five editions by the previous authors, Pamela L. Swearingen and Jacqueline D. Wright. Thanks also to the reviewers for their suggestions for this edition. We extend a special thanks to our contributors, Ruth Cody, Alicia Powell, and Sherry Ferki, who gave us helpful suggestions and insights as we developed this edition.

Julie thanks her husband, Jonathan, for his love, support, and patience during this project. She is especially thankful for the nursing students, our future nurses, whose eagerness to learn is an inspiration. Most importantly, Julie thanks God, our source of hope and strength.

Christine would also like to thank her husband, David, for his love, support, and encouragement during this endeavor. She is also thankful for the many mentors, colleagues, and students who have shaped her professional and personal growth.

**Julie S. Snyder**
**Christine A. Sump**

# About the Authors

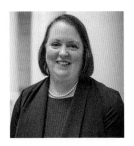

**Julie S. Snyder, MSN, RN-BC**
Julie S. Snyder received her diploma from the Norfolk General Hospital School of Nursing and her BSN and MSN from the Old Dominion University. After working in medical-surgical nursing, she worked in nursing staff development and community education. Later, she transferred to the academic setting and taught fundamentals of nursing, pharmacology, physical assessment, and adult medical-surgical nursing at a university school of nursing. Julie has recently worked as a quality initiative coordinator and a clinical nurse educator in a local hospital. She is now an adjunct instructor for the School of Nursing at Old Dominion University in Virginia Beach, Virginia. She currently holds ANCC certification in Medical-Surgical Nursing. She has worked for Elsevier as a reviewer, ancillary writer, and author since 1997. Julie is a coauthor of Elsevier's *Pharmacology and the Nursing Process* and *Clinical Reasoning Cases in Nursing*. She has also served as a consultant on various projects for local hospital education departments and has conducted pharmacology review classes for recent nursing graduates.

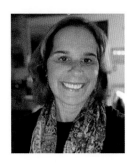

**Christine A. Sump, DNP, RN, CNE**
Dr. Christine A. Sump is an assistant clinical professor at the Old Dominion University School of Nursing in Virginia Beach, Virginia. She coordinates undergraduate health assessment, pharmacology, and adult health clinical courses. In addition to her undergraduate commitments, Dr. Sump works in the graduate program with MSN students in the lab, clinical, and classroom settings and acts as an advisor to several DNP students. Dr. Sump has worked as a bedside, charge, and cardiac rehabilitation nurse in multiple acute care facilities throughout the United States. She earned a BSN from the University of Saint Joseph, an MSN from the Old Dominion University, and a DNP from the Francis Payne Bolton School of Nursing, Case Western Reserve University.

# Contributors

## Maternity Nursing Care Plans

**Alicia Powell, MSN, RNC-OB**
Labor and Delivery Clinical Coordinator
Chesapeake Regional Medical Center
Chesapeake, Virginia

## Pediatric Nursing Care Plans

**Sherry D. Ferki, MSN, RN**
Pediatric Nursing Instructor
Suffolk, Virginia

## Psychiatric–Mental Health Nursing Care Plans

**Ruth Cody, DNP, MSN, RN-BC**
Professor, Nursing Program
Riverside College of Health Careers
Newport News, Virginia

# Reviewers

Carolyn M. Allen, DNP, AGN-BC, MS
Associate Nursing Instructor
George Washington University
Washington, DC

Family Nurse Practitioner, Associate Investigator
National Institute of Nursing Research
Bethesda, Maryland

Michael D. Bumbach, PhD, APRN, FNP-BC, MSN, RN
Clinical Assistant Professor, Family Nurse Practitioner
    Track Coordinator
University of Florida, College of Nursing
Gainesville, Florida

Jennifer Downing, MSN, RNC-OB
Associate Professor, Career-Ladder Program Coordinator
Oklahoma State University-Oklahoma City
Oklahoma City, Oklahoma

Terri Dutton, MSN, RNC-NIC, Post-Grad Certificate
    in Simulation Education
Associate Professor/Simulation Lab Coordinator
Wayland Baptist University
New Braunfels, Texas

Mary Franczek, MSN, RN, AHN-BC
Nurse Peer Reviewer With American Holistic Nursing
    Association, Associate Professor
Northern Michigan University
Marquette, Michigan

EmmaLee Greene, MSN, RN
Assistant Professor
Nashville State Community College, Nursing,
    Healthcare Professions
Nashville, Tennessee

Margaret G. Harrison, MSN, RN, CPN
Faculty III, Department of Professional Nursing,
    Baptist Health System, School of Health Professions
San Antonio, Texas

Ginger Holloway, DNP, APRN, FNP-BC, AGACNP-BC,
    CNP, CNE
Instructor
Eleanor Mann School of Nursing, University of Arkansas
Fayetteville, Arkansas

Debra F. Lett, PhD, MSN, MPA, RN
Director of Nursing, Health Sciences Division,
    Trenholm State Community College
Montgomery, Alabama

Nicole M. Lynch, DNP, MSN, CNE, RNC-OB
Curriculum and Instructor Developer/Assistant Professor
Chamberlain College of Nursing
Chicago, Illinois

Tammie McCoy, PhD, RN
Dean and Professor
Emerita of Nursing, Mississippi University for Women
Columbus, Mississippi

Melanie J. McGlone Morris, MSN, RN
Professor of Nursing, Assistant Coordinator
Maysville Community and Technical College, Licking Valley
    Campus ADN Program
Maysville, Kentucky

Mary Elizabeth McKenna-Dailey, MSN, RN, FNP-BC
Professor, Family Nurse Practitioner
North Shore Community College
Danvers, Massachusetts

Sarah Miller, EdD, DNP, APRN, FNP-C
Dean
MidAmerica Nazarene University, School of Nursing
Olathe, Kansas

Family Nurse Practitioner
Mercy Family Medicine Neosho
Neosho, Missouri

Michele Ann Pfaff, RN, MSN, DNP
Associate Professor of Nursing
Wingate University
Wingate, North Carolina

Candace Pierce, DNP, RN, CNE, COI
Contributing Faculty
Walden University
Minneapolis, Minnesota

**Kimberly Poje, NP**
Instructor
Department of Nursing, Mount Saint Mary College,
Newburgh, New York

**Mary Poston, BS, ADN, MSN**
Instructor
Nashville State Community College, Nursing,
    Academic Affairs
Nashville, Tennessee

**Laurie Robinson, DNP, APRN, FNP-C, CPNP-CP, CLC**
Assistant Professor
University of the Cumberlands
Williamsburg, Kentucky

**Linda N. Roney, EdD, RN-BC, CPEN, CNE**
Associate Professor and Director of Undergraduate Nursing,
    Egan School of Nursing
Fairfield University
Fairfield, Connecticut

**Sandy A. Salicco, MSN, RN, CCRN-K**
Adjunct Faculty
School of Nursing, Rasmussen University
Altamonte Springs, Florida

**Ellen Schoen, MSN-Ed, RN**
Instructor
Nashville State Community College, Nursing
Nashville, Tennessee

**Susan Self, DNP, RN**
Associate Professor of Nursing, College of Education
    and Health
Arkansas Tech University
Russellville, Arkansas

**Amber Shammas, PhD, RN, ACNS-BC**
Associate Professor, Senior Director, Nursing, College of
    Health Sciences
Concordia University Texas
Austin, Texas

**Barbara Sinacori, PhD, RN, CNRN, CNE**
Assistant Professor and Director, Rutgers University
New Brunswick, New Jersey

**Shannon L. Smith-Stephens, DNP, MSN, BSN; APRN-BC,
    SANE, RN; ANCC Board Certified Family Nurse
    Practitioner**
Family Nurse Practitioner/Professor of Nursing, Morehead
    State University
Olive Hill, Kentucky

**Muatasem Ubeidat, PhD**
Professor of Developmental Molecular Genetics
Department of Biological and Biomedical Sciences,
    Southwestern Oklahoma State University
Weatherford, Oklahoma

**Mary E. von Merveldt, MSN, EdS, APRN, CPNP-PC**
Director of Nursing Education, South Florida
    State College
Avon Park, Florida

# Contents

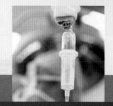

# Immobility   1

## OVERVIEW/PATHOPHYSIOLOGY

Patients who are immobile, such as those on prolonged bedrest, face many potential physiologic and psychosocial problems. Complications may include respiratory, cardiac, gastrointestinal, urinary, and musculoskeletal disorders resulting in permanent disabilities. This section reviews the most common physiologic and psychosocial problems that may occur. With patients being discharged from the hospital sooner, many health care problems are being treated in long-term care facilities or at home.

## HEALTH CARE SETTING

Acute care, extended care, home care

## Patient Problem/Analyze Cues/Prioritize Hypotheses

## Activity Intolerance

*due to* immobility or prolonged bedrest

*Desired Outcomes/Generate Solutions:* Within 48 hours of improved mobility or discontinuing bedrest, the patient exhibits cardiac tolerance to exercise or activity as evidenced by heart rate (HR) of 20 bpm or less over resting HR; systolic blood pressure (SBP) of 20 mm Hg or less over or under resting SBP; respiratory rate of 20 breaths/minute or less with normal depth and pattern (eupnea); normal sinus rhythm; warm and dry skin; and absence of crackles, new murmurs, new dysrhythmias, gallop, or chest pain. The patient rates perceived exertion (RPE) at 11 or less on a scale of 6 (no exertion) to 20 (maximum exertion). In addition, the patient maintains muscle strength and joint range of motion (ROM).

| ASSESSMENT—RECOGNIZE CUES/ INTERVENTIONS—TAKE ACTION | RATIONALES |
|---|---|
|  *Assess for orthostatic hypotension:* Prepare the patient for this change by increasing the amount of time spent in high Fowler position and moving the patient slowly in stages. | Orthostatic hypotension can occur as a result of decreased plasma volume and difficulty in adjusting immediately to postural change. For more information about orthostatic hypotension, see *Risk for Altered Blood Pressure (Orthostatic Hypotension),* later. |
| *Assess activity/tolerance:* Be alert to signs and symptoms that the cardiovascular and respiratory systems are unable to meet the demands of the low-level ROM exercises. | Excessive shortness of breath may occur if (1) transient pulmonary congestion occurs secondary to ischemia or left ventricular dysfunction, (2) lung volumes are decreased, (3) oxygen-carrying capacity of the blood is reduced, or (4) there is shunting of blood from the right to the left side of the heart without adequate oxygenation. If the cardiac output does not increase to meet the body's needs during modest levels of exercise, SBP may fall; the skin may become cool, cyanotic, and diaphoretic; dysrhythmias may be noted; crackles may be auscultated; or a systolic murmur of mitral regurgitation may occur. |
| Assess for preexisting conditions, such as arthritis and limited joint movement. | Such conditions may affect the patient's ability to perform ROM exercises and may result in pain. |
| Perform ROM exercises 2–4 times/day on each extremity. Individualize the exercise plan. | These exercises build stamina by increasing muscle strength and endurance. |

| ASSESSMENT—RECOGNIZE CUES/ INTERVENTIONS—TAKE ACTION | RATIONALES |
|---|---|
| **Caution:** Avoid isometric exercises in cardiac patients. | These exercises can increase systemic arterial BP. |
| *Mode or type of exercise:* Begin with passive exercises, moving the joints through the motions of abduction, adduction, flexion, and extension. Progress to active-assisted exercises in which you support the joints while the patient initiates muscle contraction. When the patient is able, supervise him or her in active isotonic exercises, during which the patient contracts a selected muscle group, moves the extremity at a slow pace, and then relaxes the muscle group. Have the patient repeat each exercise 3–10 times. | Beginning with passive movement, progressing to active-assisted, and continuing with active isotonic takes patients from the least exerting to the most exerting exercises over a period of time, thus increasing gradual tolerance. |
| **Caution:** Stop the exercise if the patient becomes overly short of breath, has a rapid heart rate, passes out, or experiences severe pain, dizziness, or lightheadedness. Consult with the health care provider accordingly, especially if the patient is an older adult. | These exercises need to be used with caution in any patient who is an older adult, has been recently ill, or has unexplained weight gain or swelling of a joint because these may be signs of a serious health condition. |
| **Caution:** Stop any exercise that results in muscular or skeletal pain. Consult a physical therapist (PT) about necessary modifications. | This action prevents injury in a joint too inflamed or diseased to tolerate this type of exercise intensity. |
| *Intensity:* Begin with 3–5 repetitions as tolerated by the patient. | Starting with minimal intensity and progressing step by step to greater intensity enables gradual tolerance. |
| Measure HR and BP at rest, peak exercise, and 5 minutes after exercise. | These assessments help determine tolerance to the exercise. If HR or SBP increases more than 20 bpm or more than 20 mm Hg over resting level, the number of repetitions should be decreased. If HR or SBP decreases more than 10 bpm or more than 10 mm Hg at peak exercise, this could be a sign of left ventricular failure, denoting that the heart cannot meet this workload. For other adverse signs and symptoms, see *Assess activity tolerance.* |
| *Duration:* Begin with 5 minutes or less of exercise. Gradually increase the exercise to 15 minutes as tolerated. | Starting with minimal duration and progressing to greater duration enables gradual tolerance. |
| *Frequency:* Begin with exercises 2–4 times/day. | As duration increases, the frequency can be reduced. |
| Ask the patient to rate perceived exertion (RPE) experienced during exercise, basing it on the following scale developed by Borg (1982). | Borg Scale is a simple method of RPE that can be used to gauge a person's level of exertion in training. It is a subjective measure on a 6 to 20 scale. |
| 6=No exertion<br>7<br>7.5=Extremely light<br>8<br>9=Very light<br>10<br>11=Light<br>12<br>13=Somewhat hard<br>14<br>15=Hard (heavy)<br>16<br>17=Very hard<br>18<br>19=Extremely hard<br>20=Maximum exertion | Exercises to prevent deconditioning should be performed at low levels of effort. Patients should not experience an RPE more than "very light" or "light" but can progress to higher levels of exertion as tolerated (Williams, 2017). |

## ASSESSMENT—RECOGNIZE CUES/ INTERVENTIONS—TAKE ACTION

## RATIONALES

| ASSESSMENT—RECOGNIZE CUES/ INTERVENTIONS—TAKE ACTION | RATIONALES |
|---|---|
| If the patient tolerates the exercise, increase intensity or number of repetitions each day and increase activity as soon as possible to include sitting in a chair. | Tolerance is a sign that cardiovascular and respiratory systems are able to meet the demands of this low-level ROM exercise. To promote optimal conditioning, activity should be increased to correspond to the patient's increased tolerance. |
| Monitor complete blood count (CBC) and report any abnormal value. | Disorders such as anemia can decrease the oxygen-carrying capacity of the blood and affect tolerance. |
| Progress activity in hospitalized patients is as follows:<br><br>**Level I: Bedrest**<br>• Flexion and extension of extremities 4 times/day, 15 times each extremity<br>• Deep breathing 4 times/day, 15 breaths<br>• Position change from side to side every 2 hours<br>• Use of Vollman prone positioners and kinetic therapy beds | Signs of activity intolerance include a decrease in BP more than 20 mm Hg, an increase in HR to more than 120 bpm (or more than 20 bpm above resting HR in patients receiving beta-blocker therapy), and shortness of breath (discussed earlier).<br><br>A strategy to promote lung expansion by the use of Vollman prone positioner enables postural drainage. Kinetic therapy beds provide continual rotation of more than 200 times/day, which decreases the likelihood of pressure sores and pneumonia. |
| **Level II: Out of bed to chair**<br>• As tolerated, 3 times/day for 20–30 minutes<br>• May perform ROM exercises 2 times/day while sitting in a chair<br><br>**Level III: Ambulate in room**<br>• As tolerated, 3 times/day for 3–5 minutes in a room<br><br>**Level IV: Ambulate in the hall**<br>• Initially, 50–200 ft 2 times/day, progressing to 600 ft 4 times/day<br>• May incorporate slow stair climbing in preparation for hospital discharge<br>• Monitor for signs of activity intolerance | Gradually increasing activities by working up to 20- to 30-minute sessions at least 3 to 4 times a week with the use of a walker or gait belt for support and providing nonskid footwear for ambulation promotes not only promotes conditioning but also patient safety. |
| Have the patient perform self-care activities as tolerated. | Self-care activities such as eating, mouth care, and bathing may increase the patient's activity level. |
| Instruct the patient's significant other about interventions for preventing deconditioning and their purpose. Involve him or her in the patient's plan of care. | Significant others can promote and participate in the patient's activity/ exercises when they understand the rationale and are familiar with the interventions. |
| Pay attention to nonverbal behaviors and provide emotional support to the patient and significant other as the patient's activity level is increased. | Emotional support helps allay fears of failure, pain, or medical setbacks. |

## Patient Problem/Analyze Cues/Prioritize Hypotheses

# Risk for Impaired Musculoskeletal System Function

*due to* paralysis, mechanical immobilization, prescribed immobilization, severe pain, or altered level of consciousness

**Desired Outcome/Generate Solutions:** When bedrest is discontinued, the patient exhibits complete ROM of all joints without pain, and limb girth measurements are congruent with or increased over baseline measurements.

> **Note:** *ROM exercises should be performed at least 2 times/day for all immobilized patients with normal joints. Modification may be required for patients with spinal cord injuries.*

| ASSESSMENT—RECOGNIZE CUES/ INTERVENTIONS—TAKE ACTION | RATIONALES |
|---|---|
| Assess the ROM of the patient's joints, paying special attention to the following areas: shoulder, wrist, fingers, hips, knees, and feet. | These areas are especially susceptible to joint contracture. Shoulders can become "frozen" to limit abduction and extension; wrists can "drop," prohibiting extension; fingers can develop flexion contractures that limit extension; hips can develop flexion contractures that affect the gait by shortening the limb or develop external rotation or adduction deformities that affect the gait; knees may have flexion contractures that can develop to limit extension and alter the gait; and feet can "drop" as a result of prolonged plantar flexion, which limits dorsiflexion and alters the gait. |
| Assess for footdrop by inspecting the feet for plantar flexion and evaluating the patient's ability to pull the toes upward toward the head. Document the assessment daily. | Because feet lie naturally in plantar flexion, footdrop may occur when plantar flexion is prolonged. Inability to dorsiflex (pull the toes up toward the head) is a sign of footdrop, and it requires prompt intervention to prevent permanent damage. This may necessitate the use of footboards, high-top tennis shoes, specialized boots, or foot braces to facilitate normal dorsal flexion position. |
| Ensure that the patient changes position at least every 2 hours. Post a turning schedule at the bedside. | Position changes not only maintain correct body alignment, thereby reducing strain on the joints, but also prevent contractures, minimize pressure on bony prominences, decrease venous stasis, and promote maximal chest expansion. |
| Place the patient in a position that achieves proper standing. Maintain this position with pillows, towels, waffle boots, heel lift suspension boots, foam heel positioners, footboards, high-top tennis shoes, or other positioning aids. | A position in which the head is neutral or slightly flexed on the neck, hips are extended, knees are extended or minimally flexed, and feet are at right angles to the legs achieves proper standing alignment, which helps promote ambulation when the patient is ready to do so. |
| Ensure that the patient is prone or side lying, with hips extended, for the same amount of time spent in the supine position or, at a minimum, 3 times/day for 1 hour. | These positions prevent hip flexion contractures. |
| When the head of bed is elevated 30 degrees, extend the patient's shoulders and arms, using pillows to support the position. | This position maintains proper spinal posture. |
| Allow the patient's fingertips to extend over the pillow's edge. | This position maintains normal arching of the hands. |
| Place thin pads under the angles of the axillae and lateral aspects of the clavicles. | These pads help prevent internal rotation of the shoulders and maintain the anatomic position of the shoulder girdle. |
| Ensure that the patient spends time with hips in extension (see preceding interventions). | This position helps prevent hip flexion contracture. |
| When the patient is in the side-lying position, extend the lower leg from the hip. | This position helps prevent hip flexion contracture. |
| When the patient can be placed in the prone position, move him or her to the end of the bed and allow the feet to rest between the mattress and footboard. | This prevents not only plantar flexion and hip rotation but also injury to the heels and toes. |
| Use positioning devices liberally. | Using pillows, rolled towels, blankets, sandbags, antirotation boots, splints, knee abductors, drop seats, foot supports, back wedges, back support splints, wedge cushions, pommel cushions, and orthotics helps maintain joints in neutral position, which helps ensure that they remain functional when activity is increased. |
| When using adjunctive devices, monitor the involved skin at least 3 times daily. | Assessing for alterations in skin integrity enables prompt interventions that prevent skin breakdown. |

| ASSESSMENT—RECOGNIZE CUES/ INTERVENTIONS—TAKE ACTION | RATIONALES |
|---|---|
| Instruct the patient and significant other on the rationale and procedure for ROM exercises, and have the patient give return demonstrations. Review *Activity Intolerance*, earlier, to ensure that the patient does not exceed his or her tolerance. Provide passive exercises for patients unable to perform active or active-assisted exercises. In addition, incorporate movement patterns into care activities, such as position changes, bed baths, getting the patient on and off the bedpan, or changing the patient's gown. | These actions facilitate adherence to the exercise regimen and help prevent contracture formation. |
| Provide the patient with a handout that reviews exercises and lists repetitions for each. Instruct the patient's significant other/caregiver to encourage the patient to perform exercises as required. | These actions facilitate learning and adherence to the exercise program. |
| Perform and document limb girth measurements and ROM and establish exercise baseline limits. | This assessment of existing muscle mass, strength, and joint motion enables subsequent evaluation and promotes exercise and ROM appropriate for the patient. |
| Explain to the patient how muscle atrophy occurs. Emphasize the importance of maintaining or increasing muscle strength and periarticular tissue elasticity through exercise. If there are complicating pathologic conditions, consult the health care provider about the appropriate form of exercise for the patient. | Muscle atrophy occurs because of disuse or failure to use the joint, often caused by immediate or anticipated pain. This explanation encourages patients to perform exercises because disuse eventually may result in decreased muscle mass and blood supply and a loss of periarticular tissue elasticity, which in turn can lead to increased muscle fatigue and joint pain with use. |
| Explain the need to participate in self-care as much as can be tolerated. | Self-care helps maintain muscle strength and promote a sense of participation and control. |
| For noncardiac patients needing greater help with muscle strength, assist with resistive exercises (e.g., moderate weight lifting to increase the size, endurance, and strength of the muscles). For patients in beds with overbed frames, provide a means for resistive exercise by implementing a system of weights and pulleys. | Resistance increases the force needed to perform the exercise and promotes the maintenance or rebuilding of muscle strength. |
| Determine the patient's baseline level of performance on a given set of exercises, and then set realistic goals for repetitions. | Well-planned goals provide markers for assessing the effectiveness of the exercise plan and progress made. For example, if the patient can do 5 repetitions of lifting a 5-lb weight with the biceps muscle, the goal may be to increase repetitions to 10 within 1 week, to an ultimate goal of 20 within 3 weeks, and then advance to 7.5-lb weights. |
| If the joints require rest, instruct isometric exercises. | In these exercises, the patient contracts a muscle group and holds the contraction for a count of 5 or 10. The sequence is repeated for increasing counts or repetitions until an adequate level of endurance has been achieved. Thereafter, maintenance levels are performed. **Note:** These exercises do not build strength but, rather, help to maintain strength. |
| Provide a chart to show the patient's progress, and combine this with large amounts of positive reinforcement. | Attaining progress and having positive reinforcement promote continued adherence to the exercise plan. |
| Post the exercise regimen at the bedside. Instruct the patient's significant other/caregiver in the exercise regimen, and elicit their support and encouragement of the patient's performance of the exercises. | These actions ensure consistency by all health care personnel and involvement and support of significant others. |
| As prescribed, instruct the patient about transfer or crutch-walking techniques and the use of a walker, wheelchair, or cane. Include the significant other in demonstrations, and stress the importance of proper body mechanics. | These interventions help ensure that patients can safely maintain the highest possible level of mobility while also improving circulation. |
| Employ gait belts, lifts, and bed assist devices. | These devices promote safety and help to improve movement. |
| Provide periods of uninterrupted rest between exercises/activities. | Rest enables patients to replenish energy stores. |
| Seek referral to PT or OT as appropriate. | Such a referral will help patients who have special needs or who are not in a care facility to attain the best ROM possible. |

Patient Problem/Analyze Cues/Prioritize Hypotheses

# Risk for Deep Vein Thrombosis

*due to* interrupted venous flow occurring with prolonged immobility

**Desired Outcomes/Generate Solutions:** At least 24 hours before hospital discharge, the patient has adequate distal pulses (greater than 2+ on a 0–4+ scale) in peripheral extremities.

| ASSESSMENT—RECOGNIZE CUES/ INTERVENTIONS—TAKE ACTION | RATIONALES |
|---|---|
| Assess for calf or groin tenderness, redness, unilateral swelling of a leg, warmth in the involved area, and coolness, unnatural color or pallor, and superficial venous dilation distal to the involved area. | These may be signs of deep vein thrombosis (DVT)/venous thromboembolism (VTE). |
| Measure the girth of the affected limb, comparing it to the opposite side. | If the girth of the affected limb is larger in comparison to the opposite limb, this is a sign of DVT/VTE. |
| Instruct the patient about these indicators. | A knowledgeable patient is more likely to report these indicators promptly for timely intervention. |
| In addition, assess vital signs and monitor erythrocyte sedimentation rate (ESR) results if they are available. | Additional signs of DVT/VTE may include fever, tachycardia, and elevated ESR. |
| Notify the patient's health care provider of significant findings. | If signs of DVT/VTE occur, further evaluation will be necessary to protect the patient from a pulmonary embolus or clot that could compromise the limb. For more information see "Venous Thrombosis/Thrombophlebitis," Chapter 26. |
| Perform passive ROM or encourage active ROM exercises in the absence of signs of DVT. | These exercises increase circulation, which promotes peripheral tissue perfusion. |
| Instruct the patient about calf-pumping (ankle dorsiflexion–plantar flexion) and ankle-circling exercises. | Same as above. The patient should repeat each movement 10 times, performing each exercise hourly during extended periods of immobility, as long as the patient is free of symptoms of DVT/VTE. |
| Encourage deep breathing. | Deep breathing increases negative pressure in the lungs and thorax to promote emptying of large veins and thus increase peripheral tissue perfusion. |
| When not contraindicated by peripheral vascular disease (PVD), ensure that the patient wears antiembolism hose, pneumatic foot pump devices, intermittent sequential compression devices (SCDs), or graduated compression (elastic) stockings (also known as thromboembolism-deterrent hose). | These garments/devices prevent venous stasis, the precursor to DVT/VTE. The SCDs, which provide more compression than antiembolism hose, are especially useful in preventing DVT/VTE in patients who are mostly immobile. Patients with PVD may experience rest pain, which can be precipitated by graduated compression stockings, foot pump devices, and SCDs. |
| Remove compression stockings or SCD sleeves for 10–20 minutes every 8 hours. Reapply hose after elevating the patient's legs at least 10 degrees for 10 minutes. | Removing the stockings or SCD sleeves enables inspection of underlying skin for evidence of irritation or breakdown. Elevating the legs before reapplying the devices promotes venous return and decreases edema, which otherwise would remain and cause discomfort when the hose is reapplied. |
| Instruct the patient not to cross feet at the ankles or knees while in bed. | These actions may cause venous stasis. |
| If the patient is at risk for DVT/VTE, elevate foot of the bed 10 degrees. | Elevating the foot of the bed increases venous return. |
| In nonrestricted patients, increase fluid intake to at least 2–3 L/day. Educate the patient about the need to drink large amounts of fluid (9–14 8-oz glasses) daily. Monitor the intake and output (I&O) to ensure adherence. | Increased hydration reduces hemoconcentration, which can contribute to the development of DVT/VTE. |

| ASSESSMENT—RECOGNIZE CUES/ INTERVENTIONS—TAKE ACTION | RATIONALES |
|---|---|
| Administer the anticoagulant medication as prescribed. | Patients at risk for DVT/VTE, including those with chronic infection and history of PVD and smoking, as well as patients who are older, obese, and anemic, may require anticoagulants to minimize the risk for clotting. Drugs such as aspirin, warfarin, fondaparinux, rivaroxaban, heparin, or low-molecular-weight heparin (LMWH; e.g., enoxaparin sodium) may be given. Many patients are taught how to self-administer LMWH injections after hospital discharge. |
| If the patient is on intravenous heparin, monitor activated partial thromboplastin time (aPTT) and platelet counts. For warfarin therapy, monitor prothrombin time (PT) and international normalized ratio (INR). For all patients on anticoagulant therapy, monitor the CBC. | Lab values do not need to be monitored for subcutaneous heparin, but when a patient is receiving intravenous heparin, optimal laboratory values for PTT are 60–70 seconds or 1.5–2.5 times the control value. In addition, monitor platelet counts for the development of heparin-induced thrombocytopenia. The reference range for platelet count is 150,000–400,000/mm$^3$. For warfarin therapy the INR should be within the range of 2.0–3.0 for sufficient anticoagulation. Elevated aPTT and INR, or decreased platelet counts, indicate that the patient is at an increased risk for bleeding. A decreased hemoglobin or hematocrit may indicate internal bleeding. |
| Instruct the patient to self-monitor for and report bleeding. | Anticoagulant drugs increase the risk for bleeding. It is important for the patient to know the signs of bleeding so that the patient can report them as soon as they are noted to ensure timely intervention. Possible types of bleeding include epistaxis, bleeding gums, hematemesis, hemoptysis, melena, hematuria, hematochezia, menometrorrhagia, and ecchymoses. |
| Instruct patients and their families about medication, food, and herbal interactions that can affect warfarin. | Many foods and over-the-counter herbals can prolong bleeding such as alfalfa/alfalfa sprouts, dong quai, borage, bromelain, celery, clove, coenzyme Q-10, devils claw, echinacea, fenugreek, garlic, ginger, gingko biloba, ginseng, green tea, licorice, NSAIDs, parsley, red clover, St. John's Wort, and turmeric. |
| | Examples of medications and foods that decrease the effect of anticoagulation, thus increasing the chance of blood clots, are azathioprine, antithyroid medications, carbamazepine, dicloxacillin, glutethimide, griseofulvin, nafcillin, oral contraceptives, phenobarbital, rifampin, dark green leafy vegetables, spinach, kale, collards, broccoli, asparagus, cauliflower, and Brussels sprouts (Abebe, 2019; Lilley et al., 2023). |

## Patient Problem/Analyze Cues/Prioritize Hypotheses

# Risk for Altered Blood Pressure (Orthostatic Hypotension)

*due to* interrupted arterial flow to the brain occurring with prolonged bedrest

***Desired Outcome/Generate Solutions:*** When getting out of bed, the patient has adequate perfusion to the brain as evidenced by HR less than 120 bpm and BP of 90/60 mm Hg or greater (or within 20 mm Hg of the patient's baseline range) immediately after the position change, dry skin, baseline skin color, and absence of vertigo and syncope, with return of HR and BP to resting levels within 3 minutes of position change.

| ASSESSMENT—RECOGNIZE CUES/ INTERVENTIONS—TAKE ACTION | RATIONALES |
|---|---|
| Assess for recent diuresis, diaphoresis, or change in vasodilator therapy. | These are factors that increase the risk for orthostatic hypotension because of fluid volume changes. For example, bedrest incurs a diuresis of about 600–800 mL during the first 3 days. Although this fluid decrease is not noticed when the patient is supine, the lost volume will be evident (i.e., with orthostatic hypotension) when the body tries to adapt to sitting and standing. |
| Be alert to diabetic cardiac neuropathy, denervation with advanced age or severe left ventricular dysfunction. | These are factors that increase the risk for orthostatic hypotension because of altered autonomic control. |
| Assess BP in any high-risk patient for whom this will be the first time out of bed. Instruct the patient to report immediately symptoms of lightheadedness or dizziness. | Low BP, lightheadedness, and dizziness are signs of orthostatic hypotension and necessitate a return to the supine position. |
| Assess for a drop in SBP of 20 mm Hg or greater and an increased pulse rate, combined with symptoms of vertigo and impending syncope. | These are signs of orthostatic hypotension that signal the need for a return to the supine position. |
| Explain the cause of orthostatic hypotension and measures for preventing it. | Patients who are informed as to the cause and ways of preventing orthostatic hypotension are more likely to avoid it. Measures to prevent orthostatic hypotension are discussed in subsequent interventions. |
| Apply antiembolism hose after the patient is mobilized. | Used to prevent DVT/VTE, antiembolism hose and sequential compression hose also may be useful in preventing orthostatic hypotension by promoting venous return after the patient is mobilized. |
| When the patient is in bed, provide instructions for leg exercises as described under *Risk for Deep Vein Thrombosis*, earlier. Encourage the patient to perform leg exercises immediately before mobilization. | Leg exercises promote venous return, which helps prevent orthostatic hypotension. |
| Prepare the patient for getting out of bed by encouraging position changes within necessary restrictions. | Position changes help acclimate patients to the upright position. These changes may be accomplished with the assistance of an overbed trapeze, hydraulic lift, or other assistive devices. |
| Follow these guidelines for mobilization:<br>• Have the patient dangle legs at the bedside. Be alert to indicators of orthostatic hypotension, including diaphoresis, pallor, tachycardia, hypotension, and syncope. Question the patient about the presence of lightheadedness or dizziness. Again, encourage the performance of leg exercises. | This action provides for a gradual adjustment to the possible effects of venous pooling and related hypotension in persons who have been supine or in Fowler position for some time. Dangling of the legs may be necessary until intravascular fluid volume is restored. It also provides an opportunity for leg exercises that can reduce the risk for venous stasis. |
| • If leg dangling is tolerated, have the patient stand at the bedside with two staff members in attendance. If no adverse signs or symptoms occur, have the patient progress to ambulation as tolerated. | This intervention helps ensure the patient's safety in the event of a fall. |

## Patient Problem/Analyze Cues/Prioritize Hypotheses

# Constipation

*due to* less than adequate fluid or dietary intake and bulk, immobility, lack of privacy, positional restrictions, or use of opioid analgesics

***Desired Outcomes/Generate Solutions:*** Within 24 hours of this problem, the patient verbalizes accurate knowledge of measures that promote bowel elimination. The patient relates the return of baseline pattern and character of bowel elimination within 3–5 days.

| ASSESSMENT—RECOGNIZE CUES/ INTERVENTIONS—TAKE ACTION | RATIONALES |
|---|---|
| Assess the patient's bowel history. | This assessment elicits normal bowel habits and interventions that are used successfully at home. |
| Assess and document the patient's bowel movements, diet, and I&O. | This information tracks bowel movements and factors that promote or prevent constipation. Indications of constipation include the following: fewer than the patient's usual number of bowel movements, abdominal discomfort or distention, straining at stool, and patient complaints of rectal pressure or fullness. Fecal impaction may be manifested by oozing of liquid stool and confirmed by digital examination. |
| If rectal impaction is suspected, use a gloved, lubricated finger to remove stool from the rectum. | Digital stimulation may be adequate to promote a bowel movement. Oil retention enemas may soften impacted stool. |
| Instruct the patient about the importance of a high-fiber diet (20–35 g/day) and a fluid intake of at least 2–3 L/day (unless this is contraindicated by a renal, hepatic, or cardiac disorder). | These measures increase peristalsis and the likelihood of normal bowel movements. High-fiber foods—including bran, nuts, raw and coarse vegetables, beans, and lentils—are rich in insoluble fiber. |
| | Good hydration softens the stool, making it easier to evacuate. Patients with renal, hepatic, and diverticular disease, cardiac disorders, or hemorrhoids may be on fluid restrictions. |
| Offer a bedpan; ensuring privacy; and timing medications, enemas, or suppositories so that they take effect at the time of day when the patient usually has a bowel movement. | These actions may facilitate the regularity of bowel movements. |
| Provide warm fluids before breakfast, and encourage toileting. | These measures take advantage of the patient's gastrocolic and duodenocolic reflexes. |
| Maximize the patient's activity level within limitations of endurance, therapy, and pain. | Increased activity promotes peristalsis, which helps prevent constipation. |
| Request pharmacologic interventions from the health care provider when necessary. To help prevent rebound constipation, make a priority list of interventions. | Starting with the most gentle interventions helps prevent rebound constipation and ensures minimal disruption of patient's normal bowel habits. |
| | The following is a suggested hierarchy of interventions: |
| | • bulk-building additives (psyllium), bran |
| | • mild laxatives (apple or prune juice, milk of magnesia) |
| | • stool softeners (docusate sodium, docusate calcium) |
| | • stimulant (potent) laxatives and cathartics (bisacodyl, cascara sagrada) |
| | • medicated suppositories |
| | • enemas |
| Discuss the role that opioid agents and other medications play in causing constipation. | Opioids, antidepressants, anticholinergics, iron supplements, diuretics, and muscle relaxants are known to cause constipation. Methylnaltrexone, a mu-opioid receptor antagonist, is a medication that treats opioid-induced constipation. |
|  Instruct the patient about nonpharmacologic methods of pain control. See discussion in *Acute Pain/Chronic Pain* in Chapter 5. | Nonpharmacologic methods that may decrease the need for opioid analgesics include transcutaneous electrical nerve stimulation (TENS), spinal cord stimulation (SCS), ice, massage therapy, guided imagery, music therapy, biofeedback, and acupuncture. |

## Patient Problem/Analyze Cues/Prioritize Hypotheses

# Risk for Self-Care Deficit

*due to* disease process or physical limitations that necessitate relying on others for care

***Desired Outcome/Generate Solutions:*** The patient collaborates with caregivers in planning realistic goals for independence and participates in self-care.

| ASSESSMENT—RECOGNIZE CUES/ INTERVENTIONS—TAKE ACTION | RATIONALES |
|---|---|
| Assess the patient's response to the plan of care for recovery, which includes appropriate participation in self-care. | It is important to keep the patient gradually increasing activity and becoming more involved in self-care activities. However, excessive activity may lead to fatigue and setbacks in recovery. |
| Encourage the patient to be as independent as possible within limitations of endurance, therapy, and pain. | Optimally, such encouragement will facilitate independence as much as feasible. Allow for temporary periods of dependence because they enable the individual to restore energy reserves needed for recovery. |
| Ensure that all health care providers are consistent in conveying expectations of eventual independence. | Consistency facilitates trusting relationships. |
| Alert the patient to areas of excessive dependence, and involve the patient in collaborative goal setting. | It is healthy to begin to foster a degree of independence as recovery progresses. |
| Do not minimize the patient's expressed feelings of depression. Listen to the patient's concerns. Allow expressions of emotions but provide support, understanding, and realistic hope for a positive role change. | Minimizing a patient's expressed feelings of depression can add to anger and more depression. Offering realistic goals and encouragement can provide needed emotional support in movement toward independence. |
| If indicated, provide self-help devices. Consult with occupational therapy (OT) as indicated. | These devices, such as long-handled reachers or grabbers, canes, wheelchairs, and walkers, can increase the patient's independence with self-care. The OT specialist will be able to assess the patient and suggest appropriate self-help devices. |
| Provide positive reinforcement when the patient meets or advances toward goals. | Positive reinforcement builds on the patient's strengths and promotes self-efficacy. |

## Patient Problem/Analyze Cues/Prioritize Hypotheses

# Risk for Impaired Socialization

*due to* prolonged illness and hospitalization

***Desired Outcome/Generate Solutions:*** Within 24 hours of interventions, the patient engages in diversional activities and relates improved socialization and absence of boredom.

| ASSESSMENT—RECOGNIZE CUES/ INTERVENTIONS—TAKE ACTION | RATIONALES |
|---|---|
| Assess for evidence of the patient desiring something to read or do, daytime napping, and expressed inability to perform usual hobbies because of hospitalization. | These are indicators of boredom. |
| Assess the patient's activity/exercise tolerance as described in *Activity Intolerance* earlier in this careplan. | Exercise tolerance will determine the amount of activity patients can engage in within the limits of their diagnoses. |

| ASSESSMENT—RECOGNIZE CUES/ INTERVENTIONS—TAKE ACTION | RATIONALES |
| --- | --- |
| Collect a database by assessing the patient's normal support systems and relationship patterns with significant others. Question the patient and significant others about the patient's interests. | This enables the nurse to explore diversional activities that may be suitable for the health care setting and the patient's level of activity tolerance. |
| Personalize the patient's environment with favorite objects and photographs of significant others. | This intervention provides visual stimulation. |
| Provide low-level activities to the patient's tolerance. | These activities promote mental stimulation and reduce boredom. Examples include access to WiFi, laptop computers, tablets, electronic readers, and cellular phones with Internet connections. Providing books or magazines pertaining to the patient's recreational or other interests, computer games, television, and supplying writing implements for short intervals of activity are other possible actions. |
| Initiate activities that require little concentration, and proceed to more complicated tasks as the patient's condition allows (e.g., if reading requires more energy or concentration than the patient is capable of, suggest that the significant other read to the patient or bring audiotapes of books). | Initially, the patient may find difficult tasks frustrating. Physiologic problems such as anemia and pain may make concentration difficult. |
| Encourage the discussion of past activities or reminiscence. | This could serve as a substitute for performing favorite activities during convalescence. |
| As the patient's endurance improves, obtain appropriate diversional activities such as puzzles, model kits, handicrafts, and computerized games and activities; encourage the patient to use them. Suggest that the patient's significant other bring hand held devices, iPods, computers, DVD players, Kindles, phones, TV/tapes, computer, games, crafts, and grooming and beauty products from home. | Watching television, using the computer, listening to the radio or books on tape, and playing cards or board games often are good diversions. |
| Encourage significant others to visit within the limits of the patient's endurance and to involve the patient in activities that are of interest to him or her. | Visiting and partaking in activities with loved ones likely reduce boredom. |
| As the patient's condition improves, assist him or her with sitting in a chair near a window so that outside activities can be viewed. When the patient is able, provide opportunities to sit in a solarium so that he or she can visit with other patients. If physical condition and weather permit, take the patient outside for brief periods. | New scenery, whether within the same room, such as looking out the window or into another area, can reduce boredom as can meeting and speaking with other people. Being outdoors when it is possible changes the environment and optimally combats boredom. |
| Request consultation from occupational therapist, social services, pastoral services, and psychiatric nurse. Contact volunteer services to have a member visit the patient. | Such referrals may yield other diversional activities/interventions. |
| Increase the patient's involvement in self-care to provide a sense of purpose, accomplishment, and control. | Performing in-bed exercises (e.g., deep breathing, ankle circling, calf pumping), keeping track of I&O and similar activities can and should be accomplished routinely by patients to provide a sense of purpose, accomplishment, and control, which likely will diminish boredom. |

Patient Problem/Analyze Cues/Prioritize Hypotheses

# Impaired Sexual Functioning

*due to* actual or perceived physiologic limitations on sexual performance occurring with disease, therapy, or prolonged hospitalization

***Desired Outcome/Generate Solutions:*** Within 72 hours of this problem, the patient relates satisfaction with sexuality and/or understanding of the ability to resume sexual activity.

| ASSESSMENT—RECOGNIZE CUES/ INTERVENTIONS—TAKE ACTION | RATIONALES |
|---|---|
| Assess the patient's usual sexual function, including importance placed on sex in the relationship, frequency of interaction, normal positions used, and the couple's ability to adapt or change to meet the requirements of the patient's limitations. | This assessment helps determine the patient's usual sexual function and adaptations that will be necessary under current conditions. |
| Identify the patient's problem diplomatically, and clarify it with the patient. | This assessment helps determine whether the patient suffers from sexual dysfunction resulting from lack of privacy, current illness, or perceived limitations. Indicators of sexual dysfunction can include regression, acting-out with inappropriate behavior such as grabbing or pinching, sexual overtures toward staff members, self-enforced isolation, and similar behaviors. |
| Encourage the patient and significant other to verbalize feelings and anxieties about sexual abstinence, fear of pain during sexual activity, or having to use new or alternative methods for sexual gratification. | Open communication is the foundation for maintaining a strong intimate relationship. |
| Develop strategies in collaboration with the patient and significant other. | This information will promote an understanding of ways to achieve sexual satisfaction. |
| Encourage the acceptable expressions of sexuality by the patient. | Examples of positive and acceptable behaviors may eliminate inappropriate behaviors. |
| Inform the patient and significant other that it is possible to have time alone together for intimacy. Provide that time accordingly by putting a *Do not disturb* sign on the door, enforcing privacy by restricting staff and visitors to the room, or arranging for temporary private quarters. | These actions facilitate intimacy by ensuring privacy. |
| Encourage the patient and significant other to seek alternative methods of sexual expression when necessary. | Accustomed methods of sexual expression may not work under current circumstances. Alternative methods may include mutual masturbation, altered positions, vibrators, and identification of other erotic areas for each partner. |
| Refer the patient and significant other to professional sexual counseling as necessary. | Counseling may improve communication and acceptance of alternative therapies. |

## ADDITIONAL PROBLEMS:

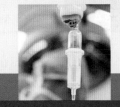

# Infection 2

## OVERVIEW/PATHOPHYSIOLOGY

An infection occurs when a pathogen causes a disease. Pathogens are microorganisms, such as bacteria, fungi, viruses, or protozoa, and can cause harm when they enter a host's body and multiply. An infection with a microorganism will result in signs and symptoms related to the specific pathogen and will also result in the stimulation of the host's immune and inflammatory responses. A local infection is contained in a small area, such as a surgical wound. A systemic infection has spread throughout the body, usually by the bloodstream, and is often more deadly and difficult to treat.

Bacteria can cause disease by entering the host and growing inside the cells, or by secreting substances known as toxins, that cause cellular damage. Examples of bacterial infections include tuberculosis, *Escherichia coli*, strep throat, gonorrhea, and *Clostridioides difficile*. Viruses are not cells; they are infectious particles that can reproduce only if they release their genetic material into the living cells of the host. Examples of viral infections include chickenpox, COVID-19, and HIV. Fungi are living, plant-like organisms that do not contain chlorophyll. In most patients, a fungal infection is usually localized such as athlete's foot (tinea pedis), but in immunocompromised patients, fungal infections can occur throughout the body and are difficult to treat. Some medications, such as inhaled corticosteroids, can cause an overgrowth of normal flora in the body and result in candidiasis of the mouth (also known as thrush); antibiotic therapy in women may result in vaginal fungal (or yeast) infections. Protozoa are single-cell organisms that usually live in soil or bodies of water, but if they enter a host's body, an infection will result. Protozoa cause diseases such as giardiasis, malaria, and toxoplasmosis (Harding et al., 2023).

If microbes can enter the body, spread throughout the body's tissues, and grow, then an infection occurs. If a patient's immune system is healthy, then infection may not occur. However, when patients are ill, there are several factors that can increase the risk for infection. Medical conditions such as diabetes and cancer decrease the effectiveness of a patient's immune system. Organ transplant recipients, the unvaccinated as well as those with chronic kidney disease or liver disease, and malnutrition are all at risk for decreased immune responses. Certain medications such as corticosteroids, antibiotics, biologic response modifiers, and cancer treatment drugs reduce the effectiveness of the immune system. Medical devices such as IV catheters, urinary catheters, and surgical incisions may provide a means of entry for microorganisms.

The Centers for Disease Control and Prevention have published guidelines for the prevention of infection: **Standard Precautions** and **Transmission-Based Precautions**. Both are designed to protect patients, health care workers, and the community from the transmission of infectious organisms. Standard Precautions apply to all patient-care situations; transmission-based precautions apply to specific infectious diseases (CDC, 2016a, 2016b, 2016c).

According to the Centers for Disease Control (2016b), Standard Precautions include measures such as

- performing hand hygiene
- using personal protective equipment whenever exposure to infectious materials is possible;
- following the principles of respiratory hygiene;
- ensure proper placement of patients when assigning rooms;
- cleaning and disinfecting patient-care equipment and devices properly, and the patient's environment;
- handle patient care linens/laundry appropriately; and
- following safe injection procedures, and ensuring that needles and other sharps are handled and disposed of properly.

The CDC (2020) also outlines procedures for effective hand hygiene. Health care workers should use an alcohol-based hand sanitizer rub or wash with soap and water in these situations:

- just before touching a patient;
- just before performing an aseptic task (such as inserting an indwelling device);
- before moving from work on a soiled body area to a clean body area, even on the same patient;
- after touching a patient or the patient's environment;
- after contacting body fluids, blood, or contaminated surfaces; and
- immediately after removing gloves.

Note that the CDC also recommends that hand hygiene be performed with soap and water when hands are visibly soiled, after exposure to spore-forming pathogens such as *C. diff*, and after using the toilet. See www.cdc.gov for specific instructions on hand hygiene.

The CDC (2016c) also recommends Transmission-Based Precautions for patients who may be infected with specific pathogens that require additional precautions. Transmission-based precautions are to be used along with Standard Precautions. Contact Precautions are used for patients who have infections (or suspected infections) that can be transmitted by direct contact. Droplet Precautions are used for patients with known or suspected infections that can be transmitted by respiratory droplets (sneezing, coughing, talking). Airborne precautions are for those who have known or suspected infections that are transmitted by the airborne route. Examples include tuberculosis and varicella (chickenpox). See www.cdc.gov for specific information.

COVID-19, the common term for illness caused by the SARS-CoV-2 virus (coronavirus 2019), first appeared in 2019 and soon became a global pandemic. Special measures are recommended to curb the spread of COVID-19 including getting vaccinated, with booster vaccinations as indicated; wearing a well-fitted mask that covers the nose and mouth, social distancing (6 feet apart) from those who do not live with you; avoiding crowds and indoor spaces that are poorly ventilated; testing if infection is suspected;

quarantining per current guidelines if testing is positive. Frequent hand washing often with soap and water, or using hand sanitizer, is essential. Guidelines are often updated; for the most recent guidance on COVID-19 protocols, see www.cdc.gov.

Nurses need to be aware of the factors that increase a patient's risk for infection and create a safe environment that emphasizes infection prevention. In addition, always monitor the patient for signs and symptoms of infection, and teaching both the patient and their caregivers about infection prevention is important for reducing infection risks.

## HEALTH CARE SETTING

Acute care, extended care, home care

### Patient Problem/Analyze Cues/Prioritize Hypotheses

# Infection

*due to* the presence of an infectious pathogen

**Desired Outcome/Generate Solutions:** After receiving appropriate treatment, the patient becomes free of infection as evidenced by orientation to person, place, and time and behavior within the patient's baseline limits; vital signs, including temperature, within the patient's baseline limits; urine that is straw colored, clear, and of characteristic odor; sputum that is clear to whitish in color; and skin that is intact and of baseline color and temperature for the patient.

| ASSESSMENT—RECOGNIZE CUES/ INTERVENTIONS—TAKE ACTION | RATIONALES |
|---|---|
| Assess and monitor for signs and symptoms of infection: redness, swelling, increasing pain, purulent drainage from wounds, incisions, skin around exit sites of tubes or drains. Also, assess for elevated temperature, changes in the color of respiratory secretions, and in the appearance of urine, and elevated white blood cell (WBC) counts. | These are all possible indicators of an infection; early detection of potential infection will allow for immediate treatment. Ongoing monitoring for these signs and symptoms will help in evaluating whether prescribed treatments are effective. |
| If infection is suspected, obtain cultures before starting any antiinfective medication therapy. | Cultures and sensitivity reports help to identify the causative organism and which antiinfectives agents would be effective as treatment. Starting medications before cultures are obtained may alter the results and reduce the effectiveness of therapy. |
| Administer antiinfectives and IV fluids as prescribed. | Antiinfectives are given for bacterial, viral, fungal, and parasitic infections. These drugs either kill the pathogen or reduce its growth. Antiinfectives are usually started before the results of cultures are available and may be changed based on culture and sensitivity reports. |
| Monitor the temperature and notify the health care provider (HCP) of a temperature greater than 101°F (38.3°C). Implement measures to reduce higher temperatures as ordered:<br>• tepid baths<br>• cool packs<br>• cooling blankets<br>• fan (if permitted by facility)<br>• antipyretics | A low-grade fever is an expected response to inflammation, stress, surgery, illness, or trauma and is considered a helpful response in fighting infection. Measures to reduce higher fevers increase patient comfort and prevent complications from hyperthermia. |

| ASSESSMENT—RECOGNIZE CUES/ INTERVENTIONS—TAKE ACTION | RATIONALES |
|---|---|
| Implement the measures to maintain hydration. | Fluids may be lost through diaphoresis. |
| Provide measures to improve patient's comfort by managing pain and fatigue as well as fever. Change linens as needed if they become wet from diaphoresis. | Promoting comfort and a quiet environment will encourage rest and improve the patient's ability to fight the infection. Keeping the linens dry also improves comfort and reduces shivering. |
| Assist the patient with maintaining adequate nutritional intake. | Patients with reduced nutritional status may be unable to have an adequate cellular/immune response to pathogens and thus may have difficulty fighting the infection. |

## Patient Problem/Analyze Cues/Prioritize Hypotheses

# Risk for Infection

*due to* the presence of an infectious pathogen, suppressed immune response occurring with long-term medication use (e.g., antiinflammatory agents, corticosteroids, chemotherapy agents) or disease process

***Desired Outcome/Generate Solutions:*** The patient remains free of infection as evidenced by orientation to person, place, and time; behavior within the patient's baseline limits; respiratory rate (RR) and pattern within the patient's baseline limits; urine that is straw colored, clear, and of characteristic odor; core temperature and heart rate (HR) within the patient's baseline limits; sputum that is clear to whitish in color; and skin that is intact and of baseline color and temperature for the patient.

| ASSESSMENT—RECOGNIZE CUES/ INTERVENTIONS—TAKE ACTION | RATIONALES |
|---|---|
| Assess for the presence of factors that increase the patient's risk for infection (see discussion above). | An assessment of risk factors can identify patients who are at a higher risk for infection. |
| Assess the baseline vital signs (VS), including level of consciousness (LOC) and orientation. Also, be alert to HR greater than 100 bpm and RR greater than 24 breaths/min. Auscultate lung fields for adventitious sounds. | Signs of infection include tachycardia and tachypnea. In older adults a change in mentation may occur. Adventitious breath sounds may be present with a respiratory illness. |
| Monitor the temperature and notify the HCP of a temperature greater than 101°F (38.3°C). | A low-grade fever is an expected response to inflammation, stress, surgery, illness, or trauma and is considered a helpful response in fighting infection. Elevated temperature is also a sign of infection. |
| Assess for and report signs and symptoms of infection (see *Infection*, above). | These are all possible indicators of an infection; early detection of potential infection will allow for immediate treatment. |
| Assess the patient's skin for tears, breaks, redness, or ulcers. Document the condition of the patient's skin, especially over pressure points, on admission and as an ongoing assessment. | Skin that is not intact is susceptible to infection. |
| Assess the quality and color of the patient's urine. Document changes when noted, and report findings to the HCP. Also be alert to urinary incontinence, which can signal urinary tract infection (UTI). | UTIs are manifested by cloudy, foul-smelling urine with or without painful urination and urinary incontinence. |
| Obtain drug history about the use of antiinflammatory or immunosuppressive drugs or long-term use of analgesics or corticosteroids. | These drugs mask fever, a sign of infection, and may make the patient more susceptible to infection by reducing immunity. |
| Always use hand hygiene and encourage the patient to practice it as well. | Reduces transmission of pathogens |

Continued

| ASSESSMENT—RECOGNIZE CUES/ INTERVENTIONS—TAKE ACTION | RATIONALES |
|---|---|
| Avoid the insertion of urinary catheters when possible. | Urinary catheter use increases the risk for infection. External urine collection devices may be used if accurate urine output is needed. |
| If infection is suspected, anticipate initiation of IV fluid therapy. | Fluid therapy will help maintain optimal hydration as well as replace losses caused by fever. |
| Anticipate orders for cultures (blood, urine, sputum, wound, etc.) and obtain them *before* antiinfective medications are started. | Cultures will isolate the infectious agent, and sensitivity reports will indicate the appropriate antiinfective medication. It is essential to obtain cultures before starting antiinfective drugs because the medications may alter the results of the cultures. |
| Anticipate WBC count. | The reference range for WBC count is 4.5–11,000/mm³ (ranges may vary with different facilities). An elevated WBC count may indicate infection. |
| Expect a chest radiographic examination if the patient's chest sounds are not clear. | This will be performed to rule out pneumonia. |
| If infection is present, prepare for initiation of broad-spectrum antibiotic therapy, oxygen therapy, and use of an antipyretic. | These interventions will eliminate infection, promote oxygenation to the brain, and decrease fever. Fever increases cardiac workload (i.e., HR rises) as the body responds to infection. |
| Protect patient from others who may have infections. | Reduces exposure to pathogens. |
| Always use sterile technique during invasive procedures such as venipuncture, catheter insertion, dressing changes. | Sterile technique reduces the introduction of pathogens to the patient's body. |

## Patient Problem/Analyze Cues/Prioritize Hypotheses

# Deficient Knowledge

*due to* not knowing how to avoid exposure to pathogens

**Desired Outcome/Generate Solutions:** The patient will demonstrate improved knowledge about infection prevention as evidenced by identifying the risk for infection, implementing measures to prevent infection, and following prescribed therapeutic regimens.

| ASSESSMENT—RECOGNIZE CUES/ INTERVENTIONS—TAKE ACTION | RATIONALES |
|---|---|
| Teach hand hygiene. Instruct the patient and caregiver to wash hands often and especially after toileting and before food preparation and meals. | This reduces the spread of potentially infectious pathogens. |
| Discuss the patient's infection risks and measures to avoid them. | Improved awareness of infection risks and how to avoid them may reduce the risk of infection. |
| Instruct the patient and caregivers about the importance of avoiding others who have infections or colds. | Infections may occur by direct contact with someone who is ill, or by indirect contact (contaminated inanimate objects) or through the air. |
| Discuss the signs and symptoms of infection and when to report them to the HCP. | Patients need to be able to recognize signs and symptoms of infection and what to report to their HCP so that treatment can begin early. |
| Recommend regular health screenings and immunizations. | Immunizations can reduce the chance of infection for certain diseases. |
| Instruct patient, and assist as necessary, to perform appropriate perineal care regularly and after each bowel movement. | The perineal area has increased bacteria content. Regular cleaning of the perineal area reduces the risk of perineal, urinary tract, or vaginal infections. |

## ASSESSMENT—RECOGNIZE CUES/ INTERVENTIONS—TAKE ACTION

| ASSESSMENT—RECOGNIZE CUES/ INTERVENTIONS—TAKE ACTION | RATIONALES |
|---|---|
| Instruct the patient to take the entire course of antiinfectives, even if they are feeling better or symptoms disappear. | Drug resistance may occur if the entire course of antiinfectives is not completed. Symptoms may reappear if the antiinfective medication is stopped too soon. |
| Instruct the patient to report signs and symptoms of superinfections, such as oral thrush, vaginal itching, or diarrhea. | Superinfections (bacterial or fungal) may occur as a result of antiinfective therapy. Early detection improves treatment. |

### ✔ PATIENT–FAMILY TEACHING AND DISCHARGE PLANNING

When providing patient–family teaching, focus on necessary information, and avoid giving excessive information, and initiate a visiting nurse referral for necessary follow-up teaching. Include verbal and written information as outlined in *Deficient Knowledge*, above. In addition:

✓ ensure that appropriate follow-up appointments with the patient's HCP have been made;

✓ provide telephone numbers to call in case questions or concerns arise about the therapy or disease after discharge;

✓ additional general information and patient education resources can be obtained by contacting the following;

✓ additional general information and patient education resources can be obtained by contacting the following:

- Infection Control: https://www.cdc.gov/ infectioncontrol/
- Top 10 Ways to Prevent Infection in the New Year: https://apic.org/monthly_alerts/top-10-ways-to-prevent-infection-in-the-new-year/
- COVID-19 Information: https://www.cdc.gov/ coronavirus/2019-nCoV/index.html

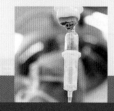

# Older Adult Care 3

## Confusion

*due to* age-related decreased physiologic reserve, renal function, or cardiac function; altered sensory/perceptual reception occurring with poor vision or hearing; or short-term memory loss occurring with decreased brain oxygenation

***Desired Outcomes/Generate Solutions:*** Optimally, acute confusion diminishes following interventions. The patient sustains no evidence of injury or harm as a result of mental status or sensory losses.

| ASSESSMENT—RECOGNIZE CUES/ INTERVENTIONS—TAKE ACTION | RATIONALES |
|---|---|
| Assess the patient's baseline level of consciousness (LOC) and mental status on admission. Obtain preconfusion functional and mental status abilities from significant other or clinical caregiver. Ask the patient to perform a three-step task. For example, "Raise your right hand, place it on your left shoulder, and then place the right hand by your right side." | A component of the Mini-Mental Status Examination, this assessment of a three-step task provides a baseline for subsequent assessments of a patient's confusion. A three-step task is complex and is a gross indicator of brain function. Because it requires attention, it can also test for delirium. |
| Use the standardized assessment tool (available online) to help identify the presence or absence of delirium, which is an acute confusional state (see "Delirium," Chapter 98). | Delirium, a potential source of confusion in older adults, often goes unrecognized. |
| Test short-term memory by showing the patient how to use the call light, having the patient return the demonstration, and then waiting at least 5 minutes before having the patient demonstrate the use of the call light again. Document the patient's actions in behavioral terms. Describe the "confused" behavior. | Inability to remember beyond 5 minutes indicates poor short-term memory. |
| Identify the cause of acute confusion (delirium). | Acute confusion is caused by physical and psychosocial conditions and not by age alone. For example, oximetry or arterial blood gas (ABG) values may reveal low oxygenation levels, serum glucose or fingerstick glucose may reveal high or low glucose level, and electrolytes and complete blood count (CBC) will ascertain imbalances and/or presence of elevated white blood cell (WBC) count as a determinant of infection. Hydration status may be determined by checking for dry, sticky mucous membranes and a furrowed tongue. |
| Assess for pain using a rating scale of 0–10. If the patient is unable to use a scale, assess for behavioral cues such as grimacing, clenched fists, frowning, and hitting. Ask the family or significant other to assist in identifying pain behaviors. | Acute confusion can be a sign of pain. |
| Treat the patient for pain, as indicated, and monitor behaviors. | If pain is the cause of the confusion, the patient's behavior should change if pain relief is successful. |

| ASSESSMENT—RECOGNIZE CUES/ INTERVENTIONS—TAKE ACTION | RATIONALES |
|---|---|
| Review cardiac status. Assess apical pulse and notify the health care provider of an irregular pulse that is new to the patient. If the patient is on a cardiac monitor or telemetry, watch for dysrhythmias; notify the health care provider accordingly. | Dysrhythmias and other cardiac dysfunctions may result in decreased oxygenation, which can lead to confusion. |
| Review current medications, including over-the-counter drugs. Note any medications that are new orders. | New medications may be the source of confusion in the elderly. Toxic levels of certain medications, such as digoxin, cause acute confusion. Anticholinergic medications can also cause confusion, as can drug interactions. |
| Monitor the intake and output (I&O) at least every 8 hours. | Optimally, the output should match the intake. Dehydration can result in acute confusion. |
| Have the patient wear glasses and hearing aids, or keep them close to the bedside and within easy reach for patient use. | Glasses and hearing aids are likely to help decrease sensory confusion. |
| Keep the patient's urinal and other routinely used items within easy reach of the patient. | A confused patient may wait until it is too late to seek assistance with toileting. |
| If the patient has short-term memory problems, take the patient to the commode or offer the urinal or bedpan every 2 hours while awake and every 4 hours during the night. Establish a toileting schedule and post it on the patient care plan and, inconspicuously, at the bedside. | A patient with a short-term memory problem cannot be expected to use the call light. |
| Check on the patient at least every 30 minutes and every time you pass the room. Place the patient close to the nurses' station if possible. Provide an environment that is nonstimulating and safe. | A confused patient requires extra safety precautions. |
| Obtain an order for a sitter to sit with the patient. | The presence of a sitter will help to prevent the patient from getting out of bed alone and improve safety. |
| Provide music but not TV. | Patients who are confused regarding place and time often think the action on TV is happening in the room. |
| Attempt to reorient the patient to his or her surroundings as needed. Keep a clock with large numerals and a large print calendar at the bedside; verbally remind the patient of the date and day as needed. | Reorientation may decrease confusion. |
| Tell the patient in simple terms what is occurring. For example, "It's time to eat breakfast," "This medicine is for your heart," "I'm going to help you get out of bed." | Sentences that are more complex may not be understood. |
| Encourage the patient's significant other to bring items familiar to the patient, including blanket, bedspread, and pictures of family and pets. | Familiar items may promote orientation while also providing comfort. |
| If the patient becomes belligerent, angry, or argumentative while you are attempting to reorient, *stop this approach*. Do not argue with the patient or the patient's interpretation of the environment. State, "I can understand why you may [hear, think, see] that." | This approach prevents escalation of anger in a confused person. |
| If the patient displays hostile behavior or misperceives your role (e.g., nurse becomes thief, jailer), leave the room. Return in 15 minutes. Introduce yourself to the patient as though you had never met. Begin dialog anew. | Patients who are acutely confused have poor short-term memory and may not remember the previous encounter or that you were involved in that encounter. |
| If the patient attempts to leave the hospital, walk with him or her and attempt distraction. Ask the patient to tell you about the destination. For example, "That sounds like a wonderful place! Tell me about it." Keep your tone pleasant and conversational. Continue walking with the patient away from exits and doors around the unit. After a few minutes, attempt to guide the patient back to the room. Offer refreshments and rest. For example, "We've been walking for a while and I'm a little tired. Why don't we sit and have some juice while we talk?" | Distraction is an effective means of reversing a behavior in a patient who is confused. |

Continued

General Care Plans

| ASSESSMENT—RECOGNIZE CUES/ INTERVENTIONS—TAKE ACTION | RATIONALES |
|---|---|
| If the patient has a permanent or severe cognitive impairment, check on her or him at least every 30 minutes and reorient to baseline mental status as indicated; however, do not argue with the patient about his or her perception of reality. | Arguing can cause a cognitively impaired person to become aggressive and combative.<br>**Note:** Individuals with severe cognitive impairment (e.g., Alzheimer's disease or dementia) also can experience acute confusional states (i.e., delirium) and can be returned to their baseline mental state. |
| If the patient tries to climb out of bed, offer a urinal or bedpan or assist to the commode. | The patient may need to use the toilet. |
| Alternatively, if the patient is not on bedrest, place the patient in chair or wheelchair at the nurses' station. | This action provides added supervision to promote a patient's safety while also promoting stimulation and preventing isolation. |
| Bargain with the patient. Try to establish an agreement to stay for a defined period, such as until the health care provider, meal, or significant other arrives. | This is a delaying strategy to defuse anger. Because of poor memory and attention span, the patient may forget he or she wanted to leave. |
| Have the patient's significant other talk with the patient by phone or come in and sit with the patient if the patient's behavior requires checking more often than every 30 minutes. | These actions by the significant other may help promote the patient's safety. |
| Use restraints with caution and according to agency policy. | Patients can become more agitated when wrist and arm restraints are used. |
| Use medications cautiously for controlling behavior. | Follow the maxim "start low and go slow" with medications because older patients can respond to small amounts of drugs.<br>Neuroleptics, such as haloperidol, can be used successfully in calming patients with dementia or psychiatric illness (contraindicated for individuals with parkinsonism). However, if the patient is experiencing acute confusion or delirium, short-acting benzodiazepines (e.g., lorazepam) are more effective in reducing anxiety and fear. Anxiety or fear usually triggers destructive or dangerous behaviors in acutely confused older patients.<br>**Note:** Neuroleptics can cause akathisia, an adverse drug reaction evidenced by increased restlessness. |

**See also** "Dementia—Alzheimer's Type," Chapter 101, as appropriate.

## Patient Problem/Analyze Cues/Prioritize Hypotheses

# Impaired Gas Exchange

*due to* decreased functional lung tissue

***Desired Outcomes/Generate Outcomes:*** The patient's respiratory pattern and mental status are at the patient's baseline level. ABG or pulse oximetry values are at the patient's baseline levels.

| ASSESSMENT—RECOGNIZE CUES/ INTERVENTIONS—TAKE ACTION | RATIONALES |
|---|---|
| Assess and document the following on admission and routinely thereafter: respiratory rate (RR), pattern, and depth; breath sounds; cough; sputum; and sensorium. | This assessment establishes a baseline for subsequent assessments of the patient's respiratory system. |
| Assess the patient for subtle changes in mentation or behavior such as increased restlessness, anxiety, disorientation, and hostility. If available, monitor oxygenation status using ABG findings (optimally $PaO_2$ 80%–95% or greater) or pulse oximetry (optimally greater than 92%). | Mentation changes such as increased restlessness, anxiety, disorientation, and hostility can signal decreased oxygenation. To adequately evaluate pulse oximetry, the hemoglobin (Hgb) must be known. Patients with low Hgb can have a higher pulse oximeter reading and yet display restlessness or acute confusion. This is due to the lack of Hgb to circulate oxygen. |

| ASSESSMENT—RECOGNIZE CUES/ INTERVENTIONS—TAKE ACTION | RATIONALES |
|---|---|
| Assess the lungs for adventitious sounds. | The aging lung has decreased elasticity. The lower part of the lung may no longer adequately aerate. As a result, crackles commonly are heard in individuals 75 years and older. This sign alone does not mean that a pathologic condition is present. Crackles that do not clear with coughing in an individual with no other clinical signs (e.g., fever, increasing anxiety, changes in mental status, increasing respiratory depth) are considered benign. |
| Encourage the patient to cough and breathe deeply. When appropriate, instruct the patient in the use of incentive spirometry. | These actions promote alveolar expansion and clear the secretions from the bronchial tree, thereby helping ensure better gas exchange. |
| Unless contraindicated by a cardiac or renal condition, encourage fluid intake to be greater than 2.5 L/day. | Hydration helps ensure less viscous pulmonary secretions, which are more easily mobilized. |
| Treat fevers promptly, decrease pain, minimize pacing activity, and lessen anxiety. | These interventions reduce the potential for increased oxygen consumption. |
| Instruct the patient in the use of support equipment such as oxygen masks or cannulas. | Knowledge helps promote adherence to therapy. |

## Patient Problem/Analyze Cues/Prioritize Hypotheses

# Risk for Aspiration

*due to* depressed cough and gag reflexes or ineffective esophageal sphincter

***Desired Outcomes/Generate Solutions:*** The patient swallows independently without choking. The patient's airway is patent and lungs are clear to auscultation both before and after meals.

| ASSESSMENT—RECOGNIZE CUES/ INTERVENTIONS—TAKE ACTION | RATIONALES |
|---|---|
| Perform a baseline assessment of the patient's ability to swallow by asking if the patient has any difficulty swallowing or if any food or fluids are difficult to swallow or cause gagging. If the patient is unable to answer, consult the patient's caregiver or significant other. Document the findings. | This assessment helps determine a patient's ability to swallow without choking and needs to be compared with subsequent assessments to document improvements or deficits. |
| Assess the patient's ability to swallow by placing your thumb and index finger on both sides of the laryngeal prominence and asking the patient to swallow. Check for the gag reflex by gently touching one side and then the other of the posterior pharyngeal wall using a tongue blade. Document both findings. | Ability to swallow and an intact gag reflex are necessary to prevent aspiration and choking before the patient takes food or fluids orally. |
| As indicated, request the evaluation by a speech therapist. | This evaluation will enable a specialized assessment of gag and swallow reflexes. |
| Place the patient in an upright position with the chin tilting down slightly while eating or drinking, and support the upright position with pillows on the patient's sides. | This position minimizes the risk for choking and aspirating by closing off the airway and facilitating the gravitational flow of food and fluids into the stomach and through the pylorus. |
| Monitor the patient when he or she is swallowing. | This assessment will help determine the patient's ability to swallow without choking. Deficits may necessitate aspiration precautions. |
| Watch for drooling of saliva or food or inability to close the lips around a straw. | These are signs of limited lip, tongue, or jaw movement. |
| Check for retention of food in sides of the mouth. | This is an indication of poor tongue movement. |

Continued

## ASSESSMENT—RECOGNIZE CUES/ INTERVENTIONS—TAKE ACTION

## RATIONALES

| ASSESSMENT—RECOGNIZE CUES/ INTERVENTIONS—TAKE ACTION | RATIONALES |
|---|---|
| Monitor the intake of food. Document consistencies and amounts of food the patient eats, where the patient places food in the mouth, how the patient manipulates or chews before swallowing, and the length of time before the patient swallows the food bolus. | Other caregivers will find this information useful during subsequent feedings. |
| Monitor the patient for coughing or choking before, during, or after swallowing. | Coughing or choking may occur up to several minutes following the placement of food or fluid in the mouth and signals aspiration of material into the airway. |
| Monitor the patient for changes in lung auscultation (e.g., crackles, wheezes), shortness of breath, dyspnea, decreasing LOC, increasing temperature, and cyanosis. | These are signs of silent aspiration. For example, some older patients, especially those in declining health, have an increased risk for silent aspiration when the esophageal sphincter fails to close completely between swallows. |
| Monitor the patient for a wet or gurgling sound when talking after a swallow. | This sound indicates aspiration into the airway and signals delayed or absent swallow and gag reflexes. |
| For a patient with poor swallowing reflex, tilt the head forward 45 degrees during swallowing. **Note:** For patients with hemiplegia, tilt the head toward the unaffected side. | This head position will help prevent inadvertent aspiration by closing off the airway. |
| Anticipate swallowing video fluoroscopy in the evaluation of the patient's gag and swallow reflexes. | This procedure is used to determine whether patients are aspirating, consistency of materials most likely to be aspirated, and aspiration cause. Using four consistencies of barium, the radiologist and speech therapist watch for the presence of reduced or ineffective tongue function, reduced peristalsis in the pharynx, delayed or absent swallow reflex, and poor or limited ability to close the epiglottis that protects the airway. |
| Based on the results of the swallowing video fluoroscopy, thickened fluids may be prescribed. Or, mechanical soft or pureed diets may be prescribed. | Agents are added to the fluid to make it more viscous and easier for patients to swallow. Similarly, mechanical soft, pureed, or liquid diets enable patients to ingest food with less potential for aspiration. |
| Provide adequate rest periods before meals. | Fatigue increases the risk for aspiration. |
| Remind patients with dementia to chew and swallow with each bite. Check for retained food in sides of the mouth. | Patients with dementia might forget to chew and swallow. |
| Ensure that the patient has dentures in place, if appropriate, and that they fit correctly. | Chewing well minimizes the risk for choking. |
| Ensure that someone stays with the patient during meals or fluid intake. | This ensures added safety in the event of choking or aspiration. |
| Provide adequate time for the patient to eat and drink. | Generally, patients with swallowing deficits require twice as much time for eating and drinking as those whose swallowing is adequate. |
| Be aware of the location of suction equipment to be used in the event of aspiration. | If the patient is at increased risk for aspiration, make sure suction equipment is available at the bedside. |
| If the patient aspirates, implement the following: | |
| • Follow American Heart Association (AHA) standards if the patient displays characteristics of complete airway obstruction (i.e., choking). | This is an emergency situation. |
| • For partial airway obstruction, encourage the patient to cough as needed. | This action will clear the airway. |
| • For partial airway obstruction in an unconscious or nonresponsive individual who is not coughing, suction the airway with a large-bore catheter such as Yankauer or tonsil suction tip. | Suctioning clears the airway. |
| • For either a complete or partial aspiration, inform the health care provider and obtain a prescription for chest radiographic examination. | Radiography will determine whether food/fluid remains in the airway. |

| ASSESSMENT—RECOGNIZE CUES/ INTERVENTIONS—TAKE ACTION | RATIONALES |
|---|---|
| • Implement nothing by mouth (NPO) status until a diagnosis is confirmed. | NPO prevents further risk to patient. |
| • Monitor the breathing pattern and RR every 1–2 hours after a suspected aspiration for alterations (i.e., increased RR). | This assessment helps determine that a change in the patient's condition has occurred. |
| • Anticipate the use of antibiotics. | There is risk for infection/pneumonia after aspiration. |
| Encourage the patient to cough and deep breathe every 2 hours while awake and every 4 hours during the night. | These measures promote the expansion of available lung tissue and help prevent infection. |

## Patient Problem/Analyze Cues/Prioritize Hypotheses

# Risk for Dehydration

*due to* the potential inability to obtain fluids because of illness or lack of access

***Desired Outcomes/Generate Solutions:*** Within 24 hours after interventions, the patient's mental status; vital signs (VS); and urine specific gravity, color, consistency, and concentration are at the patient's baseline levels. The patient's mucous membranes are moist, and there is no furrowing in the tongue. The patient's intake equals output.

| ASSESSMENT—RECOGNIZE CUES/ INTERVENTIONS—TAKE ACTION | RATIONALES |
|---|---|
| Assess the fluid intake. In nonrestricted individuals, encourage fluid intake of 2–3 L/day. Specify intake goals for day, evening, and night shifts. | These actions help ensure that the patient's hydration status is adequate. Restrictions may apply to patients with cardiopulmonary and renal disorders. |
| Assess for signs and symptoms of dehydration such as dry, sticky mouth, dark-colored urine, new-onset confusion, dizziness or lightheadedness, or fatigue.<br>**Note:** Checking skin turgor may not indicate dehydration in an older adult. | These signs and symptoms may indicate dehydration. Assessing skin turgor in an elderly person is not a reliable indicator of dehydration because the skin loses elasticity with aging. Delayed skin turgor may occur even when dehydration is not present. A furrowed tongue signals severe dehydration. |
| Assess and document the color, amount, and frequency of any fluid output, including emesis, urine, diarrhea, or other drainage. | This assessment enables the comparison of intake to output amounts. Urine that is dark in color signals concentration and thus dehydration. |
| Monitor the patient's orientation, ability to follow commands, and behavior. | Loss of the ability to follow commands, decrease in orientation, and confused behavior can signal a dehydrated state. |
| Weigh the patient daily at the same time of day (preferably before breakfast) using the same scale and bed clothing. | Using comparable measurements ensures more accurate comparisons. Wide variations in weight (e.g., 2.5 kg [5 lb] or greater) can signal increased or decreased hydration status. |
| In patients who are dehydrated, anticipate elevations in serum sodium and blood urea nitrogen (BUN). | These elevations often occur with dehydration. |
| If the patient is receiving IV therapy, assess cardiac and respiratory systems for signs of fluid overload. Assess the apical pulse and listen to lung fields during every VS assessment. | Overload could precipitate heart failure or pulmonary edema. Rising heart rate (HR), crackles, and bronchial wheezes can be signals of heart failure or pulmonary edema. |
| Carefully monitor the I&O when the patient is receiving tube feedings or dyes for contrast. Watch for evidence of third spacing of fluids, including increasing peripheral edema, especially sacral; output significantly less than intake (1:2); and urine output less than 0.5 mL/kg/hr. | These agents act osmotically to pull fluid into the interstitial tissue, which may lead to dehydration. |
| Whenever in the room, offer the patient fluids. Offer a variety of drinks the patient likes, but limit caffeine because it acts as a diuretic. | Older persons have a decreased sense of thirst and need encouragement to drink. |

Continued

| ASSESSMENT—RECOGNIZE CUES/ INTERVENTIONS—TAKE ACTION | RATIONALES |
|---|---|
| Assess the patient's ability to obtain and drink fluids by himself or herself. Place fluids within easy reach. Use cups with tops to minimize concern over spilling. | These actions remove barriers to adequate fluid intake. |
| Ensure access to the toilet, urinal, commode, or bedpan at least every 2 hours when the patient is awake and every 4 hours at night. Answer the call light quickly. | The time between recognition of the need to void and urination decreases with age. |

## Patient Problem/Analyze Cues/Prioritize Hypotheses

# Risk for Infection

Older adults are at risk for infection because of age-related changes and/or suppressed inflammatory response occurring with long-term medication use (e.g., antiinflammatory agents, corticosteroids, analgesics), slowed ciliary response, or poor nutrition. It is important to remember that older adults manifest infection differently, with cognitive and behavioral changes occurring before fever, pain, or changes in labwork. In addition, fever is not a reliable indicator of fever in an older adult; a temperature less than 98.6°F (37°C) may be normal. The shivering reflex is also diminished in older adults. A change in mentation is a leading sign of infection in older patients. Other signs of infection include tachycardia and tachypnea. Adventitious breath sounds may or may not be seen until late in the course of illness. A urinary tract infection, as manifested by cloudy, foul-smelling urine without painful urination, and possible urinary incontinence, is the most common infection in older adults.

For Desired Outcomes, Interventions, and Rationale, see *Risk for Infection* in Chapter 2.

## Patient Problem/Analyze Cues/Prioritize Hypotheses

# Altered Temperature (Hypothermia)

*due to* age-related changes in thermoregulation and/or environmental exposure

***Desired Outcome/Generate Solutions:***  Body temperature remains within the patient's baseline levels, or it returns to the patient's baseline levels at a rate of 1°F/hour, after interventions.

| ASSESSMENT—RECOGNIZE CUES/ INTERVENTIONS—TAKE ACTION | RATIONALES |
|---|---|
| Assess the patient's temperature, using a low-range thermometer if possible. | This assessment will determine whether the patient has hypothermia. Older adults can have a baseline temperature of 96°F (35.5°C). |
| **Note:** Do not take axillary temperature in the older adult. If unable to measure the temperature orally, measure tympanic or temporal temperature but note that reliability of these thermometers may be inconsistent because of improper use. | Older persons have decreased peripheral circulation and loss of subcutaneous fat in the axillary area, resulting in the formation of a pocket of air that may make readings inaccurate. |
| Assess and document the patient's mental status. | Increasing disorientation, mental status changes, or atypical behavior can signal hypothermia. |

| ASSESSMENT—RECOGNIZE CUES/ INTERVENTIONS—TAKE ACTION | RATIONALES |
|---|---|
| Be alert to use of sedatives, hypnotics (including anesthetics), and muscle relaxants. | These medications decrease shivering and therefore place patients at risk for environmental hypothermia. In addition, all older adults are at risk for environmental hypothermia at ambient temperatures of 72°F–75°F (22.22°C–23.89°C). |
| Ensure that patients going for testing, radiographic examination, or surgery are sent with enough blankets to keep warm. | This intervention will help prevent hypothermia. Low ambient air temperature combined with the older person's diminished ability to maintain thermal homeostasis can be dangerous. |
| If the patient is mildly hypothermic, initiate slow rewarming. | To reverse mild hypothermia, one method of slow rewarming is raising the room temperature to at least 75°F (23.89°C). Other methods of external warming include the use of warm blankets, head covers, and warm circulating air blankets. |
| If the patient's temperature falls below 95°F (35°C), warm the patient internally by administering warm oral fluids, or IV fluids as ordered. | To reverse moderate to severe hypothermia, patients are warmed internally by administering warm oral or IV fluids. Introduction of warmed humidified air into the airway is another method of internal warming. |
| Avoid, and be alert to signs of too rapid rewarming. | Signs of too rapid rewarming include irregular HR, dysrhythmias, and very warm extremities caused by vasodilation in the periphery, which causes heat loss from the core. |
| If the patient's temperature fails to rise 1°F/hour using these techniques, anticipate laboratory tests, including WBC count for possible sepsis, thyroid test for hypothyroidism, and glucose level for hypoglycemia. | Causes other than environmental ones may be responsible for the hypothermia. |
| As prescribed, administer antibiotics for sepsis, thyroid therapy, or glucose for hypoglycemia. | The patient's temperature will not return to baseline unless the underlying condition has been treated. |

## Patient Problem/Analyze Cues/Prioritize Hypotheses

# Risk for Impaired Skin Integrity

*due to* decreased subcutaneous fat and decreased peripheral capillary networks in the integumentary system and decreased mobility

***Desired Outcome/Generate Solutions:*** The patient's skin remains nonerythremic and intact.

| ASSESSMENT—RECOGNIZE CUES/ INTERVENTIONS—TAKE ACTION | RATIONALES |
|---|---|
| Assess the patient's skin on admission and routinely thereafter. | This assessment provides a baseline for subsequent assessments of skin integrity. |
| Note any areas of redness or any breaks in the skin surface. | Redness or breaks in skin integrity necessitate aggressive skin care interventions to prevent further breakdown and infection. |
| Ensure that the patient turns frequently (at least every 2 hours). | Turning alternates sites of pressure and pressure relief. |
| Lift or roll the patient across sheets when repositioning. | Pulling, dragging, or sliding across sheets can lead to shear (cutaneous or subcutaneous tissue) injury. |
| Monitor the skin over bony prominences for erythema. | Skin that lies over the sacrum, scapulae, heels, spine, hips, pelvis, greater trochanter, knees, ankles, costal margins, occiput, and ischial tuberosities is at increased risk for breakdown because of excessive external pressure. |

Continued

| ASSESSMENT—RECOGNIZE CUES/ INTERVENTIONS—TAKE ACTION | RATIONALES |
| --- | --- |
| Use pillows or pads around bony prominences, even when the patient is up in a wheelchair or sits for long periods. | This intervention maintains alternative positions and pads the bony prominences, thereby protecting overlying skin. The ischial tuberosities are susceptible to breakdown when a patient is in the seated position. Gel pads for the chair or wheelchair seats aid in distributing pressure. |
| Use lotions liberally on dry skin. | Lotions promote moisture and suppleness. Lanolin-containing lotions are especially useful. |
| Use alternating-pressure mattresses, air-fluidized mattresses, specialty air bed, or other pressure-sensitive mattresses for older patients who are on bedrest or unable to get out of bed. | These mattresses protect skin from injury caused by prolonged pressure. |
| Avoid placing tubes under the patient's limbs or head. Place a pillow or pad between the patient and tube for cushioning. | Excess pressure from tubes can create a pressure ulcer. |
| Get the patient out of bed as often as possible. Liberally use mechanical lifting devices to aid in safe patient transfers. If the patient is unable to get out of bed, assist with position changes every 2 hours at a minimum. | These actions promote blood flow, which helps prevent skin breakdown. |
| Establish and post a turning schedule on the patient care plan and at the bedside. | Schedules increase awareness of staff and patient/family of the turning schedule. |
| Ensure that the patient's face, axillae, and genital areas are cleansed daily. | These areas must be kept clean to avoid infection, but complete baths dry out older adults' skin and should be given every other day instead of daily |
| Use tepid water (90°F–105°F [32.2°C–40.5°C]) and superfatted, nonperfumed soaps. | Hot water can burn older adults, who have decreased pain sensitivity and decreased sensation to temperature. Superfatted soaps help decrease the dryness of skin. |
| Minimize the use of plastic protective pads under the patient. When used, place at least one layer of cloth (draw sheet) between the patient and the plastic pad to absorb moisture. For incontinent patients, check the pad at least every 2 hours. Discourage the use of adult diapers unless the patient is ambulatory, going for tests, or is up in a chair. | Pads and adult diapers trap moisture and heat and can lead to skin breakdown (maceration-associated skin damage). |
| Document the percentage of food intake with meals. Encourage the significant other/family to provide the patient's favorite foods. Suggest nutritious snacks if the patient's diet is not restricted. Obtain nutritional consultation with a dietitian as needed. | Food/snacks high in protein and vitamin C help prevent skin breakdown. |

For more information, see "Managing Wound Care," Chapter 75, for **Pressure Injury: Overview/Pathophysiology** and "Providing Nutritional Support," Chapter 76.

## Patient Problem/Analyze Cues/Prioritize Hypotheses

# Fatigue

*due to* interrupted sleep occurring with unfamiliar surroundings and hospital routines

***Desired Outcomes/Generate Solutions:*** Within 24 hours of interventions, the patient reports attainment of adequate rest. Mental status remains to baseline for the patient.

PART I: Medical-Surgical Nursing Care Plans

| ASSESSMENT—RECOGNIZE CUES/ INTERVENTIONS—TAKE ACTION | RATIONALES |
|---|---|
| Assess and document the patient's sleeping pattern, obtaining information from the patient, the patient's caregiver, or significant others. | Older adults typically sleep less than they did when they were younger and often awaken more frequently during the night. |
| Ask questions about naps and activity levels. | Individuals who take naps and have a low level of activity frequently sleep only 4–5 hours per night. |
| Determine the patient's usual nighttime routine and attempt to follow it. | Following the usual nighttime rituals may facilitate sleep. |
| Attempt to group together activities such as medications, VS, and toileting during nighttime hours. | This reduces the number of interruptions and facilitates rest and sleep. |
| Provide pain medications if needed, back rub, and pleasant conversation at sleep time. | These comfort measures may facilitate sleep. |
| Monitor the patient's activity level. | If the patient complains of being tired after activities or displays behaviors such as irritability, yelling, or shouting, encourage napping after lunch or early in the afternoon. Otherwise, discourage daytime napping, especially in the late afternoon, because it can interfere with nighttime sleep. |
| Discourage caffeinated coffee, cola, and tea after 6 p.m. | Stimulants can make it difficult to fall asleep and stay asleep as well as increase nighttime awakenings to urinate. |
| Provide a quiet environment and minimize interruptions during sleep hours. | Excessive noises, bright overhead lights, noisy roommates, and loud talking can cause sleep deprivation. The use of sound generators (e.g., of ocean waves) or white noise (e.g., fan) may promote sleep. |

## Patient Problem/Analyze Cues/Prioritize Hypotheses

# Constipation

*due to* changes in diet, decreased activity, and psychosocial factors

**Desired Outcomes/Generate Solutions:** The patient states that his or her bowel habit has returned to baseline pattern within three to four days of this problem. Stool appears soft, and the patient does not strain in passing stools.

| ASSESSMENT—RECOGNIZE CUES/ INTERVENTIONS—TAKE ACTION | RATIONALES |
|---|---|
| On admission, assess and document the patient's baseline bowel elimination pattern. Include frequency, time of day, associated habits, and successful methods used to correct constipation in the past. Consult the patient's caregiver or significant other if the patient is unable to provide this information. | This assessment establishes a baseline and determines a patient's usual bowel elimination pattern. |
| Inform the patient that changes occurring with hospitalization may increase the potential for constipation. Urge the patient to institute successful nonpharmacologic methods used at home as soon as this problem is noticed or prophylactically as needed. | Constipation is easier to treat preventively than when it is present and/or prolonged. |
| Explain the relationship between fluid intake and constipation. Unless otherwise contraindicated, encourage fluid intake that exceeds 2500 mL/day. | A high fluid intake promotes soft stool and decreases risk/degree of constipation. A high fluid volume may be contraindicated in patients with renal, cardiac, or hepatic disorders who may have fluid restrictions. |
| Encourage the patient to include roughage (e.g., raw fruits and vegetables, whole grains, nuts, fruits with skins) as a part of each meal when possible. For patients unable to tolerate raw foods, encourage intake of bran through cereals, muffins, and breads. | Eating roughage reduces the potential for constipation by promoting bulk in the stool. |

Continued

| ASSESSMENT—RECOGNIZE CUES/ INTERVENTIONS—TAKE ACTION | RATIONALES |
|---|---|
| Titrate the amount of roughage to the degree of constipation. | Too much roughage taken too quickly can cause diarrhea, gas, and distention. |
| Explain to the patient the relationship between constipation and activity level. Encourage optimal activity for all patients. Establish and post an activity program to enhance participation; include devices necessary to enable independence. | Exercise can prevent or decrease constipation by promoting peristalsis. |
| If the patient's usual bowel movement occurs in the early morning, use the patient's gastrocolic or duodenocolic reflex to promote colonic emptying. If the patient's bowel movement occurs in the evening, ambulate the patient just before the appropriate time. Drinking hot liquids in the morning, for example, may promote peristalsis. | Scheduling interventions that coincide with a patient's bowel habit is more likely to promote bowel movements. |
| Attempt to use methods the patient has used successfully in the past. Follow the maxim "go low, go slow" (i.e., use the lowest level of nonnatural intervention and advance to more powerful interventions slowly). | Aggressive interventions may result in rebound constipation and interfere with subsequent bowel movements. |
| When requesting a pharmacologic intervention, use the more benign, oral methods first. | Older persons tend to focus on the loss of habit as an indicator of constipation rather than on the number of stools. Do not intervene pharmacologically until the older adult has not had a stool for 3 days. |
| | The following hierarchy is suggested: |
| | • Bulk-building additives such as psyllium or bran. |
| | • Mild laxatives (apple or prune juice, Milk of Magnesia). |
| | • Stool softeners (docusate sodium, docusate calcium). |
| | • Potent laxatives or cathartics (bisacodyl, cascara sagrada). |
| | • Medicated suppositories (glycerin, bisacodyl). |
| | • Enema (tap water, saline, sodium biphosphate/phosphate). |
| After diagnostic imaging of the gastrointestinal tract with barium, ensure that the patient receives a postexamination laxative and drinks extra fluids as allowed. | The laxative facilitates the removal of the barium. After any procedure involving a bowel clean-out, there may be rebound constipation from the severe disruption of bowel habit. |
| **Evaluate Outcomes:** | Documentation of bowel movements provides information as to whether interventions are needed or were successful. |
| Monitor and record bowel movements (date, time, consistency, amount). | |
| Monitor hydration status for signs of dehydration. Emphasize diet, fluid, activity, and resumption of routines. If no bowel movement occurs in 3 days, begin with mild laxatives to try to regain the baseline pattern. | Dehydration can occur as a result of the osmotic agents used. Decreased fluid volume can result in hard stools, which are more difficult to evacuate. |

**See also:** "Immobility," Chapter 1 *Constipation*.

## Patient Problem/Analyze Cues/Prioritize Hypotheses

# Impaired Functional Ability

*due to* loss of independence, malnutrition, depression, cognitive impairment, impaired immune function, impact of chronic illness, and adult failure to thrive

***Desired Outcome/Generate Solutions:*** By the 24-hour period before hospital discharge, the patient exhibits or verbalizes improvement in at least one of the following: weight gain, increased appetite, increased functional ability, sense of hopefulness, peaceful death.

| ASSESSMENT—RECOGNIZE CUES/ INTERVENTIONS—TAKE ACTION | RATIONALES |
|---|---|
| Perform a thorough physical assessment. Assess the status of a chronic illness. | A complete system assessment provides a baseline for subsequent comparison. |
| Review laboratory and other studies such as CBC with differential, basic metabolic panel, thyroid-stimulating hormone, albumin, and prealbumin levels. | A review of laboratory information identifies issues in nutrients and electrolytes essential for basic body function, status of protein and thyroid function, and presence/absence of infection. |
| Perform a thorough patient history; engage caretakers as needed. Analyze critical factors such as the death of a spouse or family member. | A thorough history focusing on timing of the change in behaviors and appetite, medications, and decline in activities of daily living (ADLs) and instrumental ADLs will help identify contributing factors to the decline in function. Examples of contributing factors include hypothyroidism, dementia, decreased sense of taste or smell, and depression. |
| Encourage the patient to verbalize feelings of despair, frustration, fear, anger, and concerns about hospitalization and health. | Verbalization of feelings and the knowledge that they are normal often help minimize feelings of despair. |
| Discuss expected age changes with the patient and family. | As people age, their physiologic reserve decreases and affects multiple systems. Failure to thrive can occur from the interaction of three components: physical frailty, disability or decline in functional ability, and impaired neuropsychiatric function. Frailty is defined by decreased physiologic reserve affecting many systems. Disability is defined as difficulty or decline in completing ADLs. Neuropsychiatric impairment is a complex phenomenon that can occur from life circumstances leading to depression, physiologic disruption leading to delirium, or neurologic changes resulting in cognitive impairment. |
| As indicated, consult with other health care professionals, such as speech therapists, dietitians, physical and occupational therapists, social services, and discharge planning. | A multidisciplinary approach is necessary for this complex condition. Speech therapists and dietitians can help assess unexplained decline in eating. Physical and occupational therapists can help analyze physical limitations/strengths and the potential for improvement with a program or assistive device. Social services can help assess support networks and readiness for palliative care and end-of-life concerns (see Chapter 7). |

# Perioperative Care    4

## Problems for Patients Who Are Preoperative

### Patient Problem/Analyze Cues/Prioritize Hypotheses

## Deficient Knowledge

*due to* unfamiliarity with the surgical procedure, preoperative routine, and postoperative care

***Desired Outcomes/Generate Solutions:*** After instruction the patient verbalizes knowledge about the surgical procedure, including preoperative preparations and sensations and postoperative care and sensations, and demonstrates postoperative exercises and the use of devices before the surgical procedure or during the immediate postoperative period for emergency surgery.

| ASSESSMENT—RECOGNIZE CUES/ INTERVENTIONS—TAKE ACTION | RATIONALES |
|---|---|
| **Preoperatively:** | |
| Evaluate the patient's desire for knowledge about the diagnosis and procedure. | Some individuals find detailed information helpful; others prefer very brief and simple explanations. |
| Assess the patient's understanding about the diagnosis, surgical procedure, preoperative routine, and postoperative regimen. | Assessment needs to include the patient's primary language and whether an interpreter is needed; the patient's readiness to learn; limitations on the patient's ability to learn such as blindness or decreased hearing; and the patient's self-assessment as to which modes of learning he or she finds most helpful, such as reading, listening, visual aids, or demonstration. |
| Determine past surgical experiences and their positive or negative effect on the patient. Assess the nature of any concerns or fears related to surgery. Document and communicate these assessment data to others involved in the patient's care. | Assessing the patient's knowledge, past experiences, and concerns about the surgical procedure will enable the nurse to focus on individual areas in need of the greatest intervention. |
| Based on your assessment, clarify and explain the diagnosis and surgical procedure accordingly. When possible, emphasize associated sensations (e.g., dry mouth, thirst, muscle weakness). Provide ample time for instruction and clarification and reinforce the health care provider's explanation of the procedure. | This information provides a knowledge base from which patients can make informed therapy choices and consent for procedures and presents an opportunity to clarify misconceptions. |
| Use anatomic models, diagrams, and other audiovisual aids when possible. Provide simply written information to reinforce learning. Provide written and verbal information in the patient's native language for non–English-speaking patients. | Because individuals learn differently, using more than one teaching modality will provide teaching reinforcement of verbal information given. |
| **Note:** Evaluate the patient's reading comprehension before providing written materials. | |

## ASSESSMENT—RECOGNIZE CUES/ INTERVENTIONS—TAKE ACTION

## RATIONALES

| ASSESSMENT—RECOGNIZE CUES/ INTERVENTIONS—TAKE ACTION | RATIONALES |
|---|---|
| Document if the patient provides an advance directive. If the patient desires an advance directive, consult the facility's procedure for providing assistance. Five Wishes (https://fivewishes.org/five-wishes/individuals-families/individuals-and-families) is an available resource. | Laws about advance directives differ for each state. |
| Explain the perioperative course of events. Review the following with the patient and significant other: | These measures increase the patient's knowledge of the surgical procedure, which optimally will promote adherence and minimize stress. |
| • Procedures for required preoperative assessment and testing and when and where they will be performed. Issue written directions, phone numbers, and maps as indicated. Discuss location and proper arrival time for the surgery. | Patients will need information regarding location of the preoperative testing center, parking arrangements, and expected length of time such testing will require. |
| • Where the patient will be before, during, and immediately after surgery. | Patients may be in postanesthesia care unit, intensive care unit, or specialty unit. |
| • Clarification of sounds and other sensations (e.g., sore throat, cool temperature, hard stretcher) the patient may experience during the immediate postoperative period. If possible, take the patient to the new unit and introduce him or her to the nursing staff. | Including sensory information in patient teaching is consistent with current nursing research that has determined patient outcomes are improved when expected sensations are explained. |
| • Preoperative medications and timing of surgery (scheduled time, expected duration). | Informing the patient of what to expect can help to reduce anxiety. |
| • If indicated, preoperative bowel preparation. | Patients need to know the correct procedure if a bowel preparation is required. |
| • Pain management, including sensations to expect and methods of relief. If patient-controlled analgesia (PCA) or patient-controlled epidural anesthesia (PCEA) will be prescribed, have the patient give a return demonstration of use of the delivery device. | This information increases the likelihood of successful pain management. Some patients mistakenly expect to be pain free; others fear becoming addicted to opioids. |
| • Use of pain assessment tools such as the numeric pain rating scale or the Wong–Baker FACES pain rating scale. | Pain assessment tools aid in the evaluation of pain and effectiveness of interventions. |
| • Placement of tubes, catheters, drains, cooling systems, oxygen delivery devices, and similar devices routinely used for the patient's surgery. Show these devices to the patient when possible. | Patients may be unfamiliar with the use and purpose of these devices. Learning about them and seeing them in advance of surgery may help decrease fears and anxieties perioperatively. |
| • Use of antiembolism stockings, sequential compression devices, pneumatic foot pumps, or similar devices. | These garments/devices prevent venous stasis and decrease risk for thrombus formation. |
| • Dietary alterations and progression, including nothing by mouth (NPO) status followed by clear liquids until return of full gastrointestinal (GI) function. | Traditionally, health care providers have progressed patients from clear liquids to a regular diet after surgery for a variety of reasons, including ease of swallowing and digestion and liquid diet being more readily tolerated in the presence of an ileus. However, practices may vary according to the provider and procedure performed. |
| • Restrictions of activity and positions, as indicated by the specific surgical procedure. | For example, patients undergoing hip arthroplasty have specific positional limitations. |
| • The need to refrain from smoking during perioperative period. | Inhalation of toxic fumes/chemical irritants can damage lung tissue by decreasing ciliary function. Cilia line the respiratory tract and carry particles to the lower pharynx. Damaged lung tissue increases the likelihood of hypoxemia and lung infections, including pneumonia. |
| • Visiting hours and location of waiting room. | Families may feel less anxious when they are aware of a designated area where they can wait and receive updates on the progress of the surgery. Knowledge of visiting hours likely will reassure them they will have access to the patient after surgery. |

Continued

| ASSESSMENT—RECOGNIZE CUES/ INTERVENTIONS—TAKE ACTION | RATIONALES |
|---|---|
| **Postoperatively:** | |
| Explain postoperative activities, exercises, and precautions. Have the patient give a return demonstration of the following devices and exercises, as appropriate: | Adherence is enhanced when patients are knowledgeable about activities, exercises, and precautions. Patients gain confidence when they practice new skills before surgery and are provided feedback on their technique. |
| • Deep-breathing and coughing exercises (see *Risk for Impaired Airway Clearance*, later). | These actions help prevent atelectasis, pneumonia, and other respiratory disorders that can occur during the postoperative period. |
| **Caution:** Individuals for whom increased intracranial, intrathoracic, or intraabdominal pressure is contraindicated must not cough. | Coughing increases intracranial, intrathoracic, and intraabdominal pressure. Patients undergoing intracranial surgery, spinal fusion, eye and ear surgery, and similar procedures need to avoid vigorous coughing because it raises intracranial pressure, which could cause harm. Coughing after a herniorrhaphy and some thoracic surgeries need to be done in a controlled manner, with the incision supported carefully, to avoid raising intraabdominal and intrathoracic pressure dramatically. |
| • Use of incentive spirometry and other respiratory devices. | Incentive spirometry, when used with coughing and deep breathing, expands alveoli and mobilizes secretions, which helps prevent atelectasis, pneumonia, and other respiratory disorders. |
| • Calf-pumping, ankle-circling, and footboard-pressing exercises (see "Venous Thrombosis/Thrombophlebitis," Chapter 26, for more information). | These exercises promote circulation and help prevent thrombophlebitis/ venous thromboembolism (VTE) in the legs. |
| • Use of PCA/PCEA device. | Adequate pain management increases mobility, which decreases risk for nosocomial pneumonia and thrombosis formation and aids in the return of GI peristalsis. |
| • Movement in and out of bed. | Logrolling, raising self by using a trapeze device, and gradual movement are techniques that may be required. |
| Before the patient is discharged, explain prescribed activity precautions. | This instruction helps prevent excessive strain on the operative site. A patient who has a total hip replacement, for example, will need to follow activity precautions to prevent dislocation of the new joint. |
| | Increasing exercises gradually to tolerance, avoiding heavy lifting (more than 10 lb), and avoiding driving a car are precautions given to many surgical patients for safety because of the potential for decreased attention span and impaired reflexes resulting from opioid use. Lifting precautions may reduce stress on surgical incisions. Restrictions on sexual activity are indicated by the surgical procedure. Returning progressively to preoperative activity level promotes physical and psychosocial well-being. |
| Provide time for the patient to ask questions and express feelings of anxiety; be reassuring and supportive. Be certain to address the patient's main concerns. | Expressing feelings of anxiety and having questions answered are essential ways of reducing anxiety while learning new information. |

## Patient Problem/Analyze Cues/Prioritize Hypotheses

# Risk for Injury (Perioperative)

*due to* untoward effects of pharmacotherapy or other external factors

***Desired Outcome/Generate Solutions:*** The patient does not experience untoward effects of pharmacotherapy or other external factors.

| ASSESSMENT—RECOGNIZE CUES/ INTERVENTIONS—TAKE ACTION | RATIONALES |
| --- | --- |
| Assess need for holding, administering, or adjusting the patient's maintenance medications before or immediately after surgery. | Some medications, such as anticonvulsants, beta-blockers, and other cardiac medications, need to be continued throughout the perioperative period. Sometimes, patients need to be weaned from medications such as baclofen for the perioperative period because stopping them suddenly could result in seizures or hallucinations. Other medications may require increased dosages during surgery (e.g., hydrocortisone in place of prednisone and with increased dosage for steroid-dependent patients) or alternative routes. Individuals with diabetes will need close monitoring of blood glucose levels with possible adjustments of insulin doses. |
| Reinforce the importance of NPO status. | Maintaining NPO status reduces risk for aspiration postoperatively. NPO policies vary widely from facility to facility. |
| Verify the completion of preoperative activities and procedures, and document this on the preoperative checklist or nursing documentation. | Documentation on the patient's preoperative checklist or inpatient's medical record helps ensure communication among health care team members, continuity, and optimal patient outcomes. |
| Be sure that consent has been signed and witnessed and the patient seems to understand what the procedure involves. Answer questions, or call the health care provider to answer patient's questions. Ensure that the patient's identification bracelet, blood transfusion bracelet, and allergy alert bracelet are in place. | These interventions help ensure that all appropriate documentation is present and that all steps have been taken to provide for the patient's safety and well-being. |
| Document allergies, any evidence of skin breakdown, bruises, rashes, or wounds; and presence of dressings, drains, or ostomy. | Documentation decreases risk for untoward outcomes. Noting the patient's preexisting wounds, dressings, and drains also helps ensure appropriate intraoperative positioning. |
| Document the patient's access to care and transportation on discharge. | Surgery, pain, and analgesic medications may impede the patient's ability to care for self adequately after discharge. |
| Review the medical record to ensure that all appropriate documentation is present; report untoward findings to the health care provider. | The health care provider may not be aware of recent abnormal electrocardiogram, suspicious chest radiograph, or abnormal laboratory findings. |
| Prepare the surgical site and perform additional presurgical procedures as prescribed. | The Association of periOperative Registered Nurses recommendations state that surgical site hair removal needs to be minimal and only done when the hair interferes with the procedure Clippers or a depilatory cream are used instead of shaving, and the procedure is done in the preoperative setting to minimize contamination of the surgical suite (Edmiston et al., 2019). |
| | Additional presurgical procedures may involve bathing or showering with an antimicrobial agent, douching, enemas, or eye drops. |
| Administer the preoperative antibiotics, sedation, or other medications as prescribed and on time. | This intervention helps ensure adequate serum levels of the prescribed medication. Timing may vary with facilities and procedures, but giving antibiotics within recommended timeframes may decrease the risk of postoperative infection. |
| Make provisions for patient safety following sedative administration (e.g., bed in lowest position, side rails up, and reminding patient not to get out of bed without assistance). | Sedatives administered preoperatively may alter mental status and coordination, increasing the patient's risk for injury. |

Continued

## ASSESSMENT—RECOGNIZE CUES/ INTERVENTIONS—TAKE ACTION

Implement the preoperative verification and time-out process as follows:

1. Confirm identification of the patient by all team members by verifying the patient's armband, patient speak back, or patient caregiver if the patient has been sedated.

2. In the preoperative/holding area confirm that a mark has been made by the surgeon (who will have used a single-use surgical skin marker with a consistent mark type [e.g., surgeon's initials]) placed as close as anatomically possible to the incision site.

3. Perform a preoperative briefing in the operating room with patient involvement.

4. Perform a standardized time-out process, which occurs after the prep and drape.

5. Perform a pause between each surgical procedure that occurs within a single case to ensure that each procedure is performed accurately and according to the procedure, site, and laterality contained within the signed surgical consent.

## RATIONALES

This verification process needs to take place on admission to the facility, before the patient leaves the preoperative area, on entry to the surgical room, just before incision or start of procedure, and any time responsibility for patient care is transferred to another caregiver. If possible, involve the patient, while still awake and aware, with the verification process.

Prevention of the wrong site, wrong procedure, and wrong person surgery is accomplished by the use of a time-out procedure. A "time out" must include verification of the correct patient identity, the correct surgical site and side, and agreement on the procedure to be done.

## Problems for Patients Who Are Postoperative

### Patient Problem/Analyze Cues/Prioritize Hypotheses

# Risk for Impaired Airway Clearance

*due to* alterations in pulmonary physiology and function occurring with anesthetics, opioids, mechanical ventilation, hypothermia, and surgery; increased tracheobronchial secretions occurring with effects of anesthesia combined with ineffective coughing; and decreased function of the mucociliary clearance mechanism

***Desired Outcome/Generate Solutions:*** The patient's airway is clear as evidenced by normal breath sounds to auscultation, respiratory rate (RR) 12–20 breaths/minute with normal depth and pattern (eupnea), normothermia, baseline skin color, and $O_2$ saturation greater than 92% on room air.

## ASSESSMENT—RECOGNIZE CUES/ INTERVENTIONS—TAKE ACTION

Assess the respiratory status, including breath sounds, dyspnea, cough, and rapid, shallow respirations, every 1–2 hours during immediate postoperative period and every 8 hours during recovery.

Use pulse oximetry to assess the oxygen saturation as indicated, and report saturation 92% or less to the health care provider.

## RATIONALES

Frequent assessment for signs and symptoms of impaired airway clearance allows for early interventions and prevention of respiratory system compromise.

Pulse oximetry is a noninvasive measure of arterial oxygen saturation. Values 92% or less are consistent with hypoxia and probably signal need for oxygen supplementation or workup to determine cause of desaturation. Pulse oximetry is especially indicated in patients with chronic obstructive pulmonary disease (COPD), respiratory or cardiovascular disease, morbid obesity, cardiothoracic surgery, major surgery, prolonged general anesthesia, and surgery for a fractured pelvis or long bone, as well as in debilitated patients and older adults, all of whom are at increased risk for desaturation.

| ASSESSMENT—RECOGNIZE CUES/ INTERVENTIONS—TAKE ACTION | RATIONALES |
|---|---|
| Administer the humidified oxygen as prescribed. | This intervention prevents further drying of respiratory passageways and secretions through added humidity. |
| Keep emergency airway equipment (e.g., Ambu bag and mask, intubation tray, endotracheal tubes, suctioning equipment, tracheostomy tray) readily available. | This ensures their availability in the event of sudden airway obstruction or ventilatory failure. |
| Encourage deep breathing and coughing every 2 hours or more often for the first 72 hours postoperatively in nonambulatory patients. In the presence of fine crackles and if not contraindicated, have the patient cough to expectorate secretions. Facilitate deep breathing and coughing by demonstrating how to splint abdominal and thoracic incisions with hands or a pillow. If indicated, medicate 1/2 hour before deep breathing, coughing, or ambulation to promote adherence. | These actions expand alveoli and mobilize secretions. The effects of anesthesia and immobility may collapse alveoli and place patient at risk for nosocomial pneumonia and atelectasis. Proper positioning promotes chest expansion and ventilation of basilar lung fields.<br><br>**Note:** Turning, coughing, and deep breathing (TCDB) are less effective than ambulation. Ambulation makes TCDB unnecessary in the vast majority of patients. |
| If the patient has a weak cough or poor reserve, try the "step-cough" technique. Coach the patient to cough in rapid succession.<br><br>**Caution:** Vigorous coughing may be contraindicated for some individuals (e.g., those undergoing intracranial surgery, spinal fusion, eye and ear surgery, and similar procedures). Coughing after a herniorrhaphy and some thoracic surgeries must be done in a controlled manner, with the incision supported carefully. | A few weak coughs in a row may stimulate a larger, productive cough at the end of the cycle to clear the bronchial tree of secretions. |
| Consider whether the patient may be more motivated to perform pulmonary toilet with incentive spirometer or positive expiratory pressure (PEP) device. | Devices may be a motivating factor because the patient has a visual indicator of effectiveness of the breathing effort. |

## Patient Problem/Analyze Cues/Prioritize Hypotheses

# Impaired Gas Exchange

*due to* hypoventilation occurring with central nervous system (CNS) depression, pain, muscle splinting, recumbent position, obesity, opioids, and effects of anesthesia

***Desired Outcome/Generate Solutions:*** After interventions, the patient exhibits effective ventilation, as evidenced by relaxed breathing, RR of 12–20 breaths/minute with normal depth and pattern (eupnea), clear breath sounds, baseline skin color, and $O_2$ saturation greater than 92% on room air. $PaO_2$ of 80 mm Hg or greater, pH of 7.35–7.45, $PaCO_2$ of 3–45 mm Hg, and $HCO_3^-$ of 22–26 mEq/L.

| ASSESSMENT—RECOGNIZE CUES/ INTERVENTIONS—TAKE ACTION | RATIONALES |
|---|---|
| See the assessment/interventions under *Risk for Impaired Airway Clearance*, earlier. | |
| Review preoperative baseline assessment of the patient's respiratory system, noting rate, rhythm, degree of chest expansion, quality of breath sounds, cough, and sputum production, as well as smoking history and current respiratory medications. Note preoperative $O_2$ saturation and arterial blood gas (ABG) values if available. | Baseline assessment enables rapid detection of subsequent postoperative problems and timely intervention. |
| If appropriate, encourage the patient to refrain from smoking for at least 1 week after surgery. Explain effects of smoking on the body. | Inhalation of toxic fumes/chemical irritants can damage lung tissue, increasing likelihood of hypoxemia, and respiratory infection. |

Continued

| ASSESSMENT—RECOGNIZE CUES/ INTERVENTIONS—TAKE ACTION | RATIONALES |
|---|---|
| Monitor the $O_2$ saturation continuously by oximetry in high-risk individuals (e.g., patients with obstructive sleep apnea [OSA] or who are heavily sedated, patients with preexisting lung disease, morbidly obese patients, patients having undergone upper airway surgery, or older patients) and at periodic intervals in other patients as indicated. | Pulse oximetry is a noninvasive method of measuring saturated hemoglobin in tissue capillaries. |
| Identify factors that predispose the patient to OSA, such as<br>1. history of snoring;<br>2. history of feeling tired, fatigued, or sleepy during daytime;<br>3. history of stopping breathing during sleep;<br>4. history of hypertension;<br>5. body mass index (BMI) greater than 35;<br>6. age greater than 50 years;<br>7. neck circumference greater than 40 cm; and<br>8. male gender. | Identifying high-risk factors for OSA helps to identify individuals who may have impaired gas exchange postoperatively. |
| Notify the health care provider of $O_2$ saturation 92% or less. | $O_2$ saturation of 92% or less may signal need for supplemental oxygen. |
| Evaluate the ABG values, and notify the health care provider of low or decreasing $PaO_2$ and high or increasing $PaCO_2$. | Declining $PaO_2$ may signal hypoxemia and the need for supplemental oxygen. Hypercapnia combined with acidosis and hypoxemia may result in pulmonary vasoconstriction that may be severe and life threatening. |
| Assess for signs of hypoxia. Early signs of hypoxia include restlessness, dyspnea, tachycardia, tachypnea, and confusion. Cyanosis, especially of the tongue and oral mucous membranes, and extreme lethargy or somnolence are late signs of hypoxia. | Hypoxia may signal the need for supplemental oxygen. |
| Assist the patient with turning and deep-breathing/coughing exercises every 2 hours until the patient is ambulatory. | These activities promote expansion of lung alveoli and prevent pooling of secretions, which could lead to health care–associated pneumonia. |
| If the patient has an incentive spirometer *or* PEP device, provide instructions and ensure adherence to its use every 2 hours or as prescribed. | These devices promote expansion of the alveoli and help mobilize secretions in the airways; subsequent coughing further mobilizes and clears secretions. |
| Unless contraindicated, assist the patient with ambulation beginning on the day of surgery. | Ambulation promotes circulation and ventilation, which helps prevent formation of deep vein thrombosis and pulmonary embolus. |

**Patient Problem/Analyze Cues/Prioritize Hypotheses**

# Risk for Aspiration

*due to* decreased level of consciousness, depressed cough and gag reflexes, decreased GI motility, abdominal distention, recumbent position, presence of gastric tube, gastroesophageal reflux disease (GERD), and dysphagia (impaired swallowing) in individuals with oral, facial, or neck surgery

***Desired Outcome/Generate Solutions:*** The patient's upper airway remains unobstructed, as evidenced by clear breath sounds, RR of 12–20 breaths/minute with normal depth and pattern (eupnea), baseline skin color, and a return to preoperative $O_2$ saturation.

| ASSESSMENT—RECOGNIZE CUES/ INTERVENTIONS—TAKE ACTION | RATIONALES |
|---|---|
| If a sedated patient experiences nausea or vomiting, turn immediately into a side-lying position. | This position minimizes the potential for aspiration. |
| Encourage fully alert patients to remain in an upright position. | Maintaining a sitting position after meals decreases risk for aspiration by facilitating gravity drainage from the stomach to the small bowel. An upright position also helps prevent reflux. |
| As necessary, suction the oropharynx with Yankauer or similar suction device to remove vomitus. | Suctioning enables immediate removal of vomitus, which could be aspirated. Suctioning apparatus must be immediately available for patients who are at high risk for aspiration. |
| Administer the antiemetics, histamine-2 ($H_2$)-receptor blocking agents, omeprazole, metoclopramide, and similar agents as prescribed. | These agents decrease nausea, vomiting, and acidity of gastric contents and stimulate GI motility. $H_2$-receptor antagonists increase gastric pH, and nonparticulate antacids act as aspiration pneumonitis prophylaxis. Neutralizing gastric acidity may reduce severity of pneumonia if aspiration occurs. |
| Check the placement and patency of gastric tubes every 8 hours and before instillation of feedings and medications. Consult the health care provider before irrigating tubes for these individuals. | These actions prevent instillation of anything into the airway. |
| Use caution when irrigating and otherwise manipulating GI tubes of patients with recent esophageal, gastric, or duodenal surgery. | The tube may be displaced or the surgical incision disrupted by such activity. |
| Assess the patient's abdomen every 4–8 hours by inspection, palpation, percussion and auscultation for evidence of distention (increasing size, firmness, increased tympany, decreased bowel sounds). | A distended and rigid abdomen along with absent bowel sounds may indicate an ileus, which places patient at increased risk for vomiting and aspiration. Increased tympany or high-pitched or increased bowel sounds may signal mechanical obstruction, which also places patient at increased risk for vomiting and aspiration. |
| Notify the health care provider if distention is of rapid onset or if it is associated with pain. | Rapid abdominal distention postoperatively may indicate intraabdominal hemorrhage and can lead to a sometimes-fatal condition called *abdominal compartment syndrome*. |
| Encourage early and frequent ambulation. | Ambulation improves GI motility and reduces abdominal distention caused by accumulated gases. |
| Introduce oral fluids cautiously, especially in patients with oral, facial, and neck surgery. | Swelling and irritation in the oropharynx may cause dysphagia and pain postoperatively. Nasal packing or intranasal splint aspiration also may cause airway obstruction. |
| For additional information, see "Providing Nutritional Support," Chapter 76, *Risk for Aspiration*. | |

## Patient Problem/Analyze Cues/Prioritize Hypotheses

# Risk for Infection

*due to* inadequate primary defenses (e.g., broken skin, traumatized tissue, decrease in ciliary action, stasis of body fluids), invasive procedures, or chronic disease

***Desired Outcome/Generate Solutions:*** The patient is free of infection, as evidenced by normothermia; heart rate (HR) of 100 bpm or less; RR of 20 breaths/minute or less with normal depth and pattern (eupnea); negative cultures; urine clear and without a foul odor; clear and thin sputum; no significant mental status changes; orientation to person, place, and time; and absence of unusual tenderness, erythema, swelling, warmth, or drainage at the surgical incision.

| ASSESSMENT—RECOGNIZE CUES/ INTERVENTIONS—TAKE ACTION | RATIONALES |
|---|---|
| Monitor the vital signs (VS) for evidence of infection, such as elevated HR and RR and increased body temperature. | With onset of infection, the immune system is activated, causing symptoms of infection to appear. Sustained temperature elevation after surgery may signal the presence of pulmonary complications, urinary tract infection (UTI), wound infection, or thrombophlebitis. |
| Notify the health care provider if these are new findings. | Presence of a fever affects treatment decisions. |
| Prevent the transmission of infectious agents by washing your hands thoroughly before and after caring for the patient and by wearing gloves when contact with blood, drainage, or other body substance is likely. | Hand hygiene is an effective means of preventing microbial transmission. Wearing gloves protects the caregiver from the patient's body substances. |
| Encourage and assist the patient with coughing, deep breathing, incentive spirometry, and turning every 2–4 hours, and note quality of breath sounds, cough, and sputum. | These activities expand alveoli in the lung and mobilize secretions, which will decrease the potential for respiratory infection/pneumonia. Optimally they will promote cough and improve quality of breath sounds. |
| Evaluate intravenous (IV) sites for erythema, warmth, swelling, tenderness, or drainage. | These are signs of infection. The body may be mounting a response to ward off offending pathogens. |
| Change the IV line and site if evidence of infection is present and according to agency protocol. | These are standard infection prevention guidelines. |
| Evaluate the patency of all surgically placed tubes or drains. Irrigate, or attach to low-pressure suction as prescribed. Promptly report unrelieved loss of patency. | These actions prevent stasis and reflux of body fluids, which can result in infection. |
| Assess the stability of tubes/drains. | Movement of improperly secured tubes and drains enables access of pathogens at the insertion site. |
| Note color, character, and odor of all drainage. Report significant findings. | Foul-smelling, purulent, and abnormal drainage are indicators of infection. |
| Evaluate incisions and wound sites for unusual erythema, warmth, tenderness, induration, swelling, delayed healing, and purulent or excessive drainage. | These are indicators of localized infection. |
| Change dressings as prescribed, using "no touch" and sterile techniques. Prevent cross-contamination of wounds in the same patient by changing one dressing at a time and washing hands and changing gloves between dressing changes. | These are standard infection prevention guidelines. |
| Be alert to patient complaints of a feeling of "letting go" or to a sudden release of serous drainage on or a bulge in the dressing. | It is possible that a wound dehiscence or evisceration has occurred. Wound infection and poor wound healing put patients at risk for wound dehiscence. |
| If the patient develops evisceration, do not reinsert tissue or organs. Place a sterile, saline-soaked gauze over eviscerated tissues and cover with a sterile towel until the wound can be evaluated by a health care provider. | Keeping viscera moist with a sterile towel increases viability of tissues and reduces risk for contamination and further infection. |
| If evisceration or wound dehiscence occurs, maintain the patient on bedrest, usually in semi-Fowler position with knees slightly bent. Keep the patient NPO and anticipate need for IV therapy. | These actions provide comfort, prevent further evisceration, and prepare the patient for surgery. |
| Ensure that the urinary catheter is removed on postoperative day 1 or day 2, as soon as possible. **Note:** This does not apply to patients who have had urinary tract surgery (i.e., prostate or urethral procedures). | The risk for catheter-associated UTI increases with prolonged duration of indwelling urinary catheterization. |
| When appropriate, encourage the use of intermittent catheterization every 4–6 hours instead of indwelling catheter. | Emptying the bladder routinely prevents stasis of urine and decreases presence of pathogens. |
| Keep the drainage collection container below bladder level, avoiding kinks or obstructions in drainage tubing. | This intervention prevents both reflux of urine (and potential pathogens) into bladder and urinary stasis, either of which could lead to infection. |

| ASSESSMENT—RECOGNIZE CUES/ INTERVENTIONS—TAKE ACTION | RATIONALES |
|---|---|
| Do not open the closed urinary drainage system unless absolutely necessary, and irrigate the catheter only with the health care provider's prescription and when obstruction is the known cause. | Keeping the system closed decreases risk for contamination and infection. |
| Assess the patient for chills; fever (temperature higher than 100°F [37.7°C]); dysuria; urgency; frequency; flank, low back, suprapubic, buttock, inner thigh, scrotal, or labial pain; and cloudy or foul-smelling urine. | These are indicators of UTI, which signal that the body is mounting a response to ward off offending pathogens. |
| Encourage the intake of 2–3 L/day in nonrestricted patients. | Increasing hydration minimizes the potential for UTI by diluting the urine and maximizing urinary flow. |
| Ensure that the patient's perineum and meatus are cleansed during daily bath and the perianal area is cleansed after bowel movements. Do not hesitate to remind the patient of these hygiene measures. | Microorganisms can be introduced into the body through the catheter. Good hygiene decreases the number of microorganisms. |
| Be alert to meatal swelling, purulent drainage, and persistent meatal redness. Intervene if the patient is unable to perform self-care. | These are indicators of meatal infection and potential UTI. |
| Obtain the cultures of suspicious drainage or secretions (e.g., sputum, urine, wound) as prescribed. For urine specimens, be certain to use the sampling port, which is at the proximal end of the drainage tube. | Cultures determine whether an infection is present and direct therapy with an appropriate antibiotic if it is. |
| Cleanse the sampling port with an antimicrobial wipe and use a sterile syringe with 25-gauge needle to aspirate urine. | Larger gauge needles form larger puncture holes that increase the risk for compromising the sterile system. |
| Evaluate the mental status, orientation, and level of consciousness every 8 hours. | Consider infection the likely cause if altered mental status or loss of consciousness is unexplained, especially in older adults. |
| Refer to *Risk for Infection* in Chapter 2. | |
| Refer to *Risk for Infection* in Chapter 3 for information specific to older adults. | |

## Patient Problem/Analyze Cues/Prioritize Hypotheses

# Dehydration

*due to* active loss occurring with indwelling drainage tubes, wound drainage, or vomiting; inadequate intake of fluids occurring with nausea, NPO status, CNS depression, or lack of access to fluids; or failure of regulatory mechanisms with third spacing of body fluids and *due to* the effects of anesthesia, endogenous catecholamines, blood loss during surgery, and prolonged recumbency

*Desired Outcomes/Generate Solutions:* Following intervention, the patient becomes normovolemic, as evidenced by blood pressure (BP) of 90/60 mm Hg or higher (or within the patient's preoperative baseline), HR of 60–100 bpm, distal pulses greater than 2 on a 0–4 scale, urinary output of 30 mL/hour or more, urine specific gravity of 1.030 or less, stable or increasing weight, good skin turgor, warm skin, moist mucous membranes, and normothermia. The patient does not demonstrate significant mental status changes and verbalizes orientation to person, place, and time.

| ASSESSMENT—RECOGNIZE CUES/ INTERVENTIONS—TAKE ACTION | RATIONALES |
|---|---|
| Monitor the VS every 4–8 hours during the recovery phase. | Decreasing BP, increasing HR, and slightly increased body temperature are indicators of dehydration. |
| Monitor the urinary output every 4–8 hours. Be alert for concentrated urine. | Concentrated urine (specific gravity more than 1.030) and low or decreasing output (average normal output is 60 mL/hour or 1400–1500 mL/day) are indicators of dehydration. |
| Administer and regulate the IV fluids and electrolytes as prescribed until the patient is able to resume oral intake.  When IV fluids are discontinued, encourage the intake of oral fluids, at least 2–3 L/day in nonrestricted patients. As much as possible, respect the patient's preference in oral fluids, and keep them readily available in the patient's room. | Oral fluids usually are restricted until peristalsis returns and the nasogastric (NG) tube is removed. However, ice chips or small sips of clear liquids may be allowed. |
| Measure and record the output from drains, ostomies, wounds, and other sources. Ensure patency of gastric and other drainage tubes. Record quality and quantity of output. | Both sensible and insensible losses need to be determined to ensure complete estimation of the patient's fluid volume status. |
| Measure, describe, and document any emesis. Be alert to and document excessive perspiration along with documentation of urinary, fecal, and other drainage. | Both sensible and insensible losses need to be determined to ensure complete estimation of the patient's fluid volume status. |
| Report excessive losses. | Replacement fluids likely will be indicated. |
| Monitor the patient's weight daily. | Daily weight measurement is an effective means of evaluating hydration and nutritional status. |
| Always weigh at the same time every day, using the same scale and same type and amount of bed clothing.  **Note:** Weighing patients daily is not useful in detecting intravascular fluid loss due to third spacing. Movement of fluid from one area of the body to another will not change the total body weight. | Weighing patients at the same time and under the same conditions avoids discrepancies that could reflect inaccurate losses or gains. |
| If nausea and vomiting are present, assess for potential causes. | Potential causes include administration of opioid analgesics, loss of gastric tube patency, and environmental factors (e.g., unpleasant odors or sights). |
| Administer antiemetics, metoclopramide, or similar agents as prescribed. | These agents combat nausea and vomiting, which could impair intake and add to fluid losses. |
| Instruct the patient to request medication *before* nausea becomes severe. | Postoperative vomiting is significantly less when patients receive nausea/vomiting prophylaxis. |
| Monitor for hypokalemia and hypocalcemia.  *Hypokalemia:* Muscle weakness, lethargy, dysrhythmias, abdominal distention, and nausea and vomiting (secondary to ileus).  *Hypocalcemia:* Neuromuscular irritability, for example, positive Trousseau sign (carpopedal spasm) and Chvostek sign (facial muscle spasm), and paresthesias. | A large fluid loss may cause electrolyte imbalances leading to life-threatening cardiac dysrhythmias. |

## Patient Problem/Analyze Cues/Prioritize Hypotheses

# Risk for Hemorrhaging

*due to* invasive procedure

**Desired Outcomes/Generate Solutions:** The patient remains normovolemic, as evidenced by BP of 90/60 mm Hg or higher (or within the patient's preoperative baseline), HR of 60–100 bpm, RR of 12–20 breaths/minute with normal depth and pattern (eupnea), brisk capillary refill (less than 2 seconds), warm extremities, distal pulses greater than 2+ on a 0–4+ scale, urinary output of 0.5 mL/kg/hr or more, and urine specific gravity of less than 1.030. The patient does not demonstrate significant mental status changes and verbalizes orientation to person, place, and time.

| ASSESSMENT—RECOGNIZE CUES/ INTERVENTIONS—TAKE ACTION | RATIONALES |
|---|---|
| Assess the VS and physical indicators at frequent intervals during the first 24 hours of the postoperative period for signs of internal hemorrhage and impending shock.<br><br>Physical indicators include pallor, diaphoresis, cool extremities, delayed capillary refill, diminished intensity of distal pulses, restlessness, agitation, mental status changes, and disorientation, as well as subjective complaints of thirst, anxiety, or a sense of impending doom.<br><br>See "Cardiac and Noncardiac Shock (Circulatory Failure)," Chapter 19, for management. | There is greater potential for postoperative bleeding/hemorrhage during this period. Decreasing pulse pressure (difference between systolic BP and diastolic BP), decreasing BP, increasing HR, and increasing RR are indicators of internal hemorrhage and impending shock. |
| **!** Inspect the surgical dressing; record saturated dressings and report significant findings to the health care provider. | Rapid saturation of the dressing with bright-red blood is evidence of frank bleeding, which necessitates immediate intervention. |
| If the initial postoperative dressing becomes saturated, reinforce the dressing and notify the health care provider. | The health care provider may want to perform the initial dressing change. |
| **!** Monitor wound drains and drainage systems, and report significant findings to the health care provider. | Excessive drainage (more than 50 mL/hour for 2–3 hours) needs to be reported promptly for timely intervention. |
| Note the amount and character of drainage from gastric and other tubes at least every 8 hours.<br><br>**Note:** After gastric and some other GI surgeries, patients will have small amounts of bloody or blood-tinged drainage for the first 12–24 hours. Be alert to large or increasing amounts of bloody drainage. | If drainage appears to contain blood (e.g., bright-red, burgundy, or dark coffee-ground appearance), it will be necessary to perform an occult blood test (may be performed in the laboratory). Report results that are newly or unexpectedly positive to the health care provider for timely intervention. |
| **!** Monitor and measure the urinary output every 4–8 hours during the initial postoperative period. Report significant findings to the health care provider. | Average hourly output less than 30 mL/hour and specific gravity of 1.030 or more are indicators of decreased fluid volume, which can signal bleeding/hemorrhage. |
| **!** Review the complete blood count (CBC) values for evidence of bleeding; report significant decreases. | Evidence of bleeding may be indicated by decreases in hemoglobin (Hgb) (references for males 14–18 g/dL; females 12–16 g/dL); and decreases in hematocrit (Hct) (references for males 40%–54%; females 37%–47%). Significant decreases occur with active bleeding, which is an emergency situation. |
| Maintain a patent indwelling 18-gauge or larger IV catheter. | The gauge of this catheter will enable infusions of blood products if hemorrhagic shock develops. |

## Patient Problem/Analyze Cues/Prioritize Hypotheses

# Fluid Imbalance (Overload)

*due to* compromised regulatory mechanisms after major surgery

***Desired Outcome/Generate Solutions:*** After interventions/treatment, the patient becomes normovolemic, as evidenced by BP within range of the patient's preoperative baseline, distal pulses less than 4+ on a 0–4+ scale, presence of eupnea, clear breath sounds, absence of or barely detectable edema (1+ or less on a 0–4+ scale), urine specific gravity at least 1.010, and body weight near or at preoperative baseline.

| ASSESSMENT—RECOGNIZE CUES/ INTERVENTIONS—TAKE ACTION | RATIONALES |
|---|---|
| Assess for and report any indicators of fluid overload, including elevated BP, bounding pulses, dyspnea, crackles, and pretibial or sacral edema. | An increase in BP and an S3 galloping rhythm may indicate impending heart failure. Crackles and dyspnea may signal a shift of fluid from the vascular space to the pulmonary interstitial space and alveoli causing pulmonary edema. |
| Maintain a record of 8- and 24-hour intake and output. Note and report a significant imbalance. Monitor urinary specific gravity and report consistently low (less than 1.010) findings. | Expected 24-hour output is 1400–1500 mL, and expected 1-hour output is 60 mL/hour or 480 mL per 8 hours. Decreased urinary output could be a sign of fluid volume excess. |
| Weigh the patient daily, using the same scale and same type and amount of bed clothing. Note significant weight gain. | Weight changes reflect changes in body fluid volume. One liter of fluid equals approximately 2.2 lb. Weighing the patient at the same time and under the same conditions avoids discrepancies that could reflect inaccurate losses or gains. |
| Administer diuretics as prescribed. | Diuretics mobilize interstitial fluid and decrease excess fluid volume. |
| Monitor the patients carefully who are on diuretic therapy. | Diuretic therapy may cause dangerous potassium depletion that could result in cardiac dysrhythmias. In addition, diuretic therapy can lead to hyponatremia because of sodium losses. |
| Monitor the older adults and individuals with cardiovascular disease especially carefully. | These individuals are especially at risk for developing postoperative fluid overload. Older adults have age-related changes of decreased glomerular filtration rate (GFR). Decreased kidney function and increased probability of chronic illness such as cardiac disease may signal higher risk for postoperative excessive fluid volume. |
| Anticipate postoperative diuresis approximately 48–72 hours after surgery. | This may occur because of mobilization of third-space (interstitial) fluid. |

**Patient Problem/Analyze Cues/Prioritize Hypotheses**

# Risk for Falls

*due to* weakness, balancing difficulties, and reduced muscle coordination resulting from anesthetics and postoperative opioid analgesics

***Desired Outcome/Generate Solutions:*** The patient does not fall and remains free of trauma, as evidenced by the absence of bruises, wounds, and fractures.

| ASSESSMENT—RECOGNIZE CUES/ INTERVENTIONS—TAKE ACTION | RATIONALES |
|---|---|
| Orient and reorient the patient to person, place, and time during the initial postoperative period. Inform the patient that the surgery is over. Repeat information until the patient is fully awake and oriented (usually several hours but may be days in heavily sedated or otherwise obtunded individuals). | Orientation and repeated explanations increase mental awareness and alertness, which decrease risk for trauma caused by disorientation. These measures also help the patient cope with unfamiliar surroundings. |
| Maintain side rails on stretchers and beds in upright and locked positions. | Side rails help prevent trauma to the head and extremities. Some individuals experience agitation and thrash about as they emerge from anesthesia. |
| Secure all IV lines, drains, and tubing. | This action prevents their dislodgment. |
| Maintain the bed in its lowest position when leaving the patient's room. | This action protects the patient from major trauma in case he or she falls out of bed. |

| ASSESSMENT—RECOGNIZE CUES/ INTERVENTIONS—TAKE ACTION | RATIONALES |
|---|---|
| Place the call mechanism within the patient's reach; instruct the patient in its use. | The patient can call for help when it is needed—for example, when needing to use the toilet. This will reduce risk for falls and injury. |
| Identify patients at risk for falling. Correct or compensate for risk factors. Risk factors include the following:<br>• *Time of day:* night shift, peak activity periods such as meals, bedtime<br>• *Medications:* opioid analgesics, sedatives, hypnotics, and anesthetics<br>• *Impaired mobility:* individuals requiring assistance with transfer and ambulation<br>• *Sensory deficits:* diminished visual acuity caused by disease process or environmental factors; changes in kinesthetic sense because of disease or trauma | Risk factors that are present and identified can be corrected or compensated for, thus preventing injury. |
| Use restraints and protective devices if necessary and prescribed. May also want to add bed alarm activation and fall precautions. | These devices provide protection during an emergent state. However, because they can cause agitation, their use should be infrequent and as a last resort. Behavioral intervention or a patient sitter is preferred. |

## Patient Problem/Analyze Cues/Prioritize Hypotheses

# Risk for Impaired Skin Integrity (Skin Excoriation)

*due to* the presence of secretions/excretions around percutaneous drains and tubes

*Desired Outcome/Generate Solutions:* The patient's skin around percutaneous drains and tubes remains intact and nonerythematous.

| ASSESSMENT—RECOGNIZE CUES/ INTERVENTIONS—TAKE ACTION | RATIONALES |
|---|---|
| Assess and change dressings as soon as they become wet. (The health care provider may prefer to perform the first dressing change at the surgical incision.) Use sterile technique for all dressing changes. | These interventions protect the wound from contamination and accumulation of fluids that may cause skin excoriation. |
| Keep areas around drains as clean as possible. Sterile normal saline or a solution of saline and hydrogen peroxide or other prescribed solution may be used to clean around the drain site. | Intestinal secretions, bile, and similar drainage can lead quickly to skin excoriation (pepsin, conjugated bile acids, gastric acid, and lysolecithin all have a low [acidic] pH of 1–3). |
| If some external drainage is present, position a pectin-wafer skin barrier around drain or tube. Ointments, such as zinc oxide, petrolatum, and aluminum paste, also may be used. | Skin barriers and ointments are used to protect the skin from drainage that could cause breakdown because of caustic enzymes, especially from the small bowel. |
| Consult a wound, ostomy, continence, or enterostomal therapy nurse as indicated. | These nurses provide specialized interventions if drainage is excessive, skin excoriation develops, or a collection bag needs to be placed over drains and incisions. |
| For additional information, see "Managing Wound Care," Chapter 75. | |

## Patient Problem/Analyze Cues/Prioritize Hypotheses

# Fatigue

*due to* interrupted sleep occurring with preoperative anxiety, stress, postoperative pain, noise, and altered environment

*Desired Outcomes/Generate Solutions:* After interventions/treatment, the patient relates minimal or no difficulty with falling asleep and describes a feeling of being well rested.

| ASSESSMENT—RECOGNIZE CUES/ INTERVENTIONS—TAKE ACTION | RATIONALES |
|---|---|
| Use nonpharmacologic measures to promote sleep. Environmental stimulation should be reduced by use of minimum lighting and noise reduction. Pillows and bedding need to be comfortable, and patients should be allowed to maintain their bedtime routine as close to normal as possible. | Behavioral interventions are the preferred method for insomnia because of their established efficacy and absence of drug side effects. |
| Administer the analgesics and/or sedatives at bedtime when indicated. | This action reduces nighttime pain and augments effects of the hypnotic agent to promote sleep. |
| ! Use special care when administering sedative/hypnotic to patients with COPD. Monitor respiratory function, including oximetry, at frequent intervals in these patients. | Sedative/hypnotics could cause respiratory depression in patients who already have inadequate ventilation. |
| ! After administering the sedative/hypnotic, be certain to raise side rails, lower bed to its lowest position. | The patient will become drowsy, which necessitates these safety measures. |

## Patient Problem/Analyze Cues/Prioritize Hypotheses

# Impaired Mobility

*due to* postoperative pain, decreased strength and endurance occurring with CNS effects of anesthesia or blood loss, musculoskeletal or neuromuscular impairment occurring with the disease process or surgical procedure, sensory-perceptual impairment occurring with the disease process or surgical procedure (e.g., ocular surgery, neurosurgery), or cognitive impairment occurring with the disease process or effects of opioid analgesics and anesthetics

*Desired Outcome/Generate Solutions:* Optimally, by hospital discharge (depending on type of surgery), the patient returns to preoperative baseline physical mobility, as evidenced by the ability to move in bed, transfer, and ambulate independently or with minimal assistance.

| ASSESSMENT—RECOGNIZE CUES/ INTERVENTIONS—TAKE ACTION | RATIONALES |
|---|---|
| Review the patient's preoperative mobility, including coordination and muscle strength, control, and mass. | Preoperative/baseline assessments enable accurate measurements of postoperative mobility problems. |
| Implement medically imposed restrictions against movement, especially with conditions or surgeries that are orthopedic, neurosurgical, or ocular. | Restricting movement and certain positions can prevent disruption of the surgical repair. |
| Evaluate and correct factors limiting mobility. | Factors such as oversedation with opioid analgesics, failure to achieve adequate pain control, and poorly arranged physical environment can be corrected. |
| Initiate movement from bed to chair and ambulation as soon as possible after surgery, depending on postoperative prescriptions, type of surgery, and the patient's recovery from anesthetics. | Patients usually can tolerate a graduated progression in activity and ambulation. |
| ! Assist with moving slowly to a sitting position in bed and then standing at the bedside before attempting ambulation. For more information, see *Risk for Altered Blood Pressure (Orthostatic Hypotension)*, Chapter 1. | Many anesthetic agents depress normal vasoconstrictor mechanisms and can result in sudden hypotension with quick changes in position. |
| Encourage frequent movement and ambulation by postoperative patients. Provide assistance as indicated. | These actions reduce the potential for postoperative complications, including atelectasis, pneumonia, thrombophlebitis, skin breakdown, muscle weakness, and decreased GI motility. |
| Instruct about exercises that can be performed in bed and explain their purpose. | Exercises such as gluteal and quadriceps muscle sets (isometrics) and ankle circling and calf pumping promote muscle strength, increase venous return, and prevent stasis. |

For additional information, see "Immobility," Chapter 1, for *Activity Intolerance*.

## Patient Problem/Analyze Cues/Prioritize Hypotheses

# Impaired Oral Mucous Membrane

*due to* NPO status and/or presence of NG or endotracheal tube

***Desired Outcome/Generate Solutions:*** At the time of hospital discharge, the patient's oral mucosa is intact, without pain or evidence of bleeding.

| ASSESSMENT—RECOGNIZE CUES/ INTERVENTIONS—TAKE ACTION | RATIONALES |
|---|---|
| Provide oral care and oral hygiene every 4 hours and as needed. Arrange for patients to gargle, brush teeth, and cleanse mouth with sponge-tipped applicators as necessary. | Oral care provides comfort and prevents excoriation and excessive dryness of oral mucous membrane. |
| Use a moistened cotton-tipped applicator to remove encrustations. Carefully lubricate lips and nares with an emollient cream. | These interventions provide comfort and decrease risk for tissue breakdown caused by dry tissues. |
| If indicated, obtain a prescription for lidocaine gargling solution. | This solution provides comfort if the patient's throat tissue is irritated from the presence of an NG tube. |

## Patient Problems/Analyze Cues/Prioritize Hypotheses

# Constipation/Risk for Ileus

*due to* immobility, opioid analgesics and other medications, dehydration, lack of privacy, or disruption of abdominal musculature or manipulation of abdominal viscera during surgery

***Desired Outcome/Generate Solutions:*** The patient returns to baseline bowel elimination pattern, as evidenced by the return of active bowel sounds within 48–72 hours after most surgeries, absence of abdominal distention or sensation of fullness, and elimination of soft, formed stools.

| ASSESSMENT—RECOGNIZE CUES/ INTERVENTIONS—TAKE ACTION | RATIONALES |
|---|---|
| Assess for and document elimination of flatus or stool. | This signals return of intestinal motility. |
| Assess for abdominal distention, tenderness, absent or hypoactive bowel sounds, and sensation of fullness. Report gross distention, extreme tenderness, and prolonged absence of bowel sounds. | Gross distention, extreme tenderness, and prolonged absence of bowel sounds are signs of decreased GI motility and possible ileus. High-pitched bowel sounds may indicate impending bowel obstruction. |
| Encourage in-bed position changes, exercises, and ambulation to the patient's tolerance unless contraindicated. | These activities stimulate peristalsis, which promotes bowel elimination. |
| If an NG tube is in place, perform the following: | A malpositioned NG tube will be ineffective in relieving gastric distention and pose a threat to the patient's well-being. |
| • Follow facility procedures and protocol for checking tube placement after insertion, before any instillation, and every 8 hours. If the tube is in the trachea, the patient may exhibit signs of respiratory distress or consistently low $O_2$ saturation levels, or there may be absence of drainage. Reposition the tube immediately. When assured of placement, mark tube to easily assess tube migration, and secure tubing in place. | |
| • For patients with gastric, esophageal, or duodenal surgery, notify the health care provider before manipulating the tube. | Manipulation of NG tubes in these patients could result in disruption of the surgical anastomosis. |

Continued

General Care Plans

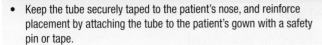

| ASSESSMENT—RECOGNIZE CUES/ INTERVENTIONS—TAKE ACTION | RATIONALES |
|---|---|
| • Keep the tube securely taped to the patient's nose, and reinforce placement by attaching the tube to the patient's gown with a safety pin or tape. | Securing the tube prevents its migration into the patient's airway. |
| • Measure and record the quantity and quality of output, including color. | Typically the color will be green. For patients who have undergone gastric surgery, output may be brownish initially because of small amounts of bloody drainage but should change to green after about 12 hours. |
| • Test reddish, brown, or black output for the presence of blood. Reposition tube as necessary. | These colors may signal GI bleeding. |
| • Gently instill normal saline as prescribed. | This action helps maintain patency of the GI tube. |
| • Ensure low, intermittent suction of gastric sump tubes by maintaining patency of the sump port (usually blue). | When the port is open and air is entering the stomach, continuous suction is safe. |
| • If the sump port becomes occluded by gastric contents, flush the sump port with air until a *whoosh* sound is heard over the epigastric area. | If the port becomes occluded, the tube essentially becomes a single-lumen tube and the continuous suction could damage the lining of the stomach. |
| • Never clamp or otherwise occlude the sump port. For patients with gastric, esophageal, or duodenal surgery, notify the health care provider before irrigating the tube. | Excessive pressure may accumulate and damage gastric mucosa or disrupt the surgical anastomosis. |
| • When the tube is removed, monitor for abdominal distention, nausea, and vomiting. | These are signs that GI motility is still decreased and requires further intervention. |
| Monitor and document the patient's response to diet advancement from clear liquids to a regular or other prescribed diet. | Poor response to diet advancement as evidenced by abdominal distention, nausea, and vomiting may signal continued decreased GI motility and need to be reported for timely intervention. Postoperatively, decreased GI motility can result from stress (autonomic), surgical manipulation of the intestine, immobility, and effects of medications. |
| When permitted, encourage oral fluid intake (more than 2500 mL/day), especially intake of prune juice. | Increased hydration, including prune juice, helps promote soft stools that will minimize need to strain. |
| Administer stool softeners, mild laxatives, and enemas as prescribed. As appropriate, encourage a high-fiber diet (fresh vegetables and fruits). Monitor and record the results. | These interventions promote bulk and softness in stools for easier evacuation. |
| Arrange periods of privacy during the patient's attempts at bowel elimination. | Privacy promotes relaxation and success with defecation. |

## ADDITIONAL PROBLEMS:

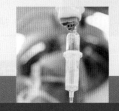

# Pain 5

**Note:** For *Chronic Cancer Pain*, see "Cancer," in Chapter 6.

## Patient Problems/Analyze Cues/Prioritize Hypotheses

## Acute Pain/Chronic Pain

*due to* the disease process, injury, or surgical procedure

***Desired Outcome/Generate Solutions:*** The patient's subjective report of pain using a pain scale, the family's report, and behavioral and/or physiologic indicators reflect that pain is either reduced or at an acceptable level within 1–2 hours.

| ASSESSMENT—RECOGNIZE CUES/ INTERVENTIONS—TAKE ACTION | RATIONALES |
|---|---|
| Obtain history about ongoing/previous pain experiences and previously used methods of pain control. Elicit what was/was not effective. Consider whether pain is acute, chronic, or acute with an underlying chronic component. | A pain history enables development of a systematic approach to pain management for each patient, using information gathered from the pain history and the hierarchy of pain measurement (self-report, pathologic conditions or procedures that usually cause pain, behavioral indicators, report of family, and physiologic indicators). **Self-report of pain is the single most reliable indicator of pain** (Kang et al., 2018). |
| Use a formal patient-specific method of assessing self-reported pain when possible, including description, location, intensity, and aggravating/alleviating factors. | The first step of effective pain management is accurate assessment of pain. Pain-rating scales identify the intensity of pain over time and assist in evaluating the effectiveness of interventions. |
| A numeric rating scale (NRS) of 0 (no pain) to 10 (worst possible pain), descriptive scales, and visual analog scale (VAS) are commonly used to assess intensity in adults who are cognitively intact. Pain-intensity scales are also available in many different languages when language barriers are present. | |
| The Wong–Baker FACES scale was developed for use in children. It is used in younger children and cognitively impaired adults. This scale is appropriate for cognitively intact and cognitively impaired older adults and for patients of various cultures. **Use the selected scale consistently**. | |
| **Note:** Although pain is multidimensional in nature, it is the subjective intensity of pain that is most often measured in clinical practice. | |

Continued

| ASSESSMENT—RECOGNIZE CUES/ INTERVENTIONS—TAKE ACTION | RATIONALES |
|---|---|
| Assess for behavioral and physiologic indicators of pain at frequent intervals [e.g., during scheduled vital signs (VS) assessments]. Document responses. | This assessment optimizes reassessment and treatment intervals. |
| *Behavioral responses:* Examples include facial expression (grimacing, facial tension, furrowed brow), vocalization (moaning, groaning, sighing, crying), verbalization (praying, counting), body action (rocking, rubbing, restlessness), and behaviors (massaging, guarding, short attention span, irritability, sleep disturbance). | Behavioral and physiologic responses are potential indicators of pain in patients who are unable to self-report. Behavioral examples may be seen in patients with impaired communication, including those who are cognitively impaired, unconscious, or conscious but unable to communicate. Physiologic indicators may reflect pain as a result of autonomic stimulation of the sympathetic and parasympathetic responses. |
| *Physiologic responses:* Examples include diaphoresis, vasoconstriction, increased or decreased blood pressure (15% or more from baseline), increased pulse rate (15% or more from baseline), pupillary dilation, change in respiratory rate (RR) (usually increased to greater than 20 breaths/minute), muscle tension or spasm, and decreased intestinal motility (evidenced by nausea, vomiting). | **Note:** Not all patients demonstrate the same response to pain, nor does the lack of response negate the presence of pain. |
| Explain to patients that pain assessment and management are not only a part of their treatment but also their right. | Patients need to know to expect appropriate assessment and management of their pain. |
| Accept the patient's report of pain and plan interventions based on this report. | A patient's self-report needs to be the primary source of pain assessment when possible. |
| Examine the patient's health history for alcohol and drug (prescribed and nonprescribed) use. Ensure that the surgeon, anesthesiologist, and other health care providers are aware of any significant findings. Consult a pain management team if available. | Other medication use could alter effective doses of analgesics or lead to undertreatment. Previous use of opioids or use of alcohol may require an adjustment in medication dosages for effectiveness (i.e., the patient may require more or less medication). |
| Develop a systematic and collaborative approach to pain management for each patient, using information gathered from pain history and the patient's rating of the pain level. | It is important to involve the patient, family, and other health care providers in data collection, formulation of outcomes, and development of the pain management plan. Self-reporting of pain is the single most reliable indicator of pain (Kang et al., 2018). |
| Use at least two identifiers (e.g., patient's name, date of birth, or medical record number) before administering medications. | Using two or more identifiers improves accuracy of patient identification in keeping with The Joint Commission (TJC, 2023) National Patient Safety Goals promoting the right patient receiving the right medication. |
| Use a preventive approach: administer as-needed pain medications before pain becomes severe as well as before painful procedures, ambulation, and bedtime. | Pain relief after administration of medications is more successful if the pain is treated before it reaches maximum intensity. Prolonged stimulation of pain receptors results in increased sensitivity to painful stimuli and the need to increase the amount of drug required to relieve pain. |
| Use a pain plan with a multimodal regimen that has been customized to the individual and the procedure. | Multimodal analgesia combines drugs with different underlying mechanisms of action and nonpharmacologic treatment (see the alternative therapy/complementary intervention later in this patient problem). |
| Recognize that the choice of analgesic agent is based on three general considerations: therapeutic goal, the patient's medical condition, and drug cost. | Individualized therapeutic goals and the stage of illness/disease process are important factors in agent selection to maximize pain relief and minimize potential of adverse side effects. The difference in cost of different agents used to accomplish the same goal may be large. Where there is no proven or expected benefit of using one medication in preference to another to accomplish a desired goal, the less costly medication should be considered. **The right medication is the one that works with the fewest side effects.** |

| ASSESSMENT—RECOGNIZE CUES/ INTERVENTIONS—TAKE ACTION | RATIONALES |
|---|---|
| Assess the patient's previous experience with a specific agent (if any) or patient's recall of side effects experienced with a specific agent, including route. | The preferred route is the one that is least invasive while achieving adequate relief. Aversion to painful routes of delivery [e.g., subcutaneous, intramuscular (IM)] may lead to underreporting of pain by patients and to undermedication by nurses. |
| | • IM analgesia is inconsistent and has unreliable absorption; it is less titratable; and it can cause complications such as hematoma, granuloma, infection, aseptic tissue necrosis, and nerve injury. The IM route should be used rarely and avoided when possible. |
| | • Oral route is least invasive, is convenient and flexible, and produces relatively steady analgesia. |
| | • Intravenous (IV) route is used for agents with quick time to onset of analgesia and for severe pain. |
| ⚠ Use acetaminophen with caution. Be alert to the total amount of acetaminophen a patient is receiving through over-the-counter and other combined medications. | Excessive doses of acetaminophen have occurred when different combination medications (especially over-the-counter formulations) are taken together. |
| | The FDA limits total daily doses of acetaminophen to 4000 mg/day, but the manufacturer of the brand name Tylenol suggests a limit of 3000 mg/day. If the patient has liver disease or a history of chronic alcohol use, amounts must not exceed 2000 mg/day. Dose adjustments are required for patients with impaired liver/renal function (Lilley et al., 2023). |
| ⚠ If the use of naloxone is necessary for an excessive opioid dose, titrate with caution. | Too much too fast can precipitate severe pain, hypertension, tachycardia, and even cardiac arrest. More than one dose is sometimes necessary because naloxone has a shorter duration than most opioids. |
| Do not administer mixed agonist–antagonist analgesics concurrently with morphine or other pure agonists. | Reversal of analgesic effects may occur, instead of pain relief. Mixed agonist–antagonist agents such as butorphanol (Stadol) and pentazocine (Talwin) produce analgesia by binding to opioid receptors, while blocking or remaining neutral to the mu (μ) receptors. |
| **Evaluate Outcomes:** | Sedative effects precede respiratory depression. Close monitoring of sedation level may prevent respiratory depression. |
| Assess patients receiving opioid analgesics for level of pain relief and potential side effects, including evidence of excessive sedation or respiratory depression (i.e., RR less than 10 breaths/minute or $SpO_2$ less than 90%–92%). In the presence of respiratory depression, reduce amount or frequency of the dose as prescribed. Have naloxone readily available to reverse severe respiratory depression. | |
| Monitor older adults and individuals with chronic obstructive pulmonary disease, obstructive sleep apnea, asthma, and other respiratory disorders closely for respiratory depression and excessive sedation when they are receiving opioid analgesics. Consider using reduced doses and titrate carefully. | Older adults who are opioid naive and patients with coexisting conditions are at higher risk for respiratory depression. The most critical time for monitoring for respiratory depression is the first 24 hours of opioid therapy in these populations. Increased tolerance to respiratory depression occurs over days to weeks. Therefore patients who are opioid naive (or have coexisting conditions) are at greater risk for respiratory depression than the patient who has been receiving an opioid for a week or more. |
| Wean patients as prescribed from opioid analgesics by decreasing dose or frequency. | In general, reduce doses by no more than 10%–20% per day with vigilant assessment for withdrawal signs and symptoms. |

Continued

General Care Plans

| ASSESSMENT—RECOGNIZE CUES/ INTERVENTIONS—TAKE ACTION | RATIONALES |
|---|---|
| **Evaluate Outcomes:** Reassess pain level and assess for side effects:<br>• Routinely at scheduled intervals (e.g., every hour for the first 12 hours of opioid therapy, every 2–4 hours with VS)<br>• With each report of pain<br>• Following administration of pain medication based on time to onset, time to peak effect, and duration of action | It is essential to evaluate whether the patient's pain has decreased. Sedative effects precede respiratory depression. Close monitoring of the level of sedation and respiratory status may prevent respiratory depression. |
| Consult with the health care provider to discuss converting to scheduled dosing with supplemental as-needed analgesics when pain exists for 12 hours out of 24 hours. | Experts recommend around-the-clock dosing for patients with continuous pain because it provides superior pain relief with fewer side effects. Prolonged stimulation of pain receptors results in increased sensitivity to painful stimuli and the need to increase the amount of drug required to relieve pain. Addiction to opioids occurs infrequently in hospitalized patients. |
| Titrate the dose to achieve the desired effect. | The initial effect and duration of action of analgesics may differ vastly in acutely ill older adults who may require lower doses, whereas higher doses may be required for those with opioid tolerance or polysubstance use. It is important to consider factors such as these that can influence the initial effect and duration of action due to variations in the metabolism of analgesics. The goal is to develop a safe and effective pain management plan. |
| Provide patient-controlled analgesia (PCA) as prescribed. | PCA is a patient-activated system for pain control that uses an infusion pump to deliver specified doses of analgesics with options of continuous infusions, bolus dosing, or both. The PCA route can be IV, subcutaneous, epidural, wound infiltration, or perineural (around a nerve). Patient selection is important because patients must be capable of understanding and activating the device and be willing to participate in their own treatment.<br><br>Morphine, fentanyl, and hydromorphone are examples of opioids available for PCA use.<br><br>Examples of local anesthetics used in wound infiltration, epidurally, or perineurally are bupivacaine and ropivacaine. |
| When administering PCA, increase patient monitoring following initiation, during the initial 24 hours, and at night when the patient may hypoventilate. Do not assume that pain is controlled; assess the patient to determine whether relief has been obtained. | Monitoring involves pain, sedation, and respiratory assessments and may include $SpO_2$ and capnography. Safety issues with PCA have been described with suggested strategies to reduce risk in Institute for Safe Medical Practices Medication Safety Alerts (2016). |
| Monitor patients in whom neuraxial analgesia is used based on drug being administered, catheter placement, and drug concentration and volume. | Neuraxial analgesia (spinal, epidural, and caudal) is a widely used option for regional analgesia. It decreases many side effects associated with IV opioids, and there is evidence that it can lead to increased mobility and postoperative recovery. Local anesthetics, opioids, steroids, and clonidine are examples of agents that may be used. |
| For local anesthetics, monitor motor examination/sensory level and pain intensity. | Assessments may include sensory level and motor examination evaluations, level of pain intensity, sedation level, VS, and side effects. Potential side effects/complications include catheter migration, occlusion, hematoma, respiratory depression, hypotension, nausea/vomiting, urinary retention, and pruritus. For local anesthetics, sensory assessments are performed bilaterally along dermatomes. |
| Assess for analgesia side effects. Side effects can include sedation, respiratory depression, nausea, vomiting, pruritus, constipation, and hypotension. | Side effects of opioids can interfere with the medication's effectiveness and cause increased discomfort. Monitoring for side effects allows for early intervention as needed to treat or prevent them. |

| ASSESSMENT—RECOGNIZE CUES/ INTERVENTIONS—TAKE ACTION | RATIONALES |
|---|---|
| For management of constipation, see *Constipation* in "Immobility," Chapter 1. Teach patients the likelihood of opioid-induced constipation (OIC). Administer peripherally acting mu (μ) opioid receptor antagonist or secretagogue (substance that stimulates secretion) as prescribed. | OIC is a change in baseline bowel habits when initiating opioid therapy. OIC can be identified by reduced frequency of bowel movements, increased straining to pass a bowel movement, or a sense of incomplete rectal evacuation. Stools are hard, dry, and infrequent. Stool softeners and stimulant laxatives are prescribed as maintenance laxatives. These agents specifically target the biologic systems that mediate OIC, providing effective alternatives to over-the-counter laxative use. |
| Augment action of the medication by advising nonpharmacologic methods of pain control, including physical therapy, cognitive behavioral therapies, acupuncture, massage, and biofeedback. Other methods include back and foot massage, range-of-motion exercises, transcutaneous electrical nerve stimulation, music, aromatherapy, distraction, relaxation exercises, and guided imagery. | Patients in whom nonpharmacologic interventions may be most successful include those who express interest in the approach, anxiety or fear, or inadequate relief with pharmacologic management (Chou et al., 2016). Many of these techniques may be taught to and implemented by the patient and significant other. |
| Maintain a quiet environment and plan nursing activities to enable long periods of uninterrupted rest at night. | Promoting rest and sleep may decrease level of pain. |
| Evaluate for and correct other sources of discomfort. | Such sources, including uncomfortable positioning, full bladder, and infiltrated IV site, can be corrected readily without resorting to drug use. |
| Carefully evaluate the patient if sudden or unexpected changes in pain intensity occur, and notify the health care provider immediately if these occur. | These may signal complications such as internal bleeding or leakage of visceral contents. |
| **Evaluate Outcomes:** Document efficacy of analgesics and other pain control interventions using a pain scale or other formalized method. | This documentation communicates level of pain relief obtained, interventions, effectiveness of the interventions, and ongoing follow-up to meet the analgesic goal. |

---

## Patient/Caretaker Problem/Analyze Cues/Prioritize Hypotheses

# Deficient Knowledge

*due to* unfamiliarity with the safe use of opioid analgesia

***Desired Outcome/Generate Solutions:*** Immediately after instruction, the patient and/or caregiver verbalize(s) accurate knowledge about the safe use, adverse events, storage, and disposal of opioids.

| ASSESSMENT—RECOGNIZE CUES/ INTERVENTIONS—TAKE ACTION | RATIONALES |
|---|---|
| Assess the patient's and caretaker's health care literacy, culture, and culturally specific needs. | This assessment helps ensure the information is selected and presented in a manner that is culturally and educationally appropriate. |
| Identify the goals of opioid therapy, along with its comfort function, in a timely manner. | Education about pain management analgesia needs to begin before surgery with the development of a realistic comfort function goal. The goals of opioid therapy are to provide enough pain control to function, participate in postoperative therapies, and perform activities of daily living. |
| Instruct patients about the importance of reducing the use of opioids as soon as possible after surgery. | Opioids are for short-term use after surgery. |

Continued

| ASSESSMENT—RECOGNIZE CUES/ INTERVENTIONS—TAKE ACTION | RATIONALES |
|---|---|
| Instruct caregivers to recognize new or unusual snoring or unusually deep sleep from which it is difficult to rouse the patient. Explain this to the patient as well. | These changes could be signs of oversedation. Patients and caregivers must be knowledgeable about reportable side effects and complications. Knowledgeable patients/caregivers are more likely to recognize signs of oversedation and report this information to the provider. |
| ⚠ Instruct patients to take opioids as prescribed and not share opioids or self-administer them for reasons other than as prescribed. | Lack of knowledge can contribute to inappropriate and nonmedical use of opioids.<br><br>Receiving a prescription for opioids places patients at risk for developing an opioid use disorder. |
| ⚠ Before discharge, explain that opioids must be stored in the original packing inside a locked cabinet, lockbox, or a location where others cannot easily gain access. Explain the necessity of disposal of leftover medicine after pain has resolved and the medication is no longer needed. | The patient and caregiver must have an adequate understanding of safe use, storage, and disposal of opioids to prevent adverse drug events in the patient and others. Safe storage and disposal minimize the risk for use by others or accidental poisoning. |

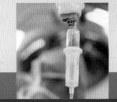

# Cancer Care   6

## OVERVIEW/PATHOPHYSIOLOGY

The term *cancer* refers to several disease entities, all of which have in common the proliferation of abnormal cells. To varying degrees, these cells have lost their ability to reproduce in an organized fashion, function normally, and die a natural death (apoptosis). As a result, they may develop new functions not characteristic of their site of origin, spread and invade uncontrollably (metastasize), and cause dysfunction and death of other cells. Cancer is the second most common cause of death in the United States, exceeded only by heart disease (American Cancer Society [ACS], 2022a). It can cause damage and dysfunction at the site of origin or regionally, or it can metastasize and cause problems at more distant body sites. Eventually, a malignancy may cause irreversible systemic damage and failure, resulting in death. Although the exact cause of many cancers remains unclear, cancers caused by cigarette smoking and heavy alcohol use could be prevented completely. Cigarette smoking is by far the most important risk factor for lung cancer. Risk increases with both quantity and duration of smoking (American Cancer Society [ACS], 2022a) states that cigarette smoking is the cause for almost 80% of lung cancer deaths in the United States. Certain cancers that are related to infectious agents such as human papillomavirus (HPV), hepatitis B virus, hepatitis C virus, human immunodeficiency virus, and *Helicobacter pylori* could be prevented through behavioral changes, vaccinations, or treatment of the infections. Skin cancer is the most common cancer diagnosed in the United States. Most cases can be prevented by protecting the skin from excessive sun exposure and avoiding indoor tanning devices (ACS, 2022a).

Early detection of cancer usually results in less extensive treatment and better outcomes. Screening has been shown to reduce the mortality rate in cancers of the breast, colon, rectum, and cervix, as well as lung cancer among long-term and/ or heavy smokers (Centers for Disease Control and Prevention [CDC], 2021b). The 5-year relative survival rate for all cancers combined has increased since the early 1960s, but the survival rate continues to be significantly lower for African Americans compared with Caucasians (ACS, 2022a). Improvement in survival rates is attributed to improvements in treatment and earlier diagnosis of some cancers. However, survival rates depend on the cancer type, the stage of the cancer at diagnosis, and the patient's age at diagnosis.

## HEALTH CARE SETTING

Medical or surgical floor in acute care; primary care, hospice, home care, long-term care outpatient infusion centers.

## CARE OF PATIENTS WITH CANCER

### Lung cancer

Lung cancer is the most common cause of cancer death among men and women in the United States (National Cancer Institute [NCI], 2021j). Both incidence and death rates from lung cancer began declining for men since the 1990s. Although exposure to known carcinogens such as secondhand smoke, radon, arsenic, asbestos, and air pollution (to name a few) may cause lung cancer, the single most important risk factor for lung cancer is smoking (ACS, 2022a). The risk increases with the amount and length of time someone smokes. Estimating a person's pack year is a helpful way to assess risk. Pack year is calculated by multiplying the number of packs of cigarettes a person smokes per day by the number of years the person has smoked. For example, the pack year is 10 for a person who has smoked two packs per day for 5 years (NCI, n.d.). The higher the pack year, the higher the risk.

Treatment for lung cancer is based on whether the tumor is small cell or non–small cell. The cell type, diagnosed by biopsy and pathologic staging, determines the appropriate treatment, which can include surgery, radiation therapy, chemotherapy, immunotherapy, and/or targeted therapy (ACS, 2021a). Lung cancer has a 5-year survival rate of 21.7% (NCI, 2021j). For patients with advanced disease for whom cure is not foreseen, palliative care (see Chapter 7) should be initiated concurrently with other treatment modalities.

***Screening.*** Annual screening with chest radiography has not been shown to reduce lung cancer mortality. Current lung cancer screening recommendations encourage shared decision making between the patient and the clinician to determine the best screening option. The American Cancer Society, while currently reviewing its 2018 guidelines for screenings for lung cancer, advises following the recently updated recommendations from the US Preventive Services Task Force (USPSTF) and other groups that recommend yearly lung cancer screening with low-dose computed tomography for those who are 50–80 years old in fairly good health AND currently smoke (or have quit smoking within the past 15 years) AND have at least a 20-pack-year smoking history (ACS, 2021b; NCI, 2021i). Shared decision making between the patient and the clinician is recommended to determine the best screening option. This discussion needs to include a description of the benefits, uncertainties, and harms associated with lung cancer screening.

See also: "Perioperative Care," for patient problems, outcomes, and interventions, Chapter 4; and *Impaired Mobility*, later in this chapter.

## Nervous system tumors

Nervous system tumors may be primary or secondary tumors of the central nervous system (CNS), which includes the brain and spinal cord. They are classified according to their cell of origin and graded according to their malignant behavior. Although histologically the tumor may be benign, the enclosed nature of the CNS may result in tumor effects causing significant damage or even death. CNS cancer has a 5-year relative survival rate of 32.6%. According to the National Cancer Institute (2022b), brain tumors account for 85%–90% of all CNS tumors.

There are relatively few known risk factors for brain and CNS cancers. Patients with exposure to radiation and vinyl chloride and those with certain genetic syndromes may be at higher risk. The primary CNS tumor may be diagnosed because of symptoms related to changes in functions of neurons, spinal cord or brain compression, or symptoms resulting from obstruction of the flow of cerebrospinal fluid (e.g., increased intracranial pressure, headache, seizures, visual changes, and mood or personality changes). Standard treatment options may include surgery, radiation therapy, chemotherapy, active surveillance, and supportive therapy (NCI, 2022b).

**Screening.** Currently, there are no recommendations for screening for CNS tumors.

See also: "Perioperative Care," Chapter 4 for patient problems, outcomes, and interventions, and "Traumatic Brain Injury," *Deficient Knowledge: Craniotomy procedure*, Chapter 45.

## Gastrointestinal malignancies

Malignancies of the gastrointestinal (GI) system include carcinomas of the stomach, esophagus, colon, anus, rectum, pancreas, liver, and gallbladder. Each disease site has its own staging criteria and prognostic factors. Most early-stage tumors of all sites are surgically treated. Many treatment plans now begin with preoperative chemotherapy and/or concurrent radiation therapy in the weeks preceding surgery. This approach may eliminate the need for extensive surgeries, increase the chances for cure, or, in the case of anorectal sparing approach, eliminate the necessity for a colostomy. Radiation therapy treatments are less common in gastric, colon, and liver tumors because of the toxicities associated with radiating these areas.

**Screening.** Currently, the colon and rectum are the only GI sites with recommended screening parameters. In the United States, colorectal cancer is the third most common cancer in men and women, with a higher incidence in men than women (ACS, 2022b). The ACS (2021b) recommends routine screening for average-risk individuals beginning at age 45 years through age 75.

After age 75, screening decisions are to be made with the health care provider. The ACS does not recommend colon cancer screening after age 85. Currently, there are several screening options that differ based on key elements such as (1) how well precancerous lesions are detected, (2) the bowel preparation needed, (3) required frequency of testing, (4) cost, and (5) potential harms (American Cancer Society, 2021b). The nurse needs to explain the benefits and potential harms of each of these methods to the patient: (1) guaiac-based fecal occult blood test or fecal immunochemical test (FIT), done annually; (2) stool DNA test every 3 years; (3) flexible sigmoidoscopy every 5 years or every 10 years in combination with FIT; (4) colonoscopy every 10 years if no increased risks for colon cancer; or (5) computed tomographic colonography (virtual colonoscopy) every 5 years. Persons at higher risk, such as those with certain other medical conditions or with first-degree relatives with colorectal cancer, should have screening earlier than age 50 years (CDC, 2022b). An abnormal test with any method other than a colonoscopy needs to be followed up with a colonoscopy.

See also: "Perioperative Care," Chapter 4 "Fecal Diversions," Chapter 58; and "Managing Wound Care," Chapter 75, for patient problems, outcomes, and interventions.

*Recommendations for colorectal cancer prevention*
Following are the recommendations for colorectal cancer prevention:
- Have regular screenings.
- Maintain a healthy weight.
- Adopt a physically activity lifestyle.
- Consume a healthy diet, low in animal fats and high in whole grains, fruits, and vegetables.
- Limit alcohol.
- Avoid tobacco.

## Neoplastic diseases of the hematopoietic system

Hematopoietic system cancers include lymphomas, leukemias, plasma cell disorders, and myeloproliferative disorders.

*Lymphomas*, including Hodgkin lymphoma (HL) and non-HL (NHL), are characterized by abnormal proliferation of lymphocytes. In addition to characteristic lymph node enlargement, involvement of other lymphoid organs such as the liver, spleen, and bone marrow occurs.

Age (young or late adulthood), gender (male), infection with the Epstein–Barr virus, or having a first-degree relative with lymphoma can affect the risk of developing the disease (ACS, 2018). Treatment involves a combination of chemotherapy and/or radiation therapy. The 5-year relative survival rate for people with NHL is 73.2%; for HL, the 5-year survival rate is 88.3% (NCI, 2021b, 2021d).

**Screening.** Currently, no routine screening is recommended for the lymphomas.

*Leukemia*, the most common blood cancer, is the abnormal proliferation and accumulation of white blood cells (WBCs). Divided into two categories, leukemia presents as either acute or chronic, depending on cellular characteristics. In both types of leukemia, abnormal cells may interfere with normal production of other WBCs, red blood cells, and platelets. Patients with chronic lymphocytic leukemia (CLL) may have compromised immunity, resulting in frequent and possibly fatal infections. The four major types of leukemia are acute lymphocytic leukemia, also called acute lymphoblastic leukemia, CLL, acute myelogenous leukemia, and chronic myelogenous leukemia. Symptoms vary depending on the type of leukemia but may include fatigue, pallor, weight loss, repeated infections, fever, bleeding or bruising easily, bone or joint pain, and swelling in the lymph nodes or abdomen (NCI, 2022a). According to NCI (2021c), the 5-year relative survival rate is 65%. Depending on the type of leukemia, treatments may include chemotherapy, targeted therapy, anticancer drugs, and stem cell transplantation (ACS, 2021a).

***Screening.*** Currently, no routine screening is recommended for the leukemias.

**See also:** "Hematologic Care Plans," Section 8, for patient problems, outcomes, and interventions for care of patients with abnormal blood cells.

## Head and neck cancers

Head and neck cancers include tumors of the tonsils, larynx, pharynx, tongue, and oral cavity. Incidence rates are double in men compared with women (ACS 2021a). By far the greatest risk factors are tobacco consumption (through smoking or smokeless tobacco) and alcohol consumption. The risk increases if alcohol and tobacco use is combined (NCI, 2021h). However, infection with cancer-causing HPV, especially HPV-16, is a risk factor for some types of head and neck cancers, particularly oropharyngeal cancers that involve the tonsils or the base of the tongue. In fact, the incidence of oropharyngeal cancers caused by HPV infection (transmitted through sexual contact) is increasing in the United States, whereas the incidence of oropharyngeal cancers related to other causes is decreasing (NCI, 2021h).

***Screening.*** Although no formal recommendations regarding screening exist, routine dental examinations are one mechanism by which early detection occurs.

**See also:** "Pneumonia," *Impaired Gas Exchange* in Chapter 13 for patient problems, outcomes and interventions.

## Breast cancer

With the exception of skin cancer, breast cancer is the most commonly occurring cancer in women, accounting for one in three cancer diagnoses in women (ACS, 2021a). Several modifiable factors (obesity, inactivity, smoking, alcohol consumption) and nonmodifiable factors (e.g., increased age, family history, genetic factors) are believed to influence breast cancer risk among women. Treatment for breast cancer involves either breast-conserving surgery or mastectomy. Surgery is often combined with other treatments such as radiation therapy. According to the American Cancer Society (2021a, 2022c), the overall 5-year relative survival rate is 90% for breast cancer in women. This rate increases to 100% for women diagnosed with stage I breast cancer, but survival rates decline to 26% for those diagnosed with stage IV disease.

***Screening.*** For women aged 45–54 years with average risk and without symptoms, the American Cancer Society (2022a) recommends annual mammography. Further, it is suggested that women aged 55 years and older may transition to biennial mammograms or continue annually.

**See also:** "Perioperative Care," Chapter 4, for patient problems, outcomes, and interventions; and *Ineffective Tissue Perfusion (peripheral)* regarding lymphedema, later in this chapter.

## Genitourinary cancers

For both men and women, genitourinary cancers include cancers of the bladder, kidney (renal cell), renal pelvis, ureter, and urethra and Wilms tumor and other childhood kidney tumors. Additional sites for men include the penis, prostate, and testicle. Sites of neoplasms of the female pelvis include the vulva, vagina, cervix, uterus, and ovaries. Selected cancers are briefly summarized in the following paragraphs.

*Bladder cancer* occurs four times more often in men than in women. Smoking is the primary modifiable risk factor for bladder cancer. Bladder cancer typically presents with gross or microscopic hematuria. When bladder cancer is suspected, the most useful diagnostic test is cystoscopy. Surgery, alone or with other treatments, is part of the treatment for most bladder cancers, with a 5-year survival rate of about 77% (ACS, 2022a; NCI, 2022c).

***Screening.*** No standards currently exist for routine screening for bladder cancer. Some providers may recommend bladder cancer tests for people at very high risk.

*Prostate cancer* is the most commonly occurring cancer in men, excluding skin cancer. Risk factors for prostate cancer include age (greater than 50 years), race (African American or African ancestry), geography (North America, northwestern Europe, Australia, and Caribbean islands), and genetic factors (ACS, n.d., b). For reasons that are not known, the incidence of prostate cancer is 73% higher in non-Hispanic Black men than in non-Hispanic White men (ACS, 2022a). Treatment varies depending on the man's age as well as the stage and grade (Gleason score) of the cancer, along with his other medical conditions. Treatments may include surgery or radiotherapy but come with a high risk of physical impairment, such as urinary incontinence, erectile dysfunction, or bowel problems (ACS, 2021a). The overall 5-year relative survival rate is 97.5% (NCI, 2021f).

In recent years, there has been much discussion, debate, and controversy surrounding the routine screening for prostate cancer using prostate-specific antigen. The American Cancer Society (2021d) recommends that beginning at age 50 years, men who are at average risk for prostate cancer and have a life expectancy of at least 10 years talk with their providers about the potential benefits and known limitations associated with testing for early prostate cancer detection and have an opportunity to make an informed decision about testing. Men at higher risk (i.e., African Americans and men with a close relative diagnosed with prostate cancer) should have this discussion at age 45 or 40 years (if a close relative was diagnosed at an early age).

*Testicular cancer* forms in tissues of one or both testicles and is most common in young or middle-aged men. Most testicular cancers begin in germ cells (cells that make sperm) and are called *testicular germ cell tumors*. Tumors are classified as seminomas and nonseminomas, depending on their cellular line of differentiation, with many consisting of a mixed cellular type. Nonseminomas tend to grow and metastasize more aggressively. Treatment options include surgery, radiation, chemotherapy, surveillance, or high-dose chemotherapy with stem cell transplantation. The 5-year relative survival rate is 94.9% (NCI, 2021g).

**Screening.** There is no standard or routine screening for testicular cancer. Some providers recommend that men self-examine their testicles monthly starting after puberty.

**See also:** "Perioperative Care," Chapter 4; "Urinary Diversions," Chapter 34; and "Benign Prostatic Hyperplasia" Chapter 28, for patient problems, outcomes, and interventions. Also see *Urinary Incontinence*, and *Impaired Sexual Function*, later in this chapter.

*Cervical cancer* incidence has decreased over the past several decades, thanks to improved screenings. Most cervical cancers are caused by persistent infections with certain types of HPV. Women who begin having sex at an early age or who have many sexual partners are at increased risk for HPV infection and cervical cancer (ACS, n.d.a). However, a woman can become infected even if she has had only one sexual partner. Preinvasive lesions may have no symptoms. Invasive lesions may cause abnormal vaginal bleeding, bleeding after menopause, and excessive vaginal discharge. Preinvasive lesions may be treated with methods to remove or destroy the abnormal cells. Invasive lesions may be treated with surgery, radiation, and chemotherapy (in some cases) (ACS, n.d.a). The 5-year relative survival rate for cervical cancer is 66.3% (NCI, 2021a).

**Screening.** The Papanicolaou (Pap) test is the most widely used screening test for cervical cancer. The American Cancer Society (2021c) recommends routine screening to begin at age 25. Those who are aged 25–65 should have a primary HPV test done every 5 years. Screening may be done with a cotest that combines HPV testing with a Pap test or a Pap test alone every 3 years (ACS, 2021c). Vaccines that target the most common types of HPV known to cause cervical cancer are available for females aged 9–26 years (CDC, 2021a).

*Ovarian cancer* is the number five cause of cancer deaths in women and causes more deaths than any other cancer of the female reproductive organs (ACS 2022d). It usually has no obvious symptoms. The most common sign is swelling of the abdomen. The most important risk factor is a strong family history of breast or ovarian cancer, and the risk increases with age. Treatment includes surgery and chemotherapy. The 5-year relative survival rate is 49.1% (NCI, 2021e).

**Screening.** Currently, there is no screening test for the early detection of ovarian cancer.

**See also:** "Perioperative Care," Chapter 4, for patient problems, outcomes, and interventions.

## Patient Problems and Interventions for General Cancer Care

> **Note:** The following patient problems, desired outcomes, and interventions relate to generalized cancer care. Those for care specific to chemotherapy, immunotherapy, and radiation therapy follow this section.

### Patient Problem/Analyze Cues/Prioritize Hypotheses
## Impaired Gas Exchange

*due to* altered oxygen supply occurring with anemia, pulmonary tumors, pneumonia, pulmonary emboli, pulmonary atelectasis, ascites, radiation, pericardial effusion, superior vena cava syndrome, hepatomegaly, and medication side effects

> **Note:** For desired outcomes and interventions, see this patient problem in "Pneumonia," Chapter 13, and in "Pulmonary Embolus," Chapter 15.

### Patient Problem/Analyze Cues/Prioritize Hypotheses
## Acute Pain

*due to* disease process, surgical intervention, or treatment effects

> **Note:** For desired outcomes and interventions, see "Pain," Chapter 5.

## Patient Problem/Analyze Cues/Prioritize Hypotheses

# Chronic Cancer Pain

*due to* direct tumor involvement such as infiltration of tumor into nerves, bones, or hollow viscus; postchemotherapy pain syndromes (peripheral neuropathy, avascular necrosis of femoral or humeral heads, or plexopathy); or postradiation syndrome (plexopathy, radiation myelopathy, radiation-induced enteritis or proctitis, burning perineum syndrome, or osteoradionecrosis)

*Desired Outcomes/Generate Solutions:* The patient participates in a prescribed pain regimen and reports that pain and side effects associated with the prescribed therapy are reduced to level three or less within 1–2 hours of intervention, based on pain assessment tool (e.g., descriptive, numeric [on a scale of 0–10], or visual scale).

| ASSESSMENT—RECOGNIZE CUES/ INTERVENTIONS—TAKE ACTION | RATIONALES |
|---|---|
| After the patient has undergone a complete medical evaluation for the causes of pain and the most effective strategies for pain relief, assess understanding of the evaluation and pain-relief strategies. | This review helps determine the patient's level of understanding and reinforces findings, thereby promoting knowledge and adherence to pain-relief strategies. It also empowers the patient as much as possible to participate in controlling his or her pain. |
| Assess the patient's cultural beliefs and attitudes about pain. *Never* ignore a patient's report of pain, taking into consideration that a patient's definition of pain may be different from that of the assessing nurse. Promptly report *any* change in pain pattern or new complaints of pain to the health care provider. | Cultural beliefs may influence how individuals describe their pain and its severity and their willingness to ask for pain medications. Pain is dynamic, and competent management requires frequent assessment at scheduled intervals. |
| Assess the patient's level of "discomfort" or abnormal sensations in addition to the usual pain queries. | Patients with *neuropathic pain* may not describe their discomfort as pain; therefore be sure to use additional terms. Neuropathic pain is caused by damage to central or peripheral nervous system tissue or from altered processing of pain in the CNS. The resulting pain is chronic, may be difficult to manage, and is often described as burning, electric, tingling, numbness, pricking, shooting. |
| Include the Following in Your Pain Assessments: • Characteristics (e.g., "burning" or "shooting" often describes nerve pain). • Location and sites of radiation. | Not all types of pain are managed solely by opioid therapy. Characterizing pain and documenting its location accurately will result in better pharmacologic intervention and help nurses develop a customized pain-management plan that incorporates nonpharmacologic measures as well. |
| • Onset and duration. | Determining precipitating factors (as with onset) and duration of pain may help prevent or alleviate pain. |
| • Severity: using a pain scale that is comfortable for the patient (e.g., descriptive, numeric, or visual scale). | Severe pain can signal complications such as internal bleeding or leaking of visceral contents. Using a pain scale provides an objective measurement that enables the health care team to assess the effectiveness of pain-management strategies. Optimally the patient's rated pain on a 0–10 scale is 3 or less. Be aware of literacy levels and/or cultural issues that may influence the patient's understanding of the pain scale. |
| • Aggravating and relieving factors. | This information may help prevent or alleviate pain. |
| • Previous use of strategies that have worked to relieve pain. | Strategies that have worked in the past may work for current pain. |
| • Assessment of the patient's and caregiver's attitudes and knowledge about the pain medication regimen. | Many patients and their families have fears related to the patient's ultimate addiction to opioids. It is important to dispel any misperceptions about opioid-induced addiction when chronic pain therapy is necessary. Fears of addiction may result in ineffective pain management. |

Continued

| ASSESSMENT—RECOGNIZE CUES/ INTERVENTIONS—TAKE ACTION | RATIONALES |
|---|---|
| Incorporate the Following Principles: | |
| • Administer nonopioid and opioid analgesics as prescribed in correct dose, at correct frequency, and by correct route. | Pharmacologic management of pain is often the mainstay of treatment of chronic cancer pain. Chronic cancer analgesia is often administered orally. Transmucosal and transdermal forms are available. If pain is present most of the day, analgesia needs to be given around the clock (at scheduled intervals) rather than as needed because prolonged stimulation of the pain receptors increases the amount of drug required to relieve pain. |
| • Recognize and report/treat side effects of opioid analgesia early, including opioid-induced constipation. | Side effects of opioids include respiratory depression, nausea and vomiting, constipation, sedation, and itching. The presence of these side effects does not necessarily preclude continued use of the drug. Consult with the care provider regarding the prophylactic use of stool softeners to prevent constipation. |
| • Use prescribed adjuvant medications. | Adjuvant medications help increase the efficacy of opioids and may minimize their objectionable side effects as well. For example, corticosteroids may be prescribed for their antiinflammatory effects, which may reduce the inflammation and swelling that may be contributing to cancer pain. Nonsteroidal antiinflammatory drugs (NSAIDs) are often used for bone pain. Antiseizure and antidepressant medications are often helpful when neuropathic pain is present because neuropathic pain may not be relieved by opioids. |
| • Assess for signs and symptoms of tolerance, and when it occurs discuss treatment with the health care provider. | Patients with chronic pain often require increasing doses of opioids to relieve their pain (tolerance). Respiratory depression occurs rarely in these individuals. |
|  • Never stop opioids abruptly in patients who have been taking them for a prolonged period. | There is potential for physical dependence in patients taking opioids for a prolonged period; therefore the medications need to be tapered gradually to prevent withdrawal discomfort. |
|  • Use nonpharmacologic approaches, such as biofeedback, relaxation therapy, imagery, application of heat or cold, and massage, when appropriate. See "Pain," Chapter 5, for details. | Nonpharmacologic approaches are often effective in enhancing the effects of opioid therapy. |

## Patient Problem/Analyze Cues/Prioritize Hypotheses

# Ineffective Tissue Perfusion (Peripheral)

*due to* interrupted blood flow occurring with lymphedema

***Desired Outcome/Generate Solutions:*** Following intervention/treatment, the patient exhibits adequate peripheral perfusion as evidenced by peripheral pulses greater than 2+ on a 0–4+ scale, baseline skin color, decreasing or stable circumference of edematous site, equal sensation bilaterally, and ability to perform range of motion (ROM) in the involved extremity.

| ASSESSMENT—RECOGNIZE CUES/ INTERVENTIONS—TAKE ACTION | RATIONALES |
|---|---|
| Assess the involved extremity for degree of edema, quality of peripheral pulses, color, circumference, sensation, and ROM. Measure the circumference of the affected and unaffected extremity for comparison. | This assessment helps determine the presence/degree of lymphedema and potential threat to the limb from hypoxia. Patients may be at risk based on a variety of disease processes, treatments, and medications. |

PART I: Medical-Surgical Nursing Care Plans

| ASSESSMENT—RECOGNIZE CUES/ INTERVENTIONS—TAKE ACTION | RATIONALES |
|---|---|
| Assess for tenderness, erythema, and warmth at edematous site. | These signs of infection need to be communicated to the health care provider for prompt intervention. A continuous supply of oxygen to the tissues through microcirculation is vital to the healing process and for resistance to infection. |
| Elevate and position the involved extremity on a pillow in slight abduction. If surgery has been performed, instruct the patient not to perform heavy activity with the affected limb during the recovery period. | As blood collects, waiting to get into the heart, pressure in the veins increases. The veins are permeable, and the increased pressure causes fluid to leak out of the veins and into the tissue. Elevating the extremity helps reduce venous pressure. |
| Encourage the patient to wear loose-fitting clothing. | Tight-fitting clothing may cause areas of constriction, reducing lymph and blood flow, as well as creating potential areas for impaired skin integrity. |
| Avoid blood pressure (BP) measurements, venipuncture, intravenous (IV) lines, and injections or vaccinations in the affected arm. As indicated, advise the patient to get a medical alert bracelet that cautions against these actions. | BP cuffs can constrict lymphatic pathways, and injections or blood draws will cause an opening in the skin, providing an entrance for bacteria. A medical alert bracelet will inform other health care providers of the need to avoid using that extremity. |
| Consult the physical therapist (PT) and health care provider about the development of an exercise plan. | Exercise increases mobility, which promotes lymphatic flow. This in turn helps decrease edema. |
| As indicated, suggest the use of elastic bandages, compression garments, or sequential compression devices. Ensure that compression garments are fitted properly and that the patient understands when and how to use them. | Elastic bandages decrease edema in mild, chronic cases of lymphedema. The other devices decrease edema in more severe cases of lymphedema. |

#### Patient/Caregiver Problem/Analyze Cues/Prioritize Hypotheses

# Health Care Associated Complication (Excessive Clotting)

*due to* interrupted venous flow, lymphedema, and treatment side effects

***Desired Outcomes/Generate Solutions:*** Before hospital discharge, the patient and/or caregivers competently administer anticoagulant therapy as prescribed and describe reportable signs and symptoms suggestive of progressive coagulopathy.

| ASSESSMENT—RECOGNIZE CUES/ INTERVENTIONS—TAKE ACTION | RATIONALES |
|---|---|
| Instruct the patient or caregiver in the technique of administration of injectable low-molecular-weight heparin, if it is prescribed. | Individuals with certain malignancies (especially brain, breast, colon, renal, pancreatic, and lung) are at higher than average risk for deep vein thrombosis (DVT) and venous thromboembolism (VTE). Other possible contributing factors include recent surgery, presence of a venous access device, sepsis, obesity, concurrent cardiac disease, and underlying increased coagulability disorders. These patients may need to self-administer injectable anticoagulants. |
| If the patient is taking oral anticoagulants, provide instructions about precautions, dietary restrictions (if any), and required lab monitoring, if indicated. | Patients need to be informed about side effects and correct administration of these medications to avoid potential complications. |
| Provide education to the patient on reportable signs and symptoms, such as unilateral edema of a limb with possible associated warmth, erythema, and tenderness. | DVT/VTE may reoccur. |
| Caution that a sudden increase in shortness of breath with or without chest pain also must be reported immediately. | DVT/VTE may progress to pulmonary embolism, which is a life-threatening condition that requires immediate intervention. |
| For additional desired outcomes and interventions, see "Venous Thrombosis/Thrombophlebitis," for *Impaired Hematologic System Function*, Chapter 26. | |

## Patient Problem/Analyze Cues/Prioritize Hypotheses

# Impaired Mobility

*due to* musculoskeletal or neuromuscular impairment occurring with bone metastasis or spinal cord compression; pain and discomfort; intolerance to activity; or perceptual or cognitive impairment

> **Note:** For desired outcomes and interventions, see this patient problem in "Osteoarthritis," Chapter 71. Also see "Managing Wound Care," Chapter 75, for discussions on care of patients at risk for pressure injury.

## Patient Problem/Analyze Cues/Prioritize Hypotheses

# Risk for Impaired Skin Integrity (Skin Lesions)

*due to* disease state or related treatments

***Desired Outcome/Generate Solutions:*** Following instruction, the patient verbalizes measures that promote comfort, preserve skin integrity, and promote competent management and infection prevention of open wounds.

| ASSESSMENT—RECOGNIZE CUES/ INTERVENTIONS—TAKE ACTION | RATIONALES |
|---|---|
| Identify whether the patient is at risk for skin lesions. | Individuals with breast, lung, colon, and renal cancers; T-cell lymphoma; melanoma; and extensions of head and neck cancers may be susceptible to skin lesions. These lesions often erode, providing challenges to wound care, patient dignity, body image, and odor control. Treatment may include radiation, systemic or local chemotherapy, cryotherapy, or excision. |
| Assess common sites of cutaneous lesions. | These sites include the anterior chest, abdomen, head (scalp), neck, and around stomas, and need to be assessed in patients at risk. |
| Assess for local warmth, swelling, erythema, tenderness, and purulent drainage. | These are indicators of infection, which can occur as a result of nonintact skin. |
| Inspect skin lesions. | The presence of skin lesions necessitates being alert to and documenting general characteristics, location and distribution, configuration, size, morphologic structure (e.g., nodule, erosion, fissure), drainage (color, amount, character), and odor so that changes can be detected and reported promptly. |
| Perform the following skin care for nonulcerating lesions and explain these interventions to the patient and significant other, as indicated: | Maintaining skin integrity reduces the risk for infection. |
| • Wash the affected area with tepid water and pat dry. | Excessively warm temperatures damage healing tissue. |
| • Avoid pressure on the area. | Pressure may further damage friable (delicate) tissue. |
| • Apply dry dressing. | This dressing will protect the skin from exposure to irritants and mechanical trauma (e.g., scratching, abrasion). |
| • Apply occlusive dressings, such as Telfa, using paper tape, if indicated, for topical medications. | An occlusive dressing promotes penetration of topical medications. |
| Perform the following skin care for ulcerating lesions and explain these interventions to the patient and significant other, as indicated: | |

| ASSESSMENT—RECOGNIZE CUES/ INTERVENTIONS—TAKE ACTION | RATIONALES |
|---|---|
| For Cleansing and Débriding: | |
| Cleanse the area with the prescribed solution, and follow with a normal saline rinse. As necessary, gently irrigate using a syringe. | The prescribed solution will irrigate and débride the lesion, and rinsing with normal saline removes the solution and residual wound debris. Gentle irrigation protects delicate granulation tissue. |
| As necessary, use wet-to-dry dressings. | These dressings will provide gentle débridement. |
| For Prevention and Management of Local Infection: | |
| Collect wound cultures, as prescribed. | A culture will determine the presence of infection and optimal antibiotic therapy. |
| Apply topical antibacterial agents (e.g., sulfadiazine cream, bacitracin ointment) to open areas, as prescribed. | These agents prevent infection in open areas that are susceptible. |
| Administer systemic antibiotics, as prescribed. | Systemic antibiotics are used for wounds that are more extensively infected. |
| To Maintain Hemostasis: | |
| Consult wound, ostomy, continence (WOC)/enterostomal therapy (ET) nurse as needed on wound-healing techniques. | A WOC/ET nurse may provide alternative suggestions to promote wound healing. |
| Instruct the patient to avoid wearing such fabrics as wool and corduroy. | These fabrics are irritating to the skin. |
| See also: "Managing Wound Care," Chapter 75, and "Providing Nutritional Support," Chapter 76. | Wound healing depends on the adequate intake of nutrients/protein for tissue synthesis. |

### Patient Problem/Analyze Cues/Prioritize Hypotheses

# Diarrhea

*due to* chemotherapeutic agents; radiation therapy; biologic agents; antacids containing magnesium; tube feedings; food intolerance; and bowel dysfunction such as Crohn disease, ulcerative colitis, tumors, and fecal impaction

> **Note:** For desired outcomes and interventions, see "Ulcerative Colitis," *Diarrhea and Risk for Impaired Skin Integrity (Perineal/Perianal Skin)* in Chapter 63; "HIV/AIDS," *Diarrhea* in Chapter 74; and "Providing Nutritional Support," *Diarrhea*, Chapter 76.
>
> For patients receiving chemotherapy (e.g., 5-fluorouracil, irinotecan), provide instructions on the necessity of having appropriate antidiarrheal medications available and other methods used to combat effects of diarrhea (fluid replacement, addition of psyllium to the diet to provide bulk to stool, perineal hygiene). Instruct patients to notify their health care providers if experiencing more than six loose stools per day.

### Patient Problem/Analyze Cues/Prioritize Hypotheses

# Constipation

*due to* treatment with certain chemotherapy agents, opioids, tranquilizers, and antidepressants; less than adequate intake of food and fluids because of anorexia, nausea, or dysphagia; hypercalcemia; neurologic impairment (e.g., spinal cord compression); mental status changes; decreased mobility; or colonic disorders

**Note:** "Immobility," *Constipation*, Chapter 1; "Perioperative Care," *Constipation*, Chapter 4; and "General Care of Patients With Neurologic Disorders," *Constipation*, Chapter 36. Patients with cancer should not go more than 2 days without having a bowel movement. Patients receiving vinca alkaloids are at risk for ileus in addition to constipation. Preventive measures, such as the use of senna products or docusate calcium with casanthranol, especially for patients taking opioids, are highly recommended. Consult with the health care provider. In addition, all individuals taking opioids need to receive a prophylactic bowel regimen. The Oncology Nursing Society published a summary of evidence and recommended guidelines for the prevention and management of constipation for opioid-induced and nonopioid-related cancer constipation. For all patients at risk for constipation, lifestyle education about mobility, high-fiber diet, and hydration is provided. For opioid-induced constipation, in addition to lifestyle education, a bowel regimen with a stimulant and stool softener is recommended. A peripherally acting mu-opioid receptor antagonist may be added. For nonopioid-related constipation, treatment with an osmotic or stimulant laxative is recommended in addition to lifestyle education (LeFebvre et al., 2020).

## Patient Problem/Analyze Cues/Prioritize Hypotheses

# Urinary Incontinence

*due to* loss of muscle tone in the urethral sphincter after radical prostatectomy

*Desired Outcome/Generate Solutions:* Within the 24-hour period before hospital discharge, the patient relates the understanding of incontinence cause and suggested regimen to promote bladder control.

| ASSESSMENT—RECOGNIZE CUES/ INTERVENTIONS—TAKE ACTION | RATIONALES |
|---|---|
| Before surgery, explain that there is potential for permanent urinary incontinence after prostatectomy but that it may resolve within 6 months. Describe the reason for the incontinence. | A knowledgeable patient is not only less anxious but also more likely to adhere to the treatment regimen. Aids such as anatomic illustrations will promote understanding. |
| Encourage the patient to maintain adequate fluid intake of at least 2–3 L/day (unless contraindicated). | Dilute urine is less irritating to the prostatic fossa, as well as less likely to result in incontinence. Paradoxically, patients with urinary incontinence often reduce their fluid intake to avoid incontinence. |
| Document time, amount voided, amount of fluid intake, timing of fluid intake followed by voiding, and related information such as degree of wetness experienced (e.g., number of incontinence pads used in a day, degree of underwear dampness) and exertion factor causing the wetness (e.g., laughing, sneezing, bending, lifting). | This helps estimate the amount of time patients can hold urine and avoid incontinence episodes. With this information, the patient can then attempt to lengthen time intervals between voidings, thus improving the management of incontinence. **N**ote: Patients need to empty their bladders at least every 4 hours to reduce the risk for urinary tract infection (UTI) caused by urinary stasis. |
| Instruct the patient to avoid caffeine and alcoholic beverages. | Caffeine and alcoholic beverages are examples of irritants that may increase stress incontinence. |
| Instruct the patient on how to perform Kegel exercises (see *Deficient Knowledge* in "Benign Prostatic Hyperplasia," Chapter 28) to promote sphincter control. Begin teaching before surgery if possible. | Kegel exercises strengthen pelvic area muscles, which will help regain bladder control. Patients must first identify the correct muscle groups to perform Kegel exercises correctly. |
| | These exercises require diligent effort to reverse incontinence and in fact may need to be done for several months before any benefit is obtained. |
| Remind the patient to discuss any incontinence problems with his health care provider during follow-up examinations. | Such a discussion will enable follow-up treatment for this problem. |

## Patient Problem/Analyze Cues/Prioritize Hypotheses

# Impaired Sexual Functioning

*due to* the disease process; psychosocial issues; radiation therapy to the lower abdomen, pelvis, and gonads; chemotherapeutic agents; or surgery

***Desired Outcomes/Generate Solutions:*** Following instruction, the patient identifies potential treatment side effects on sexual and reproductive function and acceptable methods of contraception during treatment if appropriate.

| ASSESSMENT—RECOGNIZE CUES/ INTERVENTIONS—TAKE ACTION | RATIONALES |
|---|---|
| Assess the impact of diagnosis and treatment on the patient's sexual functioning and self-concept. | Sexual dysfunction affects every individual differently. It is important not to assume its meaning but rather explore it with the individual and allow him or her to give meaning to the changes. |
| Assess the patient's readiness to discuss sexual concerns. | Gentle, sensitive, open-ended questions allow patients to signal their readiness to discuss concerns. |
| Initiate a discussion about the effects of treatment on sexuality and reproduction, using, for example, the PLISSIT model. | The PLISSIT model provides an excellent framework for discussion. This four-step model includes the following: (1) **P**ermission—give the patient permission to discuss issues of concern; (2) **L**imited **I**nformation—provide the patient with information about expected treatment effects on sexual and reproductive function, without going into complete detail; (3) **S**pecific **S**uggestions—provide suggestions for managing common problems that occur during treatment; and (4) **I**ntensive **T**herapy—although most individuals can be managed by nurses using the first three steps in this model, some patients may require referral to an expert counselor (Faghani & Ghaffari, 2016). |
| If a female patient is of childbearing age, inquire if pregnancy is a possibility before treatment is initiated. | Pregnancy will cause a delay in treatment. The patient may be referred to a fertility specialist. |
| Discuss the possibility of decreased sexual response or desire. | This may result from the side effects of chemotherapy. Informing the patient may allay unnecessary anxiety. |
| Encourage patients to maintain open communication with their partners about their needs and concerns. Explore alternative methods of sexual fulfillment, such as hugging, kissing, talking quietly together, or massage. | Encouraging open dialogue promotes intimacy and helps prevent ill feelings or emotional withdrawal by either partner. In the presence of symptoms related to therapy, such interventions as taking a nap before sexual activity or use of pain or antiemetic medication may help decrease symptoms. Other suggestions include using a water-based lubricant for dyspareunia. If fatigue is a problem, partners might consider changing the usual time of day for intimacy or using supine or side-lying positions, which require less energy expenditure. |
| Discuss the possibility of temporary or permanent sterility resulting from treatment. | This discussion could open the door to explaining the possibility of harvesting sperm or ova before treatment begins. The patient may need a referral to a fertility specialist. |
| Instruct patients about the importance of contraception during treatment, if relevant. Suggest that patients receive genetic counseling before attempting pregnancy, as indicated. | Healthy offspring have been born from parents who have received radiation therapy or chemotherapy, but long-term effects have not been clearly identified. Referral to a specialist will help to determine the safe timing of pregnancy after treatments. |

## Patient Problem/Analyze Cues/Prioritize Hypotheses

# Risk for Impaired Musculoskeletal System Function (Arm)

*due to* upper extremity immobilization resulting from discomfort, lymphedema, treatment- or disease-related injury, or infection after breast surgery

**Desired Outcomes/Generate Solutions:**  Before surgery, the patient verbalizes knowledge about the importance of and rationale for upper extremity movements and exercises. On recovery, the patient has full or baseline level ROM of the upper extremity.

| ASSESSMENT—RECOGNIZE CUES/ INTERVENTIONS—TAKE ACTION | RATIONALES |
|---|---|
| Consult the surgeon before breast surgery regarding such issues as wound healing, suture lines, and extent of the surgical procedure. | This consultation will determine the type of surgery anticipated and enable development of an individualized exercise plan in collaboration with physical and occupational therapists (OTs) specific to the patient's needs. |
| Encourage finger, wrist, and elbow movement. | Such movements aid circulation, minimize edema, and maintain mobility in the involved extremity. |
| Elevate the extremity as tolerated. | Elevation decreases edema. |
| Encourage progressive exercise by having the patient use the affected arm for personal hygiene and activities of daily living (ADLs). Initiate other exercises (e.g., clasping hands behind the head and "walking" fingers up the wall) as soon as the patient is ready. | After drains and sutures have been removed (usually 7–10 days postoperatively), patients should begin exercises that will enhance external rotation and abduction of the shoulder. Ultimately they should be able to achieve maximum shoulder flexion by touching fingertips together behind the back if they were capable of this exercise before the surgery. |
| ⚠ In patients who have had lymph node removal, avoid giving injections, measuring BP, or taking blood samples from the affected arm. Remind the patient about lowered resistance to infection and importance of promptly treating any breaks in the skin. Advise the patient to treat minor injuries with soap and water after hospital discharge and to notify the health care provider if signs of infection occur. | Loss of lymph nodes alters lymph drainage, which may result in edema of the arm and hand and also increases the risk for infection. |
| ⚠ Advise the patient to wear a medical alert bracelet that cautions against injections, BP, and venipunctures in the involved arm. | Information on this bracelet optimally will help prevent infection caused by invasive procedures or ensure that the patient receives prompt treatment if an infection occurs. |
| Advise the patient to wear a thimble when sewing and a protective glove when gardening or doing chores that require exposure to harsh chemicals such as cleaning fluids. | This information promotes patient safety/infection prevention. |
| Explain that cutting cuticles needs to be avoided and lotion should be used to keep skin soft. Use an electric razor for shaving the axilla. | This information promotes skin integrity and protects the hand and arm from injury and subsequent infection. |

## Patient/Significant Other/Caregiver Problem/Analyze Cues/Prioritize Hypotheses

# Deficient Knowledge

*due to* unfamiliarity with the purpose, type, and management of central venous access device (CVAD).

> **Note:** A CVAD can be used for venipunctures and administration of medications, fluids, and blood products. Three types of VADs are generally tunneled catheters, nontunneled catheters, and implanted ports.

1. **Nontunneled catheters (peripheral or central):** These catheters are inserted by venipuncture into the vessel of choice, usually basilic, cephalic, or medial cubital vein, near or at the antecubital area, or jugular or subclavian vein in the upper thorax. A

peripherally inserted central catheter is an example of a nontunneled catheter. Maintenance involves daily flushing after each use with normal saline and/or heparinized solution. Sterile dressing and cap changes are necessary. Refer to institutional policies for specific instructions.

2. **Tunneled central venous catheters:** These catheters are inserted into a central vein with a portion of the catheter tunneled through subcutaneous tissue and exiting the body at a convenient area, usually the chest. A synthetic cuff encircles the catheter about two inches from the exiting end of the catheter. Tissue grows into this cuff, helping prevent catheter dislodgment and decreasing the risk for microorganisms migrating along the catheter surface and entering the bloodstream. Single-lumen or multilumen catheters are available. Examples of tunneled central venous catheters include Broviac, Hickman, and Groshong. Maintenance involves flushing per institutional protocol and dressing changes until the site is healed. Cap changes are performed using sterile technique. Refer to institutional policies for specific instructions.

3. **Implanted infusion ports:** Implanted infusion ports are commonly inserted when long-term therapy is anticipated or lack of venous access is expected to be a chronic issue. They consist of a surgically implanted central catheter connected to a port or reservoir. The port, either titanium or plastic, is covered with silicone, which is self-sealing. The port is accessed with a special noncoring needle. The device is then sutured in place in a surgically created subcutaneous pocket, most commonly on the chest. These ports are embedded under the skin and may have single or dual access ports. Noncoring needles must be used to access the port, which allows the system to reseal when the needle is removed. Access may be by direct injection or through an IV infusion into the port. Flush according to facility policy.

*Desired Outcome/Generate Solutions:* Within the 24-hour period before hospital discharge, the patient and significant other/caregiver verbalize understanding regarding the CVAD, including its purpose, appropriate management measures, and reportable complications.

| ASSESSMENT—RECOGNIZE CUES/ INTERVENTIONS—TAKE ACTION | RATIONALES |
|---|---|
| Assess the patient's and caregiver's level of understanding of the CVAD that will be or has been inserted and intervene accordingly. | Determining the patient's and caregiver's current knowledge base helps the nurse devise an individualized teaching plan. Three types of VADs are generally tunneled catheters, nontunneled catheters, and implanted ports. |
| Instruct patients to carry with them the card provided by the manufacturer identifying the type of catheter and recommended flushing solution. | There is a wide variety of catheter types, and the type of catheter determines the proper flushing solution. Refer to agency policy as indicated. |
| Provide a model of the device during patient teaching. | Visual aids augment understanding. |
| Explain where the device will be inserted. | Nontunneled catheters may be inserted at the bedside or in the clinic under local anesthesia. Tunneled central venous catheters and implanted ports are inserted in the operating room under local anesthesia. |
| Explain to the patient that there may be mild discomfort, similar to a toothache, for 48 hours after the procedure, but medication can be given to reduce pain. | Explaining expected sensations and the availability of analgesics reduces anxiety and provides the patient with guidelines for reportable symptoms. |
| If possible, introduce the patient and caregiver to another individual who has this type of device. | Conversing with someone who has already undergone a procedure may increase knowledge, decrease anxiety, and provide another avenue of support. |
| Provide instructions about CVAD maintenance care. Provide both verbal and written instructions, including educational materials provided by the CVAD manufacturer. | Maintenance care likely will be done while the patient is at home, where written materials will serve as a reference. |
| Have the patient or caregiver demonstrate dressing care, flushing technique, and cap-changing routine before hospital discharge. Provide 24-hour emergency number to call in case of problems. | This demonstration will reinforce previous teaching and, when done correctly, provides emotional support that this care can be done when at home. |
| Make arrangements for a home-care nurse to visit the patient after discharge. | The home-care nurse can assess the patient's or caregiver's ability to care for the CVAD and reinforce instructions as needed. |
| Discuss potential complications associated with CVADs, along with appropriate self-management measures. | |

Continued

General Care Plans

## ASSESSMENT—RECOGNIZE CUES/ INTERVENTIONS—TAKE ACTION | RATIONALES

*Infection:*

The patient needs to be taught how to assess the exit site for erythema, swelling, local increased temperature, discomfort, purulent drainage, and fever (temperature higher than 100.4°F [38°C]).

*Bleeding:*

The patient needs to be taught how to apply pressure to the site and to notify a health care team member if bleeding does not stop in 5 minutes.

*Clot in the catheter:*

The patient needs to be taught how to flush the catheter without using excessive pressure, which could damage or dislodge the catheter (particularly an implanted port). If flushing does not dislodge the clot, the patient or caregiver must notify a health care team member.

*Disconnected cap:*

The patient needs to be taught how to tape all connections and the importance of always carrying hemostats or alligator clamps with padded blades to prevent the catheter from tearing.

*Extravasation:*

Although this is a relatively rare complication, it can cause severe damage if a chemotherapy agent with vesicant properties is involved. The patient needs to be taught to report pain, burning, and stinging in the arm, chest, clavicle, and port pocket or along the subcutaneous tunnel during medication administration.

## Patient Problem/Analyze Cues/Prioritize Hypotheses

# Deficient Knowledge

*due to* unfamiliarity with the side effects of antiandrogen therapy or bilateral orchiectomy

**Desired Outcome/Generate Solutions:** Within the 24-hour period before hospital discharge, the patient verbalizes knowledge about the extent and duration of body changes.

| ASSESSMENT—RECOGNIZE CUES/ INTERVENTIONS—TAKE ACTION | RATIONALES |
|---|---|
| Assess the patient's health care literacy (language, reading, comprehension). Assess culture and culturally specific information needs. | This assessment helps ensure that information is selected and presented in a manner that is culturally and educationally appropriate. A knowledgeable patient likely will have less stress about his treatment, adhere to the treatment regimen accordingly, and report side effects promptly for timely treatment. |
| Inform the patient of the side effects of estrogen therapy and orchiectomy. | Breast enlargement, breast tenderness, loss of sexual desire, and hot flashes can occur. |
| For patients undergoing estrogen therapy, provide instruction about symptoms related to complications of thromboembolic disorders and myocardial infarction (including shortness of breath; orthopnea; dyspnea; pedal edema; unilateral leg swelling or pain; and left arm, left jaw, or left-sided chest pain) which must be reported promptly to the health care provider. | These complications can occur with this therapy and related signs and symptoms must be reported promptly to the health care provider for timely intervention. |
| Explain that when therapy is discontinued, most side effects will resolve. | This knowledge may bring some reassurance to the patient. |

## Problems and Interventions Specific to Chemotherapy, Immunotherapy, and Radiation Therapy

### Patient Problem/Analyze Cues/Prioritize Hypotheses

# Risk for Infection

*due to* inadequate secondary defenses resulting from myelosuppression or with invasive procedures or cancer-related treatments

***Desired Outcome/Generate Solutions:*** The patient is free of infection as evidenced by oral temperature of 100.4°F (38°C) or less, BP of 90/60 mm Hg or higher, and heart rate (HR) of 100 bpm or less. The patient identifies risk factors for infection, verbalizes early signs and symptoms of infection and reports them promptly to a health care professional if they occur, and demonstrates appropriate self-care measures to minimize risk for infection.

| ASSESSMENT—RECOGNIZE CUES/ INTERVENTIONS—TAKE ACTION | RATIONALES |
|---|---|
| Assess each body system. | This assessment will help determine the potential for and actual sources of infection. Patients with severe neutropenia have a significantly increased risk for infection because of invasion of surface bacteria in the mouth, intestinal tract, and skin. These patients frequently exhibit mucosal inflammation, particularly of the gingival and perirectal areas. |
| Assess vital signs (VS), temperature, and invasive sites every 4 hours. Look for temperature of 100.4°F (38°C) or higher, increased HR, decreased BP, and the following clinical signs: tenderness, erythema, warmth, swelling, and drainage at invasive sites; chills; and malaise. | These are signs of infection and must be reported to the health care provider immediately. |
| **!** Before administering chemotherapy, ensure that blood counts and other related laboratory studies are within accepted parameters per institutional policy. | Chemotherapy causes predictable drops in WBCs, RBCs, and platelet counts because it can damage normal, healthy blood cells forming in the bone marrow. Administering chemotherapy to individuals with counts below specified parameters may put them at risk for infection, bleeding, or worsening anemia. |
| **!** Identify whether the patient is at risk for infection by reviewing the absolute neutrophil count (ANC). ANC is calculated by multiplying the percent of neutrophils by the total WBC count. | Neutropenia is a condition in which the number of neutrophils in the blood is too low. Because neutrophils are important in defending the body against bacterial and some viral infections, neutropenia places patients at increased risk for these infections. Severe neutropenia can lead to serious problems that require prompt care and attention because the patient could develop bacterial, viral, fungal, or mixed infection at any time. |
| | ANC may be used to determine whether the patient is at unacceptable risk for infection when administering chemotherapy. |
| Neutropenia is defined as ANC less than 1000/mm³. An ANC less than 500 mm³ is considered severe neutropenia. | Neutropenic precautions need to be initiated based on agency policy, and chemotherapy may be held until the risk is less severe. |
| Avoid invasive procedures when possible. | Invasive procedures increase the risk for infection. |
| **Note:** Temperature of 100.4°F (38°C) or higher may be the only sign of infection in the neutropenic patient. | A low-grade fever in a patient with neutropenia is of great importance because other signs of infection may be absent in the presence of neutropenia. Sepsis and septic shock may develop, which may result in death. |
| | **Note:** An elevated WBC will not be present if a neutropenic patient develops an infection. |

Continued

PART I: Medical-Surgical Nursing Care Plans

| ASSESSMENT—RECOGNIZE CUES/ INTERVENTIONS—TAKE ACTION | RATIONALES |
|---|---|
| Be alert to subtle changes in mental status: restlessness or irritability; warm and flushed skin; chills, fever, or hypothermia; increased urine output; bounding pulse; tachypnea; and glycosuria. | These are signs of impending sepsis, which often precede the classic signs of septic shock: cold, clammy skin; thready pulse; decreased BP; and oliguria. These signs must be reported promptly for timely intervention. |
| Place a sign on the patient's door indicating that neutropenic precautions are in effect for patients with ANC of 1000/mm³ or less. | These patients are vulnerable to infection. |
| Obtain an order for STAT blood cultures and expect an order for antibiotics to be started within 1 hour if a patient with a neutrophil count below 500 develops a low-grade fever, with or without other symptoms of an infection. | Neutropenic fever is considered a medical emergency and requires immediate intervention. |
| Instruct all persons entering patient's room to wash hands thoroughly and to follow other appropriate Centers for Disease Control and Prevention (CDC) guidelines. | Hand hygiene is the most important form of infection prevention. Current CDC guidelines also state that individuals caring for patients at high risk for infection must not wear artificial nails and need to consider keeping natural nails shorter than 1/4 inch. |
| Restrict individuals from entering who have transmissible illnesses. | Individuals with colds, influenza, chickenpox, or herpes zoster can transmit these illnesses to the patient. |
| Instruct the patient to avoid uncooked meats, seafood or eggs, and unwashed fruits and vegetables. Follow agency policy on restriction of flowers. | Some facilities do not permit fresh fruits or flowers because of a possible increased risk of transmission of microorganisms. |
| Encourage the patient to practice good personal hygiene, including good perineal care after elimination. | Proper hygiene eliminates flora or bacteria that can easily lead to infection in an immunocompromised patient. |
| Implement routine oral care. Instruct the patient to use a soft-bristle toothbrush after meals and before bed (bristles may be softened further by running them under hot water). | Gentle oral care helps prevent injury to oral mucosa that could result in infection. |
| Inspect the oral cavity daily, noting presence of lesions, erythema, or exudate on the tongue or mucous membranes. | Individuals with prolonged neutropenia are at risk for fungal, bacterial, and viral infections. |
| Encourage coughing, deep breathing, and turning. | These actions decrease the risk for pneumonia and skin breakdown, which could lead to infection. |
| Avoid use of rectal suppositories, rectal thermometer, or enemas. Caution the patient to avoid straining at stool. | These actions could traumatize the rectal mucosa, thereby increasing the risk for infection because of infectious flora in the rectum. |
| Suggest the use of stool softener. | Patients with prolonged neutropenia are at increased risk for perirectal infection and need to be monitored accordingly. Because the immune system is compromised, normal bacterial flora in the colon can be introduced to other parts of the body if perirectal abscesses are ruptured, leading to systemic infection. |
| Instruct the patient to use electric shavers rather than razor blades, avoid vaginal douche and tampons, use an emery board rather than clipper for nail care, check with the health care provider before dental care, and avoid invasive procedures. | These measures help maintain skin integrity, thereby minimizing the risk for infection. |
| Use antimicrobial skin preparations before injections, and change IV sites every 48–72 hours or per protocol. | These actions help prevent infection. |
| Instruct the patient to use water-soluble lubricant before sexual intercourse and avoid oral and anal manipulation during sexual activities. Caution the patient to abstain from sexual intercourse during periods of severe neutropenia. | These measures decrease the risk for introducing infection because of nonintact skin. |
| As prescribed, administer colony-stimulating factors. | These agents minimize the risk for myelosuppression associated with chemotherapy, especially for patients with a history of neutropenic fever. |

## Patient Problem/Analyze Cues/Prioritize Hypotheses

# Fatigue and Activity Intolerance

*due to* anemia (caused by some chemotherapeutic drugs, radiation therapy, chronic diseases such as renal failure, or surgery), or *due to* imbalance between oxygen supply and demand occurring with acute or chronic lung changes (e.g., *due to* lobectomy, pneumonectomy, pulmonary fibrosis)

*Desired Outcomes/Generate Solutions:* After treatment, the patient reports that fatigue has decreased, rates perceived exertion at 3 or less on a 0–10 scale, and exhibits tolerance to activity/exercise as evidenced by respiratory rate (RR) of 12–20 breaths/minute with normal depth and pattern (eupnea), HR of 100 bpm or less, and absence of dizziness and headaches.

| ASSESSMENT—RECOGNIZE CUES/ INTERVENTIONS—TAKE ACTION | RATIONALES |
|---|---|
| Assess for fatigue and activity intolerance, and explain that they are manifestations of decreased oxygen-carrying capacity of the blood and can be tempered by various interventions mentioned below. | Fatigue and activity intolerance are temporary side effects of chemotherapy or radiation therapy and will abate gradually when therapy has been completed. Understanding this relationship likely will help the patient cope better with the treatment. |
| Stress the importance of good nutrition. | Vitamin and iron supplements and intake of foods high in iron such as liver and other organ meats, seafood, green vegetables, cereals, nuts, and legumes likely will help reverse the effects of anemia. |
| As prescribed, administer erythropoietin and/or iron supplements. | Epoetin alfa (Epogen, Procrit) is a synthetic form of erythropoietin that stimulates the production of RBCs to treat anemia associated with cancer chemotherapy. (Erythropoietin will not be effective in patients who are iron deficient.) |
| As the patient performs ADLs, be alert for dyspnea on exertion, dizziness, palpitations, headaches, and verbalization of increased exertion level. | These are signs of activity intolerance and decreased tissue oxygenation. If these signs are present, the patient may be at risk for falls, which necessitates the implementation of safety measures. |
| Ask the patient to rate perceived exertion (RPE) per the Borg scale (1982), See, (see *Activity Intolerance* in Chapter 1). | An RPE greater than 3 is a sign of activity intolerance and usually necessitates stopping the activity. |
| Facilitate coordination of care providers to provide rest periods as needed between care activities. | Undisturbed rest periods lasting at least 90 minutes will help the patient regain energy stores. Frequent activity periods without associated rest periods may result in depleted energy stores and emotional exhaustion. |
| Assess oximetry and report significant findings. | Oxygen saturation at 92% or less indicates the need for oxygen supplementation and may be necessary only during periods of activity. |
| Administer oxygen as prescribed, and encourage deep breathing. | Augmenting oxygen delivery to the tissues will help decrease fatigue. |
| Administer blood components as prescribed. | Infusing RBCs increases hemoglobin level and treats anemia. |
| Encourage gradually increasing activities to tolerance as the patient's condition improves. Set mutually agreed-on goals with patient. | Mutually agreed-on goals promote adherence to increased activity levels, which will increase the patient's tolerance. |

## Patient Problem/Analyze Cues/Prioritize Hypotheses

# Risk for Hemorrhaging

*due to* thrombocytopenia (for all patients receiving chemotherapy and radiation therapy, as well as those with cancers involving the bone marrow)

*Desired Outcome/Generate Solutions:* The patient is free of signs and symptoms of bleeding as evidenced by negative occult blood tests, HR of 100 bpm or less, and systolic BP (SBP) of 90 mm Hg or greater.

| ASSESSMENT—RECOGNIZE CUES/ INTERVENTIONS—TAKE ACTION | RATIONALES |
|---|---|
| Monitor platelet counts; identify whether the patient is at risk for bleeding. | • In thrombocytopenia, the platelet count is decreased. A platelet count that goes below 150,000/µL is considered thrombocytopenia.<br><br>• Prolonged bleeding from injury or trauma usually does not happen until the platelet count goes below 50,000/µL.<br><br>• Platelets less than 20,000/µL put the patient at severe risk for bleeding. The patient may develop spontaneous hemorrhage that is life-threatening (i.e., intracranial bleeding). |
| Perform a baseline physical assessment; assess for evidence of bleeding, such as petechiae, ecchymosis, hematuria, hematemesis, tarry or bloody stools, hemoptysis, heavy menses, headaches, somnolence, mental status changes, confusion, and blurred vision. | These findings signal bleeding and must be reported promptly for timely intervention. |
| Assess VS at least every shift or with each appointment if the patient is not hospitalized. | Hypotension and tachycardia are signs that signal bleeding and need to be reported promptly for timely intervention. |
| Report hypotension, tachycardia, or SBP higher than 140 mm Hg. | In the presence of thrombocytopenia, the patient is at risk for intracranial bleeding when SBP is elevated. |
| Avoid invasive procedures when possible, including intramuscular (IM) injections. If present, use the patient's CVAD to obtain blood specimens. | IM injections and invasive procedures increase the risk for bleeding. If punctures are necessary, the use of smaller gauge needles and gentle pressure at the puncture site until bleeding stops will help prevent hemorrhage. The use of the patient's CVAD avoids venipuncture. |
| Avoid the use of rectal thermometer. | A rectal thermometer can damage rectal mucosa and cause rectal bleeding. |
| Test all secretions and excretions for occult blood. | Testing secretions/excretions may detect occult bleeding early. |
| For patients with platelet count less than 50,000/µL, place a sign on patient's door indicating that thrombocytopenia precautions are in effect. | Notifying all who enter the patient's room that the patient is at risk for bleeding optimally promotes the patient's safety. |
| In the presence of bleeding, begin pad count for heavy menses; measure the quantity of vomiting and stool. | These actions quantify the amount of bleeding. |
| Discourage the use of tampons. | Tampons may cause vaginal trauma during placement, resulting in bleeding. |
| Apply direct pressure and ice to site of bleeding (CVAD, venipuncture). | Applying pressure and ice promotes bleeding cessation. |
| Deliver platelet transfusions as prescribed and be alert to a transfusion reaction. | Patients may lose blood from surgery, or cancer may cause internal bleeding. In addition, both radiation and chemotherapy affect cells in the bone marrow, leading to low blood cell counts. Transfusion reactions can occur if white cells or antigens were not removed properly. |
| Initiate gentle oral care at frequent intervals. | Gentle oral care promotes the integrity of gingiva and mucosa and helps prevent bleeding and infection. |
| Advise brushing with a soft-bristle toothbrush after meals and before bed (hot water run over bristles may soften them further). | Hard bristles may damage the gingival and oral mucosa. |
| Avoid oral irrigation tools. In the presence of gum bleeding, instruct the patient to use a sponge-tipped applicator rather than a toothbrush, to avoid using dental floss, and to avoid mouthwash that contains alcohol. | **Caution:** Dental care must not be performed until the platelet count approaches normal levels. |
| Suggest the use of normal saline solution mouthwashes four times a day and water-based ointment for lubricating lips. | Alcohol-based products irritate impaired oral tissue and could promote bleeding. |

| ASSESSMENT—RECOGNIZE CUES/ INTERVENTIONS—TAKE ACTION | RATIONALES |
|---|---|
| Implement bowel program and check with the patient daily for bowel movement. | If the patient's platelet count is critically low, straining at stool must be avoided to prevent intraabdominal bleeding. Daily monitoring of bowel pattern promotes early intervention if it is needed. |
| Assess the need for stool softeners or bulk-forming laxatives, such as psyllium. | These agents help prevent constipation and straining, which could result in bleeding. |
| Encourage high-fiber foods and adequate hydration (at least 2500 mL/ day) if not contraindicated due to comorbid conditions. | Hydration and fiber promote stools that are soft with adequate bulk, both of which facilitate bowel movements without straining. |
| Avoid the use of rectal suppositories, enemas, or harsh laxatives. | These products increase risk for bleeding/infection from inadvertent trauma to rectal mucosa. |
| Implement and explain measures that the reduce risk for bleeding. | Patients need to use an electric shaver; apply direct pressure and elevation for 3–5 minutes after injections and venipuncture; and avoid vaginal douche and tampons and constrictive clothing. Alcohol is to be avoided, as are medications that could induce bleeding, such as aspirin or aspirin-containing products, anticoagulants, and NSAIDs. Patients should perform gentle nose blowing and use emery board rather than clippers for nail care. |
| Caution the patient to abstain from sexual intercourse when the platelet count is less than 50,000/µL. Otherwise, instruct the patient to use water-soluble lubrication during sexual intercourse. Caution the patient to avoid anal intercourse. | Sexual intercourse could traumatize vaginal, anal, and penile tissue, causing bleeding, or introduction of bacteria. |
| Caution the patient to avoid activities that predispose to trauma or injury, and remove hazardous objects or furniture from the patient's environment. Assist with ambulating if physical mobility is impaired. | This information reduces the possibility of trauma that could result in bleeding. |
| For severe thrombocytopenia, explain the importance of avoiding activities such as moving up in bed, straining at stool, bending at the waist, and lifting heavy objects (more than ten pounds). Suggest bedrest if the platelet count is less than 10,000/mm$^3$. | Valsalva and other maneuvers that increase intracranial pressure put the patient at risk for intracerebral bleeding. |

**See also:** "Thrombocytopenia," Chapter 67.

## Patient Problem/Analyze Cues/Prioritize Hypotheses

# Risk for Impaired Skin Integrity

*due to* treatment with chemotherapy or biotherapy

***Desired Outcomes/Generate Solutions:*** Before chemotherapy, the patient identifies potential skin and tissue side effects of chemotherapy and measures that will maintain skin integrity and promote comfort.

| ASSESSMENT—RECOGNIZE CUES/ INTERVENTIONS—TAKE ACTION | RATIONALES |
|---|---|
| **Transient Erythema/Urticaria:** | |
| Perform and document a pretreatment assessment of the patient's skin. | Pretreatment assessment enables a more accurate assessment of the posttreatment reaction. Alterations of skin or nails that occur in conjunction with chemotherapy are a result of the destruction of the basal cells of the epidermis (general) or of cellular alterations at the site of chemotherapy administration (local). Transient erythema/urticaria may be generalized or localized at the site of chemotherapy administration. |

Continued

| ASSESSMENT—RECOGNIZE CUES/ INTERVENTIONS—TAKE ACTION | RATIONALES |
|---|---|
| If a skin reaction occurs and the chemotherapy is infusing, halt the chemotherapy temporarily. Notify the health care provider. | This action may prevent further skin/tissue damage until the nature of the reaction can be ascertained. |
| Assess and document the onset, pattern, severity, and duration of the reaction after treatment. | Reactions are specific to the agent used and vary in onset, severity, and duration. Usually, they occur soon after chemotherapy is administered and disappear in several hours. |
| **Hyperpigmentation:** | |
| Inform the patient before treatment that this reaction is to be expected and may or may not disappear over the first few months when treatment is finished. | Hyperpigmentation is believed to be caused by increased levels of epidermal melanin-stimulating hormone. It can occur on the nail beds, on the oral mucosa, or along the veins used for chemotherapy administration, or it can be generalized. Hyperpigmentation is associated with many chemotherapeutic agents, but incidence is highest with alkylating agents and antitumor antibiotics. In addition, it can occur with tumors of the pituitary gland. |
| Caution the patient to wear sunscreen with a high sun protection factor (SPF) and cover exposed areas. | Sunlight may exacerbate hyperpigmentation. |
| **Telangiectasis (Spider Veins):** | |
| Inform the patient that this reaction is permanent but that the vein configuration will become less severe over time. | Telangiectasis is believed to be caused by the destruction of the capillary bed and occurs as a result of applications of topical carmustine and mechlorethamine. |
| **Photosensitivity:** | |
| Assess the onset, pattern, severity, and duration of the reaction. | Photosensitivity is enhanced when skin is exposed to ultraviolet light. Acute sunburn and residual tanning may occur with very short exposure to the sun when receiving certain chemotherapy drugs. Photosensitivity can occur during the time the agent is administered, or it can reactivate a skin reaction caused by recent sun exposure before chemotherapy. |
| Instruct the patient to avoid exposing skin to the sun. Advise wearing protective clothing and using an effective sun-screening agent (SPF of 15 or higher). Patients also need to avoid using tanning beds. | Photosensitivity is enhanced when skin is exposed to ultraviolet light. Acute sunburn and residual tanning can occur with short exposure to the sun. |
| Instruct the patient to treat sunburns with comfort measures and to consult the health care provider accordingly. | Such measures as taking a tepid bath and using moisturizing cream and aloe are usually effective. |
| **Hyperkeratosis:** | |
| For patients taking bleomycin, assess for the presence of skin thickening and loss of fine motor function of the hands. | Hyperkeratosis presents as a thickening of the skin, especially over hands, feet, face, and areas of trauma. It is disfiguring and causes loss of fine motor function of the hands. |
| In the presence of skin thickening, assess for fibrotic lung changes: dyspnea, cough, tachypnea, and crackles. | Hyperkeratosis may be an indicator of more severe fibrotic changes in the lungs that usually are not reversible. |
| Reassure the patient that skin thickening is usually reversible when bleomycin has been discontinued. | The patient will be less anxious knowing the condition is usually reversible. |
| **Acne-Like Reaction:** | |
| Working with the health care provider, suggest the use of commercial acne preparations, such as benzoyl peroxide lotion, gel, or cream, to treat blemishes. | An acne-like reaction presents as erythema, especially of the face, and progresses to papules and pustules, which are characteristic of acne and will disappear when the drug is discontinued. |

| ASSESSMENT—RECOGNIZE CUES/ INTERVENTIONS—TAKE ACTION | RATIONALES |
|---|---|
| **Instruct About Proper Skin Care:** | |
| Avoid hard scrubbing of the skin. | Scrubbing can cause skin breaks that enable bacterial entry. |
| Avoid the use of antibacterial soap. Use a mild plain soap. | Removal of nonpathogenic bacteria on the skin results in replacement by pathogens, which are implicated in the development of acne. |
| Avoid the use of oil-based cosmetics. | Oil can clog pores and trap bacteria. |
| **Skin Ulceration:** | |
| Assess for skin ulceration. | Ulceration presents as a generalized, shallow lesion of the epidermal layer and may be caused by several chemotherapeutic agents. |
| Consult with a wound care nurse to determine what to use to cleanse the ulcer. | Choosing the correct regimen for wound care promotes healing. |
| Expose the ulcer to air, if possible. | A dark, moist, warm environment may promote bacterial growth and delay healing. |
| Be alert to signs of infection at the ulcerated site. | Local warmth, swelling, tenderness, erythema, and purulent drainage may be present at the site of ulceration and need to be reported to the health care provider for treatment. |
| **Dry, Pruritic Skin:** | |
| Explain why dry, pruritic skin can occur and its signs and symptoms. | Dry, pruritic skin commonly occurs with biotherapy (e.g., interferon, interleukin-2 [IL-2]) or radiation recall reaction and needs to be treated aggressively. It may be accompanied by a rash and eventual desquamation. |
| Explain strategies for treating this condition. <br>• Apply creams and water-based lotions several times a day, avoiding perfumed products. <br>• Avoid hot bathing water and use only mild soaps. <br>• Manage pruritus with antipruritic medications such as diphenhydramine or hydroxyzine hydrochloride. | These are strategies that may lessen the severity of dry, pruritic skin. |
| Collaborate with a WOC nurse as needed. | This nurse is trained specifically and often certified in wound and ostomy care. |

*Risk for Impaired Skin Integrity*, which follows, for more details about wound care related to radiation therapy.

## Patient Problem/Analyze Cues/Prioritize Hypotheses

# Risk for Impaired Skin Integrity

*due to* radiation therapy

**Desired Outcomes/Generate Solutions:** Within 24 hours of instruction, the patient identifies skin reactions and management interventions that will promote comfort and skin integrity.

| ASSESSMENT—RECOGNIZE CUES/ INTERVENTIONS—TAKE ACTION | RATIONALES |
|---|---|
| Assess the degree and extent of the skin reaction. Erythema may start 1–24 hours after one treatment, and damage may occur cumulatively as treatments continue. | Severe skin reactions may necessitate a delay in radiation treatments. |

Continued

| ASSESSMENT—RECOGNIZE CUES/ INTERVENTIONS—TAKE ACTION | RATIONALES |
|---|---|
| Provide instructions to the patient on skin care measures for the treatment field: | These measures will help to prevent complications and promote comfort during the treatment period. |
| • Cleanse skin gently and in a patting motion, using mild soap, tepid water, and soft cloth. Rinse the area and pat it dry. | |
| • Apply a nonmedicated, nonperfumed moisturizing lotion (such as Biafine or Aquaphor). | |
| • Expose the area to air if possible. | |
| • Apply a nonabsorbent dressing if drainage is present. | |
| • Avoid tight-fitting clothes, including belts and bras, over the treatment area. | |
| • Wear lightweight clothing, preferable cotton, over the area. Avoid harsh fabrics such as wool and corduroy. | |
| • Wash clothing with gentle detergents, such as Ivory Snow or Dreft. | |
| • Avoid swimming in saltwater or chlorinated water during the treatment. | |
| • Do not apply perfumes, powders, or cosmetics unless cleared by the radiation therapist. | |
| • Use an electric razor if shaving the affected area is necessary. | |
| Instruct the patient to avoid exposure to sunlight or to use a sunscreen and protective clothing if exposure is necessary during treatment and after the treatments are completed. | Exposure to sunlight may further damage the skin over the treatment area. The healing skin will still need protection even after treatments are completed. |
| Instruct the patient to observe for and report signs of infection (redness, swelling, purulent drainage). | Affected areas are prone to infection, and early detection promoted healing. |
| Collaborate with a WOC nurse as needed. | This nurse is trained specifically and often certified in wound and ostomy care. |
| Explain the potential for altered pigmentation, atrophy, fragility, or ulceration. | These long-term skin changes are associated with radiation. |

## Patient Problem/Analyze Cues/Prioritize Hypotheses

# Risk for Health Care Associated Complication (Tissue and Vascular Trauma)

*due to* extravasation of the vesicant or irritating chemotherapy agents

***Desired Outcome/Generate Solutions:***  The patient's tissue remains intact without evidence of inflammation or tissue/vascular damage near the injection site.

| ASSESSMENT—RECOGNIZE CUES/ INTERVENTIONS—TAKE ACTION | RATIONALES |
|---|---|
|  Ensure that vesicant chemotherapy is administered by a nurse who is experienced in venipuncture and knowledgeable about chemotherapy. | Vesicant agents have the potential to produce tissue damage and therefore must be administered by a nurse skilled in venipuncture. Vesicant agents include dactinomycin, daunomycin, doxorubicin, mitomycin C, epirubicin, estramustine, idarubicin, mechlorethamine, mitoxantrone, paclitaxel, vinblastine, vincristine, vindesine, and vinorelbine. |
| | The following irritants have the potential to produce pain along the injection site with or without inflammation: amsacrine, bleomycin, carmustine, dacarbazine, doxorubicin liposome, etoposide, ifosfamide, plicamycin, streptozocin, docetaxel, and teniposide. |

| ASSESSMENT—RECOGNIZE CUES/ INTERVENTIONS—TAKE ACTION | RATIONALES |
|---|---|
| Select the IV site carefully, using a new site if possible. | Ideally, the IV site will be newly accessed for vesicant administration. A site older than 24 hours needs to be avoided because it will be difficult to ensure vessel integrity. |
| ⚠ Avoid sites such as the antecubital fossa, wrist, or dorsal surface of the hand. | In these sites, there is an increased risk for damage to underlying tendons or nerves if extravasation occurs. |
| ⚠ Assess the patency of the venous site before and during the administration of the drug. Instruct patient to report burning, itching, or pain immediately. | Extravasation of vesicants often causes immediate symptoms. Prompt reporting of these symptoms by the patient will enable early intervention to minimize tissue damage. |
| Assess the venous access site at frequent intervals. | Pain, burning, and stinging are common with extravasation, as are erythema and swelling around the needle site. Blood return should not be used as the sole indicator to ascertain that extravasation has not occurred because blood return is possible even in the presence of extravasation. |
| ⚠ Keep an extravasation kit readily available, along with institutional guidelines for extravasation management. | Not all vesicants have antidotes. When administering vesicants with known antidotes, the antidote needs to be readily available in combination with the extravasation kit. Because time is of the essence to minimize tissue destruction when extravasation occurs, institutional guidelines or extravasation kit must be readily accessible before initiating drug delivery. |
| ⚠ In the event of extravasation, follow these general guidelines: | Early intervention at the site of extravasation minimizes tissue damage. |
| • Stop the infusion immediately and aspirate any remaining drug from needle. To do this, first don latex gloves, then attach syringe to the tubing and aspirate the drug. | This action removes as much drug as possible from the extravasated site, thereby limiting tissue exposure. |
| • Consult chemotherapy infusion guidelines. | These guidelines provide specifics regarding the management of extravasation of individual drugs. |
| • Leave the needle in place if using an antidote. | The needle enables access if an antidote is to be used with the extravasated drug. |
| • Do not apply pressure to the site. Apply a sterile occlusive dressing, elevate the site, and apply heat or cold as recommended by guidelines. | Pressure may cause added tissue damage. |
| • Document the incident, noting date, time, needle insertion site, VAD type and size, drug, drug concentration, approximate amount of drug extravasated, patient symptoms, extravasation management, and appearance of the site. Review institutional guidelines regarding the necessity of photo documentation. Assess the site at frequent intervals. | Documentation of actions taken ensures accuracy in case questions arise later about how the extravasation was managed. Photos provide a reference point for evaluation. |
| • Provide the patient with information about site care and follow-up appointments for evaluation of the extravasation. If appropriate, collaborate with health care provider regarding a plastic surgery consultation. | Tissue damaged by extravasation may take a long time to heal or may deteriorate so much that plastic surgery may be necessary. Patient needs to understand these possibilities to ensure optimal extravasation management. |

## Patient Problem/Analyze Cues/Prioritize Hypotheses

# Body Weight Problem (Weight Loss)

*due to* nausea, vomiting, and anorexia occurring with chemotherapy, radiation therapy, or disease; fatigue; or taste changes

***Desired Outcome/Generate Solutions:*** At least 24 hours before hospital discharge, the patient and caregiver verbalize understanding of basic nutritional principles to prevent further weight loss.

## ASSESSMENT—RECOGNIZE CUES/ INTERVENTIONS—TAKE ACTION

## RATIONALES

| ASSESSMENT—RECOGNIZE CUES/ INTERVENTIONS—TAKE ACTION | RATIONALES |
|---|---|
| For Anorexia: | |
| See "Providing Nutritional Support," *Body Weight Problem (Weight Loss)*, Chapter 76. | |
| Weigh the patient daily. | Nausea, vomiting, anorexia, and taste changes all may contribute to weight loss. |
| Assess food likes and dislikes, as well as cultural and religious preferences related to food choices. | Providing foods on the patient's "like" list as often as feasible and avoiding foods on "dislike" list optimally will promote sufficient intake. However, keep in mind that foods previously enjoyed may become undesirable, whereas previously disliked foods may now appeal. |
| Explain that anorexia may be caused by the pathophysiology of cancer and surgery or side effects of chemotherapy and radiation therapy. | Taste and olfactory receptors have a high rate of cell growth and may be sensitive to chemotherapy and radiation therapy. |
| Consult with a dietitian for measures to increase caloric and protein intake. | Increasing calories augments energy, minimizes weight loss, and promotes tissue repair. Increasing protein facilitates the repair and regeneration of cells. |
| Suggest that the patient eat several small meals at frequent intervals throughout the day. | Smaller, more frequent meals are usually better tolerated than larger meals. |
| Encourage the use of nutritional supplements. | Adequate protein and calories are important for healing, fighting infection, and providing energy. Nutritional supplements are high in calories, protein, and other nutrients. |
| For Nausea and Vomiting: | Nausea and vomiting may occur with advanced cancer, bowel obstruction, some medications, and metabolic abnormalities. |
| Assess the patient's pattern of nausea and vomiting: onset, frequency, duration, intensity, and amount and character of emesis. | Knowledge about the pattern of nausea and vomiting enables the use of proper medication, route, and timing. |
| Explain that nausea and vomiting may be side effects of chemotherapy and radiation therapy. | The pathophysiology of nausea and vomiting is complex and involves the transmission of impulses to receptors in the brain. Various antiemetics work at different points in the nausea and vomiting cycle. This action helps ensure coverage of the expected emetogenic period of the chemotherapy agent given. |
| Instruct the patient to take the antiemetic, if prescribed, 1 hour before chemotherapy and to continue to take the drug as prescribed. Consider the duration of previous nausea and vomiting episodes following chemotherapy when recommending antiemetic administration schedule. | Nausea is better controlled when the goal is prevention. Antiemetics are most effective if taken prophylactically before the nausea onset. |
| Instruct the patient to eat cold foods or foods served at room temperature. | The odor and taste of hot food may aggravate nausea. |
| Suggest intake of clear liquids and bland foods. | Strong odors and tastes can stimulate nausea or suppress appetite. |
| Instruct the patient to avoid sweet, fatty, highly salted, and spicy foods, as well as foods with strong odors. | Any of these foods may increase nausea. |
| Minimize stimuli such as smells, sounds, or sights, all of which may promote nausea. | Previous stimuli associated with nausea may provoke anticipatory nausea. |
| Encourage the patient to eat sour or mint candy during chemotherapy. | These candies may decrease unpleasant, metallic taste. |
| If not contraindicated, instruct the patient to take oral chemotherapy with antiemetics at bedtime. | This therapeutic combination and its timing help minimize the incidence of nausea. |
| Encourage the patient to explore various dietary patterns. Suggest that the patient avoid eating or drinking for 1–2 hours before and after chemotherapy and to follow a clear liquid diet for 1–2 hours before and 1–24 hours after chemotherapy. | Some patients become nauseated in anticipation of chemotherapy. Reducing intake at this time may lessen this symptom. |

| ASSESSMENT—RECOGNIZE CUES/ INTERVENTIONS—TAKE ACTION | RATIONALES |
|---|---|
| Suggest that the patient avoid contact with food while it is being cooked and avoid being around people who are eating. | Prolonged exposure to smells can extinguish appetite or promote nausea. |
| Advise eating small, light meals at frequent intervals (five or six times/day). | Presenting large volumes of food can be overwhelming, thereby extinguishing the appetite or causing nausea. |
| Suggest that the patient sits near an open window. | Breathing fresh air when feeling nauseated may relieve nausea. |
| Help the patient find an appropriate distraction technique (e.g., music, television, reading) or to use relaxation techniques. | Helping focus on things other than nausea may be helpful in nausea management. |
| Instruct the patient to slowly sip clear liquids such as broth, ginger ale, cola, tea, or gelatin; suck on ice chips; and avoid large volumes of water. | These actions help to increase oral moisture to relieve dry mouth. |
| For Fatigue: | |
| If easily fatigued, encourage the patient to eat frequent, small meals, and document intake. | The energy required to consume and digest a large meal may exacerbate fatigue and discourage further nutritional intake. |
| Provide foods that are easy to eat. | "Finger foods" (e.g., crackers with cheese or peanut butter, nuts, chunks of fruit, smoothies) require less energy expenditure to eat and enable the patient to eat in a position of comfort rather than sitting at a table, which requires more energy. |
| If the patient wears oxygen during exertion, encourage wearing it while eating. | Food consumption requires energy. A fatigued, hypoxic person likely will consume less food. |
| Avoid offering meals immediately after exertion. | A fatigued person will be less likely to want to eat and will tire quickly while eating, which also requires energy expenditure. |
| For Taste Changes: | |
| Suggest trying foods not previously enjoyed. | Previously enjoyed foods may no longer seem attractive, whereas foods that were once undesirable may now seem pleasant. |
| Encourage good mouth care; assess mucous membrane for thrush, lesions, or mucositis. | Thrush infections can cause taste alterations yet are easily treated. A coated tongue may interfere with the ability to taste. |

## Patient Problem/Analyze Cues/Prioritize Hypotheses

# Impaired Oral Mucous Membrane

*due to* side effects of chemotherapy or biotherapy; radiation therapy to the head and neck; ineffective oral hygiene; gingival diseases; poor nutritional status; tumors of the oral cavity and neck; and infection

***Desired Outcomes/Generate Solutions:*** The patient complies with the therapeutic regimen within 1 hour of instruction. The patient's oral mucosal condition improves as evidenced by intact mucous membrane; moist, intact tongue and lips; and absence of pain and lesions.

| ASSESSMENT—RECOGNIZE CUES/ INTERVENTIONS—TAKE ACTION | RATIONALES |
|---|---|
| Assess the oral mucosa for integrity, color, and signs of infection. | Patients receiving cancer treatments are at risk for problems of the oral cavity such as dryness, lesions, inflammation, infection, and discomfort. |

Continued

| ASSESSMENT—RECOGNIZE CUES/ INTERVENTIONS—TAKE ACTION | RATIONALES |
|---|---|
| For patients with myelosuppression, caution not to floss teeth or use oral irrigators or a stiff toothbrush. Use a soft-bristled toothbrush for oral care. | The oral cavity is a prime site for infection in a myelosuppressed patient. Actions such as brushing with a stiff toothbrush and flossing could affect the integrity of the oral mucous membrane and place patients at risk for infection. Patients need to consult with a dentist as indicated. |
| Be aware that some patients may require parenteral analgesics. | Parenteral analgesics may be necessary to relieve pain and promote adequate nutritional intake in patients with moderate to severe mucositis. |
| Suggest to patients with xerostomia (dryness of the mouth from a lack of normal salivary secretion) caused by radiation therapy that they may benefit from chewing sugarless gum; sucking on sugarless candy, frozen fruit juice pops, or sugar-free popsicles; or taking frequent sips of water. Saliva substitutes are another option, although they are expensive and do not last long. | These products replenish oral hydration and promote mucous membrane integrity. A dry mouth also interferes with nutritional intake and swallowing. |
| Advise frequent dental follow-ups. | Lack of or decrease in salivary fluid predisposes patients to dental caries. Fluoride treatment may be recommended for these patients for this reason. |

## Patient Problem/Analyze Cues/Prioritize Hypotheses

# Impaired Swallowing

*due to* mucositis of the oral cavity or esophagus (esophagitis) occurring with radiation therapy to the neck, chest, and upper back; use of chemotherapy agents; obstruction (tumors); or thrush

***Desired Outcome/Generate Solutions:*** Before food or fluids are given, the patient exhibits the gag reflex and is free of symptoms of aspiration as evidenced by RR of 12–20 breaths/minute with normal depth and pattern (eupnea), baseline skin color, and the ability to speak. Following instruction, the patient verbalizes early signs and symptoms of esophagitis, alerts the health care team as soon as they occur, and identifies measures for maintaining nutrition and comfort.

| ASSESSMENT—RECOGNIZE CUES/ INTERVENTIONS—TAKE ACTION | RATIONALES |
|---|---|
| Assess for evidence of dysphagia (impaired swallowing) along with respiratory difficulties. | Esophagitis can occur with radiation therapy to the neck, chest, and upper back or be caused by chemotherapy agents, tumors, or thrush. Impaired swallowing places patients at risk for aspiration and necessitates aspiration precautions. |
| Explain the early signs and symptoms of esophagitis and of stomatitis and the importance of reporting symptoms promptly if they occur. | Patients need to report these indicators promptly to the health care team if they occur so that timely interventions can be made. |
| Sensation of a lump in the throat with swallowing, difficulty with swallowing solid foods, and discomfort or pain with swallowing occur early in esophagitis. Signs of stomatitis include a generalized burning sensation of the oral cavity, white patches on oral mucosa, ulcerations, and pain. | |
| Assess the patient's dietary intake and weight, teaching the following guidelines: | Impaired swallowing predisposes patients to nutritional deficits. Monitoring weight closely evaluates early weight loss. |

## ASSESSMENT—RECOGNIZE CUES/ INTERVENTIONS—TAKE ACTION

| ASSESSMENT—RECOGNIZE CUES/ INTERVENTIONS—TAKE ACTION | RATIONALES |
|---|---|
| • Maintain a high-protein diet. | Protein promotes healing. |
| • Eat foods that are soft and bland. | These foods minimize pain and mucosal irritation while swallowing. |
| • Add milk or milk products to the diet (for individuals without excessive mucus production). | These products coat the esophageal lining to facilitate swallowing. |
| • Add sauces and creams to foods. | These foods may facilitate swallowing. |
| • Ensure adequate fluid intake of at least 2 L/day (if not contraindicated). | Patients with impaired swallowing are at risk for dehydration because they may avoid drinking and eating to prevent pain. |
| • Implement the following measures that promote comfort, and discuss them with the patient accordingly: | Reducing pain associated with swallowing will assist in maintaining adequate nutritional intake. |
| • Use a local anesthetic or solution as prescribed to minimize pain with meals. Liquid lidocaine 2% and diphenhydramine may be taken by the patient to swish and spit or swallow before eating. Some solutions such as magic mouthwash may be prescribed by the health care provider for oral mucositis symptom relief. | The use of these products before eating may help to diminish pain and discomfort and promote intake. |
| ⚠ Advise the patient to use the solution as directed and to be aware that the gag reflex may be decreased. Foods and drinks must be swallowed carefully. | These solutions cause a decrease of the gag reflex and may increase the chance of choking on food or liquids. |
| Suggest that the patient sit in an upright position during meals and for 15–30 minutes after eating. | Esophageal reflux may occur with obstructions and can be distressing. |
| Explain the importance of taking prescribed analgesics before eating or drinking to promote proper nutrition and hydration. | Discomfort may prevent patients from maintaining adequate nutritional intake. If pain is unrelieved with mild analgesics, an opioid such as oxycodone or morphine may be necessary. |
| Encourage frequent oral care with nonalcoholic oral solutions. | Impaired mucous membranes are at risk for infection with bacteria, yeast, and viruses. Solutions that contain alcohol may cause irritation and pain. |
| Instruct the patient to avoid irritants, such as alcohol, tobacco, and alcohol-based commercial mouthwashes. | Irritants exacerbate discomfort and may prevent the intake of adequate nutrients. |
| ⚠ Have suction equipment readily available in case the patient experiences aspiration. Educate the patient about ways to manage oral secretions. | Esophageal reflux may occur with obstructions and can be distressing and cause aspiration. |
| ⚠ Suction the mouth as needed, using low, continuous suction equipment. | Suction helps manage secretions and prevent aspiration. |
| Instruct the patient to expectorate saliva into tissues, and dispose of them per institutional policy. | This intervention helps the patient manage oral secretions using proper infection-control measures. |
| **See also:** "Providing Nutritional Support," *Impaired Swallowing* in Chapter 7, for desired outcomes and interventions. | |

## Patient Problem/Analyze Cues/Prioritize Hypotheses

# Risk for Health Care Associated Problem (Hemorrhagic Cystitis and Urotoxicity)

*due to* cyclophosphamide/ifosfamide treatment or renal toxicity caused by medications, disease process, or treatments

***Desired Outcome/Generate Solutions:*** Patients receiving cyclophosphamide/ifosfamide test negative for blood in their urine, and patients receiving cisplatin exhibit urinary output of 100 mL/hour or more 1 hour before treatment and 4–12 hours after treatment. Patients with leukemia and lymphomas and those taking methotrexate exhibit urine pH of 7.5 or higher.

| ASSESSMENT—RECOGNIZE CUES/ INTERVENTIONS—TAKE ACTION | RATIONALES |
|---|---|
| Assess for and ensure adequate hydration during treatment and for 24–72 hours after treatment for patients taking cyclophosphamide, ifosfamide, methotrexate, or cisplatin. Explain the importance of drinking at least 2–3 L/day. IV hydration also may be required, especially with high-dose chemotherapy. | Adequate hydration ensures sufficient dilution of the drug by urine in the urinary system and prevents exposure of renal cells to high drug concentrations and possible toxicity. Renal failure also may ensue when cellular breakdown products deposit in the renal tubules when patients have been inadequately hydrated before the chemotherapy given for leukemia or lymphoma. |
| Administer cyclophosphamide early in the day. Encourage the patient to urinate every 2 hours during the day and before going to bed at night. | These actions help minimize the retention of metabolites in the bladder, especially during the night. |
| Test urine for the presence of blood, and report positive results to the health care provider. | Hemorrhagic cystitis can occur in patients taking cyclophosphamide/ ifosfamide and must be reported promptly to ensure timely intervention. |
| Assess input and output (I&O) at least every 8 hours during high-dose treatment for 48 hours after treatment. Be alert to decreasing urinary output. | Most chemotherapy drugs are eliminated from the body within a 48-hour period. Maintaining adequate urine output for 48 hours prevents high drug metabolite concentrations in the kidneys and bladder. |
| Ensure that mesna is administered as directed. | Mesna is cytoprotective and inhibits the hemorrhagic cystitis caused by ifosfamide/cyclophosphamide. |
| Promote fluid intake for at least 24–72 hours after treatment, especially for patients taking diuretics. Notify the health care provider promptly if urine output drops to less than 100 mL/hour. | Continual flushing of the urinary system prevents the concentration of cisplatin metabolites in the kidneys and potentially associated nephrotoxicity. Urine output should be kept at a relatively high level. |
| In patients with leukemia and lymphoma, assess I&O every 8 hours, being alert to decreasing output. Test urine pH with each voiding to ensure that it is 7.5 or higher. | If cellular breakdown products that occur from the chemotherapy effect on tumor cells are allowed to concentrate in the renal tubules, renal failure can occur. Proper hydration prevents this potential cause of renal failure. Alkaline urine promotes the excretion of uric acid that results from tumor lysis associated with the treatment of leukemia and lymphoma. |
| Assess patients with leukemia and lymphoma for the presence of urinary calculi. For more information, see "Urinary Tract Calculi," Chapter 33. | Hyperuricemia may be caused by chemotherapy treatment for leukemia and lymphoma. The rapid cell lysis and increased excretion of uric acid may result in renal calculi. |
| Provide instructions to the patient about the signs of cystitis: fever, pain with urination, malodorous or cloudy urine, blood in the urine, and urinary frequency and urgency. Instruct the patient to notify the health care professional if these signs and symptoms occur. | Cystitis can occur secondary to cyclophosphamide and ifosfamide treatment and needs to be reported to the health care provider for timely intervention. |

### Patient/Significant Other/Caregiver Problem/Analyze Cues/Prioritize Hypotheses

# Deficient Knowledge

*due to* unfamiliarity with the type of, procedure for, and purpose of radiation implant (internal radiation) and measures for preventing and managing complications

***Desired Outcomes/Generate Solutions:*** Before the radiation implant is inserted, the patient and significant other/caregiver verbalize understanding of the implant type and procedure and identify measures for preventing and managing complications.

| ASSESSMENT—RECOGNIZE CUES/ INTERVENTIONS—TAKE ACTION | RATIONALES |
|---|---|
| Assess the patient's health care literacy (language, reading, comprehension). Assess culture and culturally specific information needs. | This assessment helps ensure that materials are selected and presented in a manner that is culturally and educationally appropriate. |

| ASSESSMENT—RECOGNIZE CUES/ INTERVENTIONS—TAKE ACTION | RATIONALES |
|---|---|
| Determine the patient's and caregiver's level of understanding of the radiation implant. Explain the following, as indicated: | Knowledge level will determine the content of the individualized teaching plan. |
| • Afterloading | Implant carrier is inserted in the operating room, and radioactive source is inserted later. |
| • Preloading | Radioactive source is implanted with carrier. |
| Explain that the implant is used to provide high doses of radiation therapy to one area. | This method spares normal tissue from radiation. |
| Explain that radiation precautions are required. | These precautions protect the patient, health care team, other patients, and visitors. |
| Explain the following assessment guidelines and management interventions for specific types of implants: | |
| Gynecologic Implants: | |
| Explain that the following may occur: vaginal drainage, bleeding, or tenderness; impaired bowel or urinary elimination; and phlebitis. Instruct the patient to report any of these or any associated signs and symptoms. | An informed patient likely will report untoward signs and symptoms promptly to ensure timely treatment. |
| Explain that complete bedrest is required. HOB may be elevated to 30–45 degrees, and the patient may logroll from side to side. A urinary catheter is placed to facilitate urinary elimination. | Bedrest and other measures help prevent the displacement of implants. |
| Instruct the patient to perform isometric exercises while on bedrest. | Isometric exercises minimize the risk for contractures and muscle atrophy and promote venous return during bedrest. |
| Encourage the patient to take analgesics routinely for pain or to request analgesic before pain becomes severe. | These actions help keep pain at a minimal level. Prolonged stimulation of pain receptors results in increased sensitivity to painful stimuli and increase the amount of drug required to relieve pain. |
| Explain the importance of and rationale for wearing antiembolism hose and performing calf-pumping and ankle-circling exercises while on bedrest. If prescribed, describe rationale for and use of sequential compression devices or pneumatic foot pumps. | These actions help prevent the lower extremity venostasis, thrombophlebitis, and emboli that can occur during enforced bedrest. |
| Explain that ambulation will be increased gradually when bedrest no longer is required (see "Immobility," Chapter 1, for guidelines after prolonged bedrest). | Gradual increments in ambulation will promote return to normal body function without undue stress on the body. |
| Explain that after the radiation source has been removed, the patient will need to dilate her vagina either through sexual intercourse or a vaginal dilator. Additional lubrication may also be necessary. | Vaginal shortening related to vaginal fibrosis and loss of elasticity and lubrication may occur after treatment. |
| Head and Neck Implants: | |
| After a complete nutritional assessment, discuss measures for nutritional support during the implantation, such as a soft or liquid diet, a high-protein diet, and optimal hydration (more than 2500 mL/day). | Irradiated tissues may be swollen, irritated, and painful, which may interfere with nutritional intake. A high-protein diet promotes healing. |
| Provide instructions on the signs and symptoms of infection at the site of implantation. | Fever, pain, swelling, local increased warmth, erythema, and purulent drainage at the implantation site may occur. Patients need to report these indicators promptly to ensure timely treatment. |
| When appropriate, advise the need for careful and thorough oral hygiene while the implant is in place. | Irradiated tissues are vulnerable to infection by bacteria, yeast, and viruses. |
| | **Note:** When implants are placed within the tongue, palate, or other structures of the buccal cavity, patients must not perform oral hygiene. Oral hygiene will be specifically prescribed by the health care provider and generally accomplished by the nurse. Improper mouth care could result in dislodgment of the device, pain, or improper cleansing. |

Continued

General Care Plans

| ASSESSMENT—RECOGNIZE CUES/ INTERVENTIONS—TAKE ACTION | RATIONALES |
|---|---|
| Encourage the patient to take analgesics routinely for pain or to request analgesic before pain becomes severe. | These actions help ensure optimal pain management. Prolonged stimulation of pain receptors results in increased sensitivity to painful stimuli and increases the amount of drug required to relieve pain. |
| Advise the patient to use a humidifier. | A humidifier will aid in maintaining moist mucous membranes and secretions. The patient will need to be instructed in procedures for cleaning the humidifier to avoid introduction of bacteria. |
| Identify alternative means for communication if the patient's speech deteriorates. Consult a speech therapist as appropriate. | Patients need to be aware that cards, Magic Slate, pencil and paper, and picture boards are potential communication measures. Preparing patients before impairment likely would reduce anxiety. |
| **Breast Implants:** Provide instructions about the signs of infection that may appear in the breast. | Pain, fever, swelling, erythema, warmth, and drainage at insertion site are indicators of infection and must be reported immediately for timely treatment. |
| Provide instructions on the importance of avoiding trauma at the implant site and keeping skin clean and dry. | These actions will help maintain skin integrity, prevent infection, and promote healing. |
| Encourage the patient to take analgesics routinely for pain or to request analgesic before pain becomes severe. | Pain is more efficiently managed when pain medications are administered promptly and before it becomes severe. Prolonged stimulation of pain receptors results in increased sensitivity to painful stimuli and will increase the amount of drug required to relieve pain. |
| **Prostate Implants:** Explain the need for the patient to use a urinal for voiding. | Use of a urinal will help ensure that urinary output is measured every shift and enable inspection of urine for the presence of radiation seeds. |
| Instruct the patient or caregiver to report dysuria, decreasing caliber of stream, difficulty urinating, voiding small amounts, feelings of bladder fullness, or hematuria. | Localized inflammation from radiation may cause urinary obstruction. |
| Inform the patient that linen, dressings, and trash need to be saved. | This information helps ensure that all radiation seeds will be accounted for. |
| Encourage the patient to take analgesics routinely for pain or to request analgesic before pain becomes severe. | Pain is more efficiently managed when pain medications are administered promptly and before it becomes severe. Prolonged stimulation of pain receptors results in increased sensitivity to painful stimuli and will increase the amount of drug required to relieve pain. |
| Caution that the caregiver needs to limit the amount of time spent close to implant site. | This precaution helps ensure the caregiver's protection from the radiation source. |
| If implanted seeds are found in linens, or voided urine, follow the facility procedure for handling and storing the seeds. | These measures protect the patient and others from excessive exposure to radiation. |

## Patient/Significant Other/Caregiver Problem/Analyze Cues/Prioritize Hypotheses

# Deficient Knowledge

*due to* unfamiliarity with the purpose and procedure for external beam radiation therapy, appropriate self-care measures after treatment, and available educational and community resources

***Desired Outcomes/Generate Solutions:*** Before external radiation beam therapy is initiated, the patient and significant other/caregiver identify its purpose and describe the procedure, appropriate self-care measures, and available educational and community resources.

| ASSESSMENT—RECOGNIZE CUES/ INTERVENTIONS—TAKE ACTION | RATIONALES |
|---|---|
| See the first eight assessment/interventions under *Deficient Knowledge* (chemotherapy), which follows. | |
| Provide information about the treatment schedule, duration of each treatment, and number of treatments planned. | Outlining the plan of care reduces anxiety and helps the patient and family plan their lives and activities accordingly. |
| Radiation therapy usually is given 5 days/week, Monday through Friday. The treatment itself lasts only a few minutes; the majority of the time is spent preparing the patient for treatment. Immobilization devices and shields are positioned before treatment to ensure the proper delivery of radiation and to minimize radiation to surrounding normal tissue. | |
| ! Explain that the skin will be marked with pinpoint dots called *tattoos*. Emphasize that these markings must not be washed off. | These markings assist technicians in positioning the radiation beam accurately and ensuring precise delivery of the radiation each time. |
| ! Caution that it is important not to use skin lotions, deodorants, or soaps unless approved by the radiation therapy provider. | Some products may interfere with radiation. |
| Discuss side effects that may occur with radiation treatment and appropriate self-care measures. See other nursing problems and interventions in this section for more detail about local side effects. | Systemic side effects include fatigue and anorexia; however, the most commonly occurring side effects appear locally (e.g., side effects associated with head and neck radiation include mucositis, xerostomia, altered taste sensation, dental caries, sore throat, hoarseness, dysphagia, headache, and nausea and vomiting). |
| Provide instructions on strategies for skin care. These strategies include preventing local irritation by clothing, belts, or collars; avoiding chemical irritants such as alcohol, deodorants, or lotions; avoiding sun exposure of irradiated areas; and avoiding tape application to the radiation field. | These measures help to prevent skin breakdown. |
| Provide written materials that list radiation side effects and their management. | Supplemental written materials enhance knowledge and understanding. |
| Provide information about community resources for transportation to and from the radiation center and for skilled nursing care, as needed. | Stress associated with travel to a radiation center may interfere significantly with the lives of family members and may even give patients cause to terminate treatment. Home-care nurses can assist the patient and family at home as treatment progresses and side effects become more pronounced. |

## Patient/Significant Other/Caregiver Problem/Analyze Cues/Prioritize Hypotheses

# Deficient Knowledge

*due to* unfamiliarity with chemotherapy and the purpose, expected side effects, and potential toxicities related to chemotherapy drugs; appropriate self-care measures for minimizing side effects; and available community and educational resources

***Desired Outcomes/Generate Solutions:*** Before the nurse administers specific chemotherapeutic agents, the patient and caregiver(s) verbalize knowledge about potential side effects and toxicities, appropriate self-care measures for minimizing side effects, and available community and educational resources.

| ASSESSMENT—RECOGNIZE CUES/ INTERVENTIONS—TAKE ACTION | RATIONALES |
|---|---|
| Assess the patient's health care literacy (language, reading, comprehension). Assess culture and culturally specific information needs. | This assessment helps ensure that information is selected and presented in a manner that is culturally and educationally appropriate. |
| Establish the patient's and caregiver's current level of knowledge about the patient's health status, goals of therapy, and expected outcomes. | Understanding the knowledge level of the patient and caregiver will facilitate the development of an individualized teaching plan. |
| Assess the patient's and caregiver's cognitive and emotional readiness to learn. | To facilitate learning, teaching must be tailored to comprehensive abilities. The denial process may prevent comprehension of teaching content. |
| Assess barriers to learning. Define all terminology as needed. Correct any misconceptions about therapy and expected outcomes. | Barriers, including ineffective communication, inability to read, neurologic deficit, sensory alterations, fear, anxiety, or lack of motivation will affect learning and the teaching plan. |
| Provide written materials or refer to reputable Internet sources to reinforce information taught. | The ACS, NCI, pharmaceutical companies, and other organizations publish high-quality patient education materials (written and online) that the nurse may use to complement any verbal teaching. |
| Assess the patient's and caregiver's learning needs and establish short- and long-term goals. Identify preferred methods of learning and amount of information they would like to receive. | Identifying preferred methods of learning and amount of information they would like to receive enables the nurse to develop a teaching plan based on this information. |
| Use individualized verbal and audiovisual strategies. Give simple, direct instructions; reinforce this information often. | These strategies promote learning and comprehension. Because anxiety may interfere with comprehension, repetition will help reinforce teaching. |
| Provide an environment free of distractions and conducive to teaching and learning. | A quiet setting free of distraction facilitates learning and retention. |
| Discuss medications the patient will receive. Provide both written and verbal information. Use the Teach Back method to verify learning. | To help ensure that retention has occurred, the patients should be able to verbalize accurate knowledge about route of administration, duration of treatment, schedule, frequency of laboratory tests, most common side effects and toxicities, follow-up care, and appropriate self-care. |
| Provide emergency phone numbers. | These numbers need to be used in case the patient develops fever or side effects of chemotherapy that require emergent intervention. |
| Identify appropriate community resources to assist with transportation, costs of care, emotional support, and skilled care as appropriate. | Community resources may provide comfort for families under stress and prevent psychosocial issues from interfering with the plan of care. |

## Patient/Significant Other/Caregiver Problem/Analyze Cues/Prioritize Hypotheses
# Deficient Knowledge

*due to* unfamiliarity with immunotherapy and its purpose, potential side effects, and toxicities; appropriate self-care measures to minimize side effects; and available community and education resources

***Desired Outcomes/Generate Solutions:*** Before immunotherapy is administered, the patient and significant other/caregiver verbalize understanding of its purpose, potential side effects and toxicities, appropriate self-care measures to minimize side effects, injection technique and site rotation (if appropriate), and available community and education resources.

| ASSESSMENT—RECOGNIZE CUES/ INTERVENTIONS—TAKE ACTION | RATIONALES |
|---|---|
| See the first eight assessment/interventions under *Deficient Knowledge* (chemotherapy), earlier. | |
| Provide instructions about the proper injection technique and site rotation schedule. Explain the importance of recording the site of injection, time of administration, side effects, self-management of side effects, and any medications taken, as well as proper disposal of needles. | These patients or caregivers often give their own injections of interferon. A diary or log will facilitate self-care. |
| Provide instructions about the proper handling and storage of medication (e.g., refrigeration). As appropriate, arrange for community nursing follow-up for additional supervision and instruction. | Home-care nursing support may reinforce teaching, assist with patient monitoring, and provide emotional support to patient and family. |
| Explain the importance of being alert to the side effects of interferon. Fever, chills, and flu-like symptoms are expected side effects of interferon. | This information helps the patient to be prepared for possible side effects. |
| Suggest that the patient take acetaminophen, with health care provider's approval, to manage these symptoms, but avoid aspirin and NSAIDs. | Acetaminophen may help with the expected fever and chills, but aspirin and NSAIDs may interrupt the action of interferon. |
| Assess I&O and weight closely for hospitalized patients and explain to patients how to do these assessments. | Fluid shifts may occur with IL-2 treatment. |
| Instruct the patient to monitor and record temperature twice daily and to drink 2000–3000 mL fluid/day if not contraindicated. | These actions enable the detection of fever, an expected interferon side effect, and replace fluid losses that can occur as a result. |
| Provide information regarding nutritional supplementation. | Dose-related anorexia and weight loss are other common side effects of interferon. |
| **See also:** "Providing Nutritional Support," Chapter 76. | |

## Patient Problem/Analyze Cues/Prioritize Hypotheses

# Risk for Health Care Associated Complication (Alopecia)

*due to* radiation therapy to the head and neck or administration of certain chemotherapeutic agents

*Desired Outcomes/Generate Solutions:* The patient discusses the effects alopecia may have on self-concept, body image, and social interaction and identifies measures to cope satisfactorily with alopecia.

| ASSESSMENT—RECOGNIZE CUES/ INTERVENTIONS—TAKE ACTION | RATIONALES |
|---|---|
| Discuss the potential for hair loss before treatment, and when to expect regrowth. Higher doses of radiation may cause permanent hair loss. | Patients need to be informed about expected hair loss, depending on the type of therapy, to develop strategies for coping and adaptation. |
| Hair loss associated with chemotherapy is temporary and related to specific agent, dose, and duration of administration. Regrowth usually begins 1–2 months after last treatment, and hair often temporarily grows back a different texture. | Patients need to be informed about expected hair loss, depending on the type of therapy, to develop strategies for coping and adaptation. |
| Assess the impact hair loss has on the patient's self-concept, body image, and social interaction. | Alopecia is an extremely stressful side effect for most people. For some men, beard loss is disturbing as well. |
| Caution about the inadvisability of scalp hypothermia and tourniquet applications during IV chemotherapy. | These measures have not proved to be effective in minimizing hair loss and are contraindicated with some malignancies. |

Continued

| ASSESSMENT—RECOGNIZE CUES/ INTERVENTIONS—TAKE ACTION | RATIONALES |
|---|---|
| Suggest measures for women, such as cutting their hair short before treatment and selecting a wig before hair loss occurs that matches color and style of their own hair. Suggest wearing a hair net or turban during hair loss to help collect hair as it falls out. | These measures may help minimize the psychologic impact of hair loss. Being prepared by having head coverings available when hair loss actually occurs may reduce anxiety surrounding the event. Wearing scarves, hats, caps, turbans, makeup, and accessories may enhance self-concept. **Note:** Wigs are tax deductible and often are reimbursed by insurance with appropriate prescriptions. Some centers and communities have wig banks that provide used and reconditioned wigs at no cost. |
| Inform the patient that hair loss may occur on body parts other than the head. Areas such as the axillae, groin, legs, eyes (eyelashes and eyebrows), and face also may lose hair. Loss of facial hair makes it difficult for makeup to stay on. | Patients need to be informed about expected hair loss, depending on the type of therapy, to develop strategies for coping and adaptation. |
| Instruct the patient to keep the head covered during summer and winter. | Covering the head minimizes sunburn during summer and prevents heat loss during winter. Certain chemotherapy agents and radiation therapy may sensitize skin to sun exposure. |
| Suggest resources that promote adaptation to alopecia. For example, ACS hosts the "Look Good Feel Better" program, which provides women with encouragement and tips for managing body image changes during treatment. | These programs provide support during a time that may be difficult for the patient. |

## Patient Problem/Analyze Cues/Prioritize Hypotheses

# Sensory Deficit (Decreased Sensation)

*due to* neuropathies associated with certain chemotherapeutic drugs

**Desired Outcomes/Generate Solutions:** The patient reports early signs and symptoms of peripheral neuropathy (functional disturbance of the peripheral nervous system), and measures are implemented promptly to minimize these side effects.

| ASSESSMENT—RECOGNIZE CUES/ INTERVENTIONS—TAKE ACTION | RATIONALES |
|---|---|
| [!] Assess for the development of peripheral neuropathy. Suggest consultation with PT or OT to assist with maintaining function. Explain that the severity of symptoms may abate when treatment is halted; however, recovery may be slow and is usually incomplete. | Peripheral neuropathy can occur with several antineoplastic agents. Neurotoxicity is cumulative with some chemotherapy drugs, and therefore assessment of symptoms is done before the delivery of each dose. |
| [!] Instruct the patient to report early signs and symptoms of peripheral neuropathy. | Numbness and tingling (paresthesias) of fingers and toes occur initially and can progress to difficulty with fine motor skills, such as buttoning shirts or picking up objects. The most severely affected individuals may lose sensation at hip level and have difficulty with balance and ambulation. |
| Assess for neuropathic pain. See *Chronic Cancer Pain*, Chapter 6, for desired outcomes and assessment/interventions. | Patients with neuropathies may experience neuropathic pain, which is often described and treated differently from nociceptive pain. |

## Patient Problem/Analyze Cues/Prioritize Hypotheses

# Sensory Deficit (Hearing Ability)

*due to* ototoxicity associated with certain chemotherapeutic drugs

**Desired Outcomes/Generate Solutions:** The patient reports early signs and symptoms of ototoxicity, and measures are implemented promptly to minimize these side effects.

| ASSESSMENT—RECOGNIZE CUES/ INTERVENTIONS—TAKE ACTION | RATIONALES |
| --- | --- |
| Instruct the patient and caregivers to report early symptoms of hearing loss the patient may experience. | Cumulative doses of cisplatin can result in irreversible loss of high-frequency range hearing or tinnitus. |
| Suggest that the patient face speakers and watch their lips during conversation while being aware that background noise may interfere with hearing ability.<br><br>**Note:** Keep in mind that masks worn in health care facilities often block a patient's ability to read lips. | This information promotes skills with which to cope with hearing loss. |
| Suggest a trial of a hearing aid before purchasing it. | A hearing aid may be helpful, or it may amplify background noise and worsen speech comprehension. |
| In instances of cisplatin-induced hearing loss, refer the patient to community resources for hearing-impaired persons. | Hearing loss from cisplatin is usually irreversible. A baseline audiogram may be done before cisplatin administration. |

PART I: Medical-Surgical Nursing Care Plans

General Care Plans

# Palliative and End-of-Life Care 7

## OVERVIEW

The concept of palliative care is undergoing significant change in the United States in the face of an increasingly aging society. The number of Americans aged 65 and older is projected to be 95 million by 2060, which almost doubles 2018's number of 52 million (Population Reference Bureau, 2022). The increased number of people entering the Medicare system had prompted significant changes in approaches to health care delivery. It is also important to note that 6 in 10 adults in the United States have one chronic illness, and 4 in 10 have two or more (CDC, 2022a). To address these issues, the Affordable Care Act has provided extensive funding to almost every agency under the US Department of Health and Human Services to focus on initiatives that address chronic illness to provide better care, improve health, and reduce the cost of care to support the needs of this fastest growing patient population.

The goal of palliative care is to provide optimal symptom management. The symptom burden that accompanies chronic illness and malignancies requires the skilled use of palliative interventions. Optimally managing symptoms reduces disease exacerbations, promotes physical activity, reduces hospital use, and improves patients' quality of life.

Palliative care can be started at any time, but optimal benefits occur when it begins following the diagnosis of a serious illness, such as cancer, neurogenerative diseases, heart failure (HF), dementia, chronic kidney disease, or chronic obstructive pulmonary disease. Palliative care involves the assessment and management of pain and other symptoms, promoting comfort, supporting caregiver needs, and coordination of care. The goal is to reduce the burden of health-related suffering while improving quality of life, and the approach is patient and family centered.

As the trajectory of the disease progresses toward the end of life, palliative interventions increase in use, complexity, and intensity. Near the end of life, patients often become more symptomatic, require full assistance with activities of daily living, and are profoundly weaker and often bedbound. Physical, emotional, and spiritual symptoms may become more pronounced during this time and will require skilled and knowledgeable interventions by an interdisciplinary team of professionals (e.g., medicine, nursing, social work, clergy, ancillary support). The use of a team-based approach is essential to address and meet the multiple needs of the patient and family.

## HEALTH CARE SETTING

Primary care, outpatient clinic, rehabilitation center, surgical center, acute care, home care, long-term care, skilled hospital, and hospice

## Patient/Family Problem/Analyze Cues/Prioritize Hypotheses

## Deficient Knowledge

*due to* unfamiliarity with the optimal course of action as the patient moves from an acute curative medical model into a palliative care/symptom management plan of care

*Desired Outcome/Generate Solutions:* The patient and family effectively transition from the acute medical management of advanced disease into a palliative care approach with minimal conflict and confusion.

| ASSESSMENT—RECOGNIZE CUES/ INTERVENTIONS—TAKE ACTION | RATIONALES |
| --- | --- |
| Assess the understanding of the underlying disease pathophysiology and associated symptoms that interfere with the patient's perceived quality of life. | Individuals who gain an understanding of the disease that is nonresponsive to acute medical interventions will be better prepared to understand the transition from acute medical management to palliative care. |

| ASSESSMENT—RECOGNIZE CUES/ INTERVENTIONS—TAKE ACTION | RATIONALES |
|---|---|
| Determine whether there are conflicts associated with the transition of care from acute to palliative. | Individuals who understand the rationale for moving from being acutely managed to symptom management or to less invasive medical management will be more likely to move with greater ease along the trajectory of their disease. |
| Help the patient and family differentiate palliative care from hospice care. | Not all individuals are comfortable with or want to be referred to hospice care. Palliative care interventions do not depend on a 6-month or less prognosis, nor are they mandated by reimbursement criteria. |
| As needed, assist the patient and family members to identify supportive disciplines, such as advanced practice nurses, medical social workers, dietitians, nursing assistants, physical therapists, and spiritual advisors. | The patient and family may require support from multiple disciplines to provide needed care. |
| Promote the physical activity and social engagement and active participation in life for as long as possible. | Physical activity helps to reduce disease exacerbations, minimize depression, reduce discomfort, promote socialization, reduce isolation, and prevent complications associated with immobility. |
| Explain that palliative care can be provided along with advanced disease management by the patient's primary care provider and is reimbursed as routine medical management. | Palliative care is integrated into the management of advanced diseases with a primary focus on symptom management and is not contingent on the treatment being provided during the last months, days, or weeks of life. This enables coordinated and continuous medical management by the patient's primary care or specialty provider. |

## Caregiver Problem/Analyze Cues/Generate Hypotheses

# Caregiver Role Strain

*due to* the demands associated with the patient's physical care needs as the patient's disease progresses and contributes to physical limitations and disability

***Desired Outcome/Generate Solutions:*** Caregivers are assisted with providing care and offered frequent respite opportunities within 24–48 hours of intervention.

| ASSESSMENT—RECOGNIZE CUES/ INTERVENTIONS—TAKE ACTION | RATIONALES |
|---|---|
| Assess the specific support systems used to provide the patient with advanced disease care management. | This assessment will help determine whether an appropriate support system is in place to address the physical, emotional, and spiritual demands associated with advanced disease, illness, and disability. |
| Identify the primary caregiver and any additional caregivers who can support the patient and primary caregiver. Then determine the specific roles of the patient's family or support system. | In addition to a primary caregiver, a secondary caregiver should be identified and mobilized to reduce the potential for burn-out. Burn-out often occurs when only one person provides all the caregiving. |
| Evaluate the community-based services or supportive programs that can be used to provide caregiver respite. | Services for the aging, adult daycare, respite care, and church-specific services, as well as help provided by volunteers, friends, and neighbors, may be considered to provide respite for the primary caregiver. |
| Encourage communication between the patient and caregiver. | Communication will provide an opportunity to identify and verbalize fears and concerns regarding the demands of meeting the patient's activities of daily living. This communication will provide earlier identification of problems that require prompt attention and problem-solving to reduce caregiver burn-out. |

Continued

| ASSESSMENT—RECOGNIZE CUES/ INTERVENTIONS—TAKE ACTION | RATIONALES |
|---|---|
| Elicit interdisciplinary support to assist the caregiver in problem-solving and seeking additional supportive resources. | Social workers, spiritual advisors, and advanced practice nurses will have additional ideas and be familiar with community resources that can be facilitated to support the primary caregiver, thereby reducing the potential for burn-out. |
| Provide information about online resources for the patient and caregivers. | Organizations such as Get Palliative Care (https://getpalliativecare.org/resources/) may have useful resources for patients and caregivers. |
| If caregiving demands are increased out of proportion to the caretaker's abilities and physical reserves, reevaluate the plan of care and the expectations of both the patient and caregiver. | Progressive symptomatic disease may increase the physical demands on the caregiver. For example, a dementia patient who becomes combative and is not sleeping may require admission into a psychiatric facility, long-term care facility, or nursing home. Reevaluation should occur when it is no longer safe for the patient or the caregiver to continue to meet the many needs of the patient. |

### Patient Problem/Analyze Cues/Prioritize Hypotheses

# Risk for Multisymptom Discomfort

*due to* the pathophysiologic and psychologic consequences associated with advanced symptomatic disease and illness

**Desired Outcome/Generate Solutions:** Within 1–2 hours of intervention, the patient's discomfort level decreases as evidenced by a self-rated symptom intensity score of less than 5 on a 1–10 numeric multisymptom rating scale.

| ASSESSMENT—RECOGNIZE CUES/ INTERVENTIONS—TAKE ACTION | RATIONALES |
|---|---|
| Identify and recognize the multiple symptoms associated with progressive advanced disease, using a multisymptom, numeric self-rating scale of 1–10 (e.g., Edmonton Symptom Assessment Scale). Multiple symptoms that accompany advanced disease can include pain, dyspnea, fatigue, edema, weakness, anxiety, depression, and insomnia. | Significant evidence suggests that any symptom rated at 5 or higher interferes with the patient's perceived quality of life (Hui & Bruera, 2017). |
| Assess the multidimensional aspects of specific symptoms: modifying or aggravating factors, location, quality, character, timing, intensity, and/or relieving factors. | The use of a numeric scale captures the intensity of the symptom but does not help to determine the full impact of the symptom's influence on the patient's perceived quality of life. Obtaining a full description of the symptom helps to identify specific physiologic aspects and guide appropriate interventions. In addition, emotional and spiritual aspects can interface with and intensify symptom complaints. |
| Assess for and report the use of all medications that are used to manage specific symptoms. | The use of multiple medications (polypharmacy) may reduce or exacerbate the efficacy of specific medications prescribed to reduce symptoms. Multiple providers may have prescribed specific medications that alter the effects of other medications. It is important to report all of the medications used by the patient to the managing provider to ensure their use does not interfere with the efficacy of necessary medications. |

| ASSESSMENT—RECOGNIZE CUES/ INTERVENTIONS—TAKE ACTION | RATIONALES |
|---|---|
| **Evaluate Outcomes:** Document the patient's symptom intensity rating before an intervention and again after the intervention. | Evaluating the pre- and postsymptom intensity scores and reporting these findings in the patient health record promote standardized communication among the interdisciplinary team and help identify the efficacy of the intervention. |
| Provide early and prompt identification and assessment of pain and other symptoms—physical, psychologic, and spiritual. Refer to "Pain," Chapter 5. | Approaching the patient from a multidimensional perspective will promote a holistic approach to pain and symptom management, thereby preventing or reducing the incidence of somatization and poorly managed symptoms. |
| Recognize common symptoms associated with advanced diseases and end-of-life care such as pain, fatigue, dyspnea, and depression and discuss them with the patient and caregiver. | Providing information on what to expect preemptively prepares the patient and family regarding what to look for and how to be proactive in seeking symptom management. |
| Assess and differentiate the type of pain syndromes, including acute, chronic, neuropathic, visceral, and somatic (nociceptive). Acute pain is a normal response to injury or a warning of potential injury and resolves with healing (e.g., surgical incision). Chronic pain persists and may last for months or years (e.g., arthritis). Patients can have an acute exacerbation of chronic pain. Neuropathic pain involves nerves, visceral pain comes from stretching or pressure within solid organs, and somatic pain comes from bone, muscle, joints, and hollow organs. | The patient's verbal descriptors will help to differentiate the types of pain the patient is experiencing. For example, neuropathic pain (sharp, shooting, hot, radiating) from somatic (nociceptive) pain (dull, constant, gnawing, deep, constant). Specific analgesic interventions are based on the type of pain. |
| Explain to the patient and significant others how pain may be treated in the palliative and end-of-life care settings. | Mild pain may be managed with nonopioid analgesics. Opioids are appropriate for moderate to severe pain or persistent mild to moderate pain. |
| Follow general principles when initiation, titration, and/or discontinuation of opioid analgesics are considered: <br><br> 1. Establish the pain relief goal (e.g., 30% reduction in numeric pain score). <br><br> 2. Initiate analgesia with a short-acting, low-dose upload. <br><br> 3. Use a titration schedule based on the opioid's pharmacologic properties. <br><br> 4. Frequently monitor for analgesia and adverse effects. <br><br> These activities are carried out by the prescribing provider. | These principles promote the efficient use of opioid analgesics for the optimal relief of the patient's pain. |
| Explain the common side effects of opioid analgesics and the interventions that can help mitigate these symptoms. Common side effects include nausea, vomiting, itchiness (pruritus), and drowsiness, all of which resolve or decrease with continued use. Constipation is a common symptom and usually does not resolve with continued use, and therefore a stool softener and stimulant need to be prescribed. Respiratory depression is a rare side effect that can be avoided with correct and accurate prescribing. | Prior knowledge of expected side effects allows the patient or caregiver to implement necessary measures to resolve them as needed. |
| Explain the value of adjuvant analgesics in promoting optimal management of neuropathic and somatic (nociceptive) pain syndromes. | Adjuvant analgesics are medications that, when combined with opioid analgesics, help to reduce neuropathic and nociceptive pain. No amount of opioid alone will effectively manage these two pain syndromes. Neuropathic pain syndromes benefit from the adjuvant use of selective serotonin-norepinephrine reuptake inhibitor antidepressants, anticonvulsants, and corticosteroids. Somatic or nociceptive pain syndromes respond to nonsteroidal anti-inflammatory agents, corticosteroids, and bisphosphonates (e.g., Boniva, Fosamax). |

Continued

General Care Plans

| ASSESSMENT—RECOGNIZE CUES/ INTERVENTIONS—TAKE ACTION | RATIONALES |
|---|---|
| Assess the need for around-the-clock analgesic dosing versus as-needed dosing. | Patients who self-rate their pain intensity at a 5 or greater and are using short-acting analgesics (every 4 hours) and remain without optimal pain relief should be considered for longer acting opioid analgesics. Long-acting opioids can be administered every 8–12 hours, once daily, or every 3 days (every 72 hours, such as with fentanyl). Short-acting opioids are used for breakthrough pain and to increase therapeutic systemic opioid levels. Frequent or excessive use of rescue dosing signifies the need for a reassessment of the patient's pain and its management. |
| Assess for barriers that may affect the optimal and effective management of the patient's pain. | Barriers to optimal pain management can occur through providers, patients, families, and the health care system. Provider barriers include concerns about medication risks, lack of appropriate assessment skills, limited knowledge of treatment options, or cultural or social barriers. Patient/family barriers include cognitive communication issues, fear of side effects or influence on mentation, and cultural or social barriers. Barriers associated with the health care system include limited specialists or access to care, formulary limitations, or inventory system restrictions. |
| Provide the patient and caregiver with tips for safe opioid use. 1. Patients should not combine opioids with other central stimulating medications, including alcohol. 2. Patients should consult with their health care provider before stopping or changing an opioid dose. 3. Store medication in a locked or secure cabinet to prevent wrongful use or theft. 4. Patients need to avoid driving or performing complex tasks when initiating therapy. | Consult with the provider before taking any other medications or alcohol, with opioids, because of potential interactions. Abrupt discontinuation of opioids can precipitate withdrawal symptoms. Even though all medications must be stored securely, opioids are often the target for substance abuse. Complex tasks and driving must be avoided because opioids can cause drowsiness, impair concentration, and slow reflexes. |
| Offer the patient and caregiver resources to promote effective pain management education. | Additional resources help to promote effective pain management education. Acute and chronic pain resources include: Pain Action: www.painaction.com U.S. Pain Foundation: https://uspainfoundation.org/ American Cancer Society: www.cancer.org |

## Patient Problem/Analyze Cues/Prioritize Hypotheses

# Impaired Functional Ability

*due to* the normal process of death and dying and its effects on the human body

**Desired Outcome/Generate Solutions:** Within 24 hours of having received information, the patient and family acknowledge their acceptance of the normal process of death and dying and their understanding of the effects on the human body.

| ASSESSMENT—RECOGNIZE CUES/ INTERVENTIONS—TAKE ACTION | RATIONALES |
|---|---|
| Be proactive in assessing for and preventing or controlling distressing symptoms with the goal of the patient's peaceful death. | Patients who are in the final stages of disease and illness tolerate symptoms poorly, largely because of weakness and generalized debility. Uncontrolled symptoms, especially at this stage of the disease trajectory, can easily escalate into a crisis for both the patient and family. |

| ASSESSMENT—RECOGNIZE CUES/ INTERVENTIONS—TAKE ACTION | RATIONALES |
|---|---|
| Assess for a decrease in cardiac function as death nears, including a decreased blood pressure (BP). | The BP decreases because of the combination of these factors: the heart's ineffective pumping ability, dehydration, and renal insufficiency. |
| Assess for increased heart rate (HR), even though the pulse may be weak, thready, and irregular. | An increased HR is a compensatory mechanism that occurs when BP decreases as death approaches. |
| Monitor for cyanosis and coolness and a mottling appearance to the skin. | Cyanosis is often present and becomes progressive as death nears, resulting from ineffective delivery of blood, nutrients, and oxygen to the body's tissues. This causes the patient's skin to become cool and appear mottled. Circulatory blood is shunted to essential organs, including the heart, lungs, and brain, and is no longer adequately perfusing the periphery. |
| Monitor for changes in the patient's breathing. | Compensatory mechanisms of the pulmonary system used to regulate normal homeostasis are often seen as changes in the patient's breathing. Respirations may become increasingly shallow or deep as the dying process nears. More frequent periods of apnea are often seen as death approaches. When the patient becomes unconscious, the swallowing mechanism is impaired, which can cause secretions to pool in the back of the throat, potentially causing difficulty swallowing or clearing the airway. |
| If the patient experiences dyspnea, facilitate simple environmental comfort (e.g., use a fan, elevate head of bed, and reposition the patient from side to side, suction oral secretions). | Dyspnea is one of the most distressing symptoms for dying patients and their families. In addition to environmental comfort measures, pharmacologic interventions are often needed. These include opiates, bronchodilators, cough suppressants, diuretics (use cautiously in patients with established dehydration), anticholinergics, corticosteroids, and oxygen. |
| Assess for dyspnea, tachypnea, Cheyne–Stokes, apnea, labored breathing, and/or noisy respirations, and intervene accordingly | Dyspnea is difficulty in breathing; tachypnea is a rapid respiratory rate; and Cheyne–Stokes is an abnormal pattern of breathing characterized by progressively deeper and sometimes faster breathing, which can also be identified as labored or apneic or irregular. Noisy respirations occur close to death and are often termed "death rattle." To effectively manage these symptoms, providers may prescribe specific medications such as opiates, bronchodilators, anxiolytics, anticholinergics, and oxygen. The nurse can help to position the patient (high-Fowler position, 45-degree angle, moving the patient from side to side), minimize the patient's energy expenditure, and provide reassurance. |
| Instruct the family on how to provide good oral hygiene for the patient. | Patients who are mouth breathing will have a dry oral mucosa. Keeping the mouth and lips moist with a cool, damp washcloth, lip moisturizers, and ice chips (if the patient is still swallowing) will promote comfort. |
| Monitor for decreased or absent urine output on each daily assessment. | Absent or diminished urine output is expected in the dying process because of decreased cardiac perfusion, decreased oral intake of fluids, medications, or decreased renal function. Renal insufficiency is more pronounced in patients with renal disease, chronic diabetes, unmanaged hypertension, and HF. Urinary retention can result from an enlarged prostate, anticholinergic or opioid medications, weakness, disinterest because of depression, lack of cognitive awareness, or a full rectal vault. It is important to recognize the underlying cause and consider indwelling catheterization. Although incontinence may be manageable at the end of life, it may require frequent linen and position changes, which may be uncomfortable for the patient. |

Continued

General Care Plans

| ASSESSMENT—RECOGNIZE CUES/ INTERVENTIONS—TAKE ACTION | RATIONALES |
|---|---|
| Base your decisions regarding the need for hydration on the patient's comfort level, symptom burden, use of opioid medications, and proximity to death. | Dehydration is the common pathway of a natural death. With end-stage disease, patients have diminished oral intake because of weakness, withdrawal, and increased somnolence. As kidney function declines, opioid metabolite accumulation can occur, which can lead to nausea, confusion, restlessness, myoclonus, delirium, nightmares, hallucinations, and hyperalgesia. Sometimes mild hydration can help to relieve these symptoms. Patients who are taking opioids may need to have the dose titrated down from the original dose to lessen the accumulation of toxic metabolites. |
| Assess the changes in cognition that often occur close to death, with the most common being somnolence, delirium, difficulty communicating, labile mood, hallucinations, agitation, or restlessness. | Delirium is frequently seen near the end of life, but it is important to evaluate for a reversible etiology and provide treatment when warranted. Delirium is generally multifactorial and often can be reversible (e.g., in opiate and benzodiazepine toxicities, metabolic disorders, or dehydration). |
| Assess and evaluate the reversible causes of delirium that require prompt attention and intervention. | Treatment of reversible causes of delirium may reverse the delirium. All medications require a thorough investigation to determine whether they are contributing to delirium (e.g., opioids, benzodiazepines, antidepressants, antihistamines, anticonvulsants, nonsteroidal anti-inflammatory agents, corticosteroids, metoclopramide, ranitidine, angiotensin-converting enzyme inhibitors, and digoxin). Other causes include hypoxia, visual and hearing deficits, hypertension, infection, trauma, surgery, hepatic or renal failure, and metabolic abnormalities (e.g., hypercalcemia, hypernatremia, uremia, hypercapnia, hyponatremia, and hypoglycemia). |
| Differentiate agitation and restlessness from delirium and dementia and intervene accordingly. Educate the family that the patient may "act out" toward them during these episodes because they are "safe" targets. | Uncontrolled pain, full bladder, constipation, or emotional issues can be misinterpreted as restlessness. Adding more opiates can aggravate agitation. If pain is suspected as the cause of restlessness, administer an extra dose of pain medication per orders for breakthrough pain. If this is ineffective, the underlying cause requires further evaluation. An antipsychotic medication may be ordered (titrated to effect) if the restlessness is not reversible. |
| Monitor for dysphagia and impaired cognition. As indicated, administer medications by sublingual, rectal, transdermal, or subcutaneous routes. | Patients at the end of life can have impaired cognition and develop dysphagia resulting from progressive weakness and are unable to swallow oral medications. |
| Prepare the family for the patient's expected death awareness. Some examples of death awareness (also called Near Death Phenomena) include<br>• communicating with or seeming to experience the presence of someone who is not alive,<br>• describing a location in another realm (such as heaven),<br>• getting ready for travel or a trip, and<br>• expressing knowledge of when one's death will happen (Marks & Marchand, 2022). | Death awareness is not confusion or hallucinations but important work for the patient. It is important to listen to the patient closely to find out what the patient may be trying to communicate, address any unresolved issues, and prepare to finalize their time with the patient. |
| Identify the patient's withdrawal from close and social relationships and activities. Educate the family to expect withdrawal and not to take it personally as the patient turns inward. | The dying process is unique for each individual. The patient may shift focus and disengage from loved ones. The patient does not have the energy for relationships. |

## Patient/Family Problem/Analyze Cues/Prioritize Hypotheses

# Risk for Spiritual Distress

*due to* chronic illness, life change, impending death, or disturbances in belief and value systems that give meaning and a sense of hope

**Desired Outcome/Generate Solutions:** Before hospital discharge, the patient will be comfortable with his/her own beliefs and expresses acceptance or decreased anxiety regarding impending death.

| ASSESSMENT—RECOGNIZE CUES/ INTERVENTIONS—TAKE ACTION | RATIONALES |
|---|---|
| Be aware that not everyone has spiritual or religious beliefs. | It is important not to assume anything about a patient's belief system. |
| Assess the patient's and family's concerns about spiritual needs or pastoral care preferences. | Chronic illness or terminal illness may challenge one's beliefs, feelings about religion, and thoughts about an afterlife, resulting in spiritual distress and loss of hope. The use of an assessment tool, such as the FICA Spiritual History Tool can provide information and guidance for meeting the spiritual needs of the patient and family. The tool provides examples of questions that can be asked during a spiritual assessment. |
| | The steps of the FICA tool are as follows: |
| | F. Faith, Belief, Meaning: Determine whether or not the patient identifies with a particular belief system or spirituality at all. |
| | I. Importance and Influence: Understand the importance of spirituality in the patient's life and its influence on health care decisions. |
| | C. Community: Find out if the patient is part of a religious or spiritual community, or if they rely on their community for support. |
| | A. Address/Action in Care: Learn how to address spiritual issues with regard to caring for the patient (Puchalski, 2020). |
| | The tool is available at https://smhs.gwu.edu/spirituality-health/program/transforming-practice-health-settings/clinical-fica-tool |
| Be alert to comments related to spiritual concerns or conflicts. Listen closely to comments made. | Comments such as "I don't know why God is doing this to me" and "I'm being punished for my sins" suggest that the patient is feeling some degree of spiritual distress and helps the nurse plan how best to assist the patient. |
| Refer the patient and family to available pastoral care services, or, if preferred, contact their chosen spiritual or religious leader. | The patient's known spiritual or religious leader can provide spiritual support as needed. Professional chaplains are trained to identify and help with spiritual issues. This information increases awareness of available spiritual resources and promotes a sense of acceptance of the patient's spirituality. |
| When possible, provide privacy and opportunities for patients and families to participate in chosen rituals. | Rituals, such as prayer, meditation, readings from religious books, singing, or reflection, may provide comfort during times of illness. |
| Provide all care for patients and their families in a nonjudgmental manner that is respectful of their religious or spiritual beliefs and practices, even if they decline to discuss their beliefs or accept spiritual support. | Sometimes, patients or families are reluctant to discuss private issues or beliefs. Showing respect for their choices provides support during difficult times and creates an environment that is conducive to free expression. |

<u>Patient/Family Problem/Analyze Cues/Prioritize Hypotheses</u>

# Anticipatory Grief

*due to* the anticipatory loss of one's own life or that of the loved one

***Desired Outcome/Generate Solutions:*** The patient and family acknowledge and eventually reach a state of acceptance of the impending loss.

| ASSESSMENT—RECOGNIZE CUES/ INTERVENTIONS—TAKE ACTION | RATIONALES |
|---|---|
| Assess for signs of grieving (such as tearfulness and feelings of sadness or disbelief in the ending of life) and encourage expressions of feelings by the patient, family, and interdisciplinary health care team. | Expressions of grief can be cathartic. Anger is often substituted for grief and is considered normal. |
| Explain to the family how to differentiate normal grieving from complicated grieving. | Complicated grief may be present when an individual's ability to resume normal activities and responsibilities is continually disrupted beyond 6 months of the time of death. |
| Help the patient and family identify successful past coping strategies that have worked in stressful situations. | Building from past strategies that have worked can be encouraged for use in the current situation. |
| Respect the patient's and family's need to use denial occasionally. | Denial can be an effective coping mechanism for grief. |
| Give the family permission to express culturally specific concerns and issues about the patient's impending death. | Many cultures handle death and dying differently. |
| Encourage family members to engage in conversations that involve sensitive issues or unfinished business. Honor their wishes, for example, by contacting the spiritual advisor or people whom the patient desires to see. | Verbalizing unfinished or sensitive issues might require the integration of interdisciplinary support (social worker, spiritual advisor) to help resolve difficult or sensitive issues between the patient and family. |

## ADDITIONAL PROBLEMS:

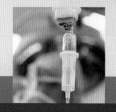

# Psychosocial Support for the Patient  8

## Patient Problem/Analyze Cues/Prioritize Hypotheses

# Fatigue

*due to* disease process, treatment, medications, depression, or stress

***Desired Outcome/Generate Solutions:*** Before hospital discharge, the patient and caregivers describe interventions that conserve energy resources. In addition, the patient verbalizes feeling less fatigued.

| ASSESSMENT—RECOGNIZE CUES/ INTERVENTIONS—TAKE ACTION | RATIONALES |
|---|---|
| Assess the patient's patterns of fatigue and times of maximum energy. (Use of a visual analog scale may be helpful in monitoring the fatigue level.) | This information helps identify areas for teaching energy conservation, relaxation, and diversional activities to reduce fatigue. |
| Assess how fatigue affects the patient's emotional status and ability to perform activities of daily living (ADLs). Suggest activity schedules to maximize energy expenditures (e.g., "After you eat lunch, take a 30-minute rest before you do your range of motion exercises"). | Developing an activity plan (e.g., rescheduling activities, allowing rest periods, asking for assistance, exercise) will help conserve energy, reduce fatigue, and maintain ADLs. |
| Assess patterns of sleep. | Disturbance in sleep pattern may influence the level of fatigue. |
| Help the patient maintain a regular sleep pattern by allowing for uninterrupted periods of sleep. Encourage rest when fatigued rather than attempting to continue activity. See *Impaired Sleep* below. | Lack of effective sleep can lead to psychosocial distress (e.g., inability to concentrate, anxiety, uncertainty, and depression). |
| Reduce environmental stimulation overload (e.g., noise level, visitors for long periods of time, lack of personal quiet time). | This action helps promote uninterrupted sleep patterns. |
| Discuss how chores can be delegated to family and friends who are offering to assist once the patient is home. | This action helps conserve energy and enables family and friends to feel a part of patient's care. |
| Encourage the patient to maintain a regular schedule after discharge, recognizing that attempting to continue previous activity levels may not be realistic. | This information helps patients engage in a realistic activity schedule to minimize fatigue and avoid frustration if physical functioning does not return to baseline levels. |
| Encourage mild exercise such as short walks and stretching, which may begin in the hospital if not contraindicated. | Such exercise will promote flexibility, muscle strength, and cardiac output and reduce stress. |
| ! Avoid exercise or use caution in patients with certain disease states. | Exercise should be used with caution and may be contraindicated in cases of anemia, bone metastases, thrombocytopenia, fever or active infection, and joint disease due to physical limitations or potential for injury. |

## Patient Problem/Analyze Cues/Prioritize Hypotheses

# Impaired Sleep

*due to* interrupted sleep occurring with environmental changes, illness, therapeutic regimen, pain, immobility, psychologic stress, altered mental status, or hypoxia

***Desired Outcomes/Generate Solutions:*** After discussion, the patient identifies factors that promote sleep. Within 8 hours of intervention, the patient attains longer periods of uninterrupted sleep and verbalizes satisfaction with the ability to rest.

| ASSESSMENT—RECOGNIZE CUES/ INTERVENTIONS—TAKE ACTION | RATIONALES |
|---|---|
| Assess the patient's usual (before and after diagnosis) sleeping patterns (e.g., bedtime routine, hours of sleep per night, sleeping position, use of pillows and blankets, napping during the day, nocturia). | Some or all of the patient's usual sleep pattern may be incorporated into the plan of care. A routine as similar to the patient's usual routine as possible will help promote sleep. |
| Assess causative factors and activities that contribute to the patient's insomnia, awaken the patient, or adversely affect sleep patterns. | Factors such as pain, anxiety, hypoxia, therapies, depression, hallucinations, medications, underlying illness, sleep apnea, respiratory disorder, caffeine, and fear may contribute to sleep pattern disturbance. Some may be ameliorated, and others may be modified. |
| As indicated, administer pain medications before sleep. | This intervention decreases the likelihood that pain will interfere with sleep. |
| Promote physical comfort by such measures as massage, back rubs, bathing, and fresh linens before sleep. | These measures may help relieve stress and promote relaxation. |
| Organize procedures and activities to allow for 90-minute periods of uninterrupted rest/sleep. Limit visiting during these periods. | Ninety minutes of sleep enables complete progression through the normal phases of sleep. |
| Whenever possible, maintain a quiet environment. If possible, provide earplugs, reduce alarm volumes, or use white noise (i.e., low-pitched, monotonous sounds: electric fan, soft music) to facilitate sleep. Provide dimmed lighting, drawn curtains/blinds, or providing sleep eye masks | Excessive noise and light can cause sleep deprivation. These measures may help to promote sleep. |
| If appropriate, limit the patient's daytime sleeping. Attempt to establish regularly scheduled daytime activity (e.g., ambulation, sitting in chair, active range of motion), which may promote nighttime sleep. | Napping less during the day will promote a more normal nighttime pattern. Physical activity causes fatigue and may facilitate nighttime sleeping. |
| Promote nonpharmacologic comfort measures that are known to promote the patient's sleep. | Nonpharmacologic comfort measures such as earplugs, anxiety reduction, and use of the patient's own bed clothing and pillows may promote sleep. |

## Patient Problem/Analyze Cues/Prioritize Hypotheses

# Anxiety

*due to* actual or perceived threat of death, change in health status, threat to self-concept or role, unfamiliar people and environment, medications, preexisting anxiety disorder, the unknown, or uncertainty

***Desired Outcome/Generate Solutions:*** Within 1–2 hours of intervention, the patient's anxiety has resolved or decreased as evidenced by the patient's verbalization of same, stabilization of vital signs if they were elevated because of anxiety (compared with the patient's baseline levels), and absence of or decrease in irritability and restlessness.

| ASSESSMENT—RECOGNIZE CUES/ INTERVENTIONS—TAKE ACTION | RATIONALES |
|---|---|
| Assess the patient's level of anxiety. Be alert to verbal and nonverbal cues. Assess for the following criteria that can contribute to anxiety: general medical condition, withdrawal from alcohol or opioids, pain, generalized anxiety disorder, panic disorder, posttraumatic stress disorder, phobic disorder, or obsessive–compulsive disorder (Cope et al., 2017). | Being aware of a patient's level of anxiety enables the nurse to provide appropriate interventions, as well as modify the plan of care accordingly. Levels of anxiety include:<br>• *Mild:* restlessness, irritability, increased questions, focusing on the environment<br>• *Moderate:* inattentiveness, expressions of concern, narrowed perceptions, insomnia, increased heart rate<br>• *Severe:* expressions of feelings of doom, rapid speech, tremors, poor eye contact. Patient may be preoccupied with the past; may be unable to understand the present; and may have tachycardia, nausea, and hyperventilation.<br>• *Panic:* inability to concentrate or communicate, distortion of reality, increased motor activity, vomiting, tachypnea. |
| Validate assessment of the anxiety with the patient. For example, "You seem distressed. Are you feeling uncomfortable now?" | Validating a patient's anxiety level provides confirmation of nursing assessment, as well as openly acknowledges their emotional state. In so doing, patients are given permission to share feelings. |
| Introduce self and other health care team members; explain each individual's role as it relates to the patient's care. | Familiarity with staff and their individual roles may increase the patient's comfort level and decrease anxiety. |
| Engage in honest communication with the patient, providing empathetic understanding. Listen closely. | These actions help establish an atmosphere that enables free expression. |
| For patients with severe anxiety or panic state, refer to psychiatric clinical nurse specialist, licensed clinical social worker, case manager, or other health care team members as appropriate. | Patients in severe anxiety or panic state may require more sophisticated interventions or pharmacologic management. |
| Approach the patient with a calm, reassuring demeanor. Show concern and focused attention while listening to the patient's concerns. Provide a safe environment and stay with the patient during periods of intense anxiety. | These actions reassure patients that you are concerned and will assist in meeting their needs. |
| Restrict the patient's intake of caffeine. | Caffeine is a stimulant that may increase anxiety in persons who are sensitive to it. Cessation of caffeine can lead to physiologic withdrawal symptoms including anxiety. |
| Assess the patient's prehospital consumption of nicotine products and alcohol. | Cessation of nicotine, and alcohol can lead to physiologic withdrawal symptoms including anxiety. |
| Avoid abrupt discontinuation of anxiolytics. | Abrupt withdrawal can cause headaches, tiredness, and irritability. |
| If the patient is hyperventilating, have him or her concentrate on a focal point and mimic your deliberately slow and deep-breathing pattern. | Modeling provides patients with a focal point for learning effective breathing technique. |
| After an episode of anxiety, review and discuss the thoughts and feelings that led to the episode. | This action validates the cause of the anxiety and explores interventions that may avert another episode. |
| Identify the patient's current coping behaviors. Review coping behaviors the patient has used in the past. Assist with using adaptive coping to manage anxiety. For example, "I understand that your wife reads to you to help you relax. Would you like to spend a part of each day alone with her?" (See *Difficulty Coping* below) | Identifying maladaptive coping behaviors (e.g., denial, anger, repression, withdrawal, daydreaming, or dependence on opioids, sedatives, or tranquilizers) helps establish a proactive plan of care to promote healthy coping skills. |
| Encourage the patient to express fears, concerns, and questions. For example, "I know this room looks like a maze of wires and tubes; please let me know when you have any questions." | Encouraging questions gives patients an avenue in which to share concerns. |
| Provide an organized, quiet environment. | Such an environment reduces sensory overload that may contribute to anxiety. |
| Encourage social support network to be in attendance whenever possible. | Many people benefit from the support of others and find that it reduces their stress level. |
| Explain relaxation and imagery techniques. | Relaxation and imagery skills empower individuals to manage anxiety-provoking episodes more skillfully and foster a sense of control. |

## Patient Problem/Analyze Cues/Prioritize Hypotheses

# Difficulty Coping

*due to* the patient's health crisis, sense of vulnerability, or inadequate support systems

**Desired Outcome/Generate Solutions:** Before hospital discharge, the patient verbalizes feelings, identifies strengths and coping behaviors, and does not demonstrate ineffective coping behaviors.

| ASSESSMENT—RECOGNIZE CUES/ INTERVENTIONS—TAKE ACTION | RATIONALES |
|---|---|
| Assess the patient's perceptions and ability to understand current health status. Discuss the meaning of disease and current treatment with the patient, actively listening with a nonjudgmental attitude. | Evaluation of the patient's comprehension enables the development of an individualized care plan. |
| Establish honest, empathetic communication with the patient. For example, "Please tell me what I can do to help you." | This promotes effective therapeutic communication. |
| Support positive coping behaviors and explore effective coping behaviors used in the past. For example, "I see that reading that book seems to help you relax." | These actions identify, reinforce, and facilitate positive coping behaviors. |
| Identify factors that inhibit the patient's ability to cope. | This enables patients to identify areas such as unsatisfactory support system, deficient knowledge, grief, and fear that may contribute to anxiety and ineffective coping and to consider modification of these factors. |
| Help the patient identify previous methods of coping with life problems. | How individuals have handled problems in the past may be a reliable predictor of how they will cope with current problems. |
| Recognize maladaptive coping behaviors. If appropriate, discuss these behaviors with the patient. For example, "You seem to be requiring more pain medication. Are you having more physical pain, or does it help you cope with your situation?" | Examples of maladaptive behaviors include severe depression; dependence on opioids, sedatives, or tranquilizers; hostility; violence; and suicidal ideation. Patients may have used substances and other maladaptive behaviors in controlling anxiety. This pattern can interfere with the ability to cope with the current situation. If appropriate, nurses need to discuss these behaviors with patients. |
| Refer the patient to psychiatric liaison, clinical nurse specialist, licensed clinical social worker, case manager, or clergy, or recommend support groups or other programs as appropriate. | Professional intervention may assist with altering maladaptive behaviors. |
| Help the patient identify or develop a support system. | Many people benefit from outside support systems in helping them cope. |
| As the patient's condition allows, assist with reducing anxiety. See *Anxiety*, earlier. | Anxiety makes effective coping more difficult to achieve. |
| Maintain an organized, quiet environment. | Such an environment helps reduce patient's sensory overload to aid with coping. |
| Encourage frequent visits by family and caregiver if visits are supportive to patient. Encourage the use of technology such as social media to stay in touch with family and friends. | Visitors and social media may help minimize a patient's emotional and social isolation, thereby promoting coping behaviors. |
| As appropriate, explain to the caregiver that increased dependency, anger, and denial may be adaptive coping behaviors used by the patient in the early stages of crisis until effective coping behaviors are learned. | Lack of understanding about the patient's maladaptive coping can lead to unhealthy interaction patterns and contribute to anxiety within the family. |
| Arrange community referrals for discharge planning, as appropriate. | Support in the home environment promotes healthier adaptations and may avert crises. |

## Patient Problem/Analyze Cues/Prioritize Hypotheses

# Risk for Spiritual Distress

*due to* chronic illness, life change, or disturbances in belief and value systems
that give meaning and a sense of hope

***Desired Outcome/Generate Solutions:*** Before hospital discharge, the patient will be comfortable
with his/her own beliefs and expresses acceptance or decreased anxiety regarding impending
death.

| ASSESSMENT—RECOGNIZE CUES/ INTERVENTIONS—TAKE ACTION | RATIONALES |
|---|---|
| Be aware that not everyone has spiritual or religious beliefs. | It is important not to assume anything about a patient's belief systems. |
| Assess the patient's spiritual or religious beliefs, values, and practices. For example, "Do you have a religious preference?" "How important is it to you?" "Are there any religious or spiritual practices in which you wish to participate while in the hospital?" See "Palliative and End-of-Life Care," Chapter 7, for the FICA Spiritual History Tool. | This assessment will assist in the development of an individualized care plan. |
| Inform the patient of the availability of spiritual resources, such as a chapel or chaplain. | This information increases awareness of available spiritual resources and promotes a sense of acceptance of the patient's spirituality. |
| Display a nonjudgmental attitude toward the patient's religious or spiritual beliefs and values. | This action creates an environment that is conducive to free expression. |
| Identify available support persons or systems that may assist in meeting the patient's religious or spiritual needs (e.g., clergy, fellow church members, support groups). | Many people derive an increased sense of hope from religious and spiritual counselors. |
| Be alert to comments related to spiritual concerns or conflicts. | Comments such as "I don't know why God is doing this to me" and "I'm being punished for my sins" may suggest that the patient is feeling some degree of spiritual distress. |
| Listen closely and ask questions. For example, "I understand that you want to be baptized. We can arrange to do that here." | These actions help the patient resolve conflicts related to spiritual issues and help the nurse plan how best to assist the patient. |
| Provide privacy and opportunities for spiritual practices such as prayer and meditation. | Many people find prayer and meditation difficult in a nonprivate setting. |
| If spiritual beliefs and therapeutic regimens are in conflict, provide honest, substantiated information. For example, "I understand your religion discourages receiving blood transfusions. We respect your position; however, it does not allow us to give you the best care possible." | Such information promotes informed decision making. |
| Refer the patient for help with decision making if he or she is struggling with treatment-related decisions. | Such help assists in resolving care dilemmas, if appropriate. Many hospitals provide assistance in the form of educational materials and counseling to help resolve such dilemmas. |

## Patient Problem/Analyze Cues/Prioritize Hypotheses

# Anticipatory Grief

*due to* actual or anticipated loss of physiologic well-being (e.g., expected loss
of body function or body part, changes in self-concept or body image, illness,
death)

***Desired Outcome/Generate Solutions:*** After interventions, the patient expresses grief, participates in decisions about the future, and discusses concerns with health care team members.

| ASSESSMENT—RECOGNIZE CUES/ INTERVENTIONS—TAKE ACTION | RATIONALES |
|---|---|
| Assess and accept the patient's behavioral response. | Reactions such as disbelief, denial, guilt, anger, and depression are normal reactions to grief. |
| Determine the patient's stage of grieving. | Comprehension of the stage of grief enables more effective therapeutic interventions. It is normal for a person to move from one stage to another and then revert to a previous stage. The time required to do so varies from individual to individual. If a patient is unable to move into the next stage, referral for professional intervention may be indicated.<br>• *Protest stage:* denial, disbelief, anger, hostility, resentment, bargaining to postpone loss, appeal for help to recover loss, loud complaints, altered sleep and appetite.<br>• *Disorganization stage:* depression, withdrawal, social isolation, psychomotor retardation, silence.<br>• *Reorganization stage:* acceptance of loss, development of new interests and attachments, restructuring of lifestyle, return to preloss level of functioning. |
| Assess the spiritual, religious, and sociocultural expectations related to loss. For example, "Is religion an important part of your life?" "How do you and your family deal with serious health problems?" See *Risk for Spiritual Distress*, earlier. | Helping individuals find meaning in their experience may facilitate the grieving process |
| Assess the patient's grief reactions and identify the potential for dysfunctional grieving reactions (e.g., absence of emotion, hostility, avoidance). | This assessment helps identify and reduce dysfunctional grieving, if present. |
| If dysfunctional grieving is present, refer the patient to a psychiatric clinical nurse specialist, licensed clinical social worker, case manager, clergy, or other sources of counseling as appropriate. | Promoting normal progression through the grieving stages may allay unnecessary emotional suffering. |
| Refer to clergy or community support groups as appropriate. | Such a referral reinforces that there are support systems and resources to help work through grief. |
| Demonstrate empathy. For example, "This must be a very difficult time for you and your family" or "Is there anything you'd like to talk about today?" | Empathetic communication (including respecting the desire not to communicate) promotes a trusting relationship and open dialog. |
| In selected circumstances, explain the grieving process. | This approach may help the patient and family better understand and acknowledge their feelings and help family members better understand behaviors and verbalizations expressed by the patient. |
| When appropriate, provide referral for bereavement care. | Such a referral helps the patient and family grieve their loss. |

**Patient Problem/Analyze Cues/Prioritize Hypotheses**

# Risk for Impaired Communication

*due to* neurologic or anatomic deficit, psychologic or physical barriers (e.g., tracheostomy, intubation), or cultural or developmental differences

***Desired Outcome/Generate Solutions:*** At the time of intervention, the patient communicates needs and feelings and reports decreased or absent feelings of frustration over communication barriers.

| ASSESSMENT—RECOGNIZE CUES/ INTERVENTIONS—TAKE ACTION | RATIONALES |
|---|---|
| Assess the patient's health literacy level. Make sure materials are at an appropriate literacy level. Also, assess digital literacy (ability to navigate websites or other technology) if they are used to provide information. | Although individuals may be able to read, their understanding of health-related materials may be low or they may have limited proficiency with computers. |
| Assess the cause of impaired communication (e.g., tracheostomy, stroke, cerebral tumor, Guillain–Barré syndrome). | Determining the cause of communication impairment will enable the nurse to develop a customized plan of care that incorporates communication skills patients can use, given their disability. |
| Involve the patient and/or caregiver in assessing the patient's ability to read, write, and understand English. If the patient speaks a language other than English, collaborate with an English-speaking family member (with the patient's permission) or an interpreter to establish effective communication. | This assessment helps establish effective communication and ensure teaching materials provided are at a level appropriate for the patient. |
| When communicating, face the patient; make direct eye contact; and speak in a clear, normal tone of voice. | A visual or hearing-impaired person often develops compensatory methods—for example, lip reading for a person who is hearing impaired. Be aware that mask requirements may prevent the patient from relying on lip reading. |
| When communicating with a deaf person about the treatment plan, arrange to have an interpreter present. | An interpreter facilitates effective communication, promotes informed consent, and enables the patient to ask questions. |
| If the patient cannot speak because of a physical barrier (e.g., tracheostomy, wired mandibles), provide reassurance and acknowledge his or her frustration. For example, "I know this is frustrating for you, but please do not give up. I want to understand you." | These actions will help decrease frustration caused by the inability to communicate verbally. |
| Provide writing board, word cards, pencil and paper, alphabet board, pictures, computers, electronic devices, voice-activated devices, or other technology to assist with communication. Adapt call system to meet the patient's needs. Document the meaning of signals used by the patient to communicate. | These actions will enable effective communication, promote continuity of care, and lessen the patient's anxiety. |
| Explain the source of the patient's communication impairment to the caregiver; instruct the caregiver about effective communication alternatives (see the previous list). | Inability to communicate with ease may cause feelings of isolation that can be intensified if patients have difficulty communicating with caregivers. |
| Be alert to nonverbal messages. Validate their meaning with the patient. | Nonverbal response, such as facial expressions, hand movements, and nodding of the head, is a valid means of communication, and its meaning must be validated to facilitate understanding. |
| Encourage the patient to communicate needs; reinforce independent behaviors. | Inability to speak may foster maladaptive behaviors, and this reinforces the need for patients to be understood. |
| Be honest with the patient; do not pretend to understand if you are unable to interpret the patient's communication. | Pretending to understand patients will only add to their frustration and diminish trust. |
| If surgery is expected to create a physical condition that will interfere with communication, begin teaching preoperatively. Facilitate postoperative referrals for speech and swallowing. | These actions will help ensure that an effective method of communication will be in place postoperatively so that the patient's needs will be met. |

## Patient Problem/Analyze Cues/Prioritize Hypotheses

# Risk for Social Isolation

*due to* altered health status, decreased socialization, inability to engage in satisfying personal relationships, altered mental status, body image change, or altered physical appearance

***Desired Outcome/Generate Solutions:*** Before hospital discharge, the patient demonstrates movement toward interaction and communication with others.

| ASSESSMENT—RECOGNIZE CUES/ INTERVENTIONS—TAKE ACTION | RATIONALES |
|---|---|
| Assess the factors contributing to the patient's social isolation. These may include:<br><br>• restricted visiting hours,<br>• inability to access social media or use other technology,<br>• absence of or inadequate support system,<br>• inability to communicate (e.g., presence of intubation/tracheostomy),<br>• physical changes that affect self-concept,<br>• denial or withdrawal, and<br>• hospital environment. | • This assessment will help determine the causes of social isolation and modify those factors. |
| Identify patients at risk for social isolation. | Individuals most at risk for social isolation include older adults and disabled, chronically ill, and economically disadvantaged persons. |
| Help the patient identify feelings associated with loneliness and isolation. For example, "You seem very sad when your family leaves the room. Can you tell me more about your feelings?" | This information facilitates interventions based on individual need. |
| Determine the patient's need for socialization, and identify available and potential support person or systems. Explore methods for increasing social contact. | Assessing the need for interaction and developing a care plan accordingly will reduce the sense of isolation surrounding the illness. Methods for increasing social contact include TV, radio, videos, use of computers and the Internet, social media, more frequent visitations, and scheduled interaction with nurse or support staff. |
| Provide positive reinforcement for socialization that lessens the patient's feelings of isolation and loneliness. For example, "Please continue to call me when you need to talk to someone. Talking will help both of us better understand your feelings." | Encouraging interaction gives patients permission to ask for social interaction from the nurse while decreasing the sense of isolation. |
| Facilitate patient's ability to communicate with others (see *Risk for Impaired Communication*, earlier). | Impaired communication may be the cause of social isolation. |

## Patient Problem/Analyze Cues/Prioritize Hypotheses

# Deficient Knowledge

*due to* unfamiliarity with current health status and prescribed therapies

**Desired Outcome/Generate Solutions:** Before procedures or hospital discharge (as appropriate), the patient verbalizes understanding regarding current health status and therapies.

| ASSESSMENT—RECOGNIZE CUES/ INTERVENTIONS—TAKE ACTION | RATIONALES |
|---|---|
| Assess the patient's health care literacy (language, reading, comprehension). Assess culture and culturally specific information needs as well as cognitive and emotional readiness to learn. | This assessment helps ensure that information is selected and presented in a manner that is culturally and educationally appropriate. |
| Assess other barriers to learning. | Barriers to learning include ineffective communication, educational deficit, neurologic deficit, sensory alterations, fear, anxiety, and lack of motivation. |
| Assess the patient's current level of knowledge regarding health status. | This assessment enables the development of an individualized teaching plan, as well as correction of misperceptions and misinformation. |

| ASSESSMENT—RECOGNIZE CUES/ INTERVENTIONS—TAKE ACTION | RATIONALES |
|---|---|
| Assess learning needs and establish short- and long-term goals. As appropriate, assess understanding of informed consent. | Well-planned goals provide markers for assessing effectiveness of the teaching plan and progress made. Patients will use the information received to make informed decisions regarding care. |
| Use individualized verbal or written information to promote learning and enhance understanding. Give simple, direct instructions. As indicated, use audiovisual tools or technology-assisted devices. | Because individuals learn differently, using more than one teaching modality will provide more opportunities to assimilate information. |
| Include the caregiver in all patient teaching, and encourage reinforcement of correct information regarding diagnosis and treatments. | Anxiety often filters the information given. Involving a spouse or other family member provides teaching reinforcement. |
| Encourage the patient's involvement in care information by planning care collaboratively. Explain the rationale for care and therapies. | Involving patients in their own care planning promotes adherence to the treatment plan and engenders a sense of control and ownership. |
| Communicate often with the patient. Request feedback regarding what has been taught. | Anxiety may interfere with reception, comprehension, and retention. Individuals in crisis often need repeated explanations before information can be understood. Creating an environment of permission in which patients feel comfortable asking questions and revealing knowledge deficits facilitates learning. |
| Provide written information appropriate to the patient's comprehension and literacy levels. Also, consider social media or other computer-assisted devices to provide verbal/visual information that can be replayed as needed. | Written and recorded material reinforces teaching and enables review at a later time. |
| **Evaluate Outcomes:** Have the patient demonstrate learning by using the Teach-Back method. | Use of the Teach-Back method helps to determine whether the patient understands the information provided, or if the instruction needs to be repeated or revised. |

## ADDITIONAL PROBLEMS:

| | |
|---|---|
| "Palliative and End-of-Life Care," as appropriate for issues facing patients who are dying | Chapter 7 |
| "Anxiety Disorders" for *Difficulty Coping* | Chapter 99 |
| "Bipolar Disorder" for *Risk for Injury* | Chapter 100 |
| "Major Depression" for *Risk for Suicide, Risk for Hopelessness, and Grief* | Chapter 102 |

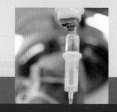

# Psychosocial Support for the Patient's Family and Significant Others

**9**

## Family/Significant Other Problem/Analyze Cues/Prioritize Hypotheses
### Anxiety

*due to* the patient's potential life-threatening condition and lack of information

***Desired Outcome/Generate Solutions:*** After interventions, significant others/family members report that anxiety has lessened.

| ASSESSMENT—RECOGNIZE CUES/ INTERVENTIONS—TAKE ACTION | RATIONALES |
|---|---|
| Assess the family's anxieties and their understanding of the patient's clinical situation. | Some anxieties may be realistic; others may not be and need clarification. |
| Evaluate the verbal and nonverbal responses. | Some family members may not readily verbalize their feelings but may give nonverbal cues such as withdrawing emotionally (evidenced by body position, facial expression, attitude of disinterest), refusing to be present during discussion, or disrupting discussion. |
| Acknowledge the family's anxieties. For example, "I understand these tubes must frighten you, but they are necessary to help nourish your son." | Simple acknowledgment and giving more information can go a long way toward decreasing anxiety. |
| Assess the family's history of coping behavior. For example, "How does your family react to difficult situations?" Awareness of maladaptive responses may assist the nurse in fostering more productive methods of coping. | How a family has coped with anxiety in the past often is a reliable predictor of how they will cope in the current situation. |
| Provide opportunities for family members to express anxieties and concerns. | Verbalizing feelings in a nonthreatening environment can help them deal with unresolved/unrecognized issues that may be contributing to the current stressor. Anger, denial, withdrawal, and demanding behavior may be adaptive coping responses during the initial period of crisis. Identifying anxieties also enables the nurse to dispel inaccuracies, which will help the family cope with the situation as it exists. |
| Provide information at frequent intervals about the patient's status, treatments, and equipment used. | This information increases the family's knowledge of the patient's health status, helping alleviate fear of the unknown. |

## ASSESSMENT—RECOGNIZE CUES/ INTERVENTIONS—TAKE ACTION

## RATIONALES

| ASSESSMENT—RECOGNIZE CUES/ INTERVENTIONS—TAKE ACTION | RATIONALES |
|---|---|
| Explain the implications of HIPAA to the family and how this affects the type of information that can be given and how it can be given (e.g., no specific information can be given by phone or email). | Protection of patient privacy is critical. Helping families understand what information can be provided and why will help alleviate anxiety. |
| Encourage the family to use positive coping behaviors by identifying anxieties, developing goals, identifying supportive resources, facilitating realistic perceptions, and promoting problem-solving. For example, "Who usually helps your family during stressful times?" | When under stress, the family may not recall sources of support without being reminded. |
| Recognize anxiety, and encourage family members to describe their feelings. For example, "You seem very uncomfortable tonight. Can you describe your feelings?" | Before family members can learn coping strategies, they must first clarify their feelings. |
| ⚠ Be alert to maladaptive responses to anxiety. Provide referrals to a psychiatric clinical nurse specialist, licensed clinical social worker, or other staff members as appropriate. | Violence, withdrawal, severe depression, hostility, and unrealistic expectations for the staff or of the patient's recovery are maladaptive responses to anxiety, and they require expert guidance. |
| Offer *realistic* hope, even if it is hope for the patient's peaceful death. | Even though family members may have feelings of hopelessness, it sometimes helps to hear realistic expressions of hope. |
| Explore the family's desire for spiritual or other counseling. See *Risk for Spiritual Distress* in "Psychosocial Support for the Patient," Chapter 8. | People often derive hope and experience a decrease in anxiety and dread from spiritual counseling. |
| Assess your own feelings about the patient's life-threatening illness. | Without personal awareness of one's beliefs, a health care provider's attitude and anxieties may be reflected inadvertently to the family. |

For other interventions, see *Difficulty Coping*, which follows.

<u>Family/Significant Other Problem/Analyze Cues/Prioritize Hypotheses</u>

# Difficulty Coping

*due to* inadequate or incorrect information or misunderstanding, temporary family disorganization and role change, exhausted support persons or systems, unrealistic expectations, fear, anxiety, or financial burden

**Desired Outcomes/Generate Solutions:** After interventions, family members begin to verbalize feelings, identify ineffective coping patterns, identify strengths and positive coping behaviors, and seek information and support from the nurse or other support persons or systems outside the family.

## ASSESSMENT—RECOGNIZE CUES/ INTERVENTIONS—TAKE ACTION

## RATIONALES

| ASSESSMENT—RECOGNIZE CUES/ INTERVENTIONS—TAKE ACTION | RATIONALES |
|---|---|
| Establish open, honest communication within the family. Help family members identify strengths, stressors, inappropriate behaviors, and personal needs. For example, "I understand your mother was very ill last year. How did you manage the situation?" "I know your loved one is very ill. How can I help you?" | These actions will help promote positive, effective communication among family members while enabling them to examine areas that contribute both to effective and ineffective coping in a nonthreatening environment. |
| Assess family members for ineffective coping and identify factors that inhibit effective coping. For example, "You seem to be unable to talk about your husband's illness. Is there anyone with whom you can talk about it?" | Ineffective methods of coping (e.g., depression, chemical dependency, violence, withdrawal) can interfere with the ability to deal with the current situation. Awareness of barriers to effective coping (e.g., inadequate support system, grief, fear of disapproval by others, and deficient knowledge) is the first step toward promoting changes and healthy adaptation. |

Continued

PART I: Medical-Surgical Nursing Care Plans

| ASSESSMENT—RECOGNIZE CUES/ INTERVENTIONS—TAKE ACTION | RATIONALES |
|---|---|
| Assess the family's knowledge about the patient's current health status and treatment. Provide information often, and allow sufficient time for questions. Reassess the family's understanding at frequent intervals. | By providing information frequently and answering questions, stress, fear, and anxiety can be attenuated. |
| Provide opportunities in a private setting for family members to talk and share concerns with nurses. If appropriate, refer the family to a psychiatric clinical nurse specialist or licensed clinical social worker for therapy. | The family may need additional assistance in working through their issues. |
| Offer realistic hope. Help the family to develop realistic expectations for the future and to identify support persons or systems that will assist them. | These actions will foster realistic expectations about the patient's future health status and promote adaptation to impending changes. |
| Help the family to reduce anxiety and caregiver strain by encouraging diversional activities (e.g., time spent outside the hospital) and interaction with support persons or systems outside the family. For example, "I know you want to be near your son, but if you would like to go home to rest, I will call you if any changes occur." | Promoting respites enhances coping and helps family members remain focused and supportive of the patient. |
| For more information, see "Palliative and End-of-Life Care," Chapter 7, for *Caregiver Problem: Caregiver Role Strain* | |

### Family/Significant Other Problem/Analyze Cues/Prioritize Hypotheses

# Difficulty Coping

*due to* unexpressed feelings, ambivalent family relationships, or disharmonious coping styles among family members

**Desired Outcomes/Generate Solutions:** Within the 24-hour period before hospital discharge, family members begin to verbalize feelings; identify sources of support as well as ineffective coping behaviors that create ambivalence and disharmony; and do not demonstrate destructive behaviors.

| ASSESSMENT—RECOGNIZE CUES/ INTERVENTIONS—TAKE ACTION | RATIONALES |
|---|---|
| Establish open, honest communication and rapport with family members. For example, "I am here to care for your mother and to help your family as well." | An atmosphere in which the family can express honest feelings and needs will help move them toward healthy coping and adaptation. |
| Identify ineffective coping behaviors. For example, "You seem to be angry. Would you like to talk to me about your feelings?" Refer to a psychiatric clinical nurse specialist, licensed clinical social worker, case manager, clergy, or support group as appropriate. | Ineffective coping behaviors (e.g., violence, depression, substance misuse, withdrawal) can interfere with learning effective strategies. Awareness of ineffective or destructive coping behaviors is the first step toward promoting change. |
| Identify perceived or actual conflicts. For example, "Are you able to talk freely with your family members?" "Are your brothers and sisters able to help and support you during this time?" | This information enables the family to examine areas that require a change in a nonthreatening environment and identify potential sources of support. |
| Assist in the quest for healthy functioning and adaptations within the family unit (e.g., facilitate open communication among family members and encourage behaviors that support family cohesiveness). For example, "Your mother enjoyed your last visit. Would you like to see her now?" | Facilitating open communication among family members and encouraging behaviors that support family cohesiveness promote skill acquisition in a nonthreatening environment and identify existing coping strengths |

| ASSESSMENT—RECOGNIZE CUES/ INTERVENTIONS—TAKE ACTION | RATIONALES |
|---|---|
| Help family members develop realistic goals, plans, and actions. Refer them to clergy, psychiatric clinical nurse specialist, social services, financial counseling, and family therapy as appropriate. | These actions help provide direction in making necessary changes and adaptations. |
| Encourage family members to spend time outside the hospital and to interact with support individuals. Respect their need for occasional withdrawal. | A life out of balance adds to stress and promotes maladaptive coping. |
| Include family members in the patient's plan of care. Offer them opportunities to become involved in patient care. | Becoming involved in the patient's care (e.g., range-of-motion exercises, patient hygiene, and comfort measures such as back rubs) may decrease feelings of powerlessness, thereby increasing coping ability. |

## Family/Significant Other Problem/Analyze Cues/Prioritize Hypotheses
# Deficient Knowledge

*due to* lack of knowledge about support persons or systems, referrals, and choosing experiences that optimize wellness

*Desired Outcomes/Generate Solutions:* After instruction, family members express intent to use support persons, systems, and resources and identify alternative behaviors that promote communication and strengths. Family members express realistic expectations and do not demonstrate ineffective coping behaviors.

| ASSESSMENT—RECOGNIZE CUES/ INTERVENTIONS—TAKE ACTION | RATIONALES |
|---|---|
| Assess family relationships, interactions, support persons or systems, and individual coping behaviors. | This assessment facilitates the development of an individualized care plan using the existing family structure. |
| Acknowledge the expressions of hope, plans, and growth among family members. | A sense of hopefulness is essential to process painful events in a healthy manner. |
| Provide opportunities in a private setting for family interactions, discussions, and questions. For example, "I know the waiting room is very crowded. Would your family like some private time together?" | Discussions and sharing of emotions in a nonpublic forum encourage the development of open, honest communication within the family. |
| Refer the family to community or support groups (e.g., ostomy support group, head injury rehabilitation group). | Many people benefit from the support of other people who have had similar experiences in learning new coping strategies. |
| Encourage the family to explore outlets that foster positive feelings. | Examples of outlets that foster positive feelings and thus promote effective coping include periods of time outside the hospital area, meaningful communication with the patient or support individuals, and relaxing activities such as showering, eating, and exercising. |

## Family/Significant Other Problem/Analyze Cues/Prioritize Hypotheses
# Deficient Knowledge

*due to* unfamiliarity with the patient's current health status or therapies

*Desired Outcome/Generate Solutions:* After instruction, family members/significant others begin to verbalize knowledge and understanding about the patient's current health status and treatment.

| ASSESSMENT—RECOGNIZE CUES/ INTERVENTIONS—TAKE ACTION | RATIONALES |
|---|---|
| Assess the family's health and digital literacy (language, reading, comprehension, ability to navigate, and use computers/Internet for information seeking). Assess culture and culturally specific education needs. | This assessment helps ensure that information is selected and presented in a manner that is culturally and educationally appropriate. |
| At frequent intervals, inform the family about the patient's current health status, therapies, and prognosis. Use individualized verbal, written, and audiovisual strategies to promote their understanding. | Being informed frequently promotes an accurate understanding of the patient's health status and allays unnecessary anxiety. In turn, this enables family members to process and plan. |
| **Evaluate Outcomes:** At frequent intervals, evaluate the family's comprehension of information provided. Assess factors for misunderstanding, and adjust teaching as appropriate. For example, "I have explained many things to you today. Would you mind summarizing what I've told you so that I can be sure you understand your husband's status and what we are doing to care for him?" | Some individuals in crisis need repeated explanations before comprehension can be ensured. |
| Encourage the family to relay the correct information to the patient. | This will reinforce comprehension for both the family and patient and promote open communication. |
| Inquire of family members if their information needs are being met. For example, "Do you have any questions about the care your mother is receiving or about her condition?" | This action reinforces understanding by family members and assures them that the information/support they desire will be met. |
| Help family members use the information they receive to make health care decisions about the patient. | Family members may require assistance in processing information and applying it appropriately (e.g., regarding surgery, resuscitation, organ donation). |

## Family/Significant Other Problem/Analyze Cues/Prioritize Hypotheses

# Grief

*due to* actual or anticipated loss of physiologic well-being (e.g., expected loss of body function or body part, changes in self-concept or body image, illness, death of family/significant other)

*Desired Outcome/Generate Solutions:* After interventions, family members/significant others express grief, participate in decisions about the future, and discuss concerns with health care team members.

| ASSESSMENT—RECOGNIZE CUES/ INTERVENTIONS—TAKE ACTION | RATIONALES |
|---|---|
| Assess and accept the individual's behavioral response. | Reactions such as disbelief, denial, guilt, anger, and depression are normal reactions to grief. |
| Determine the stage of grieving. | Comprehension of the stage of grief enables more effective therapeutic interventions. It is normal for a person to move from one stage to another and then revert to a previous stage. The time required to do so varies from individual to individual. If a patient is unable to move into the next stage, referral for professional intervention may be indicated. |
| | • *Protest stage:* denial, disbelief, anger, hostility, resentment, bargaining to postpone loss, appeal for help to recover loss, loud complaints, altered sleep and appetite |
| | • *Disorganization stage:* depression, withdrawal, social isolation, psychomotor retardation, silence |
| | • *Reorganization stage:* acceptance of loss, development of new interests and attachments, restructuring of lifestyle, return to preloss level of functioning |

| ASSESSMENT—RECOGNIZE CUES/ INTERVENTIONS—TAKE ACTION | RATIONALES |
|---|---|
| Assess spiritual, religious, and sociocultural expectations related to loss. For example, "Is religion an important part of your life?" or "How do you and your family deal with serious health problems?" See *Risk for Spiritual Distress* in "Psychosocial Support for the Patient," Chapter 8. | Helping individuals find meaning in their experiences may facilitate the grieving process. |
| Assess the grief reactions and identify the potential for dysfunctional grieving reactions (e.g., absence of emotion, hostility, avoidance). | This assessment helps identify and reduce dysfunctional grieving, if present. |
| If dysfunctional grieving is present, refer the patient to a psychiatric clinical nurse specialist, licensed clinical social worker, case manager, clergy, or other sources of counseling as appropriate. | Promoting normal progression through the grieving stages may allay unnecessary emotional suffering. |
| Refer to clergy or community support groups as appropriate. | Such a referral reinforces that there are support systems and resources to help work through grief. |
| Demonstrate empathy. For example, "This must be a very difficult time for you and your family" or "Is there anything you'd like to talk about today?" | Empathetic communication (including respecting the desire not to communicate) promotes a trusting relationship and open dialogue. |
| In selected circumstances, explain the grieving process. | This approach may help the patient and family better understand and acknowledge their feelings and help family members better understand behaviors and verbalizations expressed by the patient. |
| When appropriate, provide a referral for bereavement care. | Such a referral helps individuals grieve their loss. |

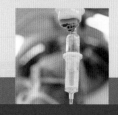

# Support for Lesbian, Gay, Bisexual, Transgender, Queer/Questioning, and Intersex Patients

**10**

This chapter provides a general overview of some of the health challenges faced by lesbian, gay, bisexual, transgender, queer, questioning, nonbinary, and intersex (LGBTQ+) patients and assists students in providing holistic care for each individual's optimal health. This care plan does not assume that every patient will require extensive care, but rather, its goal is to promote awareness and guide health care personnel in providing culturally sensitive, holistic care to help these individuals attain maximum wellness.

## OVERVIEW

Approximately 3.5% of people in the United States identify as LGBTQ+. This statistic is believed to be underreported because of incomplete surveying techniques and client concerns for safety, social stigma, lack of legal recognition, and fear of discrimination (Qureshi et al., 2017). The LGBTQ+ population has notable health challenges and disparities compared with heterosexual communities, and thus Healthy People 2030, the National Institutes of Health, and the World Health Organization (WHO) recognize the need to address and improve the health inequities and human rights violations experienced by LGBTQ+ populations worldwide.

The terms *sex* and *gender* often are used interchangeably, but to better address the needs of this diverse community, it is important to be accurate when using words and labels such as sex, gender, sexuality, and gender identity because people in the LGBTQ+ community are often isolated or marginalized by the misuse of words or labels. The WHO defines *sex* as the biologic and physiologic characteristics that define men and women. *Gender identity* is what an individual's internal sense of self is in relation to gender—being male, female, or something else. *Gender expression* refers to the way a person communicates gender identity through behavior, clothing, hairstyles, voice, or body characteristics (APA, 2015b). An individual's gender is usually assigned at birth, based on visual assessment of the external genitalia, although in some circumstances gender designation may require chromosome studies in order to assign a designation. Gender expression and sexual expression are often influenced by societal norms, genetics, and the environment, which affect an individual's physical and psychologic health.

It is important to note that people do not choose their gender identity. According to the American Academy of Pediatrics (Rafferty, 2022), children have a stable sense of their gender identity early in childhood, often before the age of 5 years. Gender identity is a unique part of each human being and is an expression of the individual. Sexual identity is also a unique part of each human being, and it is believed to form in early childhood. For example, persons may be transgender, while their sexual identities may be bisexual, gay, or straight.

***Terminology.*** People use many words to describe gender and sexual identities. This is not a comprehensive list, and these definitions may not apply to every individual who identifies with these terms.

***Lesbian:*** A female who is sexually/romantically attracted to another female: homosexual.

***Homosexual/gay:*** A male who is sexually/romantically attracted to another male.

***Bisexual:*** A male or female who is sexually/romantically attracted to people of either sex.

***Transgender:*** The person whose gender identity is different from the gender assigned at birth.

***Gender nonconforming:*** A person whose gender identity and/or gender expression does not conform to a single set of culturally specific gender norms. This might include nonbinary individuals as well as people who dress/act/present in ways perceived as contrary to their gender.

***Gender dysphoria:*** Distress caused by the discrepancy between the gender assigned a person at birth and a person's gender identity.

***Intersex:*** People who do not fit the typical definition for the male or female because of several variations of sexual characteristics. This may include chromosomal variations other than the typical XX female and XY male, genital ambiguity, and sex hormone variations.

***Agender:*** An individual who does not identify as any specific gender.

***Binary:*** A view of gender whereby a person is defined as being either male or female, often based on biologic sex.

***Nonbinary:*** An individual who does not identify strictly as male or female; gender is fluid.

*Cisgender:* An individual whose gender aligns with the gender assigned at birth.

*Transitioning:* A process transgender people undergo to align their gender identity to their physical self. This may or may not include surgery and cross-sex hormone treatments.

*Coming out:* For homosexual individuals, disclosing to family, friends, and society that they are homosexual or bisexual.

**Health care needs.** LGBTQ+ patients are at an increased risk for anxiety, mood disorders, and depression, and they experience increased suicidal ideation and attempt suicide in greater numbers than the heterosexual (non-LGBTQ+) population (Dickey et al., 2017). Contributing factors for increased mental health issues among LGBTQ+ patients include social stressors such as isolation, discrimination, increased incidences of bullying or violence, and lack of community or family support. Maladaptive coping behaviors may be adopted by LGBTQ+ individuals in response to these experiences and may influence high-risk health behaviors, which in turn can escalate feelings of isolation, lack of acceptance, and hopelessness.

Substance use disorder is another health concern common to this population. Tobacco use is higher in LGBTQ+ individuals than in the general population, including teenagers. and exposure to secondhand smoke in clubs and bars increases cancer risk (American Cancer Society, 2022e). In addition, smoking accelerates the onset of AIDS in individuals with human immunodeficiency virus (HIV).

For patients whose gender assigned at birth does not align with their gender identity, internal and external barriers to expressing their gender identity can cause significant emotional and psychologic distress. Gender identity issues may be seen in young children and adolescents in whom signs and symptoms of depression may be prevalent (Olson et al., 2015). Gender-nonconforming children may grow up to identify as cisgender, or transgender, and may be heterosexual, lesbian, gay, or bisexual as adults. Specialists agree it is important for children to feel accepted and to live in a safe physical environment. Transgender youth are more likely to be isolated, become homeless, and experience violence such as bullying, and they are two to three times more likely to attempt suicide than non-LGBTQ+ youth (Dickey et al., 2017; Healthy People, 2020; Olson et al., 2015).

Gender-nonconforming children may choose to wear clothing and hairstyles to reflect their self-identified gender and may seek medical treatment that can block the signs of puberty. A pediatric endocrinologist can be consulted to guide medical treatment. Later in adolescence or in early adulthood, these individuals may choose to take medications or undergo surgical procedures to medically "transition" to their identified gender. There are specific protocols and standards of care to guide health care professionals to assist transgender and gender-nonconforming clients to attain well-being and overall health (World Professional Association for Transgender Health [WPATH], 2011). Medically transitioning is a complex process that can include a number of specified regimens, among them initiation of cross-sex hormone treatments and surgical interventions. Psychosocial therapy is important not only to assist the transgender client in adjusting to gender and social issues but also to support members of the LGBTQ+ community in "coming out" and dealing with family, friends, coworkers, and society and developing skills to cope with the stress, anxiety, and depression that may accompany these events.

**Barriers to health care.** Compared with non-LGBTQ+ populations, LGBTQ+ individuals often experience limited access to health care. Income disparities between LGBTQ+ and non-LGBTQ+ populations can exacerbate lack of access. In addition, because most workplace policies do not cover unmarried partners, LGBTQ+ families are often left without adequate insurance. Clinics and facilities skilled in the needs of LGBTQ+ patients, staffed with health care providers knowledgeable in treatments and medication regimens (especially for transgender patients), are not readily available in all areas. Travel or transportation to facilities with these services may present a significant barrier for many LGBTQ+ individuals in accessing necessary health care. Studies confirm that LGBTQ+ patients have fewer routine screenings, such as HIV, human papillomavirus, sexually transmitted infections (STIs), cancer, and preventative wellness screenings, compared with non-LGBTQ+ clients. In addition, LGBTQ+ individuals report they are often reluctant to seek health care or disclose health-related concerns or lifestyle behaviors to health care providers because of previous negative encounters, bias, and prejudice experienced in the health care setting. These prior negative encounters can place the individual at further risk for timely intervention and treatment (Qureshi et al., 2017). Some medical programs and health organizations now include LGBTQ+ cultural competency training in their curriculums to help overcome this barrier and teach providers how to interact with these patients with sensitivity. Because LGBTQ+ individuals may not seek routine or preventative health care for the reasons outlined earlier, they may be very ill by the time they enter the health care system. Access to care, preferably in the individual's own community, in a safe, nonjudgmental atmosphere is important in improving health and well-being.

## HEALTH CARE SETTING

Primary care, outpatient care, clinics, acute care (inpatient medical and psychiatric), and possibly individual, group, and family therapy

## ASSESSMENT

Routine physical examinations, including preventative health maintenance, vaccinations, weight management, diet counseling, domestic abuse screening, and healthy lifestyle counseling, should be provided.

**Cancer screening:** The American Cancer Society recommends cancer screenings for all patients and publishes fact sheets specifically for the LGBTQ+ community, identifying risk factors and routine screening recommendations (American Cancer Society, 2022e). Preventative screenings for cancer are recommended: Papanicolaou (Pap) tests, prostate examinations, and mammograms. Preventative health screenings are especially important for the patient who is still at risk for cancers for the gender they were assigned at birth, even if they do not live as that gender. For example, patients may not be aware they are still at risk for breast or female cancers even if they have transitioned to and live as men.

**STI screening:** HIV, STIs, and identification of high-risk behaviors, especially among gay/bisexual men, where high-risk behaviors are more common than with heterosexual populations.

**Mental health support:** Screening needs to include a mental health history and assessments for depression, mood disorders, anxiety, risk behaviors, and suicidal ideation as well as identification of coping skills, support systems, and spiritual needs. Referrals to mental health counseling and support groups in the community are encouraged.

**Substance use disorders:** LGBTQ+ populations have the highest rates of tobacco, alcohol, and drug use (Healthy People, 2020). Assessment of family history, history of drug and alcohol use, and medication use and careful screening of symptoms and behavior patterns are important. (See "Substance-Related Addictive Disorders", Chapter 104.)

**Environmental and social stressors:** Living in poverty is more common among transgender people, as is discrimination, loss of family, homelessness, and acts of violence. Adequate housing, food, finances, and safety concerns need to be addressed in the primary care setting and referrals to community support systems provided to the patient.

## Patient Problem/Analyze Cues/Prioritize Hypotheses

# Risk for Suicide

*due to* depression, anxiety, mood issues, and/or issues with gender identity

***Desired Outcome/Generate Solutions:*** By discharge (if inpatient) or within 4 weeks of outpatient treatment, the patient expresses and demonstrates that they are free of suicidal thinking.

| ASSESSMENT—RECOGNIZE CUES/ INTERVENTIONS—TAKE ACTION | RATIONALES |
|---|---|
| Complete a suicide assessment. Consider using a standardized assessment tool such as SAD PERSONS suicide assessment scale. | The degree of hopelessness, depression, and planning expressed by the patient is important in assessing the risk for suicide. The more the patient has thought out a plan, the greater the risk for suicide attempt. There is a higher risk if the patient has attempted suicide previously or has a family history of suicide. This population has a greater attempted suicide rate than heterosexual populations (Qureshi et al., 2017). |
| Reassess for suicidality, especially during times of change or increased stress. Identify whether the patient has thought about suicide and if they have a suicide plan. | Changes in living situation, health status, medication/treatment plan, and personal loss may increase depression and feelings of hopelessness. The stress experienced during "coming out" or transitioning can be an intense time for the patient, causing a severe emotional reaction. This information will enable a specific plan of action for the health care staff. |
| Encourage the patient to verbalize feelings and examine the relationship between feelings and the event/stressor. | Verbalizing feelings in a nonthreatening environment can help patients identify unrecognized/unresolved feelings that may be contributing to depression. It also helps patients connect the response (feeling) to the stressor and may assist in developing coping strategies. |
| Teach the patient healthy ways to cope and identify underlying feelings of hurt, anger, and rejection. Ask about previous coping behaviors that may have been unhealthy. | Before patients can change or adopt healthy coping mechanisms, they need to identify feelings and responses as well as previously unhealthy behaviors. |
| If the patient is hospitalized, implement the following: | |
| • Monitor at least every 15 minutes for moderate risk, preferably staggering monitoring times so that the patient does not take advantage of a guaranteed time period to engage in suicidal behavior. Avoid assigning a single room. Accompany the patient with all off-unit activities. Ensure that the patient is in view of staff members at all times. | Providing close observation may prevent suicide attempts. |

| ASSESSMENT—RECOGNIZE CUES/ INTERVENTIONS—TAKE ACTION | RATIONALES |
|---|---|
| • Routinely check the environment for hazards to ensure environmental safety. | This intervention minimizes opportunities for self-harm (e.g., keeping doors, windows, and access to stairwells and roof locked and monitoring and removing cleaning, chemical, and repair supplies). |
| Initiate a safety plan with the patient. | Including the patient in creating a safety plan builds a trust relationship and promotes self-care and monitoring. The safety plan can include actions that the patient agrees to initiate when suicidal feelings increase (e.g., seeking interaction with the staff, requesting an as-needed medication, creating a list of friends or support persons the patient can contact). |

## Patient Problem/Analyze Cues/Prioritize Hypotheses

# Deficient Knowledge

*due to* unfamiliarity with preventative health care needs and the need for health maintenance visits

*Desired Outcome:* The patient verbalizes the need for preventative medical care and is being seen by a health care provider on a routine basis.

| ASSESSMENT—RECOGNIZE CUES/ INTERVENTIONS—TAKE ACTION | RATIONALES |
|---|---|
| Take a thorough medical history. Assess which preventative and screening procedures the patient has had and when the service was provided. | Recognizing that the LGBTQ+ patient may be reluctant to share information is important when building a trusting relationship. Compiling a history may take time while a trusting relationship is being built. Identifying which screenings have occurred and when they occurred will provide the health care provider with a foundation for recommending preventative care and help direct teaching for the patient. |
| Teach healthy behaviors (diet, exercise, lifestyle). Discuss recommended preventative health screenings (e.g., Pap tests, colorectal cancer screening, and mammograms), including how often these screenings need to be performed. | Patients may not be aware that they remain at risk for health problems related to the gender to which they were born, even if they have transitioned or lived as their identified gender for many years. Informed patients can make better decisions regarding their health. |
| Assess whether the patient has ever undergone specific screenings. | The provider may need to make accommodations (e.g., for a lesbian patient who has never undergone a pelvic examination). |
| Provide the patient with recommended health maintenance screenings. | An informed patient who understands the importance of routine health care may be more likely to adhere to such screenings. Prescheduling appointments and providing transportation options may enable the patient to be more adherent in health-seeking behaviors. |
| Preschedule appointments and provide information regarding transportation if this is a challenge for the patient. | |

## Transgender Patient Problem/Analyze Cues/Prioritize Hypotheses

# Risk for Social Isolation

*due to* societal rejection, significant life stressors, and social stigma or discrimination

*Desired Outcome/Generate Solutions:* Within 2 weeks of meeting with the clinical staff, the patient verbalizes feelings and identifies community resources and available support systems.

| ASSESSMENT—RECOGNIZE CUES/ INTERVENTIONS—TAKE ACTION | RATIONALES |
|---|---|
| Provide a respectful atmosphere in the clinical setting. Treat the patient as you would want to be treated. Provide staff training regarding supporting a positive atmosphere. | Providing an atmosphere that is inclusive and welcoming to all patients conveys respect. Examples of a respectful environment include promoting privacy when discussing patient information, proving non–gender-specific restrooms, and issuing intake forms that include gender options other than male or female. |
| Address patients as their preferred gender. If staff members are unsure about the preferred gender, ask patients how they wish to be addressed. For example: "By what name would you like to be called and which pronoun would you like me to use?" | Addressing patients by their preferred names and pronouns, even if you are not in their presence, conveys respect, which in turn will help patients overcome their sense of rejection and discrimination. |
| Encourage patients to verbalize their feelings. | Information sharing and communication can reduce feelings of isolation. |
| Assess and accept behavioral responses. | Patients may experience a variety of emotions (e.g., anger, grief, and shame). Encouraging them to identify and explore these feelings and the behaviors they exhibit in response to these feelings is important in the development of healthy coping mechanisms. |
| Provide referrals to community support groups. | Providing patients with psychosocial support and resources either in the community or online can reduce feelings of isolation. |
| Include friends and the patient's support systems in the patient's care. | Friends and support people can reduce feelings of isolation. |
| If available, involve Social Services in the patient's care. | Social Services provide resources and referrals for individual counseling and support groups for the patient and for partners and family, which may help participants feel less isolated. Social Services also may provide community resources nurses and staff are unaware of. |

## Transgender Patient Problem/Analyze Cues/Prioritize Hypotheses

# Deficient Knowledge

*due to* unfamiliarity with medications (including hormone treatment regimens to feminize or masculinize the body), professional mental health support, and surgical options

*Desired Outcomes/Generate Solutions:* The patient verbalizes accurate information about the medical treatment plan. The patient has verbal and written instructions/materials and identifies common side effects. The patient verbalizes the need for follow-up care.

| ASSESSMENT—RECOGNIZE CUES/ INTERVENTIONS—TAKE ACTION | RATIONALES |
|---|---|
| Assess the patient's health care literacy (language, reading, comprehension). Assess culture and culturally specific information needs. Provide verbal and written educational materials when possible. | This assessment helps ensure that information is presented in a manner that is culturally and educationally appropriate. This is especially important in the LGBTQ+ community where bias and prejudice may prevent the patient from sharing important personal information that affects health. Patients should be addressed as the gender by which they identify, not the gender assigned at birth. |
| Ask patients by which gender they wish to be addressed, for example, using the pronouns "she" or "he," or "they." | |
| Teach the patient about treatment options, including cross-sex hormone therapy and surgical options. | Increasing knowledge of options for treatment, including regimens, costs, risks, timeframes, and side effects, helps patients make educated decisions while also fostering a trusting relationship. |
| Assess whether the patient understands what has been taught using open-ended questions, for example, "Can you explain why it is important for you to complete all your medication?" | Open-ended questions encourage more dialogue. |

| ASSESSMENT—RECOGNIZE CUES/ INTERVENTIONS—TAKE ACTION | RATIONALES |
|---|---|
| Discuss the importance of psychosocial counseling and provide referrals. | Psychotherapy can be invaluable in assisting transgender and gender-nonconforming individuals to cope with gender identity and social stressors they will encounter. Gender identity issues can be explored in individual, group, and family therapy. Identification of community and peer support groups is beneficial (World Professional Association for Transgender Health [WPATH], 2017). |
| Instruct the patient on the importance of adhering to hormone treatments. Teach possible side effects and the signs and symptoms to report to the provider. | This information increases patient awareness of medication regimens. The patient who is aware of the side effects and possible complications will report to the health care provider for timely intervention. |
| Provide community and online resources for support and education. | Support groups and accurate information empower patients as they progress through this lengthy and personal journey. Patients often benefit from sharing a commonality with other individuals who have experienced similar situations. |

## ADDITIONAL PROBLEMS:

"Psychosocial Support for the Patient," Chapter 8, for *Anxiety, Difficulty Coping, and Anticipatory Grief*
"Psychosocial Support for the Patient's Family and Significant Others," Chapter 9, for *Difficulty Coping*

 **PATIENT–FAMILY TEACHING AND DISCHARGE PLANNING**

The LGBTQ+ patient faces many health challenges because of societal biases, increased risk behaviors, and mental and emotional stress, as well as fewer than optimal preventative health screenings. LGBTQ+ patients may not seek medical care until a medical condition is advanced because of previous poor experiences with the medical community, which places them at risk for having an advanced illness when they enter the health care system. Health care personnel need to be aware that LGBTQ+ patients experience higher rates of anxiety, depression, and risk for suicide than the heterosexual population. Because there is social stigma associated with being LGBTQ+, patients may be hesitant to fully disclose lifestyle, high-risk behaviors, or personal medical information to the health care provider. To provide comprehensive medical care, it is important to identify barriers to physical and emotional health, along with a complete medical history, prior preventative health screenings, vaccinations, mental health, substance use, and a complete sexual history. Providers should be aware that living in poverty is more common among transgender people, as is discrimination, loss of family, homelessness, and acts of bullying and violence. Adequate housing, food, finances, and safety concerns need to be addressed during the health interview and referrals to community support systems provided. Providers must be inclusive and take steps to provide a safe, private, and respectful environment that includes cultural competency training of the staff.

Transgender patients may seek not only preventative health care but medical treatment such as cross-sex hormone and surgical regimens to achieve gender congruence. Health professionals can provide protocols for these regimens and make referrals to provide these patients with education so that they may make informed decisions regarding their health care. Psychosocial therapy is part of a holistic approach and is helpful for patients dealing with the stress of coming out and transitioning.

When providing patient–family teaching, focus on sensory information, avoid giving excessive information, and include verbal and written information about the following:

✓ Signs and symptoms of medical complications and the importance of contacting the health care provider in a timely manner.
✓ Necessity of modifying high-risk sexual behaviors and practicing safe sex.
✓ Importance of adhering to the hormone regimen for transgender patients (if used), including possible side effects and when to call the provider.
✓ Importance of a well-balanced diet and regular exercise.
✓ Potential risk factors for cancers for the gender the patient was assigned at birth, even if gender reassignment surgery has occurred.
✓ Importance of maintaining medical follow-up appointments. See *Deficient Knowledge*, earlier.
✓ Availability of Social Services and spiritual care, including local community and support groups.
✓ Medications, including drug name, purpose, dosage, frequency, precautions, and potential side effects. Also discuss potential drug–drug, food–drug, and herb–drug interactions.

✓ Referrals to local and national support organizations, including:

- Alcoholics Anonymous: https:aa.org
- Center of Excellence for Transgender Health (at the University of San Francisco): http://www.transhealth.ucsf.edu/trans?page=org-00-00
- International Foundation for Gender Education: www.ifge.org
- LGBT Health, Centers for Disease Control and Prevention: www.cdc.gov/lgbthealth/about.htm
- Medical Advocate: http://www.advocate.com/transgender
- Narcotics Anonymous: http://www.na.org
- National Center for Transgender Equality: www.transequality.org
- National Institute on Drug Abuse: http://nida.nih.gov
- National LGBT Health Education Center: https://www.lgbthealtheducation.org
- National Suicide Prevention Lifeline: https://suicide-preventionlifeline.org/
- World Profession Association for Transgender Health: www.wpath.org

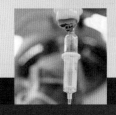

# Acute Respiratory Failure 11

## OVERVIEW/PATHOPHYSIOLOGY

Acute respiratory failure (ARF) develops when the lungs are unable to exchange $O_2$ and $CO_2$ adequately. There are two classifications of ARF. Hypoxemic respiratory failure, also known as oxygenation failure, exists when $PaO_2$ is less than 60 mm Hg with the patient at rest and breathing room air. The low $PaO_2$ may persist even when oxygen is given. Hypercapnic respiratory failure, also called ventilatory failure, occurs when the $PaCO_2$ is 50 mm Hg or more with a pH less than 7.35. Respiratory acidosis, indicated by the low pH, is a common precursor to ARF. With this type of ARF, the body cannot sufficiently remove $CO_2$, which raised the $PaCO_2$ levels. Eventually, the acidosis worsens as the body tries to compensate.

Although a variety of disease processes can lead to the development of respiratory failure, four basic mechanisms are involved.

**Alveolar hypoventilation.** This is a decrease in ventilation that results in increased $PaCO_2$. It occurs with problems that cause reduced ventilation, such as CNS conditions, acute asthma, or chest wall dysfunction. This condition reflects hypercapnic respiratory failure, but severe hypoxemia may result.

**Ventilation–perfusion mismatch.** This is considered one of the most common causes of hypoxemia. Normal alveolar ventilation occurs at a rate of 4–6 L/minute, with normal pulmonary vascular blood flow occurring at a rate of 4–6 L/minute. The normal ventilation/perfusion ratio is 0.8 : 1.2. Any disease process that interferes with either side of the equation upsets physiologic balance and can lead to respiratory failure because of the reduction in arterial $O_2$ levels. For example, if a person is experiencing severe chest or abdominal wall pain, the resulting short, shallow respirations (because deep breaths cause pain) may result in atelectasis, worsening the ventilation/perfusion ratio.

**Diffusion disturbances.** Processes that physically impair gas exchange across the alveolar-capillary membrane. Diffusion is impaired because of the increase in anatomic distance the gas must travel from alveoli to capillary and capillary to alveoli.

**Right-to-left shunt.** Occurs when the previously mentioned processes go untreated. Large amounts of blood pass from the right side of the heart to the left and out into the general circulation without adequate ventilation; therefore, blood is poorly oxygenated. This mechanism occurs when alveoli are atelectatic or fluid filled, inasmuch as these conditions interfere with gas exchange. Unlike the first three responses, hypoxemia secondary to right-to-left shunting does not improve with $O_2$ administration because the additional inspired oxygen ($FiO_2$) is unable to cross the alveolar-capillary membrane. This is also one of the most common causes of ARF.

## HEALTH CARE SETTING

Primary care; acute care resulting from complications

## ASSESSMENT

Clinical indicators of ARF vary according to the underlying disease process and severity of the failure. ARF is one of the most common causes of the impaired level of consciousness. Often, it is misdiagnosed as heart failure, pneumonia, or stroke. ARF may develop suddenly or gradually.

**Early indicators.** Restlessness, changes in mental status, anxiety, headache, fatigue, cool and dry skin, increased blood pressure, tachycardia, cardiac dysrhythmias.

**Intermediate indicators.** Confusion, increased agitation, and increased oxygen requirements with decreased oxygen saturations. Patients who have hypoventilation respiratory failure often exhibit lethargy and bradypnea. Patients with ventilation–perfusion mismatch often exhibit tachypnea.

**Late indicators.** Cyanosis, diaphoresis, coma, respiratory arrest. Note that cyanosis is a late sign of ARF, and often does not occur until the $PaO_2$ is 45 mm Hg or less.

## DIAGNOSTIC TESTS

**Arterial blood gas analysis.** Assesses the adequacy of oxygenation and effectiveness of ventilation and is the most important diagnostic tool. Typical results are $PaO_2$ of 60 mm Hg or less, $PaCO_2$ of 50 mm Hg or more, and pH less than 7.35, which are consistent with severe respiratory acidosis.

**Chest radiography.** Ascertains the presence of underlying pathophysiology or disease process that may be contributing to the failure.

**Other testing:** If a pulmonary embolus is suspected, a CT scan or V/Q lung scan may be done. Other studies may include a complete blood count, serum electrolytes, electrocardiogram, blood and sputum cultures, and urinalysis. Pulse oximetry may be done continuously to monitor oxygenation status indirectly.

## PATIENT PROBLEMS[a]:

[a]The listed disorders may be precursors to acute respiratory failure.

## PATIENT–FAMILY TEACHING AND DISCHARGE PLANNING

ARF is an acute condition that is symptomatically treated during the patient's hospitalization. Discharge planning and teaching needs to be directed at educating the patient and significant others about the underlying pathophysiology and treatment specific for that process. For patient problems that are related to precursors that relate specifically to the underlying pathophysiology contributing to the development of ARF, see chapters in the "Respiratory Care Plan" section, and other chapters as indicated.

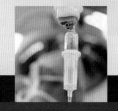

# Chronic Obstructive Pulmonary Disease 12

## OVERVIEW/PATHOPHYSIOLOGY

Chronic obstructive pulmonary disease (COPD) is the sixth leading cause in the United States (Centers for Disease Control and Prevention [CDC], 2022a). It is a disease state characterized by airflow limitation that is not fully reversible. Airflow limitation is progressive and associated with an abnormal inflammatory response of the lungs to noxious particles or gases and characterized by chronic inflammation throughout the airways, parenchyma, and pulmonary vasculature.

The chronic airflow limitation characteristic of COPD is caused by a mixture of small airway inflammation (bronchitis) and parenchymal destruction (emphysema), and the relative contributions of each vary from person to person.

## HEALTH CARE SETTING

COPD may be found in any health care setting, such as the home, primary care, hospitalized patients (medical, surgical floors, or critical care units), and long-term care facilities.

## ASSESSMENT

**Signs and symptoms, acute and chronic.** Common symptoms associated with chronic COPD include dyspnea, chronic cough, and chronic sputum production. Dyspnea that interferes with daily activities, and is possibly present at rest, is the main reason patients seek medical attention. Increased sputum production may be prominent. As lung function deteriorates and dyspnea worsens, arterial hypoxemia and hypercarbia become more pronounced, and additional complications such as weight loss, right heart failure (cor pulmonale), and respiratory failure occur.

**Key health history.** Environmental exposure is the most common cause of COPD. Cigarette smoking, or passive exposure to cigarette smoke, is the most encountered risk factor and causes 85%–90% of COPD cases (American Lung Association, 2021). Other risk factors include chronic occupational exposure to dust, chemicals, fumes, secondhand smoke, or air pollution. A deficiency in alpha-1 protein is a genetic condition that may predispose one to developing COPD. Any process that affects lung development and growth (such as low birth weight or recurrent respiratory infections) may increase the potential for developing COPD later in life. Multiple risk factors magnify the possibility of developing COPD.

Significant comorbidities include cardiovascular disease, osteoporosis, anxiety/depression, lung cancer, respiratory infections, and diabetes. All of these may have a significant impact on the COPD patient. The comorbidities are treated in the usual manner in the COPD patient.

**Physical assessment.** Prolonged expiratory phase, decreased thoracic expansion, adventitious breath sounds (especially wheezing), use of accessory muscles of respiration, development of a barrel chest, digital clubbing, dullness on percussion over areas of consolidation, ankle edema, distended neck veins.

## DIAGNOSTIC TESTS

**Spirometry.** When the common symptoms associated with chronic COPD are present, spirometry confirms the diagnosis of COPD. It is expressed as a ratio of the forced expiratory volume ($FEV_1$), or the volume of air that is forcefully exhaled in the first second, divided by the forced vital capacity (FVC), or the maximum volume of air that can be forcefully exhaled after bronchodilator use. The ratio is expressed as $FEV_1$/FVC but sometimes simply abbreviated to $FEV_1$. Clinical symptoms and a post–short-acting bronchodilator use $FEV_1$ of less than 70% are used to diagnose and classify the severity and prognosis of COPD. The lower the $FEV_1$ values, the more the airways are obstructed.

**Pulse oximetry ($SpO_2$).** A useful tool for both screening and monitoring disease progression, with the expected range for COPD patients being between 88% and 92%. Pulse oximetry readings may be done at rest and when walking. If oxygen saturation levels fall to 88% or lower at rest on room air, then supplemental oxygen will be ordered.

**Chest radiography.** Rarely diagnostic unless bullous disease is present. Radiologic changes in COPD include signs of hyperinflation (i.e., flattened diaphragm on lateral chest radiograph and increase in the volume of the retrosternal airspace).

**Arterial blood gas values.** Important in monitoring COPD during exacerbations or respiratory failure ($PaO_2$ less than 60 mm Hg with or without $PaCO_2$ greater than 50 mm Hg). Arterial blood gases (ABGs) are not diagnostic but help to identify the severity of the COPD exacerbation.

**Alpha-1 antitrypsin deficiency screen.** Performed in patients who develop COPD at a young age (younger than 45 years) or who have a strong family history of the disease.

**Complications.** Heart failure, pneumonia, or acute respiratory failure may also occur.

## Patient Problem/Analyze Cues/Prioritize Hypotheses

# Dyspnea

*due to* ineffective inspiration and expiration occurring with chronic airflow limitations

**Desired Outcome/Generate Solutions:** After treatment/interventions, the patient's breathing pattern improves as evidenced by reduction in or absence of reported dyspnea and related symptoms.

| ASSESSMENT—RECOGNIZE CUES/ INTERVENTIONS—TAKE ACTION | RATIONALES |
|---|---|
| Assess respiratory status every 2–4 hours and as indicated by the patient's condition. Report significant findings. | Restlessness, anxiety, mental status changes, shortness of breath, tachypnea, and use of accessory muscles of respiration are signs of respiratory distress, which must be reported promptly for immediate intervention. |
| Auscultate breath sounds every 2–4 hours and as indicated by the patient's condition. | A decrease in breath sounds or an increase in adventitious breath sounds (crackles, wheezes) may indicate respiratory status change and necessitate prompt intervention. |
| Administer bronchodilator therapy as prescribed. | Bronchodilators increase $FEV_1$ by altering airway smooth muscle tone, with long-acting formulations being preferred. If symptoms do not improve with a single agent, combined short- and long-acting agents are used. |
| Administer inhaled corticosteroids as prescribed. | This treatment is used for patients with $FEV_1$ at less than 30%, whose frequent exacerbations are not well controlled with long-acting bronchodilators. |
| Administer oral corticosteroids as prescribed. | Short-term corticosteroids shorten recovery time, improve lung function and arterial hypoxemia, and decrease hospital length of stay. A typical course is 10–14 days. Long-term oral corticosteroid monotherapy is not recommended because the side effects outweigh the minimal advantage oral corticosteroids provide over inhaled corticosteroids. |
| Administer combination of inhaled corticosteroids and bronchodilator therapy as prescribed. Advise the patient about the increased risk for pneumonia. Monitor for tachycardia and dysrhythmias. | Corticosteroids combined with a long-acting beta-2 agonist are more effective than any one individual treatment in reducing exacerbations and overall improvement of lung function. However, its use also carries an increased risk for pneumonia. |
| If inhaled bronchodilators and inhaled corticosteroids are to be given at the same time, administer the bronchodilator first, then administer the corticosteroid after waiting 2–5 minutes. | Administering the bronchodilator first allows the airways to open, thus making more surface area available for the inhaled corticosteroid. |
| Monitor for tachycardia and dysrhythmias. | These are side effects of bronchodilator therapy. |
| Instruct the patient to rinse the mouth with water and spit it out the water after each dose of inhaled corticosteroids. | These medications may cause oral candidiasis (thrush); rinsing the mouth after inhaled doses can prevent this infection. |
| Deliver humidified oxygen as prescribed and monitor the patient's response. | Long-term oxygenation for chronic hypoxemia has been shown to reduce mortality. Delivering $O_2$ with humidity will help minimize convective losses of moisture, decreasing dry mucous membranes and enhancing lung compliance. |
| Monitor pulse oximetry readings and titrate oxygen to keep $SpO_2$ between 88% and 92%. | $SpO_2$ saturation at 87% or less can indicate the need for initiating or increasing $O_2$ therapy. $SpO_2$ saturation at 93% or more can indicate need for decreasing $O_2$ therapy to prevent the complications of oxygen toxicity in the patient with COPD. |

Patient Problem/Analyze Cues/Prioritize Hypotheses

# Impaired Gas Exchange

*due to* altered oxygen supply occurring with small airway inflammation and parenchymal destruction or alveolar edema

**Desired Outcomes/Generate Solutions:** Optimally within 1–2 hours after treatment/interventions or by discharge, the patient has adequate gas exchange as evidenced by respiratory rate (RR) of 12–20 breaths/minute (or values consistent with patient's baseline). Before discharge from the care facility, the patient's ABG values are as follows: $PaO_2$ of 60 mm Hg or higher, $PaCO_2$ of 35–45 mm Hg, and pH of 7.35–7.45, or $SpO_2$ of 88%–92% or values consistent with the patient's baseline.

| ASSESSMENT—RECOGNIZE CUES/ INTERVENTIONS—TAKE ACTION | RATIONALES |
|---|---|
| Assess for signs and symptoms of hypoxia and report significant findings. | Hypoxia (evidenced by agitation, anxiety, restlessness, changes in mental status or level of consciousness) indicates oxygen deficiency and necessitates prompt treatment. |
| Auscultate breath sounds every 2–4 hours and as indicated by the patient's condition and report significant findings. | A decrease in breath sounds or an increase in adventitious breath sounds (crackles, wheezes) may indicate respiratory status change and necessitate prompt intervention. |
| Deliver humidified oxygen as prescribed, and monitor the patient's response. | Long-term oxygenation for chronic hypoxemia has been shown to reduce mortality. Delivering $O_2$ with humidity will help minimize convective losses of moisture, decreasing dry mucous membranes and enhancing compliance. |
| • Monitor pulse oximetry readings and titrate oxygen to keep $SpO_2$ between 88% and 92%.<br><br>**Note:** High concentrations of oxygen (over 2 L/minute) may worsen hypercapnia in acute exacerbations of COPD (McDonald, 2014). | $SpO_2$ at 87% or less can indicate the need for $O_2$ therapy. $SpO_2$ at 93% or more can indicate the need for decreasing $O_2$ therapy. See this rationale with *Dyspnea*, earlier. |
| Position the patient in high-Fowler position, with the patient leaning forward and elbows propped on the over-the-bed table. Pad the over-the-bed table with pillows or blankets. Record the patient's response to positioning. | This position promotes comfort and optimal gas exchange by enabling maximal chest expansion, using activation of accessory muscles during inspiration and gravity during expiration. |
| Administer noninvasive positive-pressure ventilation (NIPPV) as prescribed. If the patient is able to tolerate oral intake, switch the NIPPV to nasal cannula oxygen during meals | NIPPV has been shown to increase blood pH, reduce $PaCO_2$, and reduce the severity of dyspnea in the first four hours of treatment, possibly eliminating the need for mechanical ventilation in some patients. Switching the NIPPV to nasal cannula oxygen during meals facilitates eating and prevents aspiration while using NIPPV. |
| Explain, as indicated, that intubation, mechanical ventilation, pressure support, and minimal positive end-expiratory pressure (PEEP) may be necessary and this would necessitate intensive care support. Goals and possible outcomes need to be discussed with the patient and/ or significant others *before* intubation and mechanical ventilation are instituted, if possible. | Exacerbations of COPD or complications (e.g., pneumonia, surgery, trauma) may require endotracheal intubation and short-term mechanical ventilation. Pressure support provides inspirational assistance to overcome the resistance of the endotracheal tube and ventilator circuit. PEEP is limited to exert the least internal pressure on the fragile lungs. |
| Monitor serial ABG values as indicated by the patient's condition. | $PaO_2$ likely will continue to decrease as the patient's disease progresses. Patients with chronic $CO_2$ retention may have chronically compensated respiratory acidosis with a low normal pH (7.35–7.38) and a $PaCO_2$ greater than 50 mm Hg. |

Patient Problem/Analyze Cues/Prioritize Hypotheses
# Fatigue (With Decreased Exercise Tolerance)

*due to* imbalance between oxygen supply and demand occurring with inefficient work of breathing

**Desired Outcome/Generate Solutions:** The patient reports decreasing dyspnea during activity or exercise and rates perceived exertion at 3 or less on a 0–10 scale. See "Immobility," *Activity Intolerance*, Chapter 1, for a description of the Borg scale.

| ASSESSMENT—RECOGNIZE CUES/ INTERVENTIONS—TAKE ACTION | RATIONALES |
|---|---|
| Monitor the patient's respiratory response to exercise or activity, including assessment of oxygen saturations. | Exercise or activity intolerance is indicated by excessively increased RR (e.g., more than 10 breaths/minute above baseline) and depth, and use of accessory muscles of respiration. Ask the patient to rate perceived exertion. If activity intolerance is noted, instruct the patient to stop the activity and rest. Individuals with COPD may become hypoxic during increased activity and require oxygen therapy to prevent hypoxemia, which increases the risk for exacerbations of the COPD. |
| Maintain prescribed activity levels and explain rationale to the patient. | Prescribed activity levels will increase the patient's stamina while minimizing dyspnea. COPD is a progressive disease, and affected individuals can gradually become totally disabled because they must use all available energy for breathing. |
| Allow at least 90 minutes between activities for undisturbed rest. Facilitate coordination across health care providers. | Ninety minutes of undisturbed rest decreases oxygen demand and enables adequate physiologic recovery. |
| Assist with active range-of-motion (ROM) exercises. | ROM exercises help build stamina and prevent complications of decreased mobility. |
| Request consultation from pulmonary rehabilitation. | A comprehensive program includes exercise training, nutrition counseling, and education and provides benefits to patients with all stages of COPD. Pulmonary rehabilitation is strongly recommended for any patient with an $FEV_1$ of less than 50%. Pulmonary rehabilitation may help the patient experience improved quality of life and slowed disease progression. |

Patient Problem/Analyze Cues/Prioritize Hypotheses
# Body Weight Problem (Weight Loss)

*due to* decreased intake occurring with fatigue and anorexia

**Desired Outcome/Generate Solutions:** For a minimum of 24 hours before hospital discharge, the patient has adequate nutrition as evidenced by intake of at least 50% of prescribed calories/meals and stable or increased body weight.

| ASSESSMENT—RECOGNIZE CUES/ INTERVENTIONS—TAKE ACTION | RATIONALES |
|---|---|
| Assess food and fluid intake. | This assessment provides data that will determine the need for dietary consultation. |
| Provide the diet in small, frequent, high caloric meals that are nutritious and easy to consume. | Small meals are easier to consume in individuals who are fatigued. Patients with COPD expend an extraordinary amount of energy simply on breathing and require high caloric meals to maintain body weight and muscle mass. Cachexia (loss of muscle and fat despite adequate nutrition) is associated with higher mortality in individuals with COPD. |

## ASSESSMENT—RECOGNIZE CUES/ INTERVENTIONS—TAKE ACTION

| ASSESSMENT—RECOGNIZE CUES/INTERVENTIONS—TAKE ACTION | RATIONALES |
|---|---|
| Request consultation with a dietitian as indicated. | Such a consultation enables a comprehensive nutritional assessment and possible additional therapies, including nutritional counseling related to the disease process. The dietitian also may facilitate the establishment of enteral or parental nutrition in the cachectic or intubated patient or those who are not able to consume adequate nutrition orally. |
| For patients who require NIPPV and are able to eat, consult with respiratory therapy for the most appropriate device to allow the patient to eat. | Attempting oral intake while using NIPPV may result in aspiration. Changing devices for short periods to enable the patient to eat may avoid the need for enteral or parental nutrition support. |
| When not otherwise indicated, encourage fluid intake (2.5 L/day or more). | Adequate hydration helps decrease sputum viscosity for patients with chronic increased sputum production. |
| Discuss with the patient and significant others the importance of good nutrition in the treatment of COPD. | This information optimally will promote adequate nutrition and stable body weight. A knowledgeable patient is more likely to adhere to the treatment plan. |

## ✔ PATIENT–FAMILY TEACHING AND DISCHARGE PLANNING

When providing patient–family teaching, focus on sensory information, avoid giving excessive information, and initiate a visiting nurse referral for necessary follow-up teaching and/or pulmonary rehabilitation program. Include verbal and written information about the following:

✔ Use of home $O_2$, including instructions for when to use it, importance of not increasing prescribed flow rate, precautions, community resources for $O_2$ replacement when necessary, and an absolute restriction of smoking near $O_2$.

✔ Importance of respiratory therapy consultation to assist with teaching related to $O_2$ therapy, if indicated.

✔ Medications, including drug name, route, purpose, dosage, schedule, precautions, and potential side effects. Also discuss drug–drug, herb–drug, and food–drug interactions. If patient will take corticosteroids while at home, provide instructions accordingly to ensure patient takes the prescribed amount. Have the patient perform a return demonstration of the correct use of inhalers, including spacers and rinsing of the mouth after steroid inhalation.

✔ Smoking cessation: single most effective way of reducing risk for development and progression of COPD. Nicotine replacement therapy reliably decreases smoking rates.

✔ Staying alert to public health announcements about air-quality alerts. If significant COPD is present, the patient needs to avoid outdoor exercise or stay indoors during these alerts.

✔ Signs and symptoms that necessitate medical attention to such conditions as COPD exacerbation, pneumonia/infections, or heart failure:
  • Increased dyspnea, fatigue, and coughing
  • Changes in the amount, color, or consistency of sputum
  • Fever
  • Increased swelling of ankles and legs or sudden weight gain. Patients with COPD often have

right-sided heart failure and fluid retention related to the cardiac effects of the disease. For more information, see "Heart Failure," Chapter 23.

✔ Early treatment of COPD exacerbations decreases mortality and health care costs and shortens recovery.

✔ Importance of avoiding contact with infectious individuals, especially those with respiratory infections, and limiting exposure in general during seasonal outbreaks.

✔ The CDC (2022b) recommends that all adults 65 years and older, who have never received any pneumococcal conjugate vaccine receive either the PCV15 or PCV20 vaccine. If the PCV15 is given, then the PCV23 needs to be followed by a dose of PPSV23 one year later. If an immunocompromising condition, cochlear implant, or cerebrospinal leak is present, the PPSV23 dose can be given after 8 weeks. The PPSV23 dose is not needed if the PCV20 vaccine is given. The CDC also recommends pneumococcal vaccination for adults ages 19 through 64 if certain medical conditions, such as COPD, are present. See the CDC recommendations for more information.

✔ Review of sodium-restricted diet and other dietary considerations as indicated.

✔ The need to remain active and the importance of pacing activity level and taking frequent rest periods to conserve energy.

✔ Follow-up appointment with the health care provider; confirm date and time of next appointment.

✔ Introduction to pulmonary rehabilitation programs. Physical training programs may improve ventilation and cardiac muscle function, which may compensate for non-reversible lung disease.

✔ Additional resources and patient education materials may be found at:
  • American Lung Association: www.lung.org
  • Better Breathers Club: https://www.lung.org/help-support/better-breathers-club

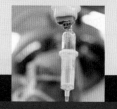

# Pneumonia 13

## OVERVIEW/PATHOPHYSIOLOGY

Pneumonia is an acute bacterial or viral infection that causes inflammation of the lung parenchyma (alveolar spaces and interstitial tissue). As a result of the inflammation involved, lung tissue becomes edematous and air spaces fill with exudate (consolidation), gas exchange cannot occur, and nonoxygenated blood is shunted into the vascular system, causing hypoxemia. Bacterial pneumonias involve all or part of a lobe, whereas viral pneumonias appear diffusely throughout the lungs.

Influenza, which can cause pneumonia, is the most serious viral airway infection for adults. Patients older than 50 years, residents of extended care facilities, and individuals with chronic health conditions have the highest mortality rate from influenza. According to the CDC (2021a), pneumonia, along with influenza, is the ninth leading cause of death in the United States.

Pneumonias generally are classified into two types: community acquired and hospital acquired (also known as nosocomial). This classification guides the health care provider in choosing the most effective antimicrobial treatment. Opportunistic pneumonia occurs in individuals with compromised immune systems.

***Community acquired.*** Community-acquired pneumonia occurs in individuals who have not been hospitalized or in a long-term care facility within 14 days and is the most common type. Individuals with community-acquired pneumonia generally do not require hospitalization unless an underlying medical condition, such as chronic obstructive pulmonary disease (COPD), cardiac disease, or diabetes mellitus, or an immunocompromised state complicates the illness.

***Hospital-acquired pneumonia.*** Hospital-acquired pneumonia (HAP) occurs in an individual 48 hours or more after admission to a hospital and was not present at admission. It usually occurs after aspiration of oropharyngeal flora or stomach contents in an individual whose resistance is altered or whose coughing mechanisms are impaired (e.g., a patient who has decreased level of consciousness [LOC], dysphagia, diminished gag reflex, or a nasogastric [NG] tube or who has undergone thoracoabdominal surgery or is on mechanical ventilation). Bacteria invade the lower respiratory tract by three routes: (1) gastric acid aspiration (the most common route), causing toxic injury to the lung; (2) obstructions (foreign body or fluids); and (3) infections (rare). Gram-negative pneumonias are associated with a high mortality rate, even with appropriate antibiotic therapy. Aspiration pneumonia is a nonbacterial (anaerobic) cause of hospital-associated pneumonia that occurs when gastric contents are aspirated.

Ventilator-associated pneumonia (VAP) is a type of HAP and defined as pneumonia occurring more than 48 hours after patients have been endotracheally intubated and receive mechanical ventilation. The risk for pneumonia increases 3- to 10-fold in patients receiving mechanical ventilation. Both HAP and VAP result in longer hospitalizations and increased mortality.

***Pneumonia in the immunocompromised individual (opportunistic pneumonia).*** Immunosuppression and neutropenia are predisposing factors in the development of nosocomial pneumonias from both common and unusual pathogens. Severely immunocompromised patients are affected not only by bacteria but also by viruses (cytomegalovirus) and fungi (*Candida, Aspergillus, Pneumocystis jirovecii*). Most commonly, *P. jirovecii* is seen in persons with human immunodeficiency virus infection or in persons who are immunosuppressed therapeutically after organ transplantation.

## HEALTH CARE SETTING

Primary care, with acute or intensive care hospitalization resulting from complications

## ASSESSMENT

Findings are influenced by patient's age, extent of the disease process, underlying medical condition, and pathogen involved. Generally, any factor that alters the integrity of the lower airways, thereby inhibiting ciliary activity, increases the likelihood of developing pneumonia.

***General signs and symptoms.*** Cough (productive and nonproductive), increased sputum (rust colored, discolored, purulent, bloody, or mucoid) production, fever, pleuritic chest pain, dyspnea, chills, headache, and myalgia. Older adults may be confused or disoriented but may present with few other signs and symptoms. They may either run a low-grade fever or be hypothermic.

***General physical assessment findings.*** Restlessness, anxiety, decreased skin turgor and dry mucous membranes secondary to dehydration, presence of nasal flaring and expiratory grunt, use of accessory muscles of respiration (scalene, sternocleidomastoid, external intercostals), decreased chest expansion caused by pleuritic pain, dullness on percussion over affected (consolidated) areas, tachypnea (respiratory rate [RR] more than 20 breaths/minute), tachycardia (resting heart rate [HR] more than 100 bpm), increased vocal fremitus, egophony ("e" to "a" change) over area of consolidation, and decreased breath sounds. Coarse or fine crackles may be heard over the affected areas. Circumoral cyanosis is a late finding.

## DIAGNOSTIC TESTS

**Chest radiography.** To confirm the presence of pneumonia which would be seen as an infiltrate over the lung fields.

**Sputum for Gram stain and culture and sensitivity tests.** Sputum is obtained from the lower respiratory tract before the initiation of antibiotic therapy to identify causative organism. It can be obtained by expectoration, suctioning, transtracheal aspiration, bronchoscopy, or open-lung biopsy.

**White blood cell count.** Will be increased (more than 15,000/mm³) in the presence of bacterial pneumonias. Normal or low white blood cell (WBC) count (less than 4000/mm³) may be seen with viral or mycoplasma pneumonias.

**Chemistry panel.** To detect the presence of hypernatremia, hyperglycemia, and/or dehydration.

**Blood culture and sensitivity.** To determine presence of bacteremia and help identify causative organism. To attain the best yield, blood cultures must be drawn before the administration of antibiotics.

**Oximetry.** May reveal decreased $O_2$ saturation (92% or less).

**Arterial blood gas values.** May vary, depending on the degree of lung involvement or other coexisting diseases. Arterial blood gases (ABGs) may demonstrate hypoxemia, hypercapnia, and/or acidosis

**Acid-fast sputum stains and cultures.** To rule out tuberculosis.

## Problem for Patients at Risk for Developing Pneumonia

### Patient Problem/Analyze Cues/Prioritize Hypotheses

# Risk for Health Care–Associated Complication (HAP)

*due to* inadequate primary defenses (e.g., decreased ciliary action), invasive procedures (e.g., intubation), immunosuppressed condition, and/or chronic disease

**Desired Outcome/Generate Solutions:** After surgery or a procedure, the patient is free of HAP as evidenced by normothermia, WBC count 11,000/mm³ or less, and sputum clear to whitish in color.

| ASSESSMENT—RECOGNIZE CUES/ INTERVENTIONS—TAKE ACTION | RATIONALES |
|---|---|
| Identify presurgical candidates who are at increased risk for HAP. | This assessment helps ensure that surgical patients remain free of infection because nosocomial pneumonia has a high morbidity and mortality rate. Factors that increase the risk for HAP in surgical patients include the following: older adult (older than 70 years), obesity, COPD, other chronic pulmonary conditions (e.g., asthma), history of smoking, abnormal pulmonary function tests (especially decreased forced expiratory flow rate), intubation, and upper abdominal/thoracic surgery. |
| Perform thorough hand hygiene before and after contact with the patient (even when gloves have been worn). | This intervention helps prevent the spread of infection by removing pathogens from the hands. |
| When appropriate, provide preoperative instructions, explaining and demonstrating pulmonary activities such as deep breathing, coughing, turning in bed, splinting wounds before breathing exercises, ambulation, maintaining adequate oral fluid intake, and use of a hyperinflation device or incentive spirometry. | These activities, when done postoperatively, are measures to prevent respiratory infection. |
| Use the Teach Back method after instructing the patient about preventative respiratory activities. Make sure the patient verbalizes knowledge of these activities and their rationales and returns demonstrations appropriately. | These actions help ensure the patient is knowledgeable and capable of performing these activities. Learning how to apply information through a return demonstration is more helpful than receiving verbal instruction alone. A knowledgeable patient is more likely to adhere to therapy. |

Continued

## ASSESSMENT—RECOGNIZE CUES/ INTERVENTIONS—TAKE ACTION

## RATIONALES

| ASSESSMENT—RECOGNIZE CUES/ INTERVENTIONS—TAKE ACTION | RATIONALES |
|---|---|
| Advise individuals who smoke to discontinue smoking, especially during preoperative and postoperative periods. Refer to a community-based smoking cessation program as needed or provide nicotine replacement therapy. | Inhalation of toxic fumes/chemical irritants can damage cilia and lung tissue and is a factor that increases the likelihood of developing pneumonia. |
| Administer analgesics 1/2-hour before deep-breathing exercises. Support (splint) the surgical wound with hands, pillows, or folded blanket placed firmly across the site of incision. | These interventions help control pain, which otherwise would interfere with lung expansion. |
| Identify patients who are at increased risk for aspiration. | Individuals with depressed LOC, advanced age, dysphagia, or an NG or enteral tube in place are at risk for aspiration, which predisposes them to pneumonia. |
| Maintain the head of bed at 30- to 45-degree elevation, and turn the patient into a side-lying position. When the patient receives enteral tube feedings, recommend continuous rather than bolus feedings. Hold feedings when the patient is lying flat. | These measures can reduce the risk of aspiration, which is a leading cause of HAP. |
| Recognize risk factors for infection in patients with tracheostomy and intervene as follows: | Risk factors include the presence of underlying lung disease or other serious illness, increased colonization of oropharynx or trachea by aerobic Gram-negative bacteria, greater access of bacteria to the lower respiratory tract, and cross-contamination caused by manipulation of the tracheostomy tube. |
| • Perform hand hygiene, and wear gloves on both hands when handling the tube or when handling mechanical ventilation tubing. | Loss of skin integrity or space around the tube would enable the ingress of pathogens by the wound or tube. |
| • Suction as needed rather than on a routine basis. | Frequent suctioning increases the risk for trauma and cross-contamination. |
| • Always wear gloves on both hands to suction. Use a sterile catheter for each suctioning procedure. Consider the use of closed suction system; replace closed suction system per agency policy. Always replace the suction system between patients. Use only sterile fluids and dispense them using sterile technique. Change breathing circuits according to agency policy. Fill fluid reservoirs immediately before use (not far in advance). | These practices further decrease the risk for contamination. |
| • Avoid saline instillation during suctioning. If the patient has tenacious secretions, increase heat and humidity. | Saline instillation can cause dislodgment of bacteria into the lower lung fields, increasing the risk for inflammation and invasion of sterile tissue. It can also stimulate coughing. |
| • Avoid the following when working with nebulizer reservoirs: introduction of nonsterile fluids or air, manipulation of the nebulizer cup, or backflow of condensate from delivery tubing into the reservoir or into the patient when tubing is manipulated. | These are ways in which nebulizer reservoirs can contaminate patients. |
| • Discard any fluid that has condensed in tubing; do not allow it to drain back into the reservoir or into the patient. | |

See also *Risk for Infection* in Chapter 2.

## Problems for Patients with Pneumonia

## Patient Problem/Analyze Cues/Prioritize Hypotheses

# Impaired Gas Exchange

*due to* altered oxygen supply and alveolar-capillary membrane changes occurring with the inflammatory process and exudate in the lungs

*Desired Outcome/Generate Solutions:* At least 24 hours before hospital discharge, the patient is experiencing PaO$_2$ at 92 mm Hg or higher and PaCO$_2$ levels between 35 and 45 mm Hg and no signs of respiratory distress.

| ASSESSMENT—RECOGNIZE CUES/ INTERVENTIONS—TAKE ACTION | RATIONALES |
|---|---|
| Monitor for and promptly report signs and symptoms of respiratory distress. Signs and symptoms of respiratory distress include restlessness, anxiety, mental status changes, shortness of breath, tachypnea, and use of accessory muscles of respiration. | Respiratory distress necessitates prompt medical intervention. |
| Auscultate breath sounds at least every 2–4 hours or as indicated by the patient's condition. Report significant findings. | Decreased or adventitious sounds (e.g., crackles, wheezes) can signal potential respiratory failure that would further aggravate hypoxia and necessitate prompt intervention. |
| Monitor and document vital signs (VS) every 2–4 hours or as indicated by the patient's condition. Report significant findings. | A rising temperature and other changes in VS (e.g., increased HR and RR) may signal the presence of worsening inflammatory response in the lungs. This could cause further hypoxia, contributing to adult respiratory distress syndrome and need for mechanical ventilation. |
| Administer antibiotics as soon as possible (following established guidelines) but after blood and sputum cultures have been obtained. Continue antibiotics as prescribed. **Note:** Do not delay antibiotic therapy if specimens cannot be obtained. | Early administration of antibiotics decreases inflammatory response in the lung, promoting healing and reducing the risk for mortality. Administration of antibiotics before cultures are obtained may alter results. Proper identification of the organism and determination of sensitivity to specific antibiotics are critical for appropriate therapy. |
| Monitor oximetry readings; report O$_2$ saturation of 92% or less. | O$_2$ saturation of 92% or less is a sign of a significant oxygenation problem and can indicate the need for O$_2$ therapy. |
| Administer oxygen as prescribed. | Oxygen is administered when O$_2$ saturation or ABG results demonstrate hypoxemia. Initially, oxygen is delivered in low concentrations, and oxygen saturation is watched closely. If O$_2$ saturation does not rise to an acceptable level (more than 92%), FiO$_2$ is increased in small increments, with concomitant checks of O$_2$ saturations or obtaining ABG values. Significant increases in oxygen requirements to maintain O$_2$ saturations greater than 92% need to be reported promptly. |
| Monitor ABG results. | Acute hypoxemia (PaO$_2$ less than 80 mm Hg) often indicates the need for oxygen therapy. Hypocarbia (PaCO$_2$ less than 35 mm Hg), with a resultant respiratory alkalosis (pH greater than 7.45) in the absence of an underlying pulmonary disease, is consistent with pneumonia. However, if pneumonia progresses to acute respiratory distress, respiratory acidosis will result. |
| Position the patient for comfort (usually semi-Fowler position). | This position provides comfort, promotes diaphragmatic descent, maximizes inhalations, and decreases work of breathing. Gravity and hydrostatic pressure when the patient is in this position promote perfusion and ventilation-perfusion matching. In patients with unilateral pneumonia, positioning on the unaffected side (i.e., "good side down") promotes ventilation-perfusion matching. |
| Facilitate coordination across the health care team to provide rest periods between care activities. Allow 90 minutes for undisturbed rest. | Rest decreases oxygen demand in a patient whose reserves are likely limited. |

## Patient Problem/Analyze Cues/Prioritize Hypotheses

# Risk for Impaired Airway Clearance

*due to* the presence of excessive tracheobronchial secretions occurring with infection

*Desired Outcomes/Generate Solutions:* After instruction, the patient demonstrates an effective cough. After interventions, the patient's airway is free of excessive secretions and adventitious breath sounds.

| ASSESSMENT—RECOGNIZE CUES/ INTERVENTIONS—TAKE ACTION | RATIONALES |
|---|---|
| Auscultate breath sounds every 2–4 hours (or as indicated by the patient's condition) and report changes in the patient's ability to clear pulmonary secretions. | This assessment determines the presence of adventitious breath sounds (e.g., crackles, wheezes). Coarse crackles are a sign the patient needs to cough. Fine crackles at lung bases likely will clear with deep breathing. Wheezing is a sign of airway obstruction, which necessitates prompt intervention to ensure effective gas exchange. |
| Inspect sputum for quantity, odor, color, and consistency; document findings. | As the patient's condition worsens, sputum can become more copious and change in color from clear/white to yellow and/or green, or it may show other discoloration characteristics of underlying bacterial infection (e.g., rust colored; "currant jelly"). |
| Ensure that the patient performs deep breathing with coughing exercises at least every 2 hours. Controlled coughing includes tightening upper abdominal muscles while coughing 2 to 3 times. | These exercises help clear airways of secretions. Controlled coughing ensures a more effective cough because it uses the diaphragmatic muscles, which increases the forcefulness of the effort. |
| Assist the patient into a position of comfort, usually semi-Fowler position. | This position provides comfort and facilitates ease and effectiveness of these exercises by promoting better lung expansion (there is less lung compression by abdominal organs) and gas exchange. |
| Assess the need for hyperinflation therapy. Instruct as needed: The patient inhales slowly and deeply two times normal tidal volume and holds the breath for at least 5 seconds at the end of inspiration. To maintain adequate alveolar inflation, 10 such breaths/hour are recommended. | The patient's inability to take deep breaths is a sign of the need for this therapy. Deep inhalation with a hyperinflation device expands alveoli and helps mobilize secretions to the airways, and coughing further mobilizes and clears the secretions. Emphasis of this therapy is on inhalation to expand the lungs maximally. |
| ❗ Report complications of hyperinflation therapy to the health care provider. | Complications include hyperventilation, gastric distention, headache, hypotension, and signs and symptoms of pneumothorax (shortness of breath, sharp chest pain, unilateral diminished breath sounds, dyspnea, cough). |
| Instruct the patient to splint the chest with pillow, folded blanket, or crossed arms, when coughing. | This action reduces pain while coughing, thereby promoting a more effective cough. |
| Instruct patients who are unable to cough effectively in a cascade cough. | A cascade cough removes secretions and improves ventilation by a succession of shorter and more forceful exhalations than are done with the usual coughing exercise. |
| Deliver oxygen with humidity as prescribed. | This intervention provides oxygenation while decreasing convective losses of moisture and helping mobilize secretions. |
| Assist the patient with position changes every 2 hours. If the patient is ambulatory, encourage ambulation to the patient's tolerance. | Movement and activity help mobilize secretions to facilitate airway clearance. |
| Suction as prescribed and indicated. | Suctioning maintains a patent airway by removing secretions. |
| When not contraindicated, encourage fluid intake (2.5 L/day or more). | Increasing hydration decreases viscosity of the sputum, which will make it easier to raise and expectorate. |

## Patient Problem/Analyze Cues/Prioritize Hypotheses

# Dehydration

*due to* increased insensible loss occurring with tachypnea, fever, or diaphoresis

***Desired Outcome/Generate Solutions:*** At least 24 hours before hospital discharge, the patient is normovolemic as evidenced by urine output of 0.5 mL/kg/hour or more, stable weight, HR less than 100 bpm, SBP greater than 90 mm Hg, fluid intake approximating fluid output, moist mucous membranes, and elastic skin turgor.

## ASSESSMENT—RECOGNIZE CUES/ INTERVENTIONS—TAKE ACTION

| ASSESSMENT—RECOGNIZE CUES/ INTERVENTIONS—TAKE ACTION | RATIONALES |
|---|---|
| Assess intake and output. Be alert to and report urinary output less than 0.5 mL/kg/hour. | This assessment monitors the trend of fluid volume. An indicator of dehydration is urinary output less than 0.5 mL/kg/hour for 2 consecutive hours. Consider insensible losses if the patient is diaphoretic and tachypneic. |
| Weigh the patient daily at the same time of day and on the same scale; record weight. Report weight changes of 1–1.5 kg/day. | These actions ensure consistency and accuracy of weight measurements. Weight changes of 1–1.5 kg/day can occur with fluid overload or dehydration. |
| Encourage fluid intake (at least 2.5 L/day in unrestricted patients). Maintain intravenous fluid therapy as prescribed. | These actions help ensure adequate hydration. |
| Promote oral hygiene, including lip and tongue care. | Oral hygiene moistens dried tissues and mucous membranes in patients with fluid volume deficit. |
| Provide humidity for oxygen therapy. | Humidity helps minimize convective losses of moisture during oxygen therapy. |

## ADDITIONAL PROBLEMS FOR PATIENTS ON MECHANICAL VENTILATION

*"General Care of Patients with Neurologic Disorders"*    Chapter 36
*for Risk for Infection, due to inadequate primary defenses occurring with intubation*

 **PATIENT–FAMILY TEACHING AND DISCHARGE PLANNING**

When providing patient–family teaching, focus on sensory information, avoid giving excessive information, and initiate a visiting nurse referral for necessary follow-up teaching. Include verbal and written information about the following:

✓ Techniques that promote gas exchange and minimize stasis of secretions (e.g., deep breathing, coughing, use of incentive spirometer, increasing activity level as appropriate for patient's medical condition, percussion, and postural drainage as necessary).

✓ Medications, including drug name, purpose, dosage, frequency or schedule, precautions, and potential side effects, particularly of antibiotics. Also discuss drug–drug, herb–drug, and food–drug interactions. Instruct patient to complete full dose of antibiotics to prevent reinfection and subsequent readmission.

✓ Signs and symptoms of pneumonia and importance of reporting them promptly to the health care professional if they recur. Inform the patient's significant others that changes in mental status may be the only indicator of pneumonia in older adults.

✓ Importance of preventing fatigue by pacing activities and allowing frequent rest periods.

✓ Importance of avoiding exposure to individuals known to have flu and colds and reducing exposure in general during seasonal outbreaks.

✓ Vaccinations: The CDC (2022b) recommends that all adults 65 years and older, who have never received any pneumococcal conjugate vaccine receive either the PCV15 or PCV20 vaccine. If the PCV15 is given, then the PCV23 needs to be followed by a dose of PPSV23 one year later. If an immunocompromising condition, cochlear implant, or cerebrospinal leak is present, the PPSV23 dose can be given after 8 weeks. The PPSV23 dose is not needed if the PCV20 vaccine is given. The CDC also recommends pneumococcal vaccination for adults ages 19 through 64 if certain medical conditions, such as COPD, are present. See the CDC recommendations for more information. Recommendation that the following individuals receive an influenza vaccination annually: all persons 6 months and older with rare exception (e.g., allergy, history of Guillain–Barré). Influenza vaccines are routinely administered from the months of October through March, but ideally should be given in October (CDC, 2021).

✓ Minimizing factors that can cause reinfection, including close living conditions, poor nutrition, and poorly ventilated living quarters or work environment.

✓ Importance of smoking cessation education and community resources to assist in cessation. Information on smoking cessation programs and information
• Smoke Free: https://smokefree.gov/
• Quit Smoking (American Lung Association): https://www.lung.org/quit-smoking/smoking-facts
• How to Quit Smoking (CDC): https://www.cdc.gov/tobacco/campaign/tips/quit-smoking/index.html

✓ Additional general information can be obtained by visiting www.lung.org

✓ Phone numbers to call in case questions or concerns arise about therapy or disease after discharge.

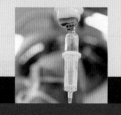

# Pneumothorax/Hemothorax 14

## OVERVIEW/PATHOPHYSIOLOGY

Pneumothorax is an accumulation of air in the pleural space that leads to increased intrapleural pressure. Risk factors include blunt or penetrating chest injury, chronic obstructive pulmonary disease (COPD), previous pneumothorax, and positive pressure ventilation. Types of pneumothorax include spontaneous, traumatic, and tension pneumothorax, as well as hemothorax.

***Spontaneous.*** Also referred to as *closed pneumothorax* because the chest wall remains intact with no leak to the atmosphere. It results from the rupture of a bleb or bulla on the visceral pleural surface, usually near the apex. Generally, the cause of the rupture is unknown, although it may result from a weakness related to a respiratory infection or from an underlying pulmonary disease (e.g., COPD, tuberculosis, malignant neoplasm). Smoking also increases the risk for spontaneous pneumothorax. Other risk factors include being tall, thin, male, and usually young (20–40 years). previously healthy or having a family history of spontaneous pneumothorax. Generally, the onset of symptoms occurs at rest rather than with vigorous exercise or coughing. There is a 15%–40% risk of recurrence for spontaneous pneumothorax (McKnight & Burns, 2021).

***Traumatic.*** Can be open or closed. An *open pneumothorax* occurs when air enters the pleural space from the atmosphere through an opening in the chest wall, such as with a gunshot wound, stab wound, or invasive medical procedure (e.g., lung biopsy, thoracentesis, or placement of a central line into a subclavian vein). A sucking sound may be heard over the area of penetration during inspiration, accounting for the classic wound description as a "sucking chest wound." A *closed pneumothorax* occurs when the visceral pleura is penetrated but the chest wall remains intact with no atmospheric leak. This usually occurs after blunt trauma that results in rib fracture and dislocation. It also may occur from the use of positive end-expiratory pressure or after cardiopulmonary resuscitation.

***Tension.*** Generally occurs with closed pneumothorax; also can occur with open pneumothorax when a flap of tissue acts as a one-way valve. Air enters the pleural space through the pleural tear when the individual inhales, and it continues to accumulate but cannot escape during expiration because the tissue flap closes. With tension pneumothorax, as pressure in the thorax and mediastinum increases, it produces a shift in the affected lung and mediastinum toward the unaffected side, which further impairs ventilatory efforts. The increase in pressure also compresses the vena cava, which impedes venous return, leading to a decrease in cardiac output and, ultimately, to circulatory collapse if the condition is not diagnosed and treated quickly. Tension pneumothorax is a life-threatening medical emergency.

***Hemothorax.*** Hemothorax is an accumulation of blood in the pleural space. Hemothorax generally results from blunt trauma to the chest wall, but it can also occur after thoracic surgery, after penetrating gunshot or stab wounds, as a result of anticoagulant therapy, after insertion of a central venous catheter, or after various thoracoabdominal organ biopsies. Mediastinal shift, ventilatory compromise, and lung collapse can occur, depending on the amount of blood accumulated.

## HEALTH CARE SETTING

Acute care, primary care

## DIAGNOSTIC TESTS

***Chest radiography.*** Will reveal the presence of air or blood in the pleural space on the affected side, pneumothorax/hemothorax size, and any shift in the mediastinum.

***Computed tomography.*** Used when a chest radiograph cannot confirm or exclude the presence of a pneumothorax or hemothorax or for the evaluation of recurrent spontaneous pneumothorax.

***Oximetry.*** Will reveal decreased $O_2$ saturation (92% or less).

***Arterial blood gas values.*** Hypoxemia ($PaO_2$ less than 80 mm Hg) may be accompanied by hypercarbia ($PaCO_2$ greater than 45 mm Hg) with resultant respiratory acidosis (pH less than 7.35).

***Complete blood count.*** May reveal decreased hemoglobin proportionate to the amount of blood lost in a hemothorax or if other trauma is present.

## Assessment

Clinical manifestations will vary, depending on the type and size of the pneumothorax or hemothorax.

| Pneumothorax | Tension Pneumothorax | Hemothorax |
|---|---|---|
| **Small pneumothorax:** mild tachycardia and dyspnea may be the only symptoms.<br>**Large pneumothorax:** respiratory distress (dyspnea, short, shallow, and rapid respirations), air hunger, decreasing PaO$_2$ levels. Breath sounds over affected area absent. | Severe dyspnea, anxiety, tachycardia, cyanosis, jugular vein distention, tracheal deviation toward the unaffected side, decreased or absent breath sounds on affected side, neck vein distention, cyanosis, profuse diaphoresis, hypotension, change in mental status | Tachypnea, pallor, cyanosis, dullness over affected side, tachycardia, hypotension, diminished or absent breath sounds, change in mental status |

## Patient Problem/Analyze Cues/Prioritize Hypothesis

# Impaired Gas Exchange

*due to* decreased lung expansion occurring with pneumothorax/hemothorax, pain, or malfunction of the chest drainage system

***Desired Outcome/Generate Solutions:*** After interventions, the patient becomes eupneic; lung expansion is noted on chest radiograph. At a minimum of 24 hours before hospital discharge, the patient's arterial blood gas (ABG) values are as follows: PaO$_2$ of 80 mm Hg or more and PaCO$_2$ of 35–45 mm Hg (or values within patient's acceptable baseline parameters), or O$_2$ saturation greater than 92%.

| ASSESSMENT—RECOGNIZE CUES/ INTERVENTIONS—TAKE ACTION | RATIONALES |
|---|---|
| Assess the patient's mental, respiratory, and cardiac status at frequent intervals (every 2–4 hours, as appropriate). Also assess the status and functioning of the chest drainage system. | This assessment monitors the patient's status while the chest drainage system is in place. The purpose of a chest drainage system is to drain air or fluid and reexpand the lung. Diminished breath sounds, along with tachycardia, restlessness, anxiety, and changes in mental status, are signs of respiratory distress that may occur as a result of chest drainage system malfunction and the chest tube insert site. If these signs are present, prompt intervention is necessary to prevent further hypoxia and distress (Light, 2017). |
| Assess and maintain the closed-chest drainage system as follows: | These actions help ensure the maintenance of the closed-chest drainage system and facilitate drainage. |
| • Tape all connections and secure the chest tube to the thorax with tape or other securement devices. | |
| • Avoid all tubing kinks, and ensure that the bed and equipment are not compressing any component of the system. Eliminate all dependent loops in tubing. | These actions help ensure the maintenance of the chest drainage system and facilitate drainage. |
| • Many closed systems come prefilled with water. Otherwise, maintain fluid in the water-seal chamber and suction chamber at appropriate levels. | The suction apparatus does not regulate the amount of suction applied to the closed-chest drainage system. The amount of suction is determined by the water level in the suction control chamber. |
| • Monitor bubbling in the water-seal chamber. | Intermittent bubbling in this chamber is normal and signals that air is leaving the pleural space. Intermittent bubbling with coughing and exhalation is also normal. Absence of bubbling indicates the system is malfunctioning and suction is not being maintained. Immediate intervention will be needed to correct the suction. |

Continued

| ASSESSMENT—RECOGNIZE CUES/ INTERVENTIONS—TAKE ACTION | RATIONALES |
|---|---|
| • Locate and seal any leak in the system if possible. | Continuous bubbling in the water-seal chamber may be a signal that air is leaking into the drainage system. |
| | Check to see whether the leak is in the equipment or patient. If the bubbling continues after suction is turned off, the leak is in the patient and not the equipment. Prepare to investigate and seal off the air leak to prevent subcutaneous air leakage at the patient's insertion site and worsening of the pneumothorax. |
| • Dial the level of dry suction per the health care provider's recommendation. | This action maintains air and fluid removal from the pleural space. |
| | **Note:** Suction aids in lung reexpansion, but removing suction for short periods, such as for transporting, will not be detrimental or disrupt the closed-chest drainage system. |
| • Monitor fluctuations in the water-seal chamber. | These fluctuations are characteristic of a patent chest tube, and the water level may rise and fall with respirations. Fluctuations stop when either the lung has reexpanded or there is a kink or obstruction in the chest tube. |
| ⚠ • Do not strip the chest tubes. | This mechanism for maintaining chest tube patency is not recommended and has been associated with creating high negative pressures in the pleural space, which can damage fragile lung tissue. |
| ⚠ Keep the following necessary emergency supplies at the bedside: | |
| • Petrolatum gauze pad | This gauze pad is applied over the insertion site if the chest tube becomes dislodged. Use of this dressing provides an airtight seal over the insertion site to prevent recurrent pneumothorax. |
| • A bottle of sterile water | Submerging the chest tube in a bottle of sterile water if it becomes disconnected from the water-seal system provides for a temporary closed-chest drainage system. Follow the facility's protocol. |
| ⚠ Never clamp a chest tube without a specific directive from the health care provider. | Clamping may lead to tension pneumothorax because air in the pleural space no longer can escape. |
| Use the sterile technique when changing the chest tube dressing. Monitor for signs of infection (redness, drainage) and report if present. | Infection is a potential complication of chest tube therapy; early detection will prompt immediate treatment for infection. |

## Patient Problem/Analyze Cues/Prioritize Hypotheses

# Impaired Gas Exchange

*due to* ventilation-perfusion mismatch

***Desired Outcomes/Generate Outcomes:*** After treatment/interventions, the patient exhibits adequate gas exchange and ventilatory function, as evidenced by respiratory rate (RR) of 20 breaths/minute or less with normal depth and pattern (eupnea); no significant mental status changes; and orientation to person, place, and time. At a minimum of 24 hours before hospital discharge, the patient's ABG values are as follows: $PaO_2$ of 80 mm Hg or more and $PaCO_2$ of 35–45 mm Hg (or values within patient's acceptable baseline parameters), or $O_2$ saturation greater than 92%.

| ASSESSMENT—RECOGNIZE CUES/ INTERVENTIONS—TAKE ACTION | RATIONALES |
|---|---|
| ⚠ Monitor serial ABG results or oximetry readings. Report significant findings to the health care provider. | These assessments detect decreasing $PaO_2$ or $O_2$ saturation and increasing $PaCO_2$, which can signal impending respiratory compromise and necessitate prompt intervention. |

| ASSESSMENT—RECOGNIZE CUES/ INTERVENTIONS—TAKE ACTION | RATIONALES |
|---|---|
| ⚠ Assess for indicators of hypoxia. Report significant findings. | Increased restlessness, anxiety, tachycardia, and changes in mental status are early indicators of hypoxia and can signal impending respiratory compromise, which would necessitate prompt intervention. |
| ⚠ Assess vital signs and breath sounds every 2 hours or as indicated by the patient's condition. Report significant findings. | These assessments monitor patient trends. Significant changes such as increased heart rate (HR), increased RR, and unilateral decreased breath sounds signal a worsening or unresolved condition. |
| ⚠ Following chest tube placement or exploratory thoracotomy, assess the patient every 15 minutes until stable. Report significant findings, such as increased RR, diminished or absent movement of the chest wall on the affected side, paradoxical movement of the chest wall, increased work of breathing, use of accessory muscles of respiration, complaints of increased dyspnea, unilateral diminished breath sounds, and cyanosis. | These assessments enable prompt detection of respiratory distress for timely intervention, including |
| ⚠ Evaluate HR and blood pressure for tachycardia and hypotension. Report significant findings. | Tachycardia, along with tachypnea, is a compensatory mechanism that results from hypoxia/hypoxemia. Tachycardia and hypotension are indicators of shock. |
| Support the patient in an optimal position (e.g., semi-Fowler). | This position provides comfort and enables full expansion of the unaffected lung, adequate expansion of the chest wall, and descent of the diaphragm. |
| Change the patient's position every 2 hours. | This intervention promotes drainage and lung reexpansion and facilitates alveolar perfusion. |
| Encourage the patient to take deep breaths, providing necessary analgesia to decrease discomfort during deep-breathing exercises. Instruct the patient in splinting the thoracotomy site with arms, a pillow, or folded blanket. | Deep breathing promotes full lung expansion and decreases the risk for atelectasis. Analgesia and splinting decrease discomfort during deep-breathing exercises. Coughing facilitates mobilization of tracheobronchial secretions, if present. |
| Deliver and monitor oxygen and humidity as indicated for patients with oxygen saturation of 92% or less. | This intervention ensures adequate oxygen levels if the patient has hypoxemia, which is likely to be present if the pneumothorax/ hemothorax is large. Humidity minimizes convective losses of moisture. |

## Patient Problem/Analyze Cues/Prioritize Hypotheses

# Acute Pain

*due to* impaired pleural integrity, inflammation, presence of a chest tube, or surgical intervention

**Desired Outcome/Generate Solutions:** Within 1 hour of intervention, the patient's subjective perception of pain decreases, as documented by a patient-reported pain scale.

| ASSESSMENT—RECOGNIZE CUES/ INTERVENTIONS—TAKE ACTION | RATIONALES |
|---|---|
| At frequent intervals, assess the patient's degree of discomfort, using the patient's verbal and nonverbal cues. Use a self-report pain scale with the patient, rating pain from 0 (no pain) to 10 (worst pain). | These assessments monitor the patient's trend of pain and help determine the success of subsequent pain interventions. |
| Medicate with analgesics as prescribed, using a pain scale to evaluate and document medication effectiveness. | These actions provide pain relief and determine the effectiveness of the analgesia. |

Continued

| ASSESSMENT—RECOGNIZE CUES/ INTERVENTIONS—TAKE ACTION | RATIONALES |
|---|---|
| Encourage the patient to request analgesics before the pain becomes severe or, alternatively, administer analgesics at scheduled intervals. | Prolonged stimulation of pain receptors results in increased sensitivity to painful stimuli and increases the amount of analgesia required to relieve pain. |
| Premedicate the patient 30 minutes before initiating coughing, exercising, or repositioning. | This intervention provides comfort during painful exercises, procedures, and repositioning and facilitates compliance. |
| Instruct the patient to splint the affected side when coughing, moving, or repositioning. | This action reduces discomfort and promotes adherence to the treatment plan. |
| Facilitate coordination among health care providers to provide rest periods between care activities. Allow 90 minutes for undisturbed rest. | Relaxation and rest decrease oxygen demand, may decrease the level of pain, and promote healing. |
| Stabilize the chest tube with tape or a securement device securely to the thorax, positioning the tube to ensure there are no dependent loops. | These actions reduce pull or drag on latex connector tubing, prevent discomfort, facilitate drainage, prevent tube dislodgment, and facilitate appropriate device functioning. |

For additional interventions, see "Pain," p. Chapter 5.

## ADDITIONAL PROBLEMS:

| | |
|---|---|
| "Psychosocial Support for the Patient" | Chapter 8 |
| "Abdominal Trauma" for *Risk for Hemorrhaging* | Chapter 53 |

 **PATIENT–FAMILY TEACHING AND DISCHARGE PLANNING**

When providing patient–family teaching, focus on sensory information, avoid giving excessive information, and initiate a visiting nurse referral for necessary follow-up teaching. Include verbal and written information about the following:
- ✓ Purpose for chest tube placement and maintenance.
- ✓ Pain management.

- ✓ Purpose for surgical intervention, if required, including risks/benefits and recovery.
- ✓ Potential for recurrence of spontaneous pneumothorax. Explain the importance of seeking medical care immediately if symptoms recur.
- ✓ Instruct the patient not to fly or scuba dive for a minimum of 2 weeks; those with occupations that involve flying or scuba diving will need to be medically cleared before returning to work (McKnight & Burns, 2021).
- ✓ Medications, including drug name, purpose, dosage, schedule, precautions, and potential side effects. Also discuss drug–drug, herb–drug, and food–drug interactions. Importance of smoking cessation to prevent further pulmonary injury.

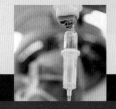

# Pulmonary Embolus 15

## OVERVIEW/PATHOPHYSIOLOGY

Pulmonary embolus (PE) is an obstruction of the pulmonary artery or one of its branches by substances (i.e., blood clot, fat, air, amniotic fluid) that originated elsewhere in the body. The most common source is a dislodged blood clot from the systemic circulation, typically the deep veins of the legs. Other sources include the pelvis (after surgery or childbirth) or the right side of the heart when atrial fibrillation is present, thrombus formation is the result of the following factors: blood stasis, alterations in clotting factors, and injury to vessel walls (see Chapter 26 for information on risk factors for venous thromboembolism [VTE]). Patients develop signs and symptoms immediately after obstruction to the pulmonary vessels. Massive acute PE causes hypotension (systolic blood pressure [SBP] less than 90 mm Hg or a greater than or equal to 40-mm Hg decrease from baseline in a 15-minute period), with accompanying right heart failure unexplained by a cardiac cause. Death occurs within the first hour in 10% of cases, but early diagnosis and intervention can reduce mortality. According to the CDC (2020), 30% of people with deep vein thrombosis or PE are at high risk for another episode. A fat embolus is the most common nonthrombotic cause of pulmonary perfusion disorders. Fat can escape into the blood from the bone marrow when a long bone is fractured or during bone surgery and form an embolus. Other less common sources of emboli include air emboli from improperly administered IV therapy; amniotic fluid; cancer; and bacterial vegetation on heart valves.

With treatment, most pulmonary emboli resolve and leave no residual deficits; however, some patients may be left with chronic pulmonary hypertension. Pulmonary infarction is another possible complication.

## HEALTH CARE SETTING

Acute care

## ASSESSMENT

Signs and symptoms often are nonspecific and variable, depending on the type, size, and extent of obstruction and whether the patient has an infarction as a result of the obstruction. Very small emboli may either go undetected or cause vague symptoms that come and go. The most common symptom is dyspnea, with mild to moderate hypoxemia. Tachypnea, cough, chest pain, hemoptysis, crackles, wheezing, tachycardia, and syncope may occur. If a massive PE is present, hypotension and a sudden change in mental status may occur. The patient may express feelings of impending doom; cardiopulmonary arrest may result.

## DIAGNOSTIC TESTS

*Arterial blood gas values.* Arterial blood gases provide important information but do not diagnose PE. Hypoxemia ($PaO_2$ less than 80 mm Hg), hypocarbia (hypocapnia) ($PaCO_2$ less than 35 mm Hg), and respiratory alkalosis (pH more than 7.45) usually are present. A normal $PaO_2$ does not rule out the presence of pulmonary emboli.

*D-Dimer.* This test measures the amount of cross-linked fibrin fragments, which are the result of clot degradation. However, the D-dimer test is not specific to PE; other conditions can cause abnormal results. If a PE is suspected and a D-dimer level is elevated, further testing is necessary to diagnose PE.

*Other testing.* Chest x-ray initial findings are normal, or an elevated hemidiaphragm may be present. After 24 hours, radiographic examination may reveal small infiltrates secondary to atelectasis that results from the decrease in surfactant. If pulmonary infarction is present, infiltrates and pleural effusions may be seen within 12–36 hours. ECG may show nonspecific ST segment and T wave changes. Serum troponin levels and b-type natriuretic peptide levels are often elevated. However, none of these tests are specific to a PE diagnosis.

*Spiral (helical) computed tomography.* This is the most common test used to diagnose PE and requires an intravenous injection of contrast media. The pulmonary blood vessels then become visible; the scanner rotates continuously around the patient during the test, and the resulting image produces a 3-D picture of all areas of the lungs and makes PEs visible.

*Pulmonary ventilation-perfusion scan.* This test is used when patients cannot receive contrast media due to an allergy or renal problems. It is used to detect abnormalities of ventilation or perfusion in the pulmonary system. It consists of two parts. The perfusion scanning involves the use of an intravenously injected radioisotope; as a result, the pulmonary circulation is assessed. The ventilation scanning requires the patient to inhale radioactive gas (such as xenon). The scanning reflects the distribution of the gas through the lungs. This portion of the test requires the patient to participate; mechanically ventilated patients cannot perform this test.

## TREATMENT

Patients with PE require immediate anticoagulation. Subcutaneous low-molecular-weight heparin such as enoxaparin, fondaparinux, or fragmin is the recommended treatment for acute PE. These drugs are considered safer and more effective than unfractionated heparin, and do not require laboratory monitoring of the activated partial thromboplastin time (aPTT). Oral drug therapy for patients with PE occurs in three phases: the initial phase: first 7 days; longer: up to 6 weeks; extended: 6 months and beyond. Oral anticoagulants include warfarin (Coumadin), apixaban (Eliquis), dabigatran (Pradaxa), and edoxaban (Savaysa). Some health care providers may treat PE with direct thrombin inhibitors or fibrinolytic agents, such as tissue plasminogen activator or alteplase (Activase).

### Patient Problem/Analyze Cues/Prioritize Hypotheses

# Impaired Hematologic System Function (Excessive Clotting)

*due to* venous stasis, hypercoagulable state, and/or vessel injury contributing to VTE

**Desired Outcome/Generate Solutions:** After treatment/interventions, the patient exhibits no new venous thromboembolic events (see descriptions under Assessment, earlier).

| ASSESSMENT—RECOGNIZE CUES/ INTERVENTIONS—TAKE ACTION | RATIONALES |
|---|---|
| Assess for risk factors relating to VTE. Examples include advanced age, surgery, smoking, hormone therapy, chemotherapeutic drugs, and immobility. | Risk factors alone or in combination increase the risk for developing VTE. |
| Provide instruction on the use of warfarin or the newer oral anticoagulants, as appropriate. | Use of warfarin is complicated by the need for frequent monitoring of the international normalized ratio (INR), dietary restrictions, and concerns about its interactions with many other drugs. |
| | The new oral anticoagulants, which include dabigatran (Pradaxa), apixaban (Eliquis), and edoxaban (Savaysa), do not require routine INR-type monitoring, have no dietary restrictions, and may have fewer drug interactions than warfarin, but there is no fixed method for determining the extent of their anticoagulant effect. In addition, they have short half-lives that increase the risk for thrombosis with missed doses, and they are not recommended for use in patients with end-stage renal disease or liver dysfunction. |
| Encourage ambulation and monitor activity. | Increased ambulation prevents venous stasis, a major risk factor for the development of VTE. |

### Patient Problems/Analyze Cues/Prioritize Hypotheses

# Dyspnea/Impaired Gas Exchange

*due to* pulmonary perfusion disorder

**Desired Outcomes/Generate Solutions:** After treatments/interventions, the patient exhibits adequate gas exchange and ventilatory function as evidenced by respiratory rate (RR) of 12–20 breaths/minute with normal pattern and depth (eupnea); no significant changes in mental status; and orientation to person, place, and time. At a minimum of 24 hours before hospital discharge, the patient has $O_2$ saturation greater than 92% or $PaO_2$ of 80 mm Hg or higher (or adjusted for altitude), $PaCO_2$ of 35–45 mm Hg, and pH of 7.35–7.45 (or values consistent with the patient's acceptable baseline parameters).

| ASSESSMENT—RECOGNIZE CUES/ INTERVENTIONS—TAKE ACTION | RATIONALES |
|---|---|
| Assess the patient for RR increased from baseline and increasing dyspnea, anxiety, restlessness, confusion, and cyanosis. Report significant findings. | These signs and symptoms of increasing respiratory distress and indicators of PE necessitate prompt intervention. |
| As indicated, monitor oximetry readings. Report O$_2$ saturation of 92% or less. | A low O$_2$ saturation may indicate the need for O$_2$ therapy. A poor response to treatment or worsening O$_2$ saturation necessitates prompt reporting for timely evaluation and further treatment. Hypoxia is common with PE, although its absence does not mean that the patient does not have a PE. |
| Instruct the patient not to cross legs when lying in bed or sitting in a chair. | Legs that are crossed impede venous return from the legs and can increase the risk for PE. |
| Pace the patient's activities and procedures. | Pacing activities and procedures decrease metabolic demands for oxygen and prevent further complications related to immobility. |
| | **Note:** It is safe for patients to ambulate after anticoagulation has been started. |
| Ensure that the patient performs deep breathing and coughing exercises 5–10 times every 2 hours. | These exercises mobilize secretions and improve ventilation. |
| Ensure delivery of prescribed concentrations and humidity of oxygen. | Supplemental oxygen helps maintain a PaO$_2$ optimally 80 mm Hg or greater. Humidifying the oxygen minimizes convective losses of moisture. |

## Patient Problem/Analyze Cues/Prioritize Hypotheses

# Risk for Hemorrhaging

*due to* anticoagulation therapy

***Desired Outcome/Generate Solutions:*** The patient is free of frank or occult bleeding and exhibits the following signs of hemodynamic stability: heart rate less than 120 bpm, SBP greater than 90 mm Hg or returned to baseline, and RR of 20 breaths/minute or less.

| ASSESSMENT—RECOGNIZE CUES/ INTERVENTIONS—TAKE ACTION | RATIONALES |
|---|---|
| Assess vital signs for indicators of profuse bleeding or hemorrhage (hypotension, tachycardia, and tachypnea). Report significant findings. | Hypotension, tachycardia, and tachypnea are signs of bleeding/ hemorrhage, which can occur with thrombolytic or anticoagulant therapy and necessitate prompt intervention. |
| At least once each shift, inspect wounds, oral mucous membranes, any entry site of an invasive procedure, and nares. | This assessment helps determine whether blood is present at any of these sites. |
| At least once each shift, inspect the torso and extremities. | The presence of petechiae or ecchymoses signals bleeding within the tissues. |
| Apply pressure to all venipuncture or arterial puncture sites until bleeding stops completely. | To ensure that all bleeding stops completely, it is necessary to apply pressure for longer than the usual amount of time. |
| • If the patient is receiving unfractionated heparin therapy, monitor serial partial thromboplastin time (aPTT). | This will confirm that aPTT is in the desired range (1.5–2.5× control). |
| • If the patient is receiving warfarin therapy, monitor serial prothrombin time (PT). | This will confirm that PT is in the desired range (1.25–1.5× control, or the INR value of 2.0–3.0) |
| • Report values outside the desired range. | This will enable prompt intervention. |

Continued

| ASSESSMENT—RECOGNIZE CUES/ INTERVENTIONS—TAKE ACTION | RATIONALES |
|---|---|
| • Consult the pharmacist about compatibility before infusing other IV drugs through heparin IV line.<br>• For patients on warfarin therapy, consult the pharmacist to obtain specific information about the patient's medication profile. | For patients on heparin therapy, the following agents decrease the effect of heparin therapy: digitalis, tetracycline, nicotine, and antihistamines.<br><br>Numerous drugs result in a decrease or increase in response to treatment with warfarin. |
| Discuss with the patient and significant others the effects of anticoagulant therapy and the importance of reporting promptly the presence of bleeding. | Hematuria, melena, frank bleeding from the mouth, epistaxis, hemoptysis, and excessive vaginal bleeding (menometrorrhagia) are potential effects of anticoagulant therapy and necessitate timely intervention to prevent further blood loss. |
| Monitor for bleeding gums. | Bleeding gums may indicate overcoagulation. |
| • If the patient is restless and combative, provide a safe environment. Use extreme care when moving the patient.<br>• Educate the patient about the risks with falls, blunt injuries, and lacerations. | These actions help prevent falls and avoid bumping extremities into side rails, which could result in severe bleeding. |
| See *Deficient Knowledge*, below, for more interventions. | |

## Patient Problem/Analyze Cues/Prioritize Hypotheses

# Deficient Knowledge

*due to* unfamiliarity with oral anticoagulant therapy, potential side effects, and foods and medications to consider during therapy

***Desired Outcome/Generate Solutions:*** Before hospital discharge, the patient verbalizes knowledge of the prescribed anticoagulant, potential side effects, and foods and medications to consider while receiving oral anticoagulant therapy.

| ASSESSMENT—RECOGNIZE CUES/ INTERVENTIONS—TAKE ACTION | RATIONALES |
|---|---|
| Assess the patient's health care literacy (language, reading, comprehension). Assess culture and culturally specific learning needs. | This assessment helps ensure that information is selected and presented in a manner that is culturally and educationally appropriate. |
| Determine the patient's knowledge of oral anticoagulant therapy. As appropriate, discuss the medication name; purpose; dose; schedule; precautions; food–drug, herb–drug, and drug–drug interactions; and potential side effects. | Knowledgeable patients are more likely to adhere to the therapeutic regimen. |
| Provide instruction on the potential side effects/complications of anticoagulant therapy: easy bruising, prolonged bleeding from cuts, spontaneous nosebleeds, bleeding gums, black and tarry or bloody stools, vaginal bleeding, and blood in urine and sputum. | This information increases patients' awareness of side effects and complications to report to their health care providers for timely intervention. |
| Discuss the importance of laboratory testing and follow-up visits with the health care provider. | Laboratory testing helps ensure that the blood clotting time stays within the therapeutic range. To promote safety, patients need close management by health care providers while undergoing anticoagulant therapy. |
| Explain the importance of informing all health care providers (including dentist) that the patient is taking an anticoagulant. Suggest the patient wear a medical alert tag or otherwise carry identification informing health care providers about the anticoagulant therapy. | These actions help ensure that patients are not given drugs or therapies that will have adverse effects on anticoagulant therapy, causing a greater risk for hemorrhaging or clotting. |

| ASSESSMENT—RECOGNIZE CUES/ INTERVENTIONS—TAKE ACTION | RATIONALES |
|---|---|
| Caution the patient that a soft-bristle rather than a hard-bristle toothbrush and electric rather than straight or safety razor needs to be used during anticoagulant therapy. | These devices minimize the risk for injury that could cause severe bleeding. |
| Instruct the patient to consult the health care provider before taking over-the-counter or prescribed medications that were used before initiating anticoagulant therapy. | Many medications, both prescribed and over-the-counter, may interfere with the action of oral anticoagulants. Prescribed medication (such as oral contraceptives, macrolides, diuretics) and over-the-counter medications, such as aspirin, acetaminophen, nonsteroidal anti-inflammatory drugs (NSAIDs, e.g., ibuprofen, naproxen), and cough and cold medications can adversely affect anticoagulant medications. |
| Inform the patient about herbal products that could affect coagulation or have an effect on anticoagulant medications. | Herbal remedies, such as gingko biloba, garlic, vitamin E, fish oil, and ginseng have been shown to adversely affect clotting. |

## ADDITIONAL PROBLEMS:

| | |
|---|---|
| "Perioperative Care" | Chapter 4 |
| "Immobility" | Chapter 1 |
| "Venous Thrombosis/Thrombophlebitis" | Chapter 26 |

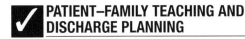

## ✓ PATIENT–FAMILY TEACHING AND DISCHARGE PLANNING

When providing patient–family teaching, focus on sensory information, avoid giving excessive information, and initiate a visiting nurse referral for necessary follow-up teaching. Include verbal and written information about the following:

**Note:** Rehabilitation and family teaching concepts for fat emboli are nonspecific.

✓ Risk factors related to the development of thrombi and embolization and preventive measures to reduce the risk.

✓ Signs and symptoms of thrombophlebitis: calf swelling; tenderness or warmth in the involved area; slight fever; and distention of distal veins, coolness, edema, and pale color in the distal affected leg.

✓ Signs and symptoms of pulmonary embolism: sudden onset of dyspnea and anxiety, nonproductive cough or hemoptysis, palpitations, nausea, syncope.

✓ Importance of preventing impairment of venous return from the lower extremities by avoiding prolonged sitting, crossing legs, and constrictive clothing.

✓ Medications, including drug name, dosage, purpose, schedule, precautions, and potential side effects. Also discuss drug–drug, herb–drug, and food–drug interactions. Patients taking warfarin need to keep their intake of Vitamin K at a consistent level and keep follow-up laboratory appointments for checking INR levels.

✓ The National Blood Clot Alliance (https://www.stopthe-clot.org/) has material for further education on the prevention of blood clots.

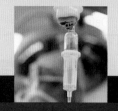

# Pulmonary Tuberculosis 16

## OVERVIEW/PATHOPHYSIOLOGY

Tuberculosis (TB) is an infectious disease caused primarily by *Mycobacterium tuberculosis. M. tuberculosis* is transmitted by the airborne route through minute, invisible particles called *small droplet nuclei.* When individuals with TB disease of the lungs or throat cough, sneeze, speak, or sing, their respiratory secretions harbor TB organisms that are expelled into the air and transform quickly into tiny droplet nuclei that can remain suspended in air for several hours, depending on the environment. To become infected, another person must breathe the air containing the droplet nuclei. Close contact and frequent or prolonged exposure is required for transmission; TB is not spread by physical contact such as kissing or sharing food utensils.

When these small droplets are inhaled, they become lodged in the bronchioles and alveoli and cause a local inflammatory reaction. This is classified as a *primary TB infection.* A calcified TB granuloma is formed as the body's defense mechanism; this granuloma "walls off" the infection to prevent further spread. When the bacillus is walled off, the infection is stopped. Most adults with competent immune systems can completely kill the TB infection and stay infection-free for the rest of their lives. In 5%–10% of cases, an active TB infection develops months or years later. The lungs are the primary location for TB because *M. tuberculosis* thrives in an oxygenated environment. However, the organism can spread to other areas through the lymphatic system and cause infections in areas such as the cerebral cortex, spine, liver, kidneys, and lymph nodes. An *active infection* occurs if the body's immune system cannot contain the organism. Those who also have an HIV infection are at a high risk for developing active TB. In some cases, a person has a positive TB skin test but no symptoms; this is known as a *latent TB infection (LTBI).* They are not infectious and cannot transmit the disease to others, but they can develop active TB later in life if certain conditions occur. Conditions that can reactivate TB include immunosuppression, diabetes, HIV, therapy with glucocorticoids, malnutrition, pregnancy, stress, and chronic disease. Treatment of LTBI is considered as important as treatment for primary TB (Harding et al., 2023).

The *M. tuberculosis* organism can develop resistance to drug therapy. *Multidrug-resistant TB* is resistant to the first-line drugs used to treat TB (isoniazid and rifampin). In rare cases, TB can be extensively drug-resistant and very difficult to treat. These resistant strains are a developing public health concern.

Drug resistance can be prevented by correct prescribing, managing care closely, and adhering to the prescribed regimen for an adequate length of time.

Worldwide, according to the World Health Organization (2021), TB is the 13th leading cause of death, and the second leading infectious killer after COVID-19 (now above HIV/AIDS). TB has been declining substantially in the United States. In 2020 the rate of TB cases in the United States was 2.2 per 10,000 persons (CDC, 2022c).

## HEALTH CARE SETTING

Primary care or long-term care, with possible hospitalization (acute care) resulting from complications or lack of adherence to the medication regimen

## ASSESSMENT

For an accurate diagnosis of TB a complete medical and psychosocial history needs to be taken along with a physical examination that includes a tuberculin skin test (TST) or an interferon-gamma release assay (IGRA) blood test (there are currently two US Food and Drug Administration–approved IGRA tests available: the QuantiFERON TB Gold In-Tube [QFT-GIT] and T-SPOT), chest radiography and/or computed tomography examinations, and sputum examination (including acid-fast bacilli [AFB] smears, cultures, and drug sensitivity studies).

***Signs and symptoms.*** Pulmonary TB symptoms may not develop until 2–3 weeks after the infection. A dry cough is the first manifestation; it often becomes productive later. Other symptoms may include fever, night sweats, chest pain, chills, loss of appetite, unintended weight loss over a short period of time, and fatigue. Dyspnea and hemoptysis are late symptoms that reflect extensive pulmonary involvement. Keep in mind that immunocompromised people (i.e., HIV) and older adults may not have a fever.

**Note:** *Close contacts of the patient require identification so that they can undergo evaluation for the presence of LTBI. TB is reportable to the Public Health Department.*

***History/risk factors for developing active tuberculosis.*** Immunocompromised state, especially HIV infection; intravenous drug use; radiographic evidence of prior, healed TB; weight loss of 10% or more of ideal body weight; and other medical conditions, including diabetes mellitus, silicosis, end-stage renal disease, organ transplants, some types of cancers, and certain immunosuppressive therapies. Persons who have emigrated from areas of the world with high rates of TB are also more likely to have LTBI than persons born in the United States.

## DIAGNOSTIC TESTS

*Tuberculin skin test or intradermal injection of antigen (purified protein derivative).* This test uses a purified protein derivative (PPD) of mycobacterial organisms that is administered intradermally and interpreted as positive or negative using measured millimeters of induration. The test is read after 48–72 hours for the presence or absence of induration, a palpable, raised, hardened area of swelling over the injection site. Redness is not considered a positive result. The induration is measured in millimeters (mm). A result over 10 mm is considered positive; for those who are immunocompromised or have an HIV infection, a positive result is any measurement over 5 mm. Those who are immunocompromised and some patients with active TB may have a negative PPD test, even in the presence of active TB disease. A positive PPD test indicates infection with TB bacteria, but additional testing must be performed to determine latent versus active disease. Some individuals born outside of the United States may have been given a vaccine called bacille Calmette–Guérin (BCG), which can cause false-positive TST results.

*Interferon-gamma release assays.* Two IGRA blood tests are currently available: the QFT-GIT test and the T-SPOT test. These test results are available in a few hours, and they are not affected by prior vaccination with BCG.

**Note:** *The TST or IGRA testing cannot differentiate between an active TB infection and LTBI. Further testing to exclude active TB must be done to diagnose LTBI.*

*Sputum culture with acid-fast stain.* Sputum culture is considered the "gold standard" for the diagnosis of TB. Three consecutive samples, collected 8–24 hours apart, are collected. At least one of the specimens needs to be an early morning collection. Detection of AFB in stained smears examined under a microscope usually provides the first bacteriologic clue of TB. Smear results should be available within 24 hours of specimen collection. It takes 6 weeks to grow the TB organism; treatment will be started while waiting for culture results in patients who are highly suspected to have TB. AFB in the smear may be mycobacteria other than *M. tuberculosis*; many patients can have TB and have a negative smear. Specimens are generally collected by asking the patient to expectorate sputum into a cup; however, tracheal washing, bronchoscopy, thoracentesis of pleural fluid, and lung biopsy are other options.

*Chest radiography.* Involvement is most characteristically evident in the apex and posterior segments of the upper lobes. Although not diagnostically definitive, it will reveal calcification at the original site, enlargement of hilar lymph nodes, parenchymal infiltrate, pleural effusion, and cavitation. Patients with HIV infection may have an atypical radiographic presentation of TB. Any abnormality on an AIDS patient's chest radiograph should be considered possible TB until ruled out.

*Gastric washings.* May reveal the presence of tubercle bacilli secondary to swallowed sputum. Gastric washings are usually used for children who cannot expectorate sputum.

## Patient Problem/Analyze Cues/Prioritize Hypotheses

# Deficient Knowledge

*due to* unfamiliarity with the spread of TB and the procedure for Airborne Isolation

*Desired Outcome/Generate Solutions:* After receiving instruction, the patient and significant others verbalize accurate information about how TB is spread and measures necessary to prevent the spread.

| ASSESSMENT—RECOGNIZE CUES/ INTERVENTIONS—TAKE ACTION | RATIONALES |
|---|---|
| Assess the patient's health care literacy (language, reading, comprehension). Assess culture and culturally specific information needs. Then explain the patient about TB and the mechanism by which it is spread (respiratory droplet nuclei). | This assessment helps ensure that information is selected and presented in a manner that is culturally and educationally appropriate. A well-informed patient is more likely to adhere to precautions against spreading the disease. |
| Educate the patient that they must be in a negative airflow room and must wear a regular surgical mask if it is necessary to leave the room until antimicrobial therapy is successful, as indicated by AFB smears. | The negative airflow ventilation dilutes and removes airborne contaminants and controls the direction of airflow. The negative pressure is monitored continuously or checked and recorded daily while the patient is isolated in this room. These actions reduce the transmission of the microbes to others. |

Continued

| ASSESSMENT—RECOGNIZE CUES/ INTERVENTIONS—TAKE ACTION | RATIONALES |
|---|---|
| Post a notice of isolation/airborne precautions on the patient's room door. Explain to the patient and significant others the rationale for isolation measures. | These measures provide guidelines for those entering the patient's room and help to reduce the transmission of the microbes to others. Providing an explanation of the measures will reduce anxiety. |
| Remind staff and visitors of the need to keep the patient's door closed. | A closed door enables the effective function of the ventilation system. |
| Explain to the staff and visitors the importance of wearing an N-95 or high-efficiency particulate air mask, including proper fit and use. Provide appropriate masks at the doorway or other convenient place. | These masks, designed to provide a tight face seal and filter particles in the 1- to 5-μm range, are worn by all individuals entering the patient's room to reduce the possibility of infection. |
| Emphasize the importance of covering the mouth and nose with tissues when sneezing or coughing and of disposing used tissues in a paper bag that is then placed in the appropriate waste container. Tissues can also be flushed down the commode. | These actions reduce the possibility of spreading infection. |

## Patient Problem/Analyze Cues/Prioritize Hypotheses

# Risk for Nonadherence

*due to* the lengthy treatment regimen

***Desired Outcome/Generate Solutions:*** Before hospital discharge, the patient verbalizes accurate information about the importance of completing the treatment regimen, including follow-up visits and testing.

| ASSESSMENT—RECOGNIZE CUES/ INTERVENTIONS—TAKE ACTION | RATIONALES |
|---|---|
| Emphasize the importance of follow-up care, including a review of all prescribed medications to ensure that all are being taken as prescribed. | Due to the side effects of medications and length of therapy, patients may become nonadherent with the medication regimen. Patients who do not display active symptomatic disease may believe that they do not need further treatment. |
| Provide education with particular attention on the risks for nonadherence and how to address any potential side effects. | Educating the patient and significant others on how to handle side effects will help promote adherence to the treatment regimen. |
| Consult with the health department if nonadherence to treatment is known or suspected. | The health department can assist with monitoring the medication regimen in high-risk cases. |

---

### ADDITIONAL PROBLEM:

See "Pneumonia" for *Impaired Gas Exchange*     Chapter 13

---

### ✓ PATIENT–FAMILY TEACHING AND DISCHARGE PLANNING

When providing patient–family teaching about TB, focus on sensory information, avoid giving excessive information, and initiate a referral to the public health department for investigation and follow-up of household members and other contacts exposed to the patient with TB. Include verbal and written information about the following:

✓ Antituberculosis medications, including drug name, purpose, dosage, schedule, precautions, and potential side effects. Also discuss drug–drug, herb–drug, and food–drug

interactions. Remind patients that medications are to be taken without interruption for the prescribed period. Remind patients of the need for continued laboratory monitoring for complications of pharmacotherapy. Describe directly observed therapy if that is the medication administration method selected.

✓ Importance of periodic reculturing of sputum.

✓ Importance of basic hygiene measures, including hand hygiene practices, covering cough with tissues, and proper disposal of contaminated items.

✓ Phone numbers to call in case questions or concerns arise about therapy or disease after discharge. Additional general information can be obtained by searching these websites for "tuberculosis":

- Centers for Disease Control and Prevention: www.cdc.gov/tb
- American Lung Association: www.lung.org
- American Thoracic Society: www.thoracic.org

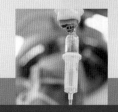

# Aneurysms 17

## OVERVIEW/PATHOPHYSIOLOGY

An aneurysm is a pathologic expansion or dilation in a section of an arterial wall. The most common cause is atherosclerosis, which alters the vessel pathology, weakens the vessel wall, and allows expansion. Additional causes include vessel wall trauma, congenital connective tissue disorders (e.g., Marfan syndrome), and infection, particularly syphilis or acquired immunodeficiency syndrome. Primary risk factors are heredity, age, and smoking. Because undiagnosed and untreated aneurysms are at risk for rupture and embolization, early diagnosis is imperative. Although aneurysms can develop in any artery, the abdominal aorta is the most common site. Abdominal aortic aneurysms (AAAs) occur more often in men and represent approximately 80% of all aneurysms. If the AAA is less then 5.4 cm and asymptomatic, conservative medical treatment and monitoring every 6–12 months is indicated. Modification of risk factors, such as hypertension, hyperlipidemia, and tobacco use, is also important. As the aneurysm enlarges, the risk for rupture increases. Aneurysms larger than 5.5 cm have the highest risk for rupture and therefore surgical repair is indicated. Ruptured aneurysms are true medical emergencies and patients die from massive hemorrhaging.

Aneurysms in the thoracic aorta are most often attributed to the modifiable risk factors of hypertension and cigarette smoking. Thoracic aneurysms are more susceptible to dissection. The atherosclerotic lesions present in *dissecting aneurysms* develop intimal tears, which allow bleeding into the layers of the vessel, causing false lumens to form that obstruct or limit blood flow in the true lumen of the vessel. This pathology is distinctly different from that of AAAs.

Early diagnosis and periodic evaluation of aneurysms are essential to protect the patient from emergent life-threatening rupture. Physical assessment, combined with ultrasound and radiologic screening of patients with risk factors, leads to diagnosis.

## HEALTH CARE SETTING

Chronic aneurysms may be monitored in primary care, with periodic radiographic or ultrasound assessment. Surgical intervention requires hospitalization and acute or intensive care during the perioperative period. Rehabilitation and home care services may be necessary during recovery.

## ASSESSMENT

*Abdominal aortic aneurysm.* A pulsatile, nontender mass may be palpated on both sides of the abdominal midline. Assessment is more difficult in obese patients. Severe acute abdominal pain of sudden onset with radiation to the back may be indicative of aneurysm rupture and is a surgical emergency. Rupture is nearly always fatal.

*Thoracic aneurysm.* Patients may be free of symptoms for years; however, pressure from the aneurysm on adjacent structures can result in dull pain in the upper back, dyspnea, cough, dysphasia, hemoptysis, tracheal deviation, and hoarseness. If there is pain associated with these aneurysms, it is more likely to be nonradiating central chest pain.

*Femoral aneurysm.* Leg or groin pain, decreased pulses, and swelling of the affected leg may occur. Femoral aneurysms may rupture or thrombose. See indicators discussed in "Peripheral Artery Disease," Chapter 18.

*Acute indicators (rupture or dissection).* Sudden onset of severe pain in the area of aneurysm with radiation, pallor, diaphoresis, and sudden loss of consciousness. Bruising in the back or flank, known as Grey Turner sign, may be present.

*Physical assessment with acute rupture.* Sudden drop of blood pressure (BP), weak and thready peripheral pulses, tachycardia, cyanosis, pale, cool and clammy skin, decreased urine output, abdominal tenderness, and altered level of consciousness. Hypovolemic shock and death may occur, depending on severity of the bleeding.

## DIAGNOSTIC TESTS

Chest x-rays may reveal abnormal widening of the thoracic aorta. An abdominal x-ray may show calcification within the aortic wall. An ECG may rule out MI, since thoracic aneurysm or dissection symptoms can mimic angina. Echocardiography assesses the function of the aortic valve. Ultrasound is useful for aneurysm screening and to monitor aneurysm size. A CT scan or MRI can diagnose and assess the location and severity of aneurysms. Angiography gives helpful information by using contrast imaging to map the entire aortic system.

A computed tomography scan (CT scan) or MRI is used to diagnose the location and severity of the aneurysm. They are used in urgent situations in which suspicion for rupture is high and the patient is stable. An ultrasound is used to evaluate the aneurysm size, shape and location, and is useful for initial and emergent screening, especially when the patient is unstable. Abdominal x-rays may detect calcifications in the vessel wall but are not used to evaluate aneurysms. Angiography with contrast dye determines the size of the aneurysm, presence of leaking, and origin of blood vessels arising from the aorta.

## Patient Problem/Analyze Cues/Prioritize Hypotheses
# Risk for Ineffective Tissue Perfusion (Multisystem)

*due to* interrupted arterial flow occurring with rupture, bleeding, or embolization following the invasive procedure

***Desired Outcome/Generate Solutions:*** The patient has adequate perfusion as evidenced by peripheral pulse amplitude greater than 2+ on a 0–4+ scale, brisk capillary refill (less than 2 seconds), and exhibits baseline extremity sensation, motor function, color, and temperature.

| ASSESSMENT—RECOGNIZE CUES/ INTERVENTIONS—TAKE ACTION | RATIONALES |
|---|---|
| Assess vital signs (VS) and peripheral pulses frequently in the perioperative period. Use Doppler ultrasound if necessary. When palpating arteries, use the following scale to rate the force of the pulse:<br><br>0=Absent<br><br>1+=Weak<br><br>2+=Normal<br><br>3+=Increased, full, bounding | This provides ongoing assessment of perfusion. Pulse amplitude of 2 or less (or other than "Normal") could signal embolization. Doppler ultrasound may be necessary for detection of a pulse that cannot be palpated. |
| Assess peripheral sensation with VS. Instruct the patient to report impaired sensation promptly. | Impaired sensation could signal impaired perfusion secondary to embolization or bleeding. The patient is the first to notice changes in sensation. |
| Assess urine output frequently, recording intake and output measurements. | Severe hypotension or renal artery occlusion can decrease renal perfusion. Optimally urine output is 0.5 mL/kg/hour or greater. |
| ⚠ Report to the health care provider immediately any changes in vital signs, extremity color, capillary refill, temperature, motor function, sensation, or increasing pain. | These are assessments of peripheral perfusion; changes from baseline (e.g., VS variance of 20% or greater; capillary refill of 3 seconds or greater; coolness, pallor, or mottling; decreased motor function or sensation, and pain) may signal embolization or bleeding. Arterial obstruction and bleeding must be treated emergently to prevent hemorrhage, ischemia, and potential loss of the extremity. |
| Maintain the patient in neutral position and on bedrest until otherwise directed. | Bedrest helps maintain BP and perfusion. The neutral position maintains integrity of the graft and minimizes risk for postprocedure embolization. |
| ⚠ Report any abdominal distention, pain, fever, or bloody diarrhea to the health care provider. | These may be signs of bowel ischemia, which requires immediate intervention. |
| As prescribed, administer beta-blockers (i.e., metoprolol, atenolol, propranolol) to decrease myocardial irritability and contractility. | These agents slow the heart rate and decrease BP, which aids in preventing dissection. |

PART I: Medical-Surgical Nursing Care Plans

##  PATIENT–FAMILY TEACHING AND DISCHARGE PLANNING

When providing patient–family teaching, focus on sensory information, avoid giving excessive information, and initiate a visiting nurse referral for necessary follow-up teaching. Include verbal and written information about the following:

- ✓ Preoperative and postoperative teaching focused on specific surgery. See "Cardiac Surgery," Chapter 20.
- ✓ Importance of regular medical follow-up to ensure graft patency, arterial integrity, and adequate perfusion.
- ✓ Reduction and/or management of risk factors (i.e., cigarette smoking, hypertension, obesity, diabetes) to prevent postoperative complications and slow the progression of atherosclerosis.
- ✓ Necessity of a regularly scheduled exercise program that may progress as the patient recovers.
- ✓ Indicators of wound infection and thrombus or embolus formation, and the need to report them promptly to the health care provider if they occur.

- ✓ Medications, including drug name, purpose, dosage, schedule, precautions, and potential side effects. Also discuss drug–drug, herb–drug, and food–drug interactions.
- ✓ Phone number of nurse or health care provider available to discuss concerns and questions.
- ✓ Importance of follow-up visits with health care provider; confirm date and time of next appointment.
- ✓ Potential need for assessment of other family members to rule out aneurysm, if heredity is a factor.
- ✓ Additional resources and patient educational materials may be found at:
  - Heart and Stroke Foundation: www.heartandstroke.com
  - American Heart Association: www.americanheart.org

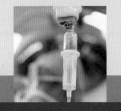

# Peripheral Artery Disease 18

## OVERVIEW/PATHOPHYSIOLOGY

Atherosclerosis is the primary etiology of peripheral artery disease (PAD). Damage to the intima of the artery occurs by the pathogenesis of atherosclerosis, which includes inflammation, plaque formation, lipid deposits, and hemorrhage. This process leads to vessel narrowing and hardening, decreasing lumen size and blood flow. Risk factors for atherosclerosis include smoking, heredity, advancing age, hyperlipidemia, hypertension, diabetes, metabolic syndrome, and a sedentary lifestyle.

Peripheral artery disease is systemic and progressive and is of grave concern when 75% or more of a cross-section of an artery becomes blocked. This disease is often associated with other comorbidities, such as coronary artery disease, hypertension, chronic obstructive pulmonary disease, and diabetes. The complexity of these comorbidities may lead to the loss of a limb or life in affected patients.

## HEALTH CARE SETTING

Acute care or primary care, rehabilitation, or long-term care

## ASSESSMENT

*Signs and symptoms.* Severe, cramping pain (intermittent claudication) with exercise that is relieved within 10 minutes by rest is the classic symptom of ischemia secondary to decreased peripheral blood flow. Additionally, decreased sensory or motor function occurs. Rest pain occurs as PAD progresses. Rest pain is present more often at night and worsens with limb elevation.

*Physical assessment.* Decreased pulse amplitude, decreased hair distribution, muscle atrophy, and cool, pale or bluish discoloration of the extremities may be present, especially if the legs are elevated. Dependent rubor may be present. Pallor, or blanching of the foot, occurs when the leg is elevated. Skin is often thin, shiny and taut, with no hair, and the nails may be thick. Audible bruits may be assessed with a stethoscope over partially occluded vessels. Capillary filling may last 2 seconds or more (with normal circulation, capillary filling occurs in less than 2 seconds); pulses may be diminished and detected only by

Doppler ultrasound examination. Critical limb ischemia occurs when chronic ischemic rest pain lasts more than two weeks, and nonhealing arterial leg ulcers or gangrene are present.

*Risk factors.* Tobacco use is the most important risk factor. Other risk factors include age over 60 years, hypertension, diabetes, hyperlipidemia, and a family history of atherosclerotic disease.

## DIAGNOSTIC TESTS

Doppler ultrasound studies use a transducer that emits sound waves through a probe to determine the amount of blood flow through arteries in which palpable pulses are difficult to obtain. Segmented blood pressures (BPs) use the Doppler ultrasound and a sphygmomanometer at the thigh, below the knee, and at the ankle level while the patient is supine. BPs are then measured at those locations; a drop in pressures that is greater than 30 mm Hg suggests PAD. Exercise or stress testing determines the amount of exercise or stress that precipitates claudication. Pulse volumes and BPs may be measured before symptom onset or after 5 minutes of exercise/stress. Ankle-brachial index (ABI) studies determine the degree of arterial occlusion and subsequent ischemia. BP is measured at the ankle (using either posterior tibial or dorsalis pedis pulse) and at the brachial artery. The pressure obtained at the ankle is divided by that at the brachial artery. Normally ABI is greater than 1.0; resting pain occurs with an ABI of 0.3 or less. However, stiffness and calcification of the lower extremity (LE) arteries may cause falsely elevated ABI readings. Angiography of the peripheral vasculature locates narrowing and obstructions and reveals the extent of vascular lesions by injecting dye into arteries and taking pictures of the arteries in a timed sequence. This imaging study is most used when angioplasty or stenting is planned. Magnetic resonance imaging demonstrates vessels in multiple projections and can be used with or without contrast. It is used widely but is not suitable for all patients. Implanted metal (e.g., pacemakers, automatic defibrillators) and prosthetic joint replacements preclude this study from being performed.

Patent Problem/Analyze Cues/Prioritize Hypotheses

# Risk for Impaired Skin Integrity (Skin Ulcerations)

*due to* altered arterial circulation occurring with atherosclerotic disease

**Desired Outcome/Generate Solutions:** Over a period of days or weeks, the patient's lower extremity circulation improves and perfusion to the tissue and skin is maximized, as evidenced by the absence/decrease in ulcerations and other skin problems.

| ASSESSMENT—RECOGNIZE CUES/ INTERVENTIONS—TAKE ACTION | RATIONALES |
|---|---|
| Assess legs, feet, and between the toes for ulcerations. | Ulcerations can occur with decreased arterial circulation. A decrease in circulation significantly decreases oxygen delivery to the tissues and subsequently impairs healing of even the most minor break in the skin. A baseline assessment enables timely interventions. |
| Provide instruction on the importance of walking and range-of-motion exercises for the hip, knee, and ankle. | Walking is the best activity, and patients can be instructed to walk until they have pain, rest until recovery, and then resume walking. Walking and exercise improve collateral circulation. This is especially useful for patients who claudicate, along with other risk factor modifications. Activity may be contraindicated for some patients with severe disease. |
| Determine the allowed activity and exercise with the health care team, and discuss this with the patient. | Exercise promotes circulation.<br><br>**Note:** Bedrest without exercise may be prescribed in acute, severe cases to decrease oxygen demand to the tissues, which optimally will decrease pain. |
| **[!]** Provide instruction on how to assess peripheral pulses, warmth, sensation, and color of the LEs. Encourage daily foot inspections by the patient or family members if the patient's vision or assessment ability is compromised. | Monitoring the status of the LEs is essential for the early identification of breaks in skin integrity because early identification and care may prevent serious complications. |
| Encourage cessation of smoking and other tobacco use. Provide smoking and tobacco cessation literature. Discuss with the health care provider use of medication for smoking cessation. | Stopping tobacco use promotes vasodilation and prevents increased vasoconstriction and progression of atherosclerosis. Nicotine affects the heart and lungs and other body organs. |
| Discuss the importance of keeping the feet warm and protected by wearing socks when walking or in bed. | Decreased circulation because of vasoconstriction results in decreased blood flow to the LEs, which promotes hypothermia. Keeping warm promotes vasodilation and a more optimal blood supply. |
| **[!]** Caution the patient about using heating pads. | Heating pads increase metabolism and may promote ischemia if circulation is limited. Also, the patient's sensitivity to temperature is often decreased and burns may result. |
| Discuss the importance of nightlights being placed in bedrooms and bathrooms. | Nightlights promote visibility and may help avoid tissue trauma if ambulating in the dark. |
| Caution the patient to avoid pressure over areas of bony prominence. | Pressure increases the risk for skin breakdown; areas over bony prominence are particularly susceptible. |
| Caution the patient to cover all exposed areas when going outside in cooler weather. | This action helps prevent hypothermia, to which patients with decreased circulation may be susceptible. Cold temperatures cause vasoconstriction, which further results in decreased tissue perfusion. |

Patient Problem/Analyze Cues/Prioritize Hypotheses

# Chronic Pain

*due to* reduced circulation and ischemia

**Desired Outcome/Generate Solutions:** Over several days or weeks, after interventions to improve perfusion, the patient's pain decreases, as documented by a pain scale.

| ASSESSMENT—RECOGNIZE CUES/ INTERVENTIONS—TAKE ACTION | RATIONALES |
|---|---|
| Assess for the presence of pain on initial contact and periodically throughout care, using a pain scale. | This assessment helps determine the degree and trend of pain. |
| Administer pain medications as prescribed. | Usually, mild analgesics are prescribed to reduce pain. Opioids may be given for acute perioperative pain. Opioids may not be effective for chronic rest pain and must be used cautiously in older adults and in all persons to avoid addiction. |
| Document pain relief obtained using a pain scale. | This documentation helps determine the effectiveness of the medication. |
| Instruct the patient to rest when claudication (severe, cramping pain) occurs. If claudication occurs at rest, encourage the patient to position the legs so that they are dependent, and ensure warmth with socks and blankets, as appropriate. | Intermittent claudication from activity is relieved by rest. Claudication at rest implies severe circulatory compromise; measures such as leg dependency and warmth may reduce pain. |
| Explore alternative methods of pain relief, such as visualization, guided imagery, biofeedback, meditation, relaxation exercises, or music. | Because the pain may be chronic and continuous, pain relief needs to be augmented with nonpharmacologic methods. |
| Institute measures to improve circulation, such as dependence of extremities, ensuring warmth, walking, and use of medications (see *Risk for Impaired Skin Integrity [Skin Ulcerations]*, earlier). | These measures increase circulation to ischemic extremities, which optimally will increase the patient's comfort level. |

## Patient Problem/Analyze Cues/Prioritize Hypotheses

# Deficient Knowledge

*due to* unfamiliarity with the potential for infection and impaired tissue and skin integrity caused by decreased arterial circulation

***Desired Outcome/Generate Solutions:*** After receiving instructions, the patient verbalizes accurate knowledge about the potential for infection and impaired tissue and skin integrity, as well as measures to prevent these problems.

| ASSESSMENT—RECOGNIZE CUES/ INTERVENTIONS—TAKE ACTION | RATIONALES |
|---|---|
| Assess the patient's health care literacy (language, reading, comprehension). Assess culture and culturally specific information needs. | This assessment helps ensure that information is selected and presented in a manner that is culturally and educationally appropriate. |
| Provide instruction on self-assessment for signs of infection or breaks in skin integrity and reporting of significant findings to the health care provider. | This information facilitates understanding of symptoms that occur with infection or impaired skin integrity and describes symptoms that must be reported for timely intervention. This includes any new or enlarging wound or ulceration, redness, swelling, increased pain, or drainage. |
| Caution about the increased potential for easily traumatizing skin (e.g., from bumping LEs). | Decreased circulation in the legs diminishes sensation and the healing process after tissue trauma. |
| Instruct the patient to inspect both feet each day for any open wounds or bruises. Suggest the use of a long-handled mirror to visualize the bottoms of both feet. Advise the patient to report any open areas to the health care provider. | Decreased circulation in the legs diminishes sensation, and therefore careful inspection is important to identify breaks in skin integrity. Open wounds can lead to infection, which must be reported promptly for timely intervention. |
| Stress the importance of wearing shoes or slippers that fit properly without areas of stress or friction. | Improper fit can lead to traumatized tissues. Bare feet in an individual with decreased sensation can lead to trauma. |
| Instruct the patient to cut toenails straight across or have them cut by a podiatrist. | Ingrown toenails can lead to infection. Cutting the skin may lead to a nonhealing wound. |
| Advise the patient to cover corns or calluses with pads. | Protection helps prevent further injury. |

| ASSESSMENT—RECOGNIZE CUES/ INTERVENTIONS—TAKE ACTION | RATIONALES |
|---|---|
| Encourage the patient to keep feet clean and dry, using mild soap and warm water for cleansing, and apply a mild lotion. Instruct patient not to apply lotion between the toes. | This promotes hygiene and prevents dryness, which could result in skin breakdown that could lead to infection. However, lotion between the toes increases the moisture and may lead to infection. |
| Advise the patient not to scratch the feet. | Abrasions can easily become infected. |
| Advise keeping the feet warm with warm soaks and loose-fitting socks. | Decreased circulation leaves patients vulnerable to hypothermia. Keeping warm promotes vasodilation and increased blood supply to the area. |
| ⚠ Caution the patient to check temperature of warm soaks and bath water carefully with an elbow before stepping into the water. | Water temperature exceeding comfort can cause burns in an individual whose temperature sensitivity is decreased. |

### Patient Problem/Analyze Cues/Prioritize Hypotheses

# Ineffective Tissue Perfusion (Peripheral)

*due to* decreased arterial flow occurring with atherosclerosis or due to acute occlusion occurring with a postsurgical graft embolus

***Desired Outcome/Generate Solutions:*** Optimally, after interventions, the patient has adequate peripheral perfusion, as evidenced by BP within 15–20 mm Hg of baseline BP and absence of the six Ps in the involved extremities: pain, pallor, pulselessness, paresthesia, poikilothermia (coolness), and paralysis.

| ASSESSMENT—RECOGNIZE CUES/ INTERVENTIONS—TAKE ACTION | RATIONALES |
|---|---|
| Assess peripheral pulses and the involved extremity for the six Ps. Report significant findings. | Sensory changes usually precede other symptoms of ischemia (i.e., pain, loss of two-point discrimination, and paresthesia). Such findings must be reported promptly for timely intervention. |
| Administer the following medications as prescribed: | Use these medications for the following reasons: |
| • Antiplatelet agents (e.g., aspirin, clopidogrel, tirofiban, or ticlopidine) | • Help prevent platelet adherence and thromboembolism. |
| • Thrombolytics (e.g., urokinase or tissue plasminogen activator) | • May be used to lyse clot formation if an embolus or thrombus is present. |
| • Blood viscosity–reducing/antiplatelet agent (e.g., pentoxifylline. cilostazol, or low-dose aspirin) | • May increase the flexibility of erythrocytes, thereby enhancing their movement through the microcirculation and preventing aggregation of red blood cells and platelets. This therapy has the potential to increase circulation at the capillary level and reduce or alleviate symptoms caused by lack of blood flow. |
| • Lipid-lowering agents (e.g., lovastatin, atorvastatin, simvastatin, and pravastatin) | • Reduce serum cholesterol levels and decrease inflammation in vessel walls. |
| • Antihypertensive agents (e.g., angiotensin-converting enzyme inhibitors, beta-blockers, diuretics, or calcium channel blockers) | • Decrease systolic and diastolic BPs, which is important in patients with peripheral arterial disease. Increased BP promotes further arterial wall damage, plaque formation, and rupture. |
| Explain the surgical intervention if one is planned. | For patients who have tissue loss, rest pain, or disabling claudication, surgical intervention may be necessary to open the occluded vessel or bypass the vessel to improve distal circulation. |
| If necessary, use a Doppler ultrasound to assess pulses, holding the probe to the skin at a 45-degree angle to the blood vessel. Record the presence or absence of pulsations, as well as rate, character, frequency, and intensity of sounds. | Doppler ultrasound evaluates the presence of blood flow in arteries in which pulses are difficult to palpate. Optimally, pulsatile blood flow will be heard as wave-like, whooshing sounds. |

Continued

| ASSESSMENT—RECOGNIZE CUES/ INTERVENTIONS—TAKE ACTION | RATIONALES |
|---|---|
| Protect legs and feet from pressure or damage. | Decreased LE sensation increases the risk for injury.Foam protectors, special mattresses, cotton socks, and blankets are useful. |
| Monitor BP. Report to the health care provider any significant increase or decrease greater than 15–20 mm Hg, or as directed. | BP is another indicator of peripheral perfusion pressure. An increase in BP may interrupt the surgical site; decreased BP may cause graft occlusion. |
| If diabetes is present, implement measures and provide teaching to maintainglycosylated hemoglobin (A1C) below 7.0%. See "Diabetes," Chapter 27. | Patients with PAD need to maintain an A1C below 7.0% because diabetes is a major risk factor for PAD. |
| For the first 48–72 hours after surgery (or as directed), prevent acute joint flexion in the presence of a graft. | Joint flexion can impede blood flow and perfusion. Mild foot elevation or light Ace bandage wrapping may help ease hyperemia of the extremity. |
| In the absence of acute cardiac or renal failure, encourage adequate fluid intake. | Adequate fluid intake enhances perfusion; inadequate fluid intake can lead to dehydration and poor perfusion. |

## ADDITIONAL PROBLEM:

| "Perioperative Care" | Chapter 4 |
|---|---|

## ✔ PATIENT–FAMILY TEACHING AND DISCHARGE PLANNING

When providing patient–family teaching, focus on sensory information, avoid giving excessive information, and initiate a visiting nurse referral for necessary follow-up teaching. Include verbal and written information about the following:

✔ Progressive exercise program as prescribed by the health care team; importance of rest periods if claudication occurs. Generally, exercise is recommended for 30–45 minutes per day, at least three times a week. Exercise can include walking or cycling.

✔ Meticulous, routine skin, and foot care.
✔ Medications, including drug name, purpose, dosage, schedule, precautions, and potential side effects. Also discuss drug–drug, food–drug, and herb–drug interactions. Referral to a smoking/tobacco cessation program if appropriate. The following Internet resources support and describe methods and reasons to advise patients to stop smoking:
  • http://smokefree.gov/
  • https://www.cancer.gov/about-cancer/ causes-prevention/risk/tobacco/cessation-fact-sheet
  • American Lung Association: https://www.lung.org/ quit-smoking

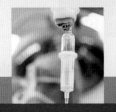

# Cardiac and Noncardiac Shock (Circulatory Failure) 19

## OVERVIEW/PATHOPHYSIOLOGY

Shock occurs when tissue perfusion is severely decreased, causing cellular metabolic collapse. Shock is a progressive event, beginning with cellular changes as perfusion decreases and extending to compensatory mechanisms to improve cardiac output. Ultimately, these measures fail and the body goes into life-threatening shock. Shock is classified according to the causative event.

**Hypovolemic shock.** Occurs when volume in the intravascular space is severely decreased and the metabolic needs of tissues cannot be met, as with severe hemorrhage or dehydration.

**Cardiogenic shock.** Occurs when cardiac pump failure results in decreased cardiac output, resulting in decreased systemic perfusion, as with severe myocardial infarction.

**Distributive shock conditions.** Characterized by a significant decrease in vascular volume. The three types are neurogenic shock, anaphylactic shock, and septic shock.

*Neurogenic shock* occurs when a neurologic event (e.g., spinal cord injury) causes loss of sympathetic tone, resulting in massive vasodilation and decreased perfusion pressures.

*Anaphylactic shock* is caused by a severe systemic response to an allergen (foreign protein), resulting in massive vasodilation, increased capillary permeability, decreased perfusion, decreased venous return, and subsequent decreased cardiac output.

*Septic shock* occurs when bacterial toxins cause an overwhelming systemic infection, resulting in severe hypotension and decreased cardiac output.

Regardless of the cause, shock results in cellular hypoxia secondary to decreased perfusion and ultimately in cellular, tissue, and organ collapse. A prolonged shock state can result in death; therefore early recognition and intervention are essential.

## HEALTH CARE SETTING

Inpatient, critical care units

## ASSESSMENT

**Early signs and symptoms.** Cool, pale, and clammy skin; decreased pulse strength; dry and pale mucous membranes; restlessness; change in the level of consciousness (LOC); hyperventilation; anxiety; nausea; thirst; weakness.

Physical assessment findings include: Rapid heart rate (HR); decreased systolic blood pressure (SBP) and increased diastolic BP secondary to catecholamine (sympathetic nervous system) response.

**Late signs and symptoms.** Decreased urinary output, hypothermia, drowsiness, diaphoresis, confusion, lethargy, and coma.

Physical assessment findings include: Thready, rapid HR; low or decreasing BP, usually with SBP less than 90 mm Hg; rapid and possibly irregular respiratory rate (RR).

## DIAGNOSTIC TESTS

No single diagnostic study determines whether the patient is in shock. Diagnosis is usually based on presenting symptoms, clinical signs, and history.

**Arterial blood gas values.** May reveal metabolic acidosis or respiratory alkalosis (bicarbonate [$HCO_3^-$] less than 22 mEq/L and pH less than 7.40) caused by anaerobic metabolism.

**Serial measurement of urinary output.** Less than 0.5 mL/kg/hour indicates decreased perfusion and decreased renal function.

**Laboratory studies.** Blood urea nitrogen (BUN) and creatinine are increased, with decreased renal perfusion. Elevated serum electrolyte levels identify renal complications. Elevated lactate levels reflect anaerobic metabolism resulting from decreased perfusion. White blood cell counts are extremely elevated in septic shock due to infection. Eosinophils may be elevated with anaphylactic shock. Hematocrit and hemoglobin may be increased in severe dehydration but decreased in the presence of hemorrhage.

**Cultures of blood, sputum, wound, and urine.** To identify the causative organism in septic shock.

Patient Problem/Analyze Cues/Prioritize Hypotheses

# Ineffective Tissue Perfusion (Multisystem)

*due to* decreased circulating blood volume or inadequate oxygenation occurring with shock

***Desired Outcome/Generate Solutions:*** After interventions, the patient has adequate perfusion and oxygenation as evidenced by peripheral pulse amplitude more than 2+ on a 0–4+ scale; brisk capillary refill (less than 2 seconds); SBP greater than 90 mm Hg; $SaO_2$ greater than 92%; mean arterial pressure of 70–100 mm Hg; HR regular and 100 bpm or less; no significant change in mental status; orientation to person, place, and time; normalized electrolytes; and urine output at least 0.5 mL/kg/hour.

| ASSESSMENT—RECOGNIZE CUES/ INTERVENTIONS—TAKE ACTION | RATIONALES |
|---|---|
| Assess and document peripheral perfusion status. Report significant findings, which include coolness and pallor of the extremities, decreased amplitude of pulses, and delayed capillary refill. | These significant findings reflect decreased peripheral perfusion, an early sign of decreased cardiac output and shock, and necessitate prompt intervention. |
| Assess BP and indicators of hypotension at frequent intervals. Indicators of hypotension include decreased SBP of greater than 20 mm Hg below the patient's baseline range, dizziness, altered mentation, and decreased urinary output. Notify the health provider promptly of significant findings. | Immediate intervention is necessary to avoid irreversible organ damage due to poor perfusion. |
| If severe hypotension is present, place the patient in a supine position. | This position promotes venous return. BP must be at least 80/60 mm Hg for adequate coronary and renal artery perfusion. |
| Assess for restlessness, confusion, mental status changes, and decreased LOC. | These are indicators of decreased cerebral perfusion/cerebral hypoxia. |
| If these indicators occur, intervene to keep the patient safe from harm; reorient as indicated and implement measures to prevent falls. | Patients with mental status changes due to decreased cerebral perfusion are at risk for falling or making inappropriate decisions regarding mobility (e.g., getting out of bed without assistance). |
| Administer $O_2$; maintain airway and prepare for mechanical ventilation if indicated. | Maintaining adequate oxygenation is essential for survival. |
| Monitor for the presence of chest pain and irregular HR. Report significant findings. | These are indicators of decreased coronary artery perfusion. Decreased coronary artery perfusion necessitates prompt intervention to prevent ischemia. |
| Monitor urinary output hourly and check weight daily; notify the health care provider of significant findings, including urine output less than 0.5 mL/kg/hour in the presence of adequate intake and/or weight gain. | Decreased urinary output is a sign of decreased cardiac output and renal perfusion. Weight gain may be a sign of fluid retention, which can occur with decreased renal perfusion. |
| Monitor laboratory results for elevated BUN and creatinine levels; report increases. | BUN of more than 20 mg/dL and creatinine of more than 1.5 mg/dL are signals of decreased renal perfusion. |
| Monitor serum electrolyte values for evidence of imbalances, particularly of lactate, $Na^+$, and $K^+$. Assess for clinical signs of hyperkalemia, such as muscle weakness, hyporeflexia, and irregular HR, and for clinical signs of hypernatremia, such as fluid retention and edema. | Hyperlactatemia (more than 2–4 mmol/L), hypernatremia ($Na^+$ more than 147 mEq/L), and hyperkalemia ($K^+$ more than 5.0 mEq/L) may be signs of renal and metabolic complications of shock as a result of decreased renal perfusion and the kidneys' inability to regulate lactate and electrolytes. |
| Notify the health care provider of significant findings. | Electrolyte imbalances and acidosis are life threatening and need immediate correction. Correction likely will include oxygen therapy, fluid resuscitation, and replacement or excretion of electrolytes. |
| Avoid the use of sedatives or tranquilizers. | LOC can be altered by these medications, and tissue hypoperfusion makes absorption unpredictable. |

| ASSESSMENT—RECOGNIZE CUES/ INTERVENTIONS—TAKE ACTION | RATIONALES |
|---|---|
| Administer fluids and medications as prescribed and according to the type of shock, the patient's clinical situation, and hemodynamic interventions. | Interventions are determined by the clinical presentation and severity of the shock state. Patients may be transferred to critical care units for invasive hemodynamic monitoring and administration of vasoactive intravenous (IV) medications to improve tissue perfusion. |
| Avoid rapid delivery of colloidal fluids in the treatment of hypovolemic shock. | Very rapid infusion of colloidal fluids may precipitate pulmonary edema. |
| For septic shock, administer antibiotic therapy within the first hour.  **Note:** Obtain blood, urine, and sputum cultures before beginning antibiotics, but do not delay the start of antibiotics within the first hour. | Early antibiotic therapy is essential for septic shock. Initial therapy is broad spectrum. After the causative organism is identified, specific antibiotic therapy will be initiated. |

## Patient Problem/Analyze Cues/Prioritize Hypotheses

# Impaired Gas Exchange

*due to* decreased cardiac output occurring with shock state

***Desired Outcome/Generate Solutions:*** Within 1–2 hours of intervention, the patient has adequate tissue perfusion and oxygenation, as evidenced by BP at least 90/60 mm Hg; HR of 70–100 bpm; RR of 12–16 breaths/minute; $SaO_2$ greater than 92%; $PaO_2$ at least 80 mm Hg; $PaCO_2$ 45 mm Hg or less; pH at or near 7.35; and improved LOC with orientation to person, place, and time.

| ASSESSMENT—RECOGNIZE CUES/ INTERVENTIONS—TAKE ACTION | RATIONALES |
|---|---|
| Monitor vital signs continuously. Report significant findings. | The presence of hypotension, tachycardia, and a change in respiratory rate signifies poor systemic perfusion and hypoxia. |
| Monitor arterial blood gases. Report significant findings. | The presence of hypoxemia (decreased $PaO_2$), hypercapnia (increased $PaCO_2$), and acidosis (decreased pH, increased $PaCO_2$, and increased lactate levels) is a sign of decreased gas exchange secondary to decreased tissue perfusion. |
| Assess for mental status changes, restlessness, irritability, and confusion. Report significant findings. | Often these are symptoms of poor tissue perfusion and hypoxia. Oxygen, mechanical ventilation, IV medications, and other interventions may be required. |

### ADDITIONAL PROBLEMS:

| | |
|---|---|
| "Psychosocial Support for the Patient" | Chapter 8 |
| "Psychosocial Support for the Patient's Family and Significant Other" | Chapter 9 |

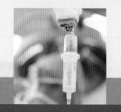

# Cardiac Surgery 20

## OVERVIEW/PATHOPHYSIOLOGY

Surgical intervention may be necessary to treat acquired or congenital heart disease. *Coronary artery bypass grafting* is performed to treat blocked coronary arteries. Veins are harvested from other areas of the patient's body and anastomosed to coronary arteries, revascularizing the affected myocardium. *Valve repair* or *replacement* is performed to treat valvular stenosis or valvular incompetence of the mitral, tricuspid, pulmonary, or aortic valve. *Aortic surgery* removes or repairs an aortic aneurysm. Other types of cardiac surgeries are performed to correct heart defects that are either acquired or congenital, such as ventricular aneurysm, ventricular or atrial septal defects, transposition of the great vessels, and tetralogy of Fallot. *Heart transplantation* may be considered for some patients diagnosed with end-stage cardiac disease. *Combined heart–lung transplantation* is performed for patients with end-stage disease affecting both organs.

## HEALTH CARE SETTING

With elective surgery patients are often admitted to the hospital on the day of surgery. Many cardiac surgeries are emergent or urgent with direct admissions from an emergency room, clinic, or medical office.

During the perioperative period, many patients may need to be in a critical care unit for monitoring and stabilization. When stable they may be transferred to a cardiac unit.

## Patient Problem/Analyze Cues/Prioritize Hypotheses

## Before Cardiac Surgery: Deficient Knowledge

*due to* unfamiliarity with the diagnosis, surgical procedure, preoperative routine, and postoperative course

***Desired Outcome/Generate Solutions:*** Before surgery, the patient verbalizes knowledge about the diagnosis, surgical procedure, and preoperative and postoperative course.

| ASSESSMENT—RECOGNIZE CUES/ INTERVENTIONS—TAKE ACTION | RATIONALES |
|---|---|
| Assess the patient's health care literacy (language, reading, comprehension). Assess culture and culturally specific information needs. | This assessment helps ensure that information is selected and presented in a manner that is culturally and educationally appropriate. |
| Assess the patient's level of knowledge about the diagnosis and surgical procedure, and provide information as necessary. Encourage questions, and allow time for verbalization of concerns and fears. | Knowledge level will vary from patient to patient. Some patients find detailed explanations helpful; others prefer brief and simple explanations. The amount of information given depends on learning needs and needs to be individualized. |
| When appropriate, provide orientation to the critical care and cardiac units and equipment that will be used postoperatively. | Familiarity with the units and equipment optimally will promote understanding and minimize stress. |
| Provide instructions for and demonstrate deep breathing and coughing techniques; ask the patient to practice with a return demonstration. | Deep breathing and coughing are essential postoperatively to reinflate the lungs and remove mucus, preventing atelectasis and pneumonia. |

156

| ASSESSMENT—RECOGNIZE CUES/ INTERVENTIONS—TAKE ACTION | RATIONALES |
|---|---|
| Reassure the patient that postoperative pain will be managed with comfort measures, positioning, and medication. Explain the types of comfort measures offered, including nonpharmacologic methods such as positioning, breathing and relaxation techniques, audio and visual distractions, massage, and pharmacologic pain relief including medication type (e.g., opioids, nonsteroidal antiinflammatory drugs [NSAIDs]) and administration method (e.g., epidural, patient-controlled analgesia, intermittent intravenous, and by mouth [PO]). | This information may aid in reducing anxiety about postoperative pain and increase understanding of the types of pain relief measures and medications available. The overall goal is to reduce postoperative pain. |
| Advise the patient that in the immediate postoperative period, speaking may not be possible and assisted methods of communication (e.g., nodding, writing, pointing) will be helpful. | An endotracheal tube may be in place postoperatively until the patient can breathe independently. Knowledge that alternate communication methods are available reduces anxiety and prepares the patient for their use. |
| Review and demonstrate safe movements and sternal precautions. Sternal precautions commonly include how to safely move in and out of the bed and chair using aids such as side rails or assistive devices and holding pressure, most often with crossed arms or a pillow against the chest. Moving cautiously and not lifting, pushing, or pulling more than 5–10 lb or driving for 4–6 weeks. | These common recommendations following cardiac surgery help to prevent injury to the sternal incision site. |

## Patient Problem/Analyze Cues/Prioritize Hypotheses

# After Cardiac Surgery: Fatigue (Decreased Exercise Tolerance)

*due to* morbidity, generalized weakness, and immobility following cardiac surgery

***Desired Outcome/Generate Solutions:*** By a minimum of 24 hours before hospital discharge, the patient rates perceived exertion at 3 or less on a 0–10 scale and exhibits cardiac tolerance to activity as evidenced by heart rate of 110 bpm or less, systolic blood pressure (SBP) within 20 mm Hg of resting SBP, and respiratory rate of 20 breaths/minute or less with normal depth and pattern (eupnea).

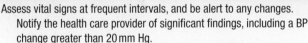

| ASSESSMENT—RECOGNIZE CUES/ INTERVENTIONS—TAKE ACTION | RATIONALES |
|---|---|
| Assess vital signs at frequent intervals, and be alert to any changes. Notify the health care provider of significant findings, including a BP change greater than 20 mm Hg. | Hypotension, tachycardia, crackles, tachypnea, and diminished amplitude of peripheral pulses are signs of cardiac complications and must be reported promptly for timely intervention. |
| Ask the patient to rate perceived exertion (RPE) during activity, and monitor for evidence of activity intolerance. Notify the health care provider of significant findings. | An RPE greater than 3, along with cool, diaphoretic skin, is a signal to stop the activity and notify the health care provider. See "Immobility," *Activity Intolerance*, Chapter 1, for a discussion of RPE. |
| Coordinate care, medical interventions, and treatments to provide adequate rest periods between care activities. | Uninterrupted rest of at least 90 minutes helps improve well-being, aids recovery, and decreases cardiac workload. |
| Assist with exercises, depending on tolerance and prescribed activity limitations. As prescribed, initiate physical therapy and/or cardiac rehabilitation. | Monitored exercise increases activity tolerance. |
| See "Immobility," *Activity Intolerance*, Chapter 1, for a discussion of in-bed exercises. | |

## ADDITIONAL PROBLEMS:

| | |
|---|---|
| "Perioperative Care" for *Risk for Infection* | Chapter 4 |
| "Pulmonary Embolus" for *Risk for Hemorrhaging,* due to anticoagulation therapy | Chapter 15 |
| "Coronary Artery Disease" for **Risk for Ineffective Tissue Perfusion (Renal)** (decreased cardiac output or reaction to contrast dye) | Chapter 21 |

 ## PATIENT–FAMILY TEACHING AND DISCHARGE PLANNING

When providing patient–family teaching, focus on sensory information, avoid giving excessive or unnecessary information, and initiate appropriate referrals for follow-up support and teaching. Include written information with verbal reinforcement and allow time for questions.

✓ Medications, including drug name, dosage, schedule, purpose, precautions, and potential side effects. Also discuss drug–drug, herb–drug, and food–drug interactions.

✓ Technique for assessing radial pulse, temperature, and weight, if required, and the importance of reporting significant changes to the health care provider.

✓ Signs and symptoms of heart failure that require immediate medical attention: chest pain, dyspnea, shortness of breath, sudden weight gain, edema, inability to urinate, nausea, vomiting, and decrease in exercise tolerance.

✓ Care of incision sites; assessing for signs of infection, such as increased incisional pain, drainage, swelling, fever, persistent redness, and local warmth and tenderness.

✓ Symptoms requiring medical attention for patients taking antiplatelet medications or anticoagulants, such as bleeding from the nose (epistaxis) or gums, hemoptysis, hematemesis, hematuria, melena, hematochezia, menometrorrhagia, and excessive bruising.

✓ Stress the importance of taking medications at the same time every day, notifying the health care provider if any signs of bleeding occur, avoiding over-the-counter and herbal medications (e.g., aspirin, NSAIDs, garlic supplements, ginkgo) unless approved by the health care provider, carrying a medical alert bracelet or card, avoiding constrictive or restrictive clothing, and using a soft-bristled toothbrush and electric razor.

✓ Importance of pacing activities to avoid undue fatigue, and allowing frequent rest periods.

✓ Referral to a cardiac rehabilitation program.

✓ Activity restrictions (e.g., no heavy lifting, pushing, or pulling anything heavier than 5–10 lb for at least 4–6 weeks); prescribed exercise program; and resumption of sexual activity, work, and driving a car, as directed.

✓ Weight maintenance or weight gain or loss if advised; nutritional education to learn foods to avoid and the importance of a healthy diet; and calorie counting. Referral to a nutritionist and obtaining daily weight may be helpful.

✓ Maintenance of a low-sodium, low-cholesterol diet. Encourage patients to use food labels to determine the calorie, sodium, fat, and cholesterol content of foods.

✓ Telephone number of the nurse and health care provider to discuss concerns and questions or clarify instructions.

✓ Importance of follow-up visits with the health care provider; confirm date and time of next appointment.

✓ Discussion of the patient's home environment and the potential need for changes or adaptations (e.g., several steps to climb or activities of daily living that are too strenuous).

✓ Introduction to local American Heart Association activities. Provide the address or telephone number for the local chapter or encourage the patient to contact the following:
  • American Heart Association: www.americanheart.org
  • United Network for Organ Sharing, as appropriate, for patients awaiting heart transplantation: www.unos.org

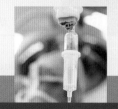

# Coronary Artery Disease 21

## OVERVIEW/PATHOPHYSIOLOGY

Coronary artery disease (CAD) is the leading cause of death in the United States (CDC, 2021b). The coronary arteries supply the myocardial muscle with oxygen and the nutrients necessary for optimal function. In CAD, the arteries are narrowed or obstructed, potentially resulting in cardiac muscle death. Atherosclerotic lesions, arterial spasm, platelet aggregation, and thrombus formation all may cause narrowing and obstruction. The most common symptom of CAD is chest pain (angina), which results from decreased blood flow and insufficient oxygen supply to the heart muscle.

Acute coronary syndrome (ACS) is an imbalance between myocardial oxygen supply and demand secondary to an acute obstruction caused by plaque disruption or erosion. ACS is an umbrella term that includes stable CAD (SCAD), unstable angina (USA), non–ST-elevation myocardial infarction (NSTEMI), and ST-segment elevation myocardial infarction (STEMI).

USA is defined as an increase in severity, frequency, or intensity of anginal pain or new onset of rest angina, lasting 10 minutes or more. NSTEMI is defined by the clinical presentation of chest pain with an elevation in cardiac biomarkers and electrocardiogram (ECG) changes that may include T-wave inversion or ST-segment depression but not ST-segment elevation. Diagnosis of STEMI is based on elevated cardiac biomarkers plus ST-segment elevation on ECG signifying ischemia. STEMI is the most serious and life-threatening presentation.

Time is essential in diagnosing and treating patients with ACS. Patients presenting with a STEMI are a high priority for intervention. An ECG is the primary assessment tool that guides the intervention strategy. Primary angioplasty is the therapy of choice for reperfusion in acute myocardial infarction (AMI). However, not all acute care hospitals in the United States can provide percutaneous coronary intervention (PCI). Time is critical in patients presenting with STEMI, and recommendations include clinical examination and ECG within 10 minutes of chest pain onset. Oxygen, aspirin (ASA), nitrates, and adequate analgesia are administered immediately, and a decision must be made by the health care provider to proceed with either thrombolytic therapy or primary PCI within 90 minutes of patient arrival. The goal for door-to-balloon time to open the artery is 90 minutes. If catheterization laboratory facilities for primary intervention are not available within this time frame, thrombolytics are administered as soon as possible, and transport needs to be arranged to a facility for primary intervention.

## HEALTH CARE SETTING

Primary care, acute care, critical care unit

## ASSESSMENT

**Signs and symptoms.** Persistent chest pain is the hallmark symptom and is described as worse than any previous angina episodes and lasts longer than 20 minutes. The pain may radiate to the jaw, back, shoulder, or arm. Other manifestations include weakness, diaphoresis, nausea, vomiting, shortness of breath, and acute anxiety also may occur. Heart rate (HR) may be abnormally slow (bradycardia) or it may be rapid (tachycardia). Stable or progressively worsening angina occurs when myocardial demand for $O_2$ is more than the supply, such as during exercise. Pain is often described as a feeling of pressure or as a crushing or burning substernal pain that radiates down one or both arms and into the neck, cheeks, and teeth. Anginal pain is often relieved by discontinuation of exercise, rest, or administration of nitroglycerin (NTG). Some patients do not have classic myocardial infarction (MI) symptoms. Some patients only describe "discomfort" along with weakness, indigestion, or shortness of breath. Women may have atypical discomfort, fatigue, or dyspnea.

Physical assessment: Anxiety, hypertension, tachycardia, tachypnea, and dynamic ECG changes with dysrhythmias are the most common symptoms of acute ischemia. Severe hypotension may occur in shock states. Temperature elevations can occur secondary to the inflammatory process. The intensity of $S_1$ and $S_2$ heart sounds may be decreased. Pulmonary congestion may occur if ventricular failure is present, and $S_3$ and $S_4$ sounds may be auscultated.

**History and risk factors.** Family history, increasing age, male gender, smoking, low high-density lipoprotein (HDL) values, hypercholesterolemia, diabetes mellitus, hypertension, and metabolic syndrome are all risk factors for CAD. Obesity, glucose intolerance, and a sedentary, stressful lifestyle also contribute to increased risk. Chest pain occurring with exertion is a primary warning sign of CAD.

## DIAGNOSTIC TESTS

**ECG.** Reveals dynamic changes in the presence of ischemia. When the ECG is performed during chest pain, characteristic changes may include ST-segment elevation or depression greater than 0.05 mV in leads over the area of ischemia. The presence of a bundle branch block also can be determined on ECG as well as dysrhythmias. If possible, comparisons to previous ECGs are done. Serial ECGs are often done on patients with acute syndromes to keep track of areas of ischemia, injury, and infarction. As ischemia advances, the muscle does not transmit electrical impulses, and the ECG helps determine the area and extent of the infarct.

**Cardiac-specific biomarkers.** There are two types of cardiac-specific troponin biomarkers: cardiac-specific troponin T (cTnT) and cardiac-specific troponin I (cTnI). These are the standard cardiac biomarkers to diagnose MI. Troponin levels increase 4–6 hours after the onset, peak at 10–24 hours, then return to baseline levels within 10–14 days. Serial sets of troponin levels are generally drawn every 6 hours in the first 24 hour. Creatinine phosphokinase a, CK-MB also measure proteins that are released in response to ischemia or MI, but they are less sensitive than troponin levels.

**C-reactive protein.** If elevated from the normal range of 0.03–1.1 mg/dL, this signals that coronary artery plaques are inflammatory, and the patient is at higher risk for an acute coronary event.

**Echocardiography.** Assesses ventricular function, chamber size, valvular function, ejection fraction (EF), wall motion, and hemodynamic measurements. Heart muscle damage may alter ventricular function, wall motion, and hemodynamic pressures. A heart muscle that moves weakly may have been damaged during an acute ischemic attack or may be receiving too little oxygen.

**Chest radiography.** May show an enlarged heart or pulmonary congestion if heart failure is present.

**Total lipid panel.** Obtained during the patient's evaluation and treatment to assess for hyperlipidemia, a risk factor in CAD. Low HDL (value less than 40 mg/dL) and high low-density lipoprotein (value greater than 100 mg/dL) are linked to atherosclerotic heart disease. (Values may change in the presence of acute ischemia and therefore are considered more valid when they are obtained before hospital discharge.)

**Stress tests.** Stress testing with concurrent imaging of the heart is the standard means of noninvasive cardiac evaluation. Stress tests are prescribed to assess coronary artery flow, valvular function, and wall motion abnormalities.

*Exercise treadmill test.* To determine the amount of exercise-induced ischemia, hemodynamic response, and ECG changes with exercise. Significant findings include 1 mm or more ST-segment depression or elevation, dysrhythmias, or a sudden decrease in blood pressure (BP).

*Stress echocardiogram.* Typically performed using either a treadmill or bicycle. Echocardiograms are obtained before and immediately after exercise. A stress-induced imbalance in the myocardial supply/demand ratio will produce myocardial ischemia and regional wall motion abnormality (the area of ischemia affects muscle contraction). Stress echocardiography is particularly useful for identifying CAD in patients with multivessel disease. Dobutamine, adenosine, or dipyridamole are medications used as stress agents with echocardiogram imaging for patients who cannot exercise.

**Cardiac nuclear imaging modalities.**

*Myocardial perfusion imaging.* Detection of CAD is found by differential blood flow through the left ventricular myocardium. Normal blood flow and normal tracer uptake are seen with unobstructed coronary arteries; diminished flow and diminished tracer uptake are found with coronary stenosis. An abnormality will be present in an area of MI resulting from a lack of blood flow.

Single-photon emission computed tomography (SPECT) is used to develop three-dimensional views of cardiac processes and cellular-level metabolism by viewing the heart from several different angles and using tomography methods to reconstruct the image. SPECT enables a clearer resolution of myocardial ischemia and better quantification of cardiac damage.

*Radionuclide angiography.* Used to evaluate left and right ventricular EF, left ventricular volume, and regional wall motion. The first-pass technique is a fast acquisition of myocardial images. Gated pool ejection or multiple-gated acquisition scan permits calculation of the amount of blood ejected with ventricular contraction and is used for risk stratification of patients after MI or with CAD.

**Computed tomography.** May be helpful in differentiating AMI from aortic dissection in patients with severe, tearing back pain and associated dyspnea and/or syncope.

**Ambulatory monitoring.** 24-hour ECG monitoring (Holter monitor) can show activity-induced ST-segment changes or ischemia-induced dysrhythmias.

**Coronary arteriography through cardiac catheterization.** Coronary arteriography is the gold standard of diagnostic testing for CAD. Arterial lesions (plaque) are located and the amount of occlusion is determined. During this test, the feasibility of a coronary artery bypass graft or PCI is determined. For details, see "Cardiac Surgery," Chapter 20.

**Intravascular ultrasound.** A flexible catheter with a miniature transducer at the tip is threaded into the coronary arteries to provide information on the interior of the coronary arteries. Ultrasound is used to create a cross-sectional image of the three layers of the arterial wall and its lumen to assess the degree of atherosclerosis.

## Patient Problem/Analyze Cues/Prioritize Hypotheses

# Acute Pain (Angina)

*due to* decreased oxygen supply to the myocardium

**Desired Outcomes/Generate Outcomes:** Within 30 minutes of the onset of pain, the patient's subjective perception of angina decreases, as documented by a pain scale. Objective indicators, such as grimacing and diaphoresis, are absent or decreased.

| ASSESSMENT—RECOGNIZE CUES/ INTERVENTIONS—TAKE ACTION | RATIONALES |
|---|---|
| Assess the location, character, and severity of the pain. Record severity on a subjective 0 (no pain) to 10 (worst pain) scale. | This assessment monitors the degree, character, precipitator, and trend of pain for the initial check and subsequent comparisons. |
| Assess HR and BP during episodes of chest pain. Be alert to and report significant findings. | Increase in HR and change in systolic blood pressure (SBP) greater than 20 mm Hg from the baseline signal increased myocardial $O_2$ demands and necessitate prompt medical intervention. |
| Administer $O_2$ as prescribed. Deliver $O_2$ with humidity. | Hypoxia is common because of decreased perfusion and additional stress to the compromised myocardium. Humidity helps prevent oxygen's convective drying effects on oral and nasal mucosa. |
| Notify the health care provider of unrelieved pain. | If pain is unrelieved or returns very quickly, emergency medical treatment is advised. |
| As prescribed, administer IV NTG and titrate to pain and blood pressure. Monitor SBP and notify the health care provider if SBP is below 90 mm Hg, HR is less than 60 bpm, or RR is less than 10 breaths/min. | NTG relieves chest pain and also lowers BP. SBP should be maintained at 90 mm Hg or higher until the pain is relieved to avoid worsening ischemia secondary to hypotension. |
| As prescribed, add IV morphine sulfate in small increments (2 mg). Monitor HR, RR, and BP. | IV morphine sulfate is added in small increments to titrate for adequate pain relief. Morphine also decreases HR, BP, RR, and anxiety. |
| Obtain ECG as prescribed. | ECG patterns may reveal ischemia, as evidenced by dynamic ST- or T-wave changes, evidence of new Q waves, or left bundle branch block. |
| Stay with the patient and provide reassurance during periods of angina. | Reassurance comforts patients and reduces anxiety, which may worsen angina. |
| Monitor for the presence of headache and hypotension after administering NTG. | These are side effects of NTG that result from vasodilation. |
| Maintain the patient in a recumbent position with the head of bed (HOB) elevated no higher than 30 degrees during angina and NTG administration. | This position minimizes the potential for headache/hypotension by enabling better blood return to the heart and head. |
| Emphasize to the patient the importance of immediately reporting angina to the health care team. | Early treatment decreases morbidity and mortality. |
| Instruct the patient to avoid activities and factors known to cause stress. | Stress may precipitate angina. |
| Discuss the value of relaxation techniques, including tapes, soothing music, or meditation. | Relaxation helps reduce stress and anxiety, which otherwise may precipitate angina. |
| Administer beta-blockers (e.g., metoprolol, atenolol, carvedilol) as prescribed. Beta-blockers must be used with caution in patients with asthma because they antagonize pulmonary vasodilation. Rising from a recumbent or seated position must be done slowly to avoid orthostatic hypotension. | These medications block beta stimulation to the sinoatrial (S-A) node and myocardium. HR, BP, and contractility are decreased, subsequently reducing the workload of the heart and myocardial oxygen demand, improving myocardial oxygenation. |
| Administer long-acting nitrates (isosorbide preparations) and/or topical nitrates as prescribed. | Nitrates are given for anginal prophylaxis, lowering BP, and decreasing $O_2$ demand. |

Continued

| ASSESSMENT—RECOGNIZE CUES/ INTERVENTIONS—TAKE ACTION | RATIONALES |
|---|---|
| Administer angiotensin-converting enzyme (ACE) inhibitor (e.g., enalapril, captopril, quinapril, ramipril) as prescribed. | ACE inhibitors reduce BP, downregulate the renin–angiotensin– aldosterone system (RAAS), and improve long-term survival. |
| Administer calcium channel blockers (e.g., nifedipine, diltiazem) as prescribed. | Calcium channel blockers decrease coronary artery vasospasm, a potential cause of ischemia and subsequent angina, and dilate coronary arteries, increasing blood flow to the myocardium. |
| Administer antithrombotic agents, including aspirin, as prescribed. | Antithrombotic agents reduce platelet aggregation, which aids in preventing coronary artery obstruction. Bleeding precautions must be reviewed (see *Risk for Hemorrhaging* in "Pulmonary Embolus," Chapter 15). |
| Administer stool softeners as prescribed. | Straining at stool or constipation can increase myocardial demand. |

## Patient Problem/Analyze Cues/Prioritize Hypotheses

# Fatigue (With Activity Intolerance)

*due to* generalized weakness and imbalance between oxygen supply and demand occurring with tissue ischemia secondary to MI.

**Desired Outcome/Generate Solutions:** During the activity, the patient rates perceived exertion at 3 or less on a 0–10 scale and exhibits cardiac tolerance to activity/exercise as evidenced by the respiratory rate of 12–20 breaths/minute, HR of 80–120 bpm or less (or within 20 bpm of resting HR), SBP within 20 mm Hg of resting SBP, and absence of chest pain and dysrhythmias.

| ASSESSMENT—RECOGNIZE CUES/ INTERVENTIONS—TAKE ACTION | RATIONALES |
|---|---|
| Assess the frequency of angina, noting alleviating and precipitating factors. Observe whether angina occurs at rest and is relieved or unrelieved by NTG. Document accordingly. | This assessment detects evidence of an imbalance between oxygen supply and demand and potential activity/exercise intolerance. |
| Angina is defined either as stable (occurs predictably, most often with exertion); unstable (occurs unpredictably, often at rest); or variant (Prinzmetal) (occurs as a result of arterial spasm). | |
| Assess the patient's response to activity/exercise and report significant findings. | Chest pain, increase in HR (greater than 20 bpm), change in SBP (20 mm Hg over or under resting BP), excessive fatigue, and shortness of breath are signs of activity/exercise intolerance that must be reported promptly for timely intervention. |
| Ask the patient to rate perceived exertion (RPE). See "Immobility," *Activity Intolerance*, Chapter 1, for details. | RPE higher than 3 is a signal to stop the activity. |
| Assist the patient with recognizing and limiting factors that increase $O_2$ demands, such as exercise and anxiety. | This helps patients recognize and attempt to control factors that increase ischemia. |
| Administer $O_2$ as prescribed for angina episodes. Deliver $O_2$ with humidity. | This measure increases the oxygen supply to the myocardium. Humidity helps prevent oxygen's convective drying effects on oral and nasal mucosa. |
| Have the patient perform range-of-motion exercises, depending on tolerance and prescribed activity limitations. | Cardiac intolerance to activity can be further aggravated by prolonged bedrest. |
| Consult the health care provider about in-bed exercises and activities that can be performed by the patient as the condition improves. Aid the patient in getting out of bed and ambulating. Consult with the cardiac rehabilitation department for progressive activity. | These interventions enable progressive pacing toward the patient's optimal activity potential. |
| For further interventions, see "Immobility," *Activity Intolerance*, Chapter 1. | |

**Patient Problem/Analyze Cues/Prioritize Hypotheses**

# Deficient Knowledge

*due to* unfamiliarity with dietary regimen (calories, sodium, fats)

***Desired Outcome/Generate Solutions:*** Within the 24-hour period before hospital discharge, the patient demonstrates knowledge of the dietary regimen by planning a 3-day menu that includes appropriate foods and excludes inappropriate foods.

| ASSESSMENT—RECOGNIZE CUES/ INTERVENTIONS—TAKE ACTION | RATIONALES |
|---|---|
| Assess body weight and body mass index (BMI). If the patient is over ideal body weight, discuss the benefits of weight loss. | Being overweight is a risk factor for CAD and puts more workload on the heart. |
| As indicated, discuss ways to decrease dietary intake of saturated (animal) fats and increase intake of polyunsaturated (vegetable oil) fats. | Reducing dietary saturated fat is effective in lowering the risk of heart and blood vessel disease in many individuals. |
| Instruct the patient to limit dietary intake of cholesterol to less than 300 mg/day. Encourage the use of food labels to determine the cholesterol content of foods. | Reducing cholesterol intake is effective in lowering the risk of heart and blood vessel disease in many individuals. |
| Instruct the patient to limit dietary intake of refined/processed sugar. | Refined sugars are empty calories that can convert to fat stores and increase weight. |
| Instruct the patient to limit dietary intake of sodium chloride (NaCl) to less than 4 g/day (mild restriction). Encourage reading food labels to determine the sodium content of foods. | Increased sodium intake can lead to water retention, which increases vascular volume and cardiac workload. |
| Instruct the patient and significant other in the use of "Nutrition Facts" (federally mandated public information on all food product labels). | This information reveals the calories, total fat, saturated fat, cholesterol, and sodium in foods. Patients need to be especially aware of the serving size listed for respective nutrients. |
| Encourage intake of fresh fruits, natural (unrefined or unprocessed) carbohydrates, fish, poultry, legumes, fresh vegetables, and grains. | These food groups ensure a healthy, balanced diet. |

**Patient Problem/Analyze Cues/Prioritize Hypotheses**

# Deficient Knowledge

*due to* unfamiliarity with the purpose, precautions, and side effects of nitrates

***Desired Outcome/Generate Solutions:*** Within the 24-hour period before hospital discharge, the patient verbalizes an accurate understanding of the purpose, precautions, and side effects of nitrates.

| ASSESSMENT—RECOGNIZE CUES/ INTERVENTIONS—TAKE ACTION | RATIONALES |
|---|---|
| Assess the patient's health care literacy (language, reading, comprehension) and culture and culturally specific information needs. | This assessment helps ensure that information is selected and presented in a manner that is culturally and educationally appropriate. |
| Provide instructions about the purpose of the prescribed nitrate (isosorbide, NTG). | These medications are given to prevent long-acting or to treat short-acting angina to increase microcirculation, venous dilation, and blood to the myocardium. A patient who is knowledgeable about the purpose of this drug will be more likely to adhere to the therapeutic regimen. |

Continued

| ASSESSMENT—RECOGNIZE CUES/ INTERVENTIONS—TAKE ACTION | RATIONALES |
|---|---|
| Instruct the patient to report to the health care provider or staff the presence of a headache associated with nitrates. | The vasodilation effect of nitrates can result in transient headaches, in which case the health care provider may alter the dose of the isosorbide. Tylenol may be recommended for the treatment of headaches if not contraindicated. |
| Instruct the patient to assume a recumbent position with HOB slightly elevated if a headache occurs. | This position may reduce pain by enabling better blood return to the heart and head. |
| Instruct the patient to rise slowly from a sitting or lying position and to remain by the chair or bed for 1 minute after standing to ensure he or she is not going to experience orthostatic changes. | Vasodilation from nitrates also may decrease BP, which can result in orthostatic hypotension and injury to the patient. |

## Patient Problem/Analyze Cues/Prioritize Hypotheses

# Deficient Knowledge

*due to* unfamiliarity with the purpose, precautions, and side effects of beta-blockers

*Desired Outcome/Generate Solutions:* Within the 24-hour period before hospital discharge, the patient verbalizes an accurate understanding of the purpose, precautions, and side effects of beta-blockers.

| ASSESSMENT—RECOGNIZE CUES/ INTERVENTIONS—TAKE ACTION | RATIONALES |
|---|---|
| Assess the patient's readiness and ability to learn. | This assessment helps ensure that information is selected and presented at a time and in a manner that is appropriate for the patient. |
| Provide instruction about the purpose of beta-blockers. | Patients who are knowledgeable about the purpose of this medication will be more likely to adhere to therapy. These medications block beta stimulation to the S-A node and myocardium. HR and contractility are decreased, subsequently decreasing the workload of the heart. Myocardial oxygen demand also is reduced. |
| Instruct the patient to be alert to depression, fatigue, dizziness, erythematous rash, respiratory distress, and sexual dysfunction. Explain the importance of notifying the health care provider promptly if these side effects occur. | Side effects may discourage patients from continuing taking the medication. |
| Explain that BP and HR are assessed before the administration of beta-blockers. | These medications can cause hypotension and excessive slowing of the heart. |
| Caution the patient not to omit or abruptly stop taking beta-blockers. | Stopping this medication abruptly may result in rebound tachycardia, potentially causing angina or MI. |

## Patient Problem/Analyze Cues/Prioritize Hypotheses

# Deficient Knowledge

*due to* unfamiliarity with the disease process and lifestyle implications of CAD

*Desired Outcome/Generate Solutions:* Within the 24-hour period before hospital discharge, the patient verbalizes an accurate understanding of the disease process of CAD and associated lifestyle implications.

| ASSESSMENT—RECOGNIZE CUES/ INTERVENTIONS—TAKE ACTION | RATIONALES |
| --- | --- |
| Explain CAD, including pathophysiologic processes of cardiac ischemia, angina, and infarction. | Increasing patients' knowledge of their health status optimally will promote adherence to the treatment regimen. |
| Assist with identifying risk factors for CAD and risk factor modification. | Risk factor identification optimally will result in risk factor modification, including:<br><br>• Diet low in cholesterol and saturated fat<br><br>• Smoking cessation<br><br>• Regular activity/exercise program<br><br>• Weight loss (if appropriate) |
| Discuss symptoms that necessitate medical attention. | Progression to USA, loss of consciousness, decreased exercise tolerance, angina unrelieved by NTG, increasing frequency of angina, and the need to increase the number of NTG tablets to relieve angina are symptoms that necessitate medical attention to treat or prevent MI. |
| Discuss guidelines for sexual activity. Resting before intercourse, finding a comfortable position, taking prophylactic NTG, and postponing intercourse for 1–1½ hours after a heavy meal are valid guidelines that help minimize oxygen demand on the heart. | Drugs for erectile dysfunction (e.g., Viagra, Cialis, Levitra) cannot be taken simultaneously with NTG because this may cause a sudden drop in BP. |
| Discuss the rationale for antihyperlipidemic therapy, which may include the following: | Increasing patients' knowledge of their medications optimally will promote adherence to the treatment regimen. |
| HMG-CoA reductase inhibitors (e.g., lovastatin, simvastatin, fluvastatin, pravastatin, atorvastatin). | These agents inhibit the enzyme involved in early cholesterol formation, thereby reducing total cholesterol levels, including LDL and triglycerides, while increasing HDL. |
| Nicotinic acid (niacin). | This vitamin lowers triglyceride and LDL levels while raising HDL levels. |
| Fibric acid derivatives (e.g., gemfibrozil, fenofibrate). | |
| Bile acid sequestrant resins (e.g., cholestyramine, colestipol). | These agents bind with bile acids in the intestine and remove LDL and cholesterol from the blood. |
| Discuss procedures such as cardiac catheterization, PCI, and CABG, if appropriate. PCI is a procedure that improves coronary blood flow by using a balloon inflation catheter to rupture plaque and dilate the artery. It is performed in the cardiac catheterization laboratory under local anesthesia and with moderate sedation, enabling patients to be awake and interact with the health care team. PCI is a common alternative to bypass surgery. Balloon angioplasty is commonly followed by stent placement. After the procedure, patients routinely are placed on antiplatelet agents (e.g., ASA and Plavix) to reduce the risk for post-PCI in-stent restenosis. Cardiac catheterization is discussed later in this section, and CABG is discussed in "Cardiac Surgery," Chapter 20. | Knowledge about the procedure and what to expect may help reduce anxiety. |

## Problems for Patients Undergoing Cardiac Catheterization Procedure

### Patient Problem/Analyze Cues/Prioritize Hypotheses

# Deficient Knowledge

*due to* unfamiliarity with the catheterization procedure and postcatheterization regimen

***Desired Outcome/Generate Solutions:*** Before the procedure, the patient verbalizes accurate knowledge about cardiac catheterization and the postcatheterization plan of care.

| ASSESSMENT—RECOGNIZE CUES/ INTERVENTIONS—TAKE ACTION | RATIONALES |
|---|---|
| Assess the patient's health care literacy (language, reading, comprehension) and culture and culturally specific information needs. | This assessment helps ensure that information is selected and presented in a manner that is culturally and educationally appropriate. |
| Assess the patient's knowledge about the catheterization procedure. As appropriate, reinforce the health care provider's explanation, and answer any questions or concerns. Describe the catheterization lab and sensations the patient may experience. | Knowledge about the procedure and what to expect may help reduce anxiety. |
| Before cardiac catheterization, have the patient practice techniques that will be used during the procedure. | Valsalva maneuver, coughing, and deep breathing may be required during cardiac catheterization, and many people are unfamiliar with the proper technique. |
| Explain that a "flushing" feeling may occur when the dye is initially injected. | Dye injection causes vasodilation, which often induces flushing. |
| Explain the postcatheterization regimen and caution that flexing the insertion site is contraindicated, often for 4–6 hours after the procedure. | After the procedure, bedrest will be required and vital signs, circulation, and the insertion site will be checked at frequent intervals to ensure integrity. Flexing the insertion site (arm or groin) is contraindicated to prevent bleeding. |
| ⚠ Stress the importance of promptly reporting signs and symptoms of concern. | Groin, leg, or back pain; dizziness; chest pain; or shortness of breath may signal hemorrhage or embolization of the stent. Prompt reporting enables rapid intervention. |

## Patient Problem/Analyze Cues/Prioritize Hypotheses

# Risk for Ineffective Tissue Perfusion (Cardiac)

*due to* interrupted arterial flow occurring with the cardiac catheterization procedure

**Desired Outcome/Generate Solutions:** Within 1 hour after the procedure, the patient has adequate perfusion, as evidenced by HR regular and within 20 bpm of baseline HR; apical/radial pulse equality; BP within 20 mm Hg of baseline BP; peripheral pulse amplitude greater than 2+ on a 0–4+ scale; baseline warmth and color in the extremities; no significant change in mental status; and orientation to person, place, and time.

| ASSESSMENT—RECOGNIZE CUES/ INTERVENTIONS—TAKE ACTION | RATIONALES |
|---|---|
| Assess BP every 15 minutes until stable on 3 successive checks, every 2 hours for the next 12 hours, and every 4 hours for 24 hours unless otherwise indicated. | These assessments monitor BP trend. |
| **Note:** If the insertion site was the antecubital space, measure BP in the unaffected arm. | This measure prevents bleeding or blood vessel injury. |
| If the femoral artery was the insertion site, maintain HOB at no greater than a 30-degree elevation. | This measure prevents acute hip joint flexion, which could compromise arterial flow. |
| ⚠ If the SBP drops 20 mm Hg or more below previous recordings, lower the HOB and notify the health care provider. | A drop in BP could signify acute bleeding or shock. Lowering the HOB aids perfusion to the heart and brain. |
| ⚠ Assess HR and notify the health care provider if dysrhythmias occur. If the patient is not on a cardiac monitor, auscultate apical and radial pulses with every BP check, and report irregularities or apical/radial discrepancies. | Dysrhythmias and apical/radial discrepancies may be signs of cardiac ischemia. |
| ⚠ Be alert to and report cool extremities, decreased amplitude of peripheral pulses, cyanosis, changes in mental status, decreased level of consciousness (LOC), and shortness of breath. | These are indicators of decreased perfusion. |

## Patient Problem/Analyze Cues/Prioritize Hypotheses

# Risk for Hemorrhaging

*due to* the possibility of arterial bleeding with failure to seal/clot at the puncture site

***Desired Outcomes/Generate Solutions:*** The patient remains normovolemic, as evidenced by HR of 80–100 bpm; BP of 90/60 mm Hg or greater (or within 20 mm Hg of baseline range); no significant change in mental status; and orientation to person, place, and time. The dressing is dry, and there is no swelling at the puncture site.

| ASSESSMENT—RECOGNIZE CUES/ INTERVENTIONS—TAKE ACTION | RATIONALES |
|---|---|
| Assess vital signs and promptly report a decrease in BP, increase in HR, and decreasing LOC. | These are indicators of hemorrhage and/or shock. Rapid reporting enables prompt intervention. |
| Inspect the dressing on the groin or antecubital space every 15 minutes for the first hour, then follow agency protocol at frequent intervals and report significant findings. | This measure detects the presence of frank bleeding or hematoma formation (fluctuating swelling), which would necessitate prompt intervention. |
| Assess for and report diminished amplitude or absence of distal pulses, delayed capillary refill, coolness of the extremities, and pallor. | These signs of decreased peripheral perfusion may signal embolization or hemorrhagic shock. |
| Caution the patient about flexing the elbow or hip more than 30 degrees for 6–8 hours, or as prescribed. | These restrictions minimize the risk of bleeding and circulation compromise. |
| If bleeding occurs, maintain pressure at the insertion site as prescribed, usually 1 inch proximal to the puncture site or introducer insertion site. | Pressure stabilizes bleeding. Typically, this is done with a pressure dressing or a 2- to 5-pound sandbag. |

## Patient Problem/Analyze Cues/Prioritize Hypotheses

# Risk for Ineffective Tissue Perfusion (Peripheral)

*due to* interrupted arterial flow in the involved limb occurring with embolization

***Desired Outcome/Generate Solutions:*** The patient has adequate perfusion in the involved limb as evidenced by peripheral pulse amplitude greater than 2+ on a 0–4+ scale; baseline color, sensation, and temperature; and brisk capillary refill (less than 2 seconds).

| ASSESSMENT—RECOGNIZE CUES/ INTERVENTIONS—TAKE ACTION | RATIONALES |
|---|---|
| Assess peripheral perfusion by palpating peripheral pulses every 15 minutes for 30 minutes, then every 30 minutes for 1 hour, then hourly for 2 hours, or per protocol. | Prompt recognition of a diminished or absent pulse is essential to prevent limb damage. |
| Be alert to and report faintness or absence of pulse; coolness of the extremity; mottling; decreased capillary refill; cyanosis; and complaints of numbness, tingling, and pain at the insertion site. Instruct the patient to report any of these indicators promptly. | These are signs of embolization in the involved limb. Prompt recognition will result in rapid intervention. |
| If there is no evidence of an embolus or thrombus formation, instruct the patient to move the fingers or toes and rotate the wrist or ankle. | These measures promote circulation in the involved limbs. |
| Ensure that the patient maintains bedrest for 4–6 hours or as prescribed. | Bedrest or immobility enables the puncture site to stabilize, thereby avoiding bleeding. |

Continued

## Patient Problem/Analyze Cues/Prioritize Hypotheses

# Risk for Ineffective Tissue Perfusion (Renal)

*due to* interrupted blood flow occurring with decreased cardiac output or reaction to contrast dye

***Desired Outcome/Generate Solutions:*** The patient has adequate renal perfusion, as evidenced by a stable blood urea nitrogen/creatinine, urinary output of at least 0.5 mL/kg/hour, specific gravity 1.005–1.030, good skin turgor, and moist mucous membranes.

| ASSESSMENT—RECOGNIZE CUES/ INTERVENTIONS—TAKE ACTION | RATIONALES |
|---|---|
| Assess for indicators of dehydration, such as poor skin turgor, dry mucous membranes, and high urine specific gravity (1.030 or more). | Contrast dye for cardiac catheterization may cause osmotic diuresis. |
| Assess intake and output. | This assessment determines whether urine output is sufficient. |
| Notify the health care provider if the urinary output is less than 0.5 mL/kg/hour in the presence of adequate intake. | A fall in urinary output is a sign of dehydration or renal insufficiency. |
| Monitor BUN and creatinine daily. | A rise in these renal markers may signify renal insufficiency or acute renal failure. |
| If the urinary output is insufficient despite adequate intake, restrict fluids. | This measure helps prevent fluid overload. |
| Be alert to and report crackles on auscultation of lung fields, distended neck veins, and shortness of breath; notify the health care provider about significant findings. | These signs are other indicators of fluid overload. Prompt detection and reporting enable rapid intervention. |
| If the patient does not exhibit signs of cardiac or renal failure, encourage daily intake of 2–3 L of fluids or as prescribed. | Increasing hydration helps flush contrast dye out of the system more quickly. |
| For more information about contrast dye, see "Appendicitis," Chapter 54. | |

### ADDITIONAL PROBLEMS

| | |
|---|---|
| "Psychosocial Support for the Patient" | Chapter 8 |
| "Psychosocial Support for the Patient's Family and Significant Others" | Chapter 9 |
| "Pulmonary Embolus," *Risk for Hemorrhaging,* due to anticoagulation therapy | Chapter 15 |
| "Cardiac Surgery" for a discussion of CABG | Chapter 20 |
| "Dysrhythmias and Conduction Disturbances" | Chapter 22 |

### ✔ PATIENT–FAMILY TEACHING AND DISCHARGE PLANNING

When providing patient–family teaching, focus on sensory information, avoid giving excessive information and initiate a visiting nurse referral for necessary follow-up teaching. Include verbal and written information about the following:

✓ Signs and symptoms necessitating immediate medical attention, including chest pain unrelieved by NTG, decreased exercise tolerance, increasing shortness of breath, increased leg edema or pain (postcatheterization), and loss of consciousness.

✓ Importance of reporting to the health care provider any change in pattern or frequency of angina.

✓ Importance of follow-up with the health care provider; confirm date and time of next appointment.

✓ Importance of getting BP checked at regular intervals (home monitoring and recording may be recommended).

✓ Importance of involvement and support of significant others in patient's lifestyle changes

✓ Pulse monitoring: how to self-measure pulse, including parameters for target HR and limits.

✓ Avoiding strenuous activity for at least 1 hour after meals to help prevent excessive O$_2$ demands.

✓ Medications, including drug name, dosage, purpose, schedule, precautions, and potential side effects. Also discuss drug–drug, food–drug, and herb–drug interactions. Instruct the patient who is taking statins to avoid grapefruits and grapefruit juice. Explain the potential for headache and dizziness after NTG administration. Caution the patient about using NTG more frequently than prescribed. Instruct the patient that up to 3 NTG tablets can be taken, 5 minutes apart, for angina, but to call emergency medical services (call 911) if one NTG tablet does not relieve the angina.

✓ Importance of reducing or eliminating the intake of caffeine, which causes vasoconstriction and increases HR.

✓ Dietary changes: low saturated fat, low sodium, low cholesterol, and need for weight loss if appropriate. Encourage the use of food labels to determine the caloric, cholesterol, fat, and sodium content of foods.

✓ Prescribed exercise program and the importance of maintaining a regular exercise schedule, with referral to a cardiac rehabilitation program, in which individualized exercise programs are outlined for the patient.

✓ Practice stress reduction techniques.

✓ Elimination of smoking and tobacco use. Refer the patient to a "stop smoking" program as appropriate. These Internet resources support and describe methods and reasons to advise patients to stop smoking:

- http://smokefree.gov/
- https://www.cancer.gov/about-cancer/causes-prevention/risk/tobacco/cessation-fact-sheet
- American Lung Association: https://www.lung.org/quit-smoking

Availability of community and medical support, such as the American Heart Association: www.americanheart.org

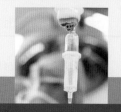

# Dysrhythmias and Conduction Disturbances 22

## OVERVIEW/PATHOPHYSIOLOGY

Dysrhythmias are abnormal rhythms of the heart caused by conditions that alter electrical conduction. Dysrhythmias originate in different areas of the conduction system, such as the sinus node, atrium, atrioventricular (A–V) node, His-Purkinje system, bundle branches, and ventricular tissue. Many conditions and diseases may cause dysrhythmias; the most common are coronary artery disease (CAD) and myocardial infarction (MI). Other causes include fluid and electrolyte imbalance, hormonal imbalance, and changes in oxygenation, medications, substance use, and drug toxicity. Cardiac dysrhythmias may result from the following mechanisms.

*Disturbances in automaticity.* May involve an increase or decrease in automaticity in the sinus node (e.g., sinus tachycardia or sinus bradycardia). Premature beats may arise from the atria, A–V junction, or ventricles. Abnormal rhythms, such as atrial or ventricular tachycardia (VT), also may occur.

*Disturbances in conductivity.* Conduction may be too rapid, as in conditions caused by an accessory pathway (e.g., Wolff–Parkinson–White syndrome), or too slow (e.g., A–V block). Reentry occurs when a stimulus re-excites a conduction pathway through which it already has passed. Once started, this impulse may circulate repeatedly. For reentry to occur, there must be two different pathways for conduction: one with slowed conduction and one with unidirectional block.

*Combinations of altered automaticity and conductivity.* Several dysrhythmias occur together, for example, a first-degree A–V block (disturbance in conductivity) and premature atrial contractions (PACs) (disturbance in automaticity).

## HEALTH CARE SETTING

Primary care, cardiac care, acute care hospitalization, and critical care unit

## ASSESSMENT

*Signs and symptoms.* Can vary from the absence of symptoms to complete cardiopulmonary collapse. General indicators include alterations in level of consciousness (LOC), vertigo, syncope, seizures, weakness, fatigue, activity intolerance, shortness of breath, dyspnea on exertion, chest pain, palpitations, sensation of "skipped beats," anxiety, and restlessness.

*Physical assessment.* Increases or decreases in heart rate (HR), blood pressure (BP), and respiration rate (RR); changes in heart rhythm; dusky color or pallor; crackles; cool skin; decreased urine output; weakened and paradoxical pulse; and abnormal heart sounds (e.g., paradoxical splitting of $S_1$ and $S_2$).

*Electrocardiogram results.* Changes with dysrhythmias include abnormalities in rate, such as sinus bradycardia or sinus tachycardia, irregular rhythm such as atrial fibrillation, extra beats such as PACs and premature junctional contractions, wide and bizarre-looking beats such as premature ventricular contractions (PVCs) and VT, a fibrillating baseline such as ventricular fibrillation, and a straight line as with asystole.

*History and risk factors.* CAD, recent MI, electrolyte disturbances, substance use disorders, drug toxicity, obesity, diabetes mellitus, obstructive sleep apnea, advanced age, genetic factors, thyroid problems, renal disease, hypovolemia, certain medications and supplements, and hypertension.

## DIAGNOSTIC TESTS

*Twelve-lead electrocardiogram.* To detect dysrhythmias and identify the possible origin.

*Serum electrolyte levels.* To identify electrolyte abnormalities that can precipitate dysrhythmias. The most common are potassium and magnesium abnormalities.

*Drug levels.* To identify toxicities (e.g., of digoxin, quinidine, procainamide) that can precipitate dysrhythmias, or to determine substance use that can affect HR and rhythm, such as cocaine use.

*Continuous ambulatory electrocardiogram monitoring (e.g., Holter monitor or cardiac event recorder).* To identify subtle dysrhythmias, associate abnormal rhythms by means of patient's symptoms, and assess response to exercise. Event monitors are used to record less frequent cardiac events.

*Electrophysiology study.* Invasive test in which two to three catheters are placed into the heart, giving it a pacing stimulus at varying sites and of varying voltages. The test determines the origin of dysrhythmia, inducibility, and effectiveness of drug therapy in dysrhythmia suppression.

*Exercise stress testing.* Used in conjunction with Holter monitoring to detect advanced grades of PVCs (those caused by ischemia) and to guide therapy. During the test, electrocardiogram (ECG) and BP readings are taken while the patient walks on a treadmill or pedals a stationary bicycle; response to a constant or increasing workload is observed. The test continues until the patient reaches the target HR or symptoms such as chest pain, severe fatigue, dysrhythmias, or abnormal BP occur.

*Oximetry or arterial blood gas values.* To document the trend of hypoxemia.

## Patient Problem/Analyze Cues/Prioritize Hypotheses

# Impaired Cardiac Function

*due to* conditions that alter electrical conduction

***Desired Outcome/Generate Solutions:*** Within 1 hour of treatment/interventions, the patient has improved cardiac output, as evidenced by BP of 90/60 mm Hg or higher, HR of 60–100 bpm, and normal sinus rhythm on ECG.

| ASSESSMENT—RECOGNIZE CUES/ INTERVENTIONS—TAKE ACTION | RATIONALES |
|---|---|
| Assess the patient's heart rhythm continuously on a monitor. | This assessment will reveal whether dysrhythmias occur or increase in occurrence. |
| Assess BP and symptoms when dysrhythmias occur. | Decreased cardiac output should be reported promptly for timely intervention because it may be life threatening. |
| Signs of decreased cardiac output include decreased BP and symptoms such as unrelieved and prolonged palpitations, chest pain, shortness of breath, weakened and rapid pulse (more than 150 bpm), sensation of skipped beats, dizziness, and syncope. Report significant findings to the health care provider. | |
| If symptoms of decreased cardiac output occur, prepare to transfer the patient to critical care. | Transfer to a critical care unit for continual monitoring is essential. |
| Document dysrhythmias with a rhythm strip, using a 12-lead ECG as necessary. | This assessment will identify dysrhythmias and their general trend. |
| Monitor the patient's laboratory data, particularly electrolyte and digoxin levels. | Serum potassium levels less than 3.5 mEq/L or more than 5.0 mEq/L can cause dysrhythmias. Digoxin toxicity may cause heart block or dysrhythmias. |
| Administer antidysrhythmic agents as prescribed; note patient's response to therapy. Refer to advanced cardiac life support (ACLS) algorithms for medications and interventions based on specific rhythm abnormalities (https://www.aclsmedicaltraining.com/acls-algorithms/). | Administer medications as prescribed for maximal therapeutic effects. Evaluate the patient's response to determine the effectiveness of treatment. |
| Monitor corrected QT interval (QTc) when initiating medications known to cause QT prolongation (e.g., sotalol, propafenone, dofetilide, flecainide). | When QTc is prolonged, it can increase the risk for dysrhythmias. QTc equals QT (in seconds) divided by the square root of the R-to-R interval (in seconds). |
| Provide humidified $O_2$ as prescribed. | $O_2$ may be beneficial if dysrhythmias are related to ischemia or are causing hypoxia. Humidity helps prevent oxygen's drying effects on oral and nasal mucosa. |
| Maintain a quiet environment and administer pain medications promptly. | Both stress and pain can increase sympathetic tone and cause dysrhythmias. |
| Prepare the patient for defibrillation or cardioversion if indicated. | Defibrillation or cardioversion is done to convert dysrhythmias to normal rhythm. This is done in a monitored environment with the patient under intravenous conscious sedation or fully sedated and intubated. After treatment, the patient will return to the unit for continual monitoring. |
| If life-threatening dysrhythmias occur, initiate emergency procedures and cardiopulmonary resuscitation (as indicated by ACLS protocol). | This action provides circulation to vital organs and restores the heart to normal or viable rhythm. |
| When dysrhythmias occur, stay with the patient; provide support and reassurance while performing assessments and administering treatment. | This action reduces stress and provides comfort, which optimally will decrease dysrhythmias. |

## Patient Problem/Analyze Cues/Prioritize Hypotheses

# Deficient Knowledge

*due to* unfamiliarity with the pathology of dysrhythmias and potential lifestyle implications

***Desired Outcome/Generate Solutions:*** Within the 24-hour period before hospital discharge, the patient and significant other verbalize accurate knowledge about the causes of dysrhythmias and implications for the patient's lifestyle modifications.

| ASSESSMENT—RECOGNIZE CUES/ INTERVENTIONS—TAKE ACTION | RATIONALES |
|---|---|
| Assess the patient's health care literacy (language, reading, comprehension). Assess culture and culturally specific information needs. | This assessment helps ensure that information is selected and presented in a manner that is culturally and educationally appropriate. |
| Discuss the etiology and pathology for dysrhythmias, including resulting symptoms. Use multiple teaching modalities, including a heart model, video or slides, written materials, or diagrams as necessary. | This information increases the patient's knowledge about health status. Multiple teaching modalities improve understanding of information. A knowledgeable patient is more likely to adhere to the therapeutic regimen. |
| Inform the patient about the signs and symptoms of dysrhythmias that necessitate medical attention. | Indicators such as unrelieved and prolonged palpitations, chest pain, shortness of breath, rapid pulse (more than 120 bpm), dizziness, and syncope are serious and should be reported promptly for timely intervention. |
| Provide instruction to the patient and significant other about how to check pulse rate for a full minute. | Checking the pulse rate for a full minute ensures a better average of rate than if it were measured for 15 seconds and multiplied by 4. |
| Provide instruction about medications that will be taken after hospital discharge, including drug name, purpose, dosage, schedule, precautions, and potential side effects. Also discuss drug–drug, food–drug, and herb–drug interactions. | The more knowledgeable the patient is, the more likely he or she is to adhere to therapy and report side effects and complications promptly for timely intervention. |
| ⚠ Stress that the patient will be taking long-term antidysrhythmic therapy and that it could be life threatening to stop or skip these medications without health care provider involvement. | Stopping or skipping these drugs may decrease blood levels effective for dysrhythmia suppression. |
| Advise about the availability of support groups and counseling; provide appropriate community referrals. Explain that anxiety and fear, along with periodic feelings of denial, depression, anger, and confusion, are expected after this experience. | Patients who survive sudden cardiac arrest may experience nightmares or other sleep disturbances at home. |
| Stress the importance of leading a productive life. If the patient has travel plans, advise taking along sufficient medication and investigating health care facilities in the travel destination area. | Patients may be fearful of life-threatening dysrhythmias and alter their lives accordingly. Planning for travel with sufficient medications and health care support may reduce stress and protect the patient from unnecessary delays if treatment is sought. |
| Advise the patient and significant other to take cardiopulmonary resuscitation classes; provide addresses for community programs. | Emergency life-saving procedures may be necessary in the future. |
| Inform the patient about the importance of follow-up care; confirm the date and time of the next appointment if known. Explain that outpatient Holter monitoring may be performed periodically. | Medical follow-up is important for the ongoing assessment and management of cardiac dysrhythmias. |
| Explain dietary restrictions that individuals with recurrent dysrhythmias should follow. Discuss the need for reduced intake of products containing caffeine, including coffee, tea, chocolate, and colas. | Caffeine is a stimulant that can cause abnormal heart rhythms. |
| Provide instruction for a general low-cholesterol diet. Encourage reading of food labels to determine the cholesterol content of foods. Refer to a dietitian as needed. | There is an overlap between dysrhythmias and CAD, often necessitating a low-cholesterol diet that decreases hyperlipidemia. |

| ASSESSMENT—RECOGNIZE CUES/ INTERVENTIONS—TAKE ACTION | RATIONALES |
|---|---|
| As indicated, provide instruction about relaxation techniques. | Such techniques enable patients to reduce stress and decrease sympathetic tone. In some types of dysrhythmias, stress can increase the incidence of occurrence. |

**If the Patient Has Had a Pacemaker or Implantable Cardioverter-Defibrillator (ICD) Inserted, Provide the Following Instructions:**

| | |
|---|---|
| • The device is programmed to deliver the electrical stimulus at a predetermined rate and/or after assessing the morphology of the ECG. Pacemakers are commonly used to correct bradycardia or heart block. First- and second-generation ICDs provide for only cardioversion or defibrillation; third-generation ICDs also provide overdrive pacing and backup ventricular pacing. | Patients need to understand the purpose of the implanted devices. |
| • Postoperative complications include atelectasis, pneumonia, seroma at the generator "pocket," pneumothorax, and thrombosis. Lead migration and lead fracture are the two most common structural problems. Interference from unipolar pacemakers and "myopotentials" (electrical interference) are common mechanical complications. | Patients should be informed of these complications and structural problems to report them promptly for timely intervention. |
| • Some procedures interfere with and may change the programming of the device. | ICDs may need to be deactivated during surgical procedures, use of electrocautery, and magnetic resonance imaging. The ICD may "see" these procedures as dysrhythmias and shock the patient during the procedure. |
| • Patients should keep a pocket card on hand stating all relevant pacemaker and ICD data. | This card ensures that medical information is available at all times in case a medical event occurs. |
| Explain the importance of follow-up care; confirm the date and time of the next appointment if known. | Regular checks will be necessary for pacemakers and ICDs. Follow-up care helps ensure the proper functioning of the device. |
| Instruct patients to avoid heavy lifting or contact sports and explain that driving must be approved by the health care provider. | These actions may alter the settings or placement of the ICD. Driving may be contraindicated if pulselessness or decreased LOC is possible. |
| Explain that home monitoring using the telephone or a transmittal device provided by the manufacturer may also be indicated and will need further instruction. | Home monitoring is an efficient and easy method of monitoring the device for many patients. |

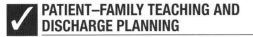

## ✓ PATIENT–FAMILY TEACHING AND DISCHARGE PLANNING

See the patient's primary diagnosis.

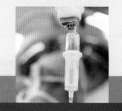

# Heart Failure 23

## OVERVIEW/PATHOPHYSIOLOGY

Heart failure (HF) occurs when the heart is unable to pump enough blood to meet the body's demands. It is caused by cardiac disease that impairs the right and/or left ventricle's (LV's) ability to fill with or eject blood. Common causes are coronary artery disease, myocardial infarction, rhythm disturbances, valvular disease, and cardiomyopathy. HF is a chronic condition that may have acute exacerbations with severe volume overload and pulmonary edema. Emergency intervention and hospitalization often are required when acute decompensation occurs. In the United States, over 6 million adults have HF (National Heart, Lung and Blood Institute, 2022a).

HF can be left-sided, right-sided, or involve both ventricles. Left-sided HF is the most common form; the LV is unable to either empty adequately during systole or to fill adequately during diastole. Left-sided HF can be divided into two types: left-sided HF with reduced ejection fraction (HFrEF), also known as systolic HF, or left-sided HF with preserved ejection fraction (HFpEF), also known as diastolic HF. Sometimes, patients may have a combination of both types. HFrEF occurs when the heart cannot pump blood effectively; common causes include MI, hypertension, heart valve disease, and cardiomyopathy. A decrease in left ventricular ejection fraction (LVEF) is the main indicator. Normal EF is 55%–65%, but patients with HFrEF usually have an EF under 40%, and it can be as low as 5%–10%. Eventually, dilation and hypertrophy of the LV occur, and the heart muscle weakens. Reduced LV function causes blood to back up into the left atrium and fluid accumulation in the lungs, resulting in pulmonary edema and congestion. With HFpEF, the ventricles become stiff and noncompliant, and are unable to relax and fill during diastole. Eventually, the decreased filling volume results in reduced stroke volume. The outcome is the same as HFrEF: fluid congestion in the lungs.

Right-sided HF occurs when the right ventricle (RV) cannot pump effectively. As a result, fluid backs up into the venous system, causing fluid to move into the tissues and organs. Patients will experience abdominal ascites, peripheral edema, jugular vein distention, and hepatomegaly. Left-sided HF is the most common cause of right-sided HF. Other causes include RV infarction, pulmonary embolism, and cor pulmonale.

Biventricular failure occurs with dysfunction of both the RV and LF. Fluid build-up and systemic engorgement occur along with decreased perfusion to vital organs due to reduced cardiac output (Harding et al., 2023).

The New York Heart Association Functional Classification system places patients in categories I–IV based on limitations of physical activities due to symptom burden. A patient's New York Heart Association (NYHA) class will change based on changes of symptoms. The American College of Cardiology Foundation and the American Heart Association use a staging system (Stages A–D) that lists the progression of HF as well as the treatment strategies. Both of these systems are available at https://www.havhrt.com/heartfailureclassification.

## HEALTH CARE SETTING

Primary care, cardiology care, acute hospitalization in cardiac unit or in a critical care unit

## ASSESSMENT

### General

***Signs and symptoms.*** Dyspnea on exertion or at rest, fatigue, decreased exercise tolerance, weakness, orthopnea (unable to lie flat; may need to sleep on pillows or sitting in a chair), paroxysmal nocturnal dyspnea, wheezing, cyanosis, irregular or rapid HR, sudden weight gain from fluid retention, lower extremity edema, abdominal distention, nausea, early satiety, and nocturia. A chronic, nonproductive cough that gets worse when lying flat is often a sign of HF and results from pulmonary congestion. Tachycardia is another early sign of HF and occurs as the body tries to compensate for reduced cardiac output by increasing the heart rate with sympathetic nervous system activation. Associated symptoms include chest/anginal pains, palpitations, near-syncope or syncope, weakness, mental status changes, and decreased urine output.

***Physical assessment.*** Decreased or elevated BP, dysrhythmias, tachycardia, tachypnea, increased venous pulsations, pulsus alternans (alternating strong and weak heartbeats), displaced apical pulse, increased central venous pressure (CVP), jugular venous distention, crackles, wheezes, decreased breath sounds, cardiac gallop and/or murmur, hepatomegaly, ascites, and pitting edema in dependent areas (lower extremities, sacrum).

***History/risk factors.*** Coronary artery disease (CAD), hypertension, diabetes, obstructive sleep apnea, chronic obstructive pulmonary disease, recent surgery, valvular disease (aortic, mitral), pregnancy, recent/current infectious illness, pneumonia, inability to follow appropriate medication or diet instructions, obesity, and hypercholesterolemia.

## Acute decompensated heart failure

**Signs and symptoms.** Increase in severity of HF symptoms and deterioration of one or more NYHA functional classes. Pulmonary edema, cardiogenic shock, and renal failure may be present.

## Acute pulmonary edema

**Signs and symptoms.** Extreme dyspnea, anxiety, restlessness, frothy and blood-tinged sputum, severe orthopnea, and paroxysmal nocturnal dyspnea. Patient exhibits "air hunger" and may thrash about and describe a sensation of drowning.

**Physical assessment.** Crackles, wheezing, decreased breath sounds, increased BP, tachycardia, tachypnea, engorged neck veins, cool and clammy skin, and cardiac gallop/murmur.

## DIAGNOSTIC TESTS

**Chest radiography.** Evaluates the lungs, heart, and vessels, potentially showing pleural or pericardial effusions, cardiomegaly, engorged pulmonary vasculature, and "Kerley-B lines" suggestive of HF.

**Electrocardiogram.** Evaluates cardiac rhythm, rate, and electrical changes caused by CAD, acute myocardial ischemia, left ventricular hypertrophy (widened QRS), and conduction defects.

**Left ventricular ejection fraction.** Determines the percentage of blood ejected from the LV during systole. Normal LVEF is 55%–65%.

**Echocardiography (transthoracic, transesophageal, tissue Doppler, 3D).** Assesses diastolic and systolic ventricular function, LVEF, degree of ventricular dilation, wall thickness, abnormal wall and septal motion, valvular function, estimated pulmonary pressure, presence of thrombus, restrictive outflow, and pericardial effusion. Three-dimensional and tissue Doppler echocardiography detail ventricular synchrony and the potential value of ventricular synchronization. Esophageal echocardiography is specific for detailing posterior cardiac structures, such as valves.

**Cardiac catheterization.** Determines coronary artery narrowing or obstruction, ischemic heart disease, and hemodynamics (left- and right-sided filling pressures, cardiac output, and systemic and pulmonary vascular resistance).

**Left ventriculography.** Evaluates LV function and LVEF.

**Endomyocardial biopsy.** Determines pathology in severe, refractory HF and is performed after heart transplantation to assess myocardial tissue. The biopsy is performed during a right-heart catheterization.

**Radionuclide stress test, stress echocardiogram.** Assesses underlying ischemic heart disease and reversible or fixed ischemic myocardium.

**Pulmonary function tests.** Determines lung capacity and function based on the patient's inspiratory and expiratory efforts.

**Oximetry/arterial blood gas values.** Oximetry assesses the percentage of oxygen in hemoglobin (Hgb). Arterial blood gases (ABGs) assess oxygen, carbon dioxide, bicarbonate, and pH levels. Hypoxemia and metabolic/respiratory alkalosis or acidosis may occur in acute myocardial ischemia, cardiac arrest, and severe HF. Overnight (sleep) oximetry evaluates obstructive sleep apnea.

**Serum blood urea nitrogen, creatinine.** Assesses kidney function. Blood urea nitrogen and creatinine are elevated in acute renal failure and chronic kidney disease.

**Serum electrolytes.** Assesses potassium, magnesium, calcium, sodium, and phosphorous, which may be elevated or decreased in several cardiac and renal diseases. Monitoring is essential to avoid cardiac dysrhythmias or arrest.

**Cardiac enzymes.** Cardiac enzymes and troponins are elevated in HF, myocardial infarction, and chronic kidney disease.

**Liver function tests, including serum aspartate aminotransferase and serum bilirubin.** Assess liver enzymes, which are elevated with hepatic congestion.

**Brain natriuretic peptide.** Evaluates the level of brain natriuretic peptide (BNP), which is released from the ventricles in response to wall stress. This test is useful in differentiating HF from other causes of dyspnea, including pulmonary disease. Negative BNP (less than 100 pg/mL) suggests non-HF etiology.

**Digoxin level.** Assesses the level of digoxin in patients taking this medication. Excessive dosing, hypokalemia, and renal failure may cause digoxin toxicity. Levels less than 1 ng/mL are expected in the presence of HF.

**Complete blood count.** Evaluates for increases or decreases in white and red blood cells, platelets, Hgb, hematocrit (Hct), and differentiated blood cells.

**Thyroid-stimulating hormone level.** Determines thyroid dysfunction (hyperthyroidism or hypothyroidism), which may contribute to HF and dysrhythmias.

## Patient Problem/Analyze Cues/Prioritize Hypotheses

# Impaired Gas Exchange

*due to* congestion or fluid in the lungs at the alveolar-capillary membrane

**Desired Outcome/Generate Outcomes:** Within 30 minutes of treatment/interventions, the patient has adequate gas exchange, as evidenced by normal breath sounds and skin color, presence of eupnea, HR of 100 bpm or less, $PaO_2$ of 80 mm Hg or higher, and $PaCO_2$ of 35–45 mm Hg.

| ASSESSMENT—RECOGNIZE CUES/ INTERVENTIONS—TAKE ACTION | RATIONALES |
|---|---|
| Assess all lung fields for breath sounds. | Decreased breath sounds signify decreased ventilation. The presence of crackles may signal alveolar congestion due to HF. Wheezing may signify associated bronchitis or asthma. |
| Monitor oximetry and ABG values and report significant findings. | Oximetry of 92% or less and the presence of hypoxemia (decreased $PaO_2$) and hypercarbia (increased $PaCO_2$) signify decreased oxygenation. |
| Assess respiratory rate (RR), lung excursion, use of accessory muscles, air hunger, mental status changes, cyanosis, and changes in HR or BP. Report significant changes. | These are signs of increasing respiratory distress that require prompt intervention. |
| Assist the patient into high-Fowler position with the head of bed (HOB) up 90 degrees. | This position decreases the work of breathing, reduces cardiac workload, and promotes gas exchange. |
| Instruct the patient to take slow, deep breaths. | Taking deep breaths increases oxygenation to the myocardium and improves prognosis. |
| Administer oxygen as prescribed. High-flow $O_2$ may be administered either by a nonrebreathing mask, positive airway pressure devices, or endotracheal intubation and mechanical ventilation. Deliver oxygen with humidity. | Once stabilized, $O_2$ is titrated to keep pulse oximetry readings higher than 92%. Humidity helps prevent oxygen's convective drying effects on oral and nasal mucosa. |
| Administer diuretics as prescribed. | Diuretics promote normovolemia by reducing fluid accumulation and blood volume. Fluid overload decreases perfusion in the lungs, causing hypoxemia. |
| Monitor potassium levels. | Hypokalemia (potassium less than 3.5 mEq/L) can occur in patients taking some diuretics, such as furosemide and metolazone. |
| Administer vasodilators as prescribed. | Vasodilators cause venous dilation and decrease pulmonary congestion, which will improve gas exchange. |
| *Hydralazine* is an oral vasodilator and afterload reducer. It is used in combination with nitrates in patients who are angiotensin-converting enzyme (ACE) inhibitor/angiotensin receptor blocker (ARB) intolerant because of renal dysfunction. It improves mortality and HF symptoms to a lesser degree than ACE inhibitors and can cause reflex tachycardia. | |
| *Nitrates* are coronary vasodilators used in conjunction with hydralazine (see earlier). They are also used in ischemic heart disease as antianginal drugs. | |
| *ACE inhibitors* (e.g., enalapril, lisinopril, benazepril, captopril, quinapril, ramipril) suppress the effects of the RAS by reducing angiotensin II and causing decreased aldosterone secretion. This lowers BP and reduces preload and afterload, decreasing the work of the LV. | |
| *ARBs* (e.g., losartan, valsartan, candesartan) are used when ACE inhibitors are not tolerated or cause adverse effects. | |
| As indicated, have emergency equipment (e.g., airway, manual resuscitation bag) available and functional. | Patients with severely decompensated HF may suffer cardiac arrest. |
| As indicated, prepare to transfer the patient to critical care. | The patient may require invasive hemodynamic monitoring, which includes measurement of pulmonary artery pressure, pulmonary artery wedge pressure, $SvO_2$, cardiac output, and CVP. |

## Patient Problem/Analyze Cues/Prioritize Hypotheses

# Fluid Imbalance (Overload)

*due to* compromised regulatory mechanisms occurring with decreased cardiac output

***Desired Outcomes/Generate Solutions:*** Within 1 hour of treatment, the patient demonstrates less shortness of breath and has increased urinary output. Within 1 day of treatment, peripheral edema is decreased. Weight loss occurs and becomes stable within 2–3 days.

| ASSESSMENT—RECOGNIZE CUES/ INTERVENTIONS—TAKE ACTION | RATIONALES |
|---|---|
| At frequent intervals assess intake and output (I&O), including insensible losses from diaphoresis and respirations. | Decreasing urinary output can signal decreased cardiac output, which decreases renal blood flow. |
| Assess daily morning weight; record and report steady losses or gains. | Weight changes identify fluid retention and fluid loss, guiding titration of diuretics. |
| Assess for edema in dependent areas such as the legs, ankles, feet, and sacrum. | The presence of weight gain and edema signifies fluid retention. Daily assessment may guide early treatment, averting a medical crisis and decreasing the potential for rehospitalization. |
| Assess lung sounds for signs of fluid retention (i.e., crackles or wheezing). Note sputum color and productivity. | Fluid retention and increased production of sputum may signify HF. |
| Monitor for jugular vein distention and ascites. | These are indicators of fluid overload. |
| Monitor laboratory results for increased urine specific gravity, decreased Hct, increased urine osmolality, hyponatremia, hypokalemia, and hypochloremia. | These are indicators of fluid imbalance. |
| Monitor intravenous (IV) rate of flow. Use an infusion control device. | These measures are essential to prevent volume overload during IV infusion. |
| Unless contraindicated, provide ice chips or ice pops. Record amount on the I&O record. Provide frequent mouth care to reduce dry mucous membranes. | This provides comfort and decreases thirst while providing minimal amounts of fluid. Small amounts of room-temperature water also relieve thirst. |
| Administer diuretics as prescribed and record the patient's response. *Loop diuretics* (e.g., furosemide, bumetanide, torsemide): these agents cause excretion of water and sodium, reduce preload, and prevent fluid retention. Loop diuretics are administered orally or by IV bolus or drip in severe HF. Loop diuretics must be given with caution in renal failure or hypokalemia. *Thiazide diuretics* (e.g., hydrochlorothiazide, metolazone): hydrochlorothiazide is administered orally for prevention or treatment of fluid retention. Metolazone is a potent diuretic often given 1/2 hour before loop diuretics. This medication potentiates diuresis and is administered in the presence of severe volume overload in HF. Hyponatremia, hypokalemia, and worsening renal dysfunction may occur, necessitating ongoing assessment. | Diuretics promote normovolemia by reducing fluid accumulation and blood volume. |
| Administer morphine sulfate if prescribed. | Morphine induces vasodilation and decreases venous return to the heart. Morphine also relieves acute anxiety and decreases RR. |
| Inform patients and families about the importance of adhering to a low-sodium diet. | Hypernatremia can increase fluid retention. A 1- to 2-g/day sodium diet is recommended. |

## Patient Problem/Analyze Cues/Prioritize Hypotheses

# Ineffective Tissue Perfusion (Cardiac and Cerebral)

*due to* decreased blood flow occurring with decreased cardiac output

***Desired Outcome/Generate Solutions:*** By at least the 24-hour period before hospital discharge, the patient has BP within 20 mm Hg of desired baseline BP; HR of 100 bpm or less with regular rhythm; RR of 20 breaths/minute or less with normal depth and pattern (eupnea); brisk capillary refill (less than 2 seconds); and significant improvement in mental status or orientation to person, place, and time.

| ASSESSMENT—RECOGNIZE CUES/ INTERVENTIONS—TAKE ACTION | RATIONALES |
|---|---|
| Assess BP every 15 minutes or more frequently if unstable. Be alert to decreases greater than 20 mm Hg over patient's baseline or associated changes such as dizziness and altered mentation. | Hypotension is a side effect of many HF medications (especially beta-blockers), as well as an effect of aggressive diuresis. Careful monitoring is essential to avoid decreased perfusion to vital organs. |
| Assess HR every 15–30 minutes. Monitor for increased or decreased HR and irregular rhythms. | These signs may signal decompensation and decreased function of the heart. |
| Assess the extremities for pulse presence and amplitude, capillary refill, color, temperature, and edema. | Decreased pulse amplitude, delayed capillary refill (more than 2 seconds), pallor, and coolness are indicators of peripheral vasoconstriction (from sympathetic nervous system (SNS) compensation). Edema is evidence of fluid overload. |
| Report any significant changes immediately to the health care provider. | Significant changes may require urgent intervention because they may be life threatening. |
| Assess for restlessness, anxiety, mental status changes, confusion, lethargy, stupor, and coma. Institute safety precautions accordingly. | These are indicators of decreased cerebral perfusion and hypoxia that must be treated promptly. |
| Administer inotropic medications and vasodilators as prescribed. Monitor effects closely and remain alert to cardiovascular changes, including hypotension and irregular heartbeats. | • Use of inotropic medications may be associated with increased mortality and ventricular dysrhythmias. Administration of inotropic medications requires transfer to the critical care unit for continual monitoring. |
| IV inotropic medications (e.g., dobutamine, dopamine, milrinone) increase the strength of ventricular contractions and are administered if signs of low cardiac output and cardiogenic shock are present. They also are administered in advanced-stage HF as a bridge to transplantation or for palliation of symptoms. | |
| IV vasodilators (e.g., nitroglycerin [NTG], nitroprusside, nesiritide) are administered to decrease cardiac workload by reducing ventricular filling pressures and systemic vascular resistance (afterload). These medications are avoided in low-output HF, cardiogenic shock, and systolic blood pressure (SBP) less than 90 mm Hg. | |
| • *NTG:* arterial and venous vasodilator. It reduces pulmonary capillary wedge pressure (PCWP) and may require continuous monitoring in critical care. Because of tachyphylaxis (drug tolerance), increased doses may be needed to achieve the desired effect. | |
| • *Nitroprusside:* potent arterial and venous vasodilator and afterload reducer. It must be administered in intensive care due to the need for continual hemodynamic monitoring. | |
| • *Morphine sulfate:* a coronary vasodilator that may be given in acute decompensated HF or acute pulmonary edema to decrease anxiety and work of breathing and to relieve angina if ischemic heart disease is present. | |

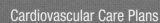

## Patient Problem/Analyze Cues/Prioritize Hypotheses

# Ineffective Tissue Perfusion (Multisystem)

*due to* decreased cardiac output

**Desired Outcomes/Generate Solutions:** By at least the 24-hour period before hospital discharge, the patient exhibits adequate cardiac output, as evidenced by SBP of at least 90 mm Hg, HR of 100 bpm or less, urinary output of at least 0.5 mL/kg/hour, stable weight, eupnea, normal breath sounds, and edema 1+ or less on a 0–4+ scale. By at least 48 hours before hospital discharge, the patient is free of new dysrhythmias, does not exhibit significant changes in mental status, and remains oriented to person, place, and time.

| ASSESSMENT—RECOGNIZE CUES/ INTERVENTIONS—TAKE ACTION | RATIONALES |
|---|---|
| Assess for jugular venous distention, extra heart sounds, changes in mental status or level of consciousness, cool extremities, hypotension, tachycardia, and tachypnea. Report any of these findings to the health care provider immediately. | These are indicators of decreased cardiac output, which must be reported promptly for timely intervention. |
| Assess lungs for adventitious breath sounds and shortness of breath. | Dyspnea, crackles, and shortness of breath signal fluid accumulation in the lungs and may be a direct indicator of ventricular failure and decreased cardiac output. |
| Monitor I&O; weigh the patient daily. | Decreasing urine output and weight gain occur as a result of decreased cardiac contractility, which causes decreased renal perfusion and fluid retention. |
| Assess for peripheral (sacral, pedal) edema. | Edema occurs with HF because of decreased cardiac output and poor renal perfusion. |
| Assist with activities of daily living and coordinate treatments and testing, promoting periods of undisturbed rest. If necessary, limit visitors. | Rest promotes well-being and decreases cardiac workload. |
| Administer medications as prescribed, such as beta-blockers, calcium channel blockers, vasodilators, and antidysrhythmic agents.<br><br>*Beta-blockers* (metoprolol XL) and *alpha/beta-adrenergic blockers* (carvedilol): block effects of SNS and toxic effects of neurohormones on the myocardium.<br><br>*Calcium channel blockers:* may be used in diastolic HF; except for amlodipine or felodipine, calcium channel blockers are avoided in LV systolic dysfunction because they decrease cardiac contractility. | *Beta-blockers* (metoprolol XL) and *alpha/beta-adrenergic blockers* (carvedilol) decrease HR and BP, decreasing cardiac workload.<br><br>*Calcium channel blockers:* may be used in diastolic HF to assist with relaxation and filling and reduce outflow tract obstruction (hypertrophic cardiomyopathy). |
| Collaborate with cardiac specialists for dysrhythmia management if required. | Dysrhythmias affect morbidity and mortality and may require rehospitalization for management. Surgical interventions may include placement of an implantable cardioverter-defibrillator (ICD) due to repeated life-threatening episodes of ventricular tachycardia, or a biventricular pacer to correct rhythm abnormalities. |
| Collaborate with cardiac specialists in preparation for placement of ventricular assistive device (VAD) or future heart transplantation if indicated. | If the patient's condition declines, placement of a VAD or a heart transplantation may be lifesaving and necessary. |
| Assist the patient into a position of comfort, usually semi-Fowler position (HOB up to 30–45 degrees). | This position decreases the work of breathing and reduces cardiac workload. |

## Patient Problem/Analyze Cues/Prioritize Hypotheses

# Fatigue (Decreased Exercise Tolerance)

*due to* imbalance between oxygen supply and demand occurring with a decrease in cardiac muscle contractility

**Desired Outcome/Generate Solutions:** During activity, the patient rates perceived exertion at 3 or less on a 0–10 scale and exhibits cardiac tolerance to activity, as evidenced by RR of 20 breaths/minute or less, SBP within 20 mm Hg of resting range, HR within 20 bpm of resting HR, and absence of chest pain and new dysrhythmias.

| ASSESSMENT—RECOGNIZE CUES/ INTERVENTIONS—TAKE ACTION | RATIONALES |
|---|---|
| Assess the patient's physiologic response to activity and report significant findings. | Chest pain, new dysrhythmias, increased shortness of breath, HR increased greater than 20 bpm over resting HR, and SBP greater than 20 mm Hg over resting SBP are significant findings of decreased cardiac output. |
| Ask the patient to rate perceived exertion (RPE) (see Chapter 1, *Activity Intolerance*, for a description). | Patients should not experience an RPE of more than 3. Decrease intensity and frequency of activity until an RPE of 3 or less is achieved during activity. |
| Assess vital signs every 4 hours and report significant findings. | Irregular HR, HR greater than 100 bpm, or decreasing BP may be signs of cardiac ischemia. |
| Provide instruction on self-measurement of HR for assessing exercise tolerance. | An elevated rate increases myocardial $O_2$ demand; a significantly decreased rate may decrease cardiac perfusion causing ischemia. |
| Assess for and report oliguria, decreased BP, decreased mentation, and dizziness. | These are indicators of acute decreased cardiac output. |
| Assess peripheral pulses and distal extremity skin temperature and color. Report significant findings. | These indicators reveal the integrity of peripheral perfusion. Changes such as decreased amplitude of pulses, coolness, pallor, or cyanosis must be reported for timely intervention. |
| Coordinate care to meet the patient's needs. Ensure that the bedside environment is organized and that necessary items are within reach. | These actions promote well-being and decrease stress and cardiac workload. |
| Facilitate coordination of treatments and tests to provide undisturbed rest periods. | Rest aids recovery and decreases cardiac workload. |
| Administer $O_2$ as prescribed. | Increasing oxygen to the myocardium promotes activity tolerance. |
| Assist with passive and active or assistive range-of-motion exercises, based on the patient's tolerance and prescribed limitations. | These exercises promote circulation and prevent complications to joints and tissue caused by prolonged immobility. |
| Facilitate participation in a post-discharge exercise or rehabilitation program, if appropriate. | This will improve the patient's quality of life, activity tolerance, heart function, and disease outcomes. |

## Patient Problem/Analyze Cues/Prioritize Hypotheses

# Anxiety

*due to* a potentially life-threatening situation

**Desired Outcome/Generate Solutions:** Within 24 hours of interventions, the patient begins to communicate anxieties and concerns and expresses ways to increase physical and psychologic comfort.

| ASSESSMENT—RECOGNIZE CUES/ INTERVENTIONS—TAKE ACTION | RATIONALES |
|---|---|
| Assess for and acknowledge the patient's anxieties and concerns and provide opportunities for the patient and significant other to express their feelings. Be reassuring and supportive. | Encouraging communication and acknowledging feelings may reduce anxieties. Empathy demonstrates support and caring. |
| Assist the patient in being as comfortable as possible, ensuring prompt pain relief and supportive positioning. | These actions promote an overall sense of well-being and positive outcomes. |
| Create and maintain a calm and quiet environment. | This action prevents or reduces the sensory overload that may cause increased anxiety. |
| Explain all treatment modalities, especially those that may be uncomfortable (e.g., $O_2$ face mask, IV therapy, invasive testing). | This reduces anxiety and enables a sense of control. |
| Remain with the patient as much as possible, especially during procedures and testing. | This provides emotional and physical support, thereby reducing anxiety. |
| For further interventions, see "Psychosocial Support," *Anxiety*, Chapter 8. | |

## Patient Problem/Analyze Cues/Prioritize Hypotheses

# Deficient Knowledge

*due to* unfamiliarity with the purpose, precautions, and side effects of diuretic therapy

*Desired Outcome/Generate Solutions:* Within the 24-hour period before hospital discharge, the patient verbalizes accurate knowledge of the precautions and side effects of diuretic therapy.

| ASSESSMENT—RECOGNIZE CUES/ INTERVENTIONS—TAKE ACTION | RATIONALES |
|---|---|
| Assess the patient's health care literacy (language, reading, comprehension). Assess culture and culturally specific information needs. | This ensures that information is selected and presented in a manner that is culturally and educationally appropriate. |
| Provide instruction about the purpose of the prescribed diuretic. | Diuretics promote urine elimination and reduce fluid accumulation. Patients who are knowledgeable about their medication's purpose are more likely to adhere to the therapeutic regimen. |
| Depending on the type of diuretic used, instruct the patient to report signs and symptoms of the following: | A knowledgeable patient will know how to monitor for and report symptoms that necessitate medical attention. |
| • *Hypokalemia*: anorexia, irregular pulse, nausea, apathy, and muscle cramps. | Use of furosemide and metolazone, which are potassium-wasting diuretics, can cause these symptoms related to hypokalemia. |
| • *Hyperkalemia*: muscle weakness, hyporeflexia, and irregular HR. | Use of amiloride and spironolactone, which are potassium-sparing diuretics, can cause these symptoms related to hyperkalemia. |
| • *Hyponatremia*: fatigue, weakness, and edema (caused by fluid extravasation). | Use of bumetanide, a diuretic that promotes the excretion of NaCl, may cause these symptoms related to hyponatremia. |
| Explain the importance of follow-up monitoring of blood levels of potassium and sodium for patients on long-term diuretic therapy. | Hypokalemia is the most common adverse effect of diuretic therapy. Hyperkalemia and sodium imbalance also may occur. |
| Provide instruction about the importance of potassium replacement with food or potassium supplements if potassium-wasting diuretics are prescribed (e.g., furosemide). | Apricots, bananas, oranges, and raisins are examples of foods high in potassium. Potassium supplements may be necessary as well. |
| Instruct the patient to rise slowly when getting up from a sitting or recumbent position. | Orthostatic hypotension may occur with diuresis. |

## Patient Problem/Analyze Cues/Prioritize Hypotheses

# Deficient Knowledge

*due to* unfamiliarity with the purpose, precautions, and side effects of digoxin therapy

***Desired Outcome/Generate Solutions:*** Within the 24-hour period before hospital discharge, the patient verbalizes an accurate understanding of the purpose, precautions, and side effects associated with digoxin therapy.

| ASSESSMENT—RECOGNIZE CUES/ INTERVENTIONS—TAKE ACTION | RATIONALES |
|---|---|
| Assess the patient's health care literacy (language, reading, comprehension). Assess culture and culturally specific information needs. | This assessment helps ensure that information is selected and presented in a manner that is culturally and educationally appropriate. |
| Provide instruction about the purpose of digoxin therapy as appropriate. Digoxin slows conduction through the atrioventricular node and increases the strength of contractility. It also may improve symptoms in classes III–IV HF patients. | A patient who is knowledgeable is more likely to adhere to the therapy. |
| Provide instruction about the technique and importance of assessing HR before taking digoxin. | Digoxin may be withheld when the HR is less than 60 bpm (or as recommended by the health care provider). |
| Instruct the patient not to take the medication if there is a 20-bpm or greater change from the normal rate and to notify the health care provider of this change. | Slowing the heart rate too much may result in cardiac arrest. |
| Explain that serum potassium levels are monitored routinely. | Low levels of potassium potentiate digoxin toxicity. |
| Explain that apical HR and peripheral pulses are assessed for irregularity. | Irregularity may signal the presence of dysrhythmias (e.g., heart block), which is associated with digoxin toxicity. |
| Instruct the patient to be alert to nausea, vomiting, anorexia, headache, diarrhea, blurred vision, yellow-haze vision, and mental confusion. Explain the importance of reporting signs and symptoms promptly to the health care provider. | These are indicators of digoxin toxicity that necessitate prompt medical attention. |

## Patient Problem/Analyze Cues/Prioritize Hypotheses

# Deficient Knowledge

*due to* unfamiliarity with the purpose, precautions, and side effects of vasodilators

***Desired Outcome/Generate Solutions:*** Within the 24-hour period before hospital discharge, the patient verbalizes accurate knowledge of the purpose, precautions, and side effects of vasodilators.

| ASSESSMENT—RECOGNIZE CUES/ INTERVENTIONS—TAKE ACTION | RATIONALES |
|---|---|
| Assess the patient's health care literacy (language, reading, comprehension). Assess culture and culturally specific information needs. | This assessment helps ensure that information is selected and presented in a manner that is culturally and educationally appropriate. |
| Provide instruction about the purpose of vasodilators. | See the discussion in *Impaired Gas Exchange*, earlier. |
| Explain that a headache can occur after the administration of a vasodilator. | Headaches can occur because of dilation of the cranial vessels or from orthostatic hypotension. |

## ASSESSMENT—RECOGNIZE CUES/ INTERVENTIONS—TAKE ACTION

## RATIONALES

| ASSESSMENT—RECOGNIZE CUES/ INTERVENTIONS—TAKE ACTION | RATIONALES |
|---|---|
| Suggest that lying down will help alleviate pain. | A supine position may help alleviate the pain by increasing blood flow to the heart and head, although blood flow to the head may worsen the headache. Pain medication and decreased dosage of the vasodilator may be necessary. |
| Provide instruction about the importance of assessment for weight gain and signs of peripheral or sacral edema. | A possible side effect of vasodilator therapy is a decrease in venous return to the right side of the heart with subsequent accumulation in the periphery. |
| For patients on long-term ACE inhibitor therapy, explain the importance of follow-up monitoring of blood levels of serum creatinine. | ACE inhibitors may cause kidney damage, resulting in decreased creatinine clearance. If this occurs, the patient may need to be taken off the medication. |
| For patients receiving ACE inhibitors, provide instruction about the importance of using care when rising from a sitting or recumbent position. | There is potential for injury caused by orthostatic hypotension, a potential side effect of ACE inhibitors. |
| For the patient receiving ACE inhibitors. Provide instructions about the technique for and importance of assessing BP before taking the medication. Explain that it is possible to purchase automatic BP machines from local pharmacies and if necessary to seek reimbursement or funding information from a social worker. | Vasodilators can cause an excessive reduction in BP. Although patients should obtain BP parameters from their health care providers, ACE inhibitors are usually withheld when BP is less than 110/60 mm Hg. |
| Instruct the patient to notify the health care provider if he or she has omitted a dose because of a low or significantly changed BP. | It may be necessary to lower the dose or change the medication. |

## ADDITIONAL PROBLEMS:

| | |
|---|---|
| "Immobility" | Chapter 1 |
| "Psychosocial Support for the Patient" | Chapter 8 |
| "Coronary Artery Disease" for *Body Weight Problem (Weight Gain)* | Chapter 21 |
| "Dysrhythmias and Conduction Disturbances," patients with HF may require an ICD. | Chapter 22 |

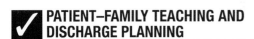

## ✔ PATIENT–FAMILY TEACHING AND DISCHARGE PLANNING

When providing patient–family teaching, focus on sensory information, avoid giving excessive information, and initiate a visiting nurse referral for necessary follow-up teaching. Include verbal and written information about the following:

✓ Medications, including drug name, purpose, dosage, schedule, precautions, and potential side effects. Also discuss drug–drug, food–drug, and herb–drug interactions.

✓ Signs and symptoms that necessitate immediate medical attention: dyspnea, decreased exercise tolerance, alterations in pulse rate/rhythm, alterations in or loss of consciousness (caused by dysrhythmias or decreased cardiac output), oliguria, and weight gain of greater than 2–3 lb over 2 days or 3–5 lb over a week.

✓ Reinforcement that HF is a chronic disease requiring lifetime treatment.

✓ Recommendation that preventive health measures be followed, including Pneumovax and flu vaccines to prevent illness.

✓ Importance of abstaining from alcohol, which increases cardiac muscle deterioration.

✓ Importance of a low-sodium diet (less than 1000 mg/ day) to prevent fluid retention.

✓ Need for physical support from family and outside agencies as the disease progresses.

✓ Availability of community and medical support, such as:
  • American Heart Association: www.americanheart .org

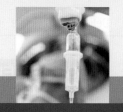

# Hypertension 24

## OVERVIEW/PATHOPHYSIOLOGY

In the United States, 48% of adults over age 18 years either have hypertension (high blood pressure [BP]), or are taking medications for hypertension (CDC, 2021a). BP is controlled by four mechanisms: (1) arterial baroreceptors control BP by altering heart rate and constricting or dilating arteries; (2) renal function regulates body-fluid volume, retaining or excreting water and electrolytes in hypotension or hypertension; (3) the renin–angiotensin system vasodilates or vasoconstricts and controls aldosterone release, causing the kidneys to reabsorb sodium and thus preventing fluid loss; and (4) vascular autoregulation maintains consistent levels of tissue perfusion. An alteration in any of these mechanisms, such as renal failure or atherosclerosis, can result in hypertension.

Determination of etiology of hypertension may include blood and urine testing to evaluate kidney function (BUN, creatinine), cortisol testing to evaluate for Cushing disease, and glucose and lipid panel to evaluate for diabetes and hyperlipidemia, which contribute to blood vessel changes and organ damage.

Risk factors include age, heredity, ethnicity (incidence is higher in African Americans), renal disease, obesity, hyperlipidemia, smoking, unhealthy diet, sleep apnea, psychosocial stress, excessive alcohol intake, and some endocrine disorders (e.g., Cushing disease, diabetes, thyroid disease, primary aldosteronism, pheochromocytoma).

Complications of hypertension include increased incidence of transient ischemic attack/stroke, retinopathy, cardiovascular disease, heart failure, aortic aneurysm, and kidney disease.

The American College of Cardiology and American Heart Association (Whelton et al., 2017) define normal BP as a systolic BP (SBP) less than 120 mm Hg and a diastolic BP (DBP) less than 80 mm Hg. An elevated BP is SBP of 120–129 mm Hg and DBP less than 80 mm Hg. For example, if a patient has an SBP of 120–129 mm Hg and a DBP of 79 mm Hg or less, that patient's BP is considered elevated based on the SBP.

Hypertension is defined as follows:

- Stage 1: SBP 130–139 mm Hg or DBP 80–89 mm Hg
- Stage 2: SBP 140 mm Hg or greater or DBP 90 mm Hg or greater
- Hypertensive crisis: SBP greater than 180 mm Hg or DBP greater than 120 mm Hg

The treatment goals of hypertension are to lower BP and prevent the complications of hypertension. Persons 65 years and older are to achieve an SBP of less than 130 mm Hg. In persons younger than 65 years and those with comorbidities including cardiac disease, chronic kidney disease, or diabetes, the treatment goal is less than 130/80 mm Hg.

## HEALTH CARE SETTING

Primary care or cardiology clinic; hospitalization may be necessary for treatment of hypertensive crisis

## Patient Problem/Analyze Cues/Prioritize Hypotheses

# Deficient Knowledge

*due to* unfamiliarity with hypertension treatment including BP evaluation, medications, activity and exercise, nutrition, and recommended lifestyle changes

*Desired Outcome/Generate Solutions:* After receiving instruction, the patient verbalizes accurate knowledge of the importance of frequent hypertension evaluation, treatments, and adhering to lifestyle changes.

| ASSESSMENT—RECOGNIZE CUES/ INTERVENTIONS—TAKE ACTION | RATIONALES |
| --- | --- |
| Assess the patient's health care literacy (language, reading, comprehension). Assess culture and culturally specific information needs. | This assessment helps ensure that information is selected and presented in a manner that is culturally and educationally appropriate. |

| ASSESSMENT—RECOGNIZE CUES/ INTERVENTIONS—TAKE ACTION | RATIONALES |
|---|---|
| Explain the importance of self-evaluation of BP at routine intervals and adherence to the prescribed medication therapy. | Frequent evaluation provides feedback on response to therapy and may help improve adherence to therapy. Self-evaluation aids in evaluating "white coat hypertension," which is defined as an increased BP when assessed by a health care provider. |
| Provide instruction on the importance of nutrition, including a low sodium diet, exercise, smoking cessation, stress reduction, weight loss, and decreased alcohol intake, as appropriate for each individual. Demonstrate food label evaluation, particularly reviewing sodium, calories, and fat in selected foods. Refer to a smoking cessation program and a nutritionist and exercise program, if appropriate. | Prevention of hypertension and primary treatment for elevated BP include promotion of lifestyle modification, which can prevent hypertension and may lower BP when adhered to. |
| Provide instructions on medication actions, administration times, side effects, adverse effects, and the importance of taking as prescribed. Include drug–drug, food–drug, and herb–drug interactions. | Knowledge about and adherence to the prescribed regimen can lower morbidity and mortality risk and improve patient outcomes. |
| Instruct the patient about the importance of seeking medical evaluation if BP reading is greater than 180/120 mm Hg or less than 90/60 mm Hg, or if headache, dizziness, lightheadedness, or blurred vision occurs. | Severe hypertension or hypotension can be life threatening, compromising perfusion to vital organs. |

## ADDITIONAL PROBLEMS:

| | |
|---|---|
| "Psychosocial Support for the Patient" | Chapter 8 |
| "Coronary Artery Disease" for *Body Weight Problem (Weight Gain)*, *Deficient Knowledge (purpose, precautions, and side effects of beta-blockers)* | Chapter 21 |

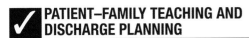

## PATIENT–FAMILY TEACHING AND DISCHARGE PLANNING

When providing patient–family teaching, focus on sensory information, avoid giving excessive information, and initiate a visiting nurse referral for necessary follow-up teaching. Include verbal and written information about the following:

✓ Signs and symptoms that necessitate immediate medical attention: elevated or decreased BP readings (greater than 180/120 mm Hg or less than 90/60 mm Hg), headache, dizziness, lightheadedness, blurred vision, chest pain, dyspnea, or syncope.

✓ Self-evaluation of BP when indicated. Monitoring machines are readily available in local stores and pharmacies or online. Evaluation of BP must be done while seated, after resting for 5 minutes, and recorded. Taking three readings 1 minute apart in the morning and evening is recommended by the American Society for Hypertension (ASH). Appropriate cuff size must be selected (AHA guidelines). Measurement of standing BP can be obtained when indicated, that is, in diabetic autonomic neuropathy, when orthostatic symptoms are present, or when a dose increase in antihypertensive therapy has been made (ASH).

✓ Medications, including name, purpose, dosage, schedule, precautions, and potential side effects. Discuss drug–drug, food–drug, and herb–drug interactions.

✓ Importance of abstaining from smoking and excessive salt and alcohol intake, which increase BP. The DASH (Dietary Approaches to Stop Hypertension) eating plan has been shown to be beneficial in lowering BP. See https://www.nhlbi.nih.gov/education/dash-eating-plan for more information.

✓ Reinforcement that hypertension is a chronic disease requiring lifetime treatment.

✓ Reinforcement of the need to keep follow-up appointments for monitoring of BP and renal function, and regular ophthalmology appointments to assess for eye complications.

✓ Need for physical support from the family and outside agencies.

✓ Availability of community and medical support:
  • American Heart Association: www.americanheart.org
  • Importance of smoking cessation education and community resources to assist in cessation. Information on smoking cessation programs and information
  • Smoke Free: https://smokefree.gov/
  • Quit Smoking (American Lung Association): https://www.lung.org/quit-smoking/smoking-facts
  • How to Quit Smoking (CDC): https://www.cdc.gov/tobacco/campaign/tips/quit-smoking/index.html
  • Additional general information can be obtained by visiting the American Lung Association www.lung.org.

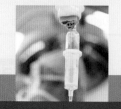

# Pulmonary Arterial Hypertension 25

## OVERVIEW/PATHOPHYSIOLOGY

Pulmonary arterial hypertension (PAH) is a chronic, progressive disease that causes right-heart failure and death as the disease advances. A diagnosis of pulmonary hypertension (PH) is confirmed by right-heart catheterization.

There are two types of PAH. The cause of idiopathic PAH (IPAH) is unknown, but it may be related to cirrhosis, HIV, and connective tissue diseases. IPAH is more common in females. Classic symptoms are fatigue and dyspnea upon exertion; syncope and dizziness may also occur. These symptoms are related to the inability of the heart to increase cardiac output in response to increased oxygen demand. As the disease progresses, dyspnea occurs at rest. The workload of the right ventricle is increased, resulting in right ventricular hypertrophy and, eventually, heart failure.

Secondary PAH (SPAH) occurs when another disease causes an increase in pulmonary artery pressures, which becomes chronic and causes changes in the pulmonary vasculature. Conditions that can lead to SPAH include chronic pulmonary embolus, interstitial lung disease, parenchymal lung disease, left ventricular dysfunction, or systemic connective tissue diseases, such as scleroderma or lupus. Symptoms of SPAH include those of the underlying disease. Symptoms related to SPAH include lethargy, fatigue, and chest pain, along with initial findings of right ventricular hypertrophy and right-sided heart failure.

There is no definitive cure for PAH. If SPAH is present, the underlying causes are treated. Treatment for both types of PAH aims to improve the quality of life and prolong life. Drug therapy is given to improve the vasodilation of the pulmonary blood vessels. Diuretics are given to remove excess fluid. Anticoagulants are given to prevent thrombus formation. Oxygen is essential and given to keep oxygen saturation levels above 92%. If a thrombus has been identified as a cause, a pulmonary thromboendarterectomy may be performed. Some patients who do not respond to drug therapy and develop severe right-sided heart failure may receive lung transplants.

## HEALTH CARE SETTING

Primary care clinic, cardiology clinic, acute hospitalization in cardiac unit or critical care unit for complications or severe exacerbations of breathing difficulties, specialty care for transplantation

## DIAGNOSTIC TESTS

***Chest radiography.*** Demonstrates enlargement of the pulmonary artery and right atrium and ventricle. Pulmonary vasculature may appear engorged.

***Echocardiography.*** Evaluation of increased right ventricular dimension, thickened right ventricular wall, and possible tricuspid or pulmonary valve dysfunction. This test indirectly measures pulmonary artery systolic pressure.

***Radionuclide imaging.*** To assess the function of the right ventricle.

***Computed tomography scan.*** Evaluates the diameter of the main pulmonary arteries, which is helpful in determining the severity of disease. High-resolution computed tomography (CT) confirms the presence of interstitial lung disease. Spiral CT helps confirm the presence of a pulmonary embolus.

***Right-heart catheterization.*** Gold standard for diagnosing PAH. It provides information regarding the severity of the disease and establishes the prognosis. Pulmonary vascular resistance will be very high, and pulmonary artery and right ventricular pressures can approach or equal systemic arterial pressures. A vasodilator challenge may be performed to assess reactivity and guide treatment.

***Pulmonary perfusion scintigraphy (perfusion scan).*** A noninvasive way to assess pulmonary blood flow. This study involves intravenous injection of serum albumin tagged with trace amounts of a radioisotope, most often technetium. The particles pass through the circulation and lodge in the pulmonary vascular bed. Subsequent scanning reveals concentrations of particles in areas of adequate pulmonary blood flow. The scan is normal in PAH. An abnormal scan suggests the presence of thromboembolic PH.

***Electrocardiogram.*** Will show evidence of right atrial enlargement and right ventricular enlargement (evidenced by right axis deviation, right bundle branch block, tall and peaked P waves, and large R waves in $V_1$) secondary to the increased pressure needed to force blood through the hypertensive pulmonary vascular bed.

***Pulmonary function test.*** May demonstrate increased residual volume, reduced maximum voluntary ventilation, and decreased vital capacity.

***Sleep study.*** Confirms diagnosis of obstructive sleep apnea as a possible etiology for SPAH.

*Exercise testing.* Symptom-limited stress test or 6-minute walk test assesses the severity of symptoms and guides response to treatment.

*Arterial blood gas test.* May show low $PaCO_2$ and high pH with hyperventilation and respiratory alkalosis or increased $PaCO_2$ with low $O_2$ and pH with respiratory acidosis. This test is essential in guiding treatment.

*Oximetry.* Evaluates $O_2$ concentration. Decreased $O_2$ saturation (92% or less) occurs with PAH.

*Blood tests to rule out secondary causes of pulmonary arterial hypertension.* Antinuclear antibody, rheumatoid arthritis, erythrocyte sedimentation rate (tests for collagen vascular disorders), HIV, and thyroid-stimulating hormone (thyroid abnormalities commonly coexist with PAH).

*Complete blood count.* Polycythemia is present with chronic hypoxemia, as a compensatory mechanism. Elevated white blood cell count may be associated with concomitant infection.

*Liver function tests.* Increased aspartate aminotransferase, alanine aminotransferase (ALT), and bilirubin may indicate biliary venous congestion.

## Patient Problem/Analyze Cues/Prioritize Hypotheses

# Impaired Gas Exchange

*due to* decreased blood flow with pulmonary capillary vasoconstriction

*Desired Outcome/Generate Solutions:* The patient has improved gas exchange by at least 24 hours before hospital discharge, as evidenced by $O_2$ saturation greater than 92% (90% or greater for patients with COPD) and $PaO_2$ 80 mm Hg or higher.

| ASSESSMENT—RECOGNIZE CUES/ INTERVENTIONS—TAKE ACTION | RATIONALES |
|---|---|
| Assess $O_2$ saturation; report $O_2$ saturation of 92% or less to the health care provider. | Low $O_2$ saturation may signal the need for oxygen supplementation. |
| Monitor arterial blood gas (ABG) results. Report significant findings to the health care provider. | ABG results can reveal signs of hypoventilation (decreased $PaO_2$, increased $PaCO_2$, and decreased pH), which can signal respiratory failure, or hyperventilation (low $PaCO_2$ and high pH), which can occur with anxiety or respiratory distress. Hypoxemia is the key gas deficit seen with pulmonary vascular vasoconstriction. Blood flow through the lungs is impaired, making it difficult to exchange $O_2$ for $CO_2$. $O_2$ becomes low (hypoxemia), and $CO_2$ becomes high (hypercarbia). Hypercarbia causes a change in pH to the acid side. Although initially respiratory in origin, hypoxemia eventually results in metabolic acidosis because of lactic acid production. Values outside of normal or acceptable range must be reported promptly for timely intervention. |
| Assess all lung fields for breath sounds every 4–8 hours or more frequently as indicated. | Adventitious sounds (especially crackles) can occur with fluid overload; diminished breath sounds are congruent with disease severity. |
| Assess respiratory rate (RR), pattern, and depth; chest excursion; and use of accessory muscles of respiration every 4 hours. | Increased RR, abdominal breathing, use of accessory muscles, and nasal flaring are signals of hypoxia and respiratory distress. |
| Inspect skin and mucous membranes for cyanosis or skin color change. | These color changes are significant late signs of decreased gas exchange. |
| Assess mental status with vital signs and report significant changes. | Changes in mental acuity or level of consciousness may be indications of hypoxemia or acid-base imbalance. |
| Assist the patient into high-Fowler position (head of bed up 90 degrees), if possible. | This position reduces the work of breathing and maximizes chest excursion. |
| Instruct the patient to take slow, deep breaths. | This promotes gas exchange. |
| Administer prescribed $O_2$ as indicated. | Oxygen treats hypoxia. |
| Use care when administering $O_2$ to patients with COPD. | High concentrations of $O_2$ may depress the respiratory drive in individuals with chronic $CO_2$ retention. |
| Deliver $O_2$ with humidity. | Humidity helps prevent oxygen's drying effects on oral and nasal mucosa. |

## Patient Problem/Analyze Cues/Prioritize Hypotheses

# Fatigue (Decreased Exercise Tolerance)

*due to* generalized weakness and imbalance between oxygen supply and demand occurring with right and left ventricular failure

**Desired Outcome/Generate Solutions:** By at least 24 hours before hospital discharge, the patient rates perceived exertion at 3 or less on a 0–10 scale and exhibits cardiac tolerance to activity as evidenced by RR of 20 breaths/minute or less, heart rate (HR) of 20 bpm or less over resting HR, and systolic blood pressure within 20 mm Hg of resting range.

| ASSESSMENT—RECOGNIZE CUES/ INTERVENTIONS—TAKE ACTION | RATIONALES |
| --- | --- |
| Assess vital signs at least every 4 hours and before and after activity. Report significant findings. | A drop in BP greater than 10–20 mm Hg signals decompensation, which must be reported for prompt intervention. |
| Ask the patient to rate perceived exertion (RPE) during activity and monitor for evidence of exercise/activity intolerance. For details, see "Immobility," Chapter 1, for *Activity Intolerance*. Notify the health care provider of significant findings. | This assessment helps determine whether activity intolerance is present (RPE higher than 3). |
| Assess for dyspnea, shortness of breath, crackles, and decreased $O_2$ saturation (92% or less). | These are signs of left (systolic) ventricular failure. |
| Measure and document intake, output, and weight, reporting any significant gains or losses. Assess for peripheral edema in arms, legs, and dependent areas; ascites; distended neck veins; and increased central venous pressure (more than 12 cm $H_2O$). | These are signs of right (diastolic) ventricular failure. |
| Administer diuretics, vasodilators, calcium channel blockers, and anticoagulants as prescribed. | *Diuretics:* decrease fluid overload. |
|  | *Vasodilators:* decrease pulmonary artery pressure. Sildenafil and tadalafil are phosphodiesterase-5 inhibitors approved for use as vasodilators in PH. |
|  | *Calcium channel blockers:* relax and dilate blood vessels, decreasing pulmonary artery pressure. They are administered in high doses for PAH. |
|  | *Anticoagulants:* decrease the risk for thromboembolization. |
| Facilitate coordination of health care providers. Allow time for undisturbed rest, limiting interruptions and visitors as necessary. | Rest helps decrease oxygen demand, improves patient's well-being, and positively affects outcomes. |
| Create a comfortable and organized bed and environment, ensuring that the call bell is within reach and essential patient items are available. | This measure increases comfort, conserves energy, and reduces oxygen demand. |
| Assist with range-of-motion exercises at frequent intervals. Plan progressive ambulation and exercise based on the patient's tolerance and prescribed activity restrictions. Provide rest from exercise as needed. | These measures help prevent complications caused by immobility, improve muscle tone, and advance independence and activity. Rest is essential to avoid overexertion. |

## Patient Problem/Analyze Cues/Prioritize Hypotheses

# Deficient Knowledge

*due to* unfamiliarity with the disease process and treatment

**Desired Outcome/Generate Solutions:** Within the 24-hour period before hospital discharge, the patient and significant other verbalize accurate knowledge of the disease, treatment plan, and measures that promote wellness.

| ASSESSMENT—RECOGNIZE CUES/ INTERVENTIONS—TAKE ACTION | RATIONALES |
|---|---|
| Assess the patient's health care literacy (language, comprehension, reading). Assess culture and culturally specific information needs. | This assessment helps ensure that information is selected and presented in a manner that is culturally and educationally appropriate. |
| Assess the patient's level of knowledge of the disease process and its treatment. | This information enables the development of an individualized teaching plan. A knowledgeable patient is more likely to adhere to the treatment. |
| Discuss the purposes of the medications: | |
| • Diuretics | Diuretics enhance renal output, reducing fluid accumulation. |
| • Vasodilators | Vasodilators decrease systemic vascular resistance, easing the workload of the heart. |
| • Calcium channel blockers | Calcium channel blockers relax and dilate blood vessels, decreasing pulmonary artery pressure when given in high doses. |
| • Anticoagulants | Anticoagulants promote improved long-term survival by preventing thromboembolic complications. |
| Provide emotional support as needed, assisting the patient in adapting to living with a chronic disease. | This action is supportive, expresses empathy, and reinforces the need to adhere to lifetime therapy. |
| Reinforce explanations of the disease process and treatment, allowing time for the patient's and family's questions. | A knowledgeable patient is more likely to adhere to the treatment regimen. Including family/support systems in teaching builds trust and promotes adherence. |
| Discuss lifestyle changes that may be necessary. | Changes may be necessary to maintain quality of life and prevent complications of the disease. |
| Explain the value of relaxation techniques, including soothing music, meditation, and biofeedback. | Relaxation can promote decreased myocardial demand, lowering HR, BP, and RR. |
| If the patient smokes, provide materials that explain the benefits of smoking cessation, such as pamphlets prepared by the American Heart Association (www.americanheart.org). Provide referrals for local smoking cessation programs (American Lung Association, www.lung.org). | Smoking increases the workload of the heart by causing vasoconstriction, in addition to causing various cancers and contributing to cardiovascular disease. |
| Confer with the health care provider about an exercise program that will benefit the patient; provide patient teaching as indicated. | Exercise improves vascular tone and strengthens muscles. In collaboration with the health care provider and physical therapist, the nurse can assist the patient in maximizing the benefits of exercise. |
| Consult with a nutritionist to ensure that a dietary plan is explained to the patient and family. | A low-sodium diet or specialty diet (i.e., low fat, low sugar, low cholesterol) may be necessary to support patient outcomes. |
| Discuss follow-up treatment of etiologic factors that are diagnosed. | This may include surgical closure of arteriovenous shunts; replacement of defective valves; or treatment of obstructive sleep apnea, pulmonary embolism, or COPD. |
| As directed by the health care provider, explain the possibility of a heart–lung transplantation and refer to appropriate team members. | Transplantation may be considered for advanced (end-stage) pulmonary vascular disease that is not responsive to medical therapy. Early referral is necessary to begin the planning stages. |

**ADDITIONAL PROBLEMS:**

## PATIENT–FAMILY TEACHING AND DISCHARGE PLANNING

When providing patient–family teaching, focus on sensory information, avoid giving too much information, and initiate a visiting nurse referral for necessary follow-up teaching. Include verbal and written information about the following:

✓ Indicators that necessitate medical attention: decreased exercise tolerance, increasing shortness of breath or dyspnea, swelling of ankles and legs, and steady weight gain.

✓ Medications, including drug name, purpose, dosage, schedule, precautions, and potential side effects. Also discuss drug–drug, food–drug, and herb–drug interactions.

✓ Support and information sites available on the Internet, which include:
  • Pulmonary Hypertension Association: https://phassociation.org/
  • American Lung Association: http://www.lung.org/lung-health-and-diseases/lung-disease-lookup/pulmonary-arterial-hypertension/
  • National Heart, Lung, and Blood Institute: https://www.nhlbi.nih.gov/health/health-topics/topics/pah/

✓ Elimination of smoking; refer patient to a local smoking cessation program as appropriate. There are many resources for programs, printed materials, and explanations of multiple ways to help patients stop smoking. Examples include:
  • American Lung Association: Quit Smoking: https://www.lung.org/quit-smoking
  • Centers for Disease Control and Prevention for smoking and tobacco use: https://www.cdc.gov/tobacco/quit_smoking/index.htm

✓ For additional information, see *Deficient Knowledge* in this chapter.

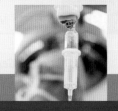

# Venous Thrombosis/ Thrombophlebitis $\quad$ 26

## OVERVIEW/PATHOPHYSIOLOGY

Venous thromboembolism (VTE) describes the conditions of vein thrombosis and pulmonary embolism (PE). Vein thromboses can be superficial, usually in the lesser or greater saphenous vein, or in a deep vein (DVT), usually the femoral and or the femoral veins. Upper extremity VTE related to invasive lines, such as a peripherally inserted central catheter, may occur. The most serious complication of DVT is embolization, causing PE.

Predisposing conditions that affect coagulation or stasis of the blood contribute to the incidence of VTE. The patient at risk for developing VTE usually has predisposing conditions to these three factors, known as Virchow's triad: Venous stasis, hypercoagulability, and damage to the endothelium, or inner lining, of the vein. Hemoconcentration, vessel trauma, and surgery also contribute to the development of VTE.

Hemoconcentration is caused by dehydration, including inadequate fluid resuscitation in the perioperative period. Patients undergoing surgery, particularly hip and knee operations, have a high incidence of DVT. Vessel trauma or inflammation may result from chemical irritation caused by intravenous (IV) solutions, direct trauma including venipuncture, and improper prolonged positioning. Pregnancy, estrogen therapy, hereditary factors, and malignancies all contribute to hypercoagulability.

Immobility resulting from prolonged bedrest, inability to move because of paralysis or stroke, and extended operating room table positioning contribute to venous stasis. Additionally, venous stasis may occur with chronic heart failure, shock states, and structural disorders of the veins; after abdominal, pelvic, or orthopedic operative procedures; and with extended air travel (National Heart, Lung and Blood Institute, 2022b).

## HEALTH CARE SETTING

Primary care, vascular care, and acute care or critical care unit because of instability related to PE

## ASSESSMENT

**Signs and symptoms.** Signs and symptoms at the site of the thrombus often include pain, tenderness, erythema, local warmth, and swelling. Distal to the thrombus, the extremity may be cool, pale or cyanotic, and edematous with prominent superficial veins. Sometimes, the condition is clinically "silent," and the late presenting sign may be PE (see "Pulmonary Embolus," Chapter 15).

**Physical assessment.** Assessment at the site of the thrombus (associated with inflammation) and distal to the clot (associated with venous congestion) is important. A knot or bump at the site of the thrombus may be palpated, along with pain upon palpation, increased warmth, redness, and edema. Distal to the site, assess pulses, limb circumference, and skin temperature. Additional findings include unilateral limb swelling, fever, and tachycardia.

**Risk factors.** Prolonged bedrest and immobility, leg trauma, recent surgery, malignancy, hormonal therapy, hypercoagulability, obesity, varicose veins.

## DIAGNOSTIC TESTS

**Blood studies.** Activated partial thromboplastin time (aPTT), international normalized ratio (INR), bleeding time, hemoglobin, hematocrit, antifactor Xa, and platelet count may be done to assess for blood dyscrasias.

**Duplex ultrasound.** Use of compression ultrasound with spectral and color flow Doppler to assess veins for compressibility and filling defects. This test helps to determine the location and extent of the thrombus and is the most widely used test for VTE.

**D-Dimer test.** A D-dimer test is indicative of fibrin breakdown, and further evaluation is warranted. A negative D-dimer test is helpful in excluding DVT if noninvasive testing also is negative.

**Computed tomography venography.** Spiral computed tomography (CT) scan is used to evaluate veins in the pelvis and lower extremities after the injection of contrast material. May also be done with CT angiography of pulmonary vessels to evaluate for PE.

---

## Patient Problem/Analyze Cues/Prioritize Hypotheses

# Impaired Hematologic System Function (Excessive Clotting)

*due to* hemoconcentration, vessel trauma or inflammation, and immobility

***Desired Outcome/Generate Solutions:*** After interventions, the patient has baseline extremity color, temperature, and sensation; respiratory rate of 12–20 breaths/minute with normal depth and pattern (eupnea); heart rate of 100 bpm or less; blood pressure (BP) within 20 mm Hg of baseline BP; $O_2$ saturation greater than 92%; and clear breath sounds.

| ASSESSMENT—RECOGNIZE CUES/ INTERVENTIONS—TAKE ACTION | RATIONALES |
|---|---|
| Assess for lower extremity pain, erythema, increased limb circumference, local warmth, distal pale skin, edema, and venous dilation. If indicators are present, maintain the patient on bedrest and notify the health care provider promptly. | These are early indicators of peripheral thrombus formation (DVT), which necessitate bedrest and prompt medical attention to prevent embolization. |
| Assess for and immediately report sudden onset of chest pain, dyspnea, tachypnea, tachycardia, hypotension, hemoptysis, shallow respirations, crackles, $O_2$ saturation 92% or less, decreased breath sounds, and diaphoresis. | These are signs of PE, a life-threatening situation. If they occur, prompt medical attention is required. See "Pulmonary Embolus," Chapter 15. |
| Monitor laboratory tests to help ensure accurate dosing:<br>• For heparin: aPTT or PTT and platelet counts<br>• For warfarin: prothrombin time (PT) and INR<br>   • Some facilities may use antifactor Xa levels to monitor dosages of unfractionated heparin or low-molecular-weight heparins. | Assessment of laboratory tests before anticoagulant administration to obtain the patient's baseline levels, and ongoing is essential to help prevent bleeding from excessive dosing. The aPTT/PTT, and PT measure the blood's clotting time. Platelet counts measure the number of platelets (the clotting component of the blood). With the INR, a calculation based on PT results, a range of 2–3 is optimal for patients on warfarin. |
| Administer anticoagulants as prescribed. | Anticoagulants prevent the extension of an existing clot. Unfractionated heparin or low-molecular-weight heparin is used during the acute phase, and long-term anticoagulation, with warfarin or other newer oral anticoagulants, is used after the acute phase. The use of warfarin necessitates frequent monitoring of the INR, dietary restrictions, and precautions about its interactions with other medications. Several new oral anticoagulants have been developed that do not require routine laboratory monitoring and have fewer dietary restrictions and drug interactions than warfarin. These include rivaroxaban (Xarelto), apixaban (Eliquis), dabigatran (Pradaxa), and edoxaban (Savaysa). Because there is no established method for determining the extent of their anticoagulant effect because of their short half-lives that increase the risk for thrombosis with missed doses, these newer anticoagulants are not recommended for use in patients who cannot adhere to a dosing schedule and are to be avoided in patients with end-stage renal disease. For information about the bleeding risk with anticoagulants, see "Pulmonary Embolus," *Imparied Hematologic System Function (Excessive Clotting)* in Chapter 15. |
| | **Note:** An inferior vena caval filter (IVC) may be surgically implanted transvenously to filter blood from distal sites to prevent PE. This is most often placed when patients cannot be anticoagulated or have had PEs while being therapeutically anticoagulated. IVCs may be left in place for several weeks and removed when the risk for clotting has passed. |
| As per the facility's policy, verify the correct parenteral anticoagulant drug and dosage with another nurse. Always use a pump for IV heparin administration. | Correct dosing is essential to avoid the adverse effects of incorrect administration. |
| Encourage early ambulation in patients with VTE. However, patients with severe edema and limb pain may initially need bedrest with the affected limb elevated. | Early ambulation after VTE helps to reduce edema and limb pain and does not increase the risk of PE in patients with VTE. |
| Apply support hose, sequential compression device, or pneumatic foot compression device as prescribed to the unaffected extremity. | These measures minimize the risk for or prevent further DVTs in the unaffected extremity. |
| Maintain elevation of the affected limb when seated or in bed. | This measure promotes venous drainage. |

## Patient Problem/Analyze Cues/Prioritize Hypotheses

# Acute Pain

*due to* the inflammatory process caused by thrombus formation

**Desired Outcomes/Generate Solutions:**  Within 1 hour of interventions, the patient's subjective perception of pain decreases, as documented by a pain scale. Objective indicators, such as grimacing, are absent.

| ASSESSMENT—RECOGNIZE CUES/ INTERVENTIONS—TAKE ACTION | RATIONALES |
|---|---|
| Assess for the presence of pain, using a pain scale from 0 (no pain) to 10 (worst pain). Administer analgesics as prescribed and document medication and relief obtained using the pain scale. | This evaluates the patient's perception of pain and determines the most effective analgesic and dosing required to relieve the pain. |
| Ensure that the patient maintains bedrest if prescribed and limb elevation during the acute phase. | These measures minimize painful engorgement, promote venous drainage, and decrease the potential for embolization. |
| Avoid flexion of hips or knees. | Flexion contributes to venous stasis and discomfort. |

## Patient Problem/Analyze Cues/Prioritize Hypotheses

# Ineffective Tissue Perfusion (Peripheral)

*due to* interrupted venous flow occurring with venous engorgement or edema

**Desired Outcome/Generate Solutions:**  After interventions, the patient has adequate peripheral perfusion, as evidenced by the absence of discomfort and the presence of baseline extremity temperature, color, sensation, and motor function.

| ASSESSMENT—RECOGNIZE CUES/ INTERVENTIONS—TAKE ACTION | RATIONALES |
|---|---|
| Assess for pain and changes in skin temperature, color, and motor or sensory function. Be alert to venous engorgement (prominence) in the lower extremities. | These are signs of inadequate peripheral perfusion. |
| Elevate the patient's legs. | Elevation promotes venous drainage. |
| As prescribed for *patients without evidence of thrombus formation*, apply antiembolic hose or use sequential compression devices. | These devices increase blood flow in the deep and superficial veins to prevent DVT and are often indicated for patients who are mostly immobile. |
| Remove the devices or hose and inspect the skin. | Removal enables skin inspection for evidence of irritation and decreased circulation. |
| Encourage the patient to perform ankle circling and active or assisted ROM exercises of the lower extremities. Perform passive ROM exercises if the patient cannot. | These exercises prevent venous stasis, which is a known cause of venous disorders. |
| If there are any signs of acute thrombus formation, such as calf hardness or tenderness, exercises are contraindicated. Notify the health care provider accordingly. | This restriction minimizes the risk for embolization. |
| Encourage deep breathing. | Deep breathing creates increased negative pressure in the lungs and thorax to assist in emptying of the large veins. |
| Assess peripheral pulses regularly. | Although arterial circulation usually will not be impaired unless there is arterial disease or severe edema compressing arterial flow, regular pulse assessment will confirm the presence of good arterial flow. |

Patient Problem/Analyze Cues/Prioritize Hypotheses

# Deficient Knowledge

*due to* unfamiliarity with the disease process of VTE and the necessary at-home treatment/management measures after hospital discharge

***Desired Outcome/Generate Solutions:*** Before hospital discharge, the patient verbalizes accurate knowledge of the disease process and treatment/management measures that are to occur after hospital discharge.

| ASSESSMENT—RECOGNIZE CUES/ INTERVENTIONS—TAKE ACTION | RATIONALES |
|---|---|
| Assess the patient's health care literacy (language, reading, comprehension). Assess culture and culturally specific education needs. | This assessment helps ensure that information is selected and presented in a manner that is culturally and educationally appropriate. |
| Discuss the process of VTE and ways to prevent thrombosis and discomfort. | Avoiding restrictive clothing and prolonged periods of standing and elevating legs above heart level when sitting promote venous return and help prevent DVT while promoting comfort. In addition, regular walking and active ankle and leg ROM exercises promote venous return, strengthen leg muscles, and facilitate the development of collateral vessels. |
| Discuss the prescribed anticoagulant therapy. (Refer to <u>Patient–Family Teaching</u>, later, and to "Pulmonary Embolus," Chapter 15.) | Most patients will be maintained on anticoagulation therapy for several months or longer. |
| Provide information about signs of venous stasis ulcers and advise the patient to report any breaks in skin to the health care provider. | Such indicators as redness and skin breakdown are signals of venous stasis ulcers, which necessitate medical attention before they lead to complications such as infection or even gangrene. |
| Stress the importance of avoiding trauma to the extremities and keeping the skin clean and dry. | Avoiding trauma decreases the risk for skin breakdown; clean and dry skin helps prevent infection that could develop in broken skin. |
| Instruct the patient to inspect both feet each day. If necessary, suggest the use of a long-handled mirror to see bottoms of the feet. Advise the patient to report any open areas to the health care provider. | Foot inspection will detect bruises or open wounds because tissues of the lower extremities may be susceptible to injury. |
| Discuss the prescribed exercise program. | Walking usually is considered the best exercise, although other exercises involving the lower extremities also prevent venous stasis, strengthen lower leg muscles, and help develop collateral vessels where circulation may be routed. |
| Provide instruction on how to apply antiembolic hose if prescribed. These hose need to be applied after the legs have been elevated above heart level for at least 1 minute to prevent entrapment of the edema in the feet and ankles. | Proper application of these hose will help to decrease venous distention and increase blood flow back to the heart. |
| ⚠ Describe indicators that necessitate medical attention. | Persistent redness, swelling, tenderness, weak or absent pulses, and ulcerations in the extremities may be signs of infection and worsening venous congestion. This must be reported to the health care provider promptly to avoid systemic infection and further compromise to the circulation. |
| Encourage long-term management of venous stasis with elastic stockings. | This measure will help prevent sequelae associated with postphlebitic syndrome and chronic venous insufficiency. |

## ADDITIONAL PROBLEMS:

"Pulmonary Embolus" for *Impaired Hematologic System Function (Excessive Clotting)* and *Risk for hemorrhaging, due to anticoagulation therapy*    Chapter 15

 **PATIENT–FAMILY TEACHING AND DISCHARGE PLANNING**

When providing patient–family teaching, focus on sensory information, avoid giving excessive information, and initiate a visiting nurse referral for necessary follow-up teaching. Include verbal and written information about the following:

✓ See *Deficient Knowledge* for topics to discuss, both verbally and through written information, with the patient and significant other.

✓ If the patient is discharged from the hospital on low-molecular-weight heparin or warfarin therapy, or has an IVC implanted, provide information about the following:

- As directed, see the health care provider for follow-up and for scheduled laboratory testing of clotting times (PT, aPTT, antifactor Xa, INR).
- Take medication at the same time each day; do not skip days unless directed to by the health care provider.
- Wear a medical alert bracelet.
- As appropriate, remain aware that the IVC will need to be surgically removed, and an appointment must be planned for this.

- Avoid alcohol consumption and changes in diet (e.g., changing to a vegetarian diet), both of which can alter the body's response to anticoagulation.
- Provide resources for smoking cessation and instruct patient to avoid all nicotine products.
- When making appointments with other health care providers and dentists, inform them that an anticoagulant is being taken.

Be alert to indicators that necessitate immediate medical attention: bloody urine or sputum, coffee-ground or bloody vomit, excessive bruising, black or bloody stools, excessive menstrual bleeding, nosebleeds, bleeding gums, dizziness, and weakness.

✓ Avoid taking over-the-counter medications (e.g., aspirin, which also prolongs coagulation time, or non-steroidal antiinflammatory drugs (NSAIDs), which may increase the possibility of GI bleeding) without consulting the health care provider or nurse.

✓ Avoid injury to self and protect skin by following bleeding precautions:

- Brush teeth with a soft-bristle toothbrush.
- Shave with an electric razor.
- Use scissors and knives cautiously.
- Avoid contact sports.
- Wear safety equipment (e.g., helmets, padding) during physical activity.

✓ Refer to online resources, such as the National Blood Clot Alliance/Stop The Clot: https://www.stoptheclot.org/about-clots/blood-clot-info/

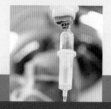

# Acute Kidney Injury 27

## OVERVIEW/PATHOPHYSIOLOGY

Acute kidney injury (AKI) is a rapid loss of renal function as a result of glomerular injury or reduced blood flow. Rapid loss of renal function is accompanied by a rise in serum creatinine, blood urea nitrogen (BUN), and potassium with or without oliguria. The kidneys lose their ability to maintain biochemical homeostasis, causing retention of metabolic wastes and dramatic alterations in fluid, electrolyte, and acid–base balance. Although alteration in renal function usually is reversible, AKI may be associated with a mortality rate of 40%–80%. Mortality varies greatly with the cause of AKI, patient's age, and comorbid conditions.

Causes of AKI are categorized according to the development of prerenal, intrarenal, and postrenal conditions. Prerenal causes cause decreased renal function secondary to decreased renal perfusion, which leads to decreased glomerular filtration. Causes of prerenal AKI include fluid volume deficit, shock, and decreased cardiac function. If hypoperfusion has not been prolonged, restoration of renal perfusion will restore normal renal function. In prerenal oliguria, there is no damage to the kidney parenchyma but can progress to intrarenal AKI if not reversed.

Intrarenal AKI is caused by direct damage to the kidney tissue, leading to decreased nephron function. Ninety percent of intrarenal AKI cases in hospitalized patients are caused by acute tubular necrosis (ATN), which results from ischemia, nephrotoxins, or sepsis. Nephrotoxin examples include aminoglycoside antibiotics and contrast media. Additional medications associated with the development of intrarenal AKI include nonsteroidal antiinflammatory drugs (NSAIDs), angiotensin-converting enzyme (ACE) inhibitors, immunosuppressants (e.g., cyclosporine), antineoplastics (e.g., cisplatin), and antifungals (e.g., amphotericin B). Other causes of intrarenal ATN include myoglobin from hemolyzed red blood cells and myoglobin released from necrotic muscle cells. The clinical course of ATN can be divided into the following three phases: oliguric (urine output of greater than 100 mL and less than 400 mL/day, lasting approximately 7–21 days), diuretic (7–14 days), and recovery (3–12 months). Causes of intrarenal AKI other than ATN include acute glomerulonephritis (GN), systemic lupus erythematosus, malignant hypertension, hepatorenal syndrome, and autoimmune syndromes. When a person does not recover from AKI, chronic kidney disease (CKD) may develop.

Postrenal AKI is caused by a mechanical obstruction to urine flow. The urine flow obstruction causes the urine to reflux into the renal pelvis, impairing kidney function. The most common postrenal causes are benign prostatic hyperplasia, prostate cancer, kidney stones, and extrarenal tumors. Early detection of prerenal and postrenal failure is essential because, if prolonged more than 48 hours, parenchymal damage may occur. Restoration of renal function in cases of postrenal failure is directly related to the removal of the obstruction.

## HEALTH CARE SETTING

Acute medical-surgical care unit

## ASSESSMENT

***Physical assessment.*** Pallor, edema (peripheral, periorbital, sacral), jugular vein distention, fine crackles, and elevated blood pressure (BP) in a patient who has fluid overload.

***Excess fluid volume.*** Oliguria, pitting edema, hypertension, pulmonary edema.

***Metabolic acidosis.*** Kussmaul respirations, lethargy, headache.

***Electrolyte disturbance.*** Muscle weakness and dysrhythmias.

***Infection.*** Urinary tract infection, septicemia, pulmonary infections, peritonitis.

***Uremia (retention of metabolic wastes).*** Altered mental state, anorexia, nausea, diarrhea, pale and sallow skin, purpura, decreased resistance to infection, anemia, fatigue.

> **Note:** *Uremia adversely affects all body systems.*

***Gastrointestinal system.*** Nausea, vomiting, diarrhea, constipation, gastrointestinal (GI) bleeding, anorexia, abdominal distention.

***History.*** Exposure to nephrotoxic substances, recent blood transfusion, prolonged hypotensive episodes or decreased renal perfusion, sepsis, administration of radiolucent contrast media, kidney stones, or prostatic hypertrophy.

## DIAGNOSTIC TESTS

***Creatinine clearance.*** Measures the kidneys' ability to clear the blood of creatinine and approximates the glomerular filtration rate. It will decrease as renal function decreases. Creatinine clearance is normally decreased in older persons.

**Note:** *Twenty-four hour urine collection: failure to collect all urine during the period of study can invalidate the test.*

**Blood urea nitrogen and serum creatinine.** Assess the progression and management of AKI. Although both BUN and creatinine will increase as renal function decreases, creatinine is a better indicator of renal function because it is not affected by diet, hydration, or tissue catabolism.

**Urinalysis.** Can provide information about the cause and location of renal disease as reflected by abnormal urinary sediment (renal tubular cells and cell casts).

**Urinary osmolality and urinary sodium levels.** To rule out renal perfusion problems (prerenal). In ATN the kidney loses its ability to adjust urine concentration and conserve sodium, producing urine $Na^+$ level greater than 40 mEq/L (in prerenal azotemia the urine $Na^+$ is less than 20 mEq/L).

**Note:** *All urine samples should be sent to the laboratory immediately after collection or should be refrigerated if this is not possible. Urine left at room temperature has greater potential for bacterial growth, turbidity, and alkalinity, any of which can distort the reading.*

**Renal ultrasound.** Provides information about renal anatomy and pelvic structures, evaluates renal masses, and detects obstruction and hydronephrosis. Because no intravenous (IV) contrast agent is used, this procedure limits the risk for further compromise to renal function.

**Renal scan.** Provides information about perfusion and function of the kidneys.

**Computed tomography scan.** Identifies dilation of renal calices in obstructive processes.

**Retrograde urography.** Assesses for postrenal causes (i.e., obstruction).

## Patient Problem/Analyze Cues/Prioritize Hypotheses
# Risk for Infection

*due to* the presence of uremia

***Desired Outcome/Generate Solutions:*** The patient is free of infection as evidenced by normothermia; white blood cell count of 11,000/mm³ or less; negative blood cultures, urine that is clear and of normal odor; clear breath sounds; eupnea; and absence of erythema, warmth, tenderness, swelling, and drainage from wounds, incisions, and tubes.

 **Note:** *One of the primary causes of death in AKI is sepsis.*

| ASSESSMENT—RECOGNIZE CUES/ INTERVENTIONS—TAKE ACTION | RATIONALES |
| --- | --- |
| Assess the temperature and secretions for indicators of infection. | Even minor increases in temperature can be significant because uremia masks the febrile response and inhibits the body's ability to fight infection. |
| Use meticulous sterile technique when changing dressings or manipulating venous catheters, IV lines, or indwelling catheters. | These measures prevent infection through the spread of pathogens. |
| Avoid long-term use of indwelling urinary catheters. Whenever possible, use intermittent catheterization instead. | Indwelling urinary catheters are a common source of infection. |
| Provide oral hygiene and skin care at frequent intervals. | Intact skin and oral mucous membranes are barriers to infection. |
| Use emollients and gentle soap. | These measures prevent drying and cracking of the skin, which could lead to breakdown and infection. |
| Rinse off all soap when bathing the patient. | Soap residue may further irritate the skin and affects its integrity. |

## Patient Problem/Analyze Cues/Prioritize Hypotheses
# Risk fo Fluid Imbalance, Electrolyte Imbalance, and Acid–Base Imbalance

*due to* the kidneys' inability to maintain biochemical homeostasis

***Desired Outcome/Generate Solutions:*** The patient is free of signs and symptoms of fluid, electrolyte, and acid–base imbalances.

## ASSESSMENT—RECOGNIZE CUES/INTERVENTIONS—TAKE ACTION

## RATIONALES

| ASSESSMENT—RECOGNIZE CUES/INTERVENTIONS—TAKE ACTION | RATIONALES |
|---|---|
| Assess for and alert the patient to indicators of alterations in fluid, electrolyte, and acid–base balance. | In AKI, the kidneys lose their ability to maintain biochemical homeostasis, causing retention of metabolic wastes and dramatic alterations in fluid, electrolyte, and acid–base balance. The following may occur: |
| | *Uremia:* Anorexia, nausea, metallic taste in the mouth, irritability, confusion, lethargy, restlessness, and itching. Uremic symptoms result from increased BUN as the kidney loses its ability to excrete nitrogenous wastes. |
| | *Hypokalemia:* Muscle weakness, lethargy, dysrhythmias, abdominal distention, and nausea and vomiting (secondary to ileus). It may occur during the diuretic phase because of urinary potassium losses. |
| | *Hyperkalemia:* Muscle cramps, dysrhythmias, muscle weakness, increased QRS duration, and peaked T waves on electrocardiogram. Hyperkalemia is a common and potentially fatal complication of AKI during the oliguric phase. It may occur if the kidney is unable to excrete potassium ions into the urine. |
| | **Caution:** A normal serum $K^+$ level is necessary for normal cardiac function. |
| | *Hypocalcemia:* Neuromuscular irritability, for example, positive Trousseau sign (carpopedal spasm) and Chvostek sign (facial muscle spasm), and paresthesias. Hypocalcemia may occur because of increased serum phosphate (there is a reciprocal relationship between calcium and phosphorus—as one rises, the other decreases). |
| | *Hyperphosphatemia:* Although usually asymptomatic, it may cause bone or joint pain and painful/itchy skin lesions. Serum phosphorus may increase because of a decreased ability of the kidneys to excrete this ion. |
| | *Metabolic acidosis:* Rapid, deep respirations; confusion. A buildup of hydrogen ions occurs in the serum because of the kidneys' inability to buffer and secrete this ion. |
| Avoid giving foods high in potassium content during oliguric phase. | This restriction helps potassium return to more normal levels. Salt substitutes also contain potassium and should be avoided, along with apricots, avocados, bananas, cantaloupe, carrots, cauliflower, chocolate, dried beans and peas, dried fruit, mushrooms, nuts, oranges, peanuts, potatoes, prune juice, pumpkins, spinach, sweet potatoes, Swiss chard, tomatoes, and watermelon. |
| Maintain adequate nutritional intake (especially calories). | If caloric intake is inadequate, body protein will be used for energy, resulting in increased end products of protein metabolism (i.e., nitrogenous wastes). A high-carbohydrate diet helps minimize tissue catabolism and production of nitrogenous wastes. |
| Prevent infections. | This measure minimizes tissue catabolism by controlling fevers. See *Risk for Infection*, earlier. |
| Avoid or use with caution the following medications: NSAIDs, ACE inhibitors, and potassium-sparing diuretics. | NSAIDs may further damage kidney function and/or cause electrolyte imbalances including hyperkalemia or hyponatremia. ACE inhibitors and potassium-sparing diuretics may cause an increase in serum potassium. |
| | **Note:** Soon after renal disease is initially diagnosed, ACE inhibitors may be prescribed for their renal protective effects. However, after CKD has developed, ACE inhibitors may require dose adjustment or may be contraindicated because of hyperkalemia risk. |
| Prepare the patient for the possibility of altered taste and smell. | Alterations in taste and smell may occur with uremia because of toxin buildup due to the inability of the kidneys to excrete nitrogenous waste. |

| ASSESSMENT—RECOGNIZE CUES/ INTERVENTIONS—TAKE ACTION | RATIONALES |
|---|---|
| Avoid the use of magnesium-containing medications. | Patients with renal failure are at risk for increased magnesium levels because of decreased urinary excretion of dietary magnesium. |
| Patients using magnesium-containing antacids such as Maalox typically are switched to aluminum hydroxide preparations such as ALternaGEL or Amphojel. Milk of Magnesia should be substituted with another, non–magnesium-containing laxative such as casanthranol. | |
| Administer aluminum hydroxide or calcium antacids as prescribed. Offer antacids in capsule form to patients who refuse liquid antacids. These medications must be administered with meals. | These agents are administered to control hyperphosphatemia. Phosphate binders vary in their aluminum or calcium content, however, and one may not be exchanged for another without first ensuring that the patient is receiving the same amount of elemental aluminum or calcium. |
| | **Note:** Aluminum-containing phosphate binders should not be used long term because of their potential to cause bone damage. |
| Administer other medications as prescribed: | |
| • Diuretics | These medications are used in nonoliguric AKI for fluid removal. For example, furosemide (Lasix) or mannitol may be given early in AKI to limit or prevent the development of oliguria. |
| • Antihypertensives | These medications are used to control BP in the presence of underlying illness, fluid overload, sodium retention, or stimulation of the renin–angiotensin system in patients with renal ischemia. |
| • Cation exchange resins (Kayexalate) | These resins are used to control hyperkalemia. Kayexalate is most effectively administered orally, but it may be administered as an enema. The resin acts in the intestinal tract through exchange of sodium ions (from the Kayexalate) for potassium ions. Kayexalate is usually administered with sorbitol to prevent constipation and fecal impaction. |
| | **Note:** Severe hyperkalemia also may be treated with *IV sodium bicarbonate*, which shifts potassium into the cells temporarily, or *glucose and insulin*. Insulin also helps move potassium into the cells, and glucose helps prevent dangerous hypoglycemia, which could result from the insulin. *IV calcium* is given to reverse the cardiac effects of life-threatening hyperkalemia. |
| • Calcium or vitamin D supplements | These supplements are given to patients with hypocalcemia. |
| • Sodium bicarbonate | This is given to treat metabolic acidosis when the serum bicarbonate level is less than 15 mmol/L. |
| Avoid or use sodium bicarbonate cautiously in patients with hypocalcemia, edema, or sodium retention. | Rapidly rising serum pH may result in muscle spasms in patients with hypocalcemia. |
| • Vitamins B and C | These vitamins replace losses if the patient is on dialysis. |
| Reassure the patient and significant other that irritability, restlessness, and altered thinking should be temporary and improve with treatment. | Reassurance may help allay added anxiety. |
| Display calendars and request that significant others bring radios and familiar objects. | These measures will help orient the patient to person, place, and time. |
| Ensure safety measures (e.g., padded side rails, airway) for patients who are confused or severely hypocalcemic. For patients who exhibit signs of hyperkalemia, have emergency supplies (e.g., manual resuscitator bag, crash cart, emergency drug tray) available. | These measures are for the patient's protection until electrolyte disturbance is reversed. |

Patient Problem/Analyze Cues/Prioritize Hypotheses

# Fluid Imbalance

*due to* compromised regulatory mechanisms occurring with renal dysfunction:
*Oliguric phase*

**Desired Outcome/Generate Solutions:** The patient is normovolemic as evidenced by decreasing or stable weight, normal breath sounds, edema 1+ or less on a 0–4+ scale, central venous pressure (CVP) 10 mm Hg or less, and BP and heart rate (HR) within the patient's baseline.

| ASSESSMENT—RECOGNIZE CUES/INTERVENTIONS—TAKE ACTION | RATIONALES |
|---|---|
| Closely assess and document the intake and output (I&O). | This assessment detects a trend of fluid volume, particularly decreasing urinary output compared with intake. Patients with AKI may/may not develop oliguria. Urine volume does not necessarily reflect renal function in patients with AKI. For example, in postrenal failure, large volumes of urine may be associated with relief of obstruction. In AKI, the kidneys lose their ability to maintain biochemical homeostasis. This causes the retention of metabolic wastes and dramatic alterations in fluid, electrolyte, and acid–base balance. For details about likely electrolyte imbalances and metabolic acidosis, see *Risk for Fluid Imbalance, Electrolyte Imbalance, and Acid–Base Imbalance,* earlier. |
| Monitor the weight daily. | The patient likely will lose 0.5 kg/day if not eating; a sudden weight gain suggests excessive fluid volume. |
| Weigh the patient at the same time each day, using the same scale and with the patient wearing the same amount of clothing. | This ensures that weight measurements are performed under the same conditions with each assessment, thereby facilitating more precise measurements of fluid volume. |
| Assess for edema, hypertension, fine crackles, tachycardia, distended neck veins, shortness of breath, and increased CVP. | These signs are indicators of fluid volume excess. In AKI, dependent edema likely will be detected in the legs or feet of patients who are ambulatory, and in the sacral area of patients who are on bedrest. Periorbital edema may also result from excessive fluid overload. Jugular veins are likely to be distended with the head of bed elevated 45 degrees because of increased intravascular volume. Crackles and shortness of breath can occur as a result of pulmonary fluid volume overload. Low serum albumin decreases colloid osmotic pressure, allowing fluid to leak into the extravascular space. Low serum albumin also may contribute to generalized edema and pulmonary edema. Hypertension, tachycardia, and increased CVP may result from sodium and fluid retention. Decreased renal perfusion also may activate the renin–angiotensin system, exacerbating these symptoms. |
| Carefully adhere to the prescribed fluid restriction. | This measure helps patients return to normovolemia. Fluids usually are restricted on the basis of "replace losses 400 mL/24 hour." Insensible fluid losses are only partially replaced to offset water formed during the metabolism of proteins, carbohydrates, and fats. |
| Provide oral hygiene at frequent intervals and offer fluids in the form of ice chips or ice pops. Spread allotted fluids evenly over a 24-hour period, and record the amount given. Instruct the patient and significant others about the need for fluid restriction. | These interventions minimize thirst during fluid restriction. Hard candies also may be given to decrease thirst. |
| | **Note:** Patients nourished by total parenteral nutrition are at increased risk for fluid overload because of the necessary fluid volume involved and its hypertonicity. |

| ASSESSMENT—RECOGNIZE CUES/ INTERVENTIONS—TAKE ACTION | RATIONALES |
|---|---|
| Monitor the results of BUN, serum creatinine, and creatinine clearance tests. | Although both BUN and creatinine will increase as renal function and renal excretion decrease, creatinine is a better indicator of renal function because it is not affected by diet, hydration, or tissue catabolism. Creatinine clearance measures the ability of the kidney to clear the blood of creatinine and approximates the glomerular filtration rate. It will decrease as renal function decreases. **Note:** Creatinine clearance is normally decreased in older persons. |
| Administer medications that promote diuresis as prescribed. | Control of fluid overload in AKI may include the use of large doses of furosemide in nonoliguric patients to induce diuresis. |
| Arrange for or administer renal dialysis as prescribed. For more information, see "Care of the Patient Undergoing Hemodialysis," Chapter 29, or, "Care of the Patient Undergoing Peritoneal Dialysis," Chapter 30, as indicated. | Hemodialysis treatments remove excess fluid through the process of ultrafiltration (removal of fluids using pressure). Peritoneal dialysis removes fluid by osmotic pressures across the peritoneal membrane. The present trend is to use dialysis early in ARF. It is done every 1–3 days (but may be done continuously in critical care). Prophylactic use of dialysis has reduced the incidence of complications and rate of death in patients with ARF. |

## Patient Problem/Analyze Cues/Prioritize Hypotheses

# Dehydration

*due to* active loss occurring with excessive urinary output: *Diuretic phase*

***Desired Outcome/Generate Solutions:*** The patient is normovolemic as evidenced by stable weight, balanced I&O, good skin turgor, CVP 4 mm Hg or greater, and BP and HR within the patient's normal range.

| ASSESSMENT—RECOGNIZE CUES/ INTERVENTIONS—TAKE ACTION | RATIONALES |
|---|---|
| Closely assess and document the I&O. | This assessment detects the trend of fluid volume. After relief of the obstruction in patients with postrenal failure, postobstructive diuresis may occur if the kidney is unable to concentrate the urine. Consequently, large volumes of solute and fluid may be lost (8–20 L/ day of urinary losses), resulting in volume depletion. |
| Monitor the weight daily. | A weight loss of 0.5 kg/day or more may reflect excessive volume loss. |
| Weigh the patient at the same time each day, using the same scale and with the patient wearing the same amount of clothing. | When weight is measured under the same conditions, more precise measurements of fluid volume can be anticipated. |
| Monitor the patient for complaints of lightheadedness, poor skin turgor, hypotension, postural hypotension, tachycardia, and decreased CVP. | These are indicators of volume depletion, which may result from loss of intravascular volume caused by urinary fluid losses and could lead to falls and other injuries. |
| As prescribed, encourage fluids in the dehydrated patient. | This intervention promotes rehydration and prevents life-threatening electrolyte abnormalities caused by the large-volume urinary and solute losses. |
| Report significant findings to the health care provider. | Although renal function usually can be reversed, there is a mortality rate of 40%–80% associated with AKI, depending on cause and the patient's age and comorbid conditions. |

Patient Problem/Analyze Cues/Prioritize Hypotheses

# Body Weight Problem (Weight Loss)

*due to* nausea, vomiting, anorexia, and dietary restrictions

*Desired Outcomes:* The patient attains optimal weight and demonstrates normal intake of food within restrictions, as indicated.

| ASSESSMENT—RECOGNIZE CUES/ INTERVENTIONS—TAKE ACTION | RATIONALES |
|---|---|
| Assess for and alert the health care provider to untoward GI symptoms and monitor BUN levels. | The presence of nausea, vomiting, and anorexia may signal increased uremia. BUN levels of 80–100 mg/dL usually require dialytic therapy. |
| Provide frequent, small meals in a pleasant atmosphere, especially controlling unpleasant odors. | Smaller, more frequent meals are usually better tolerated than larger meals. |
| Administer prescribed antiemetics as necessary. Instruct the patient to request medication before discomfort becomes severe. | Antiemetics are given to reduce nausea, which is better controlled when it is treated early. |
| Coordinate meal planning and dietary teaching with the patient, significant others, and dietitian. | Dietary restriction may include reduced protein, sodium, potassium, phosphorus, and fluid intake. |
| Provide fact sheets that list foods to restrict. | Protein is limited to minimize the retention of nitrogenous wastes. Sodium is limited to prevent thirst and fluid retention. Potassium and phosphorus are limited during the oliguric phase because of the kidney's decreased ability to excrete them. |
| Demonstrate with sample menus examples of how dietary restrictions may be incorporated into daily meals. | Sample menus show the patient how to apply this new knowledge. |
| Provide oral hygiene at frequent intervals. | Oral hygiene decreases metallic taste in the mouth associated with uremia. |

## ADDITIONAL PROBLEMS:

| | |
|---|---|
| *Constipation* | Chapter 1 |
| "Care of the Patient Undergoing Hemodialysis" | Chapter 29 |
| "Care of the Patient Undergoing Peritoneal Dialysis" | Chapter 30 |

## PATIENT–FAMILY TEACHING AND DISCHARGE PLANNING

When providing patient–family teaching, focus on sensory information, avoid giving excessive information, and initiate a visiting nurse referral for necessary follow-up teaching. Include verbal and written information about the following:

✓ Medications: Include drug name, purpose, dosage, schedule, precautions, and potential side effects. Also discuss drug–drug, herb–drug, and food–drug interactions.

✓ Diet: Include fact sheets that list foods to restrict. Provide sample menus with examples of how dietary restrictions may be incorporated into daily meals.

✓ Care and observation of dialysis access if the patient is being discharged with one. If the patient requires dialysis after discharge, coordinate discharge planning with the dialysis unit staff.

✓ Importance of continued medical follow-up of renal function.

✓ Signs and symptoms of potential complications. These should include electrolyte imbalances (see *Risk for Fluid Imbalance, Electrolyte Imbalance, and Acid–Base Imbalance* in this chapter); indicators of infection [see *Risk for Infection* in this chapter]; *Fluid Imbalance* in this chapter; and bleeding (especially from the GI tract for patients who are uremic).

✓ Telephone numbers to call in case questions or concerns arise about therapy or disease after discharge. Additional general information can be obtained by contacting the following:

• National Kidney and Urologic Diseases Information Clearinghouse: https://rarediseases.org/organizations/nihnational-kidney-and-urologic-diseases-information-clearinghouse/

• National Kidney Foundation: www.kidney.org

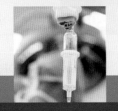

# Benign Prostatic Hyperplasia 28

## OVERVIEW/PATHOPHYSIOLOGY

The prostate is an encapsulated gland that surrounds the male urethra below the bladder neck and produces a thin, milky fluid during ejaculation. As a man ages, the prostate gland grows larger. Although the exact cause of enlargement is unknown, one theory is that hormonal changes affect the estrogen-androgen balance. While this noncancerous enlargement is common in men older than 50 years, benign prostatic hyperplasia also may result from modifiable metabolic irregularity such as diabetes, obesity, dyslipidemia, or metabolic syndrome. Prostatic enlargement can lead to lower urinary tract symptoms (LUTS) that can affect the quality of life. Treatment options include two classes of medications, alpha-adrenergic antagonists (reduce smooth muscle tone) and 5-alpha-reductase inhibitors (reduce prostate size), and surgical treatment. Watchful waiting and medical management may reduce the need for surgery. Watchful waiting is the process of active surveillance in patients with initial symptoms of LUTS. Treatment is given when symptoms of bladder outlet obstruction appear.

## HEALTH CARE SETTING

Primary care; outpatient acute (surgical) care

## ASSESSMENT

***Chronic indicators.*** Urinary frequency, hesitancy, urgency, and dribbling or postvoid dribbling; decreased force and caliber of stream; nocturia (several times each night); recurrent, severe hematuria. Scores on American Urological Association questionnaire are 0–7 (mild), 8–19 (moderate), and 20–35 (severe).

***Acute indicators/bladder outlet obstruction.*** Inability to urinate, nausea, vomiting, severe suprapubic pain, severe and constant urgency, flank pain during micturition, hematuria.

## DIAGNOSTIC TESTS

***Urinalysis.*** Checks for the presence of white blood cells (WBCs), leukocyte esterase, WBC casts, bacteria, and microscopic hematuria.

***Urine culture and sensitivity.*** Verifies the presence of an infecting organism, identifies the type of organism, and determines the organism's antibiotic sensitivities. **Note:** All urine specimens should be sent to the laboratory immediately after they are obtained, or they should be refrigerated if this is not possible (specimens for urine culture should not be refrigerated). Urine left at room temperature has a greater potential for bacterial growth, turbidity, and alkaline pH, any of which can distort test results.

***Hematocrit and hemoglobin.*** Decreased hematocrit and hemoglobin values may signal mild anemia from local bleeding.

***Blood urea nitrogen and creatinine.*** To evaluate renal and urinary function. **Note:** Blood urea nitrogen (BUN) can be affected by the patient's hydration status, and results must be evaluated accordingly: fluid volume excess reduces BUN levels, whereas fluid volume deficit increases them. Serum creatinine may not be a reliable indicator of renal function in older adults because of decreased muscle mass and decreased glomerular filtration rate; results of this test must be evaluated along with those of urine creatinine clearance, other renal function studies, and the patient's age.

***Prostate-specific antigen.*** Elevated above normal (0–4 ng/mL; normal range may increase with age); correlates well with positive digital examination findings. This glycoprotein is produced only by the prostate and reflects prostate size.

***Cystoscopy.*** Visualizes the prostate gland, estimates its size, and ascertains the presence of any damage to the bladder wall secondary to an enlarged prostate. **Note:** Because patients undergoing cystoscopy are susceptible to septic shock, this procedure is contraindicated in patients with acute urinary tract infection (UTI) because of the possible danger of hematogenic spread of Gram-negative bacteria.

***Transrectal ultrasound.*** Assesses prostate size and shape by a probe inserted into the rectum

***Maximal urinary flow rate.*** Rate less than 15 mL/second indicates significant obstruction to flow.

***Postvoid residual volume.*** Normal volume is less than 12 mL; higher volumes signal obstructive process.

## Patient Problem/Analyze Cues/Prioritize Hypotheses

# Delirium

*due to* fluid overload occurring with absorption of irrigating fluid during surgery or cerebral hypoxia occurring with sepsis

***Desired Outcome/Generate Solutions:*** The patient's mental status returns to baseline within 3 days of treatment.

| ASSESSMENT—RECOGNIZE CUES/ INTERVENTIONS—TAKE ACTION | RATIONALES |
|---|---|
| Assess the patient's baseline level of consciousness and mental status on admission. Ask the patient to perform a three-step task. | Asking patients to perform a three-step task (e.g., "Raise your right hand, place it on your left shoulder, and then place the right hand by your side.") is an effective way to evaluate baseline mental status because patients may be admitted with chronic confusion. |
| Assess the pre- and postsurgical/treatment short-term memory | Short-term memory can be tested by showing the patient how to use the call light, having the patient return the demonstration, and then waiting 5 minutes before having the patient demonstrate the use of the call light again. Inability to remember beyond 5 minutes indicates poor short-term memory. |
| Document patient's pre- and postsurgical treatment short-term memory assessment responses. | A patient's baseline status can then be compared with postsurgical status for evaluation, which will help determine the presence of acute confusion. |
| | This ensures that the patient's current/postsurgical is compared with patient's status before surgery/treatment. |
| Obtain a description of prehospital functional and mental status from sources familiar with the patient (e.g., family, friends, personnel at the nursing home or residential care facility). | The cause may be reversible. |
| Identify the cause of acute confusion as follows: | |
| • Assess the laboratory results: elevated WBCs and/or neutrophils. | Elevated WBC and/or neutrophil counts indicate sepsis, which can be caused by UTI from urinary retention. Neutrophils will be elevated before the WBC count increases. |
| • Assess the oximetry or request arterial blood gas values. | Low levels of oxygen can contribute to diminished mental status. |
| • Check serum sodium. | Dilutional hyponatremia can be caused by the absorption of irrigating fluid. |
| • Assess the hydration status by reviewing the intake and output (I&O) records after surgery. Output should match intake. | Both excess and deficient fluid volumes can affect mental status. |
| • Assess the legs for dependent edema. | Dependent edema can signal overhydration with poor venous return, which can affect mental status. |
| • Assess the cardiac and lung status. | Abnormal heart sounds or rhythms and the presence of crackles (rales) in lung bases can signal fluid excess, which could affect mental status. |
| • Assess the mouth for a furrowed tongue and dry mucous membranes. | These signs signal fluid deficit, which can affect mental status. |
| • For oximetry readings of 92% or less, anticipate initiation of oxygen therapy to increase oxygenation. | Patients usually require supplementary oxygen at these levels. Decreased levels of oxygen can adversely affect mental status. |
| • As appropriate, anticipate initiation of antibiotics in the presence of sepsis, diuretics to increase diuresis, and increased fluid intake by mouth or intravenous route to rehydrate the patient. | These interventions may help reverse acute confusion. |
| As appropriate, have the patient wear glasses and hearing aids, or keep them close to the bedside and within easy reach. | Disturbed sensory perception can contribute to confusion. |

| ASSESSMENT—RECOGNIZE CUES/ INTERVENTIONS—TAKE ACTION | RATIONALES |
|---|---|
| Keep the urinal and other commonly used items within easy reach. | Patients with short-term memory problems cannot be expected to use a call light. |
| As indicated by mental status, check on the patient frequently or every time you pass by the room. | This intervention helps ensure the patient's safety. |
| If indicated, place the patient close to the nurses' station if possible. Provide an environment that is nonstimulating and safe. | These measures provide a safer and less confusing environment for patients. |
| Provide music but avoid the use of television. | Individuals who are acutely confused regarding place and time often think the action on television is happening in the room. |
| Attempt to reorient the patient to surroundings as needed. Keep a clock and calendar at the bedside and remind him verbally of the date and place. | These orientation measures help reduce confusion. |
| Encourage the patient or significant other to bring items familiar to the patient. | Familiar items provide a foundation for orientation and can include blankets, bedspreads, and pictures of family or pets. |
| If the patient becomes belligerent, angry, or argumentative while you are attempting to reorient him, *stop this approach*. Do not argue with him or his interpretation of the environment. | Arguing with confused patients likely will increase their belligerence. State "I can understand why you may (hear, think, see) that." |
| If the patient displays hostile behavior or misperceives your role (e.g., nurse becomes thief, jailer), leave the room. Return in 15 minutes. Introduce yourself to him as though you have never met. Begin dialog anew. | Patients who are acutely confused have poor short-term memory and may not remember the previous encounter or that you were involved in that encounter. |
| If the patient attempts to leave the hospital, walk with him and attempt distraction. Ask him to tell you about his destination. For example, "That sounds like a wonderful place! Tell me about it." Keep your tone pleasant and conversational. Continue walking with him away from exits and doors around the unit. After a few minutes, attempt to guide him back to his room. | Distraction is an effective technique with individuals who are confused. |
| If the patient has permanent or severe cognitive impairment, check on him frequently and reorient to baseline mental status as indicated; however, do not argue with him about his perception of reality. | Arguing can cause a cognitively impaired person to become aggressive and combative. Patients with severe cognitive impairments (e.g., Alzheimer disease, dementia) also can experience acute confusional states (i.e., delirium) and can be returned to their baseline mental state. |

## Patient Problem/Analyze Cues/Prioritize Hypotheses

# Risk for Hemorrhaging

*due to* the invasive procedure or actions that put pressure on the prostatic capsule

***Desired Outcomes/Generate Solutions:*** The patient is normovolemic, as evidenced by a balanced I&O; heart rate (HR) of 100 bpm or less (or within the patient's normal range); blood pressure (BP) of 90/60 mm Hg or more (or within the patient's normal range); respiratory rate of 20 breaths/minute or less; and skin that is warm, dry, and of normal color appropriate for race. After receiving instruction, the patient relates actions that may result in hemorrhage of the prostatic capsule and participates in interventions to prevent them.

| ASSESSMENT—RECOGNIZE CUES/ INTERVENTIONS—TAKE ACTION | RATIONALES |
|---|---|
| On the patient's return from the recovery room, assess vital signs (VS) as his condition warrants or per agency protocol. | These assessments evaluate the trend of the patient's recovery. Increasing pulse, decreasing BP, diaphoresis, pallor, and increasing respirations can occur with hemorrhage and impending shock. |

Continued

| ASSESSMENT—RECOGNIZE CUES/ INTERVENTIONS—TAKE ACTION | RATIONALES |
|---|---|
| Monitor and document the I&O every 8 hours. Subtract the amount of fluid used with continuous bladder irrigation (CBI) from the total output. | This assessment evaluates trend of the patient's hydration status and assesses for postsurgical bleeding. |
| Assess catheter drainage closely for the first 24 hours. Watch for dark-red drainage that does not lighten to reddish pink or drainage that remains thick in consistency after irrigation. | Drainage should lighten to pink or blood tinged within 24 hours after surgery. Dark-red drainage that does not lighten to reddish pink or drainage that remains thick in consistency after irrigation can signal bleeding within the operative site. |
| Be alert to bright-red, thick drainage at any time. | This drainage can occur with arterial bleeding within the operative site. |
| Do not measure temperature rectally or insert tubes or enemas into the rectum. Instruct the patient not to strain with bowel movements or sit for long periods. | These actions can result in pressure on the prostatic capsule and may lead to hemorrhage. |
| Obtain prescription for and provide stool softeners or cathartics as necessary. Encourage a diet high in fiber and increased fluid intake. | These measures aid in producing soft stool and preventing straining. |
| Maintain traction on the indwelling urethral catheter for 4–8 hours after surgery or as directed. | The surgeon may establish traction on the indwelling urethral catheter in the operating room to help prevent bleeding. |
| | **Note:** Urethral catheters used after prostatic surgery commonly have a large retention balloon (30 mL). |

## Patient Problems/Analyze Cues/Prioritize Hypotheses

# Risk for Fluid Imbalance and Electrolyte Imbalance

*due to* the absorption of irrigating fluid during surgery (transurethral resection of the prostate syndrome)

***Desired Outcome/Generate Solutions:*** After surgery, the patient is normovolemic as evidenced by balanced I&O (after subtraction of irrigant from total output); orientation to person, place, and time with no significant changes in mental status; BP and HR within the patient's normal range; absence of dysrhythmias; and electrolyte values within normal range; and urinary output is 0.5 mL/kg/hr or more.

| ASSESSMENT—RECOGNIZE CUES/ INTERVENTIONS—TAKE ACTION | RATIONALES |
|---|---|
| Assess and record VS. | This assessment evaluates hydration status. Sudden increases in BP with corresponding decrease in HR can occur with fluid overload. |
| Assess pulse for dysrhythmias, including irregular rate and skipped beats. | Dysrhythmias, including irregular HR and skipped beats, can signal electrolyte imbalance, which can occur as a result of the high volumes of fluid used during irritation. |
| Monitor and record I&O. To determine the true amount of urinary output, subtract the amount of irrigant (CBI) from the total output. | Large amounts of fluid, commonly plain sterile water, are used to irrigate the bladder during the operative cystoscopy to remove blood and tissue, thereby enabling visualization of the surgical field. Over time, this fluid may be absorbed through the bladder wall into the systemic circulation. |
| Report discrepancies between I&O. | Differences may signal either fluid retention or fluid loss. |
| Monitor the patient's mental and motor status. Assess for muscle twitching, seizures, and changes in mentation. | These are signs of water intoxication and electrolyte imbalance, which can occur within 24 hours after surgery because of the high volumes of fluid used in irrigation. |

| ASSESSMENT—RECOGNIZE CUES/ INTERVENTIONS—TAKE ACTION | RATIONALES |
|---|---|
| Monitor electrolyte values, in particular those of Na+. | Normal range for Na+ is 137–147 mEq/L. Values less than that signal hyponatremia, which can occur with the absorption of the extra fluids and its dilutional effect. |
| Promptly report indications of fluid overload and electrolyte imbalance to the health care provider. | This intervention ensures prompt treatment, which may include diuretics. |

## Patient Problem/Analyze Cues/Prioritize Hypotheses

# Acute Pain

*due to* bladder spasms

***Desired Outcomes/Generate Solutions:*** Within 1 hour of intervention, the patient's subjective perception of pain decreases, as documented by a pain scale. Objective indicators, such as grimacing, are absent or diminished.

| ASSESSMENT—RECOGNIZE CUES/ INTERVENTIONS—TAKE ACTION | RATIONALES |
|---|---|
| Assess and document the quality, location, and duration of pain. Devise a pain scale with the patient, rating pain from 0 (no pain) to 10 (worst pain). | This assessment establishes a baseline, monitors the trend of pain, and determines subsequent response to medication. |
| Medicate the patient with prescribed analgesics, anticholinergics, opioids, and antispasmodics as appropriate; evaluate and document the patient's response, using the pain scale. | Oral anticholinergics, such as oxybutynin, are used as antispasmodics. |
| Instruct the patient to request analgesic before pain becomes severe. | Prolonged stimulation of the pain receptors results in increased sensitivity to painful stimuli and will increase the amount of drug required to relieve pain. |
| Provide warm blankets or heating pad to the affected area. | These measures increase regional circulation and relax tense muscles. |
| Monitor for leakage around the catheter. | Leakage can signal the presence of bladder spasms. |
| If the patient has spasms, assure him that they are normal. | Spasms can occur from irritation of the bladder mucosa or from a clot that results in backup of urine into the bladder with concomitant mucosal irritation. |
| Encourage fluid intake. | Adequate hydration helps prevent spasms. |
| If the health care provider has prescribed catheter irrigation for the removal of clots, follow instructions carefully. | Gentle irrigation will avoid discomfort and injury to the patient. |
| Monitor for the presence of clots in the tubing. If clots are present for a patient with CBI, adjust the rate of bladder irrigation to maintain light red urine (with clots). If clots inhibit the flow of urine, irrigate the catheter by hand according to agency or health care provider's directive. | Total output should be greater than the amount of irrigant instilled. If output equals the amount of irrigant or the patient complains that his bladder is full, the catheter may be clogged with clots. |

## Patient Problem/Analyze Cues/Prioritize Hypotheses

# Risk for Impaired Skin Integrity

*due to* wound drainage from suprapubic or retropubic prostatectomy

***Desired Outcome/Generate Solutions:*** The patient's skin remains nonerythremic and intact.

| ASSESSMENT—RECOGNIZE CUES/ INTERVENTIONS—TAKE ACTION | RATIONALES |
|---|---|
| Assess the skin and incisional dressings frequently during the first 24 hours; change or reinforce dressings as needed. | If an incision has been made into the bladder, irritation can result from prolonged contact of urine with the skin. |
| Use Montgomery straps or gauze net (Surginet) rather than tape to secure the dressing. | These measures ensure that the dressing is secure without the damage that tape can cause to the skin. |
| If drainage is copious after drain removal, apply a wound drainage or ostomy pouch with a skin barrier over the incision. | This measure provides a barrier between the skin and drainage. |
| Use a pouch with an antireflux valve. | This valve prevents contamination from reflux. |

## Patient Problem/Analyze Cues/Prioritize Hypotheses

# Deficient Knowledge (Sexual Function)

*due to* unfamiliarity with postsurgical sexual function

***Desired Outcome/Generate Solutions:*** After intervention/patient teaching, the patient discusses concerns about sexuality and relates accurate information about sexual function.

| ASSESSMENT—RECOGNIZE CUES/ INTERVENTIONS—TAKE ACTION | RATIONALES |
|---|---|
| Assess the patient's level of readiness to discuss sexual function; provide opportunities for the patient to discuss fears and anxieties. | This assessment enables the appropriate time to provide patient teaching and optimally will reveal the patient's specific fears and anxieties. |
| Assure patients who have had a simple prostatectomy that the ability to attain and maintain an erection is unaltered. | Retrograde ejaculation (backward flow of seminal fluid into the bladder, which is eliminated with the next urination) or "dry" ejaculation will occur in most patients, but this probably will end after a few months. However, it will not affect the ability to achieve orgasm. |
| Be aware of your own feelings about sexuality. | If you are uncomfortable discussing sexuality, request that another staff member take responsibility for discussing concerns with the patient. |
| As indicated, encourage the continuation of counseling after hospital discharge. Confer with the health care provider and Social Services to identify appropriate referrals. | Conferring with the health care provider and Social Services will help identify appropriate referrals. |

## Patient Problem/Analyze Cues/Prioritize Hypotheses

# Constipation

*due to* postsurgical discomfort or fear of exerting excess pressure on the prostatic capsule

***Desired Outcome/Generate Solutions:*** By the third to fourth postoperative day, the patient relates the presence of a bowel pattern that is normal for him with minimal pain or straining.

| ASSESSMENT—RECOGNIZE CUES/ INTERVENTIONS—TAKE ACTION | RATIONALES |
|---|---|
| Assess and document the presence or absence and quality of bowel sounds in all four abdominal quadrants. | A patient whose bowel sounds have not yet returned but who states that he needs to have a bowel movement during the first 24 hours after surgery may have clots in his bladder that are creating pressure on the rectum. |
| Assess for the presence of clots (see *Acute Pain*, earlier) and irrigate the catheter as indicated. | |
| Gather baseline information on the patient's normal bowel pattern and document findings. | Each patient has a bowel pattern that is normal for him. |

| ASSESSMENT—RECOGNIZE CUES/ INTERVENTIONS—TAKE ACTION | RATIONALES |
|---|---|
| Caution the patient to avoid straining when defecating. | Straining puts excess pressure on the prostatic capsule. |
| Unless contraindicated, encourage the patient to drink 2–3 L of fluids on the day after surgery. | Adequate hydration helps ensure a softer stool with less of a tendency to strain. |
| Consult the health care provider and dietitian about the need for increased fiber in the patient's diet. | Adding bulk to stools will minimize the risk for damaging the prostatic capsule by straining. |
| Encourage the patient to ambulate and be as active as possible. | Increased activity helps promote bowel movements by increasing peristalsis. |
| Consult the health care provider about the use of stool softeners for the patient during the postoperative period. | Soft stool will be less painful to evacuate following surgery and will cause less straining. |
| See "Immobility," Chapter 1, *Constipation*, for more information. | |

## Patient Problem/Analyze Cues/Prioritize Hypotheses

# Urge Incontinence of Urine

*due to* urethral irritation after removal of the urethral catheter

***Desired Outcome/Generate Solutions:*** The patient reports increasing periods of time between voidings by the second postoperative day and regains a normal pattern of micturition within 4–6 weeks after surgery.

| ASSESSMENT—RECOGNIZE CUES/ INTERVENTIONS—TAKE ACTION | RATIONALES |
|---|---|
| Before removing the urethral catheter, explain to the patient that he may void in small amounts for the first 12 hours after catheter removal. | Irritation from the catheter may cause the patient to urinate in small amounts. Initially, the patient may void every 15–30 minutes, but the interval of urination should increase toward a more normal pattern. |
| Instruct the patient to save urine in a urinal for the first 24 hours after surgery. Inspect each voiding for color and consistency. | First urine specimens can be dark red from passage of old blood. Each successive specimen should be lighter in color. |
| Note and document the time and amount of each voiding. | Initially, patients may void every 15–30 minutes, but the time interval of urination should increase toward a more normal pattern. |
| Encourage the patient to drink 2.5–3 L/day if not contraindicated. | Low intake leads to highly concentrated urine, which irritates the bladder and can lead to incontinence. |
| Before hospital discharge, inform the patient that dribbling may occur for the first 4–6 weeks after surgery. | Dribbling occurs because of disturbance of the bladder neck and urethra during prostate removal. As muscles strengthen and healing occurs (the urethra reaches normal size and function), dribbling stops. |
| Instruct patient to perform Kegel exercises (see *Deficient Knowledge (Postoperative Pelvic Exercises)* later in this chapter). | These exercises improve sphincter control. |

## Patient Problem/Analyze Cues/Prioritize Hypotheses

# Stress Incontinence of Urine

*due to* temporary loss of muscle tone in the urethral sphincter after radical prostatectomy

***Desired Outcome/Generate Solutions:*** Within the 24-hour period before hospital discharge, the patient relates the understanding of the cause of the temporary incontinence and the regimen that must be observed to promote bladder control.

| ASSESSMENT—RECOGNIZE CUES/ INTERVENTIONS—TAKE ACTION | RATIONALES |
|---|---|
| Explain that there is a potential for urinary incontinence after prostatectomy but that it should resolve within 6 months. Describe the reason for the incontinence, using aids such as anatomic illustrations. | A knowledgeable patient likely will adhere to the therapeutic regimen. Understanding that incontinence is a possibility but that it usually resolves should be encouraging. |
| Encourage the patient to maintain adequate fluid intake of at least 2–3 L/ day (unless contraindicated by an underlying cardiac dysfunction or other disorder). | Dilute urine is less irritating to the prostatic fossa and less likely to result in incontinence. |
| Instruct the patient to avoid caffeine-containing drinks. | These fluids irritate the bladder and have a mild diuretic effect, which would make bladder control even more difficult. |
| Establish a bladder routine with the patient before hospital discharge. | The goal of bladder training is to reduce the frequency of urination with small amounts of urine and thereby return the patient to a more normal bladder function. The timing of intervals between urinations is determined to estimate how long the patient can hold his urine. |
| Encourage the patient to schedule times for emptying his bladder and maintain a copy of the written schedule. An example initially would be every 1–2 hours when awake and every 4 hours at night. Then, if this is successful, the patient lengthens the intervals of urination. | |
| Provide instructions to patient on how to perform Kegel exercises. (see the next patient problem). | These exercises promote sphincter control, thereby decreasing incontinence episodes. |
| Remind the patient to discuss any incontinence problems with the health care provider during follow-up examinations. | This information helps ensure that the patient's needs are addressed and treated. |

## Patient Problem/Analyze Cues/Prioritize Hypotheses

# Deficient Knowledge (Postoperative Pelvic Exercises)

*due to* unfamiliarity with the pelvic muscle (Kegel) exercise program to strengthen perineal muscles (effective for individuals with mild to moderate stress incontinence)

***Desired Outcome/Generate Solutions:*** Within the 24-hour period after teaching, the patient verbalizes and demonstrates accurate knowledge about the pelvic muscle (Kegel) exercise program.

| ASSESSMENT—RECOGNIZE CUES/ INTERVENTIONS—TAKE ACTION | RATIONALES |
|---|---|
| Explain the purpose of Kegel exercises. | Kegel exercises strengthen pelvic area muscles, which will help regain bladder control. |
| Assist the patient with identifying the correct muscle group. | A common error when attempting to perform this exercise is contracting the buttocks, quadriceps, and abdominal muscles. |
| Teach the exercise as follows: | |
| • Attempt to shut off urinary flow after beginning urination, hold for a few seconds, and then start the stream again. | This strengthens the proximal muscle. If it can be accomplished, the correct muscle group is being used. |
| • Contract the muscle around the anus as though to stop a bowel movement. | This strengthens the distal muscle. |
| • Repeat these exercises 10–20 times, four times daily. | These exercises must be done frequently throughout the day and for 2–9 months before benefits are obtained. |

## ADDITIONAL PROBLEMS:

| | |
|---|---|
| "Perioperative Care" | Chapter 4 |
| "Delirium" | Chapter 98 |

 ## PATIENT–FAMILY TEACHING AND DISCHARGE PLANNING

When providing patient–family teaching, focus on sensory information, avoid giving excessive information, and initiate a visiting nurse referral for necessary follow-up teaching. Include verbal and written information about the following:

✓ Medications, including drug name, purpose, dosage, schedule, precautions, and potential side effects. Also discuss drug–drug, herb–drug, and food–drug interactions.

✓ Necessity of reporting the following indicators of UTI to the health care provider: chills; fever; hematuria; flank, costovertebral angle, suprapubic, low back, buttock, or scrotal pain; cloudy and foul-smelling urine; frequency; urgency; dysuria; and increasing or recurring incontinence.

✓ Care of incision, if appropriate, including cleansing, dressing changes, and bathing. Advise the patient to be aware of indicators of infection: persistent redness, increasing pain, edema, increased warmth along the incision, or purulent or increased drainage.

✓ Care of catheters or drains if the patient is discharged with them.

✓ Daily fluid requirement of at least 2–3 L/day in nonrestricted patients.

✓ Importance of increasing dietary fiber or taking stool softeners to soften stools. This will minimize the risk for damage to the prostatic capsule by preventing straining with bowel movements. Caution the patient to avoid using suppositories or enemas for the treatment of constipation.

✓ Use of a sofa, reclining chair, or footstool to promote venous drainage from legs and to distribute weight on the perineum, not the rectum.

✓ Avoiding the following activities for the period prescribed by the health care provider: sitting for long periods, heavy lifting (more than 10 lb), and sexual intercourse.

✓ Kegel exercises to help regain urinary sphincter control for postoperative dribbling. See *Deficient Knowledge (Postoperative Pelvic Exercises)*, earlier.

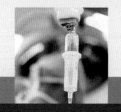

# Care of the Patient Undergoing Hemodialysis 29

## OVERVIEW/PATHOPHYSIOLOGY

During hemodialysis, substances are moved from blood across a semipermeable membrane and into a dialysis solution, called dialysate. Fluid and electrolyte imbalances are corrected and waste products in the blood are removed. Hemodialysis requires access to large vessels through arteriovenous (AV) fistulas, grafts, or temporary AV lines. Blood is removed from the vascular access, heparinized, and propelled through a dialyzer. The dialyzer is filled with fluid dialysate that is preset to filter wastes and excess fluid from the patient's blood. The blood is then returned to the patient's circulation. Hemodialysis may be a temporary treatment for patients with acute kidney injury but can also be used long term in patients with chronic kidney disease, who will need several treatments per week.

**Indications for hemodialysis.** Hemodialysis is done when the patient's uremia can no longer be adequately treated with conservative medical management, including diet, fluid restriction, and medication. This is usually when the GFR is less than 15 m/minute/1.73 m². Uremic complications such as encephalopathy, neuropathies, uncontrolled hyperkalemia, pericarditis, and accelerated hypertension are also taken into consideration as they are all indications of the immediate need for dialysis.

## HEALTH CARE SETTINGS

1. Outpatient setting in a dialysis center
2. Inpatient setting in an acute care hospital

   **Vascular access.** Access to large vessels is necessary to provide a blood flow rate of 300–500 mL/minute for an effective dialysis. Vascular access sites may include AV fistulas, AV grafts, internal jugular catheters (right side preferred), femoral vein catheters, or subclavian catheters.

## Patient Problem/Analyze Cues/Prioritize Hypotheses

# Fluid Imbalance

*due to* compromised regulatory mechanisms

**Desired Outcomes/Generate Solutions:** After dialysis the patient is normovolemic as evidenced by stable weight, respiratory rate (RR) of 12–20 breaths/minute with clear breath sounds, regular breathing pattern, and no signs of dyspnea.

The patient's heart rate and blood pressure are within the patient's baseline levels.

| ASSESSMENT—RECOGNIZE CUES/ INTERVENTIONS—TAKE ACTION | RATIONALES |
|---|---|
| Assess Central Venous Pressure (CVP), vital signs, breathing, lung sounds, neck veins, serum albumin level, jugular veins, and signs of edema. | Indicators of fluid overload include increased CVP, Blood Pressure (BP), and Respiratory Rate (RR). Other indicators are adventitious breath sounds, shortness of breath, jugular vein distention, and edema. Dependent edema likely will be detected in the legs or feet of patients who are ambulatory, whereas the sacral area will be edematous in those who are on bedrest. Periorbital edema also may result from excessive fluid overload. Low serum albumin decreases colloid osmotic pressure, allowing fluid to leak into the extravascular space. Low serum albumin also may contribute to generalized edema and pulmonary edema. Jugular veins are likely to be distended with the head of bed (HOB) elevated 45 degrees owing to increased intravascular volume. Crackles and shortness of breath can occur as a result of fluid volume overload. Hypertension, tachycardia, and increased CVP may result from sodium and fluid retention. |

| ASSESSMENT—RECOGNIZE CUES/ INTERVENTIONS—TAKE ACTION | RATIONALES |
|---|---|
| Assess the intake and output (I&O) and daily weight as indicators of fluid status. | Intake greater than output and steady weight gain indicates retained fluid. Weight is an important guideline for determining the quantity of fluid to be removed during dialysis. |
| Weigh the patient at the same time each day, using the same scale and with the patient wearing the same amount of clothing (or with the same items on the bed if using a bed scale). | Weighing patients under the same conditions helps ensure accurate measurement of fluid status. |
| Weigh the patient before and after dialysis treatment. | Weighing the patient before and after dialysis therapy assesses the effectiveness of treatment in removing fluid volume. |

## Patient Problem/Analyze Cues/Prioritize Hypotheses
# Risk for Dehydration

*due to* excessive fluid removal from dialysis

***Desired Outcome/Generate Solutions:*** After dialysis the patient is normovolemic as evidenced by stable weight, RR of 12–20 breaths/minute with normal depth and pattern (eupnea), HR and BP within the patient's baseline range, and clear breath sounds.

| ASSESSMENT—RECOGNIZE CUES/ INTERVENTIONS—TAKE ACTION | RATIONALES |
|---|---|
| After dialysis, assess for and report hypotension, decreased CVP, tachycardia, and complaints of dizziness or lightheadedness. | These are indicators of dehydration, which may result from rapid or excessive fluid losses during dialysis. It should be noted that patients with uremia may not develop compensatory tachycardia owing to autonomic neuropathy, which can occur with uremia. |
| Clarify withholding antihypertensive medications with health care provider before and during dialysis. | Antihypertensive medications usually are held before and during dialysis to help prevent hypotension during dialysis |
| Weigh the patient at the same time each day, using the same scale and with the patient wearing the same amount of clothing (or with the same items on the bed if using a bed scale). | Weighing patients under the same conditions helps ensure accurate measurement of fluid status. |

## Patient Problem/Analyze Cues/Prioritize Hypotheses
# Risk for Hemorrhaging

*due to* vascular access puncture or its disconnection and or heparinization during dialysis

***Desired Outcome/Generate Solutions:*** The patient's vascular access remains intact and connected with no excess bleeding from site.

| ASSESSMENT—RECOGNIZE CUES/ INTERVENTIONS—TAKE ACTION | RATIONALES |
|---|---|
| Monitor for postdialysis bleeding (needle sites, incisions). | This bleeding can occur due to heparinization and needle punctures during dialysis. |
| Alert the patient to the potential for bleeding from these areas. | If these signs and symptoms occur, the patient will be able to report them promptly to the staff or health care provider for timely intervention. |

Continued

| ASSESSMENT—RECOGNIZE CUES/ INTERVENTIONS—TAKE ACTION | RATIONALES |
|---|---|
| Do not give intramuscular (IM) injection for at least 1 hour after dialysis. | Avoiding IM injections for this amount of time prevents hematoma formation. |
| Test all stools for the presence of blood. Report significant findings. | Gastrointestinal bleeding is common in patients with renal failure, especially after heparinization. |
| Anchor the temporary catheter securely and tape all connections. Keep clamps at the bedside in case the line becomes disconnected. If the line is removed or accidentally pulled out, apply firm pressure to site for at least 10 minutes. | Temporary dialysis catheters are inserted into large vessels and hemorrhage can occur if the catheter becomes disconnected or dislodged. |

## Patient Problem/Analyze Cues/Prioritize Hypotheses

# Risk for Ineffective Tissue Perfusion

*due to* interrupted blood flow that can occur with clotting in the vascular access

**Desired Outcome/Generate Solutions:** The patient has adequate tissue perfusion distal to the vascular access.

| ASSESSMENT—RECOGNIZE CUES/ INTERVENTIONS—TAKE ACTION | RATIONALES |
|---|---|
| Auscultate for bruit and palpate for thrill over implanted vascular access. Notify health care provider if bruit and thrill absent. | These assessments reveal whether the patient's vascular access is patent. A bruit is a blowing sound that is made when blood moves through the access. A thrill is a vibration felt when placing a hand over the access, denoting blood flow. |
| Notify the health care provider if the extremity distal to the vascular access becomes cool or swollen, has decreased capillary refill, or has decreased pulse or is discolored. | These problems can indicate hypoxia as a result of reduced blood supply to the extremity. |
| Report complaints of severe or unrelieved pain, numbness, and tingling of the area of vascular access or extremity distal to the access. | These indicators can signal impaired tissue perfusion caused by occlusion of the vascular access. |
| Assess for postoperative swelling along the graft or fistula or area around the shunt; elevate the extremity accordingly. | Postoperative swelling along the graft or fistula or area around the shunt is expected and will diminish with extremity elevation. |
| Notify the health care provider if the extremity distal to the vascular access becomes cool or swollen, has decreased capillary refill, or has decreased pulse or is discolored. | These problems can indicate hypoxia as a result of reduced blood supply to the extremity. |
| Never use the vascular access for instillation of intravenous (IV) medications or phlebotomy. Monitor it closely and handle it with care. | The vascular access must only be used for dialysis as puncturing it for other purposes could likely compromise its patency and increase the clotting risk. |
| Explain monitoring and care procedures to the patient. | A knowledgeable patient is more likely to adhere to these principles. |
| Place a sign above HOB indicating extremity in which the fistula or graft has been placed stating not to take BP, start an IV line, or draw blood from the affected limb. Ensure that this information is clearly documented on the patient's medical record and care plan. Caution the patient to avoid tight clothing, jewelry, name bands, or restraint on affected extremity. | These procedures and precautions help prevent blood clotting in the vascular access. |

## Patient Problem/Analyze Cues/Prioritize Hypotheses

# Risk for Infection

*due to* invasive procedure (creation of vascular access for hemodialysis and frequency of site access)

***Desired Outcome/Generate Solutions:*** The patient is free of infection as evidenced by normothermia and absence of erythema, local warmth, exudate, swelling, and tenderness at the access site.

| ASSESSMENT—RECOGNIZE CUES/ INTERVENTIONS—TAKE ACTION | RATIONALES |
|---|---|
| Never use the vascular access for instillation of IV medications or phlebotomy. Monitor it closely and handle it with care. | The vascular access must only be used for dialysis as puncturing it for other purposes could likely increase infection risk. |
| Explain monitoring and care procedures to the patient. | A knowledgeable patient is more likely to adhere to these principles. |
| Cover vascular access with sterile dressing for at least eight hours after dialysis. Maintain cleanliness over vascular access area. | These interventions will decrease the risk of infection. |
| Vascular accesses include the following: | |
| Only trained dialysis nurses should access the dialysis ports. | Accessing the line for nondialysis treatments increases the risk for infection. Dialysis nurses are specially trained to appropriately access the dialysis ports. |
| Monitor for and report the presence of erythema, local warmth, exudate, swelling, and tenderness at access exit site. | These are indicators of infection. Dressing changes and cultures of any drainage should be performed only by the dialysis staff. |

## ✔ PATIENT–FAMILY TEACHING AND DISCHARGE PLANNING

When providing patient–family teaching, focus on sensory information, avoid giving excessive information, and initiate a visiting nurse referral if indicated for follow-up teaching. Include verbal and written information about the following:

- ✓ Medications, including drug name; purpose; dosage; schedule; drug–drug, herb–drug, and food–drug interactions; precautions; and potential side effects.
- ✓ Diet and fluid restrictions: Include fact sheets that list foods to limit or restrict. Review fluid restrictions. Provide sample menus with examples of how dietary restrictions may be incorporated into daily meals. Have the patient demonstrate understanding of dietary restrictions by preparing 3-day menus.
- ✓ Care of fistula or graft to prevent/detect bleeding, clotting, and infection.
- ✓ Need for and importance of monitoring daily weights, I&O, and monitoring of BP at home, if necessary.

- ✓ Importance of continued medical follow-up; confirm date and time of next health care provider and hemodialysis appointments.
- ✓ Signs and symptoms that necessitate medical attention: increased weight gain, unusual shortness of breath, edema, dizziness or fainting, fever, increased hypertension, redness around access site, decrease in bruit or thrill (fistulas, graft), prolonged bleeding from fistula or graft, discoloration or coldness distal to fistula or graft, accidental pulling on the subclavian line.
- ✓ Telephone numbers to call in case questions or concerns arise about therapy or disease after discharge. Additional general information and patient educational materials can be obtained by contacting:
  - National Kidney and Urologic Diseases Information Clearinghouse: https://rarediseases.org/organizations/nihnational-kidney-and-urologic-diseases-information-clearinghouse/
  - National Kidney Foundation: www.kidney.org

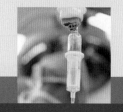

# Care of the Patient Undergoing Peritoneal Dialysis 30

## OVERVIEW

Peritoneal dialysis (PD) uses the peritoneum as the membrane through which fluid and dissolved substances are exchanged with the blood. Dialysate is instilled into the peritoneal cavity through a catheter that is surgically implanted through the anterior abdominal wall. Excess fluid, electrolytes, and toxins are removed with PD through the processes of diffusion, osmosis, and ultrafiltration as the dialysate dwells in the peritoneal space for a prescribed amount of time. At set intervals, the peritoneal cavity is drained, and new dialysate is instilled.

*Indications for peritoneal dialysis.* Episodes of renal insufficiency that cannot be managed by diet, medications, and fluid restriction; chronic kidney disease; drug overdose; hyperkalemia; fluid overload; and metabolic acidosis.

## Components of dialysis

*Catheter.* Silastic tube that is either implanted in the peritoneal space using general anesthesia as a surgical procedure for patients who will have long-term treatment or is inserted using local anesthetic at the bedside for short-term dialysis.

*Dialysate.* Sterile electrolyte solution similar in composition to normal plasma. The electrolyte composition of the dialysate can be adjusted according to individual needs. Glucose is added to the dialysate in varying concentrations to remove excess body fluid through osmosis. Insulin and other medications may be added directly to the dialysate by dialysis nurses or a pharmacist.

### Types of dialysis

*Automated peritoneal dialysis.* This is the most common form of PD. Patients are able to be dialyzed while they sleep. Dialysate is delivered via an automated device, which automatically times and controls the fill, dwell and drain phases of PD. The patient receives four or more dialysis cycles each night and although may need one more exchange during the day, is free from the PD process during most of the day.

*Continuous ambulatory peritoneal dialysis.* This is done every few hours during the day. The patient can perform PD approximately four times a day. The patient instills 2–3 L of dialysate from a plastic bag into the peritoneal cavity through a disposable administration line. The bag and line are then disconnected to allow the dialysate to dwell for several hours. When ready to drain, the line is reconnected, the dialysate is drained from the peritoneal cavity, and the process is repeated.

## HEALTH CARE SETTING

Home setting; acute care setting if the patient has complications or has been hospitalized for other medical reasons

### Patient Problem/Analyze Cues/Prioritize Hypotheses

# Risk for Infection

*due to* invasive procedure (direct access of the catheter to the peritoneum)

*Desired Outcome/Generate Solutions:* The patient is free of infection.

| ASSESSMENT—RECOGNIZE CUES/ INTERVENTIONS—TAKE ACTION | RATIONALES |
|---|---|
|  Assess for and report indications of peritonitis. | The most common complication of PD is peritonitis. Indicators include fever, extreme abdominal pain, distention, abdominal wall rigidity, rebound tenderness, cloudy dialysate outflow, nausea, and malaise. Recurrent/relapsing peritonitis is one of the most common reasons that PD treatment must be discontinued. |

| ASSESSMENT—RECOGNIZE CUES/ INTERVENTIONS—TAKE ACTION | RATIONALES |
|---|---|
| Assess the color and clarity of dialysate following outflow. | Bloody and cloudy outflow or the presence of fibrin in the outflow may be an initial sign of peritonitis.<br><br>**Note:** Gynecological-associated phenomena account for the majority of blood outflow cases in women. |
| Assess for and report redness, local warmth, edema, drainage, or tenderness at the exit site. | These are signs of infection at the exit site. |
| Culture any exudate from catheter site and report results to the health care provider. | A culture will identify any infectious organisms that are present. |
| Maintain sterile technique when making systems connections, disconnecting, and capping the system, or adding medications to the dialysate. | To minimize the risk for peritonitis and other infections, the dialysate, connection sites and catheter insertion site must remain sterile to prevent infectious organisms from entering the peritoneal cavity. |
| Follow agency policy for care of the catheter exit site. | Exit site infections may lead to the development of peritonitis. |
| Report to the health care provider if dialysate leaks around the catheter exit site. | Leakage can signal an obstruction or need for another purse-string suture around the catheter site. Leakage around the exit site has been associated with an increased risk for tunnel infections, exit site infections, and peritonitis. Organisms may track through subcutaneous tissue into the peritoneum, causing infection. |
| Instruct the patient in the preceding interventions and observations if PD will be performed after hospital discharge. | An informed patient likely will adhere to infection prevention interventions and know when to report untoward signs to the health care provider. |

## Patient Problem/Analyze Cues/Prioritize Hypotheses

# Risk for Fluid Imbalance

*due to* inadequate exchange

***Desired Outcome/Generate Solutions:*** After dialysis, the patient is normovolemic.

| ASSESSMENT—RECOGNIZE CUES/ INTERVENTIONS—TAKE ACTION | RATIONALES |
|---|---|
| Assess for and report hypertension, dyspnea, tachycardia, distended neck veins, or increased Central Venous Pressure (CVP). | These are indicators of fluid overload and should be reported promptly for timely intervention. |
| Assess the patient for respiratory distress. | Respiratory distress can occur from fluid overload or from compression of the diaphragm by the dialysate, especially when the patient is supine. |
| If respiratory distress occurs, monitor Respiratory Rate (RR) and Oxygen saturation, elevate the head of bed (HOB), and notify the health care provider. | RR and oxygen saturation will provide vital information on respiratory status. Raising the HOB helps lungs to expand and may help alleviate compression of the diaphragm because the diaphragm will be less compressed by the dialysis solution. If respiratory distress continues, the dialysis nurse should be notified because drainage of the solution may alleviate diaphragmatic pressure. |
| Assess the Intake and Output (I&O) and weight daily, using the same scale and with the patient wearing the same amount of clothing (or with the same items on the bed if using a bed scale). | The patient's weight is one of the key indicators in choosing dialysis solutions. A steady weight gain indicates fluid overload and may signal a need for increased dialysis. Weighing the patient under the same conditions helps ensure accurate measurements of fluid status. |
| Assess for the presence of incomplete dialysate returns. | Fluid retention can occur because of catheter complications that prevent adequate outflow, a severely scarred peritoneum that prevents adequate exchange, or inappropriate dialysis prescriptions. Accurate measurement and recording of outflow are critical to promptly detect these problems. |

Continued

| ASSESSMENT—RECOGNIZE CUES/ INTERVENTIONS—TAKE ACTION | RATIONALES |
|---|---|
| In the presence of outflow problems, monitor for the following:<br><br>*Full colon:* Use stool softeners, high-fiber diet, laxatives, or enemas if necessary.<br><br>*Catheter occlusion by fibrin* (usually occurs soon after insertion): Obtain the prescription to irrigate with heparinized saline.<br><br>*Catheter obstruction by omentum:* Turn the patient from side to side, elevate HOB or foot of bed, or apply firm pressure to the abdomen.<br><br>Notify the health care provider for unresolved outflow problems. | These factors are potential causes of outflow problems, and they necessitate intervention to reverse the problem. |

## Patient Problem/Analyze Cues/Prioritize Hypotheses

# Risk for Dehydration

*due to* hypertonicity of the dialysate

***Desired Outcome/Generate Solutions:*** After dialysis, the patient is normovolemic.

| ASSESSMENT—RECOGNIZE CUES/ INTERVENTIONS—TAKE ACTION | RATIONALES |
|---|---|
| Assess the I&O and weight daily, using the same scale and with the patient wearing the same amount of clothing (or with the same items on the bed if using a bed scale). | The patient's weight is one of the key indicators in choosing dialysis solutions. Weighing the patient under the same conditions helps ensure accurate measurements of fluid status. |
| ⚠ Assess for and report indicators of dehydration. | Dehydration (e.g., poor skin turgor, hypotension, tachycardia, and decreased CVP) can occur with excessive use of hypertonic dialysate and should be reported promptly for timely intervention. |

## Patient Problem/Analyze Cues/Prioritize Hypotheses

# Body Weight Problem (Weight Loss)

*due to* protein loss in the dialysate

***Desired Outcome/Generate Solutions:*** At a minimum of 24 hours before hospital discharge, the patient exhibits adequate nutrition to meet metabolic needs.

| ASSESSMENT/INTERVENTIONS | RATIONALES |
|---|---|
| Assess the patient's dietary intake of protein to ensure it is 1.2–1.5 g/kg/ day. | Protein crosses the peritoneum, and a significant amount is lost in the dialysate. An increased intake of protein is necessary to prevent excessive tissue catabolism. Protein loss increases with peritonitis. |
| Ensure that a dietary evaluation and teaching program are performed when the patient changes from one type of dialysis to the other. | Patients undergoing PD typically have fewer dietary restrictions than those on hemodialysis. Usually, sodium and potassium restrictions are less for a patient receiving PD than for one on hemodialysis. This is due, in part, to the fact that dialysis is provided continuously to PD patients versus only 3 times/week for those receiving hemodialysis. |
| Provide lists of restricted and encouraged foods with menus that illustrate their integration into the daily diet. | This information helps ensure the patient's understanding and adherence to the dietary regimen. |
| Request that the patient plan a 3-day menu that incorporates appropriate foods and restrictions. | Asking the patient to apply newly learned information to menu planning is a valid method of teaching and evaluating the patient's understanding. |

## ADDITIONAL PROBLEMS:

"Immobility" for *Constipation.*    Chapter 1
"Psychosocial Support for the Patient" for    Chapter 8
*Anticipatory Grief.*

## ✓ PATIENT–FAMILY TEACHING AND DISCHARGE PLANNING

When providing patient–family teaching, focus on sensory information, avoid giving excessive information, and initiate a visiting nurse referral if indicated for follow-up teaching. Include verbal and written information about the following:

- ✓ Medications, including drug name, purpose, dosage, schedule, drug-drug and food-drug interactions, precautions, and potential side effects.
- ✓ Diet and fluid restrictions: Include fact sheets that list foods to limit or restrict. Review fluid restrictions. Provide sample menus with examples of how dietary restrictions may be incorporated into daily meals. Have the patient demonstrate an understanding of dietary restrictions by preparing 3-day menus.
- ✓ Care and observation of exit site as per agency protocol.
- ✓ Need for and importance of monitoring daily weights, I&O, and monitoring of BP at home, if necessary.
- ✓ Importance of continued medical follow-up; confirm date and time of next health care provider appointment.
- ✓ Signs and symptoms that necessitate medical attention. For example, symptoms that may indicate a need for alteration in dialysis prescription: increased weight gain, unusual shortness of breath, edema, dizziness or fainting; symptoms that may indicate infection: fever, abdominal pain, redness or discharge from exit site, cloudy or decreased outflow, or nausea.
- ✓ Telephone numbers to call in case questions or concerns arise about therapy or disease after discharge. Additional general information and patient education materials can be obtained by contacting:
  - National Kidney Foundation: www.kidney.org

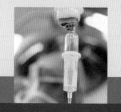

# Care of the Kidney Transplant Recipient 31

## OVERVIEW/PATHOPHYSIOLOGY

Kidney transplantation is the best treatment option that is available to patients with CKD. Transplantation reverses many of the pathophysiologic changes associated with renal disease and dependence on dialysis and dietary and lifestyle restrictions. Furthermore, after the first year, posttransplantation, it is ultimately less expensive than dialysis. However, all transplant patients must take immunosuppressive medications for the life of the graft, which have many side effects. Also, due to the large disparity between kidney supply and demand, only 17,000 kidneys are transplanted out of 100,000 people who need a transplant. Kidney donors must have compatible blood types as the recipient and may come from live or recently deceased donors. Donors include blood relatives, those who are emotionally related such as spouses and friends, and donors that are unknown to the recipient.

Postoperatively the priority of care for the kidney transplant patient is the maintenance of fluid and electrolyte maintenance. Diuresis occurs soon after blood supply to the transplanted kidney is reestablished. Rejection and infection are other complications that may occur during the postoperative period. Patients typically spend the first 12–24 hours postoperatively in the ICU to be closely monitored.

After discharge, subsequent admissions may occur for treatment of organ rejection, cardiovascular disease, infection, or medication complications. Cardiovascular disease is the leading cause of death after renal transplantation. Additionally, long-term complications that occur secondary to the use of immunosuppressive medications include hyperglycemia, electrolyte imbalance, infection, hypertension, hyperlipidemia, cardiovascular disease, chronic liver disease, bone demineralization, cataracts, gastrointestinal (GI) hemorrhage, and cancer.

### Immunosuppression

With the exception of identical twin donors, all transplant recipients must take drugs that suppress their immune system to prevent graft rejection. Each transplant center has a drug protocol outlining which combination of medications will be given to each patient. A complete list of the patient's medications, including herbal remedies, should be included on the patient's chart. Some herbs interfere with the absorption of immunosuppressive medications, causing patients to have lower levels of medications in their systems and potentially resulting in episodes of graft rejection and/or loss of the graft.

***Rejection, acute.*** Usually occurs days to weeks after transplantation; potentially reversible; treated with increased immunosuppression.

***Rejection, chronic.*** Usually classified as starting 1 year after transplantation; irreversible; managed conservatively with diet and antihypertensive agents until dialysis is required.

***Indicators of rejection.*** Oliguria, tenderness over graft site (located in iliac fossa), sudden weight gain (2–3 lb/day), fever, malaise, hypertension, and increased blood urea nitrogen (BUN) and serum creatinine. In addition, hyperglycemia will develop with combined kidney–pancreas transplants.

## Patient Problem/Analyze Cues/Prioritize Hypotheses

# Risk for Infection

*due to* immunosuppression, underlying systemic illness, invasive procedures, and exposure to infected individuals

***Desired Outcome/Generate Solutions:*** The patient is free of infection.

| ASSESSMENT—RECOGNIZE CUES/ INTERVENTIONS—TAKE ACTION | RATIONALES |
|---|---|
|  Assess for any signs and symptoms of infection. | Transplant recipients are taking large doses of immunosuppressive agents, and their immune response and thus response to infectious agents will be muted. Infections are potentially life threatening in an individual who is immunosuppressed. |

| ASSESSMENT—RECOGNIZE CUES/ INTERVENTIONS—TAKE ACTION | RATIONALES |
|---|---|
| • Assess for low-grade temperature elevation, fever, and unexplained tachycardia. | These are indicators that might signal infection in a transplant recipient. |
| • Assess for indicators of cytomegalovirus (CMV), including fever, malaise, fatigue, and muscle aches. | CMV is a common infectious agent among immunosuppressed patients. |
| ! Use sterile technique with all invasive procedures and dressing changes. | Following the sterile technique reduces the possibility of infection, which is increased with invasive procedures into the body and involving nonintact skin. |
| ! Instruct the patient to be alert to signs and symptoms of commonly encountered infections. | Infections and their indicators include *urinary tract infection*—cloudy and malodorous urine; dysuria, frequency, and urgency; pain in the suprapubic area, buttock, thighs, labia, or scrotum; *upper respiratory infection*—productive cough, malodorous, purulent, colored, and copious secretions, chest pain or heaviness; *pharyngitis*—painful swallowing; *otitis media*—malaise, earache; *impetigo*—inflamed or draining areas on the skin. |
| • Instruct patient on the importance of reporting signs and symptoms of infection to the health care provider promptly. | Prompt reporting of these indicators is essential because infections can be life threatening in a patient undergoing immunosuppression. |
| • Instruct patient to avoid exposure to individuals known to have infections and to wash hands frequently. | Consistent hand hygiene is a proven method of removing pathogens from the skin that could otherwise cause infection and is especially important in patients whose immune systems are compromised. In the absence of hand-washing opportunities, hand decontamination with an alcohol-based hand sanitizer provides adequate hand hygiene. |
| • Instruct patient that they will need to use prophylactic antibiotics for any minor invasive procedures. | Prophylactic antibiotics reduce infection risk, which can occur in even minor procedures. Some health care providers encourage antibiotics for any minor invasive procedures, including dental cleaning. |
| • Instruct patient to not work in soil for the first 6 months after transplantation. | This restriction minimizes the risk for acquiring *Aspergillus* infection. |
| • Encourage patient to abstain from smoking; provide smoking cessation literature. | Smoking increases susceptibility to respiratory infection because it damages protective mechanisms such as cilia in the lungs. Smoking also causes detrimental changes to blood pressure (BP), heart rate (HR), cholesterol levels, and clotting factors. |

## Patient Problem/Analyze Cues/Prioritize Hypotheses

# Deficient Knowledge (Medications)

*due to* unfamiliarity with signs and symptoms of rejection, side effects of immunosuppressive agents, and transplantation complications

***Desired Outcome/Generate Solutions:*** Within the 24-hour period before hospital discharge, the patient verbalizes accurate knowledge of the signs and symptoms of rejection, side effects of immunosuppressive therapy, and complications of transplantation.

| ASSESSMENT—RECOGNIZE CUES/ INTERVENTIONS—TAKE ACTION | RATIONALES |
|---|---|
| Assess the patient's health care literacy (language, reading, comprehension) as well as culture and culturally specific information needs. | This assessment helps ensure that information is selected and presented in a manner that is culturally and educationally appropriate. |

Continued

| ASSESSMENT—RECOGNIZE CUES/ INTERVENTIONS—TAKE ACTION | RATIONALES |
|---|---|
| Explain the importance of adherence to scheduled blood work including renal function monitoring as well as daily intake and output, and weight. | These tests evaluate kidney status and guide the therapeutic drug regimen and treatment plan: as renal function decreases, BUN and creatinine values will increase. |
| Educate patient on signs and symptoms of organ rejection. | Signs and symptoms of rejection necessitate prompt intervention to save the kidney. These include oliguria, tenderness over the transplanted kidney (located in iliac fossa), sudden weight gain (2–3 lb), fever, malaise, hypertension, and increased BUN (greater than 20 mg/dL) and serum creatinine (greater than 1.5 mg/dL). In addition, the patient may have body aches, swelling in the legs or hands, and a temperature greater than 100.4°F (38°C). |
| Instruct the patient to weigh self at the same time each day, using the same scale and wearing the same amount of clothing. Provide a notebook in which to record daily vital signs (VS) and weight measurements. Remind the patient to bring the notebook to all outpatient visits and to report abnormal values promptly should they occur. | The patient should record daily VS and weights and bring information to all outpatient visits. The patient should promptly report abnormal values to health care provider.These assessments monitor the trend of VS and weight measurements. Using the same standards daily ensures accuracy with weight measurements. |
| Explain the importance of scheduled lab work to monitor white blood cell (WBC) and platelet counts. | Significant decreases in WBC and platelet counts can be a side effect of immunosuppressive agents, and therefore scheduled monitoring is essential. |
| Educate patient on signs and symptoms of GI bleeding and the importance of reporting them promptly to the health care provider if they occur. | GI bleeding is a potential side effect of immunosuppressive agents and can be life threatening if it is excessive. Prompt reporting of the onset of these symptoms (e.g., tarry stools, coffee-ground emesis, orthostatic changes, dizziness, tachycardia, increasing fatigue, and weakness) enables the health care provider to adjust medications or add medications such as antacids and $H_2$-receptor blockers to treat the cause of the bleeding. |
| Educate the patient and/or significant others on how to measure BP and provide guidelines for values that would necessitate notification of the health care provider or staff member. | In a patient who has undergone renal transplantation, hypertension may develop for a variety of reasons, including cyclosporine or steroid use, rejection, or renal artery stenosis. In addition, the patient may have had hypertension before the transplantation. A value that would necessitate notification of the health care provider is BP 20% above or below the patient's "normal" BP. This value and parameters for calling the health care provider are generally agreed on before the patient leaves the hospital. |
| Educate the patient on the importance of the medication regimen, including the appropriate timing of the medication and managing missed doses. | A large portion of rejection incidence can be attributed to missing drug doses due to nonadherence (approximately 20%), lack of knowledge, side effects, and/or improved health, during which patients no longer feel the need to take their medications.Missed doses need to be carefully evaluated. Patients need to take their medications as soon as they realize a dose has been missed, unless it is time for the next dose, at which time the missed dose can be omitted.Setting up a schedule is imperative to help avoid the number of missed doses. |
| Educate the patient on the importance of adherence to scheduled medical appointments for continued medical evaluation of the transplant. | Continued evaluation will confirm that the kidney is working properly and that the patient is not undergoing rejection. |
| Verify the patient's knowledge of immunosuppressive medication precautions and dosages. | A knowledgeable patient is likely to participate more effectively in the therapeutic regimen. |

## Patient Problem/Analyze Cues/Prioritize Hypotheses

# Risk for Dehydration and Electrolyte Imbalance

*due to* rapid diuresis as the new kidney's ability to filter BUN, which acts as an osmotic diuretic, abundance of fluids administered during surgery, and initial renal tubular dysfunction

**Desired Outcome:** During the postoperative period, the renal transplant patient will be normovolemic, and electrolytes will be within normal limits.

| ASSESSMENT—RECOGNIZE CUES/ INTERVENTIONS—TAKE ACTION | RATIONALES |
|---|---|
| Assess the intake and output (I&O) and weight daily, using the same scale and with the patient wearing the same amount of clothing (or with the same items on the bed if using a bed scale). | The patient's weight is one of the key indicators in choosing dialysis solutions. Weighing the patient under the same conditions helps ensure accurate measurements of fluid status. |
| Assess for and report indicators of dehydration such as hypotension, decreased central venous pressure, and electrolyte imbalance. | Dehydration (e.g., poor skin turgor, hypotension, tachycardia, and decreased CVP), and electrolyte imbalances can occur immediately postoperatively and should be reported promptly for timely intervention. |
| Administer IV normal saline infusions, potassium, and/or sodium bicarbonate as needed as ordered by the health care provider. | Hyponatremia and hypokalemia are often associated with rapid diuresis. Sodium bicarbonate may be given if the patient develops metabolic acidosis from a delay in the return of kidney function. |

## ✔ PATIENT–FAMILY TEACHING AND DISCHARGE PLANNING

When providing patient–family teaching, focus on sensory information, avoid giving excessive information, and make appropriate referrals (e.g., visiting or home health nurse, community health resources) for follow-up teaching. Include verbal and written information about the following:

- ✔ Medications, including name; dosage; purpose; schedule; precautions; drug–drug, drug–herb, and food–drug interactions; and potential side effects. Provide guidelines for how to cope with medication side effects.
- ✔ The importance of never stopping medications, even if feeling better, because it is the medication that is keeping the kidneys functional and creating the feelings of wellness.

- ✔ Measures for preventing infection, including incision care. Stress to the patient that infections can be life threatening because of immunosuppression.
- ✔ Prescribed diet and activity level progression.
- ✔ Community resources for emotional and financial support.
- ✔ Importance of follow-up care to ensure long-term viability of the transplanted kidney.
- ✔ Telephone numbers to call in case problems or questions arise after discharge from care facility.
- ✔ Internet resources:
  - United Network for Organ Sharing: www.unos.org
  - National Kidney Disease Education Program: www.nkdep.nih.gov
  - National Kidney Foundation: www.kidney.org
  - Transplant Recipients International Organization: www.trioweb.org

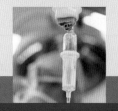

# Chronic Kidney Disease 32

## OVERVIEW/PATHOPHYSIOLOGY

Chronic kidney disease (CKD) is a progressive, irreversible loss of kidney function that develops over days to years. As CKD progresses, glomerular filtration lessens and is irreversible, and eventually, CKD can progress to end-stage renal disease (ESRD), when the glomerular filtration rate (GFR) is less than 15 mL/minute at which time renal replacement therapy (dialysis or transplantation) is required to sustain life. Before ESRD, the individual with CKD can lead a relatively normal life managed by diet and medications. The length of this period varies, depending on the cause of renal disease and the patient's level of renal function at the time of diagnosis.

The leading causes of CKD are diabetes and hypertension. In its early stages, CKD is often not recognized since the kidneys are highly adaptive to glomerular changes. As CKD progresses to ESRD, body systems become affected from retained urea, creatinine, phenols, hormones, electrolytes, and water. Alterations in neuromuscular, cardiovascular, and gastrointestinal (GI) functions are common. Renal osteodystrophy and anemia are early and common complications.

## HEALTH CARE SETTING

Primary care with possible hospitalization resulting from complications or during ESRD

## ASSESSMENT

**Anemia.** Pallor, shortness of breath on exertion, headache, persistent fatigue, dizziness.

**Fluid volume abnormalities.** Fine crackles hypertension, edema, oliguria, anuria.

**Electrolyte disturbances.** Muscle weakness, dysrhythmias, pruritus, neuromuscular irritability, tetany.

**Metabolic acidosis.** Deep respirations, lethargy, headache.

**Uremia—retention of metabolic wastes.** Weakness, malaise, anorexia, dry and discolored skin, peripheral neuropathy, irritability, clouded thinking, ammonia odor to breath, metallic taste in mouth, nausea, vomiting. **Note:** Uremia adversely affects all body systems.

## POTENTIAL ACUTE COMPLICATIONS

**Heart failure.** Crackles (rales), dyspnea, orthopnea.

**Pericarditis.** Angina, elevated temperature, presence of pericardial friction or rub on auscultation.

**Cardiac tamponade.** Hypotension, distant heart sounds, pulsus paradoxus (exaggerated inspiratory drop in systolic blood pressure [SBP]).

**Dysrhythmias.** Increased QRS duration and/or peaked T waves on electrocardiogram.

**Physical assessment.** Pallor, dry and discolored skin, edema (peripheral, periorbital, sacral); fluid overload, crackles, and elevated BP may be present.

## DIAGNOSTIC TESTS

**Glomerular filtration rate.** The best overall index of kidney function. Normal GFR varies with age, sex, and body size, but generally, GFR below 90 mL/minute denotes some kidney damage.

**Creatinine clearance.** Measures the kidney's ability to clear the blood of creatinine and approximates the GFR. Creatinine clearance decreases as renal function decreases. Creatinine clearance is determined by analyzing a 24-hour urine collection. As kidney damage progresses, serum creatinine increases and therefore creatinine clearance will decrease.

> **Note:** *Failure to collect all urine specimens during the period of study will invalidate test results.*

**Blood urea nitrogen and serum creatinine.** Both will be elevated. **Note:** Nonrenal problems, such as dehydration or GI bleeding, also can cause the blood urea nitrogen (BUN) to increase, but there will not be a corresponding increase in creatinine.

**Electrolytes.**

Potassium—Hyperkalemia can occur from decreased excretion of potassium by the kidneys. It is a serious electrolyte disorder associated with CKD as it can lead to fatal dysrhythmias.

Sodium—Hypernatremia can occur with CKD when sodium excretion is impaired. However, when large quantities of water retention occur in CKD, hyponatremia occurs because sodium is retained with water and dilution hyponatremia occurs.

Calcium and phosphate—Serum phosphate increases with CKD and binds to calcium. This will cause serum calcium levels to decrease.

Magnesium—When not excreted by the kidneys, hypermagnesemia occurs.

Patient Problem/Analyze Cues/Prioritize Hypotheses

# Impaired Nutritional Status

*due to* nausea, vomiting, anorexia, and dietary restrictions

*Desired Outcome/Generate Solutions:* The patient's intake of food is sufficient to meet metabolic needs

| ASSESSMENT—RECOGNIZE CUES/ INTERVENTIONS—TAKE ACTION | RATIONALES |
|---|---|
| See also "Acute Kidney Injury," Chapter 27, for *Body Weight Problem (Weight Loss)*. | |
| In addition: | |
| Administer multivitamins and folic acid, if prescribed. | Anorexia and nausea and vomiting may occur with increased anorexia. Vitamin supplementation assists with ensuring that patients maintain adequate nutrition. Multivitamins for patients on dialysis are specially formulated (e.g., Nephro-Vite, Dialyvite). |
| Caution against the use of over-the-counter (OTC) vitamins. | The use of OTC multivitamins is contraindicated in Chronic Kidney Disease (CKD) patients because some vitamin levels (e.g., of vitamin A) may be toxic. |
| Monitor for proteinuria and refer to the dietitian if excessive protein losses and/or low serum albumin is noted. | Proteinuria results in malnutrition. Patients with poor nutritional status at the start of dialysis have an increased risk for mortality. |

Patient Problem/Analyze Cues/Prioritize Hypotheses

# Risk for Impaired Skin Integrity

*due to* uremia, hyperphosphatemia (if severe), and edema

*Desired Outcome/Generate Solutions:* The patient's skin is intact and free of erythema and abrasions.

| ASSESSMENT—RECOGNIZE CUES/ INTERVENTIONS—TAKE ACTION | RATIONALES |
|---|---|
| Assess for the presence/degree of pruritus. | Pruritus is common in patients with uremia and occurs when accumulating nitrogenous wastes begin to be excreted through the skin, causing frequent and intense itching with scratching. Pruritus also may result from prolonged hyperphosphatemia. |
| Administer phosphate binders as ordered by the provider and encourage patient to reduce dietary phosphorus if elevated phosphorus level is a problem. | Pruritus often decreases with a reduction in BUN and improved phosphorus control. Phosphate binders are medications that, when taken with food, bind dietary phosphorus and prevent GI absorption. Calcium carbonate, sevelamer hydrochloride, aluminum hydroxide, and calcium acetate are common phosphate binders. |
| **Note:** Administer phosphate binders while food is present in the stomach. | Prolonged elevation of serum phosphorus and/or calcium absorption from ingestion of phosphate binders on an empty stomach results in an increased calcium–phosphorus product. When this product exceeds a level of 55 (normal product is approximately 40), phosphorus binds with calcium, and the resulting calcium–phosphate complex is deposited in soft tissues of the body. Deposition of these complexes in the skin produces necrotic patches. In addition, elevation in calcium–phosphate product is associated with increased risk for death, aortic calcification, mitral valve calcification, and coronary artery calcification. |

Continued

| ASSESSMENT—RECOGNIZE CUES/ INTERVENTIONS—TAKE ACTION | RATIONALES |
|---|---|
| If necessary, administer prescribed antihistamines as ordered by the provider. | Antihistamines help control itching. |
| Keep the patient's fingernails short. | If the patient is unable to control scratching, short fingernails will cause less damage. |
| Instruct the patient to monitor scratches for evidence of infection and to seek early medical attention if signs and symptoms of infection appear. | Uremia slows wound healing; nonintact skin can lead to infection. |
| Encourage the use of skin emollients and soaps with high fat content. Advise bathing every other day and to apply skin lotion immediately on exiting the bath/shower. | Uremic skin is often dry and scaly because of reduction in oil gland activity. Patients should avoid harsh soaps, soaps or skin products containing alcohol, and excessive bathing. |
| Advise the patient and significant others that easy bruising can occur. | Patients with uremia are at increased risk for bruising because of clotting abnormalities and capillary fragility. |
| Provide scheduled skin care and position changes for patients with edema. | These measures decrease the risk for skin/tissue damage resulting from decreased perfusion and increased pressure. |

## Patient Problem/Analyze Cues/Prioritize Hypotheses

# Activity Intolerance

*due to* generalized weakness occurring with anemia and uremia

**Desired Outcome/Generate Solutions:** After treatment, the patient exhibits improving endurance to activity.

> **Note:** *Anemia is better tolerated in the uremic than in the nonuremic patient.*

| ASSESSMENT—RECOGNIZE CUES/ INTERVENTIONS—TAKE ACTION | RATIONALES |
|---|---|
| Assess the patient's pulse, BP, and RR following activity (see "Immobility," Chapter 1, for *Activity Intolerance*. | This assessment evaluates the degree of exercise/activity intolerance. Optimally pulse should remain within 20 bpm of resting rate, SBP within 20 mm Hg of resting SBP, and RR within 20 breaths per minute of resting rate with a normal depth and pattern. |
| Notify the health care provider if patient has increased weakness, fatigue, dyspnea, chest pain, or further decreases in hematocrit (Hct) and hemoglobin (Hgb). | This action enables rapid treatment of anemia and dose adjustment of epoetin alfa, which induces erythrocyte production and reticulocyte production in the bone marrow. Low levels of Hgb and Hct may result in angina. Shortness of breath and shortness of breath on exertion in the long term contribute to the development of ventricular hypertrophy, increasing the risk for morbidity from cardiovascular disease (CVD), the most significant cause of death in CKD patients. |
| Administer epoetin alfa as prescribed by health care provider. | This medication is administered to treat anemia and increase activity tolerance. Current clinical practice guidelines recommend that epoetin alfa (Epogen) be started when Hgb decreases below 10 g/dL. Epoetin alfa may be contraindicated in patients with uncontrolled hypertension or sensitivity to human albumin. |

| ASSESSMENT—RECOGNIZE CUES/ INTERVENTIONS—TAKE ACTION | RATIONALES |
| --- | --- |
| Assess for increasing hypertension, dyspnea, chest pain, seizures, calf pain, erythema, swelling, severe headache, and seizures. | These are potential untoward effects of epoetin alfa (Epogen) therapy. Dose adjustment or discontinuation may be necessary. Hypertension may occur as a side effect of epoetin alfa therapy during the period in which Hct levels are rapidly rising. Headaches may accompany the rise in BP. Epoetin alfa has also been associated with increased thrombosis. Patients should be monitored for evidence of thrombotic events (i.e., symptoms of myocardial infarction, deep vein thrombosis/ venous thromboembolism, stroke, transient ischemic attack, or clotting of the vascular access in hemodialysis patients), and those symptoms should be reported immediately to the health care provider. Epoetin alfa should be used with caution in patients with a known seizure history because there is an increased risk for seizures within the first 3 months of epoetin alfa therapy. |
| Administer oral or parenteral iron if prescribed. | Iron deficiency anemia, which affects energy level, is common in CKD patients. In addition, iron is required for epoetin alfa to make new red blood cells. Thus the effectiveness of epoetin alfa requires that patients maintain their iron stores. **Note:** Anaphylaxis is a possible complication of IV iron administration, most commonly during the first dose. |
| For patients receiving oral iron, assess for signs and symptoms of constipation. | Constipation is a common side effect of oral iron. See "Immobility," Chapter 1, for *Constipation*. |
| Coordinate laboratory studies. | This intervention minimizes blood drawing. CKD patients are already at risk for anemia. |
| Provide and encourage optimal nutrition and consider referral to a renal dietitian. | Protein and phosphorus are initially restricted to slow progression of CKD and prevent early development of renal osteodystrophy. *Renal osteodystrophy* is a collective term for changes in the bone structure of patients with CKD, resulting most often in rapid bone turnover. These changes result from a combination of hyperphosphatemia, hypocalcemia, stimulation of parathyroid hormone, and alterations in the kidney's ability to convert vitamin D to its active form. Carbohydrates are increased for patients on protein-restricted diets to ensure adequate caloric intake, thereby preventing tissue catabolism, which would contribute to buildup of nitrogenous wastes. As the patient approaches End Stage Renal Disease (ESRD), sodium intake is limited to reduce thirst and fluid retention, $K^+$ intake is limited because of the kidneys' decreased ability to excrete this ion, and protein may be further restricted to limit the production of nitrogenous wastes. For patients on protein-restricted diets, protein intake should be restricted to sources primarily of high biologic value. Overrestriction of protein may lead to malnutrition; therefore referral to a renal dietitian is recommended to ensure adequate intake. |
| Do not administer ferrous sulfate at the same time as antacids. | To maximize absorption of ferrous sulfate, antacids or calcium carbonate medications are given at least 1 hour before or after ferrous sulfate. |
| Assist with identifying activities that increase fatigue and adjusting those activities accordingly. | It is important to minimize fatigue while attempting to promote tolerance to activity. |
| Assist with activities of daily living while encouraging maximum independence to tolerance. Establish realistic, progressive exercises and activity goals that are designed to increase endurance. Ensure that they are within the patient's prescribed limitations. Examples are found in "Immobility," Chapter 1, for *Activity Intolerance*. | Same as above. |
| Administer packed red blood cells as prescribed. | This measure treats severe or symptomatic anemia. |

Patient Problem/Analyze Cues/Prioritize Hypotheses

# Deficient Knowledge (Health Maintenance Regimens)

*due to* unfamiliarity with the need to adhere to health maintenance regimens in an attempt to decrease the risk of CKD complications

**Desired Outcome/Generate Solutions:** Within the 24-hour period before hospital discharge, the patient verbalizes accurate knowledge about the importance of adherence to medication, diet, and lifestyle changes necessary to decrease the risk of complications.

| ASSESSMENT—RECOGNIZE CUES/ INTERVENTIONS—TAKE ACTION | RATIONALES |
|---|---|
| Assess the patient's current level of knowledge about his or her therapy and health care literacy (language, reading, comprehension). Assess culture and culturally specific information needs. | This assessment helps ensure that information is selected and presented in a manner that is culturally and educationally appropriate. |
| Educate the patient on the importance of frequent BP checks and adherence to prescribed antihypertensive therapy. | Patients with CKD may experience hypertension because of fluid overload, excess renin secretion, or arteriosclerotic disease. Control of hypertension may slow the progression of chronic renal insufficiency and decrease the risk for CVD. |
| Educate the patient on how to manage hypertension. | In some patients, BP control can slow the progression of CKD. Measures to control hypertension include weight loss, exercise, smoking cessation, diet, and antihypertensive drugs. |
| Educate the patient about antihypertensive medications, including drug name, purpose, dosage, schedule precautions, and potential side effects. Also discuss drug–drug, herb–drug, and food–drug interactions. | These medications control BP, slow the progression of CKD, and/or reduce proteinuria/microalbuminuria. Angiotensin-converting enzyme (ACE) inhibitors and angiotensin receptor blockers (ARBs) are considered first-line medications for management of patients with CKD and coexisting diabetes, proteinuria, and/or microalbuminuria. Additional antihypertensives are often added as needed. |
| Educate the patients on ACE inhibitors or ARBs and the importance of medical follow-up. | Follow-up is important for monitoring GFR, potassium levels, and hypotension. Hypotension and cough are common side effects. ACE inhibitors and ARBs may increase serum potassium and decrease GFR. Angioedema is a potential side effect. |
| Teach the patient or caregiver how to monitor BP at home and what readings require notification of the health care provider. | This knowledge will help the patient keep BP within optimal levels by following the antihypertensive medication regimen. |
| Educate patients with DM that insulin requirements often decrease as renal function decreases. Instruct these patients to be alert to weakness, blurred vision, and headache. | Anorexia or nausea/vomiting, which occurs with uremia, may decrease dietary consumption and thereby decrease insulin requirements. These symptoms are indicators of hypoglycemia, which can occur as insulin requirements decrease. |
| Educate patients receiving diuretics about the importance of medical follow-up after discharge. | Follow-up enables monitoring for volume depletion, decreased GFR, and electrolyte abnormalities. The use of diuretics can result in dehydration and hypokalemia and may hasten loss of renal function. |
| Refer the patient and/or caregiver to a nutritionist for dietary changes required to minimize complications from CKD. | Calories protein, sodium, calcium, iron, and phosphate intake restrictions or supplements are patient specific and depend on the CKD stage and dialysis treatment (if applicable.) These measures help manage hypertension and electrolyte imbalances and slow the progression of CKD and/or prevent complications from CKD. |
| Educate the patient on the importance of limiting alcohol intake to less than 2 drinks/day for men, and less than 1 drink/day for women. | Excessive alcohol intake may increase the risk for malnutrition, hypertension, and CVD, resulting in progression of CKD and increased mortality. |
| Counsel patient on smoking cessation if applicable. | CVD is the leading cause of death in CKD patients. Smoking increases the risk for CVD and arteriosclerosis. |
| Educate the patient on the benefits of exercise and physical activity. | Thirty minutes of physical activity of moderate intensity most days of the week is recommended for hypertension management in patients with CKD. Management of hypertension may slow the progression of CKD. |

**ADDITIONAL PROBLEMS:**

| | |
|---|---|
| *Constipation* | Chapter 1 |
| *Anticipatory Grief* | Chapter 8 |

 **PATIENT–FAMILY TEACHING AND DISCHARGE PLANNING**

When providing patient–family teaching, focus on sensory information, avoid giving excessive information, and initiate a visiting nurse referral for necessary follow-up teaching. Include verbal and written information about the following:

✓ Medications, including drug name, purpose, dosage, schedule, precautions, and potential side effects. Also discuss drug–drug, herb–drug, and food–drug interactions.

✓ For patients not on dialysis but requiring epoetin alfa, educate the patient and/or significant other preparation of the medication and subcutaneous injections. Instruct patient on the importance of monitoring for and rapidly reporting to the health care provider any of the following: dyspnea, chest pain, seizures, and severe headache.

✓ Diet, including fact sheet listing foods that are to be restricted or limited. Inform the patient that diet and fluid restrictions may be altered as renal function decreases. Provide sample menus, and have the patient demonstrate understanding by preparing 3-day menus that incorporate dietary restrictions.

✓ Care and observation of the dialysis access, if applicable. (see Chapters 29 & 30).

✓ Signs and symptoms that necessitate medical attention: irregular pulse, fever, unusual shortness of breath or edema, sudden change in urine output, and unusual muscle weakness.

✓ Need for continued medical follow-up; confirm date and time of next health care provider appointment.

✓ The importance of avoiding infections and seeking treatment promptly should one develop.

✓ Telephone numbers to call in case questions or concerns arise about the therapy or disease after discharge. Additional general information and patient education resources can be obtained by contacting the following:
- National Kidney and Urologic Diseases Information Clearinghouse: https://rarediseases.org/organizations/nihnational-kidney-and-urologic-diseases-information-clearinghouse/
- National Kidney Foundation: www.kidney.org

✓ For patients with or approaching ESRD, provide data concerning various treatment options and support groups. The local chapter of the National Kidney Foundation can be helpful in identifying support groups and organizations in the area. The patient and significant others should meet with the renal dietitian and social worker before discharge.

✓ Coordinate discharge planning and teaching with the dialysis unit or facility. If possible, have the patient visit the dialysis unit before discharge.

✓ For individuals with CKD, educate them on the importance of coordinating all medical care through their nephrologist and alerting all medical and dental personnel to CKD status because of increased risk for infection and the need to adjust medication dosages. In addition, dentists may want to premedicate ESRD patients with antibiotics before dental work and avoid scheduling dental work on the day of dialysis because of the heparinization that is used with dialytic therapy.

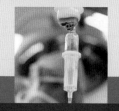

# Urinary Tract Calculi 33

## OVERVIEW/PATHOPHYSIOLOGY

Nephrolithiasis (kidney stone disease) occurs mostly in middle-aged adults. The risk of developing a calculus or stone further increases with age. Climate, diet, genetics, metabolic state, and lifestyle all play a part in the development of nephrolithiasis. Although there is no definitive cause for stone formation, it is thought that they develop when crystals precipitate in a supersaturated concentration to unite and form a stone. Key factors that increase the risk for stone formation are urinary stasis and urinary tract infections (UTIs). About 90% of all stones pass from the ureter into the bladder and out of the urinary system spontaneously.

## HEALTH CARE SETTING

Primary care; may require hospitalization for complications or surgery

## ASSESSMENT

**Signs and symptoms.** Pain (also called renal colic) that is sharp, sudden, and intense or dull and aching; located in the flank, back or lower abdominal area; and often radiating toward the groin. Men may also experience testicular pain and women may experience labial pain. This type of pain results from stretching, dilation, and spasm of the ureter in response to the obstructing stone. Nausea and vomiting may also occur during episodes of renal colic. Pain may be intermittent as the stone moves along the ureter and may subside when it enters the bladder. Fever and hematuria may indicate an infected stone or secondary UTI. Older adults may present with delirium or malaise.

**Physical assessment.** Pallor, diaphoresis, tachycardia, and tachypnea may be observed. Costovertebral angle (CVA) tenderness and guarding may be present. Bowel sounds may be absent secondary to ileus, and the abdomen may be distended and tympanic. The patient will be restless and unable to find a position of comfort.

## DIAGNOSTIC TESTS

CT scan or ultrasound of the renal system confirms the diagnosis of urinary tract calculi.

**Excretory urogram/intravenous pyelogram.** Used to visualize kidneys, renal pelvis, ureters, and bladder. It can identify the size of the stone and the presence and severity of the obstruction. This test also outlines nonradiopaque stones within the ureters. Nonradiopaque stones (e.g., uric acid calculi) are seen as radiolucent defects in the contrast media.

**Urine Tests:**

**Urinalysis.** Assesses for hematuria and crystalluria and urine pH.

**Urine culture.** To determine the presence and type of bacteria in the urinary tract.

**24-hour urinary measurement.** Calcium, phosphorus, magnesium, sodium, oxalate, citrate, cysteine, sulfate, potassium, uric acid, and total urine volume

> **Note:** *All urine samples should be sent to the laboratory immediately after they are obtained or should be refrigerated if this is not possible (specimens for culture are not refrigerated). Urine left at room temperature has greater potential for bacterial growth, turbidity, and alkaline pH, any of which can distort the reading.*

**Serum tests:**

Calcium, phosphorous, sodium, potassium, bicarbonate, uric acid, Blood Urea Nitrogen (BUN), and creatinine levels are measured.

## Patient Problem/Analyze Cues/Prioritize Hypotheses

# Acute Pain

*due to* the presence of a calculus or the surgical procedure to remove it

**Desired Outcome/Generate Solutions:** The patient will report no pain or decreased pain that is within their tolerance level.

| ASSESSMENT—RECOGNIZE CUES/ INTERVENTIONS—TAKE ACTION | RATIONALES |
|---|---|
| Assess and document the quality, location, intensity, and duration of pain. Use pain scale to document pain intensity that ranges from 0 (no pain) to 10 (worst pain). | This assessment evaluates the intensity and trend of pain and subsequent relief obtained. |
| Notify the health care provider of sudden and/or severe pain. | This is a sign that a stone is passing through the ureter. |
| Notify the health care provider of a sudden cessation of pain. Strain all urine for solid matter and send to the laboratory for analysis. | This can signal the passage of the stone. |
| Medicate the patient with prescribed opioids, NSAIDs, and alpha-1 adrenergic blockers (e.g., tamsulosin); evaluate and document the response based on the pain scale. | Opioids relieve renal colic pain. NSAIDs may also be given if renal function is normal. Adrenergic blockers such as tamsulosin relax the smooth muscle in the ureter and may aid in stone passage. |
| Encourage the patient to request medication before discomfort becomes severe. | Pain is easier to manage when it is treated before it gets too severe because prolonged stimulation of pain receptors increases sensitivity to painful stimuli and increases the amount of medication required to relieve pain. |
| Administer antiemetics (e.g., ondansetron, promethazine) as prescribed. | These agents promote comfort from nausea and vomiting. |
| Provide warm blankets or a heating pad to the affected area or supply warm baths. | These measures increase regional circulation and relax tense muscles. |
| Provide back rubs. | Back rubs are especially helpful for postoperative patients who were in the lithotomy position during surgery. |
| See "Pain," Chapter 5, for other interventions. | |

## Patient Problem/Analyze Cues/Prioritize Hypotheses

# Urinary Retention

due to urinary tract calculus

***Desired Outcome/Generate Solutions:*** The patient relates the return of a normal voiding pattern within 2 days.

| ASSESSMENT—RECOGNIZE CUES/ INTERVENTIONS—TAKE ACTION | RATIONALES |
|---|---|
| Interview patient to determine pre-urinary tract calculus voiding history and pattern. | This assessment establishes a baseline for subsequent assessment. |
| Assess the quality and color of the urine. | Optimally, urine is straw-colored and clear and has a characteristic odor. Dark urine is often indicative of dehydration, and blood-tinged urine can result from UTI or rupture of ureteral capillaries as the calculus passes through the ureter. |
| In patients for whom fluids are not restricted, encourage fluid intake of at least 2.5–3 L/day. | Increased hydration helps flush the calculus through the ureter into the bladder and out through the system. |
| Record the accurate Intake and Output (I&O); teach the patient how to record I&O. | Output that is significantly less than intake could signal an obstruction. Patients should participate in I&O documentation to ensure that all intake and output are being recorded. |
| Palpate suprapubic area for tenderness and distension. | A distended and uncomfortable suprapubic area indicates a full bladder. |
| Medicate with alpha-1 adrenergic blockers (e.g., tamsulosin) as prescribed. | Adrenergic blockers such as tamsulosin relax the smooth muscle in the ureter and may aid in stone passage. |

Continued

| ASSESSMENT—RECOGNIZE CUES/ INTERVENTIONS—TAKE ACTION | RATIONALES |
|---|---|
| Strain all urine for evidence of solid matter; teach the patient the procedure. | This intervention can detect the passage of stones. |
| Send any solid matter to the laboratory for analysis. | The laboratory will test for high levels of uric acid, cystine, oxalate, calcium, or phosphorus, which would signal the presence and type of stones. |

## Patient Problem/Analyze Cues/Prioritize Hypotheses

# Urinary Retention

*due to* obstruction of ureteral or nephrostomy catheters

***Desired Outcomes/Generate Solutions:*** After intervention, the patient has output from the ureteral catheter and is free of spasms or flank pain, which otherwise could signal obstruction or displacement of the catheter.

| ASSESSMENT—RECOGNIZE CUES/ INTERVENTIONS—TAKE ACTION | RATIONALES |
|---|---|
| If the patient has more than one ureteral catheter, label one *right* and the other *left*; keep all drainage records separate. | Occasionally, patients return from surgery with ureteral catheters. Ureteral catheters, also known as *stents*, are positioned postoperatively to enable healing and promote ureteral patency in the presence of edema. If the patient has two ureteral catheters, separate output records are used to identify how each ureter is functioning. |
| Monitor the output from the ureteral catheter. | The amount will vary with each patient and will depend on catheter dimension. |
| If drainage is scanty or absent, milk the catheter and tubing gently. If this fails, notify the health care provider. | This action will help dislodge the obstruction. |
| **Caution:** Never irrigate a catheter without specific health care provider instructions to do so. If irrigation is prescribed, use gentle pressure and sterile technique. Always aspirate with a sterile syringe before instillation. Use another sterile syringe to insert instillation amounts of 3 mL or less. | There is potential for ureteral or kidney pelvis damage and infection during irrigation caused by overdistention and/or introduction of pathogens. |
| Carefully monitor the urethral catheter for movement and ensure that it is securely attached to the patient. | Ureteral catheters are often attached to the urethral catheter after placement in the ureters. The urethral catheter should be monitored to detect movement and to ensure that it is securely attached to the patient. |
| **Note:** After ureteral or nephrostomy catheters have been removed monitor for flank pain, CVA tenderness, nausea, and vomiting. | These are indicators of ureteral obstruction, which necessitates prompt intervention. |

## Patient Problem/Analyze Cues/Prioritize Hypotheses

# Risk for Impaired Skin Integrity

*due to* flank incision after nephrolithotomy, pyelolithotomy, or ureterolithotomy

***Desired Outcome/Generate Solutions:*** The patient's skin surrounding the wound site remains nonerythemic and intact.

| ASSESSMENT—RECOGNIZE CUES/ INTERVENTIONS—TAKE ACTION | RATIONALES |
|---|---|
| Assess incisional dressings frequently during the first 24 hours for drainage and change or reinforce as needed. Assess and document the odor, consistency, and color of the drainage. | Immediately after surgery, drainage may be red. Flank approaches to the ureter or kidney require muscle-splitting incisions and result in significant postoperative oozing of blood. Because drainage will also include urine leaking from the surgical site, excoriation can result from prolonged contact of urine with the skin. |
| Use Montgomery straps or net wraps (e.g., Surginet) rather than tape to secure the dressing. | This intervention facilitates frequent dressing changes without harming the skin with tape removal. |
| If drainage is copious after drain removal, apply a wound drainage or ostomy pouch with a skin barrier over the incision. | This measure prevents contact of wound drainage with the skin. |

## Patient Problem/Analyze Cues/Prioritize Hypotheses

# Deficient Knowledge (Diet)

*due to* unfamiliarity with the dietary regimen and its relationship to calculus formation

***Desired Outcome/Generate Solutions:*** Within the 24-hour period before hospital discharge, the patient verbalizes accurate knowledge about foods and liquids to limit in order to prevent stone formation.

| ASSESSMENT—RECOGNIZE CUES/ INTERVENTIONS—TAKE ACTION | RATIONALES |
|---|---|
| Assess the patient's knowledge about diet and its relationship to stone formation. | This assessment will reveal the patient's baseline knowledge, which will enable the formulation of an individualized teaching plan. |
| Advise nonrestricted patients to maintain a urine output of at least 2.5 L/day. | Fluid intake of approximately 3 L/day produces 2.5 L/day of urine and decreases the risk for recurrent urinary tract stones in patient with a prior stone. |
| Teach the patient to maintain adequate hydration of at least 3 L/day, and more if exercising.<br>**Caution:** Patients with cardiac, liver, or renal disease require special fluid intake instructions from their health care provider. | Hydration after exercise is important because a patient's renal solute load is highest at these times. |
| Teach the technique for measuring urine specific gravity via a hydrometer. | To minimize stone formation, specific gravity should remain less than 1.010. |
| As appropriate, provide the following information. | |
| For uric acid stones: | |
| • Limit intake of foods such as lean meat, legumes, whole grains. Limit protein intake to 1 g/kg/day. | These foods are high in purines, which can lead to the formation of uric acid stones. |
| For calcium stones: | |
| • Limit intake of foods such as milk, cheese, green leafy vegetables, and yogurt. | These foods are high in calcium content and increased intake may increase the risk of calcium stones. |
| • Limit sodium intake. | A low-sodium diet helps reduce the intestinal absorption of calcium. |
| • Limit intake of refined carbohydrates and animal proteins. | These foods can cause hypercalciuria. |
| • Encourage foods high in natural fiber content (e.g., bran, prunes, apples). | These foods provide phytic acid, which binds dietary calcium. |

Continued

## ASSESSMENT—RECOGNIZE CUES/ INTERVENTIONS—TAKE ACTION | RATIONALES

| ASSESSMENT—RECOGNIZE CUES/ INTERVENTIONS—TAKE ACTION | RATIONALES |
|---|---|
| • Explain that sodium cellulose phosphate, 5 g, may be prescribed to be taken three times a day before each meal. | Sodium cellulose phosphate, when used with calcium-restricted diet, reduces the risk for stone formation by binding with intestinal calcium and thus increasing excretion of calcium. It should be used cautiously in postmenopausal women at risk for osteoporosis. |
| **For oxalate stones:** | |
| • Limit intake of foods such as chocolate, caffeine-containing drinks (including instant and decaffeinated coffees), beets, spinach, rhubarb, berries, draft beer, and nuts such as almonds, walnuts, pecans, and cashews. | These foods are high in oxalate content and increased intake may increase the risk of oxalate stones. |
| • Explain that vitamin C supplements should be avoided. | As much as half of the vitamin C is converted to oxalic acid. |
| Assess the patient's ability to plan a 3-day menu that includes or excludes appropriate foods. | This will demonstrate the patient's level of understanding of the prescribed diet and areas in which teaching should be reinforced. This effort by the patient also will reinforce learning. |

## ADDITIONAL PROBLEM:

| | |
|---|---|
| "Perioperative Care" | Chapter 4 |

## PATIENT–FAMILY TEACHING AND DISCHARGE PLANNING

When providing patient–family teaching, focus on sensory information, avoid giving excessive information, and initiate a visiting nurse referral for necessary follow-up teaching. Include verbal and written information about the following:

✓ Medications, including drug name, purpose, dosage, schedule, precautions, and potential side effects. Also discuss drug–drug, herb–drug, and food–drug interactions.

✓ Indicators of UTI that necessitate medical attention: chills; fever; hematuria; flank, CVA, suprapubic, low back, buttock, scrotal, or labial pain; cloudy and foul-smelling urine; increased frequency, urgency; dysuria; and increasing or recurring incontinence.

✓ Care of incision, including cleansing and dressing. Teach signs and symptoms of local infection, including redness, swelling, local warmth, tenderness, and purulent drainage.

✓ Care of drains or catheters if the patient is discharged with them.

✓ Importance of daily fluid intake of at least 3 L/day in nonrestricted patients.

✓ Dietary changes as specified by the health care provider. Include fact sheets that list foods to restrict or add to the diet. Provide sample menus with examples of how dietary restrictions and requirements may be incorporated into daily meals.

✓ Activity restrictions as directed for the patient who has had surgery: avoid lifting heavy objects (more than 10 lb) for the first 6 weeks, be alert to fatigue, get maximum rest, increase activities gradually to tolerance.

✓ Use of Nitrazine paper to assess pH of urine. The desired pH will be determined by the type of stone formation to which the patient is prone. Instructions for use are on the Nitrazine container.

✓ Importance of walking or other exercises to decrease the risk for stone formation.

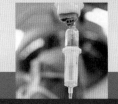

# Urinary Diversions 34

## OVERVIEW/PATHOPHYSIOLOGY

When the bladder must be bypassed or is removed, a urinary diversion is created. Urinary diversions most commonly are created for individuals with bladder cancer, neurogenic bladder, congenital anomalies, strictures, and bladder trauma. Although most urinary diversions are permanent, some act as a temporary bypass of urine, and diversion reversal can be performed if the patient's condition changes.

There are several different types of urinary diversions: incontinent urinary diversion, continent urinary diversion catheterized by the patient, orthotopic neobladder from which the patient voids through the urethra. The urinary stream may be diverted at multiple points: the renal pelvis (pyelostomy or nephrostomy), the ureter (ureterostomy), the bladder (vesicostomy), or through an intestinal "conduit."

Incontinent urinary diversion is diversion through the skin and requires a collection apparatus. A ureterostomy is a simple example of this type of urinary diversion. However, due to the risk of complications such as ureteral scarring and strictures, the ileal conduit is the most common incontinent urinary diversion.

Continent urinary diversions have an internal intrabdominal urinary reservoir that can be catheterized. The reservoir is constructed from the ileum, ileocecal segment, or ascending colon. Also, a valve is surgically created and implanted to prevent involuntary leakage from the reservoir. Patients with a continent reservoir need to self-catheterize every 4–6 hours. Typically, a small bandage should be applied over the stoma to absorb possible mucous or minimal urine drainage. Although construction of a small bowel pouch is still the most common type of urinary diversion, the neobladder or orthotopic bladder is becoming the standard of definitive care. All these procedures reconstruct a new bladder in the bladder's normal anatomic position, and drains urine through the urethra through the act of urination. The neobladder is surgically shaped from intestinal segments to make a reservoir. One possible problem with orthotopic neobladder is incontinence and may require intermittent catheterization.

***Incontinent urinary diversions.*** External collection appliances are required for urine drainage. A cutaneous ureterostomy is a surgical procedure in which the ureters are separated from the bladder and brought through the abdominal wall, and a stoma is created from which the urine drains. Another example of an incontinent urinary diversion is a nephrostomy in which a catheter is inserted into the kidney pelvis to drain urine into a collection apparatus.

***Continent urinary diversions.*** All continent urinary diversions are constructed with the following three components: a reservoir or reconstructed bladder, a continence mechanism, and an antireflux mechanism. Examples include Kock, Mainz, Indiana, and Florida pouches.

***Intestinal (ileal conduit).*** Any segment of bowel may be used to create a passageway for urine, but the ileum conduit is most commonly used. A 15- to 20-cm section of ileum is resected from the intestine to form a passageway for the urine. The proximal end is closed, and the distal end is brought out through the abdomen, forming a stoma. The ureters are resected from the bladder and anastomosed to the ileal segment. The intestine is re-anastomosed to the ileal segment, and therefore bowel function is unaffected. Occasionally, the jejunum is used for the conduit. However, jejunal-conduit syndrome (hyperkalemia, hyponatremia, hypochloremia) often occurs.

***Indiana and Kock pouches.*** Both the Indiana and Kock pouches use the ileum to create a pouch and an antireflux valve. These types of continent urostomies require the patient to perform catheterizations to remove urine from the pouch.

***Orthotopic neobladder.*** This surgery involves the use of the small intestine or small bowel–large bowel combination to create a low-pressure spherical reservoir that attaches to the patient's urinary sphincter. Similar to the Mainz and Kock techniques, the created "bladder" has the characteristics of low pressure, adequate volume, and control of urination without leakage or residual urine. The patient can sense a full bladder and urinate without catheterization. Normal continence is the goal for this procedure.

## HEALTH CARE SETTING

Surgical unit; primary care

## Patient Problem/Analyze Cues/Prioritize Hypotheses

# Anxiety

*due to* threat to self-concept, interaction patterns, or health status occurring with urinary diversion surgery

**Desired Outcomes/Generate Solutions:** Before surgery, the patient communicates anxieties and concerns, relates attainment of increased psychologic and physical comfort, and exhibits a coping demeanor.

| ASSESSMENT—RECOGNIZE CUES/ INTERVENTIONS—TAKE ACTION | RATIONALES |
|---|---|
| Assess the patient's perception of his or her impending surgery and resulting body function changes. Listen actively. | This assessment provides an opportunity for the patient to express anxieties about the upcoming surgery and for the nurse to evaluate the response |
| Acknowledge the patient's concerns. | This will help focus attention on anxieties and concerns so that they can be dealt with. |
| Provide brief, basic information regarding the physiology of the procedure and equipment that will be used after surgery, including tubes and drains. | Knowledge is one of the best means of decreasing anxiety. |
| If appropriate, show the patient the pouches that will be used after surgery. Assure the patient that the pouch usually cannot be seen through clothing and that it is odor resistant. | Patients may worry that others will be able to see and smell the pouch. |
| For the patient about to undergo a continent urostomy procedure, explain that a pouching system may be needed for a short time after surgery. Reassure the patient that continued instructions on accessing the continent urostomy will be done postoperatively in the surgeon's office or by the home care nurse. | This intervention likely will decrease anxiety by reassuring the patient that he or she will be taught necessary skills. |
| Discuss postsurgical activities of daily living (ADLs). | This information decreases anxiety that such ADLs as showers, baths, and swimming can continue and that diet is not affected after the early postoperative period. |
| As appropriate, ask the patient about the information that has been relayed by the surgeon about sexual implications of the surgery. | Patients may be very anxious about sexual implications of this surgery but afraid to ask. Asking this question will help establish an open relationship between the patient and nurse. For example, some men undergoing radical cystectomy with urinary diversion may become impotent, but recent surgical advances have enabled the preservation of potency for others. The pelvic plexus, which innervates the corpora cavernosa (allowing penile erection), may be damaged permanently as a result of autonomic nerve damage. However, sensation and orgasm are mediated by the pudendal nerve (sensorimotor) and are not affected. |
| Arrange for a visit by the wound, ostomy, and continence (WOC) nurse during the preoperative period. Collaborate with the surgeon, WOC nurse, and patient to identify and mark the most appropriate site for the stoma. | Showing patients the actual spot for placement may help alleviate anxiety by reinforcing that the impact on lifestyle and body image will be minimal. |

## Patient Problem/Analyze Cues/Prioritize Hypotheses

# Risk for Health Care Associated Complication

*due to* obstruction of ureteral stents, catheters, or drains; leak in anastomotic site; or renal failure

**Desired Outcomes/Generate Solutions:** The patient's urinary output is 30 mL/hour or greater; urine is clear and straw-colored, with normal, characteristic odor.

| ASSESSMENT—RECOGNIZE CUES/ INTERVENTIONS—TAKE ACTION | RATIONALES |
|---|---|
| Assess the intake and output and record the total amount of urine output from the urinary diversion. Differentiate and record separately amounts from all drains, stents, and catheters. Notify the health care provider of an output less than 60 mL during a 2-hour period. | This assessment checks for discrepancies between intake and output. In the presence of adequate intake, a decreased output can signal an obstruction, a leak in one of the anastomotic sites, or impending renal failure. *Ureterostomy:* Urine is drained through the stoma and/or ureteral stents. *Intestinal conduit:* Urine is drained through the stoma. Patients also may have ureteral stents and/or a conduit catheter/stent in the early postoperative period to stabilize the ureterointestinal anastomoses and maintain drainage from the conduit during early postoperative edema. *Continent urinary diversions or reservoirs:* The Kock urostomy usually has a reservoir catheter and also may have ureteral stents. The Indiana (ileocecal) reservoir usually has ureteral stents exiting from the stoma, through which most of the urine drains, and may have a reservoir catheter exiting from an incisional wound, which serves as an overflow catheter. The neobladder has a urethral catheter in place that will drain urine, which initially will be light-red to pink in color with mucus but should clear in 24–48 hours. This catheter generally remains in place for 21 days to ensure adequate healing of the anastomosis. |
| Also assess for flank pain, costovertebral angle (CVA) tenderness, nausea, vomiting, and anuria. | These are other indicators of ureteral obstruction. |
| Monitor the functioning of the ureteral stents. | Ureteral stents, which exit from the stoma into the pouch, maintain ureteral patency and assist in healing of the anastomosis. Stents may become blocked with mucus, but as long as urine is draining adequately around the stent and the volume of output is adequate, this is not a problem. Each usually produces approximately the same amount of urine, although the amount produced by each is not important as long as each drains adequately and total drainage from all sources is 30 mL/hour or greater. Urine is usually red to pink for the first 24–48 hours and becomes straw-colored by the third postoperative day. Absent or lessening amounts of urine may indicate a blocked stent or problems with the ureter. |
| If the patient has a continent urinary diversion, monitor the functioning of the stoma catheter. | Expect output from the stoma catheter to include pink or light-red urine with mucus and small red clots for the first 24 hours. Urine should become amber-colored with occasional clots within 3 postoperative days. Mucus production will continue but should decrease in volume. In continent urinary diversions, a catheter is placed in the reservoir to prevent distention and promote healing of suture lines. This new reservoir (i.e., resected intestine) exudes large amounts of mucus, necessitating catheter irrigation with 30–50 mL of normal saline, which is instilled gently and allowed to empty through gravity. |
| Monitor the functioning of the drains. | Any urinary diversion may have Penrose drains or closed drainage systems in place to facilitate healing of the ureterointestinal anastomosis. Drainage from these systems may be light-red to pink for the first 24 hours and then lighten to amber and decrease in amount. Excessive lymph fluid and urine can be removed through these drains to reduce pressure on anastomotic suture lines. In a continent urinary diversion, an increase in drainage after amounts have been low might signal an anastomotic leak, which necessitates notification of the health care provider. |
| Monitor drainage from the Foley (indwelling) catheter or urethral drain (if present). Note color, consistency, and volume of drainage, which may be red to pink with mucus. | Patients who have had a cystectomy may have a urethral drain, whereas those with a partial cystectomy will have an indwelling catheter in place. |

Continued

| ASSESSMENT—RECOGNIZE CUES/ INTERVENTIONS—TAKE ACTION | RATIONALES |
|---|---|
| Report a sudden increase or decrease in drainage to the health care provider. | A sudden increase of blood-tinged urine would occur with hemorrhage; a sudden decrease can signal blockage that can lead to infection or, with partial cystectomy, hydronephrosis. |
| Encourage an intake of at least 2–3 L/day in the nonrestricted patient. | Increased hydration keeps the urinary tract well irrigated and helps prevent infection that could be caused by urinary stasis. |

## Patient Problem/Analyze Cues/Prioritize Hypotheses

# Risk for Infection

*due to* the invasive surgical procedure and potential for ascending bacteriuria with the urinary diversion

***Desired Outcome/Generate Solutions:*** The patient is free of infection.

| ASSESSMENT—RECOGNIZE CUES/ INTERVENTIONS—TAKE ACTION | RATIONALES |
|---|---|
| Assess the patient's temperature every 4 hours during the first 24–48 hours after surgery. Notify the health care provider of fever (temperature greater than 100.4°F (38°C). | Elevated temperature is a sign that the body is mounting a defense against infection. |
| Inspect the dressing frequently after surgery. Change the dressing when it becomes wet, using the sterile technique. Use extra care to prevent disruption of the drains. | Infection is most likely to become evident after the first 72 hours. The presence of purulent or excessive drainage on the dressing signals infection and the need to notify the health care provider promptly for timely intervention. |
| Assess the condition of the incision. | Erythema, tenderness, local warmth, edema, and purulent or excessive drainage are indicators of infection at the incision line. |
| Assess and record the character of the urine at least every 8 hours. | Urine should be yellow or pink-tinged during the first 24–48 hours after surgery. Mucous particles are normal in urine of patients with ileal conduits and continent urinary diversions because of the nature of the bowel segment used. Cloudy urine, however, is abnormal and can signal infection. |
| Assess for flank or CVA pain, malodorous urine, chills, and fever. | These are indicators of urinary tract infection (UTI). |
| Note the position of the stoma relative to the incision. If they are close together, apply the pouch first to avoid overlap of the pouch with the suture line. | Overlapping the pouch with the suture line increases risk for infection. |
| If necessary, cut the pouch down on one side or place it at an angle. | This measure prevents contact of the pouch with drainage, which may loosen the adhesive. |
| Wash your hands thoroughly before and after caring for the patient. | Hand hygiene helps prevent contamination and cross-contamination. |
| Do not irrigate indwelling urethral catheters of patients with cystectomies. | Patients with cystectomies without anastomosis to the urethra may have an indwelling urethral catheter to drain serosanguineous fluid from the peritoneal cavity. Irrigation of this catheter can result in peritonitis. |
| Encourage fluid intake of at least 2–3 L/day. | Increased hydration helps flush urine through the urinary tract, removing mucus shreds and preventing stasis that could result in infection. |

Patient Problem/Analyze Cues/Prioritize Hypotheses

# Risk for Fluid Imbalance, Electrolyte Imbalance, and Acid-Base Imbalance

*due to* the presence of urine in the ileal segment

**Desired Outcomes/Generate Solutions:** Patient maintains adequate fluid balance, electrolyte levels, and acid–base balance throughout hospitalization.

| ASSESSMENT—RECOGNIZE CUES/ INTERVENTIONS—TAKE ACTION | RATIONALES |
|---|---|
| For patients with ileal conduits, assess for nausea and changes in the level of consciousness, muscle tone, and heart rhythm/rate. | Changes in neurosensory, musculoskeletal, and cardiac status are indicators of hypokalemia and metabolic acidosis that can occur in the presence of $Na^+$ and $Cl^-$ from the urine in the ileal segment, which results in compensatory loss of $K^+$ and $HCO_3^-$. |
| Monitor serum electrolyte studies and notify the health care provider of abnormal values. | $K^+$ less than 3.5 mEq/L signals hypokalemia, and $HCO_3^-$ less than 7.4 signals metabolic acidosis, which could be life threatening. |
| If the patient displays confused behavior or exhibits signs of motor dysfunction, keep the bed in the lowest position and raise the side rails. If seizures appear imminent, place patient on side and maintain patient safety. Notify the health care provider of significant findings. | These are standard safety precautions for patients who have confusion or motor dysfunction. |
| Encourage oral intake as directed and assess fluid balance. | Maintaining fluid balance will help ameliorate acid–base and electrolyte imbalances. |
| If the patient is hypokalemic and allowed to eat, encourage foods high in potassium, and administer potassium supplements as prescribed by the health care provider. | Foods high in potassium, such as potatoes, prune juice, pumpkin, spinach, sweet potatoes, Swiss chard, tomatoes, and watermelon, will help reverse hypokalemia. The health care provider may prescribe oral or intravenous fluids with potassium supplements to prevent or treat hypokalemia. |
| Encourage the patient to ambulate by the second day after surgery. | Mobility will help prevent urinary stasis, which would increase the risk for electrolyte problems. |

Patient Problems/Analyze Cues/Prioritize Hypotheses

# Risk for Impaired Skin Integrity

*due to* sensitivity to appliance materials or the presence of urine on the skin

**Desired Outcome/Generate Solutions:** The patient's peristomal skin remains nonerythematous and intact.

| ASSESSMENT—RECOGNIZE CUES/ INTERVENTIONS—TAKE ACTION | RATIONALES |
|---|---|
| For patients with significant allergy history, patch-test the skin for a 24-hour period, at least 24 hours before surgery. If erythema, swelling, bleb formation, itching, weeping, or other indicators of tape allergy occur, document the type of tape that caused the reaction and note on the chart cover "Allergic to _____ tape." Place an allergy armband on the patient. | This assessment evaluates for and documents allergies to different tapes that might be used on the postoperative appliance and will decrease the risk of using tape that may affect the patient's skin. |
| Assess the integrity of the peristomal skin with each pouch change. Question the patient about itching or burning under the adhesive or wafer. Change the ostomy collection drainage bag (per agency or surgeon preference) or immediately if leakage is suspected. | Itching or burning can signal leakage of the pouch under the protective wafer. If the seal between the adhesive backing of the wafer and skin becomes compromised, leaking onto the peristomal skin can occur. |
| | **Note:** All pouches are attached to a wafer or skin-protective device, and pouches are never placed directly over a stoma. The skin-protective device covers the skin surrounding the stoma (peristomal skin). Pouches may come already attached to a wafer (one-piece system) or come separately (two-piece system). |

Continued

| ASSESSMENT—RECOGNIZE CUES/ INTERVENTIONS—TAKE ACTION | RATIONALES |
|---|---|
| Teach the patient how often to change the wafer and/or pouch if a **one-piece system** is used. | Routine wafer/pouch change is done at least every 4–7 days. This schedule provides the consistency that usually avoids surprise leakage problems. |
| Teach the patient to monitor the skin for leakage and odor. | Leakage and odor indicate that the wafer and/or pouch must be changed. |
| Teach the patient to report signs of a rash to the health care provider. | A rash can occur with a yeast infection and will require a topical medication for treatment. |
| Assess the stoma, pouch, and skin for crystalline deposits. | These deposits are signals of alkaline urine, which can compromise skin integrity if exposure occurs. |
| In the presence of alkaline urine, instruct the patient on the following: drink fluids that leave acid ash in the urine, such as cranberry juice, or take ascorbic acid in a dose consistent with the patient's size. | These actions help decrease urine pH, which will improve the peristomal skin condition. |
| When changing the wafer, measure the stoma with a measuring guide, and ensure that the skin barrier opening is cut to the exact size of the stoma. For a patient using a **two-piece system or pouch with a wafer:** size the wafer to fit snugly around the stoma. For pouch placement, size the pouch to clear the stoma by at least 1/8 inch. | These measures protect the peristomal area from maceration caused by pooling of urine on the skin. |
| For a patient using a **one-piece "adhesive-only" pouch:** | |
| • If the pouch has an antireflux valve, size the pouch to clear the stoma and any peristomal creases. | This helps ensure that the pouch adheres to a flat, dry surface. An antireflux valve prevents pooling of urine on skin. |
| • If the pouch does not have an antireflux valve, size the pouch so that it clears the stoma by 1/8 inch. | This will help prevent stomal trauma while minimizing the amount of exposed skin. |
| Use a skin protectant film sealant wipe on the peristomal skin before applying the wafer or "adhesive-only" pouch and wafer system. | This will provide a moisture barrier and reduce epidermal trauma when the wafer is removed. |
| Wash the peristomal skin with water or a special cleansing solution marketed by ostomy supply companies. Dry the skin thoroughly before applying the skin barrier, wafer, and pouch. | Other products can dry out the skin, which would increase the risk for irritation and infection. |
| When changing the pouch or wafer, instruct the patient to hold a gauze pad or clean small towel on (but not in) the stoma. | This will absorb urine and keep the surrounding skin dry. |
| During hospitalization, after applying the pouch, connect it to a bedside drainage system if the patient is on bedrest. When the patient is no longer on bedrest, empty the pouch when it is one-third to one-half full, opening the spigot on the bottom of the pouch and draining urine into the patient's measuring container. | These interventions facilitate drainage of urine. |
| Do not allow the pouch to become too full. Instruct the patient accordingly. | An overly full pouch could break the seal of the wafer with the patient's skin. |
| Teach the patient to treat peristomal irritation as follows after hospital discharge: | |
| • Dry the skin with a hair dryer set on a cool setting. | This eliminates the necessity of wiping the skin, which would increase the irritation. |
| • Dust the peristomal skin with karaya powder or spread Stomahesive paste. | These agents absorb moisture. |
| • If desired, blot the skin with water or a sealant wipe or copolymer protectant that seals in the powder. | These agents provide a moisture barrier. |
| • Use a porous tape if tape is required. | Porous tapes prevent trapping of moisture. |
| Notify the health care provider or WOC/enterostomal therapy (ET) nurse of any severe or nonresponsive skin problems. | These problems call for skilled interventions. |

## Patient Problem/Analyze Cues/Prioritize Hypotheses

# Risk for Impaired Tissue Integrity

*due to* altered stomal circulation occurring with the urinary diversion procedure or improper appliance fit

***Desired Outcomes/Generate Solutions:*** The patient's stoma is pink or bright-red and shiny. The stoma of a cutaneous urostomy is raised, moist, and red.

| ASSESSMENT—RECOGNIZE CUES/ INTERVENTIONS—TAKE ACTION | RATIONALES |
|---|---|
| Assess the stoma at least every 8 hours and as indicated. Report significant findings to health care provider. | The stoma of an ileal conduit will be edematous and should be pink or red with a shiny appearance. The stoma formed by a cutaneous urostomy is usually raised during the first few weeks after surgery, red, and moist. A stoma that is dusky or cyanotic is indicative of insufficient blood supply and impending necrosis and must be reported to the health care provider for immediate intervention. |
| Assess the degree of swelling, if present. | The stoma should shrink considerably over the first 6–8 weeks and less significantly over the next year. The stoma formed by a cutaneous ureterostomy is usually raised during the first few weeks after surgery, red in color, and moist. |

## Patient Problem/Analyze Cues/Prioritize Hypotheses

# Deficient Knowledge (Self-Care)

*due to* unfamiliarity with self-care regarding the urinary diversion

***Desired Outcome/Generate Solutions:*** The patient or significant other demonstrates proper care of the stoma and urinary diversion before hospital discharge.

| ASSESSMENT—RECOGNIZE CUES/ INTERVENTIONS—TAKE ACTION | RATIONALES |
|---|---|
| Assess the patient's health care literacy (language, reading, comprehension). Assess culture and culturally specific information needs. | This assessment helps ensure that information is selected and presented in a manner that is culturally and educationally appropriate. |
| Assess the patient's or significant other's readiness to participate in care. | A well-thought-out teaching plan is useless if individuals are unable or unwilling to understand/learn it. |
| Collaborate with ET or WOC nurse in patient teaching if available. | An ET or WOC nurse is specially trained and skilled in teaching urinary diversion care. |
| Assist the patient with organizing the equipment and materials that are needed to accomplish home care. | Usually, patients are discharged with disposable pouching systems. Most of these patients continue using disposable systems for the long term. Those who will use reusable systems usually are not fitted until 6–8 weeks after surgery. |
| Teach patient or caregiver how to remove and reapply the pouch; how to empty it; and how to use a gravity drainage system at night, including procedures for rinsing and cleansing the drainage system. | These are the basic skills the patient will need in order to accomplish self-care after hospital discharge. |
| Teach the patient/caregiver signs and symptoms of UTI, peristomal skin breakdown, and appropriate therapeutic responses, including maintenance of an acidic urine (if not contraindicated), importance of adequate fluid intake, and techniques for checking urine pH (which should be assessed weekly). Explain that urine pH should remain at 6 or less. | Persons with urinary diversion have a higher incidence of UTI than the general public, so it is important to keep their urinary pH acidic. If it is greater than 6, advise the patient to increase fluid intake and, with health care provider approval, to increase vitamin C intake to 500–1000 mg/day, which will increase urine acidity. |

Continued

Renal-Urinary Care Plans

| ASSESSMENT—RECOGNIZE CUES/ INTERVENTIONS—TAKE ACTION | RATIONALES |
|---|---|
| Teach patients with a continent urinary diversion the technique for reservoir catheter irrigation. | In continent urinary diversions, a catheter is placed in the reservoir to prevent distention and promote healing of suture lines. This new reservoir (i.e., resected intestine) exudes large amounts of mucus, necessitating catheter irrigation with 30–50 mL of normal saline, which is instilled gently and allowed to empty by gravity. |
| Teach patients with a continent urinary diversion with urethral anastomosis signals of the urge to void. | Feelings of vague abdominal discomfort and abdominal pressure or cramping are sensations of the need to void. |
| Instruct patients with a continent urinary diversion with urethral anastomosis about the procedure to void. | Relaxing the perineal muscles and employing Valsalva maneuver help empty the diversion. |
| Emphasize the importance of follow-up visits, particularly for patients with a continent urinary diversion. | Follow-up visits, particularly for patients with continent urinary diversions who will be taught how to catheterize the reservoir and use a small dressing over the stoma rather than an appliance, help ensure that the patient can manipulate the pouch. Follow-up visits also facilitate answers to questions that ensue after hospital discharge. |
| Provide a list of ostomy support groups and ET nurses in the area. | Referrals such as this will assist the patient after hospital discharge. |
| Provide the patient with enough equipment and materials for the first week after hospital discharge. | The first postoperative visit is usually 1 week after hospital discharge. |
| Remind the patient of the importance of proper cleansing of ostomy appliances. | This knowledge will help reduce the risk for bacterial growth and UTI after hospital discharge. |

## ✓ PATIENT–FAMILY TEACHING AND DISCHARGE PLANNING

When providing patient–family teaching, focus on sensory information, avoid giving excessive information, and initiate a visiting nurse referral for necessary follow-up teaching. Include verbal and written information about the following:

- ✓ Medications, including drug name, dosage, schedule, precautions, and potential side effects. Also discuss drug–drug, herb–drug, and food–drug interactions.
- ✓ Indicators that necessitate medical intervention: fever or chills; nausea or vomiting; abdominal pain, cramping, or distention; cloudy or malodorous urine; incisional drainage, edema, local warmth, pain, or redness; peristomal skin irritation; or abnormal changes in stoma shape or color from the normal bright and shiny red.
- ✓ Maintenance of fluid intake of at least 2–3 L/day to maintain adequate kidney function.
- ✓ Importance of keeping urinary pH acidic. Individuals with urinary diversions have a higher incidence of UTI than the general public; therefore it is important to keep their urinary pH acidic. Because many fruits and vegetables tend

to make urine alkaline, the patient should drink cranberry juice rather than orange juice or other citrus juices or take vitamin C daily. (Check with the health care provider first.)

- ✓ Care of the stoma and application of urostomy appliances. Patients should be proficient in the application technique before hospital discharge.
- ✓ Care of urostomy appliances. Remind patients that proper cleansing will reduce the risk for bacterial growth, which would contaminate urine and increase risk for UTI.
- ✓ Importance of follow-up care with the health care provider and WOC/ET nurse. Confirm the date and time of the next appointment.
- ✓ Telephone numbers to call in case questions or concerns arise about therapy after discharge. In addition, many cities have local support groups. Information for these patients can be obtained by contacting the following:
  - United Ostomy Association: www.uoa.org
  - American Cancer Society: www.cancer.org
  - National Cancer Institute Cancer Information Service: www.cancer.gov/contact/contact-center

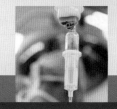

## OVERVIEW/PATHOPHYSIOLOGY

Urinary tract obstruction occurs when there is an anatomic or functional condition that blocks or impedes the flow of urine. It can result from pelvic tumors, calculi, and urethral strictures. Additional causes include neoplasms, benign prostatic hypertrophy, ureteral or urethral trauma, inflammation of the urinary tract, pregnancy, and pelvic or colonic surgery in which ureteral damage has occurred. Obstructions can occur suddenly or slowly, over weeks to months. They can occur anywhere along the urinary tract, but the most common sites are the ureteropelvic and ureterovesical junctions, bladder neck, and urethral meatus. The obstruction acts like a dam, blocking the passage of urine. Muscles in the area contract to push urine around the obstruction, and structures behind the obstruction begin to dilate. The smaller the site of obstruction, the greater the damage. Obstructions may cause damaging effects above the level of the obstruction. The severity of the effects depends on multiple factors including the duration and location of the obstruction as well as the presence of urinary stasis or infection. Obstructions in the lower urinary structures, such as the bladder neck or urethra, can lead to urinary retention and urinary tract infection (UTI). Obstructions in the upper urinary tract can lead to bilateral involvement of the ureters and kidneys, leading to hydronephrosis, renal insufficiency, and kidney destruction. Hydrostatic pressure increases, and filtration and concentration processes in the tubules and glomerulus are compromised.

## HEALTH CARE SETTING

Primary care and acute care

## ASSESSMENT

**Signs and symptoms.** Nausea, vomiting, local abdominal tenderness, hesitancy, straining to start a stream, dribbling, decreased caliber and force of urinary stream, hematuria may be seen with urinary tract obstructions. Pain may be sharp and intense or dull and aching; localized or referred (e.g., flank, low back, buttock, scrotal, labial pain). In severe cases in which the kidney function is affected, oliguria, anuria, and abnormal kidney function tests are noted.

**Physical assessment.** Bladder distention and "kettle drum" sound over the bladder with percussion (absent if the obstruction is above the bladder) and mass in the flank area, abdomen, pelvis, or rectum.

**History.** Recent fever (possibly caused by the obstruction), hypertensive episodes (caused by increased renin production from the body's attempt to increase renal blood flow).

## DIAGNOSTIC TESTS

BUN, creatinine, potassium, and sodium levels are assessed to determine renal function.

Blood urea nitrogen (BUN) and creatinine values are elevated with decreased renal-urinary function. **Note:** These values must be considered based on the patient's age and hydration status. For the older adult, serum creatinine level may not be a reliable indicator because of decreased muscle mass and a decreased glomerular filtration rate. Hydration status can affect BUN: fluid volume excess can result in reduced values, whereas volume deficit can cause higher values.

**Urinalysis.** To provide baseline data on the functioning of the urinary system, detect metabolic disease, and assess for the presence of UTI. A cloudy, hazy appearance; foul odor; pH greater than 8; and presence of red blood cells, leukocyte esterase, white blood cells (WBCs), and WBC casts are signals of UTI.

**Urine culture.** To determine the type of bacterium present in the genitourinary tract. To minimize contamination, a sample should be obtained from a midstream collection.

**Hemoglobin and hematocrit.** To assess for anemia, which may be related to the decreased renal secretion of erythropoietin.

**Kidneys, ureters, and bladder radiography.** To identify the size, shape, and position of the kidneys, ureters, and bladder and abnormalities such as tumors, calculi, or malformations. This can be done in combination with ultrasonography.

**Imaging studies.** A variety of imaging studies may be used to identify the area and cause of obstructions:

- *Ultrasonography:* This is sensitive in revealing parenchymal masses, hydronephrosis, a distended bladder, and renal calculi.
- *Computed tomography scans:* To identify the degree and location of the obstruction, as well as cause in many situations.
- *Excretory urography/intravenous (IV) pyelography:* To evaluate the cause of urinary dysfunction by visualizing the kidneys, renal pelvis, ureters, and bladder.
- *Antegrade urography:* Involves placement of a percutaneous needle or nephrostomy tube through which radiopaque contrast is injected. Antegrade urography is indicated when the kidney does not concentrate or excrete IV dye.

- *Retrograde urography:* Radiopaque dye is injected through ureteral catheters placed during cystoscopy.
- *Cystogram:* Radiopaque dye is instilled through cystoscope or catheter. This enables visualization of the bladder and evaluation of the vesicoureteral reflex.

**Bladder scanner.** Bladder scanners are designed to create a three-dimensional image of the bladder and calculate the volume based on the image. The scan is frequently used to measure postvoid residual to evaluate the need for catheterization.

**Maximal urinary flow rate.** Less than 15 mL/second indicates significant obstruction to flow.

**Postvoid residual volume.** Normal is less than 12 mL. Higher volume signals obstructive process.

**Cystoscopy.** To determine the degree of bladder outlet obstruction and facilitate visualization of any tumors or masses.

## Patient Problems/Analyze Cues/Prioritize Hypotheses

# Risk for Fluid and Electrolyte Imbalance

*due to* kidney injury

**Desired Outcomes/Generate Solutions:** Within 2 days after bladder decompression, urinary output approximates input, and electrolytes, BUN and creatinine begin to return to patient's baseline

| ASSESSMENT—RECOGNIZE CUES/ INTERVENTIONS—TAKE ACTION | RATIONALES |
|---|---|
| Using the sterile technique, insert a urinary catheter. | Catheterization will drain the bladder of the urine whose passage has been obstructed. |
| Assess the patient carefully during catheterization; clamp the catheter if the patient complains of abdominal pain. | Although research has demonstrated that rapid bladder decompression of greater than 750–1000 mL does not result in shock syndrome as previously believed, postobstructive diuresis could lead to a major electrolyte imbalance causing spasms and discomfort as a result. |
| Assess the intake and output hourly for 4 hours and then every 2 hours for 4 hours after bladder decompression. | This assessment monitors for postobstructive diuresis. |
| ⚠ Notify the health care provider if the output exceeds 200 mL/hour or 2 L over an 8-hour period. | This can signal postobstructive diuresis. If this occurs, anticipate initiation of IV infusion. |
| Anticipate the need for urine specimens for analysis of electrolytes and osmolality and blood specimens for analysis of electrolytes. | Postobstructive diuresis can lead to major electrolyte imbalances. |
| Monitor for and report the following: | |
| • Abdominal cramps, lethargy, dysrhythmias. | These are signs of hypokalemia. |
| • Diarrhea, colic, irritability, nausea, muscle cramps, weakness, irregular apical or radial pulses. | These are signs of hyperkalemia. |
| • Muscle weakness and cramps, complaints of tingling in fingers, positive Trousseau and Chvostek signs. | These are signs of hypocalcemia. |
| • Excessive itching. | This is a sign of hyperphosphatemia. |
| Monitor mentation, noting signs of disorientation. | Disorientation can occur with electrolyte disturbance. |
| Weigh the patient daily using the same scale and at the same time of day (e.g., before breakfast). | Weight fluctuations of 2–4 lb (0.9–1.8 kg) normally occur in a patient who is undergoing diuresis. Losses greater than this can result in dehydration and electrolyte imbalances.Weighing the patient in a consistent manner and under the same conditions helps ensure more precise measurements and comparisons. |

PART I: Medical-Surgical Nursing Care Plans

## Patient Problem/Analyze Cues/Prioritize Hypotheses

# Acute Pain

*due to* bladder and ureteral spasms

**Desired Outcome/Generate Solutions:** Patient verbalizes no pain or decreased pain within a tolerable level.

| ASSESSMENT—RECOGNIZE CUES/ INTERVENTIONS—TAKE ACTION | RATIONALES |
|---|---|
| Assess for and document complaints of pain in the suprapubic or urethral area. Utilize a numerical pain scale asking the patient to rate pain from 0 (no pain) to 10 (worst pain). | This assessment establishes a baseline for subsequent assessment and evaluates the degree of pain relief obtained. Spasms occur frequently with obstruction. |
| Medicate with antispasmodics or analgesics such as oxybutynin and flavoxate as prescribed. Document pain relief obtained, using the numeric pain scale. | These medications relieve spasms and pain. |
| Assess for urine leakage around Foley catheter if patient has a distended bladder (with or without bladder spasms) and check the catheter and drainage tubing for evidence of obstruction. Inspect for kinks and obstructions in the drainage tubing, compress and roll the catheter gently between your fingers to assess for gritty matter within the catheter, milk the drainage tubing to release obstructions, or instruct the patient to turn from side to side. Notify health care provider for a prescription to irrigate the catheter if these measures fail to relieve the obstruction. | These assessments detect and manage obstructions in the catheter and tubing that may be contributing to spasms. |
| In nonrestricted patients, encourage the intake of fluids to at least 2.5–3 L/day to help reduce the frequency of spasms. | Increased hydration reduces the frequency of spasms. IV fluid therapy may be indicated for acutely ill, dehydrated patients, or to increase fluids in patients with calculi. |
| Teach nonpharmacologic methods of pain relief, such as guided imagery, relaxation techniques, and distraction. | These pain relief techniques augment pharmacologic interventions. |

### ADDITIONAL PROBLEM:

| "Urinary Tract Calculi" for *Risk for Impaired Skin Integrity* | Chapter 33 |
|---|---|

 **PATIENT–FAMILY TEACHING AND DISCHARGE PLANNING**

When providing patient–family teaching, focus on sensory information, avoid giving excessive information, and initiate a visiting nurse referral for necessary follow-up teaching. Include verbal and written information about the following:

✓ Medications, including drug name, dosage, purpose, schedule, precautions, and potential side effects. Also discuss drug–drug, herb–drug, and food–drug interactions.

✓ Indicators that signal recurrent obstruction and require prompt medical attention: pain, fever, decreased urinary output.

✓ Activity restrictions as directed for the patient who has had surgery: avoid lifting heavy objects (more than 10 lb) for the first 6 weeks, be alert to fatigue, get maximum rest, increase activities gradually to tolerance.

✓ Care of drains or catheters if the patient is discharged with them; care of the surgical incision if present.

✓ Indicators of wound infection: persistent redness, local warmth, tenderness, drainage, swelling, and fever.

✓ Indicators of UTI that necessitate medical attention: chills; fever; hematuria; flank, costovertebral angle, suprapubic, low back, buttock, scrotal, or labial pain; cloudy and foul-smelling urine; increased frequency, urgency; dysuria; and increasing or recurring incontinence. In older adults, confusion may be the first sign of a UTI.

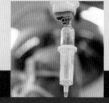

# General Care of Patients With Neurologic Disorders  36

## Care of patients with acute neurologic issues

**Health Care Setting**

Acute care

### Patient Problem/Analyze Cues/Prioritize Hypotheses

## Risk for Impaired Neurologic System Function

*due to* the positional factors, increased intrathoracic or intraabdominal pressure, fluid overload, hyperthermia, or discomfort occurring with brain injury

***Desired Outcome/Generate Solutions:*** The patient is or becomes free of symptoms of increased intracranial pressure (ICP) and herniation, as evidenced by stable or improving Glasgow Coma Scale score; stable or improving sensorimotor functioning; blood pressure (BP) within the patient's baseline range; heart rate (HR; 60–100 bpm); pulse pressure 30–40 mm Hg (difference between systolic BP and diastolic BP); oriented to person, place, and time; baseline vision acuity; PERRLA (pupils equal, round, and reactive to light and accommodation); respiratory rate (RR) 12–20 breaths/minute with eupnea (unlabored quiet breathing without diminished or increased respiratory depth); present gag, corneal, and swallowing reflexes; and absence of headache, nausea, nuchal rigidity, posturing, and seizure activity.

| ASSESSMENT—RECOGNIZE CUES/ INTERVENTIONS—TAKE ACTION | RATIONALES |
|---|---|
| Assess for and report any of the following indicators of increased ICP or impending/occurring herniation: declining Glasgow Coma Scale score; alterations in level of consciousness (LOC) ranging from irritability, restlessness, and confusion to lethargy; onset of or worsening of headache; sluggish pupils, visual disturbances, such as diplopia or blurred vision; onset of or increase in sensorimotor changes or deficits, such as weakness; onset of or worsening of nausea. | ICP is the pressure exerted by brain tissue, cerebrospinal fluid (CSF), and cerebral blood volume within the rigid, unyielding skull. An increase in any one of these components without a corresponding decrease in another will increase ICP. Normal ICP ranges from 5 to 15 mm Hg; sustained ICP greater than 20 mm Hg is considered abnormal. Cerebral perfusion pressure (CPP) is the difference between mean arterial pressure and ICP. As ICP rises, CPP may decrease. Normal CPP is 70–100 mm Hg. If CPP falls below 50 mm Hg, local tissue damage (ischemia) occurs from lack of blood flow. When CPP falls below 30 mm Hg, death occurs. |
| If changes consistent with increased ICP occur, prepare patient for possible transfer to the intensive care unit. | Insertion of ICP sensors for continuous ICP monitoring, continuous bedside cerebral blood flow (CBF) monitoring (e.g., continuous transcranial Doppler), CSF ventricular drainage, vasopressor use (e.g., dopamine), intubation, mechanical ventilation, propofol sedation, neuromuscular blocking, or barbiturate coma therapy may be necessary. Continuous cardiac monitoring for dysrhythmias also will be done. Intensive insulin therapy may be needed to maintain optimal serum glucose values. These interventions must be done in a setting that has essential staff and equipment needed for safe patient care. |

| ASSESSMENT—RECOGNIZE CUES/ INTERVENTIONS—TAKE ACTION | RATIONALES |
|---|---|
| **!** Institute preventive measures for patients at risk for increased ICP. These include assessment of arterial blood gases (ABGs), preoxygenating and limiting suctioning to 10 seconds or less, ensuring a patent airway, and delivering $O_2$ as prescribed. It may also include maintenance of mechanical ventilation as necessary. | Preventing hypoxia necessitates maintaining oxygen saturation greater than 90% or $PaO_2$ greater than 60 mm Hg. Endotracheal suctioning can result in a sudden increase in ICP and decreased CPP, and may put the patient at risk for further cerebral damage. Prevention of $CO_2$ retention (and the resulting respiratory acidosis) is essential for preventing vasodilation of cerebral arteries, which can lead to cerebral edema. |
| Assess CBF measurements, continuous jugular venous oxygen saturation ($SjO_2$), and brain tissue oxygenation ($PbtO_2$) values to assess for the effectiveness of hyperventilation if an Ambu bag or mechanical ventilation is used as a treatment. | Mechanical hyperventilation, by lowering cerebral $PaCO_2$, results in an alkalosis, which causes cerebral vasoconstriction resulting in decreased CBF and ICP. The vasoconstriction also may cause decreased cerebral oxygen delivery, which could increase injury by increasing cerebral ischemia. Hyperventilation is now generally used only in cases of acute deterioration as a "quick fix" until other interventions can be instituted (e.g., mannitol) or in cases in which increased ICP is refractory and responds to nothing else. |
| **!** Maintain head and neck alignment to avoid hyperextension, flexion, or rotation, ensure that tracheostomy, endotracheal tube ties, or $O_2$ tubing do not compress the jugular veins, and do not place patient in the Trendelenburg position. | Failure to comply with these measures will lead to a further increase in ICP. These measures promote venous blood return to the heart and therefore reduce cerebral congestion. |
| Ensure that pillows under the patient's head are flat. | This measure maintains the head in a neutral rather than flexed position and thereby prevents increased ICP by preventing backup of jugular venous outflow. |
| Keep head of bed (HOB) at whatever level optimizes CPP. | CPP needs to be at least 70 mm Hg or as prescribed to prevent ischemia. Elevating the head of the bed promotes drainage from the head and decreased the vascular congestion that can produce cerebral edema. Raising the bed above 30 degrees may decrease the CPP by lowering systemic BP. |
| **!** Take precautions against increased intraabdominal and intrathoracic pressures in the following ways:<br>• Teach the patient to exhale when turning or during activity.<br>• Provide passive range-of-motion (ROM) exercises rather than allow active or assistive exercises.<br>• Avoid extreme hip flexion.<br>• Do not place patient in prone position. | Elevated intraabdominal and intrathoracic pressures interfere with cerebral venous drainage thus adding to increased ICP.<br>Exhaling with activity and passive ROM (vs active ROM) reduce intrathoracic pressure.<br>Extreme hip flexion and prone positioning increase intraabdominal pressure. |
| • Administer prescribed stool softeners or laxatives; avoid enemas and suppositories. | These measures prevent straining at stool, which would increase intraabdominal and ICPs. |
| • Instruct the patient not to move self in bed; to allow only passive turning; and to use a pull sheet and avoid pushing against foot of bed or pulling against side rails. Avoid footboards; use high-top tennis shoes with toes removed to level of the metatarsal heads instead. | Movements involving pushing would increase intraabdominal and intrathoracic pressures. |
| • Assist the patient with sitting up and turning. | This action prevents increases in intraabdominal and intrathoracic pressures. |
| • Instruct the patient that if they need to cough or sneeze, to do so with an open mouth; provide antitussive for cough as prescribed and antiemetic for vomiting. | Coughing and sneezing with closed mouth may increase intrabdominal and intrathoracic pressures. |
| • Avoid using restraints. | Restraint application may cause straining, agitation, fear, and anxiety. This can increase ICP and BP and lead to increased ICP. |
| **!** Administer intravenous (IV) fluids with an infusion control device to prevent fluid overload. Keep accurate intake and output (I&O) and daily weight records. | IV fluids are given to maintain normovolemia and balanced electrolyte status. Fluid and electrolyte problems can have an adverse effect on ICP. I&O, accounting for insensible losses, and daily weights are important parameters in the assessment of fluid balance. |

Continued

| ASSESSMENT—RECOGNIZE CUES/ INTERVENTIONS—TAKE ACTION | RATIONALES |
|---|---|
| Help maintain the patient's body temperature within normal limits by giving prescribed antipyretics, regulating the temperature of the environment, using a fan, limiting the use of blankets, keeping the patient's trunk warm to prevent shivering, and administering tepid sponge baths or using a warming/cooling blanket or convection cooling units to reduce fever. | Hypothalamic dysfunction from swelling or injury may cause hyperthermia. In turn, fever increases the metabolic rate (5%–7% for each 1°C) and exacerbates increased ICP. |
| When using a hypothermia blanket, wrap the patient's extremities in blankets or towels, and if prescribed, administer chlorpromazine. | Both measures prevent shivering, which would increase ICP. Mild (e.g., 95°F [35°C]) hypothermia treatment also may be attempted to minimize the metabolic needs of the brain if ICP is increased. |
| Administer prescribed osmotic (e.g., mannitol) and loop diuretics (e.g., furosemide). | These agents reduce cerebral edema and blood volume, thereby lowering ICP. |
| Administer BP medications as prescribed. | These medications keep BP within prescribed limits that will promote optimal CBF without increasing cerebral edema. Hypotension is particularly detrimental inasmuch as it directly affects CBF. Hypertension may be allowed or treated first with drugs such as labetalol. Vasoactive drugs such as nitroprusside may worsen cerebral edema through vasodilation. |
| Administer prescribed analgesics promptly and as necessary. | Pain can increase ICP. Barbiturates and opioids usually are contraindicated because of the potential for masking the signs of increased ICP and causing respiratory depression. However, intubated, restless patients are usually sedated. A continuous propofol or midazolam drip can be used to decrease ICP. Lidocaine is sometimes used to block coughing before suctioning an endotracheal tube. |
| Administer antiepileptic drugs (AEDs) as prescribed. | AEDs prevent or control seizures, which would increase cerebral metabolism, hypoxia, and $CO_2$ retention, which in turn would increase cerebral edema and ICP. |
| Monitor bladder drainage tubes for obstruction or kinks. Flush as prescribed if an obstruction is suspected. | A distended bladder can increase ICP. |
| Provide a quiet and soothing environment with minimal stimulation to patient. Control noise and other environmental stimuli. Use a gentle touch and avoid jarring the bed. Coordinate with team members to minimize procedures that may cause agitation. Avoid unnecessary touch (e.g., leave BP cuff in place for frequent VS; use automatic recycling BP monitoring devices); and talk softly, explaining procedures before touching to avoid startling the patient. Try to avoid situations in which the patient may become emotionally upset. Do not say anything in the presence of the patient that you would not say if he or she were awake. Limit visitors as necessary. | A quiet, calm environment with minimal noise, stimulation, and interruptions will help decrease anxiety and irritation. This will help keep BP and metabolism within therapeutic limits. |
| Encourage significant others to speak quietly to the patient. If possible, arrange for the patient to listen to soft favorite music with earphones. | Hearing a familiar voice or listening to soft music may promote relaxation and decrease ICP. |
| Individualize care to ensure rest periods and optimal spacing of activities; avoid turning, suctioning, and taking VS all at one time. Plan activities and treatments accordingly so that the patient can sleep undisturbed as often as possible. | Multiple procedures and nursing care activities can increase ICP. For example, rousing patients from sleep has been shown to increase ICP. |
| Administer mild sedatives (e.g., diphenhydramine) or antianxiety agents (haloperidol, lorazepam, midazolam) as prescribed to a restless/ agitated patient. Attempt to identify and relieve the cause (e.g., overstimulation, pain) before medicating. | These measures decrease restlessness or decrease/control agitation that may increase ICP. |
| Administer sedation and skeletal muscle relaxants (e.g., propofol, atracurium, pancuronium) as prescribed. (This therapy requires intubation and ventilation.) | These agents decrease the skeletal muscle tension that is seen with abnormal flexion and extension posturing, which can increase ICP. |

## Patient Problem/Analyze Cues/Prioritize Hypotheses

# Risk for Aspiration

*due to* the facial and throat muscle weakness, depressed gag or cough reflex, dysphagia, or decreased LOC

***Desired Outcomes/Generate Solutions:*** The patient is free of the signs of aspiration, as evidenced by eupnea, RR of 12–20 breaths/minute, $O_2$ saturation greater than 92%, color appropriate to race, with absence of adventitious breath sounds, normothermia. Following instruction and on an ongoing basis, the patient or significant other practices measures that prevent aspiration.

| ASSESSMENT—RECOGNIZE CUES/ INTERVENTIONS—TAKE ACTION | RATIONALES |
|---|---|
| For patients with new or increasing neurologic deficit, collaborate with the speech pathologist who will perform a dysphagia screening to assess for impaired swallowing. | Dysphagia screening will identify patients at risk for aspiration. These patients should be kept nothing by mouth (NPO) until a swallowing evaluation can be performed. |
| Assess lung sounds before and after the patient eats, effectiveness of the patient's cough, and quality, amount, and color of sputum. | New onset of crackles or wheezing can signal aspiration. Patients with a weak cough are at risk for aspiration. An increase in quantity or color change of sputum may indicate an infection from aspiration. |
| Keep HOB elevated after meals or assist the patient into a right-side-lying position. | This position facilitates the flow of ingested food and fluids by gravity from the greater stomach curve to the pylorus, thereby minimizing the potential for regurgitation and aspiration. |
| If indicated, consult the health care provider about the use of an upper gastrointestinal (GI) stimulant. | Stimulating upper GI tract motility and gastric emptying help to decrease the potential for regurgitation. |
| Provide oral hygiene after meals. | Oral hygiene removes food particles that could be aspirated. |
| Assess the mouth frequently and suction as needed. | These actions assess for particles or secretions that could be aspirated and removes them. |
| If the patient has nausea or vomiting or has secretions, turn on one side. | This position facilitates secretion drainage from mouth and prevents aspiration. |
| Anticipate the need for an artificial airway if secretions cannot be cleared. | These measures help ensure a patent airway. |
| For general interventions, see this patient problem in "Older Adult Care," Chapter 3, and *Impaired Swallowing,* below in this chapter. | |

## Patient Problem/Analyze Cues/Prioritized Hypotheses (For Those Who Are Ventilated)

# Risk for Infection

*due to* inadequate primary defenses occurring with ventilator intubation in patients with neurologic disorders such as Guillain–Barré syndrome, bacterial meningitis, spinal cord injury (SCI), traumatic brain injury, and stroke

***Desired Outcome/Generate Solutions:*** The patient exhibits the absence of ventilator-associated pneumonia (VAP), as evidenced by normothermia, white blood cell count of 11,000/mm³ or less, sputum clear to whitish in color, lungs clear to auscultation, and oxygen saturation greater than 92%.

| ASSESSMENT—RECOGNIZE CUES/ INTERVENTIONS—TAKE ACTION | RATIONALES |
|---|---|
| Ensure that the ventilator bundle discussed in the following interventions has been implemented on any patient who is mechanically ventilated. | This bundle is a series of interventions that, when implemented together (rather than individually), is associated with decreased incidence of VAP. VAP is a leading cause of prolonged hospital stay and death. |
| Perform appropriate hand hygiene before and after contact with the patient (even though gloves are worn). | Hand hygiene helps prevent the spread of infection by removing pathogens from hands. Hand hygiene involves using alcohol-based waterless antiseptic agent (if hands are not visibly soiled) or soap and water. |
| Assess lung sounds, sputum characteristics, HR, temperature, oxygen saturation, ABG values, chest radiograph, and complete blood count. Report abnormal values/findings to the health care provider. | Assessing for and reporting early indicators of infection will enable prompt intervention and treatment. |
| Elevate HOB, preferably to 30 degrees if it is not contraindicated. | This elevated HOB position reduces the risk for aspirating gastric contents by promoting the stomach contents to empty into small intestine contents. This position may be contraindicated in some patients. |
| Ensure frequent position changes. | Frequent turning facilitates the drainage of secretions. |
| On a daily basis, attempt a spontaneous awakening trial ("sedation vacations") per facility protocol or as prescribed, and assess and document neurologic status and readiness to extubate. For example, "Patient awake, breathing at a sufficient rate and depth of breaths to maintain oxygenation, is able to cough and protect airway and has adequate ABG values." Note prior documentation as a basis of comparison (e.g., improvement or deterioration) and notify the care provider as appropriate (e.g., if patient does not wake or respond despite sedation being turned off). | These measures promote early extubation and minimize sedation. A spontaneous awakening trial involves reducing sedation until the patient is awake and can follow simple commands or becomes agitated. During this "awake" time, a weaning trial may be done to test the patient's ability to breathe spontaneously. The patient's unsedated neurologic status also can be tested. If sedation is reinstated, it can be titrated to the minimal amount needed to achieve a calm, relaxed state. Decreasing sedation reduces the amount of time spent on mechanical ventilation and therefore the risk for VAP. |
| Ensure a closed endotracheal suction system, ideally one that allows for continuous subglottic secretion drainage. | A closed system reduces the risk for contamination. A system that also allows for continuous subglottic secretion drainage will further reduce contamination of the lower airway by removing stagnant oropharyngeal secretions above the cuff that might otherwise be aspirated. |
| When possible, use oral tubes rather than nasal tubes. | Oral tubes reduce the risk for sinusitis and aspiration of infected secretions. |
| Provide oral hygiene every 2 hours or as recommended by facility protocol, possibly including use of a dental oral antibiotic rinse (e.g., chlorhexidine gluconate washes). | Oral hygiene reduces oral bacterial flora, which could be aspirated. Swabs and toothbrushes with built-in suction catheter capability may facilitate oral care. |
| As prescribed, implement other components that may be included in the bundle. | Many agencies also include peptic ulcer disease prophylaxis (to reduce mini-aspiration of acid secretions). |

## Patient Problem/Analyze Cues/Prioritize Hypotheses

# Impaired Tissue Integrity (Corneal)

*due to* irritation occurring with diminished blink reflex or inability to close the eyes

**Desired Outcome/Generate Solutions:** The patient's corneas become/remain clear and intact.

| ASSESSMENT—RECOGNIZE CUES/ INTERVENTIONS—TAKE ACTION | RATIONALES |
|---|---|
| If the patient has a diminished blink reflex or is stuporous or comatose, assess the eyes for irritation or presence of foreign objects such as red, itchy, scratchy, or painful eye; sensation of foreign object in eye; scleral edema; blurred vision; or mucus discharge. | The listed signs and symptoms are indicative of corneal irritation. |

| ASSESSMENT—RECOGNIZE CUES/ INTERVENTIONS—TAKE ACTION | RATIONALES |
| --- | --- |
| Instill prescribed eye drops or ointment. Instruct coherent patients to make a conscious effort to blink their eyes several times each minute. Apply eye patches or warm, sterile compresses over closed eyes. | These actions provide corneal lubrication and prevent corneal irritation. Normally, blinking occurs every 5–6 seconds. |
| If the eyes cannot be completely closed, use caution in applying an eye shield or taping eyes shut. Consider the use of moisture chambers (plastic eye bubbles), protective glasses, soft contacts, or humidifiers. | Semiconscious patients may open their eyes underneath the shield or tape and injure their corneas. |
| For chronic eye closure problems, consider the use of special springs or weights on the upper lids. | These measures help ensure closure of the eyelid. |
| Teach the patient to avoid exposing eyes to talc or baby powder, wind, cold air, smoke, dust, sand, or bright sunlight. Instruct the patient not to rub the eyes. Advise wearing glasses to protect against wind and dust and to wear tight-fitting goggles when swimming. | These are irritants that could harm the corneas. |

## Patient Problem/Analyze Cues/Prioritize Hypotheses

# Dehydration

*due to* the facial and throat muscle weakness, depressed gag or cough reflex, dysphagia, or decreased LOC affecting access to and intake of fluids

***Desired Outcome/Generate Solutions:*** Normovolemia, as evidenced by balanced I&O, stable weight, elastic skin turgor, moist mucous membranes, stable BP within the patient's baseline, HR of 100 bpm or less, normothermia, and urinary output of at least 30 mL/hour with a specific gravity of 1.030 or less.

| ASSESSMENT—RECOGNIZE CUES/ INTERVENTIONS—TAKE ACTION | RATIONALES |
| --- | --- |
| Assess gag reflex, alertness, and ability to cough and swallow before offering fluids. | These assessments demonstrate whether the patient has intact swallowing and gag reflexes, can cough, and is alert and therefore can safely ingest fluids. |
| Keep suction equipment at the bedside if indicated. | This enables immediate intervention in the event of aspiration. |
| Assess the I&O. Involve the patient or significant others with keeping fluid intake records. Obtain daily weight measurements if the patient is at risk for sudden fluid shifts or imbalances. | Patients with neurologic deficits may have difficulty attaining adequate fluid intake. Assessment of I&O values and daily weight changes will provide information on patient's fluid balance. Involving patients and significant others in record keeping optimally will keep them aware of the need for increased oral intake and influence their participation in fluid intake accordingly. |
| Alert the health care provider to a significant I&O imbalance. | This imbalance may signal the need for enteral or IV therapy to prevent dehydration. |
| Assess for and teach the patient and significant others such indicators as thirst, poor skin turgor, decreased BP, increased pulse rate, dry skin and mucous membranes, increased body temperature, concentrated urine (specific gravity more than 1.030), and decreased urinary output. | These are indicators of dehydration. Conditions such as fever and diarrhea increase fluid loss and risk for dehydration. A knowledgeable person is more likely to report these indicators promptly for timely intervention and will understand the need to increase fluid intake during conditions that increase the risk of dehydration. |
| Evaluate fluid preferences (type and temperature). Offer fluids every 1–2 hours. Establish a fluid goal. Unless contradicted, encourage a fluid intake of at least 2–3 L/day. | Patients, especially if fatigued, will be more prone to consume preferred fluids in small volumes at frequent intervals. A fluid intake of 2–3 L/ day will keep patients well hydrated. Renal and cardiac patients may have fluid restrictions. |

Continued

| ASSESSMENT—RECOGNIZE CUES/ INTERVENTIONS—TAKE ACTION | RATIONALES |
|---|---|
| Feed or assist very weak or paralyzed patients. | Such measures help ensure that fluid goals are met. |
| Instruct the patient to flex head slightly forward when swallowing. | Flexing the head forward closes the airway and helps prevent aspiration. |
| Begin with small amounts of liquid. Instruct the patient to sip rather than gulp fluids. Do not hurry the patient. | Sipping small amounts tests and promotes a patient's ability to swallow the fluid. |
| For patients at risk for aspiration, use thickened fluids. Maintain an appropriate upright position while the patient is eating/drinking the meal and for at least 30 minutes afterwards. | Thickened liquids form a cohesive bolus that can be swallowed more readily. Gravity aids swallowing, and staying upright decreases the risk for aspiration. |
| Provide periods of rest. | Rest prevents fatigue, which can contribute to decreased oral intake. |
| Provide oral care as needed. | Oral care promotes taste perception and prevents stomatitis, which otherwise may decrease oral intake. |
| If appropriate, provide assistive devices (e.g., plastic, unbreakable, special-handled, spill-proof cups or straws). | These devices promote independence, which is likely to increase fluid consumption. The individual who is with paralysis may be able to drink independently through extra-long tubing or a straw connected to a water pitcher. |
| Instruct patients with hemiparalysis or hemiparesis to tilt head toward the unaffected side. | This prevents the retention of fluids in paralyzed side and fluids will drain by gravity to the side of the face and throat over which the patient has control. |
| For patients with chewing or swallowing difficulties, see interventions under *Risk for Aspiration*, earlier in this chapter and *Impaired Swallowing*, later in this chapter. | |

## Patient Problem/Analyze Cues/Prioritize Hypotheses

# Altered Temperature (Increased)

*due to* illness or trauma affecting body temperature

***Desired Outcome/Generate Solutions:*** After interventions, the patient becomes/remains normothermic with core temperatures between 97.8°F and 100°F (36.5°C and 37.7°C).

| ASSESSMENT—RECOGNIZE CUES/ INTERVENTIONS—TAKE ACTION | RATIONALES |
|---|---|
| Assess oral, rectal, or tympanic, every 4 hours or, if the patient is in spinal shock, every 2 hours. | Infection and hypothalamic dysfunction as a result of cerebral insult (trauma, edema) are two common causes of fever. Rapid development of spinal lesions (e.g., in SCI) breaks the connection between the hypothalamus and sympathetic nervous system (SNS), causing an inability to adapt to environmental temperature. inability to perspire prevents normal cooling. **Caution:** Steroids may mask fever or infection. |
| Assess for flushed face, malaise, rash, respiratory distress, tachycardia, weakness, headache, and irritability. Monitor for complaints of being too warm, sweating, or hot and dry skin (in SCI patients, above the level of injury). | These are signs of fever. |
| Assess for parched mouth, furrowed tongue, dry lips, poor skin turgor, decreased urine output, increased concentration of urine (specific gravity greater than 1.030), and weak, fast pulse. | These are signs of dehydration that can occur as a result of fever. |

| ASSESSMENT—RECOGNIZE CUES/ INTERVENTIONS—TAKE ACTION | RATIONALES |
|---|---|
| **For fever:** Maintain a cool room temperature (68°F [20°C]). Provide a fan or air conditioning. Remove excess bedding and cover the patient with a thin sheet. Give tepid sponge baths. Place cool, wet cloths on the patient's head, neck, axilla, and groin. Administer antipyretic agent as prescribed. Use a padded hypothermia blanket (wrap hands and feet in towels or blankets to prevent shivering) or convection cooling device if prescribed. Provide cool drinks. Evaluate for a potential infectious cause. | These are measures that help prevent overheating. |
| Maintain dry skin. Change bed linens after diaphoresis. Provide careful skin care when the patient is on a hypothermia or hyperthermia blanket. | These actions prevent skin irritation and potential loss of skin integrity that could result from hyperthermia and diaphoresis. |
| Monitor the I&O and maintain adequate hydration. Unless contraindicated, encourage increased fluid intake in febrile patients (e.g., more than 3000 mL/day). | Insensible water loss from fever should be a consideration when monitoring I&O because it may affect total hydration. |
| Increase caloric intake. | Patients with fever have increased metabolic needs. |

## Patient Problem/Analyze Cues/Prioritize Hypotheses

# Altered Temperature (Decreased)

*due to* illness or trauma affecting body temperature

**Desired Outcome/Generate Solutions:** After interventions, the patient becomes/remains normothermic with core temperatures between 97.8°F and 100°F (36.5°C and 37.7°C).

| ASSESSMENT—RECOGNIZE CUES/ INTERVENTIONS—TAKE ACTION | RATIONALES |
|---|---|
| Assess oral, rectal, or tympanic temperature, every 4 hours or, if the patient is in spinal shock, every 2 hours. | Rapid development of spinal lesions (e.g., in SCI) breaks the connection between the hypothalamus and SNS, causing an inability to adapt to environmental temperature. In spinal cord shock, temperatures tend to lower toward the ambient temperature. Inability to vasoconstrict and shiver makes heat conservation difficult. |
| Assess for disorientation, confusion, drowsiness, apathy, and reduced HR and RR. Assess for complaints of being too cold, goosebumps (piloerection), and cool skin (in SCI patients, above the level of injury). | These are signs of hypothermia. |
| Increase the environmental temperature. Protect the patient from drafts. Provide warm drinks. Provide extra blankets. Provide warming (hyperthermia) blanket or convection warming device. | These are measures that help increase body temperature. |

## Problems for Patients With Subacute to Chronic Neurologic Issues

## Patient Problem/Analyze Cues/Prioritize Hypotheses

# Impaired Swallowing

*due to* decreased or absent gag reflex, decreased strength or excursion of muscles involved in mastication, perceptual impairment, or facial paralysis

**Desired Outcome/Generate Solutions:** Before oral foods and fluids are reintroduced, the patient exhibits the ability to swallow safely without aspirating.

| ASSESSMENT—RECOGNIZE CUES/ INTERVENTIONS—TAKE ACTION | RATIONALES |
|---|---|
| Assess for factors that affect the ability to swallow safely, including LOC, gag and cough reflexes, and strength and symmetry of tongue, lip, and facial muscles. | This assessment determines whether swallowing deficits are present that necessitate aspiration precautions. |
| • Assess for coughing, regurgitation of food and fluid through the nares and mouth, drooling, food trapped in buccal spaces, and development of a weak, "wet," or hoarse voice during or after eating. | These are signs of impaired swallowing. |
| • Check the swallow reflex by first asking the patient to swallow his or her own saliva. Place a finger gently on top of the larynx to determine if the larynx elevates with the attempt. Document your findings. | Inability to swallow own saliva and the presence of a stationary larynx during attempts to swallow signal the loss of the swallowing reflex. |
| **Caution:** The presence of the cough reflex is essential for the patient to relearn swallowing safely. | The cough reflex protects against aspiration and if delayed may signal silent aspiration. |
| Obtain a referral to a speech pathologist for patients with a swallowing dysfunction. | The act of swallowing is complex, and interventions vary according to the phase of swallowing that is dysfunctional. Patients with swallowing dysfunction are referred to speech pathologists for evaluation and recommendations of appropriate interventions. |
| Encourage the patient to practice prescribed exercises to facilitate swallowing. | Exercises such as tongue and jaw ROM; sound phonation such as "gah-gah-gah" to promote an elevation of the soft palate; puckering lips; and sticking the tongue out to touch the nose, chin, cheeks may be prescribed to facilitate swallowing ability. |
| Recognize that a nasogastric tube (NGT) may hinder the patient's ability to relearn to swallow. | NGTs may desensitize and impair reflexive response to food bolus stimulus. |
| Notify the health care provider of patient's swallowing impairment. | Enteral nutrition may be necessary for patients who cannot chew or swallow effectively or safely. |
| Keep suction equipment and a manual resuscitation bag with a face mask at the patient's bedside. Suction secretions in the patient's mouth as necessary. | This equipment enables immediate intervention in the event aspiration occurs. |
| Ensure that the patient is alert and responsive to verbal stimuli before attempting to swallow. Provide a rest period before meals or swallowing attempts. | Patients who are drowsy, inattentive, or fatigued have difficulty cooperating and are at risk for aspirating. |
| Initiate swallowing attempts with plain thickened liquids. Progressively add easy-to-swallow foods and liquids as the patient's ability to swallow improves. Determine and document which foods and liquids are easiest for the patient to swallow. | Generally, semisolid foods of medium consistency, such as puddings, hot cereals, and casseroles, tend to be easiest to swallow. Thicker liquids, such as nectars, tend to be better tolerated than thin liquids. |
| If indicated/prescribed, add commercially available powders (e.g., Thicket) to liquids. | Thickening foods increases their viscosity and makes them more easily swallowed. Gravy or sauce added to dry foods often facilitates swallowing as well. |
| Avoid giving peanut butter, chocolate, or milk. | Foods such as these may stick in the patient's throat or produce mucus and increase aspiration risk. |
| Avoid nuts, hard candies, or popcorn. | These foods may be aspirated. |
| Reduce stimuli in the room (e.g., turn off television, minimize conversation, and limit disruptions from phone calls). Caution the patient not to talk while eating. | These measures help the patient focus on swallowing. |
| If the patient must remain in bed, use high-Fowler position if possible. Support the shoulders and neck with pillows. | Most patients swallow best when in an upright position. Sitting in a straight-back chair with feet on the floor is ideal. |
| Ensure that the patient's head is erect and flexed forward slightly, with the chin at midline and pointing toward the chest (i.e., the "chin tuck"). | This head position minimizes the risk that food will go into the airway by forcing the epiglottis to close over the trachea and create an open path to the esophagus. |

| ASSESSMENT—RECOGNIZE CUES/ INTERVENTIONS—TAKE ACTION | RATIONALES |
|---|---|
| Maintain the patient in an upright position for at least 30–60 minutes after eating. | This position helps prevent regurgitation and aspiration by facilitating the flow of foods and fluids by gravity from the stomach to the small intestine. |
| Teach the patient to break down the act of chewing and swallowing into the following steps:<br>• Take small bites or sips (approximately 5 mL each).<br>• Place food on the tongue.<br>• Use the tongue to transfer food so that it is directly under the teeth on the unaffected side of the mouth.<br>• Chew food thoroughly.<br>• Move food to the middle of the tongue and hold it there.<br>• Flex the neck and tuck the chin against the chest.<br>• Hold the breath and think about swallowing.<br>• Without breathing, raise the tongue to the roof of mouth and swallow.<br>• Swallow several times if necessary.<br>• When the mouth is empty, raise the chin and clear the throat or cough purposefully once or twice. | Taking patients through these steps promotes concentration and focus, which will help ensure optimal swallowing. |
| Start with small amounts of food or liquid. Feed slowly. | For optimum safety, each bite should not exceed 5 mL (1 tsp). |
| Ensure that each previous bite has been swallowed. Check the mouth for pockets of food. After every few bites of solid food, provide a liquid to help clear the mouth. | Food may become pocketed in the affected side of the mouth, which could result in aspiration. |
| Avoid using a syringe. | The force of the fluid in the syringe, if sprayed, may cause aspiration. |
| Avoid the use of drinking straws. | The act of sucking may add to the complexity of swallowing and allow too much liquid to enter the mouth, thereby increasing the risk for aspiration. |
| Instruct the patient who has food that pockets in the buccal spaces to periodically sweep the mouth with the tongue or finger or to clean these areas with a napkin. Explain that applying external pressure to the cheek with a finger will help remove trapped food. | These actions help prevent the aspiration of food particles, stomatitis, and tooth decay. |
| Teach the patient who has a weak or paralyzed side to place food on the side of the face that he or she can control. | Tilting the head toward the stronger side will allow gravity to help keep food or liquid on the side of the mouth patients can manipulate. |
| Serve only warm or cool foods to individuals with loss of oral sensation. | Patients with loss of oral sensation may be unable to identify foods or fluids of tepid temperature with the tongue or oral mucosa. Verbal cues and the use of a mirror may help ensure that these patients keep their mouths clear after swallowing. |
| Encourage repeated swallowing attempts. Evaluate swallowing ability at different times of the day and reschedule mealtimes to times when the patient has improved swallowing, such as when well rested or in relationship to medications that may impact swallowing behavior (as seen in diseases such as Parkinson disease [PD]). | This is done to facilitate the movement of food. Patients with a pathology that affects swallowing such as PD and stroke have difficulty getting the tongue to move a bolus of food into the pharynx for swallowing. |
| If decreased salivation is contributing to swallowing difficulties, perform one of the following before feeding: swab the patient's mouth with a lemon-glycerin sponge; have the patient suck on a tart-flavored hard candy, dill pickle, or lemon slice; teach the patient to move the tongue in a circular motion against the inside of the cheek; or use artificial saliva. | These actions stimulate salivation, which optimally will contribute to effective swallowing. |

Continued

| ASSESSMENT—RECOGNIZE CUES/ INTERVENTIONS—TAKE ACTION | RATIONALES |
|---|---|
| Moisten food with melted butter, broth or other soup, or gravy. Dip dry foods such as toast into coffee or other liquid. | These actions moisten and soften food when salivation is decreased. |
| Investigate medications the patient is taking for the potential side effect of decreased salivation. | Drugs such as anti-Parkinson medications or those with extrapyramidal side effects may result in decreased salivation. |
| Consult with the health care provider regarding the use of tablets, capsules, and liquids for patients with swallowing difficulties. Check with the pharmacist to confirm that crushing a tablet or opening a capsule does not adversely affect its absorption or duration (i.e., slow-release medications should not be crushed). | Tablets or capsules may be swallowed more easily when added to foods such as puddings or ice cream. Crushed tablets or opened capsules also mix easily into these types of foods. Liquid forms of medications also may be available through the pharmacy. |
| For patients taking anti-Parkinson medications, assess the relationship of peak medication effect with swallowing. | Coordinating meals with peak medication effect may facilitate swallowing. |
| Teach significant others and caregivers the Heimlich or abdominal thrust maneuver. | This information helps ensure intervention in the event of a patient's choking. |

## Patient Problem/Analyze Cues/Prioritize Hypotheses

# Risk for Falls

*due to* weakness, impaired balance, or unsteady gait occurring with sensorimotor deficit

***Desired Outcomes/Generate Solutions:*** The patient is free of trauma caused by gait unsteadiness. Before hospital discharge, the patient demonstrates proficiency with assistive devices if appropriate.

| ASSESSMENT—RECOGNIZE CUES/ INTERVENTIONS—TAKE ACTION | RATIONALES |
|---|---|
| Assess gait and monitor for weakness, difficulty with balance, tremors, spasticity, or paralysis. | These are indicators of motor deficits that could lead to falls. |
| Incorporate a fall risk assessment tool into the patient's plan of care. Include appropriate interventions, specific-to-patient lifting/ transferring/mobilization aids and techniques, and the appropriate amount of assistance. Update with changes in patient status. | Assessment and documentation of the patient's fall risk provide added insurance in helping to prevent injury resulting from falls. |
| Assist the patient as needed when unsteady gait, weakness, or paralysis is noted. Instruct the patient to ask or call for assistance with ambulation. Frequently check on patients who may forget to call for assistance. Stand on the patient's weak side to assist with balance and support. Use a transfer belt for safety. Instruct the patient to use a stronger side for gripping railing when stair climbing or using a cane. | These measures minimize the risk for falls by providing assistance and surveillance. |
| Orient the patient to new surroundings. Keep necessary items (including water, snacks, phone, call light) within easy reach. | These measures minimize the risk for falls as a result of strange environment, unfamiliarity with such items as the call light, and the need to walk to get them. |
| Assess the patient's ability to use necessary items. | Patients who are very weak or partially paralyzed may require a tap bell or specially adapted call light. |
| Maintain an uncluttered environment with unobstructed walkways. Ensure adequate lighting at night (e.g., provide a night light) to help prevent falls in the dark. In addition, keep side rails up and bed in its lowest position with bed brakes on. | These measures promote safety by ensuring better sensory acuity. |

| ASSESSMENT—RECOGNIZE CUES/ INTERVENTIONS—TAKE ACTION | RATIONALES |
|---|---|
| Encourage the patient to use any needed hearing aids and corrective lenses when ambulating. | These measures minimize the risk for tripping, falls in the dark, or injury from the inability to see or hear. |
| For unsteady, weak, or partially paralyzed patients, encourage the use of low-heel, nonskid, supportive shoes for walking. Teach the use of a wide-based gait. | These measures minimize the risk for falls in patients with special needs. |
| Instruct the patient to note foot placement when ambulating or transferring. | This action ensures that the foot is flat and in a position of support before the patient ambulates and transfers. |
| Teach, reinforce, and encourage the use of an assistive device, such as a cane, walker, or crutches. | These devices provide added stability. |
| • Instruct patient about exercises that strengthen arm and shoulder muscles for using walkers and crutches. Instruct patient on the safe use of transfer or sliding boards. Instruct patients in wheelchairs on how and when to lock and unlock wheels. | These actions promote added stability and safety. |
| Demonstrate how to secure and support weak or paralyzed arms. | These actions help prevent subluxation and injury from falling into wheelchair spokes or wheels. |
| Collaborate with physical therapist (PT) to aassess patients with poor sitting balance for the potential need for a seat or chest belt, H-straps for leg positioning, and a wheelchair with an anti-tip device. | Such devices likely will prevent patients with poor sitting balance from falling or tipping the wheelchair. |
| Teach the patient to maintain a sitting position before assuming a standing position for ambulating. | Maintaining this position for a few minutes gives the patient time to get the feet flat and under self for balance and minimizes any dizziness that may occur because of rapid position changes. |
| Monitor spasticity, antispasmodic medications, and their effect on physical function. | Uncontrolled or severe spasms may cause falls, whereas mild to moderate spasms can be useful in activities of daily living (ADLs) and transfers if patients learn to control and trigger them. |
| Review with the patient and significant others potential safety needs at home. | Including the family/significant others in instructions on home safety measures will decrease the patient's fall risk at home. |
| Such measures include safety appliances (wall, bath, toilet grab rails; elevated toilet seat; nonslip surface in bathtub or shower). Loose rugs should be removed to prevent slipping and falling. Temperatures on hot-water heaters should be turned down to prevent scalding in the event of a fall in the shower or tub. Furniture in the home may need to be moved to provide clear, safe pathways that avoid sharp corners on furniture, glass cabinets, or large windows the patient could fall against. Strategically placed additional lighting also may be needed. Edges of steps in the home may require taping with brightly colored strips to provide sufficient contrast so that edges can be recognized and more safely negotiated. Beds should be modified to prevent rolling. Activity should be balanced with rest periods because fatigue tends to increase unsteadiness and potential for falls. Ramps may need to be used instead of stairs. | |
| Seek referral for a PT as appropriate. | Patients may have special needs that cannot be met by the nursing staff. |

## Patient Problem/Analyze Cues/Prioritize Hypotheses

# Risk for Injury

*due to* sensory deficit or decreased LOC

**Desired Outcomes/Generate Solutions:** The patient is free of indicators of injury caused by impaired pain, touch, and temperature sensations. Before hospital discharge, the patient and significant others identify factors that increase the potential for injury.

| ASSESSMENT—RECOGNIZE CUES/ INTERVENTIONS—TAKE ACTION | RATIONALES |
|---|---|
| Assess patient for decreased or absent vision and impaired temperature and pain sensation. | These sensory deficits could result in patient injury. |
| Document baseline neurologic and physical assessments. | These assessments enable rapid detection of deteriorating status so that changes can be detected and responded to promptly, thereby helping prevent injury. |
| Avoid the use of heating pads. Encourage the use of sunscreen when outside. Do not serve scalding hot foods and beverages. | Patients with neurosensory deficits may not be able to detect temperature. These measures protect patients from exposure to hot items and sun that can burn the skin. |
| Always check the temperature of heating devices and bath water before the patient is exposed to them. Teach the patient and significant other about these precautions. | Patients with neurosensory deficits may not recognize temperature extremes. |
| Inspect skin twice daily for evidence of irritation. Teach coherent patients to perform self-inspection and provide a mirror for inspecting posterior aspects of the body. | The patient with neurosensory deficits may not be able to feel skin irritation. |
| Use emollient lotions liberally on the patient's skin. | These lotions keep skin soft and pliable and less likely to break down. |
| Teach the patient to inspect the placement of limbs with altered sensation. | This helps ensure that limbs are in a safe and supported position and decreases the risk of skin breakdown from increased pressure on boney areas. |
| Pad wheelchair seat, preferably with a gel pad. | Padding evenly distributes weight and decreases pressure areas that could result in skin breakdown. |
| Teach the patient to change position every 15–30 minutes by lifting self and shifting position from side to side and forward to backward. Encourage frequent turning while in bed and, if tolerated and not contraindicated, periodic movement into prone position. | Changing positions and turning promote circulation and prevent pressure wounds. Patients likely will not sense the need to do this and therefore should do it on a scheduled basis. Spending time in the prone position (if not contraindicated) with hips extended helps prevent hip flexion contractures. |
| Have the patient lift, not drag, self during transfers. | This action prevents shearing damage to the skin. |
| Avoid injecting more than 1 mL into a flaccid muscle. If possible, give injections only in muscles with tone. | Injections into muscles with tone will enable better absorption with less risk for sterile abscess formation. |

## Patient Problem/Analyze Cues/Prioritize Hypotheses

# Body Weight Problem (Weight Loss)

*due to* chewing and swallowing deficits, fatigue, weakness, paresis, paralysis, visual neglect, or decreased LOC

***Desired Outcome/Generate Solutions:*** The patient achieves adequate nutrition as evidenced by energy level that meets metabolic needs, maintenance of or return to baseline body weight, appropriate BMI, serum albumin level of 3.4–5.4 g/dL, and meeting metabolic needs.

| ASSESSMENT—RECOGNIZE CUES/ INTERVENTIONS—TAKE ACTION | RATIONALES |
|---|---|
| Assess alertness, ability to cough and swallow, and gag reflexes before all meals. Keep suction equipment at the bedside if indicated. | Deficits found during this assessment signal that the patient is at risk for aspiration, which in turn could lead to imbalanced nutrition. |
| Assess for the type of diet that can be eaten safely. Request soft, semisolid, or chopped foods as indicated. | Although a pureed diet may be needed, pureed food can be unappealing and may have a negative impact on self-concept as well as decrease the patient's intake. |

| ASSESSMENT—RECOGNIZE CUES/ INTERVENTIONS—TAKE ACTION | RATIONALES |
|---|---|
| Assess food preferences and offer small, frequent servings of nutritious food. Consider cultural or religious factors that may affect eating when evaluating food preferences. Encourage significant others to bring in the patient's favorite foods if not contraindicated. Plan meals for times when the patient is rested; use a warming tray or microwave oven to keep food warm and appetizing until the patient is able to eat. Serve cold foods while they are cold. | These measures will promote food intake. |
| Reduce stimuli in the room (e.g., turn off TV or radio) during meal time. Minimize conversation and other disruptions such as phone calls. If the patient wears glasses, put them on the patient; ensure adequate lighting. As needed, redirect the patient's attention to eating. | These measures help the patient focus on eating. |
| Provide oral care before feeding. Clean and insert dentures before each meal and ensure that they fit properly. | Oral care and good dentition promote comfort and the ability to taste and chew. |
| Encourage liquid nutritional supplements if not contraindicated. Try different methods to make them more palatable (e.g., making a milkshake, serving over ice, or diluting with carbonated beverages). | Making supplements more appetizing may promote intake. |
| Cut up foods, unwrap silverware, and otherwise prepare the food tray. | This assistance helps ensure that patients with a weak or paralyzed arm can manage the tray one-handed. |
| For patients with visual neglect, place food within the unaffected visual field. Return during the meal to ensure the patient has eaten from both sides of the plate. Turn the plate around so that any remaining food is in the patient's visual field. | These actions help ensure that the patient eats all or most of the food on the plate. |
| Feed or assist very weak or paralyzed patients. If not contraindicated, position the patient in a chair or elevate HOB as high as possible. Ensure that the patient's head is flexed slightly forward. Begin with small amounts of food. Encourage chewing food on the unaffected side. Do not hurry the patient. Be sure that each bite is completely swallowed before giving another. Encourage patients with hemiplegia to consciously sweep the paralyzed side of the mouth with the tongue to clear it. | Raising the HOB helps prevent aspiration by promoting the passage of food into the stomach and through the pylorus. Assisting the patient also helps conserve his or her energy and provides social interaction, which may promote eating. Flexing the head slightly forward closes the airway. |
| If appropriate, provide assistive devices such as built-up utensil handles, broad-handled spoons, spill-proof cups, rocker knife for cutting, wrist or hand splints with clamps to hold utensils, stabilized plates, and sectioned plates. | Assistive devices promote self-feeding and independence. |
| Provide materials for oral hygiene after meals. Give oral care to patients unable to do so for themselves. | Oral care minimizes the risk for aspiration of food particles. Good oral hygiene will also help maintain the integrity of mucous membranes to the minimize risk for stomatitis, which otherwise may prevent adequate oral intake. |
| Document the assessment of the patient's appetite. Weigh the patient regularly (at least weekly) to assess for loss or gain. If indicated, notify the health care provider of the potential need for high-protein or high-calorie supplements. | The trend of the patient's weight is a good indicator of nutritional status. Calculation of weight enables the determination of the percentage below the ideal weight for height and frame. |
| Obtain dietitian consultation. | The dietician is able to develop a diet regimen that specifically meets the patient's nutritional needs. |
| For weak, debilitated, or partially paralyzed patients, assess support systems, such as family or friends, who can assist the patient with meals. Consider referral to an organization that will deliver a daily meal to the patient's home. | These actions help ensure optimal nutritional status. |
| If appropriate for the patient's diagnosis (e.g., multiple sclerosis [MS]), consider referral to a speech pathologist. | This specialist will teach exercises that enhance the ability to swallow. |

Continued

Neurologic Care Plans

| ASSESSMENT—RECOGNIZE CUES/ INTERVENTIONS—TAKE ACTION | RATIONALES |
|---|---|
| For patients with visual problems, assess their ability to see food. Identify utensils and foods and describe their location. Arrange foods in an established pattern. | These measures promote independence with eating. Poor vision has been associated with lower caloric intake. |
| For patients with diplopia, consider patching one eye. | Patching one eye may enable better vision and patient will better be able to see their food. |
| For patients with chewing or swallowing difficulties, see interventions in *Risk for Aspiration* and *Impaired Swallowing*, earlier in this chapter. | |

## Patient Problem/Analyze Cues/Prioritize Hypotheses

# Acute Pain

*due to* spasms, headache, or photophobia occurring with neurologic dysfunction

**Desired Outcomes/Generate Solutions:** The patient's subjective perception of discomfort decreases, as documented by a pain scale. Objective indicators, such as grimacing, are absent or diminished.

| ASSESSMENT—RECOGNIZE CUES/ INTERVENTIONS—TAKE ACTION | RATIONALES |
|---|---|
| Assess characteristics (e.g., quality, severity, location, onset, duration, precipitating factors) of the patient's pain or spasms. Document discomfort on a scale of 0 (no pain) to 10 (worst pain). Determine the patient's acceptable pain level and ways of coping with and relieving pain. | These assessments demonstrate the degree and type of discomfort, the trend of the discomfort, and the relief obtained after interventions. A graphic pain scale using facial expressions may be used for patients who cannot use a numeric scale. |
| Respond immediately to the patient's complaints of pain. Administer analgesics and antispasmodics as prescribed. Document the effectiveness of the medication, using a pain scale, approximately 30–60 minutes after administration. Assess for untoward effects. Consult the health care provider if a dose or interval change seems necessary. | Prolonged stimulation of pain receptors results in increased sensitivity to painful stimuli and will increase the amount of medication required to relieve pain. |
| Instruct the patient and significant others about the importance of timing the pain medication. | Providing this information helps ensure that analgesia is taken before pain becomes too severe and before major moves. |
| Instruct the patient about the relationship between anxiety and pain, as well as other factors that enhance pain and spasms (e.g., staying in one position for too long, fatigue, chilling). | This information gives patients control over some causes of pain. |
| Instruct the patient and significant others in the use of nonpharmacologic pain management techniques. | These methods promote a sense of focus and self-control. |
| Such techniques as repositioning; ROM; supporting painful extremity or part; back rubs, acupressure, massage, warm baths, and other tactile distraction; auditory distractions such as listening to soothing music; visual distractions such as television; heat applications such as warm blankets or moist compresses; cold applications such as ice massage; guided imagery; breathing exercises; relaxation tapes and techniques; biofeedback; and a transcutaneous electrical nerve stimulation device may be effective when used to supplement pharmacologic treatment. | |
| Encourage rest periods. Try to provide uninterrupted sleep time at night. | Fatigue tends to exacerbate the pain experience. Pain may result in fatigue, which in turn may cause exaggerated pain and further exhaustion. |

| ASSESSMENT—RECOGNIZE CUES/ INTERVENTIONS—TAKE ACTION | RATIONALES |
|---|---|
| If patients have photophobia, provide a quiet and dark environment. Close the door and curtains, provide sunglasses, and avoid the use of artificial lights whenever possible. | These actions eliminate painful light sources for patients with photophobia. |
| Recognize that pain in the SCI patient often is poorly localized and may be referred. | In the SCI patient, intrascapular pain may be from the stomach, duodenum, or gallbladder. Umbilical pain may be from the appendix. Testicular or inner thigh pain may be from the kidneys (e.g., with pyelonephritis). It is important to recognize this type of pain in order to seek the correct treatment. |
| If the patient's present complaint of pain varies significantly from previous pain, or if interventions are ineffective, notify the health care provider. | These situations may signal a new or acute problem and should be reported promptly for timely intervention. |
| Evaluate patients with SCI for tachycardia, restlessness, urinary incontinence when it was previously controlled, and fever. | These are signs of infection or inflammatory processes that may or may not result in discomfort in the patient with SCI but should be reported promptly for timely intervention. |

Also see "Pain," Chapter 5.

## Patient Problem/Analyze Cues/Prioritize Hypotheses

# Risk for Impaired Communication

*due to* facial/throat muscle weakness, intubation, or tracheostomy

**Desired Outcome/Generate Solutions:** The patient communicates effectively, either verbally or nonverbally, and relates decreasing frustration with communication.

| ASSESSMENT—RECOGNIZE CUES/ INTERVENTIONS—TAKE ACTION | RATIONALES |
|---|---|
| Assess the patient's ability to speak, read, write, and comprehend. | This assessment helps determine the patient's communication abilities and interventions that would promote them. |
| If appropriate, obtain a referral to a speech pathologist. Encourage the patient to perform exercises that increase the ability to control facial muscles and tongue. Such exercises may include holding a sound for 5 seconds; singing the scale; reading aloud; and extending the tongue and trying to touch the chin, nose, or cheek. | These actions assist patients in strengthening muscles used in speech. A speech pathologist will assess swallowing ability and provide exercises to enhance swallowing and prevent aspiration. |
| Provide a supportive and relaxed environment for the patient who is unable to form words or sentences or who is unable to speak clearly or appropriately. Provide enough time for the patient to articulate. Ask the patient to repeat unclear words. Observe for nonverbal cues; watch the patient's lips closely. Do not interrupt or finish sentences. Anticipate needs and phrase questions to allow simple answers, such as "yes" or "no." | Patients likely will be frustrated over the inability to communicate. Maintaining a calm, positive, reassuring attitude and continuing to speak to patients using normal volume (unless hearing is impaired) will help ease frustrations. |
| Maintain eye contact. | This will help patients maintain focus. |
| If the patient is unable to speak, provide a language board, alphabet cards, picture or letter-number board, flash cards, pad and pencil. Other systems use eye blinks, tongue clicks, or hand squeezes; bell signal taps; or gestures such as hand signals, head nods, pantomime, or pointing. Use a communication board for urgent situations. | These are alternative methods of communication. |

Continued

| ASSESSMENT—RECOGNIZE CUES/ INTERVENTIONS—TAKE ACTION | RATIONALES |
|---|---|
| Document the method of communication used. | Documentation helps ensure that other health care team members use the same method. |
| If the patient's voice is weak and difficult to hear, reduce environmental noise. | This will enhance the listener's ability to hear and comprehend the patient's words. |
| Suggest that the patient take a deep breath before speaking; provide a voice amplifier if appropriate. | These measures project the patient's voice. |
| Encourage the patient to organize thoughts and plan what he or she will say before speaking. Encourage the patient to express ideas in short, simple phrases or sentences. | These measures help make efficient use of voice strength or breath the patient does have. |
| Remind the patient to speak slowly, exaggerate pronunciation, and use facial expressions. | Patients may have a flat effect in both pronunciation and facial expression. Exaggerating both may make the patient's conversation more engaging. |
| If the patient has swallowing difficulties that result in the accumulation of saliva, suction the mouth. | Suctioning will promote clearer speech. |
| If indicated, massage facial and neck muscles before the patient attempts to communicate. | Massage promotes clearer speech in patients with muscle rigidity or spasms. |
| If the patient has a tracheostomy, ensure that a tap bell is within reach. | Tap bell sounds give patients the means to communicate and increase a sense of self-control and safety. |
| Teach patients with a temporary tracheostomy that the ability to speak will return. | This provides reassurance about the future ability to communicate. |
| For patients with a permanent tracheostomy, discuss learning alternate communication systems. | Alternate communication systems include sign language or esophageal speech, in which fenestrated tubes or covering the tracheostomy tube opening with a finger will enable speech. |
| Establish a method of calling for assistance, and make sure the patient knows how to use it. Keep a calling device where the patient can activate it (e.g., place call bell on nonparalyzed side). Depending on the deficit, use a tap bell for a weak patient, a pillow pad call light (triggered by arm or head movement), or a sip and puff device (triggered by the mouth). | These measures ensure that patients of varying abilities will be able to call for assistance. |
| Encourage patients with the ability to write to keep a diary or write letters. If the patient has a weak writing arm, evaluate the need and consult with occupational therapist (OT) for a splint or other device that will enable the patient to hold a pen or pencil. | These measures provide a means of ventilating feelings and expressing concerns. Felt-tip markers are useful because they require minimal pressure for writing. Large-barrel pens may be easier for grasping and writing. Patients also may be able to type. For patients able to speak, a computer voice recognition program may facilitate written and e-mail communication. |

## Patient Problem/Analyze Cues/Prioritize Hypotheses

# Constipation

*due to* the inability to chew and swallow a high-fiber diet, side effects of medications, immobility, and neurologic (spinal cord) involvement

**Desired Outcome/Generate Solutions:** The patient passes soft, formed stools and regains and maintains normal bowel pattern.

| ASSESSMENT—RECOGNIZE CUES/ INTERVENTIONS—TAKE ACTION | RATIONALES |
|---|---|
| Teach patients with chewing and swallowing difficulties that consuming one or two servings of applesauce with added bran, prune juice, or cooked bran cereal each day may be effective. Otherwise encourage the use of natural fiber laxatives such as psyllium (e.g., Metamucil) as prescribed. | Although a high-roughage diet is ideal for patients who are immobilized or on prolonged bedrest, individuals with chewing and swallowing difficulties may be unable to consume such a diet. |
| For patients with impaired swallowing encourage the use of polyethylene glycol (MiraLAX) as prescribed. | With **polyethylene glycol**, there is less risk for choking. |
| Encourage/promote a bowel elimination program. Keep a call bell within the patient's reach.<br><br>Elements that may be included in a successful bowel elimination program include the following: setting a regular time of day for attempting a bowel movement, preferably 30 minutes after eating a meal or drinking a hot beverage; using a commode instead of a bedpan for more natural positioning during elimination; using a medicated suppository 15–30 minutes before a scheduled attempt; bearing down by contracting abdominal muscles or applying manual pressure to the abdomen to help increase intraabdominal pressure; and drinking 4 oz of prune juice nightly. | A bowel program creates a pattern that promotes regular bowel movements. It is important to assist patient to commode or bathroom before the urge to defecate subsides. |
| As indicated, include abdominal and pelvic exercises in the patient's morning and evening routine. | These exercises will help promote bowel evacuation. |
| Assess the patient's sitting balance and ability to assume a normal toileting position and intervene accordingly. | This will help ensure the patient's safety while on the commode. |
| ⚠ SCI patients with involvement at T8 and above should use extreme caution if using an enema or suppository. If either measure is unavoidable, use large amounts of anesthetic jelly in the rectum. | Either measure can precipitate life-threatening autonomic dysreflexia (AD). Using anesthetic jelly reduces that risk. |
| Instruct patients at risk for increased ICP not to bear down with bowel movements. | This action can cause increased intraabdominal pressure, which in turn increases ICP. See *Risk for Impaired Neurologic System Function*, earlier. |
| Unless contraindicated, encourage fluid intake to at least 2500 mL/day or more, including liberal amounts of fresh fruit juices. | Adequate fluid intake helps prevent hard, dry stools that are difficult to evacuate. |
| If indicated by the patient's diagnosis (e.g., MS), provide instructions for anal digital stimulation. | This action promotes reflex bowel evacuation. |
| ⚠ Avoid the above intervention for SCI patients with involvement at T8 or above. | At this level of involvement, anal digital stimulation can precipitate life-threatening AD. |
| For other interventions, see *Constipation*, in "Immobility," Chapter 1. | |

Patient Problem/Analyze Cues/Prioritize Hypotheses

# Impaired Functional Ability

*due to* spasticity, tremors, weakness, paresis, paralysis, or decreasing LOC resulting in inability to perform self-care

***Desired Outcomes/Generate Solutions:*** The patient performs care activities independently and demonstrates the ability to use adaptive devices for the successful completion of ADLs. (Totally dependent patients express satisfaction with activities that are completed for them.)

| ASSESSMENT—RECOGNIZE CUES/ INTERVENTIONS—TAKE ACTION | RATIONALES |
| --- | --- |
| Assess the patient's ability to perform ADLs. | This assessment demonstrates performance barriers and the degree to which patients need assistance with completing ADLs. These data will enable the development of an individualized care plan. |
| As appropriate, demonstrate the use of adaptive devices, such as long- or broad-handled combs; long-handled pickup sticks, brushes, and eating utensils; dressing sticks; stocking helpers; Velcro fasteners; elastic waistbands; nonspill cups; and stabilized plates. Also consider electric toothbrush and electric razor. Consult with OT to ensure appropriate equipment, demonstration, and patient education. | Adaptive devices may assist patients in maintaining independent care. For example, a flexor-hinge splint or universal cuff may aid in brushing teeth and combing hair. |
| Set short-range, realistic goals with the patient. Acknowledge progress. Encourage continued effort and involvement (e.g., in selection of meals, clothing). | These actions help decrease frustration and improve learning. |
| Provide care to totally dependent patients. Assist those who are not totally dependent according to the degree of disability. Encourage the patient to perform self-care to the maximum ability as defined by the patient. Encourage autonomy. | Promoting autonomy and positive self-image helps prevent learned helplessness. |
| Allow sufficient time for task performance; do not hurry the patient. Involve significant others with care activities if they are comfortable doing so. Ask for the patient's input in planning schedules. Supervise activity until the patient can safely perform tasks without help. | Preserving energy by providing sufficient time for the task increases activity tolerance. |
| Encourage the use of electronically controlled wheelchair and other technical advances (e.g., environmental control system) as prescribed and appropriate for patient. | These devices help improve mobility and enable independent operation of electronic devices such as lights, radio, door openers, and window shade openers. |
| Provide privacy and a distraction-free environment. Place the patient's belongings within reach. Set out items needed to complete self-care tasks in the order they are to be used. Apply any needed adaptive devices such as hand splints. | These actions convey respect, simplify the task, and increase motivation. |
| Encourage the patient to wear any prescribed corrective eye lenses or hearing aids. | Enhanced vision and hearing may increase participation in self-care. |
| Provide prescribed analgesics before self-care activity to prevent and/or relieve pain. | Pain can hinder self-care. |
| Provide a rest period before self-care activity, or plan activity for a time when the patient is rested. | Fatigue reduces self-care ability. |
| Encourage the patient or significant others to buy shoes without laces; long-handled shoe horns; front opening garments; wide-legged pants; and clothing that is loose-fitting with enlarged arm holes, front fasteners, zipper pulls, elastic waistbands, or Velcro closures. Avoid items with small buttons or tight buttonholes. Lay out clothing in the order it will be put on. Advise the patient to sit while dressing. Suggest that the use of a dressing stick may help to pull up pants or retrieve clothing. | These products and devices facilitate dressing and undressing. |
| Place a stool in the shower. | A stool will help patients for whom sitting down will enhance self-care with bathing. |
| Explain that bathrooms should have nonslip mats and grab bars. | These mats and bars promote safety in self-care by preventing falls. |
| Suggest the use of a handheld showerhead and a long-handled bath sponge or a washer mitt with a pocket that holds soap. | These devices and products facilitate autonomy in bathing. |
| Provide a commode chair, elevated toilet seat, or male or female urinal. | These chairs, seats, and urinals promote self-care with elimination. |

| ASSESSMENT—RECOGNIZE CUES/ INTERVENTIONS—TAKE ACTION | RATIONALES |
|---|---|
| Teach self-transfer techniques. | These techniques enable patients to get to the commode or toilet independently. |
| Keep the call light within the patient's reach. Instruct the patient to call as early as possible. | Calling early provides time for the staff to respond and the patient will not have to rush because of urgency. |
| Offer toileting reminders every 2 hours after meals, and before bedtime. | Toileting schedules convey the message that continence is valued, optimally reducing episodes of incontinence. |
| Suggest the use of a long-handled grasper that can hold tissues or washcloth for perineal care. | Some patients with limited hand or arm mobility may have difficulty with perineal care after elimination. |
| For patients with hemiparesis or hemiparalysis, teach the use of the stronger or unaffected hand and arm for dressing, eating, bathing, and grooming. Instruct the patient to dress the weaker side first. | These measures simplify tasks and conserve energy. |
| For patients with visual field deficit, avoid placing items on their blind side. Encourage the patient to scan the environment for needed items by turning the head. | These measures enable visualization of the task at hand. |
| Suggest the use of splints, weighted utensils, or wrist weights for patients with tremors. | Adaptive devices increase the speed and safety of self-care and decrease exertion. |
| Teach patients to rest their head against a high-backed chair. | Resting their head against a high-backed chair may reduce head tremors. |
| Obtain referral for an OT if indicated. | This referral will help determine the best method for performing activities. |
| Provide consistent caregiver and ADL routine for patients with cognitive deficits. | Individuals with cognitive defects need simple visual or verbal cues, increased gesture use, demonstration, reminders of next step, and gentle repetition. |
| If indicated provide instruction to the patient and/or caregiver on self-catheterization. | Patients who are unable to void due to SCI will need to self-catheterize in order to fully empty their bladder. |
| Provide the following instructions: At-home intermittent catheterization usually is done with a clean (not sterile) technique and equipment. The catheter is washed after use in warm, soapy water; rinsed; and placed in a clean plastic sack. Catheter insertion guides are available commercially for females with limited upper arm mobility. Crusted catheters are soaked in a solution of half distilled vinegar and half water. | |
| Teach the patient to assess for and notify the health professional of cloudy, foul-smelling, or bloody urine; urine with sediment; chills or fever; pain in lower back or abdomen; or a red or swollen urethral meatus. | These are indicators of urinary tract infection, which necessitates timely intervention. |
| Discuss, as appropriate, modifying the home environment. | Modifying the home environment (e.g., with extended sinks, grab bars, lower closet hooks, wheelchair-accessible shower, modified phones, lowered mirrors, and lever door handles that operate with reduced hand pressure) likely will promote independence and performance of ADLs at home. |
| Listen and provide opportunities for the patient to express self and communicate that it is normal to have negative feelings about changes in autonomy. Discuss with the health care team ways to provide consistent and positive encouragement and strategies that increase independence progressively. Suggest a local support group. | Frustration can be decreased and coping skills increased when an individual expresses feelings in a supportive environment. |

## Patient Problem/Analyze Cues/Prioritize Hypotheses

# Impaired Oral Mucous Membrane

*due to* barriers to oral care (sensorimotor deficit or decreased LOC)

**Desired Outcome/Generate Solutions:** The patient or significant others demonstrate the ability to perform the patient's oral care.

| ASSESSMENT—RECOGNIZE CUES/ INTERVENTIONS—TAKE ACTION | RATIONALES |
|---|---|
| Assess the patient's ability to perform mouth care. | This assessment enables the identification of performance barriers (e.g., sensorimotor or cognitive deficits). |
| If the patient has decreased LOC or is at risk for aspiration, remove dentures and store them in a water-filled denture cup. | This action protects and prevents the loss of dentures and decreases the risk of aspiration. |
| If the patient cannot perform mouth care, clean the teeth, tongue, and mouth at least twice daily with a soft-bristle toothbrush and nonabrasive toothpaste. | This intervention promotes oral hygiene and prevents the accumulation of bacteria that can cause oral inflammation. |
| If the patient is unconscious or at risk for aspiration, turn to a side-lying position. Swab the mouth and teeth with sponge-tipped applicator (Toothette) moistened with diluted (half strength) mouthwash solution and irrigate the mouth with a large syringe. If the patient cannot self-manage secretions, use only a small amount of liquid for irrigation each time, and, using a suction catheter or Yankauer tonsil suction tip, remove secretions. | These measures provide effective oral cleansing while preventing the aspiration of oral solutions. |
| Perform this oral hygiene regimen at least every 4 hours. As appropriate, teach the procedure to significant others. | Good oral hygiene helps prevent stomatitis and tooth decay and reduces the risk for infections caused by an oral mucous membrane that is not intact. |
| Make toothbrush adaptations for patients with physical disabilities. *For patients with limited hand mobility:* Enlarge the toothbrush handle by covering it with a sponge hair roller or aluminum foil (attaching with an elastic band) or by attaching a bicycle handle grip with plaster of Paris. *For patients with limited arm mobility:* Extend the toothbrush handle by overlapping another handle or rod over it and taping them together. | These adaptations will provide the patient with the opportunity to perform oral care independently. |

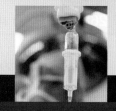

# Bacterial Meningitis 37

## OVERVIEW/PATHOPHYSIOLOGY

Bacterial meningitis is an infection that results in inflammation of the meningeal membranes covering the brain and spinal cord. Bacteria in the subarachnoid space multiply and cause an inflammatory reaction of the pia and arachnoid meninges. Purulent exudate is produced, and inflammation and infection spread quickly through the cerebrospinal fluid (CSF) that circulates around the brain and spinal cord. Bacteria and exudate can create vascular congestion, plugging the arachnoid villi. This obstruction of CSF flow and decreased reabsorption of CSF can lead to hydrocephalus, increased intracranial pressure (ICP), brain herniation, and death.

Meningitis generally is transmitted in one of four ways: (1) through airborne droplets or contact with oral secretions from infected individuals; (2) from direct contamination (e.g., from a penetrating skull wound; a skull fracture, often basilar, causing a tear in the dura; lumbar puncture [LP]; ventricular shunt; or surgical procedure); (3) through the bloodstream (e.g., pneumonia, endocarditis); or (4) from direct contact with an infectious process that invades the meningeal membranes, as can occur with osteomyelitis, sinusitis, otitis media, mastoiditis, or brain abscess. Pneumococcal meningitis, caused by *Streptococcus pneumoniae*, is the most common bacterial meningitis. Meningococcal meningitis, caused by *Neisseria meningitidis*, is the next leading cause. This organism can cause adrenal hemorrhage and insufficiency, leading to vascular collapse and death. Myocarditis also can occur. *Haemophilus influenzae* was once a very common cause of bacterial meningitis until the *H. influenzae* (Hib) vaccine became available, and consequently infection significantly decreased from that organism. Outbreaks have also been associated with the consumption of contaminated dairy or undercooked fish, chicken, and meat. The mortality rate for untreated bacterial meningitis is 50%–100%. Any bacteria can cause meningitis, and some forms of meningitis, such as that caused by *Staphylococcus aureus*, can be difficult to treat because of their resistance to antibiotic therapy.

*Risk factors.* (1) Older adults and infants; (2) institutional settings such as schools and college campuses, prisons; (3) medical conditions that either directly weakens the immune response or the treatment weakens the immune response; (4) work environments that may routinely expose one to causative pathogens; and (5) traveling to areas at higher risk for meningitis.

## HEALTH CARE SETTING

Acute care

## ASSESSMENT

*Cardinal signs.* Severe headache, fever, nuchal rigidity, change in mental status, nausea, vomiting, and photophobia.

*Increased intracranial pressure and herniation signs.* Decreased level of consciousness (LOC) (irritability, drowsiness, stupor, coma), nausea and vomiting, decreasing Glasgow Coma Scale score, vital signs changes (increased blood pressure, decreased heart rate, widening pulse pressure), changes in respiratory pattern, decreased pupillary reaction to light, pupillary dilation or inequality, severe headache, seizures.

*Meningeal irritation.* Back stiffness and pain, headache, nuchal rigidity.

## PHYSICAL ASSESSMENT

- Positive Brudzinski sign may be elicited because of meningeal irritation: when the neck is passively flexed forward, both legs flex involuntarily at the hip and knee.
- Positive Kernig sign also may be found: when the hip is flexed 90 degrees, the individual cannot extend the leg completely without pain.
- In the presence of meningococcal meningitis, a pink, macular rash; petechiae; ecchymoses; purpura; and increased deep tendon reflexes may occur. The rash signals septicemia and is associated with a 40% mortality rate, even with appropriate antibiotics. The rash can progress to gangrenous necrosis and may need debridement or even amputation.

## DIAGNOSTIC TESTS

*Lumbar puncture, CSF analysis, and Gram stain and culture.* When the patient has manifestations of bacterial meningitis, blood cultures and a computed tomography (CT) scan should be done first. An LP will also be done but only after the CT scan has ruled out an obstruction in the foramen magnum. The LP in the presence of increased ICP, can cause brain herniation and therefore the LP is done after an obstruction is ruled out. The LP is done to analyze the cerebral spinal fluid (CSF). Gram stains are done on the CSF, nasopharyngeal secretions, and sputum to detect the causative agent.

Glucose is generally decreased, usually less than 40 mg/dL, and protein is increased and can often be seen in the hundreds. Increased total lactate dehydrogenase in CSF is a consistent finding. Presence or absence of C-reactive protein (CRP) in the CSF can differentiate between bacterial (positive for CRP) and nonbacterial (negative for CRP) meningitis. Typically, CSF will be cloudy or milky because of increased white blood cells; CSF pressure will be increased because of the inflammation and exudate, causing an obstruction in the outflow of CSF from the arachnoid villi.

***Xpert enterovirus (EV) test.*** To distinguish between viral and bacterial meningitis rapidly (in less than 3 hours).

***Coagglutination tests.*** To detect microbial antigens in CSF and enable identification of the causative organism. Generally, coagglutination tests have replaced counterimmunoelectrophoresis because results are obtainable much more rapidly.

***Polymerase chain reaction.*** To analyze DNA in peripheral blood or CSF to identify causative infectious agents.

***Radioimmunoassay, latex particle agglutination, or enzyme-linked immunosorbent assay.*** To detect microbial antigens in the CSF to identify causative organism.

***Petechial skin scraping.*** For Gram-stain analysis of bacteria.

***Sinus, skull, and chest radiographic examinations.*** Taken after treatment is started to rule out sinusitis, pneumonia, and cranial osteomyelitis.

***Computed tomography with contrast.*** To rule out hydrocephalus or mass lesions such as brain abscess and detect exudate in CSF spaces.

***Magnetic resonance imaging.*** To rule out hydrocephalus or mass lesion and detect exudate in CSF spaces.

## Patient Problem/Analyze Cues/Prioritize Hypotheses

# Deficient Knowledge (Transmission-based precautions: droplet)

*due to* unfamiliarity with the rationale and procedure for transmission-based precautions: droplet

**Desired Outcomes/Generate Solutions:** Before visitation, the patient and significant other verbalize accurate knowledge about the rationale for transmission-based droplet precautions and comply with prescribed restrictions and precautionary measures.

| ASSESSMENT—RECOGNIZE CUES/ INTERVENTIONS—TAKE ACTION | RATIONALES |
|---|---|
| Assess the patient's knowledge base and explain, as indicated, the method of disease transmission through respiratory droplets generated by patients when coughing, sneezing, or talking or during the performance of cough-inducing procedures (e.g., suctioning) and by contact with oral secretions; and the rationale for a private room and droplet precautions. | Patient's knowledge base of respiratory droplet transmission must be assessed in infected patients to determine educational needs that promote participation in actions to decrease infection transmission to others. |
| Place patient on droplet precautions, until cultures are negative. Patients should be placed in a private room if possible. All health care team members and visitors must comply with the implementation of surgical masks in addition to standard precautions when within three feet of the patient. | These precautions are essential to protect the health care team and visitors as well as the patient. |
| [!] Provide instructions for covering the mouth before coughing or sneezing and properly disposing of tissue (respiratory hygiene/cough etiquette). | Infection may be spread by contact with respiratory droplets or oral secretions. |
| [!] Instruct patients with transmission-based precautions: droplet to stay in their room. If they must leave the room for a procedure or test, explain that a mask must be worn to protect others from contact with respiratory droplets. | As above. |
| [!] For individuals in contact with the patient, explain the importance of wearing a surgical mask and practicing good hand hygiene. Gloves should be worn when handling any body fluids, especially oral secretions. | As above. |
| Reassure the patient that transmission-based precautions: droplet are temporary. | These precautions will be discontinued when respiratory cultures test results are negative. |

| ASSESSMENT—RECOGNIZE CUES/ INTERVENTIONS—TAKE ACTION | RATIONALES |
|---|---|
| Instruct individuals in contact with the patient that if symptoms of meningitis develop (e.g., headache, fever, neck stiffness, photophobia, change in mental status), they should report immediately to their health care provider. | This measure helps ensure prompt treatment. The mortality rate is high (50%–100%) in persons with untreated bacterial meningitis. Prognosis improves significantly with early antibiotic treatment. |

## Patient Problem/Analyze Cues/Prioritize Hypotheses

# Acute Pain

*due to* headache, photophobia, and nuchal rigidity

**Desired Outcomes/Generate Solutions:** Within 1–2 hours of intervention, the patient's subjective perception of discomfort decreases, as documented by pain scale. Objective indicators, such as grimacing, are absent or diminished.

| ASSESSMENT—RECOGNIZE CUES/ INTERVENTIONS—TAKE ACTION | RATIONALES |
|---|---|
| Assess the patient for pain and discomfort using an appropriate pain scale. | Using a pain scale provides a common language for assessing pain and relief obtained. |
| Provide a quiet environment and darkened room or sunglasses and restrict visitors as necessary. | These measures reduce sensory stimulation and help prevent photophobia. |
| Promote bedrest and assist with activities of daily living as needed. | These measures decrease movement that may cause pain. |
| Apply an ice bag to head or cool cloth to eyes. | These actions help diminish headache. |
| Support the patient in a position of comfort. Keep the neck in alignment during position changes. Elevate head of bed to 30 degrees. | Many persons with meningitis experience pain relief with the head in extension and slightly elevated and the body slightly curled. |
| Provide a gentle passive range of motion and massage to neck and shoulder joints and muscles. If the patient is afebrile, apply moist heat to neck and back. | These measures help relieve stiffness, promote muscle relaxation, and decrease pain. |
| Keep communication simple and direct, using a soft, calm tone of voice. Avoid needless stimulation. Consolidate activities. Loosen constricting bed clothing. Avoid restraining the patient. Reduce stimulation to the minimal amount needed to accomplish required activity. | Patients tend to be hyperirritable with hyperalgesia. Sounds are loud, and even gentle touching may startle them. |
| Administer medications as prescribed. | Analgesics (e.g., acetaminophen, codeine) are given to relieve headache, myalgia, and other pain. Codeine provides some pain relief without undue sedation. Antipyretics (e.g., acetaminophen) are given for the control of fever to reduce cerebral metabolism.Mild sedatives (e.g., diphenhydramine) are given to promote rest. |
| For other interventions, see *Acute Pain* in "General Care of Patients With Neurologic Disorders," Chapter 36. | |

## Patient Problem/Analyze Cues/Prioritize Hypotheses

# Deficient Knowledge (Medications)

*due to* unfamiliarity with the purpose, side effects, and precautions for the prescribed medications

***Desired Outcome/Generate Solutions:*** Before beginning the medication regimen, the patient and significant others verbalize accurate knowledge about the purpose, potential side effects, and precautions for the prescribed medications.

| ASSESSMENT—RECOGNIZE CUES/ INTERVENTIONS—TAKE ACTION | RATIONALES |
|---|---|
| Assess the patient's and significant others' health care literacy (language, reading, comprehension). Assess culture and culturally specific information needs. | This assessment helps ensure that information is selected and presented in a manner that is culturally and educationally appropriate. |
| Assess the patient's and significant other's knowledge base regarding prescribed medication. | This information will help determine patient's and significant other's learning needs regarding prescribed medication. |
| Provide instructions to the patient and significant other on prescribed antibiotics. | Because treatment cannot be delayed until culture results are known, high doses of parenteral antibiotics are started immediately, based on Gram-stain results. The antibiotic must penetrate the blood–brain barrier into the CSF. Adjustments in therapy can be made after the coagglutination test and culture and sensitivity test results are available. Antibiotics may include the following (usually in combination): penicillin G, ampicillin, cefotaxime, ceftriaxone, ceftazidime, chloramphenicol, gentamicin, and vancomycin. Patient and/or significant education regarding drug routes, actions, and side effects will provide them with knowledge of their drug treatment plan as well as outcomes and possible side effects related to antibiotic drug therapy. |
| As appropriate, educate the patient and significant other that sometimes intrathecal (i.e., in the subarachnoid space) antibiotics are used. | Intrathecal antibiotics may be used if it is believed that systemic antibiotics alone will not be curative in the presence of particular bacteria (e.g., *Pseudomonas, Enterobacter, Staphylococcus*). Patient and significant other education will prepare them to anticipate this type of treatment. |
| ⚠ As appropriate, provide education to the patient and significant other on the rationale for giving a glucocorticosteroid (e.g., dexamethasone) and its potential side effects. | Ideally, it is given before or at same time as the first dose of antibiotics and then on an ongoing basis to reduce inflammation caused by toxic by-products released by bacterial cells as they are killed by antibiotics. In children, this therapy can reduce hearing loss caused by *H. influenzae*.<br><br>**Caution:** Steroids can have side effects that may complicate the patient's clinical condition (e.g., increased glucose may make the patient more lethargic and may exaggerate emotional responses causing agitation and/or cause psychotic/hallucination-type reactions). Patient and significant other education regarding glucocorticosteroids will provide them with knowledge of their drug treatment plan as well as outcomes and possible side effects related specifically to glucocorticosteroid treatment. |

## ADDITIONAL PROBLEMS:

## ✓ PATIENT–FAMILY TEACHING AND DISCHARGE PLANNING

The extent of teaching and discharge planning will depend on whether the patient has any residual damage. When providing patient–family teaching, focus on sensory information, avoid giving excessive information, and initiate a visiting nurse referral for necessary follow-up teaching. Include verbal and written information about the following:

✓ Referrals to community resources, such as public health nurse, visiting nurses association, community support groups, social workers, psychological therapy, vocational rehabilitation agency, home health agencies, and extended and skilled care facilities.

✓ Medications, including drug name, purpose, dosage, schedule, precautions, and potential side effects for patient's medications, as well as those for the prophylactic antibiotics taken by family and significant other. Also discuss drug–drug, herb–drug, and food–drug interactions. Close contacts taking prophylactic antibiotics should know signs and symptoms to report to the health care provider (e.g., headache, fever, neck stiffness).

✓ Vaccination: There are vaccines available against *S. pneumoniae*, *N. meningitidis*, and *H. influenzae* group B causing meningitis and other infections. *N. meningitidis* has several subgroup strains. For people at increased risk (e.g., travelers to countries with endemic infections), a meningococcal vaccine (groups A, C, Y, W135) is available, although it does not confer 100% protection. The Centers for Disease Control and Prevention recommend this meningococcal vaccine for children 11–12 years of age, adolescents at high school entry, and college freshmen living in dormitories. In the United States, the most common *N. meningitidis* is from group B, and work is progressing on a group B vaccine. *H. influenzae* group B vaccine should be incorporated as part of all routine childhood inoculations.

✓ For patients with residual neurologic deficits, teach the following as appropriate: exercises that promote muscle strength and mobility; measures for preventing contractures and skin breakdown; transfer techniques and proper body mechanics; safety measures if patient has decreased pain and sensation or visual disturbances; use of assistive devices; indications of constipation, urinary retention, or urinary tract infection; bowel and bladder training programs; self-catheterization technique or care of indwelling catheters; and seizure precautions if indicated.

✓ Obtain additional information from the following:
- Centers for Disease Control and Prevention: https://www.cdc.gov/meningitis/index.html

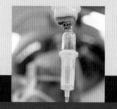

# Guillain–Barré Syndrome  38

## OVERVIEW/PATHOPHYSIOLOGY

Guillain–Barré syndrome (GBS) is an autoimmune response triggered by a bacterial or viral infection experienced by the patient a few days or weeks before its onset. Common viral and bacterial illnesses include (1) upper respiratory infection (URI), (2) gastroenteritis, (3) *Campylobacter jejuni*, (4) cytomegalovirus, (5) Epstein–Barr virus, and (6) Zika virus. Less commonly, it may also be associated with vaccinations, human immunodeficiency virus seroconversions, Hodgkin's lymphoma, systemic lupus erythematosus, sarcoidosis, thyroid disease, and lung cancer. Surgery and trauma can also trigger GBS.

GBS is a rapidly progressing polyneuritis of unknown cause. An inflammatory process enables lymphocytes to enter perivascular spaces and destroy the myelin sheath covering peripheral or cranial nerves. Posterior (sensory) and anterior (motor) nerve roots can be affected because of this segmental demyelination, and individuals may experience both sensory and motor losses. There is relative sparing of the axon. Respiratory insufficiency may occur in as many as half of affected individuals. Life-threatening respiratory muscle weakness can develop as rapidly as 24–72 hours after the onset of initial symptoms. In about 25% of cases, motor weakness progresses to total paralysis.

Peak severity of symptoms usually occurs within 4 weeks after the onset of symptoms. A plateau stage follows that usually lasts 1–2 weeks. The recovery stage starts with a return of function as remyelinization occurs, but it may take months to years for a full recovery. Fifteen percent of patients have full neurologic recovery, and another 65% have mild deficits that do not interfere with activities of daily living. Eighty percent to 90% of patients either recover completely or have only minor residual weakness or abnormal sensations, such as numbness or tingling. Of GBS patients, 5%–10% may have permanent severe disability. Deficits are the result of axonal nerve degeneration.

## HEALTH CARE SETTING

Acute care, likely in the intensive care unit (ICU) when the neurologic deficit is progressing. Acute rehabilitation when disease is in the recovery phase.

## ASSESSMENT

Progressive weakness and areflexia are the most common indicators. Typically, paresthesia, hypotonia, and weakness begin bilaterally in the legs and ascend symmetrically upward, progressing to the arms. Cranial nerve involvement manifests as facial weakness and paresthesia. Pain is also a common symptom. The most serious effect of GBS is respiratory failure. Ascending GBS is most common. Variants of GBS include acute motor axonal neuropathy (primarily a motor component, with no sensory involvement), and descending GBS, in which cranial nerves are affected first and weakness progresses downward with rapid respiratory involvement. Other variants include Miller Fisher syndrome, which is characterized by a triad of abnormal muscle coordination (ataxia), paralysis of eye muscles (ophthalmoplegia), and absence of tendon reflexes (areflexia); and pharyngeal–cervical–brachial variant (rare) involving facial, oropharyngeal, cervical, and upper limbs with no lower limb involvement. Peak severity usually occurs within 4 weeks of onset. GBS does not affect the level of consciousness (LOC), cognitive function, or pupillary function.

**Anterior (motor) nerve root involvement.** The patient develops weakness or flaccid paralysis that may progress to quadriplegia. Respiratory muscle involvement can be life threatening. There is loss of reflexes, muscle tension, and tone, but muscle atrophy usually does not occur.

**Autonomic nervous system involvement.** Sinus tachycardia, bradycardia, hypertension, hypotension, cardiac dysrhythmias, facial flushing, diaphoresis, inability to perspire, loss of sphincter control, urinary retention, adynamic ileus, syndrome of inappropriate antidiuretic hormone secretion, and increased pulmonary secretions may occur. Autonomic nervous system (ANS) involvement may occur unexpectedly and can be life threatening, but usually, it does not persist for longer than 2 weeks.

**Cranial nerve involvement.** Inability to chew, swallow, speak, or close the eyes.

**Posterior (sensory) nerve root involvement.** Presence of paresthesias, such as numbness and tingling, which usually are minor compared with the degree of motor loss. Ascending sensory loss often precedes motor loss. Muscle cramping, tenderness, or pain may occur.

**Physical assessment.** Symmetric motor weakness, impaired position and vibration sense, hypoactive or absent deep tendon reflexes, hypotonia in affected muscles, and decreased ventilatory capacity.

## DIAGNOSTIC TESTS

Diagnostic tests are performed to rule out other diseases, such as acute poliomyelitis. Diagnosis of GBS is based on clinical presentation, history of recent bacterial or viral illness, and cerebrospinal fluid (CSF) findings.

***Lumbar puncture and cerebrospinal fluid analysis.*** About 7 days after the initial symptoms, elevated protein (especially immunoglobulin G) without an increase in white blood cell (WBC) count may be present. Although CSF pressure usually is normal, in severe diseases, it may be elevated.

***Electromyography and nerve conduction studies.*** Reveal slowed nerve conduction velocities soon after paralysis that appear because of demyelinization. Denervation potentials appear later.

***Serum complete blood count.*** Will show the presence of leukocytosis early in illness, possibly as a result of the inflammatory process associated with demyelinization.

***Evoked potentials (auditory, visual, brain stem).*** May be used to distinguish GBS from other neuropathologic conditions.

## Patient Problem/Analyze Cues/Prioritize Hypotheses

# Impaired Gas Exchange

*due to* neuromuscular weakness or paralysis of the facial, throat, and respiratory muscles (severity of symptoms peaks around week 4)

*Desired Outcome/Generate Solutions:* The patient's breathing pattern improves to within baseline status after immediate and effective treatment.

| ASSESSMENT—RECOGNIZE CUES/ INTERVENTIONS—TAKE ACTION | RATIONALES |
|---|---|
| **Perform the following critical assessments:** | |
| Assess the patient's respiratory rate, rhythm, and depth. Auscultate for diminished breath sounds. | The frequency of assessment will depend on the patient's clinical condition. Accessory muscle use, nasal flaring, dyspnea, shallow respirations, diminished breath sounds, and apnea are signs of respiratory deterioration, which necessitates prompt notification of the health provider for rapid intervention. |
| On an ongoing basis, observe for changes in mental status, LOC, and orientation. | These changes may signal reduced oxygenation to the brain. |
| As indicated and at least once per shift during the acute phase, depending on the patient's clinical state, assess for ascending loss of sensation by touching the patient lightly with a pin or fingers at frequent intervals (hourly or more frequently initially). Assess from the level of the iliac crest upward toward the shoulders. Measure the highest level at which decreased sensation occurs. | Decreased sensation often precedes motor weakness; therefore, if it ascends to the level of the T8 dermatome, anticipate that intercostal muscles (used with respirations) soon will be impaired. |
| As indicated and at least once per shift during the acute phase, depending on the patient's clinical state, assess for the presence of arm drift and the inability to shrug the shoulders. Alert the health care provider to significant findings. | If present, these findings need to be reported promptly because they are known to precede respiratory dysfunction. |
| Shoulder weakness is present if the patient cannot shrug the shoulders. Arm drift is present if one arm pronates or drifts down or out from its original position. Arm drift is detected in the following way: have the patient hold both arms out in front of the body, level with the shoulders and with palms up; instruct the patient to close the eyes while holding this position. | |
| Assess the patient's ability to take fluids orally. | This assessment detects changes or difficulties that may indicate ascending paralysis. |

| ASSESSMENT—RECOGNIZE CUES/ INTERVENTIONS—TAKE ACTION | RATIONALES |
|---|---|
| Assess for dysphagia and decreased cough and gag reflexes every 8 hours and before oral intake for cough reflexes, gag reflexes, and difficulty swallowing. | Dysphagia and decreased cough and gag reflexes likely will necessitate parenteral feedings to prevent aspiration until reflexes return to normal. |
| As prescribed, keep patients with impaired reflexes and swallowing nothing by mouth (NPO). | |
| Monitor the effectiveness of breathing by checking serial vital capacity and negative inspiratory force results on pulmonary function tests. | To prevent further deterioration in patient's status. |
| If vital capacity is less than 1000 mL or is rapidly trending downward or if the patient exhibits signs of hypoxia such as tachycardia, increasing restlessness, mental dullness, cyanosis, decreased pulse oximetry readings, or difficulty handling secretions, these findings must be reported immediately to the health care provider. If present, intubation is probable. Vital capacity initially is measured every 2–4 hours and then more frequently if deterioration is present. | |
| Assess the arterial blood gas levels and pulse oximetry as per standard operating procedures or as prescribed. | These assessments detect hypoxia or hypercapnia ($PaCO_2$ more than 45 mm Hg), a signal of hypoventilation. $PaO_2$ less than 80 mm Hg or $O_2$ saturation 92% or less usually signals the need for supplemental oxygen. |
| **!** *Perform the following critical interventions:* | |
| **!** Raise the head of bed | This position promotes optimal chest excursion by taking pressure of abdominal organs off the lungs, which may increase oxygenation. This position also will reduce aspiration risk. |
| **!** At least every 4 hours and as indicated, encourage coughing and deep breathing to the best of the patient's ability. | These actions mobilize and enable the expectoration of secretions to optimize breathing pattern. |
| **!** Prepare the patient emotionally for life-saving procedures or for the eventual transfer to ICU or transition care unit for closer monitoring. | The patient may require tracheostomy, endotracheal intubation, or mechanical ventilation to support respiratory function. |
| For other interventions, see *Risk for Aspiration* in "Older Adult Care," Chapter 3. | |

## Patient Problem/Analyze Cues/Prioritize Hypotheses

# Risk for Altered Blood Pressure

*due to* ANS involvement

**Desired Outcomes/Generate Solutions:** The patient exhibits systolic blood pressure (BP) at least 90 mm Hg and less than 160 mm Hg; no significant mental status changes; and orientation to person, place, and time.

| ASSESSMENT—RECOGNIZE CUES/ INTERVENTIONS—TAKE ACTION | RATIONALES |
|---|---|
| **!** As indicated, but no less frequently than every 4 hours, assess LOC and BP, noting wide fluctuations. Report significant findings to the health care provider. | LOC will help determine the state of the patient's cerebral perfusion. Changes in BP that result in severe hypotension or hypertension may occur because of unopposed sympathetic outflow or loss of outflow to the peripheral nervous system, causing changes in vascular tone. The health care provider may prescribe a short-acting vasoactive agent for persistent hypotension or hypertension. |
| On an ongoing basis, assess carefully for changes in heart rate and BP during activities such as coughing, suctioning, position changes, or straining at stool. | These are events that can trigger BP changes. |

## Patient Problem/Analyze Cues/Prioritize Hypotheses

# Body Weight Problem (Weight Loss)

*due to* NPO status occurring with adynamic ileus

***Desired Outcome/Generate Solutions:*** The patient's nutritional status will meet their metabolic needs.

| ASSESSMENT—RECOGNIZE CUES/ INTERVENTIONS—TAKE ACTION | RATIONALES |
|---|---|
| Assess the gastrointestinal system, noting abdominal contour and tenderness, nausea and vomiting, and stool output. Auscultate the bowel sounds, noting presence, absence, or changes from baseline that may signal the onset of ileus. Notify the health care provider of significant findings. <br><br> Bowel sounds are auscultated in all four quadrants for at least 2 minutes before determining that bowel sounds are not present. Report abnormal findings to health care provider. | Decreased or absent bowel sounds, abdominal distention or tenderness, nausea and vomiting, and absence of stool output are signals of the onset of ileus. Also, GBS has been associated with *C. jejuni*, an infection that manifests as gastroenteritis. Timely interventions are imperative to prevent further complications. |
| Initiate gastric, gastrostomy, or parenteral feedings as prescribed. | Patients with adynamic ileus generally require gastric decompression with a nasogastric tube. If the patient cannot chew or swallow effectively because of cranial nerve involvement, gastric, gastrostomy, or parenteral feedings may be initiated. The patient is advanced to a solid diet on return of the gag reflex and swallowing ability. See "Providing Nutritional Support," Chapter 76. |
| On return of the gag reflex and swallowing ability, provide a high-fiber diet as prescribed. | Fiber provides bulk, which helps prevent constipation. |
| For general interventions, see *Body Weight Problem (Weight Loss)* in "General Care of Patients With Neurologic Disorders," Chapter 36. | |

## Patient Problem/Analyze Cues/Prioritize Hypotheses

# Anxiety

*due to* threat to biologic integrity and loss of control

***Desired Outcomes/Generate Solutions:*** The patient verbalizes acceptance of changes in life events, states anxiety is lessened or under control, and exhibits fewer symptoms of increased anxiety (e.g., less apprehension, decreased tension).

| ASSESSMENT—RECOGNIZE CUES/ INTERVENTIONS—TAKE ACTION | RATIONALES |
|---|---|
| Assess the need and arrange for transfer to a room close to the nurses' station for patients with progressing neurologic deficit. | This action will decrease the feeling of isolation and help alleviate the anxiety of being suddenly incapacitated and helpless. |
| Ensure the call light is within easy reach, and frequently assess the patient's ability to use it. Consider an easy-touch call bell to ensure the patient can call for help as needed. | These measures that promote patient's safety also will help allay anxiety. |
| Provide the continuity of patient care through assignment of staff and use of care plan. | Familiarity may help reduce anxiety. |
| Perform the assessments at frequent intervals and provide care in a calm and reassuring manner. | Calm begets calm. Frequent assessments also promote in the patient a sense of security that they are not isolated. |

Continued

Neurologic Care Plans

| ASSESSMENT—RECOGNIZE CUES/ INTERVENTIONS—TAKE ACTION | RATIONALES |
|---|---|
| Allow time for the patient to vent concerns; provide realistic feedback regarding what the patient may experience. Determine past effective coping behaviors. | Unexpressed concerns can contribute to frustration and stress. Information helps reduce anxiety caused by a lack of knowledge. Knowing past effective coping behaviors facilitates problem solving for ways in which these behaviors, or others, may prove useful in the current situation. |
| For other interventions, see *Anxiety*, Chapters 8 and 9. | |

## Patient Problem/Analyze Cues/Prioritize Hypotheses

# Deficient Knowledge

*due to* unfamiliarity with the therapeutic plasma exchange (plasmapheresis) procedure

*Desired Outcome/Generate Solutions:* Before the scheduled date of the procedure, the patient verbalizes accurate information about the plasma exchange procedure.

| ASSESSMENT—RECOGNIZE CUES/ INTERVENTIONS—TAKE ACTION | RATIONALES |
|---|---|
| Assess the patient's health care literacy (language, reading, comprehension). Assess culture and culturally specific information needs. | This assessment helps ensure that information is selected and presented in a manner that is culturally and educationally appropriate. |
| Determine whether the patient is taking angiotensin-converting enzyme (ACE) inhibitor medication and notify the health care provider accordingly. | ACE inhibitor use is associated with flushing, hypotension, abdominal cramping, and other gastrointestinal symptoms while on plasmapheresis. These medications usually are held for 24 hours before the procedure to prevent these problems. |
| Determine the patient's level of understanding of the health care provider's explanation of the plasma exchange procedure. | Before the plasma exchange procedure, the health care provider explains the reason for the procedure, its risks, and anticipated benefits or outcome and obtains a signed consent. The nurse's assessment of the patient's understanding provides an opportunity to clarify or reinforce information accordingly. |
| Clearly describe the plasma exchange procedure to the patient. | The procedure is similar to hemodialysis. Blood is removed from the patient and separated into its components. The plasma is discarded; other blood components (e.g., red blood cells, WBCs, platelets) are saved and returned to the patient with donor plasma or replacement fluid. Multiple exchanges over a period of weeks can be expected. |
| Explain that if started within 1–2 weeks of GBS symptoms, the exchange process seems to decrease disease duration and severity. | Antibodies to the patient's peripheral and cranial nerve tissue are reduced by the removal of the blood's plasma portion, which contains the circulating antibodies. |
| Assess the patient's experience with plasmapheresis, positive or negative effects, and nature of any fears or concerns. Document and communicate this information to other caregivers. | This will clarify the nurse's understanding of the patient's perspective, which in turn will enable further information gathering and clarification, optimally decreasing fears and concerns. |
| Explain that the patient can expect the procedure to take 2–4 hours, although it may take considerably longer. | The length of time will depend on the condition of the patient's veins, blood flow, and hematocrit level. |

| ASSESSMENT—RECOGNIZE CUES/ INTERVENTIONS—TAKE ACTION | RATIONALES |
|---|---|
| Explain to the patient that they can expect preprocedure and postprocedure blood work. | Blood will be assessed for clotting factors and electrolyte levels, particularly of potassium and calcium, which may decrease during this exchange procedure. |
| Explain that weight and vital signs (VS) will be taken before and after the procedure, with frequent VS checks during the procedure. | Hypotension and shift in fluid volume are possible. |
| Advise that calcium gluconate or potassium may be administered, based on laboratory values of calcium or potassium. | These agents will correct electrolyte imbalances. |
| Encourage the patient to report any unusual feelings or symptoms during plasma exchange. | Patients may experience chills, fever, hives, sweating, or lightheadedness, which may signal a reaction to donor plasma.<br><br>Thirst, faintness, or dizziness can occur with hypotension or hypovolemia. Patients should take oral fluids during the procedure if possible.<br><br>Numbness or tingling around lips or in the hands, arms, and legs; muscle twitching; cramping; or tetany can occur with hypocalcemia.<br><br>Fatigue, nausea, weakness, or cramping may signal hypokalemia. |
| Inform the patient that medications (e.g., plasma-bound drugs) may be held until after the procedure. | Medications otherwise would be removed from the blood during the plasma exchange. |
| If the patient does not have a urinary catheter, remind him or her to void before and during the procedure, if necessary. | This measure prevents the mild hypotension caused by a full bladder. |
| Explain that intake and output will be monitored closely during the procedure. | Decreased urine output may signal hypovolemia. |
| Explain that the patient's temperature will be checked during the procedure and warm blankets will be provided. | These measures assess for and prevent hypothermia. |
| Explain that the patient probably will feel fatigued 1–2 days after the procedure. Encourage extra rest, a high-protein diet, and milk products during this time. | Fatigue could result from the decreased plasma protein level that occurs during the exchange. |
| Instruct the patient to monitor the IV access site for warmth, redness, swelling, or drainage and to report significant findings. | These are signs of local infection. |
| Instruct the patient to monitor for signs of bruising or bleeding. Caution the patient about avoiding cutting self or bumping into objects and to sustain pressure over cuts. Inform the patient that black, tarry stools usually signal the presence of blood and should be reported. | The anticoagulant citrate dextrose is used in the extracorporeal machine circuitry to prevent clotting. This may cause excessive gastrointestinal bleeding and bleeding from minor bumps and cuts. A pressure dressing may be kept in place over the access site for 2–4 hours after the procedure. |

## Patient Problem/Analyze Cues/Prioritize Hypotheses

# Acute Pain

*due to* muscle tenderness; hypersensitivity to touch; or discomfort in the shoulders, thighs, and back

***Desired Outcomes/Generate Solutions:*** Within 1–2 hours of intervention, the patient's subjective perception of discomfort decreases, as documented by pain scale. Objective indicators, such as grimacing, are absent or diminished.

PART I: Medical-Surgical Nursing Care Plans

| ASSESSMENT—RECOGNIZE CUES/ INTERVENTIONS—TAKE ACTION | RATIONALES |
|---|---|
| For patients with hypersensitivity, assess the amount of touch that can be tolerated, and incorporate this information into the plan of care. | This assessment facilitates the development of an individualized plan of care and helps ensure that the patient is not touched more than necessary by all staff members. |
| For patients with muscle tenderness, consider the use of massage, moist heat packs, cold application, or warm baths. | These measures may be very soothing for tender muscles. |
| Reposition the patient at frequent intervals. | Repositioning will help decrease muscle tension and fatigue. Some individuals find that a supine "frog-leg" position is particularly comfortable. |
| Provide the passive range of motion and advise gentle stretching. | These measures reduce joint stiffness. |
| Administer the pain medications as prescribed. | Opioids are often the most effective means of pain control, and a continuous morphine drip may be needed. Other medications that may be used to relieve uncomfortable paresthesias include anticonvulsants such as gabapentin and carbamazepine and tricyclics such as amitriptyline. |
| For other interventions, see *Acute Pain* in "General Care of Patients With Neurologic Disorders," Chapter 36. | |

## ADDITIONAL PROBLEMS:

| | | | |
|---|---|---|---|
| *Activity Intolerance* | Chapter 1 | *Altered Temperature (Decreased)* | Chapter 36 |
| *Risk for Deep Vein Thrombosis* | Chapter 1 | *Risk for Impaired Communication* | Chapter 36 |
| *Impaired Cardiac Function* | Chapter 22 | *Impaired Functional Ability*, with inability to | Chapter 36 |
| *Ineffective Tissue Perfusion (Multisystem)* | Chapter 23 | perform self-care | |
| *Impaired Swallowing* | Chapter 36 | *Constipation* | Chapter 36 |
| *Risk for Falls*, due to unsteady gait | Chapter 36 | *Decreased Tissue Perfusion (Cardiac and Cerebral)* | Chapter 23 |
| *Risk for Injury*, due to sensory deficit, decreased LOC | Chapter 36 | *Risk for Impaired Skin Integrity* | Chapter 3 |
| *Impaired Tissue Integrity (Corneal)* | Chapter 36 | **For patients on mechanical ventilation, see** | |
| *Dehydration* | Chapter 36 | *Risk for Health Care–Associated Complications* | Chapter 13 |
| *Altered Temperature (Increased)* | Chapter 36 | *Risk for Infection*, due to inadequate primary defenses | Chapter 36 |

## ✔ PATIENT–FAMILY TEACHING AND DISCHARGE PLANNING

Most patients with GBS eventually recover fully or nearly so, but because the recovery period can be prolonged, the patient often goes home with some degree of neurologic deficit. Discharge planning and teaching will vary according to the degree of disability. When providing patient–family teaching, focus on sensory information, avoid giving excessive information, and initiate a visiting nurse referral for necessary follow-up teaching. Include verbal and written information about the following:

✓ Disease process, expected improvement, and importance of continuing in rehabilitation or physical therapy (PT) program to promote as full a recovery as possible.

✓ Safety measures relative to sensorimotor deficit.

✓ Exercises that promote muscle strength and mobility, measures for preventing contractures and skin breakdown, transfer techniques and proper body mechanics, and use of assistive devices.

✓ Indications of constipation, urinary retention, or urinary tract infection; implementation of bowel and bladder training programs; and, if appropriate, care of indwelling catheters or self-catheterization technique.

✓ Indications of URI; measures for preventing regurgitation, aspiration, and respiratory infection.

✓ Medications, including drug name, purpose, dosage, schedule, precautions, and potential side effects. Also discuss drug–drug, herb–drug, and food–drug interactions.

✓ Importance of follow-up care, including visits to the health care provider, PT, and occupational therapy.

✓ Referrals to community resources such as public health nurse, visiting nurse association, community support groups, social workers, psychologic therapy, home health agencies, and extended and skilled care facilities.

✓ Obtain additional information from the following:
- GBS/CIDP Foundation International: www.gbs-cidp.org

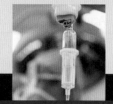

# Intervertebral Disk Disease 39

## OVERVIEW/PATHOPHYSIOLOGY

The intervertebral disk is a semi–fluid-filled fibrous capsule that facilitates movement of the spine and acts as a shock absorber. The disk's ability to withstand stressors is not unlimited and diminishes with aging. Pressure on the disk eventually may force elastic material from the center of the disk, called the *nucleus pulposus*, to break (herniate) through the fibrous rim of the disk, called the *annulus*. Herniation usually occurs posteriorly because the posterior longitudinal ligament is inherently weaker than the anterior longitudinal ligament. The bulging or rupture (protrusion or extrusion) of an intervertebral disk causes its typical symptoms by pressing on and irritating the spinal nerve roots or spinal cord. Herniated nucleus pulposus usually is the result of injury or a series of insults to the vertebral column from lifting or twisting. When the disk ruptures without a known discrete injury, degenerative changes are the likely cause. Deterioration usually occurs suddenly with rupture, but it may happen gradually, with symptoms appearing months or years after the initial injury. Almost all herniated disks occur in the lumbar spine, with 90% of the problems occurring at L4–5 and L5–S1. Research is investigating the role of certain genes and environmental influences on lumbar disk disease. The spinal cord ends around L1, so lumbar herniated disks impinge on spinal nerves, which are more resilient than actual spinal cord tissue. The spinal nerves usually bounce back and function normally after the problem is relieved. Cervical disk problems most often occur at C5–6 and C6–7 and generally are caused by degenerative changes or trauma, such as whiplash or hyperextension. Cervical herniations may compress spinal nerves or impinge on the spinal cord. Thoracic disk problems are rare because of the rigid structure of the thoracic spine.

Herniated disks account for about 4% of back pain. Most back pain is related to muscle and ligament strain. Spondylolisthesis (slippage between two vertebrae) and degenerative changes such as stenosis; osteophyte (e.g., bone spur) formation, which can cause spinal nerve root compression; osteoporosis, which can lead to compression fractures; and osteoarthritis of the facet joints are other causes of nondisk back pain. Neoplasm and infection also can be sources of back pain.

## HEALTH CARE SETTING

Primary care or acute care neurosurgery, neurology, or orthopedics; pain clinics

## ASSESSMENT

***General indicators.*** Onset can be sudden, with intense unilateral pain or with pain that is dull, diffuse, deep, and aching. Symptoms vary according to the level of injury and nerves involved. Usually, pain is increased with movement or activities that increase intraabdominal or intrathoracic pressure, such as sneezing, coughing, and straining. Often, pain is improved by lying down. **Note:** Immediate medical attention is essential if there is any weakness or paralysis, extreme sensory loss, or altered bowel or bladder function, which indicates spinal cord compression in the lumbar back (e.g., cauda equina syndrome) and need for emergency decompression surgery. Indicators of cervical spinal cord compression (and need for early surgical treatment) include balance problems, unsteadiness when standing with eyes closed (Romberg sign), hyperreflexes, and generalized numbness in the feet and legs.

***Cervical disk disease.*** Pain or numbness in the upper extremities, shoulders, thorax, occipital area, or back of the head or neck. Pain can radiate down the forearms and into the hands and fingers. Interscapular aching or suboccipital headaches are commonly associated with cervical disk disease. Usually, the neck has restricted mobility, and there can be cervical muscle spasm and loss of normal cervical lordosis. Patients may have upper extremity muscle weakness with abnormal biceps or triceps reflexes.

***Lumbar disk disease.*** Pain in the lumbosacral area with possible radiculopathy (sciatica) to the buttock, down the posterior surface of the thigh and calf, and to the lateral border of the foot and toes. Sensory distribution for the L5 nerve root is the medial portion of the foot and the great toe, whereas sensory distribution for S1 is the lateral aspect of the foot, fifth toe, and sole of the foot. Often mobility is altered, as evidenced by decreased ability to stand upright, listing to one side, asymmetric gait, limited ability to flex forward, and restricted side movement caused by pain and muscle spasms. The individual walks cautiously, bearing little weight on the affected side, and often finds sitting or climbing stairs particularly painful. Reflex muscle spasms can cause bulging of the back with concomitant flattening of the lumbar curve and possible scoliosis at the level of the affected disk. Usually, patellar and Achilles tendon reflexes are depressed owing to nerve impingement. Sciatica usually is associated with intervertebral disk herniation.

***Physical assessment.*** Possible findings include depressed reflexes, muscle atrophy, paresthesias (described as "pins and needles"), or anesthesia (numbness) in the dermatome of the involved nerves. The straight leg–raising test and sciatic nerve test are two of several that are performed to confirm the presence of lumbar disk disease.

**Risk factors.** Repetitive bending or lifting involving a twisting motion, continuous vibration, smoking, poor physical condition (especially weak abdominal muscles), poor posture, obesity, above-average height, osteoporosis, prolonged sitting, depression, severe scoliosis, spondylolisthesis, or genetic predisposition.

## DIAGNOSTIC TESTS

In the absence of serious symptoms, diagnostic testing may not be done until 3 months have passed and symptoms persist (90% of back pain resolves in less than 1 month). Diagnostic testing should be done for pain that is constant, severe, unrelieved by rest or position, and not calmed by antiinflammatory medication inasmuch as these symptoms may indicate the presence of neoplasm or infection. Thoracic back pain also should be investigated because it may be caused by medical problems (e.g., aortic aneurysm).

**Magnetic resonance imaging (MRI).** May reveal a disk impinging on the spinal cord or nerve root, or may show a related pathologic condition, such as a tumor or spondylosis. An MR neurogram helps image nerves after they leave the spinal column and can show compressions as they travel through the spinal foramina. An MR myelogram helps view the cerebrospinal fluid (CSF) sac without having to use a needle puncture. MRI has replaced computed tomography (CT) scan and myelogram as the test of choice in diagnosing herniated nucleus pulposus and is considered the gold standard.

**Computed tomography of the spine.** May reveal disk protrusion/prolapse or a related pathologic condition, such as a bone spur, tumor, spondylosis, or spinal stenosis.

**Radiographic examination of the spine.** May show narrowing of the vertebral interspaces in affected areas, loss of spine curvature, bone spur formation, and spondylosis.

**Diskography.** Identifies degenerated or extruded disks or annulus tear by means of contrast medium injected into the disk space using fluoroscopy. Often it is done in combination with CT and may differentiate between disk infection and rupture.

**Myelogram.** May show characteristic deformity and filling defect or a related pathologic condition; it is usually done in conjunction with a CT scan.

**Electromyography.** May show denervation patterns of specific nerve roots to indicate the level and site of injury.

**Evoked potential studies.** For example, somatosensory studies may show slowed conduction due to nerve root compromise and can localize specific nerve root.

## LABORATORY TESTS

Serum alkaline and acid phosphatase, glucose, calcium, erythrocyte sedimentation rate, and white blood cell count may rule out metabolic bone disease, metastatic tumors, diabetic mononeuritis, and disk space infection.

## Patient Problem/Analyze Cues/Prioritize Hypotheses

# Deficient Knowledge (Pain Control)

*due to* unfamiliarity with pain control measures

**Desired Outcome:** After instruction during outpatient treatment session or within the 24-hour period before hospital discharge, the patient verbalizes accurate knowledge about pain control measures and demonstrates the ability to initiate these measures when appropriate.

| ASSESSMENT—RECOGNIZE CUES/ INTERVENTIONS—TAKE ACTION | RATIONALES |
|---|---|
| Teach the methods of controlling pain and their individual applications. | Methods include distraction, use of counterirritants, massage, hydrotherapy, aquatherapy, acupressure, dorsal column stimulation, use of transcutaneous electrical nerve stimulation, behavior modification, relaxation techniques, hypnosis, music therapy, imagery, biofeedback, and diathermy. Whole-body vibration exercise and spinal manipulation may be considered for uncomplicated back problems with no radiculopathy. |
| | In addition, applying intermittent heat may reduce muscle spasm, whereas icing may prevent further inflammatory swelling and provide some topical anesthesia. Icing should be done frequently, especially for the first 24–48 hours after surgery, and is often recommended after exercise. Continuous low-level heat wrap therapy reduces pain and improves function. Heat may be applied by warm/hot showers or heating pads. Cold can be achieved by freezing water in a paper cup, tearing off the top of the cup to expose the ice, and massaging in a circular motion, using the remaining portion of the cup as a handle. A bag of frozen peas or corn may be used to apply continuous cold to the lower back. With any of these methods, a layer of cloth should be used so that ice does not touch the skin. A 20-minute application of cold 4–6 times per day is recommended. |

Continued

| ASSESSMENT—RECOGNIZE CUES/ INTERVENTIONS—TAKE ACTION | RATIONALES |
|---|---|
| Suggest the patient use a stool to rest the affected leg when standing. | This measure will help relieve sciatica. |
| Advise the patient to sit in a straight-back chair that is high enough to get out of easily, including toilet seats that are raised. | Higher seats facilitate ease of movement in and out of chairs and provide comfort. Straddling a straight-back chair and resting arms on the chair back is comfortable for many individuals. |
| Encourage the use of a moderately firm to firm mattress and extra pillows as needed for positioning. | These measures support normal lumbar curvature. Some patients find the normal bed height too low and use blocks to raise it to a more comfortable height. |
| Instruct the patient on bedrest to roll rather than lift off the bedpan. | This action prevents straining of the back. The patient may find a fracture bedpan more comfortable than a regular bedpan. |
| Caution the patient to avoid sudden twisting or turning movements. Explain the importance of logrolling when moving from side to side. | These measures prevent movements that could induce further back injury. Orthotics (e.g., splints, braces, girdles, cervical collars) also may be used to limit the motion of the vertebral column. Temporary use of a back brace or corset may enable an earlier return to activity with lumbar disk disease. Generally, long-term use of braces is discouraged because it prohibits the development of necessary supporting musculature. |
| Advise the patient to avoid staying in one position too long, fatigue, chilling, and anxiety. | These factors can cause back spasms. |
| Suggest lying on the side with knees bent or lying supine with knees supported on pillows. Advise the patient that a small pillow supporting the nape of the neck may be helpful with cervical pain. Teach the patient to avoid prolonged periods of sitting, which stress the back. | These measures promote spinal comfort. |
| If appropriate, teach the patient to apply a heating pad to the back for 15–30 minutes before getting out of bed in the morning. | Heat will help allay stiffness and discomfort after a night in bed. Heating pads should be used only for short intervals and only if the patient's temperature sensations are intact. |
| Remind the patient to place a towel or cloth between the heating pad and skin. | This measure will help prevent burns. |
| Encourage the patient to rest when tired or stressed and not to exercise when in pain. | Tired muscles are more susceptible to injury. Usually, patients resume normal activity as soon as possible, but pain is an indicator to limit the offending activity. |
| Teach the use of cervical traction if prescribed. | Although infrequently prescribed, it may be used to help a cervical disk that has been bulging to slip back into place and unload the neck muscles and ligaments. Traditional method is a neck/head harness attached to a pulley and weight. A device for home use may include an inflatable collar that expands to push the head away from the shoulders. |
| Encourage a high-bulk diet, adequate or increased fluids, and stool softeners. | These measures prevent constipation, which would cause straining and pain. |
| Teach the purpose and potential side effects of the following medications for acute pain: | |
| • Combination analgesics (e.g., acetaminophen and tramadol, and opioid combinations such as hydrocodone and acetaminophen or oxycodone and acetaminophen) | Sufficient medication is given to achieve pain relief or adequate pain reduction. |
| • Teach the patient and their significant others about the possibility of acetaminophen toxicity and opioid addiction. Assess risk factors for addictive behaviors. | Acetaminophen may cause a serious skin reaction, liver failure, and death. Many opioids are combination medications with acetaminophen as well as over-the-counter drugs. |

| ASSESSMENT—RECOGNIZE CUES/ INTERVENTIONS—TAKE ACTION | RATIONALES |
|---|---|
| • Nonsteroidal antiinflammatory drugs (NSAIDs) and salicylates | These medications reduce inflammation and relieve pain. Initial dosing usually is scheduled to obtain a sustained antiinflammatory as well as analgesic effect. Side effects include blood thinning and serious gastrointestinal (GI) adverse events and dyspepsia. Kidneys may be affected if these drugs are taken for a long time, including renal failure, and there is an increased risk for serious cardiovascular events with prolonged use. |
| • Misoprostol or stomach protectants such as sucralfate or famotidine | These agents may be considered for use to reduce gastric irritation caused by stress, medications, and steroids (if used). |
| • Muscle relaxants (e.g., cyclobenzaprine, carisoprodol, methocarbamol, diazepam) | These medications decrease muscle spasms, thereby reducing pain. Common side effects are drowsiness, fatigue, dizziness, dry mouth, and GI upset. |
| • Corticosteroids (e.g., dexamethasone, prednisone, prednisolone) | Steroids may be given for a short period to reduce cord edema, if present, but use is controversial. |
|  | These medications can have significant side effects such as increased blood sugar, agitation, and hallucinations. They need to be tapered while being discontinued. |
| Teach the patient about the following medications used for chronic pain: |  |
| • Analgesics (e.g., NSAIDs, gabapentin, amitriptyline) | Nonnarcotic analgesics such as NSAIDs are used for chronic pain. (See NSAID side effects, earlier.) Tricyclic antidepressants (e.g., amitriptyline, desipramine, doxepin), as well as serotonin-norepinephrine reuptake inhibitors (e.g., duloxetine and venlafaxine), may help with chronic pain. Anticonvulsants such as gabapentin, carbamazepine, phenytoin, and levetiracetam help with neuropathic pain caused by nerve injury. |
| • Local injection of anesthetic (lidocaine or bupivacaine) and/or cortisone into epidural spaces, facet joints, sacroiliac joint, or trigger points | These medications reduce pain and muscle spasms and increase function by decreasing inflammation. |
| • Botulinum toxin injection into paravertebral regions | This injection relieves pain, probably through decreased muscle spasm, and improves function for 3–8 weeks |
| Teach the patient about the following techniques that may be effective in controlling chronic pain: |  |
| • Souchard global postural reeducation | This French physical therapy technique has been effective in restoring function and relieving long-term chronic pain. It consists of a series of maneuvers in which patients are in supine, sitting, and standing positions and involves stretching the paraspinal muscles and those of the abdominal wall so that joints are relieved of the compression that is typically the source of pain. |
| • Percutaneous electrical nerve stimulation | This device uses acupuncture-like needle probes positioned in soft tissue and/or muscles to stimulate peripheral sensory nerves to relieve persistent back pain. |
| • Implantable epidural spinal cord stimulator | This stimulator may be used to aid in the control of chronic pain when all other measures (e.g., PT, medications, surgery) have failed. |
| Suggest alternative/complementary therapies such as chiropractic, acupuncture, and cranial-sacral massage. | Many people achieve pain relief from these therapies. |

## Patient Problem/Analyze Cues/Prioritize Hypotheses

# Deficient Knowledge (Back Injury Prevention)

*due to* unfamiliarity with proper body mechanics and other measures that prevent back injury

***Desired Outcome/Generate Solutions:*** Within the treatment session (outpatient) or within the 24-hour period before hospital discharge, the patient verbalizes accurate knowledge of measures that prevent back injury and demonstrates proper body mechanics.

| ASSESSMENT—RECOGNIZE CUES/ INTERVENTIONS—TAKE ACTION | RATIONALES |
|---|---|
| Teach the patient proper body mechanics: | Using proper body mechanics avoids movements such as twisting, lifting with the back, and straining to reach that can cause back injury. |
| • Stand and sit straight with chin and head up and pelvis and back straight; avoid slouching. | |
| • Bend at knees and hips (squat) rather than at the waist, keeping back straight (not stooping forward). | |
| • When carrying objects, hold them close to the body, avoiding twisting when lifting or reaching. Spread feet for a wider base of support. Lift with legs, not the back. | |
| • Turn using the entire body instead of twisting. | |
| • Do not strain to reach things. If an object is overhead, raise oneself to its level, or move things out of the way if they are obstructing the object. | |
| • Avoid lifting anything heavier than 10–20 lb. | |
| • Encourage the use of long-handled pickup sticks to pick up small objects. | |
| • Have the patient demonstrate proper body mechanics, if possible, before hospital discharge. | |
| Teach about the following measures for keeping the body in alignment: | Keeping the body in proper alignment avoids strain on the back, thereby helping to prevent recurring back injury. |
| • Sit close to the pedals when driving a car and use a seat belt and firm back rest to support the back. | |
| • Support feet on a footstool when sitting so that knees are elevated to hip level or higher. | |
| • Obtain a firm mattress or bed board; use a flat pillow when sleeping to avoid strain on neck, arms, and shoulders; sleep in a side-lying position with knees bent or in a supine position with knees and legs supported on pillows; avoid sleeping in a prone position. | |
| • Avoid reaching or stretching to pick up objects. | |
| • Avoid sitting on furniture that does not support the back. | |
| Encourage the patient to achieve and/or maintain a proper weight for age, height, and gender; continue the exercise program prescribed by the health care provider; use thoracic and abdominal muscles when lifting; when standing for any length of time, stand with one foot on a step stool; sit in a firm chair for support. | Being overweight or obese can cause back strain and alteration in the center of balance, which can result in back pain and pressure. Exercise strengthens abdominal, thoracic, and back muscles. Using thoracic and abdominal muscles when lifting keeps a significant portion of weight off vertebral disks. Standing with one foot on a step stool helps relieve sciatica. Sitting in a firm chair provides support to the back. |
| Teach the rationale and procedure for Williams back exercises: | |
| • *Pelvic tilt:* Tighten stomach and buttock muscles and tilt the pelvis while keeping the lower spine flat against the floor; that is, the hips and buttocks are kept on the floor. | To strengthen abdominal muscles. |

| ASSESSMENT—RECOGNIZE CUES/ INTERVENTIONS—TAKE ACTION | RATIONALES |
|---|---|
| • *Knee-to-chest raise:* Start with a pelvic tilt. Raise each knee individually to the chest and return to the starting position. Then raise each knee individually to the chest and hold them there (both knees on chest together). | To help make a stiff back limber. |
| • *Nose-to-knee touch:* Raise the knee to the chest, and then pull the knee to the chest with the hands. Raise the head and try to touch nose to knee. Keep the lower back flat on floor. | To stretch hip muscles and strengthen abdominal muscles. |
| • *Half sit-ups:* Slowly raise head and neck to top of the chest. Reach both hands forward to the knees and hold for a count of 5. Repeat, keeping the lower back flat on the floor. | To strengthen abdomen and back. |
| Instruct the patient to wear supportive shoes with a low or moderate heel height for walking. | This measure helps maintain proper alignment of back and hips. |
| Encourage smoking cessation. | Smoking causes vasoconstriction, thus reducing circulation to disks. |
| Teach the following technique for sitting up at the bedside from a supine position: <br>• Logroll to the side, then rise to sitting position by pushing against the mattress with the hands while swinging legs over the side of the bed. Instruct the patient to maintain alignment of the back during the procedure. | This technique prevents strain on the back and promotes good body alignment. |
| Caution the patient that pain is the signal to stop or change an activity or position. | This precaution helps prevent additional back injury. |
| Encourage the patient to continue with a regular exercise and stretching program, including PT as indicated, walking, and exercising in water. | PT and a graded exercise program are initiated after acute symptoms subside and are the mainstay of therapy for low back pain. Exercise strengthens abdominal, thoracic, and back muscles to help prevent subsequent back injury. High-impact activities such as running may be limited until the injury is well healed. |
| Instruct the patient that the following indicators necessitate medical attention: increased sensory loss, increased motor loss/weakness, and loss of bowel and bladder function. | These indicators signal disk herniation, which necessitates timely intervention to prevent further damage. |

## Problems for Patients Undergoing Diskectomy With Laminectomy or Fusion Procedure

### Patient Problem/Analyze Cues/Prioritize Hypotheses

# Deficient Knowledge (Surgical Procedure)

*due to* unfamiliarity with diskectomy with laminectomy or fusion procedure

**Desired Outcomes/Generate Solutions:** Before surgery, the patient verbalizes accurate knowledge about the surgical procedure, preoperative routine, and postoperative regimen. The patient demonstrates activities and exercises correctly.

| ASSESSMENT—RECOGNIZE CUES/ INTERVENTIONS—TAKE ACTION | RATIONALES |
|---|---|
| For general interventions, see *Deficient Knowledge* in "Perioperative Care," Chapter 4. | Surgery is performed without delay if signs of spinal cord compression are present, such as significant motor or sensory loss or loss of sphincter control. Otherwise, surgery is considered only after symptoms fail to respond to conservative therapy. |

Continued

| ASSESSMENT—RECOGNIZE CUES/ INTERVENTIONS—TAKE ACTION | RATIONALES |
|---|---|
| Instruct the patient to expect the surgical team to confirm verbally and then mark the correct spinal level and correct side (e.g., anterior, posterior, right, left) of the surgical site. | These confirmations ensure that the appropriate surgery will be performed. |
| Reinforce the surgeon's explanation about the following: | |
| • Microdiscectomy | The herniated portion of the disk and small parts of the lamina are removed, using microsurgical techniques. Patients are usually out of bed the first day and may be released as outpatients or discharged the next day. |
| • Diskectomy with laminectomy | An incision is made, enabling the removal of part of the vertebra (laminectomy) so that the disk's herniated portion can be removed (diskectomy). If multiple intervertebral disk spaces are explored, a wound drain may be present after surgery. |
| • Percutaneous lumbar disk removal | Ultrasonic Nucleotome cannula or fiberoptic arthroscopic cannula can be inserted into the intervertebral space by fluoroscopy to enable fragmentation of the disk and its aspiration. A laser may be used to aid in disk excision. This is a relatively less invasive method of relieving pain from herniated disk, is done under local anesthesia, and may be performed on an outpatient basis. |
| • Spinal fusion | Fusion may be indicated for patients with recurrent low back or neck pain, spondylolisthesis, subluxation of the vertebrae, or multilevel disease. Bone chips are harvested from the iliac crest or tibia and placed between vertebrae in the prepared area of the unstable spine to fuse and stabilize the area. |
| | Internal fixation (e.g., rods, wiring, pedicle screws, lateral mass screws, fusion cages, interbody implants, bone rings, and plates) may be necessary to provide added stability until the fusion has healed fully. If the patient's own bone quality or quantity is inadequate, allograft (e.g., cadaver) bone or use of a recombinant human osteogenic protein preparation ("bone putty") as a bone graft substitute or supplement may be considered. |
| • Intradiskal electrothermal treatment (IDET) | IDET employs a probe that uses electricity to heat and shrink collagen tissue within the annulus wall to seal up painful tears. After healing, the disk toughens and desensitizes. |
| • Total intervertebral disk replacement with artificial disks such as the Charité | This procedure may help reduce the need for spinal fusions and avoid premature degeneration at adjacent levels of the spine. |
| • Discoplasty | This procedure reduces or reshapes a bulging disk through a small puncture, threading a probe into the center of the disk, and using a laser or radiofrequency to remove/evaporate the disk's center. |
| Teach the technique for deep breathing. Also teach the use of incentive spirometry. | Deep breathing and incentive spirometry are performed immediately after surgery to help expand the alveoli and aid in mobilizing lung secretions. Coughing may be contraindicated in the immediate postoperative period to prevent disruption of the fusion or surgical repair. |
| Document baseline and serial neurovascular checks, including color, capillary refill, pulse, warmth, muscle strength, movement, and sensation. | Vital signs and neurologic status are assessed at frequent intervals after surgery and compared with baseline to monitor trend. |
| Instruct the patient on the following signs and symptoms and importance of reporting them promptly: paresthesias, weakness, paralysis, radiculopathy, and changes in bowel or bladder function. | These indicators of impairment necessitate immediate attention by the health care staff because they signal the presence of autonomic stimulation—signs of cord compression caused by bleeding or hematoma formation. |

| ASSESSMENT—RECOGNIZE CUES/ INTERVENTIONS—TAKE ACTION | RATIONALES |
|---|---|
| Instruct the patient on the following signs and symptoms and importance of reporting them promptly: increased heart rate, thirst, faintness, or dizziness. | These are signs, along with decreased blood pressure, of hypovolemia and may occur because of blood loss. Patients undergoing fusion lose more blood during surgery than do those undergoing laminectomy. |
| Explain that the surgical dressing will be inspected for excess drainage or oozing at frequent intervals and that a closed wound drainage device may be present for 1–3 days postoperatively with a fusion procedure. | Bleeding with a laminectomy usually is minimal. Patients with a fusion may have slight bloody oozing postoperatively. Serous drainage usually is checked with a glucose reagent strip. Presence of glucose is a signal of CSF leakage. Bulging in the area of the wound may also signal CSF leakage or hematoma formation and should be reported promptly. |
| Advise that dressings will be inspected for increased drainage after the patient has been up, and lumbar dressings will be checked after each bedpan use. Inform the patient undergoing fusions that he or she will have a second dressing at the donor site. | Wet or contaminated dressings require prompt changing to prevent infection. |
| Instruct the patient to report any nausea or vomiting. | This helps ensure that antiemetics are given promptly. Vomiting could cause increased intraspinal pressure, which would result in pain. |
| Explain that the patient will be assessed for bowel and bladder dysfunction after the procedure. | Nerve injury during surgery can contribute to paralytic ileus. The abdomen will be checked for bowel sounds and distention. Patients may be asked to void within 8 hours of the procedure to check for urinary retention. |
| Caution the patient to avoid straining of stool. | Straining could cause increased intraspinal pressure, which would result in pain. Stool softeners may be given for that purpose. |
| Explain that fever may occur during the first few days postoperatively but that this does not necessarily signal an infection. | Early fever may be caused by drainage and contamination of CSF. Patients will be assessed for other indicators of infection, such as heat, redness, irritation, swelling, or drainage at wound site. |
| Instruct the patient to report headache, neck stiffness, or photophobia. | These are possible signs of meningeal irritation. |
| Inform the patient that pain may take days or weeks to resolve and does not indicate that surgery was unsuccessful. | Postoperative pain or tingling (paresthesia) often is caused by nerve root irritation and edema. Spasms are common on the third or fourth postoperative day and should not discourage the patient. |
| Teach the patient to request medication for pain as needed and not let pain get out of control. Instruct in use of 0–10 pain scale. | Pain is easier to manage before it becomes severe. Prolonged stimulation of pain receptors results in increased sensitivity to painful stimuli and will increase the amount of analgesic required to relieve pain. Patients who have had a fusion may expect significant pain from the bone graft donor site (commonly the iliac crest). The donor site may have extra padding. Muscle relaxants may be prescribed to supplement pain control. Patient-controlled analgesia and NSAIDs also may be used for postoperative pain control. Use of the pain scale enables a more accurate assessment of relief obtained. |
| Explain that in the immediate postoperative period the patient will follow the surgeon's activity restrictions and that new techniques and stabilization devices may enable earlier mobilization (some the same day) and fewer activity restrictions. | Patients may be required to lie supine for several hours to minimize the possibility of wound hematoma formation. After this period, the head of bed (HOB) of laminectomy patients usually can be raised to 20 degrees to facilitate eating and bedpan use. Patients undergoing spinal fusion may be kept flat and on bedrest longer than patients with laminectomies. Activity progression for spinal fusion patients is usually more cautious and slower than for laminectomy patients. The best practice regarding trapeze use is to restrict it during the initial 24–48 hours after lumbar and cervical procedures and avoid its use after thoracic procedures because of the torque and weight strain trapeze use can have on the spine. |

Continued

## ASSESSMENT—RECOGNIZE CUES/INTERVENTIONS—TAKE ACTION

## RATIONALES

| ASSESSMENT—RECOGNIZE CUES/INTERVENTIONS—TAKE ACTION | RATIONALES |
|---|---|
| Teach the following logroll technique for turning: position a pillow between legs, cross arms across chest while turning, and contract long back muscles to maintain shoulders and pelvis in straight alignment. Explain that, initially, the patient will be assisted in this procedure. | Only the logroll method is used for turning. This method stabilizes the spine and maintains alignment to enable healing and prevent dislodgment of the bone graft if a fusion is done. A turning sheet and sufficient help are used when logrolling patients. |
| Teach the following technique for getting out of bed: logroll to side, splint back, and rise to a sitting position by pushing against the mattress while swinging legs over side of bed. | This technique facilitates ease of getting out of bed and prevents disruption of the bone graft for fusion patients. |
| Explain that initially the patient will be helped to a sitting position and should not push against the mattress. Teach the patient with a cervical laminectomy not to pull self up with arms. When assisting patients with cervical laminectomy to a sitting position, caution them not to put their arms on the nurse's shoulders. | While in hospital with an electric bed, the HOB may be raised to facilitate a sitting position. These restrictions prevent neck flexion, extension, and hyperextension and strain on the operative site and incision. Pillows can be used to support arms for comfort. |
| Explain that antiembolism hose and possibly sequential compression devices (SCDs) will be applied after surgery. | These garments and devices promote venous return and prevent thrombus formation while patient is on bedrest. SCDs or hose should be worn until the amount of time out of bed ambulating is equal to the amount of time in bed. |
| Teach techniques for ankle circling and calf pumping. | These techniques promote blood circulation in the legs. |
| Teach the patient to report calf pain, tenderness, or warmth. | These are signs of deep vein thrombosis. |
| Advise the patient that the health care provider will prescribe certain postoperative activity restrictions. | Sitting is commonly restricted or allowed for only limited, prescribed periods in a straight-back chair. |
| Teach the patient not to sit for long periods on edge of the mattress. | A mattress does not provide enough support to the spine. |
| Explain that weakness, dizziness, and lightheadedness may occur on a first walk. | These problems may occur secondary to orthostatic hypotension. For management, see the discussion in *Risk for Altered Blood Pressure (Orthostatic Hypotension)* in "Immobility," Chapter 1. |
| Explain that the patient will be encouraged to walk progressively longer distances. | This action will promote endurance. |
| Instruct the patient to avoid stretching, twisting, flexing, or jarring the spine. Explain that the spine should be kept aligned and in a neutral position and that lifting and pulling/pushing objects are to be avoided. | These restrictions help prevent vertebral collapse, shifting of bone graft, or a bleeding episode. |
| If the patient is scheduled for a cervical laminectomy or fusion, caution not to pull with arms on objects such as side rails and avoid twisting, flexion, and extensions of the neck. | These restrictions prevent torque and strain on the spine that could cause misalignment. |
| Explain that a cervical collar may be worn postoperatively. | The collar aids in immobilizing the cervical spine. |
| Teach the use of braces or corsets if prescribed. | Persons undergoing a fusion procedure often wear a supportive brace or corset for 3 months or less to keep the operative site immobile so that the graft will heal and not dislodge. Braces should be applied while in bed. |
| Explain the importance of wearing cotton underwear under the brace, powdering the skin lightly with cornstarch, or providing additional padding under braces. | These measures help protect skin from irritation. Skin should be inspected daily for irritation or breakdown. |
| Explain that driving or riding in car (may be restricted for 6–8 weeks up to several months), sexual activity, lifting and carrying objects, tub bathing (generally, soaking the incision is avoided until about 1 week after sutures are out), going up and down stairs, amount of time to spend in and out of bed, back exercises, and expected time away from work will be discussed by the health care provider before discharge. | These guidelines and activity restrictions promote patient safety and an uneventful recovery after he or she is at home. |

| ASSESSMENT—RECOGNIZE CUES/ INTERVENTIONS—TAKE ACTION | RATIONALES |
|---|---|
| Explain that the patient should call the health care provider for symptoms such as increased weakness and numbness or change in bowel or bladder function. | These are indicators of spinal cord or nerve compression. |
| Teach the importance of reporting the following to the health care provider: swelling, discharge, drainage, persistent redness, local warmth, fever, and pain. | These signs and symptoms of postoperative wound infection require timely intervention. |
| Caution the patient to keep the incision dry and open to the air. | Moisture can promote infection. Wet dressings should be changed promptly. After 24–48 hours, the incision is usually undressed to promote "air" drying. |

## Problems for Patients Undergoing Anterior Cervical Fusion

### Patient Problem/Analyze Cues/Prioritize Hypotheses

# Risk for Impaired Swallowing

*due to* postoperative edema or hematoma formation following cervical disk surgery

**Desired Outcome/Generate Solutions:** The patient regains uncompromised swallowing and speaking ability (usually by the third postoperative day), as evidenced by normal breath sounds and absence of food in the oral cavity or choking/coughing.

| ASSESSMENT—RECOGNIZE CUES/ INTERVENTIONS—TAKE ACTION | RATIONALES |
|---|---|
| Include preoperative instructions regarding swallowing and secretion management to the patient scheduled to have an anterior cervical fusion. Instruct patient to promply report problems with swallowing and management of secretions. Explain that a soft diet and throat lozenges may be prescribed for 2–3 days postoperatively. | Postoperative edema or bleeding causing difficulty with swallowing is related to retraction of the trachea and esophagus during surgery to gain access to the disk. A sore throat can be expected after this surgery as a result of surgical manipulation and/or endotracheal tube. An informed individual likely will report postoperative difficulties with swallowing promptly for timely intervention. |
| After surgery, assess for edema of the face or neck or tracheal compression or deviation that could compromise respiratory function. Assess for complaints of excessive pressure in the neck or severe, uncontrolled incisional pain. Promptly report significant findings. | These indicators may be signs of hematoma or bleeding at the operative site that could cause airway compromise and therefore necessitate immediate intervention. |
| Listen for hoarseness. Encourage voice rest and facilitate alternative communication (e.g., provide storyboards, pen and pencil, flash cards). | Hoarseness can indicate laryngeal nerve irritation and signal ineffective cough or swallowing difficulty and necessitate choking and aspiration precautions. For most patients with hoarseness, the voice usually will return to normal as inflammation around the laryngeal nerve subsides. |
| Report immediately any respiratory distress, stridor, inability to speak, worsening hoarseness, or voice change. | These may be signs of aspiration, laryngeal nerve involvement/irritation, or increased edema or hematoma formation affecting the laryngeal nerve and vocal cords, any of which can be life threatening and necessitate immediate intervention. |
| Assess for and report diminished breath sounds compared with the patient's normal or preoperative status. | Diminished breath sounds could signal that aspiration has occurred and may result in pneumonia. |
| As indicated, assess oximetry as a quantitative measure of systemic oxygenation. | Values of 92% or less may signal the need for supplemental oxygen. |

Continued

| ASSESSMENT—RECOGNIZE CUES/ INTERVENTIONS—TAKE ACTION | RATIONALES |
|---|---|
| Monitor closed-suction devices and recharge suction device/chamber as indicated. | Recharging the closed-suction device facilitates wound drainage. |
| Check for gag and swallowing reflexes before oral intake. | Absence of gag and swallowing reflexes indicates that patient cannot begin oral intake. A postoperative diet with clear fluids and progression to more solid foods may begin only after patient demonstrates the ability to ingest fluids safely. |
| Position the patient in Fowler position, or semi-Fowler position at minimum, when initiating fluid intake. | These positions minimize the risk for aspiration by promoting the movement of fluids by gravity to the stomach and into the pylorus. |
| If not prohibited by surgery, encourage the use of the chin tuck to lessen the potential for aspiration. | A chin tuck forces the trachea to close and the esophagus to open, thereby decreasing the risk for aspiration. |

Also see *Risk for Aspiration* in "Older Adult Care," Chapter 3.

## ADDITIONAL PROBLEMS:

| | |
|---|---|
| *Acute Pain/Chronic Pain* | Chapter 5 |
| *Impaired Mobility* | Chapter 4 |
| "Immobility" | Chapter 1 |
| *Risk for Injury* due to sensory deficit, decreased level of consciousness | Chapter 36 |
| *Risk for Injury (Perioperative)* | Chapter 4 |

## ✔ PATIENT–FAMILY TEACHING AND DISCHARGE PLANNING

When providing patient–family teaching, focus on sensory information, avoid giving excessive information, and initiate a visiting nurse referral for necessary follow-up teaching. Include verbal and written information about the following:

✓ Prescribed exercise regimen, including rationale for each exercise, technique for performing the exercise, number of repetitions of each, and frequency of exercise periods. If possible, ensure that the patient demonstrates an understanding of exercise regimen and proper body mechanics before hospital discharge.

✓ Wound incision care. Indicators of postoperative wound infection that necessitate medical attention include swelling, discharge, persistent redness, local warmth, fever, and pain.

✓ Review of use and application of cervical collar for patients who have had a cervical fusion and importance of wearing collar at all times.

✓ Use and care of a brace or immobilizer if appropriate.

✓ Medications, including drug name, rationale, dosage, schedule, precautions, and potential side effects. Also discuss drug–drug, herb–drug, and food–drug interactions.

✓ Anticonstipation routine, which should be initiated during hospitalization.

✓ Pain control measures.

✓ Telephone number of a resource person in case questions arise after hospital discharge.

✓ Postsurgical activity restrictions as directed by the health care provider. These may affect the following: driving and riding in a car, returning to work, sexual activity, lifting and carrying, tub bathing, going up and down steps, and amount of time spent in or out of bed.

✓ Signs and symptoms of worsening neurologic function and the importance of notifying health care provider immediately if they develop. These include numbness, weakness, paralysis, and bowel and bladder dysfunction.

✓ Obtain additional information from the following:
  • Spine Health www.spine-health.com

# Multiple Sclerosis 40

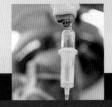

## OVERVIEW/PATHOPHYSIOLOGY

Multiple sclerosis (MS) is a chronic autoimmune disorder driven by activated T cells. It is a neurodegenerative condition of the central nervous system (CNS) causing scattered and sporadic demyelination (plaques) and axonal damage (atrophy and black holes). Although the cause is unknown, it is thought to develop in a genetically susceptible person after an environmental exposure, such as geographic location infection, physical or emotional stress, pregnancy, or low vitamin D. Common genetic factors have been found in families with more than one affected member. MS is most common among people who have lived in cool, temperate climates before puberty. African Americans have half the incidence of White Americans. More females than males are affected (3:1). Onset ranges from pediatric ages to geriatric ages.

In healthy individuals, myelin permits nerve impulses to travel quickly through the nerve pathways of the CNS. In response to the inflammation seen with MS, the myelin nerve sheaths scar, degenerate, or separate from the axon cylinders. This demyelination interrupts electrical nerve transmission and causes a wide variety of symptoms that impair neuromuscular function. As less severe inflammation resolves, myelin function may regenerate, enabling electric nerve impulse transmission to be restored. If the inflammation is severe and/or repetitive, it causes irreversible destruction of myelin or axon degeneration. Involved areas are replaced by dense glial scar tissue that forms patchy areas of sclerotic plaque, which permanently damage conductive pathways of the CNS. Axon nerve fibers may degenerate. Axonal degeneration starts early in the disease process along with demyelination. Axonal damage is speculated to cause permanent and progressive disability. Deficits presenting after 3 months usually are permanent.

The course of MS is highly variable. Multifocal presentation and frequent attacks during the first year may imply a more aggressive course. Presently, four forms of MS are considered:

| Types of MS | Description |
| --- | --- |
| Relapsing remitting (RRMS) | Up to 85% of MS patients. Marked by relapse/exacerbations followed by a period of partial or complete remission. |

| Types of MS | Description |
| --- | --- |
| Primary progressive | About 10% of MS patients are first diagnosed with this type of MS. Patients have gradual worsening neurologic function over time with some minor improvements but no distinct relapses or remissions. |
| Secondary progressive | Most people with RRMS progress to this type of MS. Begins with relapse and remissions and this is followed by the progression of the disorder with or without minor remissions or plateaus. |
| Progressive relapsing | Acute relapses occur with or without full recovery, but disease progression continues between events. Five percent of people with MS are diagnosed with this type of MS. |

Typically, an increasing number of symptoms occur with each exacerbation, with less complete clearing of symptoms and with deficits becoming cumulative. Over time, the relapsing-remitting form usually transitions to the secondary-progressive form in which neurologic impairment progresses continuously with or without superimposed relapses. A small portion of patients (10%–20%) initially begin with the primary progressive form, characterized by gradual ongoing accumulation of symptoms and deficits, with absence of clear-cut exacerbations and remissions. The progressive-relapsing form (5%) is characterized by a progressive disease course from onset, with clear acute exacerbations. Progression continues during the periods between disease exacerbations.

There are no diagnostic tests that alone definitively determine the diagnosis of MS. However, patients with the combination of the following three criteria are diagnosed with MS: (1) at least two inflammatory demyelinating lesions are found in at least two different locations within the CNS; (2) damage or attack to the CNS that occurs at different times (usually one month or more apart); and (3) all other possible diagnoses are ruled out.

## HEALTH CARE SETTING

Primary care, neurology clinic, physiatry/rehabilitation, psychiatry/mental health, pain clinic, or long-term care, with possible hospitalization resulting from complications.

## ASSESSMENT

The onset of MS can be extremely rapid, or it can be insidious, with exacerbations and remissions. Signs and symptoms vary widely depending on lesion sites and the extent of pathology and can change from day to day. Early symptoms can be vague, including fatigue, weakness, heaviness, clumsiness, numbness, and tingling. Optic neuritis is the most common presentation for MS diagnosis. Trigeminal neuralgia is also fairly common.

**Damage to motor nerve tracts.** Weakness, paralysis, and spasticity can occur. Fatigue is common. Diplopia may occur secondary to ocular muscle involvement.

**Damage to cerebellar or brainstem regions.** Signs and symptoms are intention tremor, nystagmus, or other tremors; incoordination, ataxia; and weakness of facial and throat muscles resulting in difficulty chewing, dysphagia, dysarthria, dizziness, nausea, and vomiting.

**Damage to sensory nerve tracts.** Often, only sensory symptoms occur in the beginning and may include altered perception of pain, touch, and temperature; allodynia (pain caused by simple touch); paresthesias such as numbness and tingling ("pins and needles") or burning sensations; decrease or loss of proprioception; and decrease or loss of vibratory sense. Optic neuritis is a common early symptom, potentially causing partial or total loss of vision, visual clouding or shimmering, and pain with eye movement.

**Damage to cerebral cortex (especially frontal lobes).** Mood swings, inappropriate affect, euphoria, apathy, irritability, depression, hyperexcitability, poor memory, judgment, foresight and planning, and abstract reasoning may occur. There is often difficulty with word finding, concentration, attention, and processing or learning new information.

**Damage to motor and sensory control centers.** Urinary frequency, urgency, or retention; urinary and fecal incontinence; constipation may occur.

**Lower cord lesions (low thoracic and lumbar).** Impotence may occur due to diminished sensations that result in inhibited sexual response.

**Physical assessment.** Motor or sensory impairment occurs as discussed previously. Lhermitte sign may be present, in which an electrical sensation runs down the back and legs during neck flexion. Ophthalmoscopic inspection may reveal temporal pallor of optic disks. Reflex assessment may show increased deep tendon reflexes and diminished abdominal skin and cremasteric reflexes.

## DIAGNOSTIC TESTS

**Magnetic Resonance Imaging (MRI) studies.** MRIs reveal the presence of plaques and demyelination in the CNS. This is the test of choice when MS is suspected. Expanding MRI technology is becoming ever more sensitive and capable of identifying current sites of inflammation and demyelination and showing changes associated with disease progression. T1-weighted MRI may show hypointense lesions including black holes, which correlate with axonal loss and indicate old lesions. T2-weighted MRI can show old and new lesions and is most commonly used to follow response to treatment by many clinicians. Gadolinium enhancement shows areas of active demyelination. Fluid-attenuated inversion recovery (FLAIR) is very helpful in detecting cerebral lesions specific to MS. All other forms of MRI are used strictly for research related to MS and can include MRI diffusion tensor imaging and magnetic resonance (MR) spectroscopy, which frequently reveal the involvement of otherwise normal-appearing white matter. Magnetization transfer imaging may show indirect evidence of axonal loss. MR spectroscopy can measure a decline in a brain chemical called $N$-acetylaspartate as a marker of axonal damage and appears to predict disease severity. Functional MRI can show new lesions, and short tau inversion recovery is useful in detecting demyelination.

**Electrophysiology studies.** Results may be slow or absent because of interference of nerve transmission from demyelination or plaque formation. Visual electrophysiology studies are most commonly used to evaluate optic nerve demyelination.

**Lumbar puncture and cerebrospinal fluid analysis.** This exam evaluates cerebrospinal fluid (CSF) levels of oligoclonal bands and free kappa chains of immunoglobulin G (IgG), protein, gamma globulin, myelin basic protein, and lymphocytes, any of which may be elevated in the presence of MS. During acute MS attacks, destruction of the myelin sheath releases myelin basic protein into the CSF. Oligoclonal bands of IgG are seen in 85%–95% of patients with MS. This and the finding of free kappa chains in the CSF support a diagnosis of MS.

**Computed tomography scan.** Demonstrates the presence of plaques and rules out mass lesions. This technique is less effective than MRI in detecting areas of plaque and demyelination and is no longer commonly used as part of the diagnostic workup if MRI is available.

## Patient Problem/Analyze Cues/Prioritize Hypotheses

# Pain

*due to* motor and sensory nerve tract damage

**Desired Outcomes/Generate Solutions:** Within 1–2 hours of intervention, the patient's subjective evaluation of pain and spasms improves, as documented by pain scale. Objective indicators, such as grimacing, are absent or reduced.

| ASSESSMENT—RECOGNIZE CUES/ INTERVENTIONS—TAKE ACTION | RATIONALES |
|---|---|
| Maintain a comfortable room temperature. Advise patients to keep the environment cool in warm weather and avoid hot baths or showers. | Heat tends to aggravate MS symptoms by increasing core body temperature. |
| Provide a passive, assisted, or active range of motion every 2 hours and periodic stretching exercises. Provide instructions on these exercises to the patient and caregivers, and encourage their performance several times daily. Explain that sleeping in a prone position may help decrease flexor spasm of the hips and knees and that splints or cones for hands with elastic bands may help control hand spasms. | These interventions reduce muscle tightness and spasms, maintain joint function, and prevent contractures. Physical therapy (PT), occupational therapy (OT), and assistive devices or braces may be prescribed to maintain mobility and independence with activities of daily living (ADLs). Placing weights on the affected limbs may help with mild tremors. |
| Administer muscle relaxants as prescribed. | These agents help decrease muscle spasms, thus ultimately decreasing pain. In addition, there may be a secondary benefit with a decrease in neuropathic pain. Classically used are baclofen and tizanidine. Dantrolene is an older medication that is still sometimes used, but it can cause sedation. |
| Administer sedatives (e.g., diazepam) as prescribed. | These medications may be given for both their anxiety-reducing and muscle-relaxant effects, which may help spasms and tremors. |
| Administer analgesics (e.g., nonsteroidal antiinflammatory drugs [NSAIDs], acetaminophen), antidepressants, and neuropathic pain medications as prescribed. | Nonopioid analgesia such as NSAIDs is used for chronic pain. (See NSAID side effects in "Intervertebral Disk Disease.") |
| | Tricyclic antidepressants and serotonin-norepinephrine reuptake inhibitors may increase neurotransmitters in the spinal cord that reduce pain signals. |
| | Anticonvulsants such as gabapentin, target neuropathic pain caused by nerve injury. (See "Seizures and Epilepsy," Chapter 42, for side effects/precautions.) Patients with uncontrolled pain may be referred to pain management for opioid-based interventions or interventional pain techniques such as nerve blocks or surgical intervention. |
| For other interventions, see *Acute Pain* in "General Care of Patients With Neurologic Disorders," Chapter 36. | |

## Patient Problem/Analyze Cues/Prioritize Hypotheses

# Deficient Knowledge (Disease Management)

*due to* unfamiliarity with MS symptoms and factors that affect MS pathology

***Desired Outcome/Generate Solutions:*** By day 3 (or before hospital discharge), the patient and significant other/caregiver verbalize factors that exacerbate, prevent, and ameliorate symptoms of MS.

| ASSESSMENT—RECOGNIZE CUES/ INTERVENTIONS—TAKE ACTION | RATIONALES |
|---|---|
| Assess the patient's health care literacy (language, reading, comprehension). Assess culture and culturally specific information needs. Determine the patient's knowledge base about MS. | This assessment helps ensure that materials are selected and presented in a manner that is culturally and educationally appropriate. |
| Instruct the patient/significant other/caregiver to avoid heat, both external (hot weather, bath) and internal (fever). | Heat tends to aggravate weakness, pain, and other symptoms of MS. |
| Provide instructions on preventive measures, such as avoiding hot baths or showers and using acetaminophen or aspirin to reduce fever, if present. Also suggest body cooling products such as vests, wrist wraps, or neck wraps, drinking cold water, and using fan/air conditioning if available. | These measures aid in maintaining homeostasis of core body temperature when the temperature is elevated. |

Continued

| ASSESSMENT—RECOGNIZE CUES/ INTERVENTIONS—TAKE ACTION | RATIONALES |
|---|---|
| Caution the patient to avoid exposure to persons known to have significant infections and take precautions against developing an infection. | Infection often precedes exacerbations. Some MS medications can make the patient more susceptible to infections. |
| Provide instructions in the proper technique for hand washing and hand antisepsis and the importance of avoiding vaccinations with live attenuated viruses, which could trigger an exacerbation. | |
| Review with the patient/significant other/caregiver indicators of common infections and the importance of seeking prompt medical treatment in case they occur. Instruct all involved with patient care to check for typical signs/symptoms of urinary tract infection (UTI) (increased frequency, urgency, or incontinence) and to check urine for changes in odor or presence of cloudiness or blood. Advise that an acute increase in spasticity can often signal an infection in MS. Also provide instructions on how to monitor for more serious infections such as pyelonephritis (e.g., fever, costovertebral angle tenderness, chills, flank pain). | A person with MS is especially susceptible to UTI because of bladder dysfunction. Because of the disease process, patients may not feel any pain with urination and therefore need to be alert to other signs of UTI. See "Care of the Kidney Transplant Recipient," Chapter 31, for a discussion of common infections. <br><br> Untreated UTI organisms can also ascend to the kidney and lead to a kidney infection. |
| Review with all involved in patient care the relationship between stress/ fatigue and MS exacerbations. Encourage the patient to reduce the factors that cause stress. Encourage the use of stress reduction techniques such as progressive relaxation, self-coaching, and guided imagery. | Avoiding stress and fatigue may prevent exacerbations. While there is no definitive relationship between stress and MS exacerbation, chronic stress may cause alterations in endogenous glucocorticoids, affecting the body's ability to regulate inflammatory pressure. Although each person responds differently to triggers that may worsen the disease, stress may be a trigger in some patients with MS. |
| Provide instructions to the patient/significant other/caregivers on the signs and symptoms of depression. If the patient is depressed, suggest that he or she discuss use of antidepressants (e.g., selective serotonin reuptake inhibitors, NSRIs) and counseling with a health care provider. | Depression rates in MS patients are significantly higher with a higher risk for suicide than in the general population. It has an intrinsic cause from cerebral lesions resulting in a decrease in neurochemicals. It can also be caused by extrinsic factors such as loss of self-esteem and role within the family unit or career. Depression can compound fatigue, cognitive function, and sleep issues in MS. |
| Encourage the patient to get sufficient rest, stop activity short of fatigue, schedule activity and rest periods, and conserve energy in ADLs. | Eighty percent of people with MS have fatigue. Patients can conserve energy and manage their fatigue during ADLs by sitting while getting dressed, rather than standing; sliding heavy objects along work surfaces, rather than lifting them; using a wheeled cart to transport items; having work surfaces at the proper height; and using assistive devices and delegating. |
| Suggest that the patient ask the health care provider about antifatigue medications and discuss possible contributing factors to fatigue such as depression, sleep difficulties, or metabolic issues. | Fatigue is the most common complaint in MS and does not correlate with the level of disability. Often comorbidities such as thyroid issues, low B12, anemia, sleep apnea, and depression, may intensify fatigue. <br><br> Some drugs are used off label to treat. <br><br> MS-related fatigue (e.g., amantadine, fluoxetine) and modafinil (a wakefulness-promoting agent) <br><br> help relieve fatigue associated with MS. See "Parkinsonism," Chapter 41, for side effects and precautions when using amantadine. |
| Encourage the patient to plan each day, break projects into smaller tasks, distribute tasks throughout the day, rest before difficult tasks, take planned recovery time after tasks, identify priorities, and eliminate nonessential activities. | Conserving energy and decreasing fatigue are effective strategies for improving quality of life. |
| Discuss the need for family planning with both men and women. Provide information about birth control measures to female patients who desire counseling. | Patients are often on multiple medications. Disease-modifying therapies (DMTs) are contraindicated in pregnancy, and some of these medications can affect males as well as females. There may be a decreased relapse rate during pregnancy but increased exacerbations postpartum. Those planning a pregnancy should consult and work with their health care providers before pregnancy. |
| Encourage exercise, continued activity, and normal lifestyle even when limitations are necessary. | Deconditioning can contribute to a decreased functional level and quality of life. Exercise often decreases many MS symptoms, and a planned exercise program can be incorporated into a scheduled activity/rest plan. |

## Patient Problem/Analyze Cues/Prioritize Hypotheses

# Deficient Knowledge (Medications)

*due to* unfamiliarity with MS exacerbations and its medication management

**Desired Outcome/Generate Solutions:** By day 3 (or before hospital or clinic discharge), the patient verbalizes accurate information about the prescribed medications.

| ASSESSMENT—RECOGNIZE CUES/ INTERVENTIONS—TAKE ACTION | RATIONALES |
|---|---|
| Assess the patient's health care literacy (language, reading, comprehension). Assess culture and culturally specific information needs. Determine the patient's knowledge base about MS. | This assessment helps ensure that materials are selected and presented in a manner that is culturally and educationally appropriate. |
| Assess the patient's knowledge base about the prescribed medications. As indicated, provide verbal instructions and language-appropriate written handouts that describe the name, purpose, dose, and schedule of the prescribed medications. Also discuss drug–drug, herb–drug, and food–drug interactions. | A well-informed patient is likely to follow the prescribed medication regimen, recognize side effects, and report those that necessitate prompt attention. |
| Provide instructions to the patient/significant other/caregiver on disease-modifying therapies (DMTs): *glatiramer injections, interferon injections, infusion treatments, or oral therapies.* | DMTs are prescribed to help manage the disease process by reducing relapse rates, progression to disability, and MRI lesion accumulation. DMT treatment is long-term therapy and needs to be taken as prescribed on an ongoing basis. |
| **!** • Provide instructions on the side-effect profile consistent with the patient's DMT. | DMTs have potentially very serious side effects. Patients and significant others need to know what and how to monitor for these and also when to notify their health care provider. Each DMT has specific resources available for this type of education. There are also many MS organizations that can help with this information. |
| Assess for and notify the health care provider of any and all DMT side effects. | Side effects need to be evaluated to determine the next course of action. Many side effects can be managed with minimal intervention. Some side effects can be serious and warrant immediate discontinuation of the medication. |
| Provide specific DMT administration instructions to the patient/significant other/caregiver as appropriate. | Each DMT has very specific issues in maintaining efficacy, potency, and safety. For example, frequency, timing, and route of administration; screening/monitoring of blood work and other surveillance protocols; seriousness of nonadherence, which varies with DMTs and can be potentially fatal with certain DMTs. |
| Encourage the patient/significant other/caregiver to become educated about MS, MS exacerbations, and MS symptoms. Encourage the patient and those who are involved in their care to obtain knowledge and support from reputable websites, MS organizations, and support groups, lectures by MS experts; MS publications subscriptions (most are free). | MS is a complicated and dynamic disease process. Patients, significant others, and caregivers should understand the difference between MS symptoms and exacerbation, DMT's role in managing the disease, and the difference between DMTs and medications to manage symptoms and medications to treat exacerbations. Education helps maintain better adherence to treatments and interventions. |
| Instruct the patient/significant other/caregiver about exacerbation treatment: use of high-dose steroids (i.e., prednisone, methylprednisolone, dexamethasone [Decadron]) or similar products (e.g., adrenocorticotropic hormone). | The purpose of medications used to treat exacerbation is to reduce symptoms by decreasing inflammation and associated edema of the myelin, thereby hastening the reduction of presenting symptoms. |
| • Educate the patient/significant other/caregiver about the side effects of associated high-dose steroid treatments. | Usually, exacerbations are treated in the home environment. Therefore it is essential that side effects are understood and recognized so that they can be reported to the health care provider promptly. |
| **!** Explain that tapering rather than abruptly stopping high-dose steroids when they are discontinued may be appropriate for some patients. | Tapering helps maintain the body's own cortisone sources. Abrupt discontinuation may result in adrenal crisis or psychosis. |

Continued

## ASSESSMENT—RECOGNIZE CUES/ INTERVENTIONS—TAKE ACTION

## RATIONALES

| Assessment/Interventions | Rationales |
|---|---|
| • When steroids are prescribed: Instruct the patient/significant other/caregiver on symptoms of potassium deficiency, such as anorexia, nausea, and muscle weakness, and encourage the patient to eat foods high in potassium. | Hypokalemia is a common side effect of steroid use. Potassium supplements also may be prescribed. |
| • When steroids are prescribed: Instruct the patient to eat a diet low in sodium and monitor for and report unusual weight gain or swelling of extremities. | A low-sodium diet minimizes the potential for fluid retention, which is a common occurrence with steroids. Diuretics may be prescribed to reduce fluid retention. |
| • When steroids are prescribed: Instruct the patient/significant other/caregiver to measure the patient's blood pressure daily. | Hypertension is another side effect of steroid medications. Home blood pressure kits are available at most drug stores. Antihypertensives may be prescribed. |
| • When steroids are prescribed: Instruct the patient/significant other/caregiver to monitor the patient's blood glucose for hyperglycemia, report elevations, and as indicated, control glucose level with diet, oral agents, or insulin. | Hyperglycemia is a side effect of steroid use. In patients with known diabetes mellitus, antidiabetic medication doses may need to be adjusted. |
| • When steroids are prescribed: Instruct the patient/significant other/caregiver to monitor the patient's stool for any changes in color and report gastrointestinal (GI) symptoms and change in stool, specifically very dark (tarry) stool. | Gastric ulcers are a common side effect of steroid use, which would manifest in changes in the stool color (tarry stools), which is a sign of occult blood. |
| • When steroids are prescribed: Instruct the patient to take the medication with food, milk, or buffering agents and to avoid aspirin, indomethacin, caffeine, or other GI irritants while taking steroid medication. | These measures help prevent stomach upset and gastric irritation. In addition to antacids, $H_2$-receptor blockers may be prescribed to prevent gastric ulcer. |
| • When steroids are prescribed: Instruct the patient/significant other/caregiver to monitor the patient for injuries and report wounds that are slow in healing. | Steroids can impair wound healing. |
| • Caution the patient who is taking steroids to avoid contact with persons known to have infections and to monitor for and report fever, prolonged sore throat, and colds or other infections. | Steroids can mask infections, making them appear less severe; therefore follow-up with the care provider is important. |
| • Advise the patient who is taking steroids to be alert for and to report mood changes. | Antipsychotropic agents may be prescribed to help with mood changes associated with steroid use. |

## ADDITIONAL PROBLEMS:

## ✓ PATIENT–FAMILY TEACHING AND DISCHARGE PLANNING

There are different forms of MS, and the patient with MS may have a wide variety of symptoms. MS can cause disability ranging from mild to severe. When providing patient–family teaching, focus on treatment in terms of managing the disease with DMTs, treatment of exacerbation with steroids, and treatment of symptoms. Avoid giving excessive information, and initiate a visiting nurse referral for necessary follow-up teaching. Include verbal and written information about the following:

- ✓ Exacerbation aspects of the disease process and progression. Explain the effects of demyelination and neuronal injury on sensory and motor function and factors that aggravate symptoms. Explain that DMTs are proactive treatments that interfere with the natural history of the disease and have a positive impact on exacerbation rates, disability progression, and lesion activity. Additional treatment is symptomatic and supportive.
- ✓ Safety measures relative to decreased sensation, visual disturbances, and motor deficits.
- ✓ Medications, including drug name, purpose, dosage, frequency, precautions, and potential side effects. Also discuss drug–drug, herb–drug, and food–drug interactions.
- ✓ Exercises that promote muscle strength and mobility and measures that reduce spasticity and increase strength, promote quality of life, and maintain safety. For more severe disabilities, preventing contractures and skin breakdown, transfer techniques and proper body mechanics, and use of assistive devices and other measures to maximize health and wellness are incorporated.
- ✓ Measures for relieving pain, muscle spasms, or other discomforts.
- ✓ Indications of constipation, urinary retention, or UTI; implementation of bowel and bladder training programs; and self-catheterization technique or care of indwelling urinary catheters.
- ✓ Indications of upper respiratory infection; implementation of measures that help prevent regurgitation, aspiration, and respiratory infection.
- ✓ Measures for managing fatigue.
- ✓ Measures for fall prevention.
- ✓ Dietary adjustments that may be appropriate for neurologic deficit (e.g., soft, semisolid foods for patients with chewing difficulties or a high-fiber diet for patients experiencing constipation).
- ✓ Importance of follow-up care, including visits to the health care provider, PT, and OT, as well as speech, sexual, or psychologic counseling to help the patient and significant other cope and adapt to real or potential lifestyle changes functionally, emotionally, economically, and socially that are either a direct or an indirect result of the disease process.
- ✓ Referrals to community resources, such as local and national Multiple Sclerosis Society chapters, public health nurse, visiting nurse association, community support groups, social workers, psychologists, vocational rehabilitation agencies, home health agencies, extended and skilled care facilities, and financial counseling. Additional general information can be obtained by contacting the following:
  - National Multiple Sclerosis Society: www. nationalmssociety.org
  - Multiple Sclerosis Association of America: www. mymsaa.com
  - MS Views & News: www.msviewsandnews.org
  - MS World: www.msworld.org
  - Multiple Sclerosis International Federation: www. msif.org
  - MS Perspectives: www.MSperspectives.com

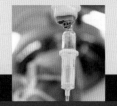

# Parkinson's Disease 41

## OVERVIEW/PATHOPHYSIOLOGY

Parkinson's disease (PD) is a slowly progressive degenerative disorder of the central nervous system (CNS) affecting the brain centers that regulate movement and balance. For unknown reasons, cell death occurs in the substantia nigra of the midbrain. When healthy, the substantia nigra projects dopaminergic neurons into the corpus striatum and releases the neurotransmitter dopamine in that area. Degeneration of these neurons leads to an abnormally low concentration of dopamine in the basal ganglia. The basal ganglia control muscle tone and voluntary motor movement through a balance between two main neurotransmitters, dopamine and acetylcholine. The deficit of dopamine, which has an inhibitory effect, allows the relative excess of acetylcholine. The excitatory effect of acetylcholine causes overactivity of the basal ganglia, which interferes with normal muscle tone and control of smooth, purposeful movement, causing the characteristic symptoms of PD: muscle rigidity, tremors, and slowness of movement. Nerve cell loss in the substantia nigra and accumulation of Lewy bodies in the brainstem and pigmented areas of the brain are the pathologic hallmarks of PD. Lewy bodies are tiny abnormal spherical alpha-synuclein protein deposits that accumulate inside the damaged nerve cells and disrupt the brain's normal functioning. Symptoms start when cell loss reaches about 80%.

Approximately 1% of all individuals older than 60 years have this disease. PD is usually progressive, and death can result from aspiration pneumonia or choking. *Neuroleptic malignant syndrome*, a medical emergency, is usually precipitated by failure to take the prescribed medications. *Acute akinesia*, sometimes referred to as *parkinsonian crisis*, is another medical emergency and seems associated with infections or surgical procedures.

## HEALTH CARE SETTING

Primary care, neurology clinic, rehabilitation facility, long-term care facility, and possible acute care hospitalization resulting from complications as the disease progresses

## ASSESSMENT

Initially, symptoms are mild and include stiffness or slight hand tremors. They gradually increase and can become disabling. Cardinal features are tremors, rigidity, and akinesia/bradykinesia and postural disturbances/loss of reflexes. Presentation is ipsilateral and will become bilateral with progression. Clinical features most suggestive of idiopathic PD include unilateral onset, presence of resting tremor, and a clear-cut response to treatment with levodopa. Assessment findings vary in degree and are highly individualized. PD is sometimes categorized as either tremor-dominant type or postural instability and gait disturbance–dominant type.

***Tremors.*** Increase when the limb is at rest and completely supported against gravity and stop with voluntary movement and during sleep (nonintentional "resting" tremor). "Pill-rolling" tremor of the hands and "to-and-fro" tremor of the head are typical.

***Bradykinesia.*** Slowness of movement, stiffness of muscles, gait difficulty, and difficulty initiating movement. Patients may have a mask-like, blank facial expression; "unblinking" stare; difficulty chewing and swallowing; drooling caused by decreased frequency of swallowing; and a high-pitched, monotone, weak voice. Speech may be slow and slurred. The patient also has loss of automatic associated movements, such as the normal arm-swing movement, difficulty getting out of a chair, and a small-step or shuffling gait when walking. Episodes of freezing are common and can be seen with gait initiation, in tight areas such as doorways, and in interrupted gait fluidity. Handwriting becomes progressively smaller, cramped, and tremulous (micrographia).

***Increased muscle rigidity.*** Limb muscles become rigid on passive motion. Typically, this rigidity results in jerky ("cogwheel") motions or steady resistance to all movement ("lead-pipe" rigidity).

***Loss of postural reflexes.*** Causes the typical stooped, forward-leaning, shuffling, propulsive gait with short, rapidly accelerating steps; stumbling; and difficulty maintaining or regaining balance, which makes the individual prone to stumbling and falling. Abnormal gait in which the body is bent backward (retropulsion) also may be present.

***Autonomic.*** Excessive diaphoresis, seborrhea, postural hypotension, decreased libido, hypomotility of the gastrointestinal (GI) tract (causing constipation), and urinary hesitancy. Vision may blur as a result of lost accommodation.

***Mental health/psychiatric.*** Dementia (e.g., forgetfulness, irritability, paranoia, hallucinations) is commonly associated with PD. However, not all patients develop impaired intellectual and mental functioning. Mental status testing may be complicated by the patient's movement disorder. Some patients may experience akathisia, a condition of motor restlessness, which can be as mild as a feeling of inner distress to a compelling need to

Risk for Falls | Parkinson's Disease | 299

PART I: Medical-Surgical Nursing Care Plans

walk about constantly. Depression is common. Psychosis is often drug-induced.

***Neuroleptic malignant syndrome.*** The classic triad of symptoms includes fever (100%), rigidity (90%), and cognitive changes (e.g., drowsiness, confusion progressing to stupor and coma). Other symptoms include tremor, tachypnea, diaphoresis, and occasionally dystonia and chorea. Symptoms are associated with discontinuation or reduction in dopaminergic medications. This sudden and severe increase in muscle rigidity can cause inability to swallow or maintain a patent airway.

***Acute akinesia.*** This sudden decrease in motor performance or inability to move ("frozen") lasts for more than 48 hours and is transiently unresponsive to dopaminergic rescue medication (e.g., apomorphine) or increases in dopaminergic medications. Triggering factors include infections, surgery, fractures, GI disease, and drug manipulations.

***Oculogyric crisis.*** Fixation of eyes in one position, generally upward, sometimes for several hours. This is relatively rare.

***Physical assessment.*** Usually, a positive glabellar blink reflex (Myerson sign) is elicited by tapping a finger between the patient's eyebrows. Normally individuals will blink several times before the reflex is extinguished. In PD the patient cannot extinguish the response and continues to blink until the stimulus (tapping) is removed. A positive palmomental (palm-chin) reflex can be elicited (ipsilateral muscles of the chin and corner of mouth contract when the patient's palm is stroked). Diminished postural reflexes are present on neurologic examination; however, there is a risk for injury with this test because patients may quickly lose balance and fall.

***History/risk factors.*** PD has many possible causes. Metabolic causes such as hypothyroidism need to be ruled out. Long-term therapy with large doses of medications, such as haloperidol, phenothiazines, metoclopramide, methyldopa, reserpine, or chlorpromazine, can produce extrapyramidal side effects known as pseudoparkinsonism. If caused by these medications, symptoms will disappear when the drug is discontinued, although it may take up to several months. The recreational drug "ecstasy" and an improperly synthesized heroin-like substance, 1-methyl-4-phenyl-1,2,3,6-tetrahydropyridine, also have induced parkinsonism. Other causes include toxins (e.g., heavy metals, pesticides, lacquer thinner, and carbon monoxide), cerebrovascular disease, head injury (especially repeated injury), and viral encephalitis. Living in a rural area is associated with increased PD risk, while nicotine intake is associated with decreased PD risk. Most cases of PD occur without an apparent or known cause, although genetic susceptibility is believed to play a role. Genetic factors appear to be more predominant when the disease begins before the ages of 45–50 years, with the most commonly known forms of hereditary parkinsonism caused by mutations in the parkin gene (*PARK2*) and alpha-synuclein gene (*SNCA*).

***Unified PD rating scale.*** May be used as a standardized assessment tool and includes evaluation of self-reported disability (i.e., inability to perform activities of daily living) as well as clinical scoring by a health care provider.

***Hoehn and Yahr stage scale.*** Simple and popular scale that establishes PD severity. The different stages of disease are classified from I (mild) to V (severe).

## DIAGNOSTIC TESTS

Diagnosis usually is made on the basis of physical assessment of the characteristic symptoms, a ruling out of other causes of pathology, and a positive response to levodopa therapy.

---

**Patient Problem/Analyze Cues/Prioritize Hypotheses**

# Risk for Falls

*due to* unsteady gait occurring with bradykinesia, tremors, rigidity, and postural and autonomic instability

***Desired Outcomes/Generate Outcomes:*** After instruction, the patient demonstrates safe and effective ambulatory techniques and preventive measures against falls and remains free of trauma.

| ASSESSMENT—RECOGNIZE CUES/ INTERVENTIONS—TAKE ACTION | RATIONALES |
|---|---|
| Assess the ambulation and movement for deficit(s). | This assessment will help the nurse tailor interventions specific to the patient's deficit(s). |
| During ambulation, encourage the patient to deliberately swing the arms and raise the feet. | These actions assist gait, thereby helping to prevent falls. |
| Advise the patient to step over an imaginary object or line, practice taking long steps, and avoid shuffling. | This will help raise the feet higher and increase the stride, which will help prevent falls. |

Continued

| ASSESSMENT—RECOGNIZE CUES/ INTERVENTIONS—TAKE ACTION | RATIONALES |
|---|---|
| Have the patient practice movements that are especially difficult (e.g., turning). Teach the patient to walk in a wide arc ("U-turn") rather than pivot when turning. | These actions prevent crossing of one leg over the other and causing a fall. |
| Provide instructions on head and neck exercises. | These exercises promote good posture, which in turn helps the gait. |
| Remind the patient repeatedly to maintain an upright posture and look up, not down, especially when walking. | This is particularly important for patients with bifocal glasses inasmuch as a stooped posture promotes looking down through the reading portion of the bifocal lens where distant items are blurred. |
| Advise the patient to stop or consciously slow down periodically. Teach the patient to concentrate on listening to the feet as they touch the floor and to count cadence to prevent too fast a gait. | This will slow the walking speed, which is less likely to result in falls. |
| Encourage the patient to lift the toes and to walk with the heels touching the floor first. | This action keeps soles of the feet flat on the floor, which is less likely to cause tripping. |
| Remind the patient to maintain a wide-based gait. | This gait improves balance. |
| Provide a clear pathway while the patient is walking. Teach the patient to avoid crowds, scatter rugs, uneven surfaces, fast turns, narrow doorways, and obstructions. | These actions minimize the risk for tripping and falling. |
| Encourage range-of-motion and stretching exercises daily. | Exercising promotes flexibility, strength, gait, and balance, thereby decreasing the risk for falls. Routine exercises, along with the prescribed medications, may prevent or delay disability. |
| Advise the patient to wear leather-soled or smooth-soled shoes but to test shoes to ensure they are not too slippery. | Rubber-soled or crepe-soled shoes tend to catch on floors, especially carpeted floors, and may cause falls. |
| Encourage males to keep a urinal at the bedside. A commode at the bedside may be helpful for females. | Slowness of gait and inability to get to the bathroom fast enough may cause incontinence or falls in an effort to get there. |
| Ask the physical therapy department to suggest exercises that improve balance. | Tai chi, for example, uses slow, graceful movements to relax and strengthen muscles and joints and may be encouraged as an option for some patients. |
| If hospitalized, place the patient on Fall Precautions per the facility's fall prevention protocol. This includes but is not limited to the following precautions: the bed alarm is activated, call light and frequently used items are in place, sign is placed on doorway to alert staff, and if possible, patient is placed in a room near the nurses' station. | This will ensure that the appropriate safety measures will be in place to decrease the patient's risk of falling. |
| For other interventions, see *Risk for Falls* in "General Care of Patients With Neurologic Disorders," Chapter 36. | |

## Patient Problem/Analyze Cues/Prioritize Hypotheses

# Impaired Mobility

*due to* difficulty initiating and/or maintaining movement

**Desired Outcome/Generate Solutions:** After instruction, the patient demonstrates measures that enhance their ability to initiate desired movement.

| ASSESSMENT—RECOGNIZE CUES/ INTERVENTIONS—TAKE ACTION | RATIONALES |
|---|---|
| Assess the mobility and movements. | This assessment will enable the nurse to tailor interventions to the patient's specific needs. |

| ASSESSMENT—RECOGNIZE CUES/ INTERVENTIONS—TAKE ACTION | RATIONALES |
|---|---|
| For patients having difficulty initiating movement, provide instructions about measures that may help with movement such as<br><br>• rocking from side to side;<br>• marching in place a few steps before resuming forward motion;<br>• relaxing back on the heels and raising the toes;<br>• tapping the hip of the leg to be moved;<br>• bending at the knees and straightening up;<br>• raising the arms in a sudden, short motion;<br>• change directions of movement;<br>• move sideways; and<br>• thinking of something else besides movement. | Patients with PD often have difficulty initiating movement because their disease affects the brain centers that regulate movement and balance. |
| Instruct the patient to get out of a chair by getting to edge of seat, placing hands on arm supports, bending forward slightly, moving the feet back, and then rhythmically rocking in the chair a few times before trying to get up. | The deficit of dopamine, which has an inhibitory effect, allows the relative excess of acetylcholine. The excitatory effect of acetylcholine causes overactivity of the basal ganglia, which interferes with normal muscle tone and the control of smooth, purposeful movement, causing the characteristic symptoms of PD: muscle rigidity, tremors, and slowness of movement. These combined problems make it difficult to get out of a chair. |
| Advise the patient to sit in chairs that have backs and arms and to purchase elevated toilet seats or sidebars in the bathroom. | These items will assist with rising from a sitting position and help prevent falls. |
| Instruct the patient on measures that may help with getting out of bed: rocking to a sitting position and elevating the head of bed. | See the previous discussion regarding getting out of a chair. |
| Provide the patient and significant others with instructions on how to recognize situations that can cause "freezing" episodes. | "Freezing" (sometimes called motor block) is **a sudden, brief inability to start the movement or to continue rhythmic, repeated movements**. "Freezing" is variable and can fluctuate with stress or emotional state. For example, attempting two movements simultaneously, such as trying to change direction quickly while walking, can cause freezing. Distracting environmental, visual, or auditory stimuli also can precipitate a freezing episode. Doorways, narrow passages, or a change in floor color, texture, or slope can pose problems for many patients. |
| Provide a referral to an organization that provides service dogs to assist the patient with their physical disabilities. | Specially trained dogs (e.g., Canine Partners for Life) can help patients walk and get up after a fall and are trained to help break a "freeze" by tapping on the individual's foot. |
| Suggest that sexual relations be planned for when the prescribed drug is working to good effect and the person is rested. Being flexible about time; experimenting with positions; use of manual, oral, and vibrator stimulation; and use of sildenafil have proved beneficial. | PD makes it more difficult to move, which can affect intimacy. |

## Patient Problem/Analyze Cues/Prioritize Hypotheses

# Deficient Knowledge (Medications)

*due to* unfamiliarity with the side effects of and precautionary measures for taking anti-Parkinson medications

***Desired Outcome/Generate Solutions:*** After instruction and before hospital discharge, the patient and significant other verbalize accurate knowledge about the side effects of and necessary precautionary measures for taking anti-Parkinson medications.

**Note:** *Instruct the patient and significant other to report adverse side effects promptly because many side effects are dose related and can be controlled by a dosage adjustment.*

| ASSESSMENT—RECOGNIZE CUES/ INTERVENTIONS—TAKE ACTION | RATIONALES |
|---|---|
| **Issues Common to Most Anti-Parkinson Medications** | |
| Assess the patient's understanding of the anti-Parkinson medications. As indicated, stress the importance of taking medication on schedule and not forgetting a dose. Advise the patient to carry extra dose(s) when leaving home. | Missing a dose may adversely affect mobility. The patient and health care provider can adjust the dose schedule so that the medication peaks at mealtime or at times when the patient needs mobility most. |
| Instruct the patient/significant other/caregiver on how to premeasure doses in segmented or separate containers labeled with the date and time of dose. | This assists patients who are having difficulty with self-medication and ensures that the patient takes the correct dose each day. |
| Encourage patients with anorexia to eat frequent small, nutritious snacks and meals. | Eating smaller meals rather than three larger meals is usually better tolerated in patients who are anorexic. Megestrol is used and approved for use as an appetite stimulant and can be used off label in PD. |
| Advise the patient to elevate the head of bed and make position changes slowly and in stages. Teach the patient to dangle legs a few minutes before standing. Antiembolism hose may help as well. Advise avoiding dehydration, especially in warm weather, by increasing fluid intake to include 4–8 oz/day of a sport drink if not contraindicated by cardiac comorbidity. Give tips for reducing morning orthostatic hypotension, including not limiting late evening fluid intake and keeping a glass of water at the bedside at night so it is available to drink in the morning before getting up. Encourage males to urinate from a sitting rather than standing position if possible. Provide a bedside commode for female patients. Suggest increasing dietary salt intake if not contraindicated by cardiac comorbidity. | These measures counteract orthostatic hypotension, which is a potential side effect of these medications. (Orthostatic hypotension also may be a result of the autonomic neuropathy from the disease process.) Fludrocortisone or midodrine may be prescribed to prevent or reduce orthostatic hypotension. |
| Instruct the patient to report dizziness to the health care provider. | This may be an indication of orthostatic hypotension. Medication adjustment may be needed. |
| Advise the use of sugarless chewing gum or hard candy, frequent mouth rinses with water, or artificial saliva products. | These measures ease dry mouth, a common side effect of these medications, and help maintain the integrity of oral mucous membrane. In the presence of drooling, however, an anticholinergic such as hyoscyamine or glycopyrrolate has a beneficial side effect of a reduction in secretions. |
| Advise the patient to report any urinary hesitancy or incontinence. | Urinary hesitancy and incontinence may signal urinary retention. Individuals taking anticholinergics may find that voiding before taking the medication eliminates this problem. |
| Instruct the patient on how to counteract constipation. For interventions, see *Constipation* in "Immobility," Chapter 1. | Constipation is a common problem with these medications as well as with the disease. Administration of laxatives and/or stool softeners and reduction in anticholinergic medications may help. |
| Advise the patient/significant other/caregiver to promptly report mental status changes to the health care provider. | Many of these drugs can cause or aggravate changes in mental status such as confusion; mental slowness or dullness; and even agitation, paranoia, and hallucinations. The health care provider may adjust the dose. |

| ASSESSMENT—RECOGNIZE CUES/ INTERVENTIONS—TAKE ACTION | RATIONALES |
|---|---|
| Advise the patient to report feelings of depression to the health care provider promptly. | Depression can be a side effect of some drugs as well as a normal response to disability. It is also caused by the disease process as a result of alteration in neurochemical balance. Counseling or psychotherapy may help patients and significant others adapt to the disability and deal with emotions and feelings such as depression that are either a direct or an indirect result of the disease process or drug therapy. Antidepressants may be prescribed to treat depression and to help with some PD symptoms (may help to block the reabsorption of dopamine and have some anticholinergic properties). |
| Implement the safety measures for patients with vision problems: orient to surroundings, identify self when entering room, keep walkways unobstructed, and encourage patients to ask for assistance when ambulating. | Blurred vision is a side effect of many anti-Parkinson medications. |
| Instruct the patient about the measures that promote sleep. See *Fatigue due to impaired sleep* in "Psychosocial Support for the Patient," Chapter 8. | Patients with PD are already at risk for sleep disorders and additionally, insomnia is a side effect of many of the drugs used to treat PD. Reducing the evening dose may help promote sleep. Modafinil may be prescribed to reduce daytime sleepiness. |
| **Provide information to the patient on the side effects specific to dopamine replacement therapy (Levodopa)** | Levodopa, the metabolic precursor of dopamine, crosses the blood–brain barrier and restores dopamine levels in the extrapyramidal centers in the brain. Before levodopa crosses the blood–brain barrier, much of it is converted into dopamine by the peripheral metabolism (GI tract and liver), causing many of the drug's side effects. Levadopa is given in increasing amounts until symptoms are reduced or the patient's tolerance to side effects is reached. It may be used as initial therapy or later when other medications can no longer control symptoms. |
| • Instruct the patients with advanced PD that levodopa should be taken with a full glass of water on an empty stomach 30 minutes before meals or 2 hours after meals. | Levodopa is a protein-bound medication. Taking it with a high-protein meal will decrease absorption. |
| • Instruct the patient to report muscle twitching, spasmodic winking, or other abnormal muscle movements. | These are signs of medication toxicity. |
| • Explain the signs and symptoms of neuroleptic malignant syndrome and acute akinesia (see Assessment). Instruct the patient that to avoid neuroleptic malignant syndrome, it is necessary to take levodopa as scheduled and not to stop this medication abruptly. | There is a need for immediate medical intervention with these crises because respiratory and cardiac support may be necessary. In neuroleptic malignant syndrome, the dopaminergic drug needs to be restarted immediately and measures to be taken to treat fever and renal dysfunction. In acute akinesia, the triggering cause must be found and treated, and the patient medically supported until this is resolved. |
| • Explain the signs of on–off response, end-of-dose wearing-off phenomenon, other complications of therapy, interventions, and importance of working with the health care provider on fine-tuning the medication regimen. | On–off response is a rapid fluctuation or change in patient's condition. The individual is "on" one moment, in a state of relative mobility, and "off" the next, in a state of decreased mobility ranging from mild reduction in function to complete or nearly complete immobility. Although the cause is uncertain, it is believed that it is related to fluctuating dopamine blood levels in the brain. "End-of-dose" wearing-off phenomenon is the return of symptoms (bradykinesia, tremors, rigidity) before the next dose is given. Other complications include choreiform or involuntary, spasmodic, jerking movements (e.g., facial grimacing, tongue protrusion, restlessness), and vivid dreaming. Medication adjustments usually help with these side effects. Dose redistribution, use of adjunctive medications such as dopamine agonist (DA), catechol-*O*-methyltransferase (COMT) inhibitor, and medication preparations in extended-release forms and transdermal forms should help downregulate these problems. |

Continued

| ASSESSMENT—RECOGNIZE CUES/ INTERVENTIONS—TAKE ACTION | RATIONALES |
|---|---|
| • Instruct the patient/significant other/caregiver to monitor for behavioral changes and report them to the health care provider promptly. | Severe depression with suicidal overtones can be caused by Levadopa and should be reported immediately. Patients can also develop severe obsessive behavior (e.g., gambling, impulsive buying, hypersexuality). The health care provider may prescribe a dose reduction. |
| • Explain that Levadopa may cause changes in urine (dark or orange-colored). | Knowing what to expect may eliminate anxiety if this side effect occurs. |
| • Caution the patient to avoid alcohol. | Alcohol impairs the effectiveness of levodopa and worsens base symptoms related to gait and balance as well as worsens mental health and cognitive issues. |
| **Provide information to the patient on the side effects specific to DAs (amantadine, apomorphine [Apokyn]).** | Although amantadine is less effective than levodopa, it has fewer severe side effects. It may be used as initial therapy or as an adjunct. Effects diminish after a time; therefore this drug may be used intermittently. |
| • Instruct the patient to take this medication early in the day. | This may prevent insomnia, which is one of its side effects. |
| • Instruct the patient/significant other/caregiver to monitor for and report any shortness of breath, peripheral edema, significant weight gain, or change in mental status. | These signs often signal heart failure, a possible side effect of amantadine. |
| • Instruct the patient not to stop taking amantadine abruptly. | Doing so may precipitate parkinsonian crisis (acute akinesia), a severe worsening of symptoms that can be life threatening. |
| • Instruct the patient that a change in skin color may occur while taking amantadine but reassure them that the condition is simply a cosmetic side effect. | A diffuse, rose-colored mottling of the skin, usually confined to the lower extremities, may develop. The condition may subside with continued therapy and will disappear in a few weeks to months after the drug is discontinued. Exposure to cold or standing for long periods may make the color more prominent. |
| • Instruct the patient to monitor and promptly report to the health care provider a loss of seizure control. | Patients with a history of seizures may have an increase in the number of seizures while taking amantadine. |
| • Caution the patient to avoid alcohol and CNS depressants. | These agents potentiate the effects of amantadine. |
| • Explain that most side effects of amantadine are dose related. | Many side effects can be controlled by an adjustment in dosage. |
| • Instruct the patient that despite its name, apomorphine does not contain morphine and is not addictive. Explain that an antiemetic should be taken before taking apomorphine, ideally on a prophylaxis basis 3 days before initiation of therapy. Presently, it is only available in a subcutaneous or sublingual formulation. | Apomorphine is a DA given subcutaneously as a "rescue" drug for acute, intermittent treatment of hypomobility ("off" episodes). It needs to be initiated and titrated under monitored conditions. It frequently causes severe nausea and vomiting, although tolerance usually develops after about 8 weeks. |
| Explain that the following can occur with apomorphine: injection site reactions including bruising, itching, and lumps that typically resolve on their own. Yawning, dyskinesia, somnolence, rhinorrhea, hallucination, and extremity edema also can occur. | These are common side effects. |
| Explain that erections in men can occur spontaneously with apomorphine and should be reported to the health care provider if they last longer than 4 hours. | This side effect of apomorphine may be beneficial for selected patients. |
| **Provide information to the patient on the side effects specific to a dopamine receptor agonists (pramipexole [Mirapex], ropinirole, [Requip], rotigotine [Neupro transdermal patch]).** | These medications are administered with a concomitant reduction of dopamine replacement dosage or as initiation therapy independent of dopamine replacement. They may be used to reduce levodopa-induced dyskinesia (such as involuntary movements) and the frequency of "on–off" responses. |
| • Caution the patient to avoid alcohol when taking these medications. | Alcohol tolerance will be lessened. |
| • Caution patients taking DAs against driving or using machinery until they know how they respond to the medications. | DAs are associated with the abrupt onset of somnolence without warning. |

| ASSESSMENT—RECOGNIZE CUES/ INTERVENTIONS—TAKE ACTION | RATIONALES |
|---|---|
| • Instruct the patient to implement safety precautions when taking apomorphine. | Dizziness or postural hypotension can occur. |
| **Explain to the patient the side effects specific to anticholinergic medications (trihexyphenidyl [Artane], benztropine [Cogentin], profenamine [Parsidol], procyclidine [Kemadrin], biperiden [Akineton]).** | As a class, these medications are used less often because of side effects, mild to moderate efficacy, and availability of other medication choices. They are often used in conjunction with dopamine replacement therapy but may be used alone if the patient's symptoms are mild or if the patient cannot tolerate levodopa. They may improve tremors and rigidity but often do little for bradykinesia or balance problems. |
| • Explain that the patient should avoid strenuous exercise and keep cool during summer to avoid heat stroke. | These medications may decrease perspiration. |
| • Teach the patient not to stop taking these medications abruptly. | Doing so can result in parkinsonian crisis (acute akinesia), a severe worsening of symptoms that can be life threatening. |
| • Teach the patient to monitor for tachycardia or palpitation and to report either condition. | Many side effects such as these can be controlled by an adjustment in dosage. |
| • Teach the patient and significant others to monitor for memory dysfunction and confusion and urinary hesitancy and retention (especially in older males) and to report symptoms to the health care provider. | As above. |
| **Side effects specific to monoamine oxidase (MAO) type B inhibitor (rasagiline [Azilect], safinamide [Xadago], selegiline [Eldepryl]).** | This medication is used as an early intervention or as an adjunct with levodopa to inhibit the breakdown of levodopa, resulting in less fluctuation in blood levels. |
| • Stress the importance of taking these medications only in prescribed dose and following dietary modifications to reduce intake of tyramine-containing foods. | Safinamide and rasagiline are MAO-B selective inhibitors but are in the MAO class. Therefore it is recommended to avoid foods containing tyramine at more than 150 mg. |
| • Suggest the avoidance of opioids. | At recommended doses, no drug interactions have been noted. However, fatal drug interactions have occurred in patients taking other nonselective MAO inhibitors and could conceivably occur if higher than recommended doses are taken. |
| • Instruct the patient to take the medication early in the day. | This may help prevent insomnia, a potential side effect. |
| **Side effects specific to a COMT inhibitor (e.g., entacapone [Comtan], tolcapone [Tasmar]).** | These medications reduce levodopa degradation in the GI tract, kidneys, and liver to minimize fluctuation in serum levels. |
| • Explain to the patient that this medication might cause urine discoloration (brownish orange), but this is not clinically important. | An informed patient is not likely to become anxious if urine discoloration occurs. |
| • Explain that hallucinations, increased dyskinesia, persistent nausea, abdominal pain, and diarrhea should be reported promptly. | Many side effects are dose related and can be controlled by adjustment in dosage. |

## Patient Problem/Analyze Cues/Prioritize Hypotheses

# Deficient Knowledge (Disease Management)

*due to* unfamiliarity with facial and tongue exercises that enhance verbal communication and help prevent choking

***Desired Outcomes/Generate Solutions:*** By the 24-hour period before hospital discharge, the patient demonstrates facial and tongue exercises and states the rationale for their use.

| ASSESSMENT—RECOGNIZE CUES/ INTERVENTIONS—TAKE ACTION | RATIONALES |
|---|---|
| Assess the patient's understanding of facial and tongue exercises. As indicated, explain that special exercises can help strengthen and control facial and tongue muscles, which in turn will improve verbal communication and help prevent choking. Refer the patient to a speech pathologist to design and individualize a speech program. | Routine exercises of facial and tongue muscles, along with prescribed medications, may prevent or delay disability. |
| Teach exercises that will improve verbal communication and help prevent choking. Have the patient return the demonstration. | Teaching, followed by return demonstration, is an effective way of helping patients understand and retain knowledge. Teaching patients how to hold a sound for 5 seconds; sing the scale; recite the alphabet and days of the week; practice vowel breaths (ah, oh, oo) and nonsense syllables (ma, me, mi, pull, pill, pie), read aloud, and extend the tongue and try to touch the chin, nose, and cheek will help improve verbal communication skills and prevent choking. |
| Encourage the patient to practice increasing voice volume. Suggest that the patient read newspapers out loud and determine how many words can be said in one breath before volume decreases. Advise that the voice should vary from soft to loud. | This exercise will help combat monotone speech while promoting speech quality and understandability. This may be accomplished by having patients take a deep breath before speaking, open the mouth to let sound come out more, use shorter sentences, exaggerate the sound of every syllable, speak louder than others may think necessary, and use a tape recorder for feedback. Patients should practice reading or reciting out loud, focusing on breathing, and using a strong voice. |
| Instruct the patient to raise the voice with a question and lower it with an answer. | These actions improve speech understandability. |
| Instruct the patient to do these tongue exercises: stick out the tongue as far as possible and hold; move the tongue slowly from corner to corner; stretch the tongue to the nose and then chin and then cheek; stick out the tongue and put it back in the mouth as quickly as possible; move the tongue in circles as quickly as possible. | These exercises will improve articulation. |
| Instruct the patient to open and close the mouth slowly and then quickly; close the lips and press tightly; stretch the lips in a wide smile and hold; then pucker the lips and hold. | These are effective lip and jaw exercises for improving articulation. |
| Advise the patient to practice in front of a mirror. | This will enable the patient to see and evaluate lip and tongue movement. |
| Provide a written handout that lists and describes the preceding exercises. Encourage the patient to perform them hourly while awake. | These measures reinforce the patient's knowledge. |
| Emphasize the importance of stating feelings verbally. Encourage the use of a mirror to practice expressing emotions such as happiness and displeasure. | Monotone speech and lack of facial expression impede nonverbal communication. |
| Advise patients to face the people to whom they are speaking and speak for themselves and not let others speak for them. | Individuals who have difficulty speaking often remain quiet and let others talk for them. |

## Patient Problem/Analyze Cues/Prioritize Hypotheses

# Deficient Knowledge (Disease Treatment)

*due to* unfamiliarity with deep brain stimulation (DBS)

**Desired Outcome/Generate Solutions:** After the explanation, the patient verbalizes an accurate understanding of the DBS procedure and general follow-up care.

| ASSESSMENT—RECOGNIZE CUES/ INTERVENTIONS—TAKE ACTION | RATIONALES |
|---|---|
| Assess the patient's understanding of DBS. As indicated, explain that the neurostimulator is an implantable pulse generator powered by a small battery that is implanted subcutaneously near the clavicle. The stimulation parameter is set to optimize symptom management with minimum adverse effects. | Deep brain electrostimulation is used preferentially over ablative procedures (e.g., stereotactic pallidotomy) because it is reversible and programmable. DBS is most effective when patients are carefully selected and screened (Harding, 2020). |
| Stimulation of the thalamus helps with tremors. Globus pallidus stimulation works better in controlling rigidity and balance and reduces medication side effects, leading to better tolerance, but it does not usually reduce the amount of medication given. Stimulation of the subthalamic nucleus (STN) helps with all parkinsonian symptoms and enables a reduction in medication. This does not replace oral medication management, but sometimes the medications can be reduced, although medication reduction should not be an expectation. The patient can switch stimulation to on/off with a magnet. | |
| Explain that health care provider follow-up is necessary. | Adverse effects may include paresthesias, muscle contractions, double vision, and mood disturbances, all of which are usually transient. It is seldom possible to alleviate completely all PD symptoms with the stimulator alone. Therefore medication may be needed and adjustments made by the provider for the first few months. |
| Advise that the sudden appearance of additional parkinsonian symptoms may be the only indicator of battery failure. | There are handheld devices that enable the determination of the on/off status of the neurostimulator as well as battery charge status. |
| Advise that turning the neurostimulator off at night to conserve the battery is not recommended. | Some symptoms, such as rigidity, respond only to continuous stimulation. |
| Explain that ineffective stimulation may signal incorrect lead placement, poor anchoring, and drifting of leads. | This may necessitate removal for accurate repositioning of the electrodes. |
| Instruct the patient that adverse effects resulting from stimulation of nearby structures are corrected by adjusting the stimulation parameters. | Adverse effects include tingling of the head or hand, depression, slurred speech, loss of balance or muscle tone, and double vision. Patients should see health care providers for adjustments. |
| Explain that excessive STN stimulation may cause disabling dyskinesia. | This would be a valid reason for turning off the device until reprogramming can be performed. |
| ⚠ Caution that some devices, such as theft detectors and screening devices found in airports, department stores, and public libraries, can cause the neurostimulator to switch on or off. Ultrasonic dental equipment and electrocautery also may affect the device. | Usually, this only causes an uncomfortable sensation. However, symptoms could worsen suddenly. Patients always should carry the identification card given with the device and use it to request assistance to bypass those devices. Magnets and home programmers also should be carried in case the stimulator is accidentally switched off by such devices. The patient can then do a self-assessment and turn it back on if needed. Computers and cellular phones do not interfere with the device. |
| Caution patients to avoid activities that may result in blunt trauma to the implanted device area. | This will help prevent the loss of function of the implanted generator or leads. |
| ⚠ Caution patients that they cannot undergo magnetic resonance imaging (MRI) because of possible movement of the leads or diathermy (shortwave or microwave). | MRI can heat up the wires and leads, resulting in serious injury or death. |
| Provide instructions on the use of a magnet to activate and deactivate the stimulator. | Magnets may damage televisions, credit cards, and computer disks and therefore should be kept at least 1 foot away from these items. |

## ADDITIONAL PROBLEMS:

## ✓ PATIENT–FAMILY TEACHING AND DISCHARGE PLANNING

When providing patient–family teaching, focus on sensory information, avoid giving excessive information, and initiate a visiting nurse referral for necessary follow-up teaching. Include verbal and written information about the following:

✓ Referrals to community resources, such as local and national Parkinson's Society chapters, public health nurse, visiting nurses association, community support groups, social workers, psychologic therapy, vocational rehabilitation agency, home health agencies, and extended and skilled care facilities. Additional general information can be obtained by contacting the following organizations:
  - Parkinson's Foundation: www.parkinson.org

✓ Importance of avoiding certain medications that can worsen extrapyramidal symptoms. Examples include phenothiazines, prochlorperazine, metoclopramide, chlorpromazine, methyldopa, tetrabenazine, haloperidol, and reserpine. An exception is ethopropazine, which is a phenothiazine derivative that does not increase extrapyramidal effects and is used to treat PD symptoms.

✓ Speech therapy tips for communication related to dysarthria and for swallowing precautions.

✓ Related safety measures and fall prevention for patients with bradykinesia, muscle rigidity, and tremors.

✓ Emphasis that disability may be prevented or delayed through exercises and medications.

✓ Evaluation of home environment and tips for home accident prevention.

✓ Measures to prevent or lessen postural hypotension.

✓ Signs and symptoms of neuroleptic malignant and acute akinesia and the need for immediate medical attention.

✓ For other interventions, see "Patient–Family Teaching and Discharge Planning" (3rd through 10th entries only), in "Multiple Sclerosis," Chapter 40.

# Seizures and Epilepsy 42

## OVERVIEW/PATHOPHYSIOLOGY

Seizures result from an abnormal, uncontrolled, and excessive electrical discharges from the neurons of the cerebral cortex in response to a stimulus. If the activity is localized in one portion of the brain, the individual will have a partial seizure, but when it is widespread and diffuse, a generalized seizure occurs. Symptoms vary widely, depending on the involved area of the cerebral cortex. Seizures are generally manifested as an alteration in sensation, behavior, movement, perception, or consciousness lasting from seconds to several minutes. A seizure can be an isolated incident that may not recur after the underlying cause is corrected (e.g., fever, alcohol withdrawal). *Epilepsy* and *seizure disorder* are the terms used for recurrent, unprovoked seizures. When there is no underlying problem in a person who has two or more seizures more than 24 hours apart, they may have seizure disorder. The cause of seizure disorder is unknown in most people with this disorder.

*Seizure threshold* refers to the amount of stimulation needed to cause neural activity. Although anyone can have a seizure if the stimulus is sufficient, the seizure threshold is lowered in some individuals, and this may result in spontaneous seizures. Potential causes for lowered seizure threshold include congenital defects; craniocerebral trauma, particularly that from a penetrating wound; subarachnoid hemorrhage; stroke; intracranial tumors; infections, such as meningitis or encephalitis; exposure to toxins, such as lead; hypoxia; alcohol or other drug withdrawal; and metabolic and endocrine disorders, such as hypoglycemia, hypocalcemia, uremia, hypoparathyroidism, excessive hydration, and fever. Phenothiazine antidepressants and alcohol use increase the risk for seizure by lowering the seizure threshold. For susceptible individuals, triggers may include emotional tension or stress; physical stimulation, such as loud music, bright flashing lights, and some videos; lack of sleep or food; fatigue; menses or pregnancy; and excessive drug or alcohol use.

Although a seizure generally is not fatal, individuals can be injured by hitting their heads or breaking bones if they lose consciousness and fall to the ground. Seizure activity increases cerebral $O_2$ consumption by 60% and cerebral blood flow by 250%. Instances of prolonged and repeated generalized seizures, *status epilepticus (SE)*, can be life threatening because apnea, hypoxia, acidosis, cerebral edema, dysrhythmias, and cardiovascular collapse can occur.

## HEALTH CARE SETTING

Primary care, neurology clinic, and possible acute care hospitalization for complications of therapy, continuous diagnostic video electroencephalogram (EEG) monitoring during pharmacologic or surgical interventions, or intensive care unit (ICU) for SE

## ASSESSMENT

It is important to obtain an accurate description of seizure characteristics and duration, as well as any antecedent events, precipitating factors, and postictal phase. There are many clinical types of seizures, but the following are the most serious or common.

**Tonic–clonic (formally called grand mal).** Caused by bilateral electrical activity and can be symmetric from onset, but in adults, it is usually preceded by an aura, indicating an initial focal onset followed by generalization. This is referred to as focal with secondary generalization. Tonic–clonic seizures always involve loss of consciousness. A possible prodromal phase of increased irritability, tension, mood changes, or headache may precede the seizure by hours or days. Patients may experience an aura (a sensory warning, such as a sound, odor, or flash of light) immediately preceding the seizure by seconds or minutes. The seizure activity, known as the ictal phase, usually does not last more than 2–5 minutes and includes the following:

- *Tonic phase (rigid/contracted muscles/extended limbs):* Often lasts only 15 seconds, usually subsiding in less than 1 minute. Symptoms include loss of consciousness, clenched jaws (potential for tongue to be bitten), apnea (may hear a cry as air is forced out of the lungs), and cyanosis. The patient may be incontinent, and pupils may dilate and become nonreactive to light.
- *Clonic phase (rhythmic contraction and relaxation of extremities and muscles):* May subside in 30 seconds but can last 2–4 minutes. Eyes roll upward, and excessive salivation results in foaming at the mouth. During this phase, the potential is greatest for biting the tongue. Incontinence may occur during this phase.
- *Postictal phase:* The first few minutes after the seizure, the individual may be limp and nonresponsive. Pupils begin to react to light and return to their normal size. After about 5 minutes, patients may be sleepy, semiconscious, confused,

unable to speak clearly, and uncoordinated; have a headache; complain of muscle aches; and have no recollection of the seizure event. This phase usually lasts less than 15 minutes but can last for several hours. Temporary weakness, Todd paralysis (postictal paralysis), dysphasia, or hemianopia lasting up to 48 hours after the seizure may be experienced.

**Generalized-onset nonmotor (absence) seizures.** Patients have momentary loss of awareness and consciousness with abrupt cessation of voluntary muscle activity. Patients may appear to be daydreaming with a vacant stare and may experience facial, eyelid, or hand twitching and then have sudden recovery. Patients usually do not lose general body muscle tone and so do not fall. The individual resumes previous activity when the seizure ends. There is usually no memory of the seizure, and patients may have difficulty reorienting after the seizure event. This type of seizure can last less than 10–20 seconds, may occur up to 100 times/day, and usually resolves by puberty.

**Generalized myoclonic.** Sudden, very brief contraction or jerking of muscles or muscle groups. Individuals may have a very brief, momentary loss of consciousness with some postictal confusion.

**Focal-onset seizures (partial focal seizures).** An irritative focus located in the motor cortex of the frontal lobe causes clonic movement in a particular part of the body, such as the hands or face. Sensory, motor, cognitive, or emotional manifestations occur that are based on the area of the brain that is affected. The seizure usually lasts several seconds to minutes. There is no loss of consciousness. Other simple focal-onset seizures include those with somatosensory symptoms (e.g., smells, sounds), autonomic symptoms (e.g., tachycardia, tachypnea, diaphoresis, goosebumps [piloerection], pallor, flushing), or psychic symptoms (e.g., fear, déjà vu).

**Focal nonmotor seizure.** Generally lasts for 1–4 minutes and involves impaired consciousness and a postictal state of confusion lasting several minutes. However, the individual does not fall to the ground, is able to interact with the environment, exhibits purposeful but inappropriate movements or behavior, and has no memory of the event. The individual will perform such automatisms as lip smacking, chewing, facial grimacing, picking, or swallowing movements. These patients may experience and remember various sensory or emotional hallucinations or sensations that occur immediately before the seizure, such as smells; ringing or hissing sounds; or feelings of déjà vu, fear, or pleasure.

**Status epilepticus.** State of continuous seizure activity lasting more than 5 minutes, or two or more recurring seizures, in which the individual does not completely recover baseline neurologic functioning between seizures. Individuals who suddenly stop taking their antiepileptic medication are likely to develop this condition. Other common causes are drug withdrawal (e.g., alcohol, sedatives) and fever. This is a medical emergency, especially with tonic–clonic seizures, resulting in such potential complications as cerebral anoxia and edema, aspiration, rhabdomyolysis, hyperthermia, and exhaustion. Brain injury may occur in 20–30 minutes, and irreversible damage may occur in 60 minutes. Death may ensue. SE can occur in the absence of movement. The patient does not regain consciousness. Nonconvulsive SE may not be life threatening, but it can cause brain damage and will require continuous EEG monitoring. Expect patients in SE to be transferred to the ICU or specialty seizure monitoring unit.

**Other classifications.** Seizures also can be classified according to the epileptic syndrome (e.g., generalized epilepsies, idiopathic with age-related onset). Establishing the correct diagnosis of seizure type and, when possible, epilepsy syndrome will help tailor effective antiepileptic drugs (AEDs) and treatment.

## DIAGNOSTIC TESTS

A variety of problems can precipitate seizures, and therefore testing may be extensive. A comprehensive description of seizures and the patient's health history is the most helpful diagnostic tool. However, there are several tests that are done for initial workup including the following:

**Laboratory tests.** To rule out metabolic causes, such as hypoglycemia, hyponatremia, or hypocalcemia; kidney and liver problems; toxicology screens; and AED level.

**Electroencephalogram—both sleeping and awake.** To reveal abnormal patterns of electrical activity, particularly with such stimuli as flashing lights or hyperventilation. Ambulatory EEGs may record brain activity for 48–72 hours, and 24 hours of continuous EEG monitoring with video recording may show an association of brain activity with the observed seizure. Generalized tonic–clonic seizures show up as high, fast-voltage spikes in all leads. A normal EEG does not rule out seizures.

**Magnetic resonance imaging.** To show structural lesions causing seizures; also may reveal a space-occupying lesion such as a tumor or hematoma. Fast fluid-attenuated inversion recovery magnetic resonance imaging may be particularly sensitive in finding tumors.

**Computed tomography.** To check for the presence of a space-occupying lesion, such as a tumor or hematoma.

**Skull radiographic examination.** To reveal fractures, tumors, calcifications, or congenital anomalies (pineal shift, ventricular deformity).

**Serum tests.** Complete blood count (CBC), serum chemistries, liver and kidney function tests, and urinalysis are done to detect metabolic problems.

## Patient Problem/Analyze Cues/Prioritize Hypotheses

# Risk for Injury

*due to* seizure activity

**Desired Outcomes/Generate Solutions:** The patient exhibits no signs of oral, musculoskeletal, airway, or cardiac compromise during or after the seizure. Before hospital discharge, the patient's significant others verbalize accurate knowledge of actions necessary during seizure activity.

| ASSESSMENT—RECOGNIZE CUES/ INTERVENTIONS—TAKE ACTION | RATIONALES |
|---|---|
| **Seizure Precautions** | |
| Assess the patient's environment. Pad side rails with blankets or pillows. Keep the side rails up and bed in its lowest position when the patient is in bed. Keep bed, wheelchair, or stretcher brakes locked. | These actions promote safety and protect the patient from trauma in case a seizure occurs. |
| Insert a saline lock as prescribed for intravenous (IV) access for high-risk patients. | Some AEDs must be administered by IV route, especially as a loading dose or in case of sustained seizure activity. |
| Use the electronic tympanic thermometers for patients at high risk for seizure. If only breakable thermometers are available, take temperature by the axillary or rectal route. | Glass or other breakable oral thermometers should be avoided when taking a patient's temperature because of the harm they could cause the patient if they break. |
| Caution patients to lie down and push the call button if they experience prodromal or aural warning. Keep the call light within reach. | Prodromal or aural warnings precede seizures in many patients. |
| Instruct patient that they are not allowed to smoke when not supervised. | This restriction prevents fire damage to the patient and surroundings if a seizure occurs. |
| Evaluate the need for and provide protective headgear as indicated. | This protects the patient's head in case of a seizure. |
| Obtain the serum laboratory tests as prescribed. | Electrolyte disorders such as hyponatremia and hypocalcemia can trigger a seizure. |
| **During the Seizure** | |
| Remain with the patient and stay calm. Assess for, record, and report type, duration, and characteristics of seizure activity and any postseizure response. | Seizure activity should be documented in detail to aid in the management and differentiation of seizure type and identification of triggering factors. This should include, as appropriate, precipitating event, aura, initial location and progression, automatisms, type and duration of movement, changes in the level of consciousness, eye movement (e.g., deviation, nystagmus), pupil size and reaction, bowel and bladder incontinence, head deviation, tongue deviation, or teeth clenching. |
| Never force anything between patient's clenched teeth. Remove or loosen the tight clothing. | Placing or forcing anything inside the patient's mouth while they are seizing could cause teeth and jaw damage. Tight clothing, especially around the neck could impede respirations. |
| Ensure the priority administration of prescribed IV lorazepam or diazepam within 3–10 minutes. | Initially, the medication is given as a slow bolus. Sublingual lorazepam or rectal diazepam gel may be given if there is no IV access. If the seizure stops, this may be the extent of the interventions if the patient is already on AEDs. |
| Prevent or break the fall and ease the patient to the floor if a seizure occurs while the patient is out of bed. | These actions promote the patient's physical safety. |
| Keep the patient in bed if a seizure occurs while there, and lower the head of the bed to a flat position. | Flattening the patient's position reduces the risk for falling out of bed during seizure activity. |

Continued

| ASSESSMENT—RECOGNIZE CUES/ INTERVENTIONS—TAKE ACTION | RATIONALES |
|---|---|
| Do not restrain the patient but rather guide the patient's movements gently. | This action helps prevent injury caused by flailing. |
| Administer AEDs as prescribed. | IV administration of the prescribed AED can shorten the length and prevent reoccurrence of seizures. |
| **After the Seizure** | |
| During the postictal phase, reassure and gently reorient the patient. Check neurologic status and vital signs (VS). | During the postictal period that follows the seizure, the patient will need to be reoriented and reassured because some memory lapse will have occurred during the event. |
| Ask the patient if an aura preceded seizure activity. Record this information and postictal characteristics. | An aura is a sensory warning such as a sound, odor, or flash of light. It can be used in the future to warn the patient of an impending seizure. |
| Provide a quiet, calm environment. Keep talk simple and to a minimum. Speak slowly and with pauses between sentences. | Sounds and stimuli can be confusing to the awakening patient. Repetition may be necessary if the patient is confused. |
| Use the room light that is behind, not above, the patient. | This prevents additional seizures triggered by the light and promotes comfort. |
| Check the patient's tongue for lacerations and the body for injuries. Assess for weakness or paralysis, dysphasia, or visual disturbances. | These are potential occurrences during a seizure. |
| Assess the urine for red or cola color. If the patient has been incontinent, provide perineal care. | Rhabdomyolysis or myoglobinuria may occur from muscle trauma. This will help prevent skin irritation. |
| Check the fingerstick blood glucose. | Hypoglycemia is a potential metabolic cause of the seizure. |

## Patient Problem/Analyze Cues/Prioritize Hypotheses

# Risk for Impaired Respiratory Function

*due to* seizure activity

***Desired Outcomes/Generate Solutions:*** The patient exhibits no signs of airway compromise after the seizure. Before hospital discharge, the patient's significant others verbalize accurate knowledge of actions necessary to protect the patient's airway during seizure activity.

| ASSESSMENT—RECOGNIZE CUES/ INTERVENTIONS—TAKE ACTION | RATIONALES |
|---|---|
| Assess the patient's environment. Pad side rails with blankets or pillows. Keep the side rails up and bed in its lowest position when the patient is in bed. Keep the bed, wheelchair, or stretcher brakes locked. | These actions promote safety and protect the patient from trauma in case a seizure occurs. |
| Keep the suction and oxygen equipment readily available. | These measures enable a patent airway, prevent hypoxia, and protect patients from trauma in case a seizure occurs. |
| Encourage the patient to empty the mouth of dentures or foreign objects. | This helps prevent choking in case a seizure occurs. |
| Never insert anything into the patient's airway during a seizure. | Forcing objects into the patient's mouth can break teeth, lacerate the oral mucous membrane, or block the airway. |
| Be sure the patient's head position does not occlude the airway. Turn the patient into a side-lying position or turn the head to the left. Remove from the environment objects (e.g., chairs) that the patient may strike. Pad floors to protect the patient's arms and legs. Remove the patient's glasses. | These measures protect the patient's airway from occlusion and the body from injury during the seizure. A towel folded flat or hands may be used to cushion the head from striking the ground. |

| ASSESSMENT—RECOGNIZE CUES/ INTERVENTIONS—TAKE ACTION | RATIONALES |
|---|---|
| Implement the ABCs: Assess airway, breathing, and circulation. Initiate O₂ therapy, oral airway suctioning, and intubation as needed. | These actions help maintain the airway and prevent hypoxia. |
| Place the patient in a side-lying position. | Positioning on the side reduces aspiration risk in case of vomiting. |
| Assess VS, pulse oximetry, heart rhythm, and arterial blood gas values. | This assessment enables early detection of hypoxia, dysrhythmias, and overall hemodynamics. |
| Determine whether the patient has had SE: that is, the seizure is continuous (longer than 5 minutes) or is longer than the patient's usual length of time by 1 or 2 minutes, or the patient has two or more seizures without recovering baseline neurologic functioning between seizures. | This condition is life threatening and can cause cerebral anoxia and edema, aspiration, hyperthermia, and exhaustion. Anticipate transfer to the ICU but do not delay initial interventions, including administration of prescribed IV lorazepam or diazepam. |
| If the patient vomited during the seizure, notify the health care provider. | This is a sign that aspiration can occur with subsequent seizures. |
| Stay with patient for 15–20 minutes after the seizure. | Sudden unexplained death in epileptic patients is not well understood, but it may be related to central respiratory apnea that can occur with a seizure. |
| Assess for the signs of respiratory depression. | This is a possible side effect of benzodiazepines and phenobarbital. |
| Do not offer food or drink during the postictal phase until the patient is fully awake. | This prevents vomiting/aspiration. |

## Patient Problem/Analyze Cues/Prioritize Hypotheses

# Deficient Knowledge (Disease Management)

*due to* unfamiliarity with life-threatening environmental factors and preventive measures for seizures

***Desired Outcomes/Generate Solutions:*** Before hospital discharge, the patient verbalizes accurate information about measures that may prevent seizures and environmental factors that can be life threatening in the presence of seizures. The patient exhibits health care measures that reflect this knowledge.

| ASSESSMENT—RECOGNIZE CUES/ INTERVENTIONS—TAKE ACTION | RATIONALES |
|---|---|
| Assess the patient's knowledge of measures that can prevent seizures and environmental hazards that can be life threatening in the presence of seizure activity. Provide or clarify information as indicated. | This assessment enables nurses to provide or clarify information as indicated and facilitates the development of an individualized teaching plan. |
| Advise the patient to check into state regulations about automobile operation. | Most states require 3 months to 2 years seizure-free before an individual can obtain/regain a driver's license. |
| ⚠ Caution the patient to refrain from operating heavy or dangerous equipment, swimming, climbing excessive heights, and possibly even tub bathing until he or she is seizure-free for an amount of time specified by the health care provider. | These restrictions prevent injury that can result while performing these activities in case a seizure occurs. |
| ⚠ Advise the patient that some activities, such as climbing or bicycle riding, require careful risk/benefit evaluation. The patient who decides to ride a bike should wear a helmet and avoid heavy traffic. Contact sports should be avoided. | These are high-risk activities when the patient who has a seizure may be injured. |
| ⚠ Caution the patient never to swim alone regardless of the amount of time he or she has been seizure-free. | This makes rescue easier if a seizure occurs. Patients should swim only in shallow water and in the company of a strong swimmer. |

Continued

| ASSESSMENT—RECOGNIZE CUES/ INTERVENTIONS—TAKE ACTION | RATIONALES |
|---|---|
| Advise the patient to turn the temperature of hot water heaters down. | This prevents scalding if a seizure occurs in the shower. |
| Encourage the stress management, progressive relaxation techniques, and diaphragmatic respiratory training. | These measures help control emotional stress and hyperventilation, which can trigger seizures. |
| Encourage the vocational assessment and counseling. | The patient's epilepsy may place others at risk in some occupations, such as bus driver or airline pilot. |
| Advise female patients that seizure activity may change (increase or decrease) during menses or pregnancy (especially at 3–4 months of gestation). | Estrogen and progesterone level changes that occur with pregnancy and during menses may increase the risk of seizures in a woman with seizure disorder. |
| Provide the birth control information if requested. | Oral contraceptive effectiveness may be reduced by many AEDs. Intrauterine devices or other methods may be needed. When seizures in women worsen with hormonal changes, suppressing ovulation with medication may be recommended. Women wanting to get pregnant should consult with their health care provider. |
| Instruct patients that the use of stimulants (e.g., caffeine) and depressants (e.g., alcohol) should be avoided. | Their use can change the seizure threshold, and withdrawal from stimulants and depressants can increase the likelihood of seizures. |
| Instruct patients that getting adequate amounts of rest, avoiding physical and emotional stress, maintaining a nutritious and balanced diet and hydration status, and avoiding certain stimuli may help prevent seizure activity. | Meals should be spaced throughout the day to prevent hypoglycemia. Overhydration may precipitate seizure activity. Stimuli such as flashing lights, video or computer games, or loud music appear to trigger seizures, and patients should avoid environments that are likely to have these stimuli. TVs with poor signals may trigger seizures and should be fixed. Patients should monitor for and treat fever early during an illness. |
| Encourage the individuals who have seizures that occur without warning to avoid chewing gum or sucking on lozenges. | They may be aspirated during a seizure. |
| Encourage the patient to wear a medical alert bracelet or similar identification or to carry a medical information card. | They provide information to health care professionals if the patient is unable to. |
| Provide significant others and caregivers with verbal and written information for the preceding interventions. | Significant others and caregivers are likely to be in the patient's presence during subsequent seizures. If well informed, they will be able to protect the patient from trauma and life-threatening complications. |

## Patient Problem/Analyze Cues/Prioritize Hypotheses

# Deficient Knowledge (Medications)

*due to* unfamiliarity with the purpose, precautions, and side effects of AEDs

**Desired Outcome/Generate Solutions:** Before hospital discharge, the patient verbalizes accurate knowledge about the prescribed AED.

| ASSESSMENT—RECOGNIZE CUES/ INTERVENTIONS—TAKE ACTION | RATIONALES |
|---|---|
| Stress the importance of taking the prescribed AED regularly and on schedule, and not discontinuing medication without health care provider guidance. | Seizures will stop with drug treatment for 60% or more individuals with this disorder. Missing a scheduled dose can precipitate a seizure several days later. Abrupt withdrawal of any AED can precipitate seizures, and discontinuing these medications is the most common cause of SE. |

| ASSESSMENT—RECOGNIZE CUES/ INTERVENTIONS—TAKE ACTION | RATIONALES |
|---|---|
| Assist the patients in finding methods that will help them remember to take their medication and monitor their drug supply to avoid running out. | AEDs may be necessary for the duration of the patient's life. Medications cannot be taken "as-needed," and absence of seizures does not mean the medication is unnecessary. |
| Explain the concept of drug half-life and steady blood levels. | It is important to maintain a therapeutic blood level of the AED to manage seizures. |
| Caution patients to consult the health care provider before changing from a trade name to a generic medication and to avoid abrupt withdrawal. | Medications differ in the amount of time they remain in the body and reach peak activity, and there may be differences in bioavailability. Medications are usually withdrawn slowly over 1–2 weeks rather than abruptly stopped, which could result in seizures. |
| Stress the importance of informing the health care provider about side effects and keeping appointments for periodic laboratory work. | Laboratory tests will reveal whether blood levels of AEDs are therapeutic. Many side effects are dose related, and medication can be adjusted based on AED blood levels and symptoms. |
| Instruct the patient to report immediately any bruising, bleeding, jaundice, or rash. | Many AEDs can cause blood dyscrasias or liver damage. |
| Advise the patient to supplement with vitamin K, vitamin D, and folic acid if prescribed. | Certain AEDs, such as phenytoin, decrease absorption of folic acid and metabolism of vitamins D and K, which can lead to deficiencies. For pregnant women, folic acid supplementation is critical to prevent birth defects. Vitamin K may be given to pregnant women 1 month before and during delivery to prevent neonatal hemorrhage. |
| Instruct the patient to avoid grapefruit juice. | It can inhibit hepatic metabolism of many AEDs and affect drug level. |
| Advise that calcium supplementation and antacids should not be taken within about 2 hours of AEDs. | AEDs taken at the same time as calcium supplements and antacids may decrease the absorption and effects of both medicines. Vitamin D and calcium supplementation are used to prevent osteomalacia (soft bone) associated with some AEDs such as phenytoin, valproic acid, and carbamazepine. Periodic bone density monitoring is recommended. |
| Advise the patient to avoid activities that require alertness until the central nervous system (CNS) response to the medication has been determined. | AEDs may make people drowsy. Splitting the dose or giving the main dose at bedtime may help. |
| Instruct the patient to take the AED with food. | Ingesting AEDs with food will decrease the risk of nausea and vomiting, which are common side effects of most AEDs. |
| Advise patients taking valproic acid that this medication may produce a false-positive test for urine ketones. | It is important for patients, especially those with diabetes, to know this because ketone assessment is one aspect of managing their diabetes. |
| Advise the patient that any visual changes or pain should be reported immediately. | With valproic acid, a visual change may signal ocular toxicity. With topiramate, blurred vision or difficulty seeing may indicate glaucoma. Patients on vigabatrin must have periodic visual field testing because irreversible damage to the retina can occur. Prompt reporting and timely intervention may preserve vision. |
| Instruct the patient to notify the health care provider if a significant weight gain or weight loss occurs. | A change in dose or scheduling may be necessary. |
| Instruct the patient to avoid alcoholic beverages and over-the-counter (OTC) medications containing alcohol. | Long-term alcohol use stimulates the body to metabolize phenytoin more quickly, thus lowering the seizure threshold because of decreased plasma phenytoin levels. |
| Caution patients taking phenobarbital or primidone to avoid alcohol. | Alcohol potentiates the CNS depressant effects of these medications. |
| Caution the patient to avoid OTC medications. | AEDs are potentiated or inhibited by many other drugs, including aspirin and antihistamines, and may affect the potency of other medications as well. |

Continued

**Neurologic Care Plans**

| ASSESSMENT—RECOGNIZE CUES/ INTERVENTIONS—TAKE ACTION | RATIONALES |
|---|---|
| Instruct the patient to report uncoordinated movement (ataxia), diplopia, nystagmus, and dizziness. | These are other side effects common to AEDs that may necessitate drug, dosage, or schedule change. |
| Instruct patients who take carbamazepine, ethosuximide, or zonisamide to report immediately fever, mouth ulcers, sore throat, peripheral edema, dark urine, bruising, or bleeding. | These are possible side effects that may necessitate drug, dose, or schedule change. |
| Advise patients taking phenytoin to perform frequent oral hygiene with gum massage and gentle flossing and brush teeth 3–4 times/day with a soft-bristle toothbrush. Teach the patient to report immediately any measles-like rash. | Phenytoin can cause gingival hypertrophy and rash. |
| Caution patients taking phenytoin that there are two types of this drug and neither should be substituted for the other. | It is important not to confuse extended-release phenytoin (e.g., Dilantin Kapseal) with prompt-release phenytoin (e.g., Dilantin). Doing so may cause dangerous underdose or overdose. |
| Caution that generic phenytoin should not be substituted for Dilantin Kapseal. | Dilantin Kapseal is absorbed more slowly and is longer acting. |
| Instruct patient to monitor for increased body hair when taking phenytoin. | Excess body hair growth is a side effect of phenytoin. Hair removal creams can be used if increased hair is a problem. |
| Monitor for hyperglycemia with phenytoin. | Phenytoin blocks the release of insulin, which may cause increased blood sugar levels. Persons with diabetes in particular may need adjustments in their diabetic medications. |
| Encourage the patient to keep a drug and seizure chart diary. | This will help detect the trend of the seizures, which will enable the health care provider to determine whether the current treatment is at a therapeutic level. |

## Patient Problem/Analyze Cues/Prioritize Hypotheses

# Nonadherence

*due to* denial of the illness, financial constraints, or perceived negative consequences of the treatment regimen

***Desired Outcome/Generate Solutions:*** Before hospital discharge, the patient verbalizes knowledge about the disease process and describes the experience that lead to nonadherence of prescribed regimen, describes appropriate treatment of side effects or appropriate alternatives, and exhibits health care measures that reflect this knowledge, following an agreed-on plan of care.

| ASSESSMENT—RECOGNIZE CUES/ INTERVENTIONS—TAKE ACTION | RATIONALES |
|---|---|
| Assess the patient's understanding of the disease process, medical management, and treatment plan. Explain or clarify information as indicated. | This assessment enables nurses to explain or clarify information as indicated and facilitates the development of an individualized care plan that promotes adherence. |
| Assess for causes of nonadherence, such as financial constraints, inconvenience, forgetfulness or memory problems, medication side effects, misunderstanding of instructions, or difficulty making significant lifestyle changes or following medication schedule. | After the causes are identified, the nurse can then focus the care plan accordingly. |

| ASSESSMENT—RECOGNIZE CUES/ INTERVENTIONS—TAKE ACTION | RATIONALES |
|---|---|
| Explain drug half-life and the concept of a steady blood level. Explain the importance of health care provider guidance if the medication is stopped for any reason. Instruct and provide written instructions for how to contact the health care provider and the importance of health care provider and laboratory follow-up. Explain what to do if a dose is missed and how to refill a prescription if the medication is lost or depleted. | Intermittent medication use may be informal experimentation or an effort to gain control. Explanation of consequences of nonadherence helps ensure awareness that medication discontinuation can be life threatening (e.g., can cause SE). |
| Encourage the patient's expression of feelings (e.g., dependence, powerlessness, embarrassment, being different). In addition, evaluate the patient's perception of the effectiveness or ineffectiveness of treatment. | This will help clarify the patient's perception of vulnerability to the disease process and signs of denial of the illness. |
| Confront myths and stigmas. Provide realistic assessment of risks, and counter misconceptions. | This will help determine whether a value, cultural conflict, or spiritual conflict is causing nonadherence. |
| Discuss the methods of dealing with common problems, such as obtaining insurance and job or workplace discrimination. | Helping to eliminate barriers and problems optimally will promote adherence. |
| Assess the patient's support systems. | This will help determine whether a family disruption pattern (whether it is caused by the patient's illness) is making adherence difficult and "not worth it." |
| After the reason for nonadherence is found, intervene accordingly. If it appears that changing the medical treatment plan (e.g., in scheduling medications) may promote adherence, discuss this possibility with the health care provider. Provide the patient with information about interventions that can minimize drug side effects (e.g., taking drug with food or large amounts of liquid to minimize gastric distress). | All may help facilitate adherence. |
| Encourage the involvement with support systems such as the local epilepsy centers and national organizations. | Many people appreciate the support of others with the same condition. Feeling less alone and supported by others may promote adherence. |
| If indicated, suggest counseling or psychotherapy. | This may help patients with poor self-concept or coping difficulties related to the diagnosis that may be a cause of the nonadherence. |

## ADDITIONAL PROBLEMS:

## ✓ PATIENT–FAMILY TEACHING AND DISCHARGE PLANNING

✓ When providing patient–family teaching, focus on sensory information, avoid giving excessive information, and initiate a visiting nurse referral for necessary follow-up teaching. Include verbal and written information about the following:

✓ Reinforcement of knowledge of the disease process, pathophysiology, symptoms, and precipitating or aggravating factors.

✓ Medications, including drug name, purpose, dosage, schedule, precautions, and potential side effects. Also discuss drug–drug, herb–drug, and food–drug interactions and importance of adhering to medication routine. Some herbs (ginkgo, valerian root, evening primrose, ephedra) may be proconvulsant and should be avoided.

✓ Importance of follow-up care and keeping medical appointments. Stress that the use of AEDs necessitates periodic monitoring of blood levels to ensure therapeutic medication levels and assessment for side effects. Instruct patient to keep emergency contact numbers for the health care provider.

✓ Seizure first aid. An uncomplicated convulsive seizure in an individual known to have epilepsy is not necessarily a medical emergency. On average, these people can continue their business after a rest period. An ambulance should be called or medical attention sought if the seizure happens in water; if the individual is injured, is pregnant, or has diabetes; if the seizure lasts longer than 5 minutes; if a second seizure starts; if consciousness does not begin to return; or if there is any question the seizure may have been caused by something other than epilepsy.

✓ Environmental factors that can be life threatening in the presence of seizures, measures that may help prevent seizures, and safety interventions during seizures. Review the state and local laws that apply to individuals with seizure disorders. Review the home and personal safety tips.

✓ Employment or vocational counseling as needed. Discuss the need to avoid overprotection and maintain, as possible, normal work and recreation. Review or provide information regarding the Americans With Disabilities Act.

✓ Risks of using AEDs during pregnancy. Provide birth control information or genetic counseling referral as requested.

✓ Benefits of joining local support groups. Provide the following addresses as appropriate:

- Epilepsy Foundation: www.epilepsyfoundation.org
- Epilepsy Information Page: National Institute of Neurological Disorders and Stroke: www.ninds.nih.gov/disorders/epilepsy/epilepsy.htm
- Antiepileptic Drug Pregnancy Registry: www.aed-pregnancyregistry.org
- American Epilepsy Society: www.aesnet.org

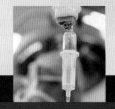

# Spinal Cord Injury  43

## OVERVIEW/PATHOPHYSIOLOGY

Spinal cord injuries (SCIs) are caused by vertebral fractures or dislocations that sever, lacerate, stretch, or compress the spinal cord and interrupt neuronal function and transmission of nerve impulses. Concussive trauma can cause damage from bruising, swelling, and inflammation. When blood supply to the spinal cord is interrupted, the spinal cord swells in response, and this, along with hemorrhage, can cause additional compression, ischemia, and compromised function. Neurologic deficits resulting from compression may be reversible if the resulting edema and ischemia do not lead to spinal cord degeneration and necrosis. Common causes of injury include motor vehicle collisions, diving or other sporting accidents, falls, and gunshot wounds. SCIs are classified in a number of different ways according to mechanism of injury (compression, hyperflexion, hyperextension, rotational, penetrating), level of injury (level of spinal cord involved), and degree of spinal cord function loss (complete, incomplete). A *spinal cord concussion* involves a transient loss of cord function caused by a traumatic event, resulting in immediate flaccid paralysis that resolves completely in a matter of minutes or hours.

*Prognosis.* Any evidence of voluntary motor function, sensory function, or sacral sensation below the level of injury (the lowest level in which motor function and sensation remain intact) indicates an incomplete SCI, with the potential for partial or complete recovery. After an acute injury, the spinal cord usually goes into a condition called *spinal shock*, in which there can be total loss of spinal cord function below the level of injury. During spinal shock, there is no reflex activity. Resolution of spinal shock with return of reflexes usually occurs within days to weeks. If there is no evidence of returning motor function after local reflexes have returned, the spinal cord is considered irreversibly damaged. Generally, SCI does not cause immediate death unless it is at C1 through C3, which results in respiratory muscle paralysis. Individuals who survive these injuries require a ventilator for the rest of their lives. If the injury occurs at C4, respiratory difficulties may result in death, although some individuals who have survived the initial injury have been successfully weaned from the ventilator. Injuries below C4 also can be life threatening because of ascending cord edema, which can cause respiratory muscle paralysis. Immediately after injury, common complications that require treatment include hypotension (systolic blood pressure [SBP] less than 80 mm Hg), bradycardia, paralytic ileus, urinary retention, pneumonia, and

stress ulcers. Other long-term, life-threatening complications of SCI include autonomic dysreflexia (AD), pneumonia, decubitus ulcers, sepsis, urinary calculi, and urinary tract infection (UTI).

## HEALTH CARE SETTING

Acute care, subacute care, rehabilitation center

## ASSESSMENT

There are a variety of neurologic assessment and functional outcome scales, including the American Spinal Injury Association Impairment Scale (https://www.icf-casestudies.org/introduction/spinal-cord-injury-sci/american-spinal-injury-association-asia-impairment-scale), in which the impairment is described by whether it is complete, incomplete, or normal, with further differentiations for incomplete injuries.

*Acute indicators.* Loss of sensation, weakness, or paralysis below level of injury, localized pain or tenderness over site of injury, headache, hypothermia or hyperthermia, and alterations in bowel and bladder function.

*Cervical injury.* Possible alterations in level of consciousness (LOC); weakness or paralysis in all four extremities (tetraparesis or tetraplegia); and paralysis of respiratory muscles or signs of respiratory problems, such as flaring nostrils and use of accessory muscles for respirations. C4 and above injuries require ventilator support. Any cervical injury can result in low body temperature (to 96°F [35.5°C]), slowed pulse rate (less than 60 bpm) caused by vagal stimulation of the heart, hypotension (SBP less than 80 mm Hg) caused by vasodilation, and decreased peristalsis.

*Thoracic and lumbar injuries.* Paraparesis/paraplegia or altered sensation in the legs; hand and arm involvement in upper thoracic injuries.

*Acute spinal shock.* Spinal shock results from loss of sympathetic nerve outflow and reflex function in all segments below the level of injury. Indicators depend on injury severity and include total loss of spinal cord function, loss of skin sensation, flaccid paralysis or absence of reflexes below the level of injury, paralytic ileus and constipation secondary to atonic bowel, bladder distention secondary to atonic bladder, bradycardia, low/falling BP secondary to loss of vasomotor tone and decreased venous return, and anhidrosis (absence of sweating and loss of temperature regulation) below the level of injury. Autonomic instability is more dramatic in higher

319

(e.g., cervical) lesions. Resolution of spinal shock is indicated by return of both the bulbocavernosus reflex (slight muscle contraction when glans penis is squeezed or urinary catheter is pulled, causing scrotal retraction) and the anal reflex (anal puckering on digital examination or gentle scratching around the anus). Remaining reflexes may take weeks to return.

**Chronic indicators.** As spinal shock resolves, muscle tone, reflexes, and some functions may return, depending on severity and level of injury. Return of reflexes usually results in muscle spasticity. Chronic autonomic dysfunction may be manifested as fever; mild hypotension; anhidrosis; and alterations in bowel, bladder, and sexual function. Chronic neural pain may occur after SCI and tends to occur as either diffuse pain below the level of injury or pain adjacent to the level of injury. Injuries at or below L1 may result in permanent flaccid paralysis. Orthostatic hypotension is more typical of lesions above T7.

**Upper motor neuron involvement.** Upper motor neurons (UMNs) are nerve cell bodies that originate in high levels of the central nervous system and transmit impulses from the brain down the spinal cord. Injury interrupts this impulse transmission, causing muscle or organ dysfunction below the level of injury. However, because the injury does not interrupt reflex arcs coming from those muscles or organs to the spinal cord, hypertonic reflexes, clonus paralysis, and spastic paralysis are seen. The patient will have a positive Babinski reflex.

**Lower motor neuron involvement.** Lower motor neurons (LMNs) are anterior horn cell bodies that originate in the spinal cord. LMNs transmit nerve impulses to muscles and organs and are involved in reflex arcs that control involuntary responses. Damage to LMNs will abolish voluntary and reflex responses of muscles and organs, resulting in flaccid paralysis, hypotonia, atrophy, and muscle fibrillations and fasciculations. The patient will have an absent Babinski reflex. The spinal cord ends at the T12–L1 level. Below that level, a bundle of nerve roots from the spinal cord, called the *cauda equina*, fills the spinal canal. Injuries at or below L1 that damage nerve fiber after it leaves the spinal cord result in flaccid paralysis because of interrupted reflex arc activity.

**Bowel and bladder dysfunction.** Usually, conscious sensation of the need to void or defecate is lost. UMN bowel and bladder involvement results in reflex incontinence. Flaccid LMN bladder involvement causes urinary retention with overflow incontinence. Flaccid LMN bowel involvement causes fecal retention/impaction.

**Sexual dysfunction.** Degree of dysfunction varies according to degree of completeness and whether injury is UMN or LMN. Males with complete UMN injuries have a loss of psychogenic erection but may have reflex erections. Ejaculation rates with complete UMN injuries are as low as 4%. Females have a loss of psychogenic lubrication but may have reflex lubrication. With complete LMN injuries, about 25% of males will have psychogenic erections but none will have reflex erections. About 50% of both sexes (by questionnaire) say they can experience orgasm regardless of injury level (possibly through other erogenous zones). Incomplete injuries will result in better sexual functioning that may include both erections and ejaculations.

**Autonomic dysreflexia.** Also known as *autonomic hyperreflexia*, AD is the exaggerated and unopposed sympathetic response to noxious stimuli below the SCI lesion and can be life threatening as reflex activity returns. AD is seen most commonly in patients with injuries at or above T6, but it has been reported with injuries as low as T8. Signs and symptoms include gross hypertension (BP more than 20 mm Hg above baseline, but BP can be as high as 240–300/150 mm Hg), pounding headache, blurred vision, bradycardia, nausea, and nasal congestion. Above the level of injury, flushing and sweating may occur. Below the level of injury, piloerection (goosebumps) and skin pallor, which signal vasoconstriction, may be present. Seizures, subarachnoid hemorrhage, stroke, or retinal hemorrhage also may occur.

## PHYSICAL ASSESSMENT

**Acute (spinal shock).** Absence of deep tendon reflexes (DTRs) below the level of injury, absence of cremasteric reflex (scratching or light stroking of inner thigh for male patients causes testicle on that side to elevate) for T12 and L1 injuries, absence of penile or anal sphincter reflex.

**Chronic.** Generally, increased DTRs occur when the spinal cord lesion is of the UMN type.

## DIAGNOSTIC TESTS

Complete spine immobilization with a rigid cervical collar and backboard or other firm surface is essential until diagnostic tests rule out injury.

**Radiographic examination of spine.** To delineate fracture, deformity, displacement of vertebrae, and soft tissue masses such as hematomas.

**Magnetic resonance imaging.** To reveal changes in spinal cord and surrounding soft tissue. Magnetic resonance imaging evaluation is preferred and considered the gold standard for the evaluation of degree of injury in patients who can tolerate it.

**Computed tomography.** This is the preferred imaging study to diagnose the location and degree of the injury and the degree of spinal canal compromise. It reveals changes in spinal cord, vertebrae, and soft tissue surrounding the spine.

**Cervical x-rays.** Done when no availability of a computed tomography scan.

**Arterial blood gas/pulmonary function tests.** To assess the effectiveness of respirations and detect the need for $O_2$ or mechanical ventilation.

**Deep vein thrombosis studies (e.g., venogram, duplex Doppler ultrasound, impedance plethysmography).** To monitor for the development of deep vein thrombosis (DVT).

## Patient Problem/Analyze Cues/Prioritize Hypotheses

# Risk for Disease (Autonomic Dysreflexia)

*due to* exaggerated unopposed autonomic response to noxious stimuli for individuals with SCI at or above T6

***Desired Outcomes/Generate Solutions:*** On an ongoing basis, the patient is free of AD symptoms as evidenced by BP within the patient's baseline range, heart rate (HR) of 60–100 bpm, and absence of headache and other clinical indicators of AD. After receiving instruction, the patient and significant others verbalize factors that cause AD, treatment and prevention, and when immediate emergency treatment is indicated.

| ASSESSMENT—RECOGNIZE CUES/ INTERVENTIONS—TAKE ACTION | RATIONALES |
|---|---|
| ⚠ Assess for indicators of AD, including hypertension (BP more than 20 mm Hg above baseline, but may go as high as 240–300/150 mm Hg), pounding headache, bradycardia, blurred vision, nausea, nasal congestion, flushing and sweating above the level of injury, and piloerection (goosebumps) or pallor below the level of injury. | AD is a medical emergency that can occur after spinal shock resolution in patients with injuries at or above T6, but cases have been reported in patients with injuries as low as T8. |
| ⚠ If AD is suspected, raise the head of bed (HOB) immediately to 90 degrees or assist the patient into a sitting position. | These actions lower the patient's BP and decrease venous return. Seizures, subarachnoid hemorrhage, myocardial infarction, stroke, or retinal hemorrhage can occur if severe hypertensive episode continues. |
| ⚠ Call for someone to notify the health care provider; stay with the patient, and systematically search to identify and relieve the noxious stimulus. Speed is essential. | The noxious stimulus (e.g., distended bladder) must be found and alleviated as quickly as possible in order to remove the stimulus triggering AD. |
| Assess the BP every 3–5 minutes during hypertensive episode. | This assesses the trend of the BP values. |
| Remain calm and supportive of the patient and significant other. | The patient will be very anxious. |
| ⚠ Assess the following sites for causes and implement measures for removing the noxious stimulus. | |
| **Bladder:** Distention, UTI, calculus and other obstructions, bladder spasms, catheterization, or bladder irrigations performed too quickly or with too cold a liquid. | Problems with the bladder are the most likely cause of AD. |
| Do not use Credé method for a distended bladder. | The increased bladder pressure could further stimulate the reflex and worsen the condition. |
| Catheterize the patient (ideally using anesthetic jelly) if there is a possibility or question of bladder distention. Consult the health care provider immediately. | Bladder distention is a potential cause of AD and requires immediate intervention. Anesthetic jelly prevents skin stimulation, which could trigger AD. |
| If a catheter is already in place, check the tubing for kinks and lower drainage bag. For obstruction, such as sediment in tubing, slowly irrigate the catheter as indicated, using 30 mL or less of normal saline. | These interventions enable checking for catheter tube patency. Obstruction is a potential cause of AD. |
| If the bladder is not distended, check for cloudy urine, hematuria, and positive laboratory or radiographic examination results. | These are signs of UTI and/or urinary calculi—two potential causes of AD. |
| Obtain a urine specimen. | Culture and sensitivity studies will show whether a UTI, a potential cause of AD, is present. |
| Instill tetracaine or lidocaine into the bladder if prescribed. | These agents will reduce bladder excitability. |
| Institute preventive measures as prescribed to prevent UTI and urinary calculi. | Future episodes may be caused by these factors. |

Continued

| ASSESSMENT—RECOGNIZE CUES/ INTERVENTIONS—TAKE ACTION | RATIONALES |
|---|---|
| **Bowel:** Constipation, impaction, insertion of suppository or enema, or rectal examination. | Problems with the bowel are the second most likely cause of AD. A good bowel regimen is a key factor in preventing the noxious stimuli that constipation may cause. |
| Do not attempt rectal examination without first anesthetizing the rectal sphincter and anal canal with anesthetic jelly. | Anesthetic jelly prevents skin stimulation, which could trigger AD. |
| Use large amounts of anesthetic jelly in the anus and rectum before disimpacting the bowel to remove potential stimulus. | Bowel impaction is a potential cause of AD. |
| Wait 5 minutes and check BP before disimpacting. | A lowered BP is a sign that anesthetic jelly has become effective. |
| **Skin:** Pressure, infection, injury, heat, pain, or cold. | These are possible causes of AD. A good skin integrity program is another key factor in preventing these noxious stimuli. |
| Loosen clothing and remove antiembolism hose, leg bandages, abdominal binder, or constrictive sheets as appropriate. For male patients, check for pressure on penis, scrotum, or testicles and remove pressure if present. | Pressure on the skin is a potential cause of AD. Removal of hose, bandages, etc., also enables assessment of the skin for redness and other signs of pressure. |
| Check skin surfaces below the level of injury. Monitor for the presence of a pressure area or sore, infection, laceration, rash, sunburn, ingrown toenail, or infected area, or check the skin for contact with a hard object. If indicated, apply a topical anesthetic. | Skin infection, pain, and injury are potential causes of AD. |
| Observe for and remove sources of heat or cold (e.g., ice pack, heating pad). | Topical heat and cold are two potential causes of AD. |
| Turn the patient on his or her side and ensure that bed linen is free of wrinkles. Consider adhering to a more frequent turning schedule. | These measures relieve other possible sources of pressure. |
| **Additional causes:** Surgical manipulation, incisional pain, sexual activity, menstrual cramps, labor, vaginal infection, or intraabdominal problems such as appendicitis. | |
| Administer antihypertensives as prescribed. | These medications lower BP. |
| Instruct patient that use of erectile dysfunction medications are contraindicated when using nitrates for hypertension. | Erectile dysfunction medications are contraindicated for people who are taking nitrates (e.g., nitroglycerin) because of the additive hypotensive effect. |
| On resolution of the crisis, answer the patient's and significant others' questions about AD. Discuss signs and symptoms, treatment, methods of prevention, and need for regular assessment of causative agents. | Prevention is the best way to deal with AD. A bowel regimen and skin integrity program are key factors in preventing the noxious stimuli that constipation and pressure areas may cause. |
| Encourage the patient to wear a medical alert bracelet or tag. | These items inform health care providers of the patient's condition in case the patient is unable to do so during AD. |
| Encourage keeping an AD kit on hand that includes a glove, lubricant jelly, straight catheter, electronic BP machine, and alert card. | This kit will help relieve and monitor this medical emergency when it occurs. |

## Patient Problem/Analyze Cues/Prioritize Hypotheses

# Impaired Gas Exchange

*due to* neuromuscular paralysis/weakness; or *due to* the restriction of chest expansion occurring with halo vest obstruction

**Desired Outcome/Generate Solutions:** After intervention, the patient's oxygen saturation is 95% or above and $PaCO_2$ is 35–45 mm Hg, respiratory rate (RR) is 12–20 breaths/minute with normal depth and pattern (eupnea) with absence of adventitious breath sounds.

| ASSESSMENT—RECOGNIZE CUES/ INTERVENTIONS—TAKE ACTION | RATIONALES |
|---|---|
| ⚠ Monitor the ventilation capability by checking vital capacity, tidal volume, and pulmonary function tests. Monitor the serial arterial blood gas values and/or pulse oximetry readings. | If vital capacity is less than 1 L or if the patient exhibits signs of hypoxia ($PaO_2$ less than 80 mm Hg, $O_2$ saturation 92% or less, tachycardia, increased restlessness, mental status changes or dullness, cyanosis), the health care provider should be notified immediately. |
| Provide oxygen as indicated. | Oxygen will help keep saturation greater than 92%. |
| ⚠ Assess for difficulty with expectoration of secretions, coughing, and respirations. Also assess the HR for bradycardia, BP changes, and increased motor and sensory losses at a higher level than baseline findings. | These signs may signal ascending cord edema secondary to the effects of contusion or bleeding. If present, the patient may require increased respiratory support. |
| ⚠ Assess for loss of previous ability to bend arms at the elbows (C5–6) or shrug shoulders (C3–4). If these findings are noted, notify the health care provider immediately. | Changes from baseline or previous assessment may signal problems such as contusion, compression, bleeding, or damage to the blood supply, and they necessitate prompt intervention. |
| ⚠ Keep the patient's head in neutral position, and suction as necessary. Be aware that suctioning may cause severe bradycardia in the patient with autonomic dysfunction. If indicated, prepare the patient for a tracheostomy, endotracheal intubation, and/or mechanical ventilation to support respiratory function. If appropriate, arrange for transfer to intensive care unit for continuous monitoring. | These actions maintain a patent airway and support respiratory function. Patients with injuries above C5 are intubated and put on a ventilator. Nasal intubation or tracheostomy may be used to prevent neck extension (and thus further damage) during intubation. |
| If the patient is wearing halo vest traction, assess respiratory status at least every 4 hours or more frequently as indicated. | This action ascertains whether the vest is restricting chest expansion. |
| Assess the ability to swallow for the patient in halo traction. | Inability to swallow may indicate improper position of the neck and chin or changes in cranial nerve function caused by cranial pin compression or irritation. |
| Instruct patients who are breathing independently on the use of incentive spirometry. | Spirometry promotes adequate ventilation and assesses the quality of inspiratory abilities. |
| ⚠ Assess for shortness of breath, hemoptysis, tachycardia, sudden shoulder pain, and diminished breath sounds | These are indicators of venous thromboembolism (VTE)/pulmonary embolus (PE), which can occur because of impaired ventilation, altered vascular tone, and decreased mobility. Pain may or may not be present with VTE/PE, depending on the level of SCI. Sudden shoulder pain may be referred pain from VTE/PE. |
| Encourage coughing exercises. If the patient's cough is ineffective, implement the following technique, known as *assisted coughing*: place the heel of your hand under patient's diaphragm (below xiphoid process and above navel). Have the patient take several deep breaths, hold a deep breath, and then cough. As the patient exhales forcibly, quickly push up into the diaphragm to assist in producing a more forceful cough. | This technique enables the production of a more forceful cough. An insufflation-exsufflation cough machine may be used to deliver breaths to patients in order to produce a more effective mechanically assisted cough.<br><br>**Caution:** Assisted coughing may be contraindicated in patients with spinal instability. |
| Provide instructions to the patient regarding intermittent positive pressure breathing, nebulizer treatments, and chest physiotherapy, if prescribed. | These therapies prevent and treat atelectasis. Respiratory therapy is ongoing past the acute stage. Noninvasive positive pressure ventilation may be used with some patients. |
| ⚠ Feed patients in Stryker frames, Foster beds, or similar mechanical beds in the prone position. Raise stable patients in halo traction to high-Fowler position if it is not contraindicated. | These actions minimize the potential for aspiration. |
| For additional information, see "General Care of Patients With Neurologic Disorders," Chapter 36, for *Risk for Aspiration*. | |

## Patient Problem/Analyze Cues/Prioritize Hypotheses

# Ineffective Tissue Perfusion (Cerebral and Cardiac)

*due to* relative hypovolemia occurring with decreased vasomotor tone

**Desired Outcomes/Generate Solutions:** By at least 24 hours before hospital discharge (or as soon as vasomotor tone improves), the patient has adequate cardiac and cerebral tissue perfusion, as evidenced by SBP of 90 mm Hg or higher and orientation to person, place, and time. For a minimum of 48 hours before hospital discharge, the patient is free of dysrhythmias.

| ASSESSMENT—RECOGNIZE CUES/ INTERVENTIONS—TAKE ACTION | RATIONALES |
|---|---|
| Assess for hypotension (drop in SBP more than 20 mm Hg, SBP less than 90 mm Hg), lightheadedness, dizziness, fainting, and confusion. | Low/falling BP can occur secondary to loss of vasomotor tone and decreased venous return. |
| Assess the oxygen saturation; administer the oxygen as indicated. | Supplemental oxygen will help keep saturation at a level greater than 92%. |
| Assess the HR and rhythm. Document dysrhythmias. | Sinus tachycardia/bradycardia may develop because of impaired sympathetic innervation or unopposed vagal stimulation. Atropine may be prescribed for symptomatic bradycardia. |
| Assess the intake and output. | Adequate hydration and elimination are necessary to maintain stable hemodynamics. |
| Administer prescribed intravenous fluids cautiously. | Impaired vascular tone can make the patient sensitive to small increases in circulating volume. Intravascular volume expanders or vasopressors (e.g., dopamine) may be required for hypotension. |
| Implement and instruct patient to change positions slowly | This prevents episodes of decreased cardiac output caused by postural hypotension. Decreased cardiac output compromises cerebral and peripheral circulation. Postural hypotension is seen frequently in SCI, but it can be prevented and managed. |
| Perform exercises to increase range of motion (ROM) every 2 hours. Prevent the patient's legs from crossing, especially when in a dependent position. | This prevents venous pooling and contractures. |
| If indicated, ensure that patients with SCI at higher levels, especially above T6, wear an abdominal binder in addition to antiembolic hose, leg wraps, and sequential compression devices or pneumatic foot pumps. | This helps prevent venous pooling. These individuals are prone to more severe hypotensive reactions, even with minor changes such as raising the HOB. |
| Work with the physical therapist to implement a gradual sitting program that will help the patient progress from a supine to an upright position. | The goal is to increase the patient's ability to sit upright while avoiding adverse effects, such as hypertension, dizziness, and fainting. This may include a bed that can rotate gradually from a horizontal position to a vertical position or a chair that has multiple positions progressing from flat to sitting. |
| Administer the salt tablets and fludrocortisone as prescribed if nonmedication methods are ineffective. | These agents prevent orthostatic hypotension. |
| For additional information, see *Risk for Altered Blood Pressure (Orthostatic Hypotension)* in "Immobility," Chapter 1. | |

## Patient Problem/Analyze Cues/Prioritize Hypotheses

# Risk for Ineffective Tissue Perfusion

*due to* venous stasis with corresponding risk for thrombophlebitis and VTE/ PE occurring with immobility and decreased vasomotor tone

***Desired Outcome/Generate Solutions:*** For at least 24 hours before hospital discharge and on an ongoing basis, the patient has adequate tissue perfusion as evidenced by absence of heat, erythema, and swelling in calves and thighs; HR of 100 bpm or less; RR of 20 breaths/minute or less with eupnea and $PaO_2$ of 80 mm Hg or more or $O_2$ saturation greater than 92%.

| ASSESSMENT—RECOGNIZE CUES/ INTERVENTIONS—TAKE ACTION | RATIONALES |
|---|---|
| Assess for erythema, warmth, and swelling over lower extremities, coolness, pallor, decreased pulse amplitude. | Erythema, warmth, and swelling may indicate inflammation and venous dilation. Coolness, pallor, and decreased pulse amplitude may indicate thrombophlebitis. |
| Measure the calves and thighs daily while the patient is supine or before activity and monitor for increased circumference. | An increase of 1.5 cm or more in 1 day is significant for thrombophlebitis, as is calf diameter greater than 3 cm larger than the opposite calf. |
| Recognize that low-grade fever may be a more reliable signal of thrombophlebitis than pain. Notify the health care provider about significant findings. | The presence of pain or tenderness depends on the level of SCI. |
| Protect the patient's legs from injury during transfers and turning and position them so they do not cross. Avoid intramuscular injections in the legs and do not massage the legs. | SCI patients are prone to DVT, which can occur in the lower extremities because of immobility and changes in vascular tone. |
| Provide ROM to the legs four times daily; elevate legs 10–15 degrees. | These measures promote venous drainage. |
| Assess for tachycardia, shortness of breath, hemoptysis, decrease in $PaO_2$, $O_2$ saturation of 92% or less, decreased or adventitious breath sounds, and chest or shoulder pain. Notify the health care provider about significant findings. | All are indicators of VTE/PE. Presence of pain depends on the level of injury. Sudden shoulder pain may represent referred pain from VTE/PE. |
| Consult the health care provider about the use of antiembolism hose, sequential compression devices, pneumatic foot pumps, or prophylactic pharmacotherapy (e.g., acetylsalicylic acid, warfarin, low-molecular-weight or low-dose heparin). | These measures help prevent VTE/PE. |
| If indicated, explain the use of a vena cava filter. | This filter helps prevent emboli from reaching the lungs in the presence of VTE/PE. |
| For other interventions, see *Risk for Deep Vein Thrombosis* in "Immobility," Chapter 1. | |

## Patient Problem/Analyze Cues/Prioritize Hypotheses

# Impaired Urinary Elimination (Retention)

*due to* neurologic impairment (flaccid and spastic bladder type)

***Desired Outcomes/Generate Solutions:*** After instruction, the patient demonstrates triggering mechanisms that promote urination and gains some control over voiding without incontinence. The patient empties the bladder with residual volumes of less than 50 mL by the time of hospital discharge.

| ASSESSMENT—RECOGNIZE CUES/ INTERVENTIONS—TAKE ACTION | RATIONALES |
|---|---|
| **General Guidelines for Individuals With Bladder Dysfunction—Both Flaccid and Spastic** | |
| Assess for evidence of bladder dysfunction or monitor cystometric test results. | Bladder dysfunction is complicated and should be assessed by cystometric testing to determine the best type of bladder program. |

Continued

| ASSESSMENT—RECOGNIZE CUES/ INTERVENTIONS—TAKE ACTION | RATIONALES |
|---|---|
| If intermittent catheterization is used and episodes of incontinence occur or more than 500 mL of urine is obtained, catheterize the patient more often. | Initially, during acute spinal shock, patients will have an indwelling urinary catheter or scheduled intermittent catheterizations. As spinal reflexes return, intermittent catheterization or other bladder-emptying technique is used. Indwelling catheters are avoided because of the potential for UTI. |
| Instruct the patient/significant other/caregiver on the procedure for intermittent catheterization, care of indwelling catheters, and indicators of UTI (e.g., fever, chills, cloudy and/or foul-smelling urine, malaise, anorexia, restlessness, increased frequency or urgency, incontinence). | This instruction helps ensure readiness for self-care or assisted care when discharged from the acute or rehabilitation facility. |
| Instruct the patient/significant other/caregiver that the habit/bladder scheduling program consists of gradually increasing the time between catheterizations or periodically clamping indwelling catheters. | The goal is a gradual increase in bladder tone. When the bladder can hold 300–400 mL of urine, measures to stimulate voiding are attempted. A bladder scan may be used to determine fullness and aid in retraining. |
| Ensure the patient ingests fluids at evenly spaced intervals throughout the day. | This promotes adequate hydration and increased bladder tone. |
| Restrict fluids before bedtime and avoid diuretic-type fluids several hours before sleep. | This helps prevent nighttime incontinence. Alcohol and caffeine-containing foods and beverages (e.g., cola, chocolate, coffee, tea) have a diuretic effect and may cause incontinence. In addition, caffeine-containing products may increase bladder spasms and reflex incontinence. |
| Instruct patients using bladder-emptying techniques to void at least every 3 hours. | Maintaining a regular schedule prevents bladder distention. Using an alarm or reminder device such as found on smartphones or wristwatches can help patients maintain this schedule. |
| To obtain postvoid residual urine, catheterize or perform a bladder scan on the patient after an attempt to empty the bladder. | Residual amounts greater than 100 mL usually indicate the need for a return to a scheduled intermittent catheterization program. |
| Assess the response to measures that promote bladder training and continence and obtain urinary specialist consult as appropriate. | A urinary diversion may be considered for patients whose bladders cannot be retrained. An artificial urinary sphincter or continent vesicostomy may be used to promote bladder continence. An external sphincterectomy may be done to reduce sphincter resistance, thereby producing continuous bladder emptying. |
| **Guidelines for Patients With LMN-Involved Flaccid Bladders** | |
| Explain to the patient that they may be able to empty the bladder manually well enough to avoid catheterization. | The need for catheterization can be determined by checking residual urine volume (see general guidelines, previously). |
| If Credé method is prescribed, teach the technique to the patient. | Credé method is a technique for increasing intraabdominal pressure. It is performed as follows: the ulnar surface of the hand is placed horizontally along or just below the umbilicus, while the patient bears down with the abdominal muscles, the hand is pressed downward and toward the bladder in a kneading motion until urination is initiated. This is continued for 30 seconds or until urination ceases. The patient then waits a few minutes and repeats the procedure to ensure complete emptying of the bladder. |
| Suggest alternative measures if the patient's bladder cannot be trained to empty completely. | Intermittent catheterization or external collection devices usually are indicated, and the patient may be a candidate for an artificial inflatable sphincter device or urinary diversion. |

PART I: Medical-Surgical Nursing Care Plans

## Patient Problem/Analyze Cues/Prioritize Hypotheses

# Impaired Urinary Elimination (Reflex Incontinence)

*due to* neurologic impairment (spastic bladder type)

***Desired Outcomes/Generate Solutions:*** After instruction, the patient demonstrates triggering mechanisms that stimulate reflex voiding and gains some control over voiding without incontinence. The patient empties the bladder with residual volumes of less than 50 mL by the time of hospital discharge.

| ASSESSMENT—RECOGNIZE CUES/ INTERVENTIONS—TAKE ACTION | RATIONALES |
|---|---|
| *See "General Guidelines for Individuals With Bladder Dysfunction" in the previous patient problem.* | |
| **Guidelines for Patients With UMN-Involved Spastic Reflex Bladder** | |
| Explain to these patients that eventually they may be able to empty the bladder automatically and therefore may not require catheterization. | Lesions above the conus medullaris (located at the lower two levels of the thoracic region, where the cord begins to taper) generally leave the S2, S3, and S4 spinal cord nerve segments intact. If this spinal reflex arc is intact, the patient will have UMN-involved bladder, resulting in a spastic bladder. This bladder has tone and occasional bladder contractions and periodically will empty on its own, resulting in reflex incontinence. The UMN-involved bladder is "trainable" with techniques that stimulate reflex voiding. |
| Instruct the patient to tap the suprapubic area with the fingers, gently pulling pubic hair, digitally stretching the anal sphincter, stroking the glans penis, stroking the inner thigh, light pulsating pressure in the abdominal area just proximal to the inguinal ligaments, or using a hand-held vibration device against the lower abdomen. Advise the patient to perform the selected technique for 2–3 minutes or until a good urine stream has started. Explain that the patient should wait 1 minute before trying another stimulation technique. | These techniques, which are described below, stimulate the voiding reflex and should be taught to patients accordingly. Stimulating reflex trigger zones accidentally may result in incontinence. Incontinence briefs will help control accidents. |
| *Bladder tapping:* The patient positions self in a half-sitting position. Tapping is performed over the suprapubic area, and the patient may shift the site of stimulation within that area to find the most effective site. Tapping is performed rapidly (7–8 times/second) with one hand for approximately 50 single taps. The patient continues tapping until a good stream starts. Explain that when the stream stops, the patient should wait about 1 minute and repeat tapping until the bladder is empty. One or two tapping attempts without response indicate that no more urine will be expelled. | |
| *Anal stretch technique (contraindicated in individuals with lesions at T8 or above because of the potential for AD):* The patient positions self on a commode or toilet, leans forward on the thighs, and inserts 1 or 2 lubricated fingers into the anus to the anal sphincter. The patient then dilates the anal sphincter gently by spreading the fingers apart or pulling in a posterior direction. The patient maintains the stretching position, takes a deep breath, and holds the breath while bearing down to void. The patient relaxes and repeats until the bladder is empty. | |
| Administer antispasmodics, anticholinergics, or tricyclic antidepressant (TCA) medications if prescribed. | Antispasmodics inhibit bladder smooth muscle contraction and may increase bladder capacity. Anticholinergics inhibit involuntary bladder contractions. TCAs have an anticholinergic and direct muscle relaxant effect on the urinary bladder. |

Patient Problem/Analyze Cues/Prioritize Hypotheses

# Risk for Impaired Gastrointestinal System Function—Paralytic Ileus

*due to* immobility, atonic bowel, and loss of sensation and voluntary sphincter control

**Desired Outcome/Generate Hypotheses:** The patient has bowel movements that are soft and formed every 1–3 days or within the patient's preinjury pattern.

| ASSESSMENT—RECOGNIZE CUES/ INTERVENTIONS—TAKE ACTION | RATIONALES |
|---|---|
| Assess the patient's bowel function by auscultating for bowel sounds; inspecting for the presence of abdominal distention; and monitoring for nausea, vomiting, and fecal impaction. Notify the health care provider of significant findings. | During the acute phase of spinal shock, which usually resolves in 1–6 weeks, constipation and paralytic ileus are common. |
| Manage a flaccid bowel with increased intraabdominal pressure technique (see later), manual disimpaction, and small-volume enemas. | Lesions below the conus medullaris (T12) may injure S3, S4, and S5 nerve segments, resulting in disruption of the reflex arc and causing LMN flaccid bowel and loss of anal tone. |
| Administer the small-volume enemas only. | The atonic intestine distends easily, and therefore only small volumes are recommended. In the presence of fecal impaction, gentle manual removal or a small cleansing enema may be prescribed. |
| Avoid the long-term use of enemas. | Enemas may disrupt normal flora and affect peristalsis and sphincter tone. |
| For UMN reflex bowel, after bowel activity returns, teach the patient to attempt bowel movements 30 minutes after a meal or warm drink. | This regimen will enable the patient's gastrocolic and duodenocolic mass peristalsis reflexes to assist with evacuation. Lesions above the conus medullaris (located at the lower two levels of the thoracic region, where the cord begins to taper) generally leave S3, S4, and S5 spinal cord nerve segments intact. |
| In addition, teach the patient to sit, bear down, bend forward, or apply manual pressure to the abdomen. If allowed, provide a bedside commode. Check the patient's ability to maintain balance on a commode. If the patient is bedridden, turn the patient onto the side and use a pad rather than a bedpan to catch bowel movement. An abdominal belt may be used if the patient is unable to strain at stool. Massaging the abdomen in a clockwise, circular motion also may help promote bowel evacuation. | These measures promote bowel movements by increasing intraabdominal pressure. |
| For patients with injuries at T8 or above, promote adequate fluid intake (more than 2500 mL/day) and use of stool softeners and a high-fiber diet. | These measures facilitate bowel evacuation by adding bulk and moisture to the stool. |
| ❗ Use prescribed suppositories and enemas only when essential and with extreme caution. Use anesthetic jelly liberally when performing a rectal examination or inserting a suppository or an enema. | Their use can precipitate AD. Anesthetic jelly prevents skin stimulation, which could otherwise trigger AD. |
| Instruct patients who are not at risk for AD and who have hand mobility on the technique for suppository insertion and digital stimulation of the anus. | These measures promote reflex bowel evacuation. Suppository inserters and rectal stimulation devices are available for patients with limited hand mobility. |
| For digital stimulation, instruct the patient to insert a lubricated finger about 1½ inches into the rectum and gently rotate in a slow, circular motion, gently stretching the sphincter for about 30 seconds (but no longer than 1 minute at a time) until the internal sphincter relaxes. Restart the circular motion if the sphincter tightens and remove the finger if the bowel movement begins. Stop if sphincter spasms are felt or if signs of AD occur. Repeat every 5–10 minutes several times until adequate evacuation occurs. If unsuccessful after 20–30 minutes of stimulation, insert a suppository if prescribed. | Digital stimulation stretches and relaxes the internal sphincter to facilitate bowel movement. |
| Instruct the patient to keep fingernails cut short. | This helps prevent injury to the rectal mucosa. |
| For other interventions, see *Constipation* in "Immobility," Chapter 1. | |

## Patient Problem/Analyze Cues/Prioritize Hypotheses

# Impaired Mobility

*due to* paralysis, immobilization, or spasticity

***Desired Outcomes/Generate Solutions:*** After stabilization of the injury, the patient exhibits complete or maximum ROM of all joints. By the time of discharge, the patient demonstrates measures that enhance mobility, reduce spasms, and prevent complications.

| ASSESSMENT—RECOGNIZE CUES/ INTERVENTIONS—TAKE ACTION | RATIONALES |
|---|---|
| After the injury is stabilized, assist the patient with position changes on a regular schedule. | This action alternates sites of pressure relief and decreases the risk for contracture formation. For example, a prone position, if not contraindicated, helps prevent sacral pressure ulcers and hip contractures. |
| For patients with spasticity, use hand splints or cones, keeping the fingers extended. | These devices assist with maintaining a functional grasp. |
| If the patient has spasticity, fit them with splints or high-top tennis shoes that are cut off at the toes so that each shoe ends just proximal to the metatarsal head. | This helps prevent foot contractures for patients with spasticity. These shoes help keep feet dorsiflexed but prevent contact of the balls of the feet with a hard surface, which can cause spasticity. |
| Avoid footboards for these patients. | Their hard surface may trigger spasticity and promote plantar flexion. |
| Advise the patient that some factors that trigger spasms are cold temperatures, anxiety, fatigue, emotional distress, infections (especially UTI), bowel or bladder distention, ulcers, pain, tight clothing, and lying too long in one position. | Controlling these factors may reduce the number of spasms experienced. |
| Provide instructions to patients with spasticity on techniques such as proper positioning, ROM, and daily sustained stretching exercises. | Steady, continuous, directional stretching several times daily is especially important because it may decrease spasticity for several hours. Cooling and icing techniques, heat, light-pressure stroking massage, vibration therapy, and transcutaneous electrical nerve stimulation of spastic muscles also may be helpful. |
| When touch is necessary, do it in a firm, gentle, steady manner. Instruct caregivers that touch may need to be limited. | Tactile stimulation may trigger spasms. |
| Administer the prescribed muscle relaxants and antispasmodics. | These medications decrease spasms. |
| Encourage participation in a physical therapy (PT) or occupational therapy (OT) program. | A therapy program is ongoing throughout the patient's rehabilitation. |
| Passive ROM is started on all joints. After the injury is stabilized, an aggressive rehabilitation program is initiated, including muscle strengthening and conditioning exercises. a sitting program; massage; instruction in adaptive devices, equipment, and transfer techniques as appropriate; and instruction in orthotics and braces or splints. | The rehabilitation program will help to develop alternative muscle groups needed for independence and prevent contractures. Patients with sacral injuries have the potential to walk and should be instructed in the use of braces, crutches, or cane as appropriate. Functional electrical stimulation of paralyzed muscles assists some paraplegic patients with walking. |
| Assess for pain, swelling, warmth, and decreased ROM function around joints, especially the hips. | These indicators may signal heterotopic ossification (HO), which is the abnormal formation of true bone within the extraskeletal soft tissues. After HO has formed, resection usually is necessary. |

## Patient Problem/Analyze Cues/Prioritize Hypotheses

# Impaired Sexual Function

*due to* altered body function and lack of information

***Desired Outcome/Generate Solutions:*** Within the 24-hour period before hospital discharge, the patient discusses concerns about sexuality and verbalizes knowledge of alternative methods of sexual expression.

| ASSESSMENT—RECOGNIZE CUES/ INTERVENTIONS—TAKE ACTION | RATIONALES |
|---|---|
| Evaluate your own feelings about sexuality. Refer the patient to someone (e.g., knowledgeable staff member, professional sexual therapy counselor) who can address the patient's sexual concerns if you are uncomfortable discussing these issues or unable to answer specific concerns and questions. | Nurses may not be able to answer all the patient's questions or may be uncomfortable discussing sexual issues. The nurse's discomfort would add to the patient's discomfort. |
| Provide a supportive, nonjudgmental environment. express sexual concerns. Elicit/assess the patient's knowledge, concerns, and questions. | This gives the patient permission to freely express sexual concerns. |
| Expect acting-out behavior related to the patient's sexuality. | This is a possible response to anxiety about sexual performance prognosis. Such behaviors may include asking personal questions, sexual jokes or innuendoes, self-deprecating remarks, or flirting with the staff. |
| Provide information about the normal sexual response and changes caused by SCI. | Sexual functioning may be different but still possible with SCI. The general rule for men is the higher the lesion, the greater the chance of retaining the ability to have an erection (but with a lesser chance of ejaculation). Women may have problems with lubrication, and orgasm may be difficult to achieve because of decreased sensation. Women may also have a transient loss of ovulation; however, ovulation usually returns, and women can become pregnant and deliver vaginally. |
| | Sperm quality decreases in men after SCI, but they may still be capable of fathering a child naturally. Use of vibromassage or electroejaculation through electrical stimulation in the area of the prostate to obtain sperm, in utero insemination, in vitro fertilization, or intracytoplasmic sperm injection has improved fertility. |
| Provide information about birth control and oral contraception for women who desire it. | Uterine contractions of labor in women with SCI lesion at T8 or above may cause AD. Oral contraceptives may be contraindicated because of the risk for thrombophlebitis. |
| Provide specific suggestions that may provide gratification, including oral-genital sex, digital stimulation, vibrator stimulation, cuddling, mutual masturbation, anal eroticism, and massage. Provide specific suggestions for managing common problems, including decreasing fluid intake 2–3 hours before sexual encounter, emptying bladder and bowels (if necessary) before a sexual encounter, (for men) folding back indwelling catheter along the penis and holding it in place with a condom, (for women) taping catheter to the abdomen and leaving it in place, taking a warm bath before sexual activity to reduce spasticity, planning sexual activity for a time of day in which both partners are rested, experimenting with a variety of positions, and applying topical anesthetics to areas that are hypersensitive to touch. | Sexual activity may seem impossible to the SCI patient. These and the suggestions that follow may provide gratification and facilitate the act. Males who have taken erectile dysfunction medications and experience erections lasting longer than 4 hours should seek medical attention. Erection assistive techniques and devices (e.g., vacuum suction pump, penile prosthesis or implant) may help men with SCI attain erections. |
| Explain that water-soluble lubricants are useful, if needed, but that petroleum-based lubricants should be avoided. | Petroleum-based lubricants can cause UTIs. |
| Explain that adductor spasms in women may pose a barrier but can be overcome if a rear entry is acceptable. Suggest that prolonged foreplay with stroking and light massage may also relax muscles. If AD occurs during sexual activity, suggest that the patient consult the health care provider about preventive measures. | These are guidelines for managing less common problems that can occur during a sexual encounter. |
| Suggest that the patient's partner be included in the discussion about sexual concerns. | Explaining the physical condition caused by SCI and preparing the partner for scars, lack of muscle tone, atrophy, and the presence of a catheter will provide the partner with an opportunity to discuss sexual concerns. |

For additional interventions, see *Impaired Sexual Function* in "Immobility," Chapter 1.

PART I: Medical-Surgical Nursing Care Plans

## Problems for Patients in Halo Vest Traction

### Patient Problem/Analyze Cues/Prioritize Hypotheses

# Risk for Injury

*due to* incorrect neck position, irritation of cranial nerves, impaired lateral vision, and balancing difficulties

**Desired Outcome/Generate Solutions:** At the time of discharge (and ongoing during the use of halo traction), the patient exhibits no adverse changes in motor, sensory, or cranial nerve function and is free of symptoms of injury caused by impaired vision or balancing difficulties.

| ASSESSMENT—RECOGNIZE CUES/INTERVENTIONS—TAKE ACTION | RATIONALES |
|---|---|
| Assess the position of the patient's neck in relation to the body. Alert the health care provider to the presence of flexion or hyperextension. Caution the patient not to turn his or her head from side to side. | To ensure proper alignment and optimal healing, the patient's neck should be in a neutral position. |
| Assess any difficulty with swallowing. | Swallowing difficulty may signal improper position of neck and chin. |
| Keep a torque screwdriver in a secure place nearby the patient. | This ensures that the health care provider can readily adjust tension on the bars to return the patient's neck position to neutral. |
| Evaluate the degree of sensation and movement of the upper extremities and assess cranial nerve function. Notify the health care provider of sudden changes in motor, sensory, or cranial nerve function (e.g., weakness, paresthesias, ptosis, difficulty chewing or swallowing). | Changes in cranial nerve function can occur if cranial pins compress or irritate a nerve. **Note:** Jaw pain may occur when chewing is attempted, and this needs to be differentiated from cranial nerve problems. A diet of soft foods, cut into small pieces, will help jaw pain. |
| Assess the pins, bolts, and vest structure for looseness at least daily. Notify the health care provider if pins become loose or dislodged. | Clicking sounds may signal a loose pin, and if this occurs, it will be necessary to stabilize the patient's head to prevent misalignment. |
| Never use the superstructure of halo traction in turning or moving the patient. Avoid putting pillows under support bars when the patient is lying down (e.g., to sleep). | This could result in misalignment of the patient's affected area. |
| Instruct the patient to avoid pulling clothes over the top of the halo apparatus but rather to step into clothes and pull them up over feet and legs. Advise the patient to buy strapless bras, tube tops, or clothes that are several sizes too large, or to modify neck openings (e.g., with Velcro closures, ties). | These measures help prevent loosening of pins. |
| Avoid loosening a buckle without the health care provider's directive. | The device must be worn correctly to maintain alignment, prevent skin breakdown, and prevent nerve injury. Buckle holes or straps should be marked so that they are always cinched correctly to the appropriate snugness. |
| If the patient is ambulatory, collaborate with PT to teach him or her to walk initially with assistance of two people and how to survey the environment while walking, either by using a mirror, by turning eyes to their extreme lateral positions, or by turning the entire body. | The halo vest impairs lateral vision. |
| If indicated, suggest the use of a cane. | A cane will help determine the height of curbs and detect unseen objects or uneven walking surfaces. |
| Explain that trunk flexibility is limited and that achieving balance can be difficult. Teach the patient that bending over can be hazardous. | The vest's weight is top-heavy. Ambulating with a walker initially may help patients learn to adjust. Abdominal- and back-strengthening exercises may aid balance and walking. |
| Collaborate with OT to instruct patient to walk only in low-heeled shoes, use long-handled assistive devices to reach or pick up objects, and realize that extra space allowance may be needed when passing through doorways and to avoid bumping into objects. | These measures prevent falls and other injuries caused by wearing the vest. |

Continued

| ASSESSMENT—RECOGNIZE CUES/ INTERVENTIONS—TAKE ACTION | RATIONALES |
|---|---|
| Advise that a shower chair that rolls usually can fit over a toilet seat, providing an extra 3–6 inches in height. | This is the best method to promote safety and avoid straining to raise and lower the body onto a toilet seat. |
| Instruct the patient to get out of bed by rolling onto their side at the edge of the bed and then drop the legs over the side of the bed while pushing up the trunk sideways. | This technique promotes good alignment and body mechanics to prevent injury. |
| Recommend backing into car seat with the body bent forward when getting into a car. | This prevents hitting pins and device on car doorframe. |
| Caution the patient against driving. | Patients will have a limited field of vision when wearing the vest. |
| Instruct the patient to use high tables and swivel chairs at home. | A high table will help bring objects into view and a swivel chair will permit easier visualization of the environment. |
| Explain to the patient that they will need the assistance of another person to shampoo their hair safely. | This promotes safety and helps prevent falling if water spills on the floor. |
| Advise that shampooing a short haircut is easiest, and hair should be blown dry. | Toweling hair may loosen the pins. |
| Provide instructions to caregivers and significant others on how to release the vest in an emergency such as need for external cardiac compression. | Most vests have side straps that, when released, enable the vest to be opened to midline. If a wrench is required, it should be kept with the jacket (e.g., attached with Velcro). |

## Patient Problem/Analyze Cues/Prioritize Hypotheses

# Risk for Impaired Tissue Integrity

*due to* altered circulation and mechanical factors with halo vest traction

**Desired Outcome/Generate Solutions:** At the time of discharge and on an ongoing basis, the patient's skin surrounding the halo vest has no erythema, is intact, and blanches appropriately.

| ASSESSMENT—RECOGNIZE CUES/ INTERVENTIONS—TAKE ACTION | RATIONALES |
|---|---|
| Assess the skin around vest edges for erythema and other signs of irritation. Keep the skin dry. | These are signs of impaired circulation caused by the vest. The skin is kept dry to prevent irritation. |
| Gently massage the nonerythematous areas routinely. | Massage promotes circulation and helps prevent breakdown. |
| Provide instructions to the patient/significant other/caregiver on how to inspect the patient's skin, which may require the use of a mirror, flashlight, or another person. | For timely intervention, the patient should alert medical personnel if breakdown, sensitive spots, odor, dirty vest liner, or loose pins are present. |
| Investigate complaints of discomfort or uncomfortable fit. Pad the vest as needed until it can be properly adjusted or trimmed by the health care provider. Protect the vest from moisture and soiling. A finger should be able to fit between the vest and the patient's skin. | Discomfort or pain around the halo vest may indicate skin damage from an ill-fitting apparatus. Moist and soiled skin increases the risk of skin breakdown. Weight loss or gain can affect fit. |
| Be alert to a foul odor from in or around the cast openings and to serosanguineous drainage on a pillowcase slipped through the vest from one side to another. | A foul odor can signal pressure necrosis beneath the vest, and serosanguineous drainage may indicate an area of skin breakdown. |
| Instruct/assist the patient with changing body position every 2 hours Support the vest while the patient is in bed and use the logroll technique with sufficient help. | Changing positions promotes circulation and prevents skin and tissue breakdown by alternating sites of pressure relief. |

## ASSESSMENT—RECOGNIZE CUES/ INTERVENTIONS—TAKE ACTION

## RATIONALES

| ASSESSMENT—RECOGNIZE CUES/ INTERVENTIONS—TAKE ACTION | RATIONALES |
|---|---|
| Use soft padding. Use a small pillow under the patient's head at sleep time. | Padding helps prevent pressure on prominent body areas such as the forehead or shoulder, and a small pillow promotes comfort and support for the neck. |
| Wash the skin under the vest with soap and warm water. Thoroughly dry the skin. | This will keep the skin free of moisture and debris, which would increase the risk of skin breakdown. Usually, releasing one vest belt at a time as the patient is lying down is allowed for washing. |
| Avoid the use of lotion and powder under the vest. | These products can cake under the vest and lead to skin breakdown. |
| Replace the soiled linens promptly. Dry perspiration with a hair dryer on a cool setting. | These actions prevent skin irritation and breakdown caused by moisture. |
| Inspect under both sides of the vest for redness, swelling, bruising, or chafing. Close the open side and repeat on the opposite side. | If a rash appears, the patient may be allergic to the vest's lining. A synthetic liner, knitted body stockinette, or T-shirt may correct this problem. |
| In the event of skin breakdown, keep the skin cleansed, dried, and covered with a transparent dressing. Notify the health care provider, wound, ostomy, and continence/enterostomal therapy (WOC/ET) nurse, and orthotist accordingly. | At the first sign of skin breakdown, a WOC/ET nurse can implement a wound care regimen. An orthotist can make a brace adjustment to prevent further breakdown. |
| Place the rubber corks over tips of the halo device. | This will diminish annoying sound vibrations if the apparatus is bumped and prevent lacerations from sharp edges. |
| Check tong placement (e.g., Crutchfield, Vinke, Gardner-Wells) and assess for pain along the area of the device. If slippage has occurred, the patient's head should be immobilized with a sandbag and health care provider notified | This will help prevent misalignment of neck. Pain may signal erosion of bone and displacement into muscle. |
| Check drainage from tong sites for the presence of cerebrospinal fluid (CSF) (see Chapter 37). | The presence of CSF indicates the tong has penetrated through the skull, and risk for meningitis and neurologic damage is possible. |
| Ensure that tong traction weights are hanging freely. | This helps ensure that traction is maintained as prescribed. |
| For a discussion of pin care, see "Fractures," Chapter 69, for *Deficient Knowledge* (function of external fixation, pin care, and signs and symptoms of pin site infection). | |

## ADDITIONAL PROBLEMS:

| | | | |
|---|---|---|---|
| *Risk for Impaired Skin Integrity* | Chapter 3 | *Deficient Knowledge* (diskectomy with laminectomy or fusion procedure) | Chapter 39 |
| *Dehydration* | Chapter 36 | | |
| *Risk for Falls*, due to unsteady gait | Chapter 36 | *Risk for Impaired Swallowing*, for patients undergoing diskectomy with laminectomy or spinal fusion | Chapter 39 |
| *Risk for Injury*, due to sensory deficit and decreased LOC | Chapter 36 | | |
| *Body Weight Problem-Weight Loss* | Chapter 36 | ***For patients on mechanical ventilation, see the following:*** | |
| *Acute Pain* | Chapter 36 | *Risk for Health Care–Associated Complication* | Chapter 13 |
| *Impaired Functional Ability* (inability to perform self-care) | Chapter 36 | *Risk for Infection*, due to inadequate primary defenses | Chapter 36 |

**PATIENT–FAMILY TEACHING AND DISCHARGE PLANNING**

When providing patient–family teaching, focus on sensory information, avoid giving excessive information, and initiate a visiting nurse referral for necessary follow-up teaching. Include verbal and written information about the following:

✓ Spinal cord functioning and the effects trauma has on how the body works.

✓ Referrals to community resources, such as public health nurse, visiting nurses association, community support groups, social workers, psychologic therapy, vocational rehabilitation agency, home health agencies, and extended and skilled care facilities. Additional general information can be obtained by contacting the following organizations:

• Christopher and Dana Reeve Foundation: www. christopherreeve.org
• Paralyzed Veterans of America: www.pva.org
• Cure Paralysis Now: www.cureparalysis.org
• Brainline: www.brainline.org/resource-directory
• Paralinks: www.unitedspinal.org/resource-center/askus/?pg=kb.page&id-420
• DisABILITY Information and Resources: www. makoa.org

✓ Safety measures relative to decreased sensation, motor deficits, orthostatic hypotension and symptoms, preventive measures, and interventions for AD.

✓ Use and care of a brace or immobilizer, medical equipment, and mobility aids as appropriate.

✓ What patient can expect if transferred to rehabilitation center.

✓ Techniques and devices for performing activities of daily living, including bathing, grooming, turning, feeding, and other self-care activities to patient's maximum potential. The patient may need a home accessibility evaluation and a driving evaluation and training.

✓ Indicators of urinary tract calculi and dietary measures to prevent their formation (see Chapter 33).

✓ Indicators of VTE/DVT and measures to prevent it (see Chapter 26).

✓ Importance of participation in counseling and psychotherapy to help patient and significant other adjust to the disability. This should include addressing sexual functioning and vocational rehabilitation.

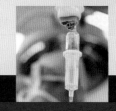

## OVERVIEW/PATHOPHYSIOLOGY

A stroke, cerebrovascular accident, or brain attack is the sudden disruption of $O_2$ supply to the brain. This can be due to a rupture in one or more of the blood vessels that supply the brain (hemorrhagic stroke) or loss of cerebral perfusion, often resulting from hypoperfusion or reduction of $O_2$ supply (ischemic stroke).

*Hemorrhagic stroke* causes neural tissue destruction because of the infiltration and accumulation of blood. Ischemia and infarction may occur distal to the hemorrhage because of interrupted blood supply. Although a cerebral hemorrhage usually results from hypertension or an aneurysm, trauma also can cause hemorrhagic stroke. Bleeding may spread into the brain tissue, causing an intracerebral hemorrhage, or into the subarachnoid space. Usually, there is a large rise in intracranial pressure (ICP) with a hemorrhagic stroke because of cerebral edema and the mass effect of blood.

*Ischemic stroke* has three main mechanisms: thrombosis, embolism, and systemic hypoperfusion. Thrombosis or embolism results in a blockage of blood supply to the brain tissue. The resulting ischemia, if prolonged, causes brain tissue necrosis (infarction), cerebral edema, and increased ICP. Most thrombotic strokes are caused by the blockage of large vessels as a result of atherosclerosis. Thrombi in small penetrating arteries result in "lacunar" strokes. Most embolic strokes are cardiogenic and the result of emboli produced from valve disease or during atrial fibrillation of the heart. Ischemic stroke caused by systemic hypoperfusion usually is the result of decreased cerebral blood flow owing to circulatory failure. Some causes of circulatory failure include hypovolemia, hypotension, and dysrhythmias. Hypoxia from any cause also can produce this syndrome.

A stroke may be classified as a *progressive stroke in evolution*, in which deficits continue to worsen over time, or as a *completed stroke*, in which maximum deficit has been acquired and has persisted for longer than 24 hours. Progressive strokes usually are the result of thrombus formation and often take 1–3 days to become "completed." Embolic strokes typically have a sudden onset with maximal deficits. Presentation may be variable depending on the scatter of the emboli. *Stroke syndromes* classically have been described according to the distribution of the vessels (middle cerebral artery, anterior cerebral artery, posterior cerebral artery, vertebral, basilar) that supply particular regions of the brain and will have typical assessment findings. Stroke is the fifth most common cause of death and the most common cause of serious long-term disability. Long-term disabilities may include paralysis, inability to walk, complete or partial dependence for activities of daily living (ADLs), aphasia, and depression. Half the survivors are left permanently disabled or experience another stroke. Improvement may continue for 1–2 years but deficits at 6 months usually are considered permanent.

A *brain attack*, also sometimes called a *code stroke* or *stroke alert*, is a sudden event and medical emergency with the same urgency as a heart attack. After the onset of a stroke, immediate medical attention is crucial to decrease disability and the risk for death. If the stroke is ischemic and the patient qualifies, the sooner the patient can be treated, the better the outcome. To achieve this, all people should be educated to recognize warning signs of stroke and immediately call 911. Rapid transport to a hospital, preferably a stroke center, should occur, with the emergency medical technician starting the medical history, especially the time of symptom onset, and alerting the hospital before arrival so that the stroke team (if available) can be assembled.

For appropriate patients with new onset ischemic stroke, treatment with recombinant tissue plasminogen activator (tPA), must occur within 3–4 1/2 hours of symptom onset. tPA is administered intravenously to break down the clot and therefore reestablish circulation through the blocked artery to prevent cell death. Patients must be screened carefully with an Magnetic Resonance Imaging (MRI) or Computed Tomography (CT) scan to rule out hemorrhagic stroke before TPA treatment. Screening is also done for blood clotting disorders, recent history of gastrointestinal bleeding, head trauma, and recent major surgery, which may contraindicate TPA treatment. Blood pressure (BP) must be closely monitored and controlled during this time. Intraarterial infusion of tPA may be used when mechanical thrombectomy is not possible. It must be administered within 6 hours of stroke symptoms onset in order to be affective.

Several surgical and medical interventions are available to treat hemorrhagic stroke, including immediate evacuation of an aneurysm-induced hematoma or cerebellar hematoma larger than 3 cm, ventriculostomy to decrease ICP, clipping or coiling the aneurysm, and administration of the calcium channel blocker nimodipine to treat cerebral vasospasms.

Stroke care can be differentiated into these basic types: thrombolytic ischemic stroke care, nonthrombolytic ischemic stroke care (including *transient ischemic attack* [TIAs]), and hemorrhagic stroke care. Care differences center mostly around BP management, use of anticoagulant and antiplatelet agents, and management of ICP. Most hospitals, especially stroke centers, have protocols for stroke management.

Risk factors that are associated with stroke can be classified as nonmodifiable and modifiable causes. Nonmodifiable risk factors include age, genetics, gender, and race. Stroke risk doubles each decade after age 55 and two-thirds of all strokes occur in people over age 65. Males are more at risk for strokes, but women are more likely to die from strokes. Heredity factors such as vascular and cardiac disease also play a role in stroke risk. Stroke incidences are doubled in Blacks and additionally lead to higher death rates compared to any other ethnic group. Modifiable risk factors include smoking, alcohol use, and obesity, all of which can lead to hypertension, heart disease, and diabetes, which ultimately cause approximately 90% of all strokes.

History of a *TIA* is also considered a risk factor for stroke. A TIA is a temporary neurologic deficit that resolves completely without permanent damage and occurs when the artery cannot deliver enough blood to meet the $O_2$ requirement of the brain. Restoration of blood flow is timely enough to make the ischemia (and deficits) transient, thereby avoiding infarction and permanent damage. TIAs usually are associated with thrombosis but may be caused by any of the ischemic mechanisms just mentioned. TIAs may precede a permanent ischemic stroke by hours, days, months, or years. TIAs are a warning sign, and treatment may prevent a stroke. Most TIAs last an average of 5–10 minutes, although some can last longer than an hour. Many patients understand these as "mini strokes."

## HEALTH CARE SETTING

Critical care unit, step-down unit, acute rehabilitation unit, outpatient rehabilitation program

## ASSESSMENT

**Note:** *Because of the narrow 3-4 1/2-hour window during which it may be possible to reverse permanent neurologic damage, it is critical to teach patients not to ignore symptoms and to call 911 without delay for the following:*

- Sudden numbness or weakness of the face, arm, or leg, especially on one side of the body
- Sudden confusion, trouble speaking or understanding
- Sudden trouble seeing in one or both eyes
- Sudden trouble walking, dizziness, loss of balance or coordination
- Sudden, severe headache with no known cause

A history to determine the time of symptom onset is critical inasmuch as this may determine eligibility for treatment. Time of onset is when patient was last known to be "normal," so if the patient woke up after sleeping with symptoms, time of onset

would be when the patient went to bed "normal" and not when he or she woke up symptomatic.

*General findings.* Classically, symptoms appear on the side of the body opposite the damaged site. For example, a stroke in the left hemisphere of the brain will produce symptoms in the right arm and leg. However, when the stroke affects the cranial nerves, symptoms of cranial nerve deficit will appear on the same side as the site of injury. Similarly, an obstruction of an anterior cerebral artery can produce bilateral symptoms, as will severe bleeding or multiple emboli. Hemiplegia is fairly common.

*Signs and symptoms.* Vary with the size and site of injury and may improve in 2–3 days as the cerebral edema decreases. Changes in mentation, including apathy, irritability, disorientation, memory loss, withdrawal, drowsiness, stupor, or coma; bowel and bladder incontinence; numbness or loss of sensation; weakness or paralysis on part or one side of the body; aphasia; headache; neck stiffness and rigidity; vomiting; seizures; dizziness or syncope; ataxia; and fever may occur. A brainstem infarct leaving the patient completely paralyzed with intact cortical function is called *locked-in syndrome*. With *cranial nerve involvement*, visual disturbances include diplopia, blindness, and hemianopia. Inequality or fixation of the pupils, nystagmus, tinnitus, and difficulty chewing and swallowing also occur.

*Transient ischemic attack.* Typical symptoms include temporary episodes of slurred speech, weakness, numbness or tingling, blindness in one eye, blurred or double vision, dizziness or ataxia, and confusion.

*Risk factors.* TIAs; hypertension; atherosclerosis; high serum cholesterol or triglycerides; high homocysteine levels; diabetes mellitus; gout; smoking; obesity; cardiac valve diseases, such as those that may result from rheumatic fever, valve prosthesis, and atrial fibrillation; cardiac surgery; blood dyscrasias; anticoagulant therapy; neck vessel trauma; oral contraceptive use; cocaine or methamphetamine use; family predisposition for arteriovenous malformation (AVM); aneurysm; advanced age; or previous stroke.

*Assessment scales (e.g., Glasgow Coma Scale and National Institutes of Health Stroke Scale).* The Glasgow Coma Scale is helpful for quickly assessing the level of consciousness (LOC). The National Institutes of Health Stroke Scale (NIHSS) not only assesses LOC but also assesses deficits and provides a standardized approach to neurologic assessment. It is used to evaluate and document the neurological status in acute stroke patients. The interdisciplinary team can use the tool at the bedside to help plan patient care by rating the patient's ability to answer questions and perform activities. Scores range from 0 to 42 with higher scores indicating greater severity. The NIHSS score also strongly predicts the likelihood of recovery, with higher scores resulting in more disability and poorer outcomes.

## DIAGNOSTIC TESTS

Selection, sequence, and urgency of the following tests will be determined by the patient's history and symptoms. For example, a patient whose symptoms have resolved from a TIA will have a different set or sequence of tests compared with the patient who is in coma. Because the usage of tPA is time limited, speed is essential in determining the type of stroke (ischemic vs hemorrhagic) and other contraindications to tPA. Obtaining a CT scan to determine the type of stroke is a top priority along with laboratory tests to assess for contraindications.

*CT.* To reveal the site of infarction, hematoma, and shift of brain structures. CT scan is of particular value in identifying blood released early during hemorrhagic strokes. CT scan is the test of choice for unstable patients. Generally, identifying ischemic areas is difficult until they start to necrose at about 48–72 hours. Xenon-enhanced CT may be done to study cerebral blood flow; CT angiography may be performed to evaluate blood vessels.

*MRI.* To reveal the site of infarction, hematoma, shift of brain structure, and cerebral edema. MRI diffusion and perfusion-weighted studies are of particular value in identifying ischemic strokes early and in differentiating between acute and chronic lesions. Other magnetic resonance (MR) techniques include MR angiography to evaluate vessels and MR spectrography for additional data analysis.

*Laboratory tests.* Certain tests (e.g., serum electrolytes, complete blood count including differential and platelet count, prothrombin time with international normalized ratio, and partial thromboplastin time) should be done immediately to assess for contraindications such as hypoglycemia or clotting abnormalities if the patient is a candidate for thrombolytic therapy. Other tests will be done depending on the patient (e.g., toxicology screen, pregnancy test, blood culture and erythrocyte sedimentation rate for endocarditis or vasculitis process, hemoglobin $A_{1C}$ for diabetics). Lipid panel, C-reactive protein, and homocysteine levels also may be obtained.

*Electrocardiogram.* To evaluate for atrial fibrillation and myocardial ischemia.

*Phonoangiography/Doppler ultrasonography.* To identify the presence of bruits if the carotid blood vessels are partially occluded. B-mode imaging and duplex scanning also may be done to evaluate the carotids to detect occlusive disease. Dimensional ultrasound improves three-dimensional visualization and includes the potential for quantitative monitoring of plaque volume changes in all three directions—circumferential, length, and thickness.

*Transcranial Doppler ultrasound.* To provide information (noninvasively) about pressure and flow in the intracranial arteries.

*Swallowing examination/videofluoroscopy.* All patients should be screened for dysphagia. Videofluoroscopy identifies the problem or pathology, determines the most appropriate treatment, and enables the teaching of proper swallowing technique. This test is not performed for individuals known to aspirate saliva because it involves swallowing a barium-containing liquid, semisolid, and/or solid.

*Single photon emission CT.* To identify cerebral blood flow.

*Electroencephalograph.* To show abnormal nerve impulse transmission and indicate the amount of brain wave activity present.

*Cerebral and carotid angiography.* If surgery is contemplated, this procedure is done to pinpoint the site of rupture or occlusion and identify collateral blood circulation, aneurysms, or AVM.

*Digital subtraction angiography.* To visualize cerebral blood flow and detect vascular abnormalities, such as stenosis, aneurysm, and hematomas.

*Echocardiography (e.g., transthoracic and transesophageal).* To evaluate valvular heart structures for thrombus and myocardial walls for mural thrombi that may provide a source of emboli.

## Patient Problem/Analyze Cues/Prioritize Hypotheses

# Impaired Mobility

*due to* neuromuscular impairment with the limited use of upper and/or lower limbs

*Desired Outcomes/Generate Solutions:* By at least 24 hours before hospital discharge, the patient demonstrates techniques that promote ambulating and transferring. The patient does not exhibit evidence of shoulder subluxation or shoulder–hand syndrome.

| ASSESSMENT—RECOGNIZE CUES/ INTERVENTIONS—TAKE ACTION | RATIONALES |
| --- | --- |
| Assess for the subluxation of the shoulder (e.g., shoulder pain and tenderness, swelling, decreased range of motion [ROM], altered appearance of bony prominences). | Shoulder subluxation occurs when the weight of the affected arm is unable to be supported by the weakened shoulder muscles, causing separation of the shoulder joint. |

Continued

| ASSESSMENT—RECOGNIZE CUES/ INTERVENTIONS—TAKE ACTION | RATIONALES |
| --- | --- |
| • Provide the following measures to prevent subluxation:<br>• Never pull on the affected arm.<br>• Guide the upper extremity movement from the scapula and not from the arm.<br>• Use a lift sheet to reposition in bed.<br>• Ensure that the arm has a firm support surface when the patient is sitting.<br>• When the patient is in bed, position the shoulder slightly forward to counteract shoulder rotation.<br>• The affected arm should be placed in external rotation when the patient is supine or lying on affected side. | These measures help prevent partial or complete dislocation of the humerus from the glenoid (the cup-like socket). |
| Provide patient/caregiver/significant other with instructions on methods for turning and moving, using the stronger extremity to move the weaker extremity.<br><br>For example, to move the affected leg in bed or when changing from a lying to a sitting position, slide the unaffected foot under the affected ankle to lift, support, and bring the affected leg along in the desired movement. | Moving the stronger extremity to move the weaker one provides the patient with independence with movement and support for the weaker extremity. |
| Encourage the patient to make a conscious attempt to look at extremities and check the position before moving. | These are safety measures to prevent falling. For example, remind the patient to make a conscious effort to lift and then extend the foot when ambulating. |
| Instruct the patient with impaired sense of balance to compensate by leaning toward the stronger side as an attempt to ensure proper upright posture. | The tendency is to lean toward the weaker or paralyzed side. For example, the patient may need to be reminded to keep body weight forward over the feet when standing. |
| Recommend wearing well-fitting shoes with nonslip soles. | This will help prevent slipping on hard surfaces. |
| Prevent shoulder–hand syndrome with regular, gentle joint ROM exercises and proper arm positioning. Never place the arm under the body. When the patient is in bed, place the arm on the abdomen or pillow for support. Encourage repeated shoulder movement, elevation of the arm above cardiac level, and regular fist clenching and reclenching. | Shoulder–hand syndrome is a neurovascular condition characterized by pain, edema, and skin and muscle atrophy caused by impairment of the circulatory pumping action of the upper extremity. |
| Protect the impaired arm with a sling. | The sling will support the arm and shoulder when the patient is out of bed. |
| Position the patient in correct alignment and provide a pillow or lapboard for support. Encourage active/passive ROM to improve muscle tone. | These measures will help maintain anatomic position. |
| Instruct the patient to do the following:<br>• Weight bear on the stronger side.<br>• Pivot on the stronger side and use the stronger arm for support.<br>• Transfer toward the unaffected side<br>• Place the unaffected side closest to the bed or chair to which they wish to transfer.<br>• When transferring, place the affected leg with the foot flat on the ground.<br>• Position a braced chair or locked wheelchair close to the patient's stronger side. | These are general principles to follow when transferring patients with impaired physical mobility. These transfer principles emphasize using the stronger or unaffected side to help support patients for safe transfers to reduce the risk for falling. |
| If the patient requires assistance from a staff member, instruct the patient not to support self by pulling on or placing hands around the assistant's neck. | Staff members should use their own knees and feet to brace the feet and knees of patients who are very weak. |
| Obtain physical therapy and occupational therapy referrals as appropriate. Reinforce the special mobilization techniques per the patient's individualized rehabilitation program. | These techniques may vary from the general principles mentioned for functional movement. |

**Patient Problem/Analyze Cues/Prioritize Hypotheses**

# Impaired Communication (Aphasia)

*due to* cerebrovascular insult

Desired Outcome/Generate Solutions: At least 24 hours before hospital discharge, the patient demonstrates improved self-expression and relates decreased frustration with communication.

| ASSESSMENT—RECOGNIZE CUES/ INTERVENTIONS—TAKE ACTION | RATIONALES |
|---|---|
| Assess the nature and severity of the patient's aphasia. When doing so, avoid giving nonverbal cues. Assess the patient's ability to speak clearly without slurring words, use words appropriately, point or look toward a specific object, follow simple directions, understand yes/ no questions, understand complex questions, repeat both simple and complex words, repeat sentences, name objects that are shown, demonstrate or relate purpose or action of objects, fulfill written requests, write requests, and read. When evaluating for aphasia, be aware that the patient may be responding to nonverbal cues and may understand less than you think. Document this assessment with simple descriptions and specific examples of aphasia symptoms. Use it as the basis for a communication plan. | Aphasia is the partial or complete inability to use or comprehend language and symbols and may occur with dominant (left) hemisphere damage. It is not the result of impaired hearing or intelligence. There are many different types of aphasias. Generally, patients have a combination of types that vary in severity. Fluent aphasia (e.g., Wernicke, sensory, or receptive aphasia) is characterized by the inability to recognize or comprehend spoken words. It is as if a foreign language were being spoken or the patient has word deafness. The patient often is good at responding to nonverbal cues. In nonfluent aphasia (e.g., Broca, motor, or expressive aphasia) the ability to understand and comprehend language is retained but the patient has difficulty expressing words or naming objects. Gestures, groans, swearing, or nonsense words may be used. |
| Ask the patient to repeat unclear words by speaking slowly in short phrases. Do not pretend you understand. If this is unsuccessful, ask the patient to use another word or give a nonverbal clue. | This will help patient to formulate words. And instill trust that you are listening to them. Nonverbal cues, pointing, flash cards of basic needs, pantomime, paper/pen, spelling, or picture board may help communication. |
| Obtain referral to a speech therapist or pathologist as needed. Provide the therapist with a list of words that would enhance the patient's independence and/or care. In addition, ask for tips that will help improve communication with the patient. | Patients may need the expertise of a specialist to facilitate the ability to communicate. |
| When communicating with the patient, try to reduce distractions in the environment, such as television or others' conversations. | This focuses the patient's attention on communication. |
| Ensure that the patient is well rested. | Fatigue affects the ability to communicate. |
| Communicate with the patient as much as possible. Use gestures, facial expressions, and pantomime to supplement and reinforce your message. Give short, simple directions, and repeat as needed to ensure understanding. Use concrete terms (e.g., "water" instead of "fluid" or "leg" instead of "limb"). If the patient does not understand after repetition, try different words. | These are general principles for patients who need time to process what they hear or may not recognize or comprehend the spoken word. |
| Face the patient and establish eye contact, speak slowly and clearly, give the patient time to process your communication and answer, keep messages short and simple, stay with one clearly defined subject, avoid questions with multiple choices but rather phrase questions so that they can be answered "yes" or "no," and use the same words each time you repeat a statement or question (e.g., "pill" vs "medication" and "bathroom" vs "toilet"). | |
| When helping the patient regain the use of symbolic language, start with nouns first and progress to more complex statements as indicated, using verbs, pronouns, and adjectives. | Progression from simple to complex helps facilitate comprehension. Using the same words will provide terminology continuity. |
| Plan to keep at the bedside a record of words to be used (e.g., "pill" rather than "medication"). | |

Continued

| ASSESSMENT—RECOGNIZE CUES/ INTERVENTIONS—TAKE ACTION | RATIONALES |
|---|---|
| Treat the patient as an adult. Be respectful. | It is not necessary to raise the volume of your voice unless the patient is hard of hearing. |
| When the patient has difficulty expressing words or naming objects, encourage the patient to repeat words after you. Begin with simple words such as "yes" or "no," and progress to others, such as "cup." Progress to more complex statements as indicated. | These measures enable practice in verbal expression. |
| Listen and respond to the patient's communication efforts. If the patient makes an error, do not criticize the patient's effort but rather compliment it by saying, "That was a good try." Praise accomplishments. | To prevent patient frustration and to encourage patient to keep trying. |
| Be prepared for labile emotions. Do not react negatively to emotional displays. Address and acknowledge the patient's frustration over the inability to communicate. Maintain a calm and positive attitude. | These patients become frustrated and emotional when faced with their impaired speech. |
| When improvement is noted, let the patient complete your sentence (e.g., "This is a _____."). Keep a list of words the patient can say and add to the list as appropriate. Avoid finishing the patient's sentences. | This list then can be used when formulating questions that the patient is known to be able to answer. |
| Avoid labeling the patient as "belligerent" or "confused" when the problem is aphasia and frustration. Listen for errors in conversation and provide feedback. | Patients who have lost the ability to monitor their verbal output may not produce sensible language but may think they are making sense and not understand why others do not comprehend or respond appropriately to them. |
| Avoid instructing the patient to "wait 5 minutes" because this may not be meaningful. | Patients who have lost the ability to recognize number symbols or relationships will have difficulty understanding time concepts or telling time. |
| Point to an object and clearly state its name. Watch signals the patient gives you. | This facilitates practice in receiving word images. |
| Bring patients with nondominant (right) hemisphere damage back to the subject by saying, "Let's go back to what we were talking about." | Patients with nondominant (right) hemisphere damage often have no difficulty speaking; however, they may use excessive detail, give irrelevant information, and get off on a tangent. These patients tend to respond better to verbal, rather than nonverbal, encouragement. |
| Observe for nonverbal cues and anticipate the patient's needs. Allow time to listen if the patient speaks slowly. | This validates the patient's message without rushing him or her, which would cause frustration. |
| Ensure that the call light is available, and that the patient knows how to use it. | The call light is the first step in communicating a need for assistance. |
| For additional interventions for patients with dysarthria, see *Risk for Impaired Communication* in "General Care of Patients With Neurologic Disorders," Chapter 36. | Dysarthria can complicate aphasia. |

**Patient Problem/Analyze Cues/Prioritize Hypotheses**

# Risk for Unilateral Neglect

*due to* ischemic damage affecting the right or left hemisphere

**Desired Outcome/Generate Solutions:** After interventions and on an ongoing basis, the patient scans the environment and responds to stimuli on the affected side.

PART I: Medical-Surgical Nursing Care Plans

| ASSESSMENT—RECOGNIZE CUES/ INTERVENTIONS—TAKE ACTION | RATIONALES |
|---|---|
| Assess the patient's ability to recognize objects to the right or left of his or her visual midline; perceive body parts as his or her own; perceive pain, touch, and temperature sensations; judge distances; orient self to changes in the environment; differentiate left from right; maintain posture sense; and identify objects by sight, hearing, or touch. Document the specific deficits. | This assessment enables the nurse to develop a plan of care individualized for the patient. Neglect of and inattention to stimuli on the affected side occur more often with right hemisphere injury. Neglect cannot be totally explained on the basis of loss of physical senses (e.g., both ears are used in hearing, but with auditory neglect, patients may ignore conversations or noises that occur on the affected side). |
| Arrange the environment by keeping necessary objects, such as call light, on the patient's unaffected side. | This will facilitate the performance of ADLs. |
| Perform the activities on the unaffected side unless you are specifically attempting to stimulate the patient's neglected side. | Communicating and performing activities on the patient's unaffected side will engage and be less confusing to the patient. |
| If you must approach the affected side, announce yourself first. | This announcement avoids startling the patient. |
| Inform significant others about the patient's deficit and compensatory interventions. | This enables significant others to be informed participants in the patient's care plan. |

**Patients With Visual Neglect:**

| | |
|---|---|
| Continuously cue the patient to the environment. Initially place the patient's unaffected side toward the most active part of room, but as compensation occurs, reverse this. As the patient begins to compensate, place additional items out of his or her visual field, thereby gradually increasing stimuli on the affected side. Place the patient's food on the neglected side, encouraging the patient to look to the neglected side and name the food before eating. | While communicating with the patient, physically moving across the patient's visual boundary and standing on that side will shift the patient's attention to the neglected side. Encouraging patients to turn their head past the midline and scan the entire environment, especially while ambulating, will help to prevent injury from falls or bumping into things. |

**Patients With Self-Neglect:**

| | |
|---|---|
| Periodically refer to the patient's body parts on the neglected side. Encourage the patient to touch or massage and look at the affected side and make a conscious effort to care for neglected body parts first when performing ADLs. | This promotes the patient's self-recognition. For example, have the patient use the unaffected arm to perform ROM on the affected side and provide a mirror so the patient can watch self while shaving and brushing teeth and hair. |
| Encourage patient to consciously monitor the affected side for position and checking for exposure to sharp objects, irritants, and hot or cold items. | This helps prevent contractures and skin breakdown or injury. For example, position the affected arm on the bedside table or wheelchair lapboard with the hand or arm past the midline, where the patient can see it. |
| Provide structured tactile stimulation on the affected side. Stimulate with a warm washcloth, cold ice chip, rough or soft-surfaced cloth, or similar items. | Tactile exploration provides the patient with important sensory information about objects because specialized sensory touch receptors perceive information about pressure, vibration, and movement during structured and repeated activities. |
| When the patient is in bed or sitting up in a chair, provide the side rails and restraints. | These are necessary safety measures because the patient is unaware of the affected side and may attempt to get up. |

**Patients With Auditory Neglect:**

| | |
|---|---|
| Move across the auditory boundary while speaking and continue speaking from the patient's neglected side to bring the patient's attention to that area. | This stimulates the patient's attention to the affected side. |

## Patient Problem/Analyze Cues/Prioritize Hypotheses

# Risk for Injury

*due to* impaired sensory reception, transmission, and/or integration

***Desired Outcome/Generate Solutions:*** After intervention and on an ongoing basis, the patient interacts appropriately with his or her environment and does not exhibit evidence of injury caused by sensory/perceptual deficit.

| ASSESSMENT—RECOGNIZE CUES/ INTERVENTIONS—TAKE ACTION | RATIONALES |
|---|---|
| Assess the type and degree of hemisphere injury the patient exhibits. | This provides the nurse with information to promote patient safety. |
| Remind patients who have a dominant (left) hemisphere injury to scan their environment. | These patients may lack or have decreased pain sensation and position sense and have visual field deficit on the right side of the body. They may need reminders to scan their environment but usually do not exhibit unilateral neglect. |
| Give short, simple messages or questions and step-by-step directions. Keep the conversation on a concrete level (e.g., say "water," not "fluid"; "leg," not "limb"). | These individuals may have poor abstract thinking skills. They tend to be slow, cautious, and disorganized when approaching an unfamiliar problem and benefit from frequent, accurate, and immediate feedback on performance. They may respond well to nonverbal encouragement, such as a pat on the back. |
| Encourage patients with nondominant (right) hemisphere injury to slow down and check each step or task as it is completed. | Patients with nondominant (right) hemisphere injury also may have decreased pain sensation and pain sense and visual field deficit but typically are unconcerned or unaware of or deny deficits or lost abilities. They tend to be impulsive and too quick with movements. |
| | Typically, they have impaired judgment about what they can and cannot do and often overestimate their abilities. These individuals are at risk for burns, bruises, cuts, and falls and may need to be restrained from attempting unsafe activities. They also are more likely to have unilateral neglect than individuals with dominant (left) hemisphere injury |
| Have patients with apraxia return your demonstration of the task. Assess if they are able to be talked through a task or may be able to talk themselves through a task step by step. | Patients with apraxia have an inability to carry out previously learned motor tasks, although they may be able to describe them in detail. |
| Encourage making a conscious effort to scan the rest of the environment by turning head from side to side. | Patients may have visual field deficits in which they can physically see only a portion (usually left or right side) of the normal visual field (homonymous hemianopsia). |
| Patients with nondominant (right) hemisphere injury: | |
| • Direct the patient's attention to a particular sound (e.g., if a cat meows on the television, state that it is the sound a cat makes and point to the cat on the screen). | Patients may impaired ability to recognize, associate, or interpret sounds (e.g., voice quality, animal noises, musical pieces, types of instruments). |
| • Provide a structured, consistent environment. Mark the outer aspects of the patient's shoes or tag inside the sleeve of a sweater or pair of pants with "L" and "R." | *Visual–spatial misconception:* The patient may have trouble judging distance, size, position, rate of movement, form, and how parts relate to the whole. For example, the patient may underestimate distances and bump into doors or confuse the inside and outside of an object, such as an article of clothing. These patients may lose their place when reading or adding up numbers and therefore never complete the task. |
| • Assist these individuals with eating. Monitor the environment for safety hazards and remove unsafe objects such as scissors from the bedside. | *Difficulty recognizing and associating familiar objects:* Patients may not know the purpose of silverware. These patients may not recognize dangerous or hazardous objects because they do not know the purpose of the object or may not recognize subtle distinctions between objects (e.g., the difference between a fork and spoon may become too subtle to detect). |
| • Provide these patients with a restraint or wheelchair belt for support. | They may not know if they are standing, sitting, or leaning. |
| • Teach the patient to concentrate on body parts (e.g., by watching feet carefully while walking). Provide a mirror to help the patient adjust. | These patients may not perceive their foot or arm as being a part of their body. |
| • Keep the patient's environment simple to reduce sensory overload and enable concentration on visual cues. Remove distracting stimuli. | These patients rely more on visual cues. |

## Problem for Patients Having Carotid Procedure/Analyze Cues/Prioritize Hypotheses

# Deficient Knowledge: Treatment Procedure

*due to* unfamiliarity with carotid endarterectomy or carotid angioplasty/stent procedure

***Desired Outcome/Generate Solutions:*** Before surgery, the patient verbalizes accurate understanding of the carotid endarterectomy procedure, including the purpose, risks, expected benefits or outcome, and postsurgical care.

| ASSESSMENT—RECOGNIZE CUES/ INTERVENTIONS—TAKE ACTION | RATIONALES |
|---|---|
| After the health care provider has explained the procedure to the patient, assess the patient's level of understanding. | This enables the development of an individualized teaching plan in the preoperative stage that the patient understands. |
| If necessary, utilize an interpreter or language-appropriate written materials; and reinforce or clarify information as needed. | |
| Obtain the baseline neurologic and cranial nerve function test results. | These assessments will be the basis of comparison postoperatively. |
| **For Patients Undergoing Carotid Endarterectomy** | |
| As indicated, reinforce procedure information that was provided to the patient by the surgeon. Carotid endarterectomy is removal of plaque in the obstructed artery to increase blood supply to the brain. | This will help the patient to understand the procedure that will be done and may relieve patient anxiety of the unknown. |
| Describe the following postsurgical assessments and their purposes. | To prepare patient for assessment procedures postoperatively and promote patient adherence. |
| • Hourly vital signs (VS) and neurologic status. PEARLA, and hands and legs strength for weakness and equality. | This provides the nurse with patient neurological status information. |
| • Patient will be asked to swallow, move the tongue, smile, speak, and shrug shoulders to determine facial drooping, tongue weakness, hoarseness, speech difficulty, dysphagia, shoulder weakness, or loss of facial sensation. | Deficits in these abilities are signs of cranial nerve impairment. Stretching of the cranial nerves during surgery can occur, causing edema, and may leave a temporary deficit. |
| Patient will be asked to report any numbness, tingling, or weakness. | These signs may indicate carotid occlusion. |
| Superficial temporal and facial pulses will be assessed by palpating for strength, quality, and symmetry. | This will evaluate the patency of the external carotid artery. |
| Assessments will be done on the neck for edema, hematoma, bleeding, or tracheal deviation from midline. Instruct the patient to report immediately any respiratory distress, difficulty managing secretions, or sensation of neck tightness. | Any bleeding or excess edema at the surgical site can cause neck edema, which can deviate the trachea and compromise the airway. This can result in an emergent situation that necessitates airway management and surgical evacuation of the hematoma. |
| Oxygen saturation will be monitored with a pulse oximeter. | Manipulation of the carotid sinus may cause temporary loss of normal physiologic response to hypoxia. |
| If needed, oxygen will be provided even if the patient does not have respiratory distress or airway compromise. | |
| BP will be monitored frequently and vasoactive medications will be administered as ordered by the provider. Patient will be monitored for orthostatic hypotension when first getting up. | Temporary carotid sinus dysfunction may cause BP problems (usually hypertension). Vasoactive drugs may be given to keep systolic BP within a specified range (usually 100–150 mm Hg) to maintain cerebral perfusion while preventing disruption of graft or sutures as well as hyperperfusion syndrome. |
| The head of bed (HOB) will be positioned in the prescribed position (flat or elevated) with the patient positioned off the operative side. | HOB may be elevated to promote wound drainage, particularly if a closed-suction drain is left in place. (A closed drainage system with suction may be left in the neck for a day.) Positioning also enables visibility of the wound site and promotes comfort. |

Continued

| ASSESSMENT—RECOGNIZE CUES/ INTERVENTIONS—TAKE ACTION | RATIONALES |
|---|---|
| Ice packs may be applied to the incision site if appropriate. | Ice will reduce edema and pain. |
| Anticoagulant/antiplatelet therapy will be administered as prescribed. | Anticoagulant/antiplatelet therapy (e.g., aspirin, warfarin) may be instituted for 3–6 months after the procedure and may continue longer, depending on the patient's needs. For more information about warfarin and other anticoagulants, see "Pulmonary Embolus," Chapter 15. |
| Include home instructions for the following: incision care (wash gently with soap and water), signs of infection (incision red, swollen, and painful; drainage, fever greater than 100.4°F [38°C]); activity restrictions (no heavy lifting, no driving while neck turning is uncomfortable), and changes in neurologic status (alterations in speech, swallowing, vision, and numbness or weakness in arm or leg, especially on the opposite side). | Following these instructions will decrease the risk for infection and promote the patient's physiologic safety. |

**For Patients Undergoing Carotid Angioplasty and Stenting**

| | |
|---|---|
| • Reinforce information about the procedure that was provided to the patient by the provider. Angioplasty is the opening of a stenosed artery through a slender catheter that is passed through the narrow spot with balloon inflation to open up the obstruction. A stent, which will physically hold the newly unblocked vessel open, also may be placed. | Reinforcement will promote patient's understanding. |
| • Explain that frequent VS and neurology checks (as described previously) will be performed. | Cranial nerve problems are less frequent with this procedure because nerves have not been stretched, but they still will be included in the neurologic examination. |
| • BP medications may be given to keep BP within specified parameters. | Temporary carotid sinus dysfunction may cause BP problems (usually hypertension), but this is less common than with endarterectomy. Maintaining systolic BP at less than 150 mm Hg may prevent hyperperfusion syndrome. |
| • Advise the patient that groin and distal pulses will be assessed for bleeding and patency. | The femoral artery is the usual vessel accessed. |
| • Explain that the HOB is usually elevated after a predetermined period of time immediately after the procedure and that this requires the patient to lie flat. | This position may help prevent headache. |
| • Advise that patients are usually discharged the next day and go home on anticoagulants such as aspirin or ticlopidine. | Anticoagulants will help prevent clots from forming in the stent and angioplasty area. |

## ADDITIONAL PROBLEMS:

## ✔ PATIENT–FAMILY TEACHING AND DISCHARGE PLANNING

When providing patient–family teaching, focus on sensory information, avoid giving excessive information, and initiate a visiting nurse referral for necessary follow-up teaching. Include the verbal and written information about the following:

✓ Symptoms that necessitate prompt attention: sudden weakness, numbness (especially on one side of the body), vision loss or dimming, trouble talking or understanding speech, unexplained dizziness, unsteadiness, or severe headache. To help families remember, teach the "FAST" acronym whereby "F"=face (have patient smile, look for weakness/numbness), "A"=arms (check for arm drift/strength/numbness), "S"=speech (have the patient say a simple sentence and watch for slurred or difficulty speaking/understanding), and "T"=Time (call 911 if any of these is present because "time is tissue"). **Note:** http://www.stroke.org/site/PageServer?pagename=symp. This site lists more information in relation to FAST and is intended to be a layperson's assessment.

✓ Interventions for safe swallowing and aspiration prevention.

✓ Importance of minimizing or treating the following risk factors: diabetes mellitus, hypertension, high cholesterol, high sodium intake, obesity, inactivity, smoking, prolonged bedrest, and stressful lifestyle.

✓ Interventions that increase effective communication in the presence of aphasia or dysarthria. Additional patient information can be obtained by contacting the National Aphasia Association at www.aphasia.org.

✓ Referrals to the following as appropriate: public health nurse, visiting nurses association, psychologic therapy, vocational rehabilitation agency, home health agencies, and extended and skilled care facilities.

✓ For patient information pamphlets, contact the National Institute of Neurological Disorders and Stroke at www.ninds.nih.gov.

✓ Additional general information can be obtained by contacting the following organizations:
  • American Stroke Association: www.strokeassociation.org
  • Stroke Center: www.strokecenter.org
  • National Stroke Association: www.stroke.org

**See also:** Teaching and discharge planning (3rd through 10th entries only) under "Multiple Sclerosis," Chapter 40.

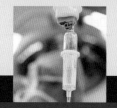

# Traumatic Brain Injury  45

## OVERVIEW/PATHOPHYSIOLOGY

Traumatic brain injury (TBI) can cause varying degrees of damage to the skull and brain tissue. Primary injuries occur at the time of impact and include skull fracture, concussion, contusion, scalp laceration, brain tissue laceration, and tear or rupture of cerebral vessels. Most deaths occur instantaneously after the injury either from the direct head trauma or from hemorrhage and shock. Secondary problems that arise soon after and are the result of the primary injury include hemorrhage and hematoma formation from tearing or rupturing of the vessels, ischemia from interrupted blood flow, cerebral swelling and edema, infection (e.g., meningitis or abscess), and increased intracranial pressure (IICP) or herniation, any of which can interrupt neuronal function. These secondary injuries or events increase the extent of initial injury and result in poor recovery and high risk for death. Cervical neck injuries are commonly associated with TBIs. Because of the potential for spinal cord injury, all TBI patients should be assumed to have cervical neck injury until it is conclusively ruled out by cervical spine radiographic examination.

Most TBIs result from direct impact on the head. Depending on force and angle of impact, the brain may suffer injury directly under the point of impact (coup) or in the region opposite the point of impact (contrecoup) because of brain rebound action within the skull. Tissue tearing or shearing may also occur elsewhere because of the rotational action of the brain within the cranial vault. TBI may be classified by location, severity, extent, or mechanism (contact, acceleration, deceleration, rotational). Common causes include motor vehicle collisions, assaults, falls, and sports-related injuries such as those occurring in football or boxing. Acts of violence, such as gunshot or stab wounds, often result in missile or impalement TBIs. This is especially true related to war-related TBIs. This population represents a special subset of TBI patients because recovery also includes managing comorbid states such as posttraumatic stress syndrome (PTSD). These patients are often managed by the Veterans Administration (VA), but because of changes in the health care arena, this population is sometimes being managed outside the VA.

## HEALTH CARE SETTING

Mobile intensive care units, flight units, acute care (trauma center, intensive care, neurology floors, medical-surgical floors), rehabilitation unit

## ASSESSMENT

The Glasgow Coma Scale (GCS) standardizes observations for objective assessment of a patient's level of consciousness (LOC). GCS score of 13–15 is mild, 9–12 is moderate, and 3–8 is severe. This or some other objective scale should be used to prevent confusion with terminology and to quickly detect changes or trends in the patient's LOC. LOC is the most sensitive indicator of overall brain function.

**Concussion.** Mild diffuse head injury in which there is temporary, reversible neurologic impairment and may involve loss of consciousness and possible amnesia of the event. No damage to brain structure is visible on computed tomography (CT) scan or magnetic resonance imaging (MRI) examination.

After concussion, patients may have headache, dizziness, nausea, lethargy, difficulty focusing, and irritability, especially to bright lights or loud noises. Although full recovery usually occurs in a few days, a postconcussion syndrome with headache; dizziness; irritability; emotional lability; lethargy; sleep disturbance; and decreased attention, judgment, concentration, and memory abilities may continue for several weeks or months.

**Diffuse axonal injury.** Diffuse brain injury may occur after a mild, moderate, or severe TBI. The head trauma changes the function of the axon, resulting in axon swelling and disconnection. It takes approximately 12–24 hours for this process to develop, but the injury may persist longer. No distinct focal lesion, such as infarction, ischemia, contusion, or intracerebral bleeding, is noted, but patients have an immediate and prolonged unconsciousness duration of at least 6 hours. CT scan may show small hemorrhagic areas in the corpus callosum, cerebral edema, and small midline ventricles. Brainstem injury may be associated with diffuse axonal injury (DAI), resulting in autonomic dysfunction. With a mild DAI, coma will last 6-24 hours and the patient will begin to follow commands within 24 hours. Full recovery is expected. *Moderate DAI* is coma lasting longer than 24 hours but without prominent brainstem signs. *Severe DAI* is prolonged coma with prominent brainstem signs, such as decortication or decerebration, and usually predicts severe disability, possible vegetative state, or death.

**Contusion.** Bruising of brain tissue, which produces a longer lasting neurologic deficit than concussion. It is usually associated with a closed head injury and often occurs at a fracture site. The size and severity of bruising vary widely. The CT scan may show infarction, necrosis, edema, and diffuse venous hemorrhage. Contusions occur at the direct impact site of the brain on the skull as well as at a second area of damage on the opposite side away from injury. These *Contrecoup* injuries tend to be more severe, and the prognosis depends on the amount of bleeding around the contusion site. Loss of consciousness is common, and it is generally more prolonged than that with concussion. Changes in behavior, such as agitation or confusion, can last for several hours to days. Headache, nausea, lethargy, motor paralysis, and paresis can occur as well. When the injury involves the frontal or temporal lobes seizures may also occur. The extent of damage determines the prognosis and can lead to either full recovery, permanent neurologic deficit, or death.

**Brain laceration.** Actual tearing of the brain's cortical surface, resulting in direct mechanical disruption of neural function and causing focal deficits. Blood vessel tearing causes hemorrhage, resulting in contusion, edema, or hematoma formation. Seizures often occur as well. Brain lacerations usually result from depressed skull fractures, penetrating injuries, missile or impalement injuries, or rotational shearing injuries within the skull. Shock waves from a bullet's high energy produce additional damage. A knife or other impalement object should be supported and left in the wound to control bleeding until it can be removed during surgery. Contusions and lacerations often are found together. The consequences of a laceration usually are more serious than those with a contusion because of the increased severity of trauma.

**Skull fracture.** Can be *closed* (simple, with skin intact) or *open* (compound), depending on whether the scalp is torn, thereby exposing the skull to the outside environment. Skull fractures are further classified as *linear* (hairline), *comminuted* (fragmented, splintered), or *depressed* (pushed inward toward the brain tissue). A blow forceful enough to break the skull is capable of causing significant brain tissue damage, and therefore close observation is essential. With a penetrating wound or basilar fracture (discussed next), there is potential for cerebrospinal fluid (CSF) leakage, meningitis, encephalitis, brain abscess, cellulitis, or osteomyelitis.

- *Basilar fractures:* Fractures of the base of the skull do not show up easily on skull/cervical radiographic examination. Indicators include blood from the nose, throat, ears; serous or serosanguineous drainage from the nose (rhinorrhea), throat, ears (otorrhea), eyes; Battle sign (bruising noted behind the ear); "raccoon's eyes" (bruising around eyes in the absence of eye injury); and bleeding behind the tympanum (eardrum) noted on otoscopic examination. Glucose in serous drainage signals the presence of CSF. CSF leakage indicates a tear in the dura, making the patient particularly susceptible to meningitis. Basilar fractures may damage the internal carotid artery and cranial nerves. Hearing loss also may occur.
- *Temporal fractures:* May result in deafness or facial paralysis.
- *Occipital fractures:* May cause visual field and gait disturbances.
- *Sphenoidal fractures:* May disrupt the optic nerve, possibly causing blindness.

### Rupture of cerebral blood vessels.

- *Epidural (extradural) hematoma or hemorrhage:* Slow (venous origin) or rapid (arterial origin) development of bleeding between the dura mater (outer meninges) and inner surface of the skull causes hematoma formation. It is a neurologic emergency. Pressure occurs on the underlying brain and produces a local mass effect, causing increased ICP and shifting of tissue, which leads to brainstem compression and herniation. Indicators are primarily those of increased ICP: altered LOC, headache, vomiting, unilateral pupil dilation (on the same side as the lesion), and possibly hemiparesis. Although some individuals never regain consciousness, most patients lose consciousness for a short period immediately after injury, regain consciousness, and then experience decreased LOC. If the origin is arterial, there will be a rapid rise in ICP leading to a rapid decrease in LOC. The bleeding site often is the middle meningeal artery or vein because of temporal bone fracture. These patients are at risk for brainstem herniation. A unilateral dilated fixed pupil is a sign of impending herniation and is a neurosurgical emergency. Patients should not be left alone because respiratory arrest may occur at any time. Rapid surgical intervention to evacuate the hematoma and prevent cerebral herniation as well as increased ICP management are crucial to improve patient outcomes.
- *Subdural hematoma or hemorrhage:* Accumulation of venous blood between the dura mater (outer meninges) and arachnoid membrane (middle meninges) that is not reabsorbed that is usually a result of an injury to the brain tissue and its blood vessels. Hematoma formation creates pressure on the underlying brain and produces a local mass effect, causing increased ICP and shifting of tissue, leading to brainstem compression and herniation. The size of the hematoma determines the patient's signs and symptoms and prognosis. This type of hematoma is classified as acute, subacute, or chronic depending on how quickly indicators arise. In acute subdural hematomas, indicators appear within 24–48 hours, symptoms progress rapidly and result from focal neurologic deficit (hemiparesis, pupillary dilation) and increased ICP (decreased LOC, falling GCS score, nausea, vomiting, headache). When indicators occur 2–14 days later, the hematoma is considered subacute and mental status decline occurs as the hematoma develops. The progression of symptoms is dependent on the size and location of the hematoma. When indicators occur more than 2 weeks after the injury, it is considered chronic. Indicators are nonspecific and progress at different rates although a progressive change in LOC occurs. Patients with cerebral atrophy (e.g., older persons, long-term alcohol users) are more prone to subdural hematoma formation.
- *Intracerebral hemorrhage:* Arterial or venous bleeding into the brain's white matter. Signs of increased ICP may develop early if the bleeding causes a rapidly expanding space-occupying lesion. If the bleeding is slower, signs of increased ICP can take 36–72 hours to develop. Indicators depend on hematoma location and size and can include altered LOC,

headache, aphasia, hemiparesis, hemiplegia, hemisensory deficits, pupillary changes, and loss of consciousness. The size and the location of the hematoma are determining factors in predicting patient outcome.

- *Subarachnoid hemorrhage:* Bleeding into the subarachnoid space below the arachnoid membrane (middle meninges) and above the pia mater (inner meninges next to brain). The patient often has a severe headache. Other general indicators include vomiting, restlessness, seizures, and loss of consciousness. Signs of meningeal irritation include nuchal rigidity and positive Kernig and Brudzinski signs (see Chapter 37). This patient may be a candidate for a shunt because of hemorrhagic interference with CSF circulation and reabsorption and is at particular risk for cerebral vasospasm.

### Indicators of Increased Intracranial Pressure.

- *Early indicators:* Alteration in LOC ranging from irritability, restlessness, and confusion to lethargy (LOC is the most sensitive, reliable indicator of neurologic dysfunction); possible onset or worsening of headache; beginning pupillary dysfunction, such as sluggishness; visual disturbances, such as diplopia or blurred vision; onset of or increase in sensorimotor changes or deficits, such as weakness; onset or worsening of nausea.

- *Late indicators:* Continued deterioration of LOC leading to stupor and coma; projectile vomiting; hemiplegia; posturing; alterations in vital signs (VS) (typically increased systolic blood pressure [BP], widening pulse pressure, decreased pulse rate); respiratory irregularities, such as Cheyne–Stokes breathing; pupillary changes, such as inequality, dilation, and nonreactivity to light; papilledema; and impaired brainstem reflexes (corneal, gag, swallowing).

> **Note:** *The single most important early indicator of increased ICP is a change in LOC. Late indicators of increased ICP usually signal impending or occurring brainstem herniation. Signs generally are related to brainstem compression and disruption of cranial nerves and vital centers. Hypotension and tachycardia in the absence of explainable causes, such as hypovolemia, usually are seen as a terminal event in TBI. Increased ICP usually peaks about 72 hours after initial insult and then gradually subsides over 2–3 weeks.*

**Brain herniation.** Brain herniation occurs when increased ICP causes displacement of brain tissue from one intracranial compartment to another, resulting in compression, destruction, and laceration of brain tissue. See late indicators of increased ICP for signs of impending or initial herniation. In the presence of actual brain herniation, the patient is in a deep coma, pupils become fixed and dilated bilaterally, posturing may progress to bilateral flaccidity, brainstem reflexes generally are lost, and respirations and VS deteriorate and may cease.

**Brain death.** Criteria for determining brain death may differ between states, and institutions may have differing guidelines.

General criteria include absent brainstem reflexes (e.g., apnea, fixed, dilated pupils), absence of corneal reflex, oculovestibular reflex, and cortical activity (as measured by electroencephalogram [EEG] readings spaced over time); and coma irreversibility over a specific timeframe.

## DIAGNOSTIC TESTS

*Cervical spine and skull radiographic examinations.* To locate neck and skull fractures. Because of the close association between TBIs and spinal or vertebral injuries, cervical immobilization is essential until cervical radiographic examination rules out fracture and potential spinal cord injury.

*Computed tomography.* Used with acute injury to identify the type, location, and extent of injury, such as accumulation of blood or a shift of midline structure caused by increased ICP.

*Magnetic resonance imaging.* To identify the type, location, and extent of injury. Although not usually performed in acute, unstable patients, this test is the study of choice for subacute or chronic TBI. It is superior to CT for detecting isodense chronic subdural hematomas or evaluating contusions and shearing injuries, especially in the brainstem area. MRI techniques such as fluid-attenuated inversion recovery are particularly sensitive to detecting DAI and small hemorrhages.

*Cerebral blood flow studies (transcranial Doppler, xenon inhalation–enhanced computed tomography).* To determine focal areas of low blood flow or spasm, possibly indicating ischemic areas, by noninvasively measuring cerebral blood flow velocities.

*EEG.* To reveal abnormal electrical activity indicating neuronal damage caused by ischemia or hemorrhage. EEG may be used to establish brain death in conjunction with other tests and may be done serially to assess the development of pathologic waves.

*Evoked potentials.* To evaluate the integrity of the anatomic pathways and connections of the brain. Stimulation of a sense organ, such as an ear, triggers a discrete electrical response (i.e., evoked potential) along a neurologic pathway to the brain. Measurement of the brain's response to auditory, visual, and/or somatosensory stimulation also aids in predicting neurologic outcome.

*Single-photon emission computed tomography.* To determine low cerebral blood flow and areas at risk for ischemic tissue perfusion.

*Infrared spectroscopy.* To continuously and noninvasively assess cerebral $O_2$ saturation.

*Cerebral angiography.* To reveal the presence of a hematoma and the status of blood vessels secondary to rupture or compression. Angiography usually is performed only if CT or MRI is unavailable or to evaluate possible carotid or vertebral artery dissection.

*Cisternogram.* To identify dural tear site with basilar skull fracture.

*Cerebral spinal fluid analysis.* To evaluate for infection, if indicators are present.

## Patient Problem/Analyze Cues/Prioritize Problems

# Deficient Knowledge (Caregiver Knowledge)

*due to* unfamiliarity with the responsibilities for observing a patient who is sent home with a concussion

**Desired Outcome/Generate Solutions:** After instruction, the caretaker verbalizes an accurate understanding about the observation regimen and of patient presentations that necessitate a return to the hospital for evaluation.

| ASSESSMENT—RECOGNIZE CUES/ INTERVENTIONS—TAKE ACTION | RATIONALES |
|---|---|
| Assess the caregiver's health care literacy (language, reading, comprehension). Assess the culture and culturally specific information needs. | This assessment helps ensure that materials are selected and presented in a manner that is culturally and educationally appropriate. |
| Give the following instructions: | |
| • Manage headache pain by stratified protocol: give the mildest analgesic prescribed to manage the level of pain. Do not exceed the maximum dose or strength. | A possible exception is codeine for pain control. Otherwise, opioids and other medications that alter mentation are avoided because they can mask neurologic indicators of increased ICP and cause respiratory depression. Aspirin is usually contraindicated because it can prolong bleeding if it occurs. |
| • Assess the patient at least every 1–2 hours for the first 24 hours or as prescribed, and as follows: awaken the patient; ask the patient's name, location, and the caretaker's name; monitor for twitching or seizure activity. | This information gives the caregiver the necessary information for returning the patient to the hospital. Timely medical care is crucial to patient outcome. |
| The caregiver should return the patient to the hospital immediately if the patient becomes increasingly difficult to awaken; cannot answer questions appropriately; cannot answer at all; becomes confused, restless, or agitated; develops slurred speech; develops twitching or seizures; develops or reports worsening headache or nausea/ vomiting; has visual disturbances (e.g., blurred or double vision); develops weakness, numbness, or clumsiness or has difficulty walking; has clear or bloody drainage from nose or ear; or develops a stiff neck. | |
| • Ensure that the patient rests and eats lightly for the first day or so after concussion or until he or she feels well. | Nausea and vomiting occur with increased ICP. |
| • Over the next several days, caution the patient to avoid activities that are physically taxing or take a high degree of concentration. Avoid alcohol and taking medication for headache or nausea without calling the health care provider. Examples of activities to avoid are driving, contact sports, swimming, using power tools. | These restrictions help ensure the patient's safety. There is potential for neurologic deterioration at this time. For this reason the patient should return to a full schedule slowly. |
| Explain that some individuals may have postconcussion syndrome. Instruct the caregiver on the importance of reporting these problems to the health care provider, especially if they worsen. | These problems should be reported promptly for timely evaluation and intervention. Additional testing may be done to ensure other processes (e.g., chronic subdural hematoma) are not occurring, and medications may be prescribed to help with some symptoms (e.g., pain, sleep problems). |
| Some individuals may continue to have headaches, dizziness, or lethargy for several weeks or months after a concussion. Patients also may experience sleep disturbance, difficulty concentrating, poor memory, irritability, emotional lability, difficulty with judgment or abstract thinking; and may be very distractible with hypersensitivity to noise and light. | |

## Patient Problem/Analyze Cues/Prioritize Hypotheses

# Risk for Infection

*due to* inadequate primary defenses occurring with basilar skull fractures, penetrating or open TBIs, or surgical wounds

***Desired Outcomes/Generate Solutions:*** The patient is free of symptoms of infection as evidenced by normothermia; stable or improving LOC; and absence of headache, photophobia, or neck stiffness. The patient verbalizes an accurate understanding about the signs and symptoms of infection and the importance of reporting them promptly.

| ASSESSMENT—RECOGNIZE CUES/ INTERVENTIONS—TAKE ACTION | RATIONALES |
|---|---|
| Assess the injury site or surgical wounds for indicators of infection. Notify the health care provider of significant findings. | Persistent erythema, local warmth, pain, hardness, and purulent drainage are indicators of localized infection that can occur as a result of loss of skin integrity. |
| Assess for indicators of meningitis or encephalitis. | Meningitis or encephalitis (fever, chills, malaise, back stiffness and pain, nuchal rigidity, photophobia, seizures, ataxia, sensorimotor deficits) can occur after a penetrating, open TBI, or cerebral surgical wound. For more details, see "Bacterial Meningitis," Chapter 37. |
| ⚠ When examining scalp lacerations and assessing for foreign bodies or palpable fractures, wear sterile gloves and follow the sterile technique. Cleanse the area gently, and cover scalp wounds with sterile dressings. | These measures reduce the possibility of infection, which can be serious if the TBI has created a breach directly into the nervous system. |
| ⚠ Document the drainage and its amount, color, and odor. | If the patient has clear or bloody drainage from the nose, throat, or ears, it should be assumed that the patient has a dural tear with CSF leakage until proven otherwise, and the health care provider should be notified accordingly. Complaints of a salty taste or frequent swallowing may signal CSF dripping down the back of the throat. Bending forward may produce nasal drainage that can be tested for CSF. |
| • Inspect the dressing and pillowcases for a halo ring (blood encircled by a yellowish stain). | A halo ring may indicate CSF drainage. |
| • Test clear drainage with a glucose reagent strip. Drainage may be sent to the laboratory to test for Cl⁻. | The presence of glucose and Cl⁻ (CSF Cl⁻ is greater than serum Cl⁻) in nonsanguineous drainage indicates that the drainage is CSF rather than mucus or saliva. |
| ⚠ If CSF leakage occurs, do not clean the ears or nose unless prescribed by the health care provider. Position the patient so that fluids can drain. Place a sterile pad over the affected ear or under the nose to catch drainage, but do not pack them. Change dressings when they become damp, using the sterile technique. | These measures prevent introducing bacteria into the nervous system from the breach created by the TBI. |
| If not contraindicated, place the patient in semi-Fowler position. | This position helps reduce cerebral congestion and edema and promotes venous drainage. |
| ⚠ With CSF leakage or possible basilar fracture, avoid nasal suction. | Nasal suction could introduce bacteria into the nervous system. |
| ⚠ Instruct the patient to avoid Valsalva maneuver, straining with bowel movement, and vigorous coughing. Caution the patient not to blow nose, sneeze, or sniff in nasal drainage. | These actions could tear the dura and increase CSF flow. |
| ⚠ Be aware that if the gastric tube is to be placed nasally, the health care provider usually performs the intubation. | Nasogastric (NG) tubes have been known to enter the fracture site and curl up into the cranial vault during insertion attempts. **Note:** The tube for gastric decompression may be placed through the mouth for patients with basilar skull fractures to avoid passing the tube through the nose, through the fracture area, and into the brain. |

| ASSESSMENT—RECOGNIZE CUES/ INTERVENTIONS—TAKE ACTION | RATIONALES |
| --- | --- |
| Check the tube placement by radiograph before applying suction. Visually check the back of the patient's throat for the NG tube to help confirm placement. | These measures help confirm the tube's proper placement and avoid causing harm to the patient. |
| As prescribed, keep individuals with basilar skull fractures flat in bed and on complete bedrest. | This position helps decrease pressure and the amount of CSF draining from a dural tear. |
| Administer the antibiotics as prescribed. | Patients are given antibiotics to prevent infection and are observed for healing and sealing of the dural tear within 7–10 days. |
| Instruct the patient that a CSF leak will be a source of infection until healed or repaired and that most CSF leaks from dural tears heal themselves in 5–10 days. | This provides the patient with vital information about his condition and will promote their compliance with restrictions needed to prevent infection. |
| • For patients with a lumbar drain, explain that they will be on bedrest with the head of bed (HOB) elevated to 15–20 degrees. Teach the patient to call for assistance and not to cough, sneeze, or strain. Explain that VS and neurologic checks will be monitored for any deterioration and the patient should call for problems such as new-onset weakness, numbness, difficult swallowing, and headache. | Deterioration of neurologic signs may indicate possible meningitis (see Chapter 37) or a pneumocranium resulting from too-rapid drainage of CSF, which causes air to siphon in through the dural tear, creating an intracranial mass effect. |
| • If neurologic signs deteriorate, the care provider should be called promptly. | |
| • Clamp the lumbar drain tubing and place the patient in a flat or in a slight Trendelenburg position with supplemental $O_2$. | This will promote absorption of intracranial air. |

## Patient Problem/Analyze Cues/Prioritize Hypotheses

# Risk for Fluid and Electrolyte Imbalance

*due to* compromised regulatory mechanisms with increased antidiuretic hormone (ADH); and increased renal resorption occurring with syndrome of inappropriate ADH secretion (SIADH)

***Desired Outcome/Generate Solutions:*** By hospital discharge (or within 3 days of injury), the patient is normovolemic as evidenced by stable weight; balanced intake and output (I&O); urinary output of 30 mL/hour or more; urine specific gravity of 1.010–1.030; BP within the patient's baseline limits; absence of fingerprint edema over the sternum; and orientation to person, place, and time.

| ASSESSMENT—RECOGNIZE CUES/ INTERVENTIONS—TAKE ACTION | RATIONALES |
| --- | --- |
| Differentiate between the syndrome of ineffective ADH (SIADH) and cerebral salt wasting (CSW) syndrome, whose treatments are different. | Although both syndromes involve hyponatremia (Na+ less than 137 mEq/L), SIADH results in hypervolemia and CSW results in hypovolemia. In CSW syndrome, the kidneys are unable to conserve Na+, and a true serum hyponatremia occurs with decreased plasma volume, weight loss, high blood urea nitrogen level, decreased serum osmolality, and hypernatremia. CSW is treated with fluid replacement (intravenous normal saline), volume expanders, salt tablets, and occasionally fludrocortisone to inhibit Na+ excretion and induce Na+ retention. If serum Na+ is very low, a hypertonic saline may be used. |
| | Usually, both syndromes resolve in 1–2 weeks. |

Continued

| ASSESSMENT—RECOGNIZE CUES/ INTERVENTIONS—TAKE ACTION | RATIONALES |
|---|---|
| Monitor the serum Na⁺, I&O, and weight and notify the health care provider of significant findings. | In the presence of SIADH, a potential complication of TBI, the patient will have very concentrated and decreased urine excretion, causing excessive water retention and a dilutional hyponatremia. Expect seizure activity when the serum Na⁺ level drops below 118 mEq/L. Serum Na⁺ level less than 115 mEq/L may result in loss of reflexes, coma, and death. Seizure activity would increase the metabolic rate in the central nervous system and further compromise the patient's neurologic status. |
| Assess for fingerprint edema over the sternum. | This reflects cellular edema. Because fluid is not retained in the interstitium with SIADH, peripheral edema will not necessarily occur. |
| Be aware that depending on the serum Na⁺ value, fluids may be restricted to an amount as low as 500–1000 mL/24 hour. Intervene accordingly and as prescribed. | Fluid restriction helps achieve homeostasis by increasing osmolarity, thereby decreasing the risk for hyponatremia. |
| If indicated and prescribed, enable the free use of salt or salty foods in the patient's diet. | This measure helps normalize the Na⁺ level. |
| For other interventions, see these patient problems in "Syndrome of Inappropriate Antidiuretic Hormone," Chapter 52. | |

## Patient Problem/Analyze Cues/Prioritize Hypotheses

# Acute Pain

*due to* headaches occurring with TBI and/or joint discomfort

**Desired Outcomes/Generate Solutions:** Within 1 hour of interventions, the patient's subjective perception of pain decreases, as documented by a pain scale. Nonverbal indicators are absent.

| ASSESSMENT—RECOGNIZE CUES/ INTERVENTIONS—TAKE ACTION | RATIONALES |
|---|---|
| Assess and document the duration and character of the patient's pain, rating it on a scale of 0 (no pain) to 10 (worst pain). Assess for nonverbal indicators of pain such as facial grimacing, muscle tension, guarding, restlessness, increased or decreased motor activity, irritability, anxiety, or sleep disturbance. | This assessment provides a baseline for subsequent comparison and quantifies the degree of pain and pain relief obtained. |
| Administer the analgesics as prescribed. | Patients with TBI generally do not have much pain, and it is usually relieved by analgesics, such as acetaminophen. Sometimes, codeine is prescribed, but as a rule, other opioids are contraindicated because they can mask neurologic indicators of increased ICP and cause respiratory depression. |
| Assess for pain, swelling, warmth, and decreased range of motion (ROM) around joints, especially the hips. | These signs may indicate heterotopic ossification (HO), which is abnormal formation of true bone within the extraskeletal soft tissues and can occur after a fracture. Etidronate, nonsteroidal antiinflammatory drugs (such as indomethacin), ROM exercises, and external beam radiation are prevention therapies. After forming HO, resection usually is necessary. |
| For additional interventions, see *Acute Pain* in "General Care of Patients With Neurologic Disorders," Chapter 36. | |

## Patient Problem/Analyze Cues/Prioritize Hypotheses

# Deficient Knowledge (Patient Undergoing Craniotomy)

*due to* unfamiliarity with the craniotomy procedure

***Desired Outcome/Generate Solutions:*** After the explanation, the patient verbalizes an accurate understanding of the craniotomy procedure, including presurgical and postsurgical care, risks, and expected outcomes.

| ASSESSMENT—RECOGNIZE CUES/ INTERVENTIONS—TAKE ACTION | RATIONALES |
|---|---|
| After the health care provider's explanation of the procedure, assess the patient's level of understanding of the purpose, risks, and anticipated benefits or outcomes. Reinforce the health care provider's explanation as appropriate. Provide and review the language-appropriate printed material if available. | This assessment enables development of an effective teaching plan. A craniotomy is a surgical opening into the skull to remove a hematoma or tumor, repair a ruptured aneurysm, apply arterial clips or wrap the involved vessel to prevent future rupture, control hemorrhage, remove bone fragment or foreign objects, debride necrotic tissue, elevate depressed fractures, or decompress the brain. Trephination ("burr" holes) may be used to evacuate hematomas or insert intracranial monitoring devices. Cranioplasty is done to repair traumatic or surgical defects in the skull. |
| Obtain the informed consent. Encourage questions and discuss fears and anxiety as they relate to the risks of the procedure discussed in the informed consent. | There is the possibility of cognitive and behavioral changes related to the site of surgery, which frequently diminish or disappear in 6 weeks to 6 months. |
| As appropriate, explain that the bone flap may be left open postoperatively. | This enables the accommodation of cerebral edema and prevents compression. When the bone is removed, the procedure is called a *craniectomy*. |
| Explain that before surgery, antiseptic shampoos may be given and the patient may be started on corticosteroids, such as dexamethasone, and antiepilepsy drugs. | Hair can be a major source of microorganisms. Dexamethasone may be given for cerebral edema; antiepilepsy drugs may be given prophylactically. |
| Explain that a baseline neurologic assessment will be performed. | This provides a basis for comparison with postoperative neurologic checks. |
| During the immediate postoperative period, the patient is in the intensive care unit (ICU). Explain the following considerations and interventions that are likely to occur: | |
| VS and neurologic status will be assessed at least hourly. Emphasize the importance of performing these tasks to the best of the patient's ability. | Patients will be asked to perform a variety of actions to assess neurological condition. Examples include squeezing the tester's hand, moving the extremities, extending the tongue, and answering questions. |
| Changes in body image can occur because of loss of hair, presence of a head dressing, and potential for and expected duration of facial edema. | Patients may consider the use of a headpiece, scarf, or wig for concerns regarding changes in body image. |
| Presence of sequential compression devices on the legs and possibly an arterial line for continuous BP monitoring as well as other devices such as ICP monitoring equipment and external ventriculostomy. | This equipment will be used to prevent thrombophlebitis and pulmonary emboli, for continuous BP monitoring, and to detect changes in ICP. Typically, patients are on a cardiac monitor for 24–48 hours because dysrhythmias are not unusual after posterior fossa surgery or when blood is in CSF. |
| Possible need for respiratory and airway support, including $O_2$, intubation, or ventilation. | Respirations will be monitored for irregularity (a sign of bleeding and brainstem compression). |
| Presence of a large head dressing and drains. Stress the importance of not pulling or tugging on the dressing or drains. Advise that the patient should report a sweet or salty taste in mouth because this may indicate a CSF leak. | Dressing and incisions will be inspected periodically for bleeding or CSF leakage, which will be reported to the health care provider for prompt intervention. |

Continued

| ASSESSMENT—RECOGNIZE CUES/ INTERVENTIONS—TAKE ACTION | RATIONALES |
|---|---|
| The patient will be given nothing by mouth (NPO) for the first 24–48 hours. | There is a risk for vomiting and choking. Patients may experience a dry throat at this time and will be assessed for swallowing difficulties, which may signal cranial nerve compression from increased ICP. |
| Possible presence of periorbital swelling and interventions if it is present. | This usually occurs within 24–48 hours of supratentorial surgery. Relief is obtained with applications of cold or warm compresses around the eyes. Having HOB raised with patient lying on the nonoperative side also may help reduce edema. |
| Insertion of an indwelling urinary catheter. | This enables accurate measurement of I&O and monitors for potential problems such as diabetes insipidus (DI). |
| Measurement of core temperature (e.g., rectal, tympanic, bladder) at frequent intervals. | A rectal probe or bladder catheter temperature probe may be used for continuous monitoring so that fever can be evaluated and treated promptly. Oral temperatures are avoided during the period in which cognitive function is decreased. |
| Teach the patient that postsurgical positioning is a key factor during recovery, as discussed in the following procedures: | Patients usually are maintained with the HOB elevated to 30 degrees (or as prescribed). Patients are assisted with turning and usually will be kept off the operative site, especially if the lesion was large. The head and neck are kept in alignment. |
| • Supratentorial craniotomy.<br><br>HOB is kept flat or as prescribed.<br><br>Pressure usually is kept off the operative site, especially with a craniectomy; therefore the patient will be kept off their backs for 48 hours.<br><br>Patient may have on a soft cervical collar and be given a small pillow for their head. | Sitting may increase the risk for venous air embolus with posterior fossa surgery. In posterior fossa surgery the supporting neck muscles are altered. Patients are logrolled to alternate sides, keeping the head in alignment with the neck and torso. A soft cervical collar may be used to prevent anterior or lateral angulation of the neck. A small pillow may be used for comfort. |
| Infratentorial craniotomy (for cerebellar or brainstem surgery).<br><br>Patient will not be placed on operative side immediately after surgery. | Placement on operative side could cause shifting inside the space. |
| For areas of evacuation causing large intracranial space.<br><br>Turning onto the side from which bone was removed is avoided. Staff will label on the chart and bed the location of the missing bone. | To protect brain tissue. |
| After craniectomy.<br><br>Patient's HOB may be elevated gradually.<br><br>For example, HOB may be flat for 24 hours, 15 degrees for the next 24 hours, 30 degrees for the next 24 hours, 45 degrees for the next 24 hours, and then 90 degrees. | To prevent cerebral hemorrhage. |
| Ventricular shunts and chronic subdural hematomas.<br><br>HOB may be flat while the drain is in place and for 24 hours after removal | To prevent air from being pulled into the subdural space. |
| *If a subdural drain is placed:* | |
| Explain that bedrest is usually maintained for the first 24 hours. | Bedrest enables the effects of anesthesia to wear off fully, reduces activity that may increase ICP, and helps ensure the stability of VS. |
| Explain that patients having supratentorial surgery near the area of the pituitary gland or hypothalamus may develop transient DI. | Supratentorial surgery may cause localized edema around the pituitary stalk, which could cause DI. See "Diabetes Insipidus," Chapter 46, for details. |

| ASSESSMENT—RECOGNIZE CUES/ INTERVENTIONS—TAKE ACTION | RATIONALES |
|---|---|
| Teach patients undergoing infratentorial surgery that they are likely to experience the following: | |
| A longer period of bedrest. | These patients are likely to experience an extended period of dizziness and hypotension. |
| Nausea, which should be reported as soon as it is noted. | This ensures that antiemetics (e.g., metoclopramide, trimethobenzamide) are given promptly. |
| Swallowing difficulties, extraocular movements, or nystagmus, any of which should be reported promptly. | These problems are the result of cranial nerve edema. |
| Provide instructions to the patient on the following precautions that are taken to prevent increased intraabdominal and intrathoracic pressure: exhaling when being turned; not straining at stool; not moving self in bed, but rather letting staff members do all moving; importance of deep breathing and avoiding coughing and sneezing (if coughing and sneezing are unavoidable, they must be done with an open mouth to minimize pressure buildup); and avoiding hip flexion and lying prone. | Increased intraabdominal and intrathoracic pressures can cause increased ICP, which could result in brain edema and ischemia, neurologic changes, and brain herniation. For additional precautions against IICP, see *Risk for Increased Intercranial Pressure*, Chapter 52. |
| Explain that precautions are taken for seizures. | See *Risk for Impaired Respiratory Function due to seizure activity*, Chapter 42. |
| Provide the patient with instructions on wound care and indicators of infection: fever; redness; drainage from surgical site, nose, or ears; and increased headache. | To prevent infection and provide education to patient about signs and symptoms of infection so that they can report any that may occur to the health care team. For more information, see *Risk for Infection*, earlier. |
| Generally, a surgical cap is worn after the removal of the head dressing. Patients must avoid scratching the wound, staples, or sutures and must keep the incision dry. When sutures or staples are removed, hair can be shampooed, being careful not to scrub around the incision line. Hair dryers are avoided until hair is regrown to prevent tissue damage caused by heat. | |
| Explain that patients undergoing acoustic neuroma excision may have nausea; hearing loss; facial weakness or paralysis; diminished or absent blinking; eye dryness; tinnitus; vertigo; headache; and occasionally swallowing, throat, taste, or voice problems. | Acoustic neuromas can wrap around cranial nerve VII, and surgery may damage this cranial nerve and cause localized edema. Other cranial nerves whose nuclei are in the brainstem also may be affected. |
| Explain that nausea and dizziness may be profound problems after surgery and that prescribed antiemetics will be given. | Contralateral routing of signal hearing aids may improve hearing by directing sound from the deaf ear to the hearing ear through a tiny microphone and transmitter. Background music or other white noise may mask tinnitus. |
| Patients should be turned and moved slowly. Patients should be spoken to on the unaffected side for best hearing, and the phone and call light should be placed on that side of the bed. Use of eye drops may be necessary. | Awareness of tinnitus eventually should lessen. Balance exercises and walking with assistance will start the compensation process by the functioning vestibular system. |
| Encourage: | Watching television or reading may be difficult because of vertigo; listening to books on tape or the radio are good alternatives. Eye dryness, from impaired eyelid function, may require the use of eye drops or ointment. |
| • background music or other white noise may mask tinnitus, | |
| • balance exercises, and | |
| • books on tape. | |
| Discourage: | |
| • television. | |
| For additional interventions, see this patient problem in "Perioperative Care," Chapter 4. | |

Patient Problem/Analyze Problems/Prioritize Hypotheses

# Deficient Knowledge (Patients Undergoing Ventricular Shunt Procedure)

*due to* unfamiliarity with the ventricular shunt procedure

**Desired Outcome/Generate Solutions:** After explanation, the patient verbalizes an accurate understanding about the ventricular shunt procedure, including presurgical and postsurgical care.

| ASSESSMENT—RECOGNIZE CUES/ INTERVENTIONS—TAKE ACTION | RATIONALES |
|---|---|
| Assess the patient's understanding of the procedure after the health care provider's explanation, including purpose, risks, and anticipated benefits or outcomes. Intervene accordingly. Also assess the patient's facility with language; provide an interpreter or language-appropriate written materials as indicated. | This assessment enables the development of an effective teaching plan. A ventricular puncture, or ventriculostomy, is a temporary procedure used to remove excess CSF. |
| As indicated, reinforce the purpose of the procedure. | This will promote patient understanding of the procedure. A ventricular shunt procedure is performed to enable permanent drainage of CSF when flow is obstructed (e.g., because of the presence of a tumor or blood) through a one-way pressure gradient valve. |
| Explain that the patient may have a cranial dressing, as well as a dressing on the neck, chest, or abdomen. | This will promote patient compliance and promote patient understanding of postoperative treatment. Shunt types vary but can extend from the lateral ventricle of the brain to one of the following: subarachnoid space of the spinal canal, right atrium of the heart, a large vein, or the peritoneal cavity. |
| Explain that it is important to avoid lying on the insertion site after the procedure. | Patient understanding of their positioning restrictions will promote compliance. This restriction prevents pressure on the shunt mechanism, which could decrease CSF drainage. |
| Advise that the head and neck are kept in alignment. | Patient understanding of their positioning restrictions will promote compliance. This prevents kinking and compression of the shunt catheter. |
| Explain that there is a shunt valve for controlling CSF drainage or reflux. | This explanation will aid patient to understand postoperative treatments. Most shunts have a valve that is preset to open at a particular pressure to permit CSF flow and does not require "pumping." There also are valves that have adjustable programmable opening pressures that are adjusted externally by using a magnet or programming device. Pumping is usually contraindicated for these new shunts, depending on manufacturer recommendations. |
| Reassure the patient and significant other that before hospital discharge, specific instructions will be given about shunt care, recognition of shunt site infection and malfunction, and steps to take should they occur. Teach signs and symptoms of IICP (i.e., headache; change in LOC such as drowsiness, lethargy, irritability, nausea, personality changes) that should be reported to the health care provider and may indicate shunt malfunction. | This explanation will aid patient to understand postoperative and discharge instructions and treatments. Kinked tubing, obstructed tubing or valve, and movement of the cannula can result in inadequate drainage of the ventricles. Cannula movement also can result in abdominal viscus perforation or subdural hematoma formation. For ventriculoatrial shunts, emboli or endocarditis may occur. For ventriculoperitoneal shunts, ascites may occur. |
| For additional interventions, see *Risk for Infection*, earlier, and *Deficient Knowledge* in "Perioperative Care," Chapter 4. | |

PART I: Medical-Surgical Nursing Care Plans

## ADDITIONAL PROBLEMS:

| | |
|---|---|
| *Immobility* for patients with varying degrees of immobility | Chapter 6 |
| "Psychosocial Support for the Patient" | Chapter 6 |
| *Difficulty Coping* | Chapter 8 |
| *Difficulty Coping* (Family) | Chapter 9 |
| *Risk for Impaired Neurologic System Function* | Chapter 36 |
| *Impaired Tissue Integrity (Corneal)* | Chapter 36 |
| *Dehydration* | Chapter 36 |
| *Impaired Swallowing* | Chapter 36 |
| *Risk for Falls* | Chapter 36 |
| *Risk for Injury,* due to sensory deficit or decreased LOC | Chapter 36 |
| *Body Weight Problem* (Weight Loss) | Chapter 36 |
| *Altered Temperature* (Increased) | Chapter 36 |
| *Altered Temperature* (Decreased) | Chapter 36 |
| *Constipation* | Chapter 36 |
| *Impaired Functional Ability* (inability to perform self-care) | Chapter 36 |
| *Impaired Communication* | Chapter 41 |
| *Risk for Injury* (altered sensory reception, transmission, and integration) | Chapter 36 |
| *Risk for Impaired Skin Integrity,* due to excessive tissue pressure | Chapter 3 |
| ***For patients on mechanical ventilation, see the following:*** | |
| *Risk for Infection,* due to inadequate primary defenses | Chapter 36 |

## ✓ PATIENT–FAMILY TEACHING AND DISCHARGE PLANNING

The patient with TBI can have varying degrees of neurologic deficit, ranging from mild to severe. When providing patient–family teaching, focus on sensory information, avoid giving excessive information, and initiate a visiting nurse referral for necessary follow-up teaching. Include verbal and written information about the following:

✓ Referrals to community resources, such as cognitive retraining specialist, head injury rehabilitation centers, visiting nurses association, community support groups, social workers, psychologic therapy, vocational rehabilitation agency, home health agencies, and extended and skilled care facilities. Additional general information can be obtained by contacting the following organizations:
  - Brain Injury Association of America: www.biausa.org
  - Brain Trauma Foundation: www.braintrauma.org
  - BrainLine: all about brain injury and PTSD: www.brainline.org/resource-directory

✓ Safety measures related to decreased sensation, visual disturbances, motor deficits, and seizure activity.

✓ Measures that promote communication in the presence of aphasia.

✓ Wound care and indicators of infection. Instruct patient to avoid scratching sutures and to shampoo only after sutures are out.

✓ Indicators of ICP, which include change in LOC, lethargy, headache, nausea, and vomiting, should be reported to health care provider promptly.

✓ Measures that deal with cognitive or behavioral problems. As appropriate, include home evaluation for safety. Caution significant other that personality can change drastically after TBI. Patient may demonstrate inappropriate social behavior, inappropriate affect, hallucination, delusion, and altered sleep pattern.

✓ Cognitive rehabilitation goals for appropriate patients to promote the highest level of cognitive functioning. Family can be instructed in and participate in coma stimulation techniques (usually for short periods 2–4v times/day). Most cognitive recovery occurs in the first 6 months.

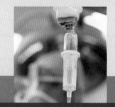

# Diabetes Insipidus 46

## OVERVIEW/PATHOPHYSIOLOGY

Diabetes insipidus (DI) is a metabolic disorder that affects free water regulation and can result from one of several problems. *Central (neurogenic) DI*, the most common form, is caused either by a defect in the synthesis, transport, or release of antidiuretic hormone (ADH) by the pituitary gland.

Although there is an adequate amount of circulating ADH in patients with Nephrogenic DI, the renal tubules do not respond adequately to ADH, causing impaired renal conservation of water. Causes of nephrogenic DI include familial X-linked trait, pyelonephritis, renal amyloidosis, Sjögren syndrome, sickle cell anemia, myeloma, potassium depletion, effects of certain drugs such as lithium or demeclocycline, or chronic hypercalcemia. Although the manifestations of nephrogentic DI are similar to central DI, fluid loss is less dramatic.

*Primary DI* is due to a structural lesion in the thirst center or psychologic disorder that triggers excess water intake.

The primary problem for all DI disorders is excessive urinary output (2–20 L daily) with very low urine-specific gravity (less than 1.005) and urine osmolality of less than 100 mOsm/kg. Serum osmolality increases (greater than 295 mOsm/kg) because of hypernatremia (serum sodium greater than 145 mg/dL). This is caused by water loss in the kidneys. When an individual cannot adequately respond to stimulation of the thirst center by drinking adequate fluids to replace fluid loss from polyuria, both intracellular and extracellular dehydrations ensue, resulting in hypernatremia.

Fatigue and weakness due to excess fluid loss and hypernatremia are common symptoms of DI. Untreated hypernatremia can also cause brain shrinkage and intracranial bleeding. *Central DI* may be idiopathic (about 30% of cases), result from a brain or pituitary tumor (25% of cases), or occur after brain surgery (20% of cases) or head trauma (16% of cases). Central DI from head trauma is often self-limiting and improves with treatment of the underlying problem. There are three phases to central DI that occurs after brain surgery: (1) acute phase that occurs abruptly with polyuria, (2) an interphase when urine volume normalizes, and (3) when central DI may become permanent.

DI must be differentiated from other syndromes resulting in polyuria. History, physical examination, and simple laboratory procedures assist in diagnosis. Other causes of polyuria include recent lithium or mannitol administration, renal transplantation, renal disease, hyperglycemia, hyperosmolality (early), hypercalcemia, and potassium depletion, including primary aldosteronism.

## HEALTH CARE SETTING

Acute care (either medical-surgical or intensive care unit) or outpatient care depending on the seriousness of the condition

## ASSESSMENT

**Signs and symptoms.** Polydipsia, polyuria (2–20 L/day) with dilute urine (specific gravity less than 1.005).

**Physical assessment.** Usually within normal limits, but the patient may show signs of dehydration if fluid intake is inadequate. Individuals with cranial injury, disease, or trauma may exhibit impairment of neurologic status, including the altered level of consciousness (LOC) and sensory or motor deficits associated with hypernatremia. Cranial nerve examination may reveal nerve palsies. Older adults are most likely to be confused, disoriented, or agitated. In extreme cases, coma and seizures are possible.

**History.** Cranial injury, especially basilar skull fracture, meningitis, primary or metastatic brain tumor, surgery in the pituitary area, cerebral hemorrhage, encephalitis, syphilis, or tuberculosis (TB). Familial incidence rarely is a factor.

## DIAGNOSTIC TESTS

**Urine osmolality.** Decreased (less than 100 mOsm/kg) in the presence of disease.

**Specific gravity.** Decreased (less than 1.005) in the presence of disease.

**Serum osmolality.** Increased (295 mOsm/kg or greater) in the presence of disease.

**Serum sodium.** Increased (greater than 145 mEq/L) in the presence of disease. Other electrolytes may be elevated resulting from hemoconcentration secondary to dehydration.

**Plasma antidiuretic hormone level (vasopressin level).** Normal value is less than 2.5 pg/mL or less than 2.3 pmol/L and varies depending on the type of DI present: central DI—decreased; nephrogenic DI—normal or increased.

**Vasopressin (DDAVP) challenge test.** After administration of vasopressin subcutaneously or desmopressin by nasal spray, urine is collected every 15–30 minutes for 2 hours. Quantity and specific gravity are then measured. Normally, individuals will show a concentration of urine but not as pronounced as that of persons with DI; a person with kidney disease will have a lesser response to vasopressin. **Note:** One serious side effect of this test is the precipitation of heart failure in susceptible individuals.

*Water deprivation test.* This is an older technique sometimes used as a marker. Baseline measurements of body weight, serum and urine osmolalities, and urine-specific gravity are obtained. Fluids are not permitted for 8–12 hours and measurements are repeated hourly. Then patients are given desmopressin acetate subcutaneously or nasally. Patients with central DI have a dramatic increase in urine osmolality and a significant decrease in urine volume. The patient with nephrogenic

DI will not be able to increase urine osmolality to greater than 300 mOsm/kg. Because the most serious side effect of this test is severe dehydration, the test should be performed early in the day so that patients can be more closely monitored. Before a firm diagnosis of DI can be made from an abnormal water deprivation test, it is also necessary to demonstrate that the kidneys can respond to vasopressin.

*Magnetic resonance imaging of the brain or pituitary gland.* Magnetic resonance imaging is used to identify pituitary lesions that may have caused the DI. If the patient has the "bright spot" or hyperintense emission from the posterior pituitary gland, the patient likely has primary polydipsia associated with dipsogenic and psychogenic DI. If the bright spot is small or absent, the patient likely has central DI.

## Patient Problem/Analyze Cues/Prioritize Hypotheses

# Dehydration

*due to* active fluid loss occurring with polyuria

***Desired Outcome/Generate Solutions:*** The patient becomes normovolemic within 3 days of onset of symptoms as evidenced by stable weight, balanced intake and output (I&O), elastic skin turgor, pink and moist mucous membranes, blood pressure (BP) of 90–120/60–80 mm Hg (or within the patient's normal range), heart rate (HR) of 60–100 bpm, urine-specific gravity greater than 1.010, sodium level of 137–147 mEq/L, serum osmolality of 275–300 mOsm/L, urine osmolality of 300–900 mOsm/24 hour, and central venous pressure (CVP) of 2–6 mm Hg.

| ASSESSMENT—RECOGNIZE CUES/ INTERVENTIONS—TAKE ACTION | RATIONALES |
|---|---|
| Assess for dehydration by monitoring I&O, specific gravity, mental status, and vital signs (VS) hourly. Check the weight daily. | Signs of dehydration include weight loss, inadequate fluid intake to balance output, thirst, poor skin turgor, decreased specific gravity, furrowed tongue, hypotension, and tachycardia. Hypernatremia, which can cause altered mental status, is associated with dehydration. |
| If available, monitor the CVP. | CVP may decrease to less than 2 mm Hg in the presence of profound dehydration. |
| Immediately report the following to the health care provider: (1) urinary output more than 200 mL in each of 2 consecutive hours, (2) urinary output more than 500 mL in any 2-hour period, or (3) urine-specific gravity less than 1.002. | These are signs of extreme diuresis. Diuresis may result in hypotension, hypokalemia, and dehydration leading to highly viscous blood. The patient is at increased risk for hypovolemic shock, stroke, dysrhythmias, and heart attack. |
| Provide unrestricted fluids: keep the water pitcher full and within easy reach of the patient. Explain the importance of consuming as much water as can be tolerated. | The chief danger to patients with DI is dehydration from the inability to take in adequate fluids to balance the excessive output of urine. Water is the best replacement, and patients should avoid excessive ingestion of salt, sugar, and artificial sweeteners. |
| Administer the vasopressin and antidiuretic agents for central DI and gestational DI (or thiazide diuretic for patients with nephrogenic DI) as prescribed. | These measures are instituted to prevent extreme diuresis. Several vasopressin preparations are available, and it is important to read package inserts carefully to ensure proper administration. Potential side efvfects of exogenous vasopressin include hypertension secondary to vasoconstriction, myocardial infarction secondary to constriction of coronary vessels, uterine cramps, and increased peristalsis of the gastrointestinal tract. |

Continued

| ASSESSMENT—RECOGNIZE CUES/ INTERVENTIONS—TAKE ACTION | RATIONALES |
|---|---|
| | A mild antidiuretic effect may be achieved with thiazide diuretics (e.g., hydrochlorothiazide), nonsteroidal antiinflammatory drugs (NSAIDs), and other medications that increase the action (desired effect for nephrogenic DI) or release of ADH (desirable for central DI). |
| | **Note:** Although it may seem counterintuitive to treat diuresis with a diuretic, one of the side effects of the thiazide diuretics and NSAIDs in patients with DI is reducing the excretion of free water. |
| For unconscious patients, administer intravenous (IV) fluids as prescribed. Unless otherwise directed, for every mL of urine output, deliver 1 mL of IV fluid. | To promote rehydration, lost water is replaced with IV hypotonic (e.g., 0.45% NaCl) solution. Initial replacement is rapid, necessitating close monitoring of BP, HR, and urine output to prevent overhydration. IV normal saline may be used following initial fluid resuscitation. |

## Patient Problem/Analyze Cues/Prioritize Hypotheses

# Risk for Fluid Imbalance

*due to* the side effects of vasopressin

**Desired Outcomes/Generate Solutions:** Optimally, the patient demonstrates normal mental acuity; verbalizes orientation to person, place, and time; and is free of signs of injury caused by side effects of vasopressin. As appropriate, the patient or significant other demonstrates administration of coronary artery vasodilators by the time of hospital discharge.

| ASSESSMENT—RECOGNIZE CUES/ INTERVENTIONS—TAKE ACTION | RATIONALES |
|---|---|
| Assess VS and report significant changes. | Significant changes such as systolic BP (SBP) elevated more than 20 mm Hg over baseline SBP or HR increased more than 20 bpm over baseline HR are signs of vasoconstriction, which is an undesirable effect when vasopressin is used solely as an ADH. |
| Assess for changes in mental status or LOC, confusion, weight gain, headache, convulsions, and coma. | These are signs of water intoxication caused by fluid retention. |
| ⚠ If these signs develop, stop the vasopressin, restrict fluids, and notify the health care provider. Institute safety measures accordingly, and reorient the patient as needed. | Water intoxication causes significant dilution of circulating electrolytes, resulting in effects seen with such electrolyte disorders as hyponatremia, hypokalemia, and hypochloremia. |
| ⚠ For older adults or persons with vascular disease, keep prescribed coronary artery vasodilators (i.e., nitroglycerin) at the bedside for use if angina occurs. Teach patients and significant others how to administer these medications. | Angina may result from coronary vasoconstriction induced by vasopressin. Vasopressin dose should be reduced if angina occurs. |

✓ **PATIENT–FAMILY TEACHING AND DISCHARGE PLANNING**

Include verbal and written information about the following:

✓ Importance of medical follow-up; confirm the date and time of the next visit to the health care provider. The patient should be taught an accurate method for measurement of urine-specific gravity, the importance of recording test results, and to bring the test results to the follow-up visit with the health care provider.

✓ Medications, particularly exogenous vasopressin, including drug name, purpose, dosage, schedule, precautions, and potential side effects. Also discuss drug–drug, food–drug, and herb–drug interactions. If the patient had a transsphenoidal hypophysectomy, additional medications may be required if the anterior pituitary gland was damaged or removed during the surgery.

✓ Importance of seeking immediate medical attention if signs of dehydration or water intoxication occur. Altered mental status is common, resulting from elevations or decreases in levels of sodium associated with loss of free water regulation. See the two patient problems earlier in this care plan.

✓ Recommendations for fluid replacement: guidelines on the type and amount of replacement fluids prescribed for the patient.

✓ Additional information available from:
- Diabetes Insipidus Foundation: www.diabetesinsipidus.org

- National Institutes of Health National Institute of Diabetes and Digestive and Kidney Diseases: https://www.niddk.nih.gov/health-information/kidney-disease/diabetes-insipidus
- Mayo Clinic: http://www.mayoclinic.org/diseases-conditions/diabetes-insipidus/symptoms-causes/dxc-20182410

# Diabetes Mellitus 47

## OVERVIEW/PATHOPHYSIOLOGY

Diabetes mellitus (DM) is a chronic multisystem disease. According to a 2021 report by the Centers for Disease Control and Prevention (CDC), 37 million people in the United States have diabetes and 96 million adults (approximately 1/3 of the United States population) have prediabetes (Centers for Disease Control and Prevention).

DM is characterized by hyperglycemia that is caused by decreased insulin production and/or use. Metabolic, vascular, and neurologic disorders develop from dysfunctional glucose transport into body cells. Insulin is needed to facilitate glucose transport into cells for oxidation and energy production. Food intake, glycogen breakdown, and gluconeogenesis increase the serum glucose level, which stimulates the beta islet cells of the pancreas to release needed insulin for the transport of glucose from the bloodstream into the cells. At the cellular level, insulin receptors play a vital role in controlling the rate of transport of glucose into the cells and subsequently facilitate the passage of glucose from the blood to the cells. This process ensures sufficient glucose in the cells to be used for energy.

Normal glucose range is approximately 74–106 mg/dL. Individuals with DM have impaired glucose transport because of insufficient or absent insulin secretion and/or defective cellular insulin receptors. Carbohydrate, fat, and protein metabolism are abnormal, and patients are unable to store glucose in the liver and muscle as glycogen, store fatty acids and triglycerides in adipose tissue, or transport amino acids into cells normally.

The American Diabetes Association (ADA) recognizes four classes of diabetes: type 1 diabetes, type 2 diabetes, gestational diabetes, and diabetes from other causes. Type 1 diabetes, in which the body makes little to no insulin, can develop at any age and there is no known way to prevent it.

## Type 1 diabetes

Type 1 diabetes accounts for 5%–10% of all diagnosed cases of diabetes. It can occur at any age but generally affects people under the age of 40. It is autoimmune disorder in which the body develops antibodies against insulin and/or the pancreatic beta cells that synthesize, store, and release insulin. Certain human leukocyte antigens have been strongly associated with type 1 DM. Other factors that may contribute to the development to type 1 diabetes are genetic predisposition and exposure to a virus. These individuals depend on insulin for survival and prevention of life-threatening diabetic ketoacidosis (DKA). All type 1 diabetics require insulin to manage their blood sugar.

## Type 2 diabetes

Type 2 diabetes, the most common form of diabetes, accounts for 90%–95% of all diagnosed cases of diabetes, can develop at any age, and is mostly preventable. People with type 2 diabetes may not produce enough insulin and/or are not able to use their insulin properly. Type 2 diabetes risk factors include obesity, family history, physical inactivity, and older than 45 years. Those with type 2 diabetes may be able to control their blood sugar levels with healthy eating and exercise, but others will need medication to manage blood sugar levels. Untreated hyperglycemia can result in hyperglycemic hyperosmolar state.

## Gestational diabetes (GD)

Gestational diabetes is first diagnosed during pregnancy, and although it is unknown why some women get gestational diabetes and others do not, risk factors include hormone level changes, being overweight, inactivity, polycystic ovary syndrome, and family history of diabetes. There is a 50% risk for GD turning to type 2 DM later in life if lifestyle changes are not made. Diabetes poses significant risks to maternal and fetal morbidity and mortality. Incidence of diabetes in pregnancy has increased because more women are delaying pregnancy until relatively late into their reproductive years. Currently the incidence of gestational diabetes is 2-10% (CDC, 2021).

## DM from other causes

Diabetes from other causes constitutes a very small fraction of diabetics. Pancreatitis and cystic fibrosis are conditions that may lead to a diabetes diagnosis. Additionally, long term glucocorticoid use may also increase blood sugar levels.

Long-term complications associated with uncontrolled diabetes can be devastating. They include heart disease, blindness, stroke, kidney failure, and nontraumatic lower limb amputations.

## Prediabetes

People who are diagnosed with prediabetes have impaired glucose tolerance and impaired fasting glucose. Glucose levels are elevated but not high enough to meet the diagnostic criteria for diabetes. Therefore they are at risk for the development of type 2 diabetes. The failing ability of pancreatic beta islet cells to compensate for insulin resistance because of excess body weight or metabolic syndrome is associated with the development of prediabetes. Weight loss is the primary goal for managing prediabetes. Some long-term damage to the body, especially the heart and circulatory system, already may be occurring during prediabetes. If blood glucose is controlled by weight loss, pharmacotherapy, lifestyle therapy, and bariatric surgery when prediabetes is identified, the development of type 2 DM can be prevented, along with an improving lipid profile and blood pressure (BP).

## HEALTH CARE SETTING

Primary care, with possible hospitalization to treat complications

## ASSESSMENT

**Metabolic signs of chronic hyperglycemia.** Fatigue, weakness, overweight or obesity for type 2, weight loss for type 1, paresthesias, mild dehydration, and symptoms of hyperglycemia (polyuria, polydipsia, polyphagia). Chronic inflammation may be present. When patients develop a severe illness or are exposed to another stressor, the inflammatory/stress response is activated. Hyperglycemia can worsen and reach crisis level resulting from the response.

## COMPLICATIONS

**Type 1 crisis—diabetic ketoacidosis.** Profound dehydration and hyperglycemia, electrolyte imbalance, metabolic acidosis caused by ketosis, altered mental status, Kussmaul respirations (paroxysmal dyspnea), acetone breath, possible hypovolemic shock (hypotension, weak and rapid pulse), abdominal pain, and possible stroke-like symptoms.

**Type 2 crisis—hyperglycemic hyperosmolar state.** Severe dehydration, hypovolemic shock (hypotension, weak and rapid pulse), severe hyperglycemia, shallow respirations, altered mental status, slight lactic acidosis or normal pH, possible stroke-like symptoms, and abdominal pain.

**Potential for long-term complications.** The most important factor in delaying progression to long-term complications is the stabilization of blood glucose levels to normal range.

**Macroangiopathy.** Patients are at higher risk for heart attack and stroke caused by vascular disease affecting the coronary arteries and larger vessels of the brain and lower extremities (peripheral vascular disease [PVD]). Risk factors are hyperglycemia, hypertension, hypercholesterolemia, smoking, aging, and extended duration of DM.

**Microangiopathy.** Patients are at higher risk for blindness and renal failure caused by thickening of capillary basement membranes resulting in retinopathy and nephropathy. Early signs and symptoms include vision loss, increased leakage of retinal vessels, and microalbuminuria.

**Neuropathy.** Patients are at higher risk for gastroparesis (impaired gastric emptying), lack of sensation (especially in the feet), and neurogenic bladder caused by deterioration of peripheral and autonomic nervous systems, resulting in impaired or slowed nerve transmission.

**Morning hyperglycemia.** Blood glucose elevation found on awakening. Causes include each of the following or a combination of the effects of their interactions.

*Dawn phenomenon.* At approximately 3:00 a.m., the release and effect of nocturnal growth may elevate glucose in people with type 1 DM. It may be corrected by changing time of the evening insulin dose.

*Somogyi phenomenon.* If the diabetic patient becomes hypoglycemic during the night, compensatory mechanisms to raise glucose levels are activated and result in overcompensation and leads to elevated glucose levels. It may be corrected by decreasing the evening dose of insulin and/or eating a more substantial bedtime snack.

**Problems with insulin therapy.**

*Insulin resistance.* Many people with type 2 diabetes and prediabetes experience this problem. Insulin resistance occurs when the cells stop responding to insulin. These people typically have increased circulating insulin as the body tries to compensate for increased serum glucose levels. With increased insulin, the liver and muscles are prompted to store increased amounts of blood glucose. Eventually, the maximum amount of stored glucose is reached, and the excess blood sugar is sent to fat cells to be stored as body fat leading to weight gain. Insulin resistance in people with prediabetes further increases their risk to develop type 2 diabetes. Type 2 diabetics with insulin resistance typically need antidiabetic drugs including increased amounts of exogenous insulin to manage their increased blood glucose levels.

*Lipodystrophy.* Local disturbance in fat metabolism resulting in loss of fat (lipoatrophy) or development of abnormal fatty masses at the injection sites (lipohypertrophy). Lipoatrophy rarely has been seen since the development of 100 U and human source insulins. Rotation of injection sites helps prevent lipohypertrophy. Individuals experiencing lipohypertrophy should use alternate injection sites until the condition resolves.

## DIAGNOSTIC TESTS

DM is diagnosed in persons of any age who have one of the following four test results:

- A1C level 6.5% or higher.
- Fasting plasma glucose level of 126 mg/dL or greater.
- A 2-hour plasma glucose.

  Glucose level of 200 mg/dL or greater during an oral glucose tolerance test, using a glucose load of 75 g.
- Classic symptoms of hyperglycemia (polyuria, polydipsia, polyphagia, unexplained weight loss) or hyperglycemic crisis, a random plasma glucose level of 200 mg/dL or greater.
- All diagnostic tests are repeated in patients without classic symptoms to rule out laboratory error.

**Hemoglobin A/glycosylated hemoglobin (glycohemoglobin).** This value is measured to assess control of blood glucose over a preceding 2- to 3-month period. The larger the percentage of glycosylated hemoglobin (Hgb), the poorer the blood glucose control. Normal range is 4%–6%. The ADA identifies an A1C goal of less than 7.0% in patients with diabetes. When the

A1C is maintained at near-normal levels, the risk for developing microvascular and macrovascular complications is greatly reduced. The ADA defines normal A1C level at below 5.7%, levels between 5.7% and 6.5% are in the prediabetes range, and an A1C more than 6.5% is in the diabetes range.

### After the diagnosis of diabetes mellitus is made

***Fasting lipid profile.*** If total and low-density lipoprotein cholesterol values are elevated, the triglyceride value is elevated, or if the high-density lipoprotein cholesterol level is decreased, the patient is at high risk for developing cardiovascular disease.

***Urinalysis for the presence of microalbuminuria, ketones, protein, and sediment.*** If present, may indicate early renal disease caused by hyperglycemia. This test should be performed with routine checkups every 3 months.

***Serum creatinine.*** If elevated, may indicate renal disease.

***12-Lead electrocardiogram.*** If the patient has symptoms of cardiovascular disease, an electrocardiogram can identify areas of myocardial ischemia, infarction, and active injury.

### Patient Problem/Analyze Cues/Prioritize Hypotheses

# Risk for Altered Blood Glucose Level

*due to* inadequate blood glucose monitoring, periodic illness or other stressors, variable dietary intake, inconsistent levels of exercise, and/or ineffective medication management

***Desired Outcomes/Generate Solutions:*** Optimally, the patient has a blood glucose reading no more than 180 mg/dL at all times; and fasting blood glucose readings 80–130 mg/dL when hospitalized; hemoglobin A1C level less than 7%; adequate tissue perfusion as evidenced by warmth, sensation, brisk capillary refill time (less than 2 seconds), and peripheral pulses greater than 2+ on a 0–4+ scale in the extremities; BP within their optimal range; urinary output of at least 30 mL/hour; baseline vision; good appetite; and absence of nausea and vomiting. The patient demonstrates adherence to the therapeutic regimen (essential for promoting optimal tissue perfusion).

| ASSESSMENT—RECOGNIZE CUES/ INTERVENTIONS—TAKE ACTION | RATIONALES |
|---|---|
| Assess the blood glucose before meals and at bedtime. | This monitors the effectiveness of blood glucose control at times when the patient's glucose is not increased by food being digested. |
| | The ADA and American Association of Clinical Endocrinologists (2017) have determined that both morbidity and mortality could be reduced for thousands of patients if hyperglycemia were diagnosed by A1C levels upon hospital admissions. The ADA recommends A1C levels be less than 7%, but endocrinologists recommend A1C levels should be less than 6.5%. It is believed that the A1C level discrepancies are driven by other comorbidites such as heart disease (https://pro.aace.com/disease-state-resources/diabetes/depth-information/type-2-diabetes-glucose-management-goals). |
| | According to the ADA (2022) Preprandial (before meals) capillary plasma glucose should be maintained between 80-130 mg/dL. However, glycemic control goals may be individualized according to patients' comorbidities, life expectancy, age, and duration of Diabetes. |
| ⚠ Assess for changes in mentation, apprehension, erratic behavior, trembling, slurred speech, staggering gait, and seizure activity. Treat hypoglycemia as prescribed. | These are signs of hypoglycemia. Patients with hypoglycemia may experience vasodilation and diminished myocardial contractility, which decrease cerebral circulation and impair cognition. |
| In addition to sensation, assess the capillary refill, temperature, peripheral pulses, and color. | This assessment monitors the patient's peripheral perfusion to detect macroangiopathy or PVD. |
| Administer the basal, prandial, and correction doses of insulin as prescribed. | Adherence to the therapeutic regimen is essential for promoting optimal tissue perfusion. Progression of vascular disease and neuropathy, including blindness, kidney failure, gastroparesis, heart attack, and stroke, is the root cause of all complications of DM. By keeping serum glucose within the appropriate range, the vascular endothelium receives better nourishment within the cells and will be less likely to deteriorate. |

| ASSESSMENT—RECOGNIZE CUES/ INTERVENTIONS—TAKE ACTION | RATIONALES |
|---|---|
| Encourage and teach the patient how to perform regular home blood glucose monitoring. Blood glucose is generally monitored before meals, at bedtime, and possibly during the night (3:00 a.m.) | To assess whether a correction dose of short-acting insulin is needed. Self-monitoring by patients is extremely useful in reducing complications. |
| Check BP every 4 hours. Alert the health care provider to values outside the patient's normal range. Administer the antihypertensive agents as prescribed and document response. | Hypertension is commonly associated with diabetes. Careful control of BP is critical in preventing or limiting the development of heart disease, stroke, retinopathy, and nephropathy. |
| **!** Monitor for orthostatic hypotension after administering BP medications. For more information, see discussion later in this patient problem. | Orthostatic hypotension is a potential side effect of antihypertensive agents and of autonomic neuropathy in which the patient's compensatory mechanisms may be impaired. |
| Protect patients with impaired peripheral perfusion from injury caused by sharp objects or heat (e.g., avoid the use of heating pads; always wear shoes outdoors and slippers at home). | Patients may experience decreased sensation in the extremities because of peripheral neuropathy. |
| Teach the patient to avoid pressure at the back of the knees by not crossing legs or "gatching" bed under the knees. Caution the patient to avoid garments that constrict circulation to the extremities and lower body. For additional information, see *Risk for Impaired Skin Integrity* later. | These actions could cause venous stasis and reduction in arterial perfusion in patients with macroangiopathy or impending PVD. |
| As indicated, orient the patient to locations of such items as water, tissues, glasses, and call light. | This orientation provides necessary information and a safe environment for patients with diminished eyesight caused by diabetic retinopathy. |
| Monitor the laboratory values for changes in renal function. Laboratory values that would signal changes in renal function include increases in blood urea nitrogen (more than 20 mg/dL) and creatinine (more than 1.5 mg/dL). | Approximately half of all persons with type 1 DM develop chronic kidney disease (CKD) and end-stage renal disease. Proteinuria (protein more than 8 mg/dL in a random sample of urine) or microalbuminuria are early indicators of developing CKD. (See "Chronic Kidney Disease," Chapter 32, for more information.) |
| Monitor the urine output, especially after exposure to contrast medium. Observe these patients for indicators of acute renal failure (ARF). (See "Acute Kidney Injury," Chapter 27, for more information.) | Individuals with DM and with reduced renal function are at significant risk for dehydration and development of ARF after exposure to contrast medium. |
| In addition, assess for the following: | Individuals with DM may experience multiple problems resulting from autonomic neuropathy. |
| *Orthostatic hypotension:* | |
| **!** • Check BP while the patient is lying down, sitting, and then standing. Alert the health care provider to significant findings. | BP decreased from the patient's normal, along with lightheadedness, dizziness, diaphoresis, pallor, tachycardia, and syncope, are signals of orthostatic hypotension. A drop in systolic BP of 20 mm Hg or more signals the need to return the patient to a supine position. |
| • Instruct patients to not get up suddenly and to ask for assistance when getting up especially after prolonged recumbency. | This action helps prevent falls caused by orthostatic hypotension. |
| *Gastroparesis/impaired gastric emptying with nausea and vomiting:* | Progressive autonomic neuropathy may cause a delay in gastric emptying, resulting in nausea and vomiting. |
| *Neurogenic bladder:* | Neurogenic bladder is caused by deterioration of peripheral and autonomic nervous systems, resulting in impaired or slowed nerve transmission. |
| • Encourage the patient to void every 3–4 hours during the day. Intermittent catheterization may be necessary in severe cases of neurogenic bladder secondary to autonomic neuropathy. | Encouraging a consistent urination schedule will aid patient and provider to assess the ability to void and determine the need for a straight catheterization. |
| • Avoid the use of indwelling urinary catheters. | Infection risk is increased with the use of indwelling catheters. |

## Patient Problem/Analyze Cues/Prioritize Hypotheses

# Risk for Infection

*due to* chronic inflammation or chronic disease process (e.g., hyperglycemia, neurogenic bladder, poor circulation)

*Desired Outcome/Generate Solutions:* The patient does not develop an infection, as evidenced by normothermia, negative cultures, and white blood cell (WBC) count of 11,000/mm³ or less.

| ASSESSMENT—RECOGNIZE CUES/ INTERVENTIONS—TAKE ACTION | RATIONALES |
| --- | --- |
| Assess the temperature every 4 hours. Alert the health care provider of temperature elevation, positive cultures, and WBC count above 11,000/mm³. | Infection is the most common cause of DKA. Fever can signal the presence of an infection. |
| Maintain the meticulous sterile technique when changing dressings, performing invasive procedures, or manipulating indwelling catheters. | Nonintact skin and invasive procedures and catheters place patients at risk for ingress of bacteria. |
| Monitor for indicators of infection, including the following: | |
| • Fever, chills, cough productive of sputum, coarse crackles, dyspnea, and sore throat. | These are indicators of upper respiratory infection. |
| • Burning or pain with urination, cloudy or malodorous urine, tachycardia, diaphoresis, nausea, vomiting, and abdominal pain. | These are indicators of urinary tract infection (UTI). Patients with DM often have a neurogenic bladder, which increases the chance of UTI caused by urinary stasis. |
| • Hypothermia, flushed skin, and hypotension. | These are indicators of systemic sepsis. |
| • Erythema, swelling, purulent drainage, and warmth at intravenous (IV) sites and areas of impaired skin integrity. | These are indicators of localized infection. |
| Consult the health care provider about obtaining culture specimens for blood, sputum, and urine during temperature spikes or for wounds that produce purulent drainage. | Infection can be present in blood (sepsis), urine, sputum (lungs/ respiratory tract), or wounds. Occult infection also can be present outside these sources. |

## Patient Problem/Analyze Cues/Prioritize Hypotheses

# Risk for Impaired Skin Integrity

*due to* altered circulation and sensation occurring with peripheral neuropathy and vascular pathology

*Desired Outcomes/Generate Solutions:* The patient's lower extremity skin remains intact. Within the 24-hour period before hospital discharge, the patient verbalizes and demonstrates knowledge of proper foot care.

| ASSESSMENT—RECOGNIZE CUES/ INTERVENTIONS—TAKE ACTION | RATIONALES |
| --- | --- |
| Assess the integrity of the skin and evaluate reflexes of the lower extremities by checking knee and ankle deep tendon reflexes, proprioceptive sensations, two-point discrimination, and vibration sensation (using a tuning fork on the medial malleolus). | These assessments monitor the presence/degree of neuropathy and vascular pathology. In addition to higher risk areas on the extremities and pressure points, skin on the legs is at the highest risk and typically is the first to exhibit problems. If sensations are impaired, the patient likely will be unable to respond appropriately to stimuli. |
| Assess the peripheral pulses, comparing quality bilaterally. | Peripheral pulses 2+ or less on a 0–4+ scale signal poor circulation that could compromise skin integrity. |

| ASSESSMENT—RECOGNIZE CUES/ INTERVENTIONS—TAKE ACTION | RATIONALES |
|---|---|
| Use a foot cradle on the bed, heel and elbow protectors, and pressure-relief mattress when appropriate. Encourage position changes every 2 hours. If patient is unable to independently change positions, turn every 2 hours. | These measures prevent pressure points and promote patient comfort. |
| Incorporate the progressive passive and active exercises into the daily routine. Discourage the extended rest periods in the same position. | These measures alleviate acute discomfort while preventing hemostasis. |
| Provide the patient with instructions on the following steps for foot care: | |
| • Wash feet daily with mild soap and warm water; check water temperature with water thermometer or elbow. | Patients with decreased sensation are at risk for burns if they are unaware that water temperature is too hot. Hot water and strong soaps also can promote dry skin, which can become irritated and break down. |
| • Inspect the feet daily for the presence of erythema, discoloration, or trauma, using mirrors as necessary for adequate visualization. | These signs indicate the need for vigilant assessment and preventive care. When the skin is no longer intact, the patient is at risk for infection that eventually can lead to amputation. |
| • Alternate between at least two pairs of properly fitted shoes. | This measure eliminates the potential for pressure points that can occur by wearing one pair only. |
| • Change the socks or stockings daily and wear white cotton or wool blends. | These measures prevent infection from moisture or dirt in contact with nonintact skin. The white fabric enables patients more readily to see any blood or exudates from nonintact skin. |
| • Use gentle, unscented moisturizers. | These products soften and lubricate dry skin. Moisturizers with scent contain alcohol, which may increase skin dryness. |
| • Avoid putting moisturizer between the toes. | Moisturizer between the toes may macerate the skin, causing skin breakdown. |
| • Instruct patient or caregiver to cut toenails straight across after softening them during a bath. File nails with an emery board. Encourage patient to see podiatrist for preventative foot care. If patient is hospitalized, consult with a podiatrist to cut patient's toenails. | These actions help prevent ingrown toenails, which could lead to infection. |
| • Do not self-treat corns or calluses; visit a podiatrist regularly. Do not go barefoot indoors or outdoors. | These measures minimize the risk for trauma, which could lead to infection and ultimately to amputation. |
| • Attend to any foot injury immediately and seek medical attention. | Diabetes can cause slow wound healing. Prompt care can prevent a small injury from becoming worse. |

## Patient Problem/Analyze Cues/Prioritize Hypotheses

# Deficient Knowledge (Diabetes Treatment)

*due to* unfamiliarity with proper insulin administration, dietary precautions, and exercise for promoting normoglycemia

***Desired Outcome/Generate Solutions:*** Within the 24-hour period before hospital discharge, the patient verbalizes and demonstrates an accurate knowledge of proper insulin administration, symptoms and treatment of hypoglycemia, the prescribed dietary regimen, and the role of exercise in promoting normoglycemia.

| ASSESSMENT—RECOGNIZE CUES/ INTERVENTIONS—TAKE ACTION | RATIONALES |
|---|---|
| Assess the patient's health care literacy (language, reading, comprehension). Assess the culture and culturally specific information needs. | This assessment helps ensure that information is selected and presented in a manner that is culturally and educationally appropriate. |
| Instruct the patient to check the expiration date on the insulin vial and to avoid using it if outdated. Instruct the patient to date the insulin vial when it is first accessed. | Insulin may lose potency if the bottle has been open for more than 30 days. |
| Provide instructions on the proper storage of insulin and the importance of avoiding temperature extremes. | Extreme temperatures destroy insulin. |
| Instruct the patient to use U-100, U-200, U-300, or U-500 insulins with the appropriate syringe for the type of insulin. | The patient must be made aware there are differences in strengths of insulin suspensions, and each strength must be given using the appropriate insulin syringe or pen. |
| Suggest that the patient ask their health care provider if the prescribed insulin is available in an insulin pen. | An insulin pen eliminates the chance for errors because the pen is a self-enclosed dosing system, wherein the patient applies a new needle and sets the dose using a dial on the pen. |
| If the patient is prescribed intermediate- and long-acting insulin that requires mixing, demonstrate rolling the insulin vial between the palms of the hands to mix contents. | Insulin additives separate when the bottle is stationary and must be remixed to ensure appropriate concentration throughout the vial. |
| Explain that long-acting analogue insulins (glargine/Lantus, detemir/Levemir, degludec/Tresiba) need to be administered only once or twice daily, depending on the dose. | Long-acting insulin analogs do not have a profound peak action. After glargine is injected and absorbed, the action is consistent over 24 hours, detemir is approximately 20 hours, and degludec up to 42 hours. |
| Caution the patient to avoid shaking the vial of insulin. | Shaking produces air bubbles that can interfere with accurate dose measurement. |
| Explain that regular prandial insulin (e.g., NovoLin or HumuLin) should be injected 30 minutes before eating a meal; insulin analogs (NovoLog, HumaLog, Apidra) may be injected immediately before eating. | Time of onset/peak of regular insulins is slightly delayed compared with that of the newer insulins. |
| Explain that either making a change in insulin type or withholding a dose of insulin may be required under various circumstances. | These instances include the following: when fasting for studies or surgery, when not eating because of nausea/vomiting, or when hypoglycemic. Stress from illness or infection can increase insulin requirements (or necessitate insulin therapy for one whose condition is normally controlled with oral hypoglycemics), and increased exercise will necessitate additional food intake to prevent hypoglycemia when no change is made in insulin dose. Adjustments are always individually based and require clarification with the patient's health care provider. |
| Provide a chart that depicts injection site rotations. Explain that injection sites should be at least 1 inch apart. | Injections in or near the same site each time may result in the development of lipodystrophy, which will delay and/or decrease insulin absorption. |
| Depending on the amount of subcutaneous fat, explain the importance of inserting the needle at a 45- to 90-degree angle to the skin. | This ensures subcutaneous administration of insulin. |
| Ensure the patient understands and demonstrates the technique and timing for home monitoring of blood glucose using a commercial kit. | A commercial kit provides ongoing data reflecting the degree of control and may identify necessary changes in diet and medication before severe metabolic changes occur. Self-monitoring by patients is extremely useful in reducing complications. Self-monitoring also enables the patient's self-control and psychologic security. |

| ASSESSMENT—RECOGNIZE CUES/ INTERVENTIONS—TAKE ACTION | RATIONALES |
|---|---|
| Instruct the patient on the importance of following a diet that is controlled in simple carbohydrates, consistent in complex carbohydrates, low in fat, and high in fiber. | Adequate nutrition, along with controlled carbohydrates and calories, is essential to maintaining normoglycemia in these individuals. A diet low in fat and high in fiber is an effective means of controlling blood fats, especially cholesterol and triglycerides. Complex carbohydrates are metabolized more slowly than simple carbohydrates. Consistent consumption of complex carbohydrates prevents "spikes" in blood glucose following consumption. Diet is the sole method of control for many individuals with type 2 DM. Typically, three daily meals and an evening snack are prescribed. Some fat and protein should be present in all meals and snacks to slow down the elevation of postprandial blood glucose. Adding 10–15 g of fiber will slow the digestion of monosaccharides and disaccharides. For all types of diabetes, refined and simple sugars and carbohydrates (white bread, any crackers made with processed flour) should be reduced and complex carbohydrates (whole grain products including breads, cereals, pasta, legumes, beans, and lentils) encouraged. Carbohydrate counting is encouraged. Weight control and weight loss for overweight individuals are of the highest priority when managing DM. |
| Provide the patient with instructions on how to count carbohydrates. The "magic number" used for counting carbohydrates generally is 15 because 15 g of carbohydrates=one serving of carbohydrates. Many carbohydrate-controlled diets allow four servings of carbohydrates per day. Complex carbohydrates are preferred to simple carbohydrates because they have a lower glycemic index; thus complex carbohydrates raise blood glucose more gradually than do simple carbohydrates. | This promotes self-management regarding the patient's food intake. |
| For patients who experience low blood glucose at night, discuss commercially available long-acting carbohydrate sources. | Long-acting carbohydrate sources may decrease the risk for nighttime low blood glucose levels. |
| Instruct the patient to be alert to changes in mentation, apprehension, erratic behavior, trembling, slurred speech, staggering gait, and seizure activity. | These are indicators of hypoglycemia. |
| Explain that the use of oral antidiabetic agents should be discussed with the provider before planned surgery or diagnostic procedures associated with IV contrast. Provide instructions to the patient on treatment of hypoglycemia as prescribed. | Metformin has been associated with the development of lactic acidosis in rare cases resulting from procedures involving the use of contrast, and in patients with heart failure, kidney disease, or liver disease. Hypoglycemia involving some of the oral antidiabetic agents can be severe and persistent. Monitoring must be diligent. Any condition, situation, or medication that enhances the hypoglycemic effects of these drugs requires close monitoring of blood glucose when symptoms of hypoglycemia arise. Common factors in the development of hypoglycemia are fasting for diagnostic purposes, skipping meals, unplanned increase in activity, malnourishment related to illness or nausea and vomiting, and other medication therapy (any of which adds to the hypoglycemic action of the oral hypoglycemics). Use of oral antidiabetic agents in hospitalized patients is discouraged because the potential for unstable blood glucose is great. Inpatient hyperglycemia may be best managed with insulin until the patient stabilizes. |
| Provide patient with information on signs, symptoms, and causes, of hyperglycemia. Hyperglycemia can occur with increased food intake, too little insulin, decreased exercise, infection or illness, and emotional stress. Signs and symptoms of hyperglycemia (polydipsia, polyuria, polyphagia, fatigue, fruity smelling breath) can appear within hours or even several days. Hyperglycemia can be detected during routine self-testing of blood glucose. | Patient will then be aware of warning signs and test for hyperglycemia during self-testing. Increased blood glucose can then be corrected, or health care provider would be notified before levels are out of control. |

Continued

Endocrine Care Plans

| ASSESSMENT—RECOGNIZE CUES/ INTERVENTIONS—TAKE ACTION | RATIONALES |
|---|---|
| Instruct that the following herbal remedies may cause changes in blood glucose levels and should only be used with health care provider permission: aloe vera, banaba, bitter melon, chia, cinnamon longa, fenugreek, ginseng, *Gymnema sylvestre*, milk thistle, nopal, and *Salacia oblonga*. | All herbal remedies listed promote lowering of the blood glucose level, which may cause hypoglycemia if taken with antidiabetic drugs. |
| Explain the importance of adequate sleep and exercise in maintaining optimal blood glucose levels. | Exercise and sleep are as important as diet, use of oral hypoglycemic agents, and insulin in treating DM. Exercise lowers blood glucose levels, helps maintain normal cholesterol levels, and decreases insulin resistance at the sites of muscle receptors. At least 150 minutes per week of walking, stair climbing, or other aerobic exercise is recommended. Adequate sleep lowers the stress experienced by the body, which helps to control the stress response. About 7 hours of sleep nightly is recommended. These effects increase the body's ability to metabolize glucose and help reduce the therapeutic dose of insulin for most patients. The exercise program must be consistent and individualized (especially for individuals with type 1 DM). Patients should be given a complete physical examination and encouraged to incorporate acceptable activities as part of their daily routine. |

## ADDITIONAL PROBLEMS:

| | |
|---|---|
| *Difficulty Coping* | Chapter 8 |

## ✓ PATIENT–FAMILY TEACHING AND DISCHARGE PLANNING

The American Association of Diabetes Care & Education Specialists (ADCES) recommends that all patients with diabetes have access to self-management information, focusing on the ADCES7 Self-Care Behaviors: (1) healthy eating, (2) being active, (3) monitoring, (4) taking medication, (5) problem solving, (6) healthy coping, and (7) reducing risks.

- ✓ Focus on sensory information, avoid giving excessive information, and initiate a visiting nurse referral for necessary follow-up teaching. Ask about existing knowledge of the disease, ability for self-management, and acceptance of the disease during initial assessment. Include verbal and written information about the following:
- ✓ Importance of carrying a diabetic identification card, wearing a medical alert bracelet or necklace, and having identification card outline diagnosis and emergency treatment. For information, contact MedicAlert Foundation at www.medicalert.org.
- ✓ Recognizing warning signs of both hyperglycemia and hypoglycemia, treatment, and factors that contribute to both conditions. Emphasize the importance of disclosing all alternative and complementary health practices being used because some may affect blood glucose or possibly lead to adverse drug reactions. Remind the patient that stress from illness or infection can increase insulin

requirements (or necessitate insulin therapy for one who is normally controlled with oral hypoglycemics) and that increased exercise will necessitate additional food intake to prevent hypoglycemia when no change is made in insulin dosage under normoglycemic conditions. Blood glucose at a level greater than 250 mg/dL at the beginning of exercise may make the exercise a stressor that elevates rather than decreases the glucose level.

- ✓ Drugs that cause hyperglycemia: estrogens, corticosteroids, thyroid preparations, beta-adrenergic agonists (many respiratory aerosols or inhalers), diuretics, phenytoin, glucagon, drugs containing sugar (e.g., cough syrup), and certain antibiotics. Drugs that cause hypoglycemia: salicylates, sulfonamides, tetracyclines, methyldopa, anabolic steroids, acetaminophen, monoamine oxidase inhibitors, ethanol, haloperidol, and marijuana. Beta-adrenergic blocking agents may mask the signs of and inhibit recovery from hypoglycemia. For a list of herbal remedies that affect blood glucose, see *Deficient Knowledge*, previously.
- ✓ Home monitoring of blood glucose using commercial kits, which provide ongoing data reflecting degree of control and may identify necessary changes in diet and medication before severe metabolic changes occur. These tests also provide a means for the patient's self-control and psychologic security. In addition, kits for monitoring glycohemoglobin (hemoglobin A1C) are available for home use and may assist patients in determining the overall effectiveness of their diabetes management regimen. New, smaller lancets allow more frequent blood glucose testing by decreasing pain from fingersticks. Stress the need for careful control of blood glucose as a means of decreasing risk for or minimizing long-term complications of DM.

Encourage the patient to rotate sites as much as possible to avoid possibility of injuring any one site. There are also the discs, like freestyle libre and dexcom, that allow testing without fingersticks (CGM).

✓ Importance of daily exercise, sleep, maintenance of normal body weight, smoking cessation, and yearly medical evaluation. Explain that sleep and exercise are as important as diet in treating DM. Exercise lowers blood glucose, helps maintain normal cholesterol levels, and increases circulation. Approximately 7 hours of nightly sleep helps to lower the overall stress level and reduce the occurrence of the stress response. These effects increase the body's ability to metabolize glucose and help reduce the therapeutic dose of insulin for most patients.

✓ Stress that each exercise program must be individualized (especially for persons with type 1 DM) and implemented consistently. The patient should have a complete physical examination and then be encouraged to incorporate acceptable exercise activities into his or her daily routine. Smoking cessation is a health habit well recognized to reduce the incidence of cardiovascular disease.

✓ Review of diet that is consistent in carbohydrates, low in fat, and high in fiber as an effective means of controlling blood fats, especially cholesterol and triglycerides. Stress that diet is the sole method of control for many individuals with type 2 DM. Adequate nutrition with controlled carbohydrates and calories is essential to maintain normoglycemia in these individuals. Patients who gained weight before developing type 2 DM are sometimes able to normalize their blood glucose by losing weight and maintaining optimal body weight.

✓ Use of syringe magnifiers that can be used by patients with poor visual acuity. Other products that permit safe and accurate filling of syringes are also available.

✓ Rotating injection sites and injecting insulin at room temperature. Provide a chart showing possible injection sites and describe the system for site rotation.

✓ Importance of daily meticulous skin, wound, and foot care.

✓ Necessity of annual eye examination for early detection and treatment of retinopathy.

✓ Scheduling dental checkups at least every 6 months to help prevent periodontal disease, a major problem for individuals with DM. The mouth often is the primary site of origination for low-grade infections.

✓ Medications, including purpose, dosage, schedule, precautions, interactions, and potential side effects for all medications used. Also discuss drug–drug, food–drug, and herb–drug interactions.

✓ Identifying available resources for ongoing assistance and information, including nurses, dietitian, the patient's health care provider, and other individuals with DM in patient care unit. Other resources include the local chapter of ADA, the local chapter of the ADCES, and local library for free access to current materials on diabetes. The following is a list of resources available to patients:

- American Diabetes Association: www.diabetes.org
- ADCES: www.diabeteseducator.org
- American Association of Diabetes Educators Patient Resources: https://www.diabeteseducator.org/patient-resources
- Joslin Diabetes Center: www.joslin.org
- National Institute of Diabetes and Digestive and Kidney Diseases: https://www.niddk.nih.gov/health-information/diabetes
- American Heart Association, National Center: www.americanheart.org

✓ The following is a list of journals available for patients:

- Diabetes Forecast: http://forecast.diabetes.org/
- Diabetes Health Magazine: www.diabeteshealth.com
- Diabetes Self-Management: www.diabetesselfmanagement.com

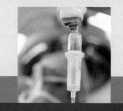

# Diabetic Ketoacidosis 48

## OVERVIEW/PATHOPHYSIOLOGY

Diabetic ketoacidosis (DKA) is a life-threatening condition and complication associated with type 1 diabetes. It is caused by a devastating lack of effective insulin resulting in severe hyperglycemia, ketoacidosis, and dehydration. Abnormal carbohydrate, fat, and protein metabolism results in the production of ketones. The intracellular environment is unable to receive necessary glucose for oxidation and energy production without insulin to facilitate the transport of glucose from the bloodstream across the cell membrane. Impairment of glucose uptake results in hyperglycemia, while the intracellular environment continues to lack the necessary nutrients for normal metabolism. Glucagon secretion is then triggered in an attempt to provide cell nourishment, which further contributes to elevated ketones. Impaired amino acid transport, protein synthesis, and protein degradation facilitate protein catabolism with a resultant increase in serum amino acids, whereas fat breakdown results in elevated free fatty acids (FFAs) and glycerol. The liver converts the newly available amino acids, fatty acids, and glycerol into glucose (gluconeogenesis) in an attempt to provide nourishment for the cells, but intracellular nourishment is not possible without the ability for glucose to be transported into the cells. Glucose remains outside the cells in the bloodstream, and hyperglycemia worsens because of the lack of insulin. The liver also produces ketone bodies from available FFAs, causing mild to severe acidosis. As ketone bodies increase in the extracellular fluid, the hydrogen ions within the ketones are exchanged with K ions from within the cells. Intracellular $K^+$ is released into the extracellular fluid and therefore to circulating fluid, where it is excreted by the kidneys into the urine. Hyperglycemia creates an environment wherein excessive glucose in the bloodstream acts as an osmotic diuretic, causing severe fluid and electrolyte losses, leading to hypovolemic shock and death if untreated.

## HEALTH CARE SETTING

Acute care (intensive care unit), diabetes units

## ASSESSMENT/DIAGNOSTIC TESTS

*Clinical findings.* Signs and symptoms are a result mainly of hyperglycemia, intracellular hypoglycemia, hypotension or impending hypovolemic shock, and fluid–electrolyte imbalance with possible acid–base imbalance.

*Neurologic:* Altered level of consciousness (LOC) (confusion, lethargy, irritability, coma), stroke-like symptoms (unilateral/bilateral weakness, paralysis, numbness, paresthesia), fatigue

*Respiratory:* Deep, rapid Kussmaul respirations

*Cardiovascular:* Tachycardia, hypotension, electrocardiogram (ECG) changes

*Metabolic/gastrointestinal (GI)/endocrine:* Polyuria, polyphagia, polydipsia, fruity "acetone" breath, abdominal pain, weight loss, fatigue, generalized weakness, nausea, vomiting

*Integumentary:* Dry, flushed skin; poor turgor; dry mucous membranes

*Vital signs (VS):* blood pressure (BP) low (more than 20% below normal), heart rate (HR) more than 100 bpm, central venous pressure (CVP) less than 2 mm Hg (less than 5 cm $H_2O$), temperature normal

**Diagnostic tests/laboratory values:** Values reflect dehydration/metabolic acidosis (ketosis) secondary to hyperglycemia, abnormal lipolysis, and osmotic diuresis; fluid loss 6.5 L or more.

*Anion gap:* more than 10 mEq/L

*Hemoglobin/Hematocrit:* elevated

*Serum BUN/creatinine:* elevated

*Serum electrolytes:* decreased sodium, potassium, chloride, magnesium, and phosphate

*Serum glucose:* 250 mg/dL and higher (+ ketones)

*Serum ketones:* elevated

*Arterial blood gases (ABGs):* pH less than 7.30, $HCO_3$ less than 16 mEq/L

*Serum osmolality:* 300–350 mOsm/L

*Urine glucose/acetone:* positive/positive

## Patient Problem/Analyze Cues/Prioritize Hypotheses

# Dehydration

*due to* the failure of regulatory mechanisms and decreased circulating volume occurring with hyperglycemia

*Desired Outcomes/Generate Solutions:* The patient becomes normovolemic within 12 hours of treatment, as evidenced by BP of 90/60 mm Hg or more (or within the patient's normal range), HR of 60–100 bpm, CVP of 6–8 mm Hg, elastic skin turgor, moist and pink mucous membranes, specific gravity no higher than 1.020, balanced intake and output (I&O), and urinary output at least 0.5 mL/kg/hour. Electrolyte levels are within normal limits.

| ASSESSMENT—RECOGNIZE CUES/ INTERVENTIONS—TAKE ACTION | RATIONALES |
|---|---|
| • Assess for signs and symptoms of profound dehydration, which can lead to hypovolemic shock. Check for changes in VS every 15 minutes until the patient remains stable for 1 hour. Notify the health care provider promptly of significant findings. | Hyperglycemia acts as an osmotic diuretic, causing severe fluid and electrolyte losses that can lead to hypovolemic shock if untreated. HR greater than 120 bpm, BP less than 90/60 mm Hg or decreased 20 mm Hg or more from baseline, and CVP less than 2 mm Hg are signs of hypovolemia and will need prompt intervention. |
| Assess for poor skin turgor, dry mucous membranes, sunken and soft eyeballs, tachycardia, and orthostatic hypotension. | These are physical indicators of hypovolemia and will need prompt intervention. |
| Measure I&O accurately and weigh the patient daily. Monitor urine specific gravity and report findings of more than 1.020 in the presence of other indicators of dehydration. Report to the health care provider if urine output is less than 30 mL/hour or less than 0.5 mL/kg/hour for 2 consecutive hours. | Decreasing urinary output may signal diminishing intravascular fluid volume or impending renal failure. Loss of weight and output that exceeds intake may signal dehydration. However, loss of weight is unlikely in the setting of aggressive rehydration. To ensure accuracy, weight should be measured on the same scale at the same time of day each day. |
| Administer the intravenous (IV) fluids as prescribed. | This ensures adequate rehydration. |
| Usually, normal saline or 0.45% saline is administered until plasma glucose falls to 200–300 mg/dL. After that, dextrose-containing solutions usually are given to prevent rebound hypoglycemia. Initially, IV fluids are administered rapidly (i.e., up to 2000 mL infused during the first 2 hours of treatment and 150–250 mL/hour thereafter until BP stabilizes). | |
| Closely monitor the correction of fluid and electrolyte loss during the first hour of treatment. | Rehydration is followed by gradual correction of hyperglycemia and acidosis. Correction of fluid loss may resolve acidosis. Any signs of dehydration may indicate more than 3 L of fluid was lost. Low fluid volume in the vasculature increases the risk for blood clotting due to the low flow of thicker blood, putting the patient at risk for stroke, myocardial infarction (MI), and deep vein thrombosis (DVT). It is essential to maintain extreme vigilance for any concomitant process such as infection, cerebrovascular accident, MI, sepsis, or DVT. |
| ❗ Be alert to indicators of fluid overload when rapidly rehydrating, particularly in elders or in patients with a history of heart failure or renal failure. | Indicators of fluid overload (jugular vein distention, dyspnea, crackles, CVP more than 12 mm Hg) can occur with rapid infusion of fluids. |
| Administer the insulin as prescribed. | Insulin usually is given by continuous IV infusion for rapid action and because poor tissue perfusion caused by dehydration sometimes makes the subcutaneous route less effective. |
| Numerous protocols for IV insulin infusion are available and vary widely in the dosing regimen. Infusion protocols usually require a dosage increase when the blood glucose fails to decrease. Safer, more effective protocols should take into consideration the patient's level of insulin sensitivity and/or insulin resistance. The continuous infusion is administered through a separate IV tubing and controlled with an infusion control device. Computerized insulin dosing systems, dosing tables, and dosing algorithms are available. Dosage is adjusted based on serial glucose levels and the resolution of ketosis. | When formulas are used, the insulin sensitivity number is reflected as a variable multiplier that increases with higher levels of insulin resistance. |
| When the blood glucose level stabilizes, pH is greater than 7.3, bicarbonate is more than 18 mEq/L, and the patient is allowed to eat a meal, anticipate transitioning insulin administration to a subcutaneous dose. | Hospital discharge is delayed until a return to the patient's daily insulin regimen without a recurrence of ketosis. |

Continued

Endocrine Care Plans

| ASSESSMENT—RECOGNIZE CUES/ INTERVENTIONS—TAKE ACTION | RATIONALES |
|---|---|
| Before initiating treatment, flush the tubing with at least 30 mL of the insulin-containing IV solution. | Insulin, when added to IV solutions, may be absorbed by the container and plastic tubing. Flushing the tubing ensures that maximum absorption of the insulin by the container and tubing has occurred before it is delivered to the patient. |
| If connecting the insulin infusion into another IV line, use the port closest to the patient to avoid unnecessary insulin dosage increases. | Using the port closest to the patient ensures the insulin is entering the bloodstream, rather than making the journey down lengthy tubing when "point of care" blood glucose readings are done. |
| Monitor laboratory results for abnormalities. Promptly report to the health care provider serum $K^+$ levels less than 3.5 mEq/L. Observe for clinical manifestations of the electrolyte, glucose, and acid–base imbalances associated with DKA as follows:<br><br>• *Hypokalemia:* Muscle weakness, hypotension, anorexia, drowsiness, hypoactive bowel sounds.<br><br>• *Hyponatremia:* Headache, malaise, muscle weakness, abdominal cramps, nausea, seizures, coma.<br><br>• *Hypophosphatemia:* Muscle weakness, progressive encephalopathy possibly leading to coma.<br><br>• *Hypomagnesemia:* Anorexia, nausea, vomiting, lethargy, weakness, personality changes, tetany, tremor or muscle fasciculations, seizures, confusion progressing to coma.<br><br>• *Hypochloremia:* Hypertonicity of muscles, tetany, depressed respirations.<br><br>• *Hypoglycemia:* Headache, impaired mentation, agitation, dizziness, nausea, pallor, tremors, tachycardia, diaphoresis.<br><br>• *Metabolic acidosis:* Lassitude, nausea, vomiting, Kussmaul respirations, lethargy progressing to coma. | Before treatment, there is a risk for hyperkalemia from excess transport of intracellular $K^+$ to extracellular spaces as a result of the acidosis. $Na^+$ and $Cl^-$ are replaced with IV normal saline. $K^+$ must be monitored and corrected carefully. After initiation of treatment, $K^+$ returns to the intracellular compartment through accelerated transport into cells through insulin and after correction of acidosis, and therefore the patient is at risk for becoming hypokalemic. Proper rehydration and insulin dosing should correct ketoacidosis and lactic acidosis resulting from hypoperfusion due to hypovolemia and/or hypovolemic shock. |

## Patient Problem/Analyze Cues/Prioritize Hypotheses

# Risk for Infection

*due to* inadequate secondary defenses (suppressed inflammatory response) occurring with protein depletion

***Desired Outcome/Generate Solutions:*** The patient is free of infection as evidenced by normothermia, HR of 100 bpm or less, BP within the patient's normal range, white blood cell (WBC) count of 11,000/mm³ or less, and negative culture results.

| ASSESSMENT—RECOGNIZE CUES/ INTERVENTIONS—TAKE ACTION | RATIONALES |
|---|---|
| Assess for evidence of infection. Monitor the laboratory results for increased WBC count; culture the purulent drainage as prescribed. | Infection is the most common cause of DKA in adults, whereas nonadherence to treatment regimen is more likely responsible for DKA in children and teenagers. Indicators of infection include fever, chills, pain with urination, vomiting, erythema and swelling around IV sites, and increased WBC count. |
| Use meticulous hand hygiene when caring for the patient. | Patients are at increased risk for bacterial infection because of suppressed inflammatory response. |

| ASSESSMENT—RECOGNIZE CUES/ INTERVENTIONS—TAKE ACTION | RATIONALES |
|---|---|
| Manage invasive lines carefully. Schedule dressing changes according to agency policy. Peripheral IV sites should be rotated at least every 96 hours (or as per facility policy) and dressings changed, depending on agency policy. Central lines should be discontinued as soon as feasible, as prescribed, and when in place should be kept clean. | These measures help prevent infection from peripheral or central IV sites. |
| Inspect insertion sites for erythema, swelling, or purulent drainage. Document the presence of any of these indicators and notify the health care provider. | These are signs of local infection that should be reported promptly for timely intervention. |
| Provide thorough skin care. | Intact skin is the first line of defense against infection. |
| Provide a pressure-relief mattress or pressure redistribution surface on the patient's bed. | These surfaces help prevent skin breakdown, which could lead to infection. |
| Use the meticulous sterile technique when caring for or inserting indwelling urinary catheters. | This minimizes the risk for bacterial entry into the body. |
| **Note:** Limit the use of indwelling urethral catheters to patients who are unable to void in a bedpan or when continuous assessment of urine output is essential. | There is an increased risk for infection with indwelling catheters. Nationally recognized nurse-sensitive indicators recommend that, if an indwelling catheter is inserted, every effort be made to remove it within 48 hours. |
| Encourage hourly use of incentive spirometry while the patient is awake, along with deep-breathing and coughing exercises. When the patient stabilizes, encourage and enable the patient to get out of bed. | Deep inhalations with incentive spirometry along with deep-breathing exercises expand alveoli and help mobilize secretions to the airways. Coughing further mobilizes and clears the secretions. These exercises help prevent pulmonary infection. Activity also helps mobilize secretions. |

## Patient Problems/Analyze Cues/Prioritize Hypotheses

# Risk for Impaired Cognition

*due to* altered cerebral function occurring with dehydration or cerebral edema associated with DKA

***Desired Outcomes/Generate Solutions:*** The patient verbalizes orientation to person, place, and time and does not demonstrate a significant change in mental status; clear breath sounds are auscultated over the patient's airway.

| ASSESSMENT—RECOGNIZE CUES/ INTERVENTIONS—TAKE ACTION | RATIONALES |
|---|---|
| Assess the patient's mental status; orientation; LOC; and respiratory status, especially airway patency, at frequent intervals. | With DKA, cerebral function may be altered because of dehydration or cerebral edema. |
| Keep an appropriate-sized oral airway, manual resuscitator and mask, and supplemental oxygen at the bedside. | In older patients the increased work of breathing may exceed their ability to compensate, and this can result in respiratory arrest. In very rare instances, increased intracranial pressure caused by cerebral edema may impinge on the brainstem, prompting respiratory arrest. |
| Maintain the bed in the lowest position, monitor the patient closely, and keep side rails up at all times. | These measures reduce the likelihood of injury from falls resulting from the patient's altered cerebral function. |
| Elevate the head of the bed to 45 degrees. | This elevation minimizes the risk for aspiration. |

Patient Problem/Analyze Cues/Prioritize Hypotheses
# Risk for Impaired Tissue Perfusion

*due to* interrupted venous or arterial flow occurring with increased blood viscosity, increased platelet aggregation/adhesiveness, and patient immobility

**Desired Outcomes/Generate Solutions:** Optimally, the patient has peripheral pulses greater than 2+ on a 0–4+ scale; warm skin; brisk capillary refill (less than 2 seconds); and absence of swelling, bluish discoloration, erythema, and discomfort in the calves and thighs. Alternatively, if signs of excessive clotting appear, they are detected and reported promptly.

| ASSESSMENT—RECOGNIZE CUES/ INTERVENTIONS—TAKE ACTION | RATIONALES |
|---|---|
| Assess for hemoconcentration by monitoring hematocrit results. | With proper fluid replacement, results should return to normal within 24 hours. |
| Assess for increasing urine output and a reduction in BUN and creatinine values. | Normal BUN value is 7–21 mg/dL. Normal creatinine is 0.6–1.1 mg/dL for women and 0.7–1.3 mg/dL for men. An increasing or normalizing urine output, coupled with decreasing BUN and creatinine values, is an indicator of improved renal perfusion. |
| Assess peripheral pulses every 2–4 hours and report significant findings. | Significant decreases in amplitude or absence of pulse should be reported to the health care provider promptly because it may signal DVT/venous thromboembolism (VTE) or other causes of perfusion deficit (e.g., dehydration). |
| [!] Be alert to erythema, pain, tenderness, warmth, and swelling over area of thrombus and bluish discoloration, paleness, coolness, and dilation of superficial veins in distal extremities, especially lower extremities. | These are indicators of DVT/VTE. For more information, see "Venous Thrombosis/Thrombophlebitis," Chapter 26. |
| [!] Also be alert to pain, paresthesias (especially loss of sensation of light touch and two-point discrimination), cyanosis with delayed capillary refill, mottling, and coolness of the extremity. | These are indicators of arterial thrombosis, which can lead to profound limb ischemia and tissue hypoxia and eventually to tissue anoxia and death. |
| Report significant findings to the health care provider immediately. | When untreated, limb ischemia may result in the loss of limb and/or digits. |
| Encourage the patient to exercise extremities every 2 hours. | Exercise increases blood flow to the tissues. Calf pumping and ankle circles should be encouraged at least every 2 hours in patients susceptible to DVT/VTE. |
| Unless contraindicated, encourage the fluid intake to more than 1000 mL/ day. | Increased hydration decreases the potential for hemoconcentration, which could lead to DVT/VTE. |
| Apply pneumatic alternating pressure stockings or pneumatic foot pumps as prescribed. | These garments and devices promote venous return and aid in the prevention of thrombosis. |

Patient Problem/Analyze Cues/Prioritize Hypotheses
# Deficient Knowledge (Disease Management)

*due to* unfamiliarity with the cause, prevention, and treatment of DKA

**Desired Outcome/Generate Solutions:** Within the 24-hour period before hospital discharge, the patient verbalizes an accurate understanding of the cause, prevention, and treatment of DKA.

## ASSESSMENT—RECOGNIZE CUES/ INTERVENTIONS—TAKE ACTION

## RATIONALES

| ASSESSMENT—RECOGNIZE CUES/ INTERVENTIONS—TAKE ACTION | RATIONALES |
|---|---|
| Assess the patient's health care literacy (language, reading, comprehension). Assess culture and culturally specific information needs. | This assessment helps ensure that information is selected and presented in a manner that is culturally and educationally appropriate. |
| Determine the patient's knowledge about DKA and its treatment. | This will enable, as needed, further explanation of the disease process of DM and DKA and common early symptoms of worsening hyperglycemia, including polyuria, polydipsia, polyphagia, dry and flushed skin, and increased irritability. |
| Assess the patient's ability to engage in self-management of blood glucose monitoring and control. Explore whether the patient psychologically accepts the disease as a significant health challenge. | This information will enable individualized teaching that will facilitate adherence to the prescribed management regimen designed to maintain normoglycemia. |
| Stress the importance of maintaining a consistently controlled carbohydrate diet, exercise, and insulin regimen. | This regimen helps ensure optimal control of serum glucose levels and prevention of adverse physical effects of DM, such as peripheral neuropathies and increased atherosclerosis. |
| Explain the importance of blood glucose monitoring during episodes of stress, injury, and illness. Caution that DKA necessitates professional medical management and cannot be self-treated. | Increased stress affects the metabolism of carbohydrates, fats, and proteins, causing increased blood glucose. |
| Discuss "sick day management," which includes continuing the same insulin regimen: *not* stopping insulin or skipping doses, testing urine ketones if ill or vomiting, and increasing the frequency of blood glucose testing to monitor more closely for hyperglycemia. | Testing urine ketones may be advised. Blood glucose greater than 250 mg/dL and the appearance of large amounts of urine ketones should be reported to the health care provider so that insulin dose can be increased. |
| Remind the patient of the importance of maintaining adequate oral fluid intake during illness despite anorexia or nausea. | Anorexia or nausea may limit food intake, but patients should make every effort to continue fluid intake to avoid dehydration, hypovolemia, and possible hypotension. |
| Review the testing and insulin administration procedure as indicated. | Insulin or insulin analog must be taken 1–4 times/day as prescribed, and lifetime insulin therapy is necessary to achieve control of blood glucose. |
| ⚠ Educate the patient about the importance of receiving prompt treatment if such indicators as dizziness, impaired mentation, irritability, pallor, and tremors occur. | These are signs of insulin or insulin analogue excess (hypoglycemia). The American Diabetes Association (ADA) promotes the 15-15 rule when treating hypoglycemia: 15 g of carbohydrate to raise blood sugar and then check it after 15 minutes. If below 79 mg/dL, have another serving. |
| ⚠ Caution the patient to get prompt treatment if the following indicators occur: polyuria, polydipsia, polyphagia, or increasingly dry and flushed skin. | These are signs of hyperglycemia. |
| Explain the consequences of not receiving prompt treatment. | If untreated, these conditions could lead to coma and death. |
| Explain the importance of dietary changes as prescribed by the health care provider. | Typically, patients are put on a consistent carbohydrate diet. Counting carbohydrates and prescribing insulin dosage according to the amount of carbohydrates consumed is a strategy of blood glucose management. |
| Advise that fats should be polyunsaturated and proteins chosen from low-fat sources. | Reducing saturated fat intake reduces the risk for developing coronary artery and peripheral vascular disease. |
| Provide instructions on the importance of eating three meals per day at regularly scheduled times and a bedtime snack. | Such a diet affords the best opportunity for maintaining a physiologically normal blood glucose level rather than "roller coaster" values of alternating hyperglycemia and hypoglycemia. |
| Meals and insulin administration must be linked together, especially when insulin analogues such as HumaLog, NovoLog, or Apidra are given before meals and in conjunction with snacks. Analogues are quicker acting than regular insulins. | |
| Refer patient to a dietician for more information. | |

Continued

| ASSESSMENT—RECOGNIZE CUES/ INTERVENTIONS—TAKE ACTION | RATIONALES |
|---|---|
| Explain the causes for adjustments in insulin dose. Instruct the patient to monitor blood glucose and urine ketone levels closely during periods of increased emotional stress and periods of increased or decreased exercise and to adjust insulin dose accordingly. | Adjustments in insulin dose include increased or decreased food or carbohydrate intake and any physical (e.g., exercise) or emotional stress. Exercise and emotional stress may increase the release of glucose from the liver or increase insulin resistance. |
| • Remind the patient that alternative and complementary health strategies may alter blood glucose levels and prompt a need for adjustment of medications. | For a list of herbal remedies that alter blood glucose, see *Deficient Knowledge* in "Diabetes Mellitus," Chapter 47. |
| • For example, certain herbal preparations can alter metabolism and may increase or decrease blood glucose. All methods used should be reported to the health care provider. | |
| Explain that good hygiene and meticulous daily foot care are necessary to prevent infection. Stress the importance of avoiding exposure to communicable diseases and explain that the following indicators of infection necessitate prompt medical treatment: fever, chills, increased HR, diaphoresis, nausea, and vomiting. In addition, teach the patient and significant other to be alert to wounds or cuts that do not heal, burning or pain with urination, and a productive cough. | Persons with diabetes are susceptible to infection because of decreased immune response. |
| **!** Instruct the patient to implement the following therapy when ill for any reason: | |
| • Do not alter insulin (NovoLin, HumuLin), insulin analog (HumaLog, NovoLog, Apidra), or oral diabetes or hyperglycemia medication dosage unless the health care provider has prescribed a supplemental regimen. | Altering the insulin regimen increases the risk for hypoglycemia if the medication dosage is increased. |
| • Perform blood glucose monitoring at least before every meal and at bedtime, and promptly report glucose greater than 250 mg/dL and positive ketones to the health care provider. | If the insulin dose is decreased for persistent incidences of hypoglycemia, the blood glucose should increase to the normal range with proper dosage. The stress associated with illness alters metabolism and glucose uptake. Hyperglycemia can ensue quickly when patients become ill. |
| • Eat small, frequent meals of soft, easily digestible, nourishing foods if regular meals are not tolerated. | If carbohydrate intake falls significantly, insulin dosage may need to be reduced to prevent hypoglycemia. Smaller, more frequent meals may help maintain a more normal intake. |
| • Maintain an adequate hydration, particularly if diarrhea, vomiting, or fever is persistent. | Dehydration can lead to hypovolemia, which in turn can lead to shock if left untreated. |
| • Use a balance of sugar-containing beverages and water to ensure adequate calories yet prevent hyperosmolality caused by sugars in the beverages. | Intake of carbohydrates must be maintained unless insulin dose is altered to avoid hypoglycemia. Water must be consumed to maintain intravascular volume. There are too many carbohydrates in juice or soda to use either as a primary source of volume. If carbohydrate intake is not appropriately balanced with water intake, glucose may increase, prompting polyuria, which increases the risk for hypovolemia or, if severe, hypovolemic shock. |
| Provide the address of the website for the ADA (www.diabetes.org) See "Diabetes Mellitus," Chapter 47, for a complete listing of organizations that can supply information regarding DM. | The ADA website is the original source of information for pamphlets and magazines related to the disease, its complications, and appropriate treatment. Other sources of information are now available. |

## ADDITIONAL PROBLEM:

| Difficulty Coping (patient) | Chapter 8 |
|---|---|

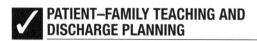

## PATIENT–FAMILY TEACHING AND DISCHARGE PLANNING

See *Deficient Knowledge*, earlier, due to unfamiliarity with cause, prevention, and treatment of DKA.

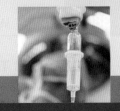

# Hyperglycemic Hyperosmolar Syndrome 49

## OVERVIEW/PATHOPHYSIOLOGY

Hyperglycemic hyperosmolar syndrome (HHS) is a life-threatening emergency resulting from a lack of effective insulin, or severe insulin resistance, causing extreme hyperglycemia. Often HHS is precipitated by a stressor such as trauma, injury, or infection that increases insulin demand. It occurs in people with type 2 diabetes who have enough circulating insulin to prevent acidosis and the formation of ketone bodies at the cellular level but not enough insulin to facilitate the transportation of all the glucose into the cells. Thus glucose molecules accumulate in the bloodstream, causing serum hyperosmolality with resultant osmotic diuresis and simultaneous loss of electrolytes, most notably potassium, sodium, and phosphate. HHS occurs most commonly in older people (over 60) with type 2 diabetes mellitus (DM), but due to more younger adults and children who are diagnosed with type 2 diabetes, HHS may occur in all ages.

**Caution:** Patients may lose up to 25% of their total body water. Fluids are pulled from individual body cells by increasing serum hyperosmolality and extracellular fluid loss, causing intracellular dehydration and body cell shrinkage. Neurologic deficits (e.g., slowed mentation, confusion, seizures, stroke-like symptoms, coma) can occur as a result. Loss of extracellular fluid stimulates aldosterone release, which facilitates sodium retention and prevents further loss of potassium. However, aldosterone cannot halt severe dehydration. As extracellular volume decreases, blood viscosity increases, causing slowing of blood flow. Increased blood viscosity, enhanced platelet aggregation and adhesiveness, and decreased mobility increase the risk for thrombus formation. Cardiac workload is increased and may lead to myocardial infarction. Renal blood flow is decreased, potentially resulting in renal impairment or failure. Stroke may result from thromboemboli or decreased cerebral perfusion. The mortality rate of HHS is high, although mortality data are difficult to interpret because of the high incidence of coexisting diseases or comorbidities. The main goals in the treatment of HHS are rehydration, correction of hyperglycemia and electrolyte imbalance, management of underlying diseases, and monitoring/support of organs affected by highly viscous blood. Increased blood viscosity creates high risk for myocardial infarction, circulatory collapse, stroke, thromboembolism, acute respiratory failure, and acute kidney failure.

The cascade of events in HHS begins with osmotic diuresis. Glycosuria impairs the ability of the kidney to concentrate urine, which exacerbates the water loss. Normally, the kidneys eliminate glucose above a certain threshold and prevent a subsequent rise in blood glucose level. In HHS the decreased intravascular volume or possible underlying renal disease decreases the glomerular filtration rate, causing the glucose level to increase. More water is lost than sodium, resulting in hyperosmolarity. Insulin is present, but not in adequate amounts to decrease blood glucose levels, and with type 2 DM, significant insulin resistance may be present.

Unlike DKA, in which ketoacidosis produces severe symptoms requiring fairly prompt hospitalization, symptoms of HHS develop more slowly and often are nonspecific. The anion gap is normal because there is no ketone production. The cardinal symptoms of polyuria and polydipsia are noted first but may be ignored by older persons or their families. Neurologic deficits may be mistaken for dementia. The similarity of these symptoms to those of other disease processes common to this age group may delay differential diagnosis and treatment, allowing the progression of pathophysiologic processes with resultant hypovolemic shock and multiple organ failure. As shock progresses, lactic acidosis may ensue because of poor perfusion.

## HEALTH CARE SETTING

Acute care (usually intensive care), diabetes specialty unit

## ASSESSMENT/CLINICAL FINDINGS

Symptoms are a result mainly of hyperglycemia, intracellular hypoglycemia, hypotension or impending hypovolemic shock, and fluid–electrolyte imbalance.

*Neurologic*: Altered level of consciousness (LOC) (confusion, lethargy, irritability, coma), stroke-like symptoms (unilateral/bilateral weakness, paralysis, numbness, paresthesia), fatigue, possible seizures, and tremors

*Respiratory*: Shallow, rapid (tachypneic) breathing

*Cardiovascular*: Tachycardia, hypotension, electrocardiogram (ECG) changes

*Metabolic/GI/endocrine*: Polyuria, polyphagia, polydipsia, fatigue, generalized weakness, nausea, vomiting

*Integumentary*: Dry, flushed skin; poor turgor; dry mucous membranes

*Vital signs:* Blood pressure (BP) low (more than 20% below normal), heart rate (HR) more than 100 bpm, central venous pressure (CVP) less than 2 mm Hg (less than 5 cm $H_2O$), temperature possibly elevated

379

## DIAGNOSTIC TESTS

Values reflect dehydration secondary to hyperglycemia, osmotic diuresis, and possible lactic acidosis from hypoperfusion; fluid loss 9 L or more.

*Anion gap:* normal
*Hemoglobin/Hematocrit:* elevated
*Serum BUN/creatinine:* elevated
*Serum electrolytes:* decreased
*Serum glucose:* greater than 600 mg/dL
*Serum ketones:* normal
*ABGs:* within normal limits

*Serum osmolality:* more than 350 nOsm/L
*Urine glucose/acetone:* positive/negative

## COMPLICATIONS

Complications of HHS include arterial thrombosis, stroke, renal failure, heart failure, respiratory failure, coma, multiple organ failure, cerebral edema, malignant dysrhythmias (due to fluid volume deficiency, which prompts poor end-organ perfusion), and Gram-negative sepsis (from infection that may have caused the problem to ensue).

## Patient Problem/Analyze Cues/Prioritize Hypotheses

# Deficient Knowledge (Disease Management)

*due to* unfamiliarity with causes, prevention, and treatment of HHS

**Desired Outcome/Generate Solutions:** Within the 24-hour period before hospital discharge, the patient and significant other verbalize understanding of causes, prevention, and treatment of HHS.

| ASSESSMENT—RECOGNIZE CUES/ INTERVENTIONS—TAKE ACTION | RATIONALES |
|---|---|
| Assess the patient's health care literacy (language, reading, comprehension). Assess the culture and culturally specific information needs. | This assessment helps ensure that information is selected and presented in a manner that is culturally and educationally appropriate. |
| Determine the patient's understanding of HHS and its treatment. Enable verbalization of fears and feelings about the diagnosis; correct any misconceptions. | This enables the nurse to reinforce, as needed, information about the disease process of DM and HHS and common early symptoms of worsening DM, including polyuria, polydipsia, polyphagia, dry and flushed skin, and increased irritability. |
| Caution the patient that fluid resuscitation may be a critical component in his or her recovery from HHS. | Aggressive fluid resuscitation is the primary treatment strategy for HHS in order to avoid circulatory collapse and support the perfusion of end organs. Fluid deficits in adults average 9 L, which equates to 25% of their total body water. Fluids are pulled from individual body cells by increasing serum hyperosmolality and extracellular fluid loss, causing intracellular dehydration and body cell shrinkage. For details, see "Diabetic Ketoacidosis," Chapter 48, for *Dehydration*. |
| Instruct the patient and caregiver on the importance of testing blood glucose levels as prescribed before meals and at bedtime. As indicated, review the testing procedure with the patient. | Blood glucose monitoring is essential for calculating appropriate basal, mealtime, and supplemental insulin dosages. |
| Explain that fasting morning blood glucose greater than 140 mg/dL should be reported to the health care provider and treated as prescribed. | Reporting this value enables prompt adjustment in insulin dose based on blood glucose levels. |
| Stress the importance of dietary changes as prescribed by the health care provider. Provide a referral to a dietitian as needed. | Adherence to a diabetic diet will decrease the risk of complications. |
| Typically, the person with type 2 DM is obese and will be on a reduced-calorie diet with fixed amounts of carbohydrate, fat, and protein. Fats should be polyunsaturated and proteins chosen from low-fat sources. | |
| Explain the importance of eating three meals per day at regularly scheduled times and a bedtime snack and information related to the type of insulin being administered. | Mealtime insulin should be administered within 30 minutes before a meal (regular insulin) or 15 minutes before or after a meal (analog short-acting insulins such as HumaLog, NovoLog, or Apidra). If meals are not spaced appropriately, patients may experience hyperglycemia or hypoglycemia between meals. |

| ASSESSMENT—RECOGNIZE CUES/ INTERVENTIONS—TAKE ACTION | RATIONALES |
|---|---|
| Explain that increased or decreased food intake will necessitate the adjustment in insulin dosage. | Mealtime insulin dose is calculated based on the average amount of carbohydrates in the patient's diet. If meal consumption changes, the insulin dose may need to be changed to align with blood sugar levels to ensure adequate control of blood glucose. |
| Emphasize to the patient the importance of adhering to oral antidiabetic drug regimen as prescribed. | Oral antidiabetic drugs must be taken as prescribed to maintain acceptable blood glucose levels. |
| Explain that exogenous insulin or insulin analogs may be required during periods of physical and emotional stress and that blood glucose levels should be monitored closely during these times. | Increased stress creates insulin resistance, which may prompt hyperglycemia even though the patient's food intake remains constant. |
| Explain the benefits of regular exercise for maintaining blood glucose levels. | Exercise increases insulin effectiveness and reduces serum triglyceride and cholesterol levels, thus also decreasing the risk for atherosclerosis. Aerobic exercises, such as walking or swimming, are most effective in lowering blood glucose levels. |
| Caution the patient to always monitor blood glucose levels before exercise. | A level greater than 250 mg/dL is indicative of inadequate blood glucose management. In this case, exercise could be a stressor in patients not used to exercise, resulting in further elevation of blood glucose. |
| Explain the need for measures to prevent infection, such as good hygiene and meticulous daily foot care. Stress the importance of avoiding exposure to communicable diseases. Explain that the following indicators of infection necessitate prompt medical treatment: fever, chills, tachycardia, diaphoresis, and nausea and vomiting. In addition, teach the patient and caregiver to be alert to wounds or cuts that do not heal, burning or pain with urination, and cough that is productive of sputum. | Immune system dysfunction results from the lack of energy production at the cellular level of all components of the immune system. Hyperglycemia indicates glucose has not been transported from the bloodstream into the cells. Without normal levels of intracellular glucose, cellular energy production is impaired. All body system functions, including the immune system, are dysfunctional because cells involved with cellular and humoral immunity are unable to do 100% of the work required. The inability of glucose to "power" the cells suppresses the immune system, thereby increasing the risk for infection. |
| Provide the following address of the American Diabetes Association: www.diabetes.org. | Patients may acquire pamphlets and magazines related to diabetes, its complications, and treatment. |
| See "Diabetes Mellitus," Chapter 47, for a complete listing of information sources. | |

## ADDITIONAL PROBLEMS:

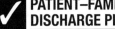

## PATIENT–FAMILY TEACHING AND DISCHARGE PLANNING

See *Deficient Knowledge*, due to unfamiliarity with causes, prevention, and treatment of HHS, earlier.

Endocrine Care Plans

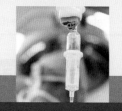

# Hyperthyroidism 50

## OVERVIEW/PATHOPHYSIOLOGY

Hyperthyroidism is a clinical syndrome caused by excessive synthesis and release of thyroid hormones. Because thyroid activity affects all body systems, excessive thyroid hormone exaggerates normal body functions and produces a hypermetabolic state. Hyperthyroidism occurs most frequently in 20- to 40-year olds and is more common in women than men.

*Graves disease* accounts for approximately 75% of reported cases of hyperthyroidism. It is characterized by spontaneous exacerbations and remissions that appear to be unaffected by therapy. Graves disease is triggered by an autoimmune response, wherein the immune system synthesizes antibodies that cross-react with endogenous proteins. The thyrotropin receptor antibodies or thyroid-stimulating immunoglobulins (TSIs) prompt cellular hypermetabolism. The antibodies bind to receptors on the surface of thyroid gland cells, resulting in the overproduction and release of thyroid hormones.

The most severe form of hyperthyroidism is *thyrotoxic crisis*, or *thyroid storm*, which results from a sudden surge of large amounts of thyroid hormones into the bloodstream, causing an even greater increase in body metabolism. This is a *medical emergency*. Precipitating factors include infection, trauma, and emotional stress, all of which increase demands on body metabolism. Thyrotoxic crisis also can occur after thyroidectomy because of manipulation of the gland during surgery.

## HEALTH CARE SETTING

Primary care with possible hospitalization resulting from complications

## ASSESSMENT

*Signs and symptoms.* Nervousness, irritability, alteration in appetite, weight loss or gain, rapid pulse (usually noted by the patient), irregular heartbeats, menstrual irregularities, fatigue, heat intolerance, increased perspiration, frequent defecation or diarrhea, anxiety, restlessness, tremor, and insomnia. Patients bordering on thyroid storm may be confused, possibly psychotic, and have chest pain or discomfort.

*Physical assessment.* Palpation of the thyroid gland may reveal a goiter (an irregular growth of the thyroid gland). Large goiters may also be seen on inspection. A bruit may be heard when auscultating directly over the thyroid. Tachycardia, palpitations, hypertension, widened pulse pressure, exophthalmos, diplopia, hyperpyrexia, enlargement of the thyroid gland, dependent lower extremity edema, muscle weakness, hyperreflexia, fine tremor, fine hair, thin skin, hypercholesterolemia, impaired glucose tolerance, and stare and/or lid lag. Occasionally males may present with gynecomastia.

*Thyrotoxic crisis (thyroid storm).* Acute exacerbation of some or all the previous signs, marked tachycardia, hyperpyrexia, central nervous system irritability, hypertension, possibly severe chest pain, and sometimes coma or heart failure. Cardiovascular collapse and shock are occasionally how patients present. Various clinical syndromes also produce hyperthyroidism, but thyroid storm is most often associated with Graves disease.

*History/risk factors.* Family history of hyperthyroidism is a significant factor for the development of this disorder. Another important factor is the presence of thyroid nodules or nodular toxic goiters in which one or more thyroid adenomas hyperfunction autonomously. Patients should have thyroid studies done before medication is initiated and be monitored serially afterward. For thyrotoxic crisis, patients with hyperthyroidism resulting from Graves disease, thyroid nodules, or toxic goiter may have undergone a recent stressful experience, including severe infection, trauma, major surgery, thromboembolism, diabetic ketoacidosis, preeclampsia, pregnancy, labor, and/or delivery.

## DIAGNOSTIC TESTS

*Serum thyroid-stimulating hormone (thyrotropin).* Most commonly used test to detect thyroid dysfunction. It is decreased in the presence of disease.

*Serum $T_4$ (thyroxine) or free $T_4$.* Elevated in the presence of disease. It may be more accurate than thyroid-stimulating hormone (TSH) if patients have been recently treated for hyperthyroidism or if receiving high doses of thyroid replacement therapy. Thyroxine should be monitored along with TSH for the first year of therapy, especially in older adults.

*Serum $T_3$ (thyroxine triiodothyronine) radioimmunoassay or free $T_3$.* Elevated in the presence of disease.

*Serum thyroid autoantibodies.* Can detect TSH receptor antibodies and TSIs, which may be present if autoimmune disease is present.

*Thyroid binding globulin.* Measures the level of the protein that binds with circulating thyroid hormones. Abnormal $T_4$ or $T_3$ measurements are often caused by binding protein abnormalities rather than abnormal thyroid function.

PART I: Medical-Surgical Nursing Care Plans

***Thyroid scan[123]I (preferably) or [99m]Tc pertechnetate.*** Helps determine the cause of the hyperthyroidism. The scan also may be useful in assessing the functional status of any palpable thyroid irregularities or nodules associated with a toxic goiter.

***Doppler ultrasonography.*** To diagnose the size of the gland and abnormal densities, which can indicate the presence of nodules.

***Radioiodine([131]I) uptake and thyroid scan.*** Clarify the gland size and detect the presence of hot or cold nodules.

## Patient Problem/Analyze Cues/Prioritize Hypotheses

# Risk for Disease (Thyroid Storm/Thyrotoxic Crisis)

*due to* the emotional stress, trauma, severe infection, excessive ingestion of thyroid hormone, preeclampsia, labor and/or delivery, or surgical manipulation of the gland

**Desired Outcomes/Generate Solutions:** The patient is free of symptoms of thyroid storm, as evidenced by normothermia; blood pressure within the optimal range as directed by the health care provider; heart rate (HR) of 100 bpm or less; and orientation to person, place, and time. If thyroid storm occurs, it is detected promptly and reported immediately.

| ASSESSMENT—RECOGNIZE CUES/ INTERVENTIONS—TAKE ACTION | RATIONALES |
|---|---|
| Assess for hyperthermia and report rectal or core temperature greater than 101°F (38.3°C). | An increased temperature often is the first sign of impending thyroid storm. |
| Assess for signs of heart failure. Immediately report significant findings to the health care provider and prepare to transfer the patient to the intensive care unit if they are noted. | Signs of heart failure (jugular vein distention, crackles, decreased amplitude of peripheral pulses, peripheral edema, and hypotension) can occur as an effect of thyroid storm. If not aggressively monitored and managed, thyroid storm can lead to lethal cardiac and hemodynamic compromise. |
| Assess vital signs hourly in patients in whom thyroid storm is suspected. | These assessments may reveal evidence of hypotension and increasing tachycardia and fever, which may reflect the increasing severity of heart failure associated with thyroid storm. |
| Provide a cool, calm, protected environment. Reassure the patient and explain all procedures before performing them. Limit the number of visitors. | These measures minimize emotional and physical stress, which can precipitate thyroid storm. |
| Ensure good hand hygiene and meticulous aseptic technique for dressing changes and invasive procedures. Advise visitors who have contracted or been exposed to a communicable disease either not to enter the patient's room or to wear a surgical mask, if appropriate. | These measures reduce the risk for infection, which is a precipitating factor in the development of thyroid storm. |
| **In the Presence of Thyroid Storm** | |
| Assess for hyperthermia and administer acetaminophen as prescribed. | Acetaminophen will decrease temperature secondary to the fever associated with thyroid storm. |
| Avoid giving aspirin. | Aspirin is contraindicated because it releases thyroxine from protein-binding sites and increases free thyroxine levels, which would exacerbate symptoms of thyroid storm. |
| Provide cool sponge baths or apply ice packs to the patient's axilla and groin area. If the high temperature continues, obtain a prescription for a hypothermia blanket. | These actions will decrease the fever caused by thyroid storm. |
| Administer the antithyroid drugs as prescribed. | Antithyroid drugs will prevent further synthesis and release of thyroid hormones. |

Continued

| ASSESSMENT—RECOGNIZE CUES/ INTERVENTIONS—TAKE ACTION | RATIONALES |
|---|---|
| Monitor the complete blood count values, particularly the white blood cell counts. | The most severe side effect of antithyroid drugs is leukopenia, which increases the possibility that patients may acquire an infection. |
| Administer the beta-adrenergic blockers as prescribed. | Beta-adrenergic blockers will block sympathetic nervous system (SNS) effects. They decrease tachycardia, nervousness, irritability, and tremors, which are elevated as a result of hyperthyroidism. |
| Administer intravenous (IV) fluids as prescribed. | Fluid volume deficit may occur because of increased fluid excretion by the kidneys or excessive diaphoresis. IV fluids will provide adequate hydration and prevent vascular collapse. |
| Carefully monitor the intake and output (I&O) hourly. | Hourly assessment of I&O will reveal fluid overload or inadequate fluid replacement, either of which necessitates prompt intervention. Decreasing output with normal specific gravity may indicate decreased cardiac output, whereas decreasing output with increased specific gravity can signal dehydration. |
| Administer the prescribed supplemental $O_2$ as necessary. | $O_2$ demands are increased as metabolism increases. |

## Patient Problem/Analyze Cues/Prioritize Hypotheses

# Body Weight Problem (Weight Loss)

*due to* the hypermetabolic state and/or inadequate nutrient absorption

**Desired Outcomes/Generate Solutions:** By a minimum of 24 hours before hospital discharge, the patient has adequate nutrition, as evidenced by stable weight and a positive nitrogen balance. Within 24 hours of the instruction, the patient lists the types of foods that are necessary to restore a normal nutritional state.

| ASSESSMENT—RECOGNIZE CUES/ INTERVENTIONS—TAKE ACTION | RATIONALES |
|---|---|
| Assess for weight loss by weighing the patient daily and report significant losses to the health care provider. Assess the daily nutritional intake. | Daily weight assessment is a useful indicator of nutritional status. Weight loss may indicate the patient is not receiving appropriate nutritional support for the accelerated metabolic rate. The patient's needs (e.g., as indicated by continued weight loss) will help determine the amount and type of nutritional intake. |
| Assess for and manage diarrhea with prescribed antidiarrheal medications. | These medications increase the absorption of nutrients from the gastrointestinal tract. |
| Provide foods high in calories, protein, carbohydrates, and vitamins. Teach about foods that will provide optimal nutrients. | This will help restore a normal nutritional state for patients with hyperthyroidism. |
| Provide between-meal snacks. | Snacks will help maximize the patient's consumption and provide needed calories. |
| Administer the vitamin supplements as prescribed and explain their importance to the patient. | Vitamins provide essential nutrients to facilitate appropriate digestion/ absorption of foods that contribute to energy production. |

## Patient Problem/Analyze Cues/Prioritize Hypotheses

# Fatigue

*due to* disturbed sleep pattern occurring with accelerated metabolism

**Desired Outcome/Generate Solutions:** Within 48 hours of hospital admission, the patient relates the attainment of sufficient rest and sleep.

| ASSESSMENT—RECOGNIZE CUES/ INTERVENTIONS—TAKE ACTION | RATIONALES |
|---|---|
| Assess the patient's sleep pattern and adjust care activities to the patient's tolerance. | It may be necessary to alter the care regimen to comply with the patient's rest/sleep disturbance. |
| Assess activity tolerance and provide frequent rest periods of at least 90-minute durations. If possible, arrange for the patient to have bedrest in a quiet, temperature-controlled room with nonexertional activities such as reading, watching television, working crossword puzzles, or listening to soothing music. | Patients will have difficulty relaxing. Therefore all efforts must be made to provide a calm, quiet environment to promote rest/sleep. Setting the temperature of the room to the patient's comfort level will assist with relaxation. |
| Assist with activity or other exertional activities if needed. | If the patient is fatigued, more assistance is needed until rest/sleep pattern normalizes. |
| • Administer sedatives as prescribed. | These medications promote rest. |
| • After administering these agents, raise the side rails if the patient is hospitalized. | This will help protect the patient, who will be drowsy after taking these sedatives. |
| Provide a calm and quiet environment with cool temperature and away from high-traffic noisy areas. | Increased metabolism and sensitivity of the SNS cause sleep problems. |

## Patient Problem/Analyze Cues/Prioritize Hypotheses

# Anxiety

*due to* SNS stimulation

***Desired Outcomes/Generate Solutions:*** Within 24 hours of hospital admission, the patient is free of harmful anxiety as evidenced by HR of 100 bpm or less, respiratory rate (RR) of 12–20 breaths/minute with normal depth and pattern (eupnea), and absence of or decrease in irritability and restlessness. The patient and significant others verbalize accurate knowledge about the causes of the patient's behavior.

| ASSESSMENT—RECOGNIZE CUES/ INTERVENTIONS—TAKE ACTION | RATIONALES |
|---|---|
| Assess for signs of anxiety; administer as prescribed. Assess the effectiveness of sedatives in controlling the anxiety. | Sedatives reduce anxiety. |
| Administer the beta-adrenergic blockers as prescribed. | Beta-adrenergic blockers reduce anxiety, tachycardia, and tremors. |
| Provide a quiet environment away from loud noises or excessive activity. | This will help reduce stress and anxiety. |
| Limit the number of visitors and the amount of time they spend with the patient. Advise significant others to avoid discussing stressful topics and refrain from arguing with the patient. | These measures will help reduce stress and anxiety. |
| Inform significant others that the patient's behavior is physiologic and should not be taken personally. | Reassuring family members helps them regain emotional control and reduces their stress regarding the patient's unusual behaviors. |
| Reassure the patient that anxiety symptoms are related to the disease process and that treatment decreases their severity. | Reassurance helps patients regain emotional control and reduces emotional stress through a better understanding of the cause and treatment. |

## Patient Problem/Analyze Cues/Prioritize Hypotheses

# Impaired Tissue Integrity (Corneal Tissue)

*due to* dryness that can occur with exophthalmos in patients with Graves disease

**Desired Outcome/Generate Solutions:** Within 24 hours of admission, the patient's corneas are moist and intact.

| ASSESSMENT—RECOGNIZE CUES/ INTERVENTIONS—TAKE ACTION | RATIONALES |
|---|---|
| Assess for dry eyes and administer lubricating eye drops as prescribed. | Eye drops will supplement lubrication and decrease SNS stimulation, which can cause lid retraction. |
| Instruct the patient to wear dark glasses. | This will help protect the corneas. Dark glasses also protect individuals who are photosensitive. |
| If appropriate, apply eye shields or apply paper tape over the eyelids to keep the eyes shut at bedtime. | Hyperthyroidism can result in severe exophthalmos that prevents eyelids from closing fully, making the corneas vulnerable to injury. |
| Administer the antithyroid drugs as prescribed. | Antithyroid drugs maintain a normal metabolic state and halt progression of exophthalmos. |

## Patient Problem/Analyze Cues/Prioritize Hypotheses

# Negative Self Image

*due to* exophthalmos or surgical scar on the neck

**Desired Outcome/Generate Solutions:** Within the 24-hour period before hospital discharge, the patient verbalizes measures for disguising exophthalmos or the surgical scar.

| ASSESSMENT—RECOGNIZE CUES/ INTERVENTIONS—TAKE ACTION | RATIONALES |
|---|---|
| Assess for indicators of a negative self-image. | Patients may exhibit nonverbal indicators (avoiding looking at self in the mirror, keeping eyes fully or partially closed when speaking, bowing head when speaking to minimize exposure of the throat) or verbal indicators (expressing negative feelings about facial appearance or surgical scar on throat/neck). |
| Advise the patient to wear dark glasses. | Dark glasses will disguise exophthalmos while also protecting the corneas from photosensitivity. |
| Suggest measures that can disguise the scar. | Customized jewelry, high-necked clothing such as turtlenecks, and loose-fitting scarves are examples of measures that will help disguise the scar. |
| Suggest that after the incision has healed, the patient can use makeup colored in his or her skin tone. | This will decrease the visibility of the scar. |
| Caution the patient that creams are contraindicated until the incision has healed completely and even then may not minimize scarring. | This is standard postoperative teaching for most surgical procedures. Patients are advised by some health care providers to increase vitamin C intake by up to 1 g/day to promote healing. Some surgeons also advise against direct sunlight to the operative site for 6–12 months to avoid hyperpigmentation of the incision. Instruct the patient accordingly. |

## Patient Problem/Analyze Cues/Prioritize Hypotheses

# Deficient Knowledge (Medications)

*due to* unfamiliarity with the potential for side effects from antithyroid drugs or abruptly stopping antithyroid drugs.

***Desired Outcome/Generate Solutions:*** Within the 24-hour period before hospital discharge, the patient verbalizes knowledge about the potential side effects of the prescribed medications, signs and symptoms of hypothyroidism and hyperthyroidism, and the importance of following the prescribed medical regimen.

| ASSESSMENT—RECOGNIZE CUES/ INTERVENTIONS—TAKE ACTION | RATIONALES |
|---|---|
| Assess the patient's health care literacy (language, reading, comprehension). Assess the culture and culturally specific information needs. | This assessment helps ensure that materials are selected and presented in a manner that is culturally and educationally appropriate. |
| Explain the importance of taking antithyroid medications daily, in divided doses, and at regular intervals as prescribed. | A knowledgeable patient is more likely to adhere to the treatment regimen. |
| Provide information on indicators of hypothyroidism and the signs and symptoms that necessitate medical attention. | Hyperthyroid treatment may lead to hypothyroidism. Providing information about the signs and symptoms of hypothyroidism to the patient will allow them to recognize the signs and symptoms and seek appropriate medical care. |
| Indicators of hypothyroidism (e.g., early fatigue, weight gain, anorexia, constipation, menstrual irregularities, muscle cramps, lethargy, inability to concentrate, hair loss, cold intolerance, and hoarseness) may occur from excessive medication. | |
| Signs and symptoms that necessitate medical attention because the medications that cause them may require dose adjustment include cold intolerance, fatigue, lethargy, and peripheral or periorbital edema. | |
| • Provide the patient with information regarding the side effects of antithyroid drugs and symptoms that necessitate medical attention. | This necessitates medical attention to adjust the dose or change the medication. |
| • Appearance of a rash, fever, or pharyngitis can occur in the presence of agranulocytosis, a recognized side effect of antithyroid drugs. | |
| Alert patients taking iodides to signs of worsening hyperthyroidism and the need to report them promptly. | Signs of worsening hyperthyroidism (high body temperature, palpitations, rapid HR, irritability, anxiety, and feelings of restlessness or panic) may signal need for medication dosage adjustment to manage the problem and should be reported promptly for timely intervention. |

## Problems for Patients Who Have Undergone Subtotal Thyroidectomy

## Patient Problem/Analyze Cues/Prioritize Hypotheses

# Acute Pain

*due to* subtotal thyroidectomy surgical procedure

***Desired Outcomes/Generate Solutions:*** Within 2 hours of surgery, the patient's subjective perception of pain decreases, as documented by a pain scale. Objective indicators, such as hesitation before turning or moving the head, are absent or diminished.

| ASSESSMENT—RECOGNIZE CUES/ INTERVENTIONS—TAKE ACTION | RATIONALES |
|---|---|
| Assess and document the degree and character of the patient's pain, including precipitating events. Devise a pain scale with the patient, rating pain on a scale of 0 (no pain) to 10 (worst pain). | This assessment will enable the nurse to determine the trend of the pain and the degree of pain relief obtained. |
| Advise the patient to clasp hands behind the neck when moving. | This measure will minimize stress on the incision. |
| After the health care provider has removed surgical clips and drain, teach the patient to perform gentle range of motion (ROM) exercises for the neck. | While the surgical clips and drain are in place, mobility of the neck is limited, leading to tight neck muscles. After removal of these devices, gentle ROM is done to help relax the neck muscles and decrease pain. |
| For other interventions, see "Pain," Chapter 5. | |

## Patient Problem/Analyze Cues/Prioritize Hypotheses

# Risk for Impaired Swallowing

*due to* edema or laryngeal nerve damage resulting from the surgical procedure

***Desired Outcomes/Generate Solutions:*** The patient reports swallowing with minimal difficulty, has minimal or absent hoarseness, and is free of symptoms of respiratory dysfunction as evidenced by RR of 12–20 breaths/minute with normal depth and pattern (eupnea) and absence of inspiratory stridor. Laryngeal nerve damage, if it occurs, is detected promptly and reported immediately.

| ASSESSMENT—RECOGNIZE CUES/ INTERVENTIONS—TAKE ACTION | RATIONALES |
|---|---|
| Assess for dysphagia by monitoring for inability to swallow, choking, and coughing while drinking or eating and respiratory status for dyspnea and inspiratory stridor. | These are signs of postsurgical edema. Edema in the neck may impinge on the pharynx or esophagus, making swallowing more difficult. |
| ⚠ Assess the patient's voice. Promptly report persisting hoarseness. | Although slight hoarseness is normal after surgery, hoarseness that persists is indicative of laryngeal nerve damage and should be reported to the health care provider promptly. If bilateral nerve damage is present, upper airway obstruction and dysphagia can occur. |
| Elevate the head of bed (HOB) by 30–45 degrees. | Elevating HOB enables gravity to facilitate swallowing and promotes edema reduction. |
| Support the patient's head with flat or cervical pillows so that it is in a neutral position with the neck (does not flex or hyperextend). | This position minimizes incisional stress and reduces the chance of choking and dysphagia. |
| ⚠ Keep a tracheostomy set and $O_2$ equipment at the bedside at all times. | This equipment will be used for emergency treatment in the event upper airway obstruction occurs. |
| Gently suction the upper airway as needed. | Patients can aspirate retained secretions if edema and/or laryngeal nerve problems are present. Using gentle, rather than aggressive, suctioning avoids stimulating laryngospasm. |
| Administer the analgesics promptly and as prescribed. | This will minimize pain and anxiety and enhance the patient's ability to swallow. |

## ADDITIONAL PROBLEMS:

## ✔ PATIENT–FAMILY TEACHING AND DISCHARGE PLANNING

When providing patient–family teaching, focus on sensory information, avoid giving excessive information, and initiate a visiting nurse referral for necessary follow-up teaching. Part of the initial assessment should include asking about existing knowledge of the disease, ability for self-management, and psychologic acceptance. Include verbal and written information about the following:

- ✔ Diet high in calories, protein, carbohydrates, and vitamins. Inform the patient that as a normal metabolic state is attained, the diet may change.
- ✔ Medications, including drug name, purpose, dosage, schedule, precautions, and potential side effects. Also discuss drug–drug, food–drug, and herb–drug interactions.
- ✔ Changes that can occur as a result of therapy, including weight gain, normalized bowel function, increased strength of skeletal muscles, and a return to normal activity levels.
- ✔ Importance of continued and frequent medical follow-up; confirm date and time of next appointment.
- ✔ Indicators that necessitate medical attention, including fever, rash, or sore throat (side effects of thioamides) and symptoms of hypothyroidism (see "Hypothyroidism," Chapter 51) or worsening hyperthyroidism.
- ✔ For patients receiving radioactive iodine, importance of not holding children to the chest for 72 hours after therapy because children are more susceptible to the effects of radiation. Explain that there is a negligible risk for adults.
- ✔ Importance of avoiding physical and emotional stress early in the recuperative stage and maximizing coping mechanisms for dealing with stress.
- ✔ Additional information and educational information:
  - American Thyroid Association: www.thyroid.org
  - Hormone Foundation: www.hormone.org

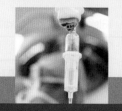

# Hypothyroidism 51

## OVERVIEW/PATHOPHYSIOLOGY

Hypothyroidism is a condition in which there is an inadequate amount of circulating thyroid hormone, causing a decrease in metabolic rate that affects all body systems.

*Primary hypothyroidism* accounts for 90% of cases of hypothyroidism and is caused by pathologic changes in the thyroid. The most common cause of the disease in the United States is chronic autoimmune thyroiditis (Hashimoto disease). Postpartum thyroiditis and granulomatous thyroiditis related to inflammatory conditions or viral syndromes also occur.

*Secondary hypothyroidism* is caused by dysfunction of the anterior pituitary gland, which results in decreased release of thyroid-stimulating hormone (TSH).

When hypothyroidism is untreated, or when a stressor such as infection affects an individual with hypothyroidism, a life-threatening condition known as *myxedema coma* can occur. Hypothyroidism is eight times more likely to occur in women than men, and it frequently presents in the later years; older women are the most likely candidates to present with myxedema. The clinical picture of myxedema coma is that of exaggerated hypothyroidism, with dangerous hypoventilation, hypothermia, hypotension, and shock. Coma and seizures can occur as well. Myxedema coma usually develops slowly, has a greater than 50% mortality rate, and requires prompt and aggressive treatment.

## HEALTH CARE SETTING

Primary care with possible hospitalization resulting from complications

## ASSESSMENT

Signs and symptoms can progress from mild early in onset to life threatening.

***Signs and symptoms.*** Early fatigue, weight gain from fluid retention, anorexia, lethargy, cold intolerance, hoarseness, ataxia, memory and mental impairment, decreased concentration, menstrual irregularities or heavy menses, infertility, constipation, depression, and muscle cramps. Signs and symptoms may be life threatening in a patient with a history of hypothyroidism who has experienced a recent stressful event.

***Physical assessment.*** Possible presence of goiter, bradycardia, hypothermia, deepened voice, hyperlipidemia, and obesity. Skin may appear yellow and dry, cool, and coarse, and hair may be thin, coarse, and brittle. The tongue may be enlarged (macroglossia), and reflexes may be slowed.

***Myxedema coma.*** Hypoventilation, hypoglycemia, hypothermia, hypotension, hyponatremia, bradycardia, and shock.

***History and risk factors.***

*Primary hypothyroidism.* Dietary iodine deficiency, thyroid gland radioablation for hyperthyroidism management, thyroid atrophy or fibrosis of unknown cause, radiation therapy to the neck, surgical removal of all or part of the gland, drugs that suppress thyroid activity including propylthiouracil and iodides, thyroid tumor or invasion of the thyroid gland by tumor (e.g., lymphoma), drugs including lithium and interferon, or a genetic dysfunction resulting in an inability to produce and secrete thyroid hormone.

*Secondary hypothyroidism.* Pituitary tumors, postpartum necrosis of the pituitary gland, hypophysectomy.

## DIAGNOSTIC TESTS

***Thyroid-stimulating hormone.*** Most commonly used test to detect thyroid dysfunction. It will be elevated unless the disease is long-standing or severe.

***Free thyroxine index and $T_4$ (thyroxine) levels.*** Decreased with hypothyroidism.

***$^{131}I$ scan and uptake.*** Will be less than 10% in a 24-hour period. In secondary hypothyroidism, uptake increases with the administration of exogenous TSH.

***Doppler ultrasonography.*** To diagnose gland size and abnormal densities, which may be present if nodules are present.

***Thyroid autoantibodies.*** Presence of thyroperoxidase autoantibodies or antithyroglobulin autoantibodies signals chronic autoimmune thyroiditis.

***Thyroid-binding globulin.*** Measures the level of the protein that binds with circulating thyroid hormones. Abnormal $T_4$ or $T_3$ measurements often occur because of binding protein abnormalities rather than abnormal thyroid function.

***Thyroid scan $^{131}I$ and radioactive iodine uptake.*** Identifies thyroid nodules. In primary hypothyroidism, uptake will be less than 10% in a 24-hour period. In secondary hypothyroidism, uptake increases with the administration of exogenous TSH.

***Electrolyte values.*** Abnormal calcium level is possible resulting from parathyroid dysfunction occurring with hypothyroidism. Sodium, potassium, and magnesium levels also may be abnormal.

## Patient Problem/Analyze Cues/Prioritize Hypotheses

# Impaired Gas Exchange

*due to* upper airway obstruction occurring with enlarged thyroid gland and/or decreased ventilatory drive caused by greatly decreased metabolism

**Desired Outcome/Generate Solutions:** By a minimum of 24 hours before hospital discharge, the patient returns to an effective breathing pattern, as evidenced by a respiratory rate (RR) of 12–20 breaths/minute with normal depth and pattern, normal skin color, $O_2$ saturation of 95% or more, and absence of adventitious breath sounds.

| ASSESSMENT—RECOGNIZE CUES/ INTERVENTIONS—TAKE ACTION | RATIONALES |
|---|---|
| Assess the rate, depth, and quality of breath sounds. | This enables the nurse to be alert to the presence of adventitious sounds (e.g., from developing pleural effusion) or decreasing or crowing sounds (e.g., from swollen tongue or glottis). |
| ⚠ Assess for signs of inadequate ventilation. Immediately report significant findings to the health care provider. | Decreased RR, shallow breathing, and circumoral or peripheral cyanosis are signs of inadequate ventilation. Ventilatory insufficiency in a patient with hypothyroid condition can indicate the onset of heart failure secondary to impending myxedema coma or hypothyroid crisis. |
| ⚠ Assess for hypoxemia by measuring $O_2$ saturation intermittently or continuously in patients with increased work of breathing or decreased RR or depth. Administer oxygen as prescribed. | Decreasing $O_2$ saturation (92% or less) may signal the need for oxygen supplementation in symptomatic patients. |
| Provide instructions to the patient on coughing, deep breathing, and use of the incentive spirometer. Suction upper airway as needed. | These measures help clear secretions that may increase with hypoventilation. |
| ⚠ For the patient experiencing respiratory distress, be prepared to assist the health care provider with intubation or tracheostomy and maintenance of mechanical ventilatory assistance or transfer to the intensive care unit (ICU). | The patient likely will need emergency treatment and intensive care. |

## Patient Problem/Analyze Cues/Prioritize Hypotheses

# Fluid Imbalance

*due to* compromised regulatory mechanisms occurring with hypothyroidism-associated adrenal insufficiency

**Desired Outcome/Generate Solutions:** At least 24 hours before hospital discharge, the patient is normovolemic with a urinary output 30 mL/hour or more, stable weight, nondistended jugular veins, eupnea, and peripheral pulse amplitude at least 2+ on a 0–4+ scale.

| ASSESSMENT—RECOGNIZE CUES/ INTERVENTIONS—TAKE ACTION | RATIONALES |
|---|---|
| Assess the intake and output hourly for evidence of decreasing output. | Decreasing output signals fluid retention leading to fluid overload. |
| Assess for weight gain by weighing the patient at the same time every day, with the same clothing, and using the same scale. Report increasing weight to the health care provider. | Increasing weight signals fluid retention, which can lead to hypervolemia/ fluid overload. Weighing the patient at the same time each day and under the same conditions avoids discrepancies that could reflect inaccurate losses or gains. |

Continued

| ASSESSMENT—RECOGNIZE CUES/ INTERVENTIONS—TAKE ACTION | RATIONALES |
| --- | --- |
| • Assess for indicators of heart failure. Report significant findings to the health care provider. <br><br> Indicators of heart failure include jugular vein distention, crackles, shortness of breath, dependent edema of extremities, and decreased amplitude of peripheral pulses. | Lack of thyroid hormones can decrease the heart rate (HR) and force of contractions, leading to heart failure. Associated fluid retention worsens the problem. |
| Restrict the fluid and sodium intake as prescribed. | This helps prevent fluid retention that could lead to fluid overload. |
| Use a rate control device to administer intravenous (IV) fluids. | This will prevent accidental fluid overload. |

## Patient Problem/Analyze Cues/Prioritize Hypotheses

# Activity Intolerance

*due to* the weakness occurring with slowed metabolism and decreased cardiac output caused by pericardial effusions, atherosclerosis, and decreased adrenergic stimulation

***Desired Outcome/Generate Solutions:*** During activity/exercise, the patient rates perceived exertion at a level of 3 or less on a 0–10 scale and exhibits tolerance to activity/exercise with an HR of less than 20 bpm over resting HR; systolic blood pressure (SBP) less than 20 mm Hg over or under resting SBP; warm and dry skin; and absence of crackles, murmurs, chest pain, and new dysrhythmias.

| ASSESSMENT—RECOGNIZE CUES/ INTERVENTIONS—TAKE ACTION | RATIONALES |
| --- | --- |
|  Assess for complications of a decreased metabolic rate by taking vital signs and auscultating the heart and lungs at frequent intervals. | This enables the nurse to be alert to hypotension, slow pulse, dysrhythmias, decreasing urine output, and changes in mentation, which along with complaints of chest pain or discomfort, labored breathing, or adventitious breath sounds may signal heart failure/ impending pulmonary edema. |
| Assess the activity tolerance by asking the patient to rate perceived exertion (RPE). See *Activity Intolerance* "Immobility," Chapter 1, for details. | An RPE more than 3 on a 0–10 scale is a signal of cardiac intolerance during exertion and also a sign that the patient should stop or modify the activity causing the exertion. |
| Promptly report the significant changes to the health care provider. | This will help prevent the progression of heart failure to cardiac arrest. |
| As prescribed, administer the IV isotonic solutions such as normal saline. | Isotonic solutions help prevent or ameliorate hypotension. Hypotension ensues as a result of reduced sympathetic nervous system stimulation, which causes decreased cardiac output and hypotension. |
| Balance the activity with adequate rest. | Rest decreases workload of the heart. |
| Assist the patient with a range of motion and other in-bed exercises and consult with the health care provider about the implementation of exercises that require greater cardiac tolerance. For details, see *Activity Intolerance* in "Immobility," Chapter 1. | Exercise prevents problems caused by immobility. |

## Patient Problem/Analyze Cues/Prioritize Hypotheses

# Risk for Infection

*due to* compromised immunologic status occurring with alterations in adrenal function

***Desired Outcome/Generate Solutions:*** The patient is free of infection, as evidenced by normothermia, absence of adventitious breath sounds, normal urinary pattern and characteristics, and well-healing wounds.

| ASSESSMENT—RECOGNIZE CUES/ INTERVENTIONS—TAKE ACTION | RATIONALES |
|---|---|
| Assess for early indicators of infection. Notify the health care provider of significant findings. | Fever; erythema, swelling, or discharge from wounds or IV sites; urinary frequency, urgency, or dysuria; cloudy or malodorous urine; presence of adventitious sounds on auscultation of lung fields; and changes in color, consistency, and amount of sputum are early indicators of infection. Prompt assessment and treatment can halt their progression to prevent complications such as myxedema coma, a life-threatening condition. |
| Assess for the appropriateness of a urinary catheter, if present, and remove as soon as possible. If present, provide meticulous perineal care, cleansing the catheter from proximal to distal direction. | This minimizes the risk for urinary tract infection. Guidelines recommend indwelling urinary catheters be removed within 48 hours of insertion. |
| Use the sterile technique when performing dressing changes and invasive procedures. | Nonintact skin and invasive procedures can lead to bacterial ingress. |
| Provide good skin care. | Open sores are sites of ingress for bacteria. |
| Advise visitors who have contracted or been exposed to a communicable disease not to enter the patient's room or to wear a surgical mask, if appropriate. | This will minimize the risk for systemic infection in patients who are immunocompromised. |

## Patient Problem/Analyze Cues/Prioritize Hypotheses

# Body Weight Problem (Weight Gain)

*due to* slowed metabolism

***Desired Outcome/Generate Solutions:*** Within the 24-hour period before hospital discharge, the patient verbalizes an accurate understanding of the rationale and measures for the dietary regimen and demonstrates weight loss.

| ASSESSMENT—RECOGNIZE CUES/ INTERVENTIONS—TAKE ACTION | RATIONALES |
|---|---|
| Assess for weight gain by weighing the patient at the same time every day, with the same clothing, and using the same scale. Report increasing weight to the health care provider. | Increasing weight may signal fluid retention or excessive calorie intake for activity level and decreased metabolic rate. Weighing patients at the same time and under the same conditions avoids discrepancies that could reflect inaccurate losses or gains. |
| Provide a diet that is high in protein and low in calories. | This diet will promote weight loss. |
| As prescribed, restrict or limit sodium intake and foods high in sodium content. | This measure decreases edema caused by fluid retention. |
| Instruct the patient on a diet that supports/improves metabolism, including foods to increase and foods to limit or avoid. | Foods high in protein and low in calories and sodium will help with weight control while the patient is in a hypometabolic/fluid-retaining state. |

Continued

| ASSESSMENT—RECOGNIZE CUES/ INTERVENTIONS—TAKE ACTION | RATIONALES |
|---|---|
| Provide small, frequent meals of appropriate foods the patient particularly enjoys. | This promotes weight control and decreases the chance of patients overeating if allowed to get too hungry. |
| Encourage the intake of high-fiber foods (e.g., fruits with skins, vegetables, whole-grain breads and cereals, nuts). | Adding bulk to the diet improves gastric motility, which will help elimination that may be decreased as a result of slowed metabolism. |
| Administer the vitamin supplements as prescribed. | Vitamins will help patients who are unable to consume appropriate recommended daily allowance minimum requirements on their restricted diets. |

## Patient Problem/Analyze Cues/Prioritize Hypotheses

# Constipation

*due to* inadequate dietary intake of roughage and fluids, prolonged bedrest, and/or decreased peristalsis occurring with slowed metabolism

*Desired Outcome/Generate Solutions:* Before hospital discharge, the patient has a bowel movement at least every third day with no evidence of abdominal distention.

| ASSESSMENT—RECOGNIZE CUES/ INTERVENTIONS—TAKE ACTION | RATIONALES |
|---|---|
| Assess for decreasing bowel sounds and the presence of distention and increases in abdominal girth. | These indicators can occur with ileus or fecal impaction and lead to an obstructive process, which is fairly common in hypothyroidism, especially in older adults. |
| Encourage the patient to maintain a diet with adequate fiber and fluids. Ensure that fluid intake in persons without underlying cardiac or renal disease is at least 2–3 L/day. | Such foods as fruits with skins, fruit juices, cooked fruits, vegetables, whole-grain breads and cereals, and nuts provide bulk, which will promote bowel elimination by increasing peristalsis and, coupled with increased fluid intake, add moisture to keep stool moving through the intestines/colon. |
| Administer the stool softeners and laxatives as prescribed. | These agents minimize constipation by moistening stool and increasing peristalsis. **Caution:** Suppositories are contraindicated because of the risk for stimulating the vagus nerve, which would further decrease HR and BP. |
| Advise the patient to increase the amount of exercise. | Exercise promotes regularity by increasing peristalsis. Exercise also tones gastrointestinal muscles to hold intestines/colon in place, which seems to facilitate bowel elimination. |

## Patient Problem/Analyze Cues/Prioritize Hypotheses

# Risk for Impaired Cognition

*due to* impaired sensory reception, transmission, or integration occurring with cerebral retention of water

*Desired Outcomes/Generate Solutions:* The patient verbalizes orientation to person, place, and time. Alternately, if signs of myxedema coma appear, they are detected, reported, and treated promptly.

| ASSESSMENT—RECOGNIZE CUES/ INTERVENTIONS—TAKE ACTION | RATIONALES |
|---|---|
| Assess the patient's mental status at frequent intervals by assessing orientation to person, place, and time. | Increasing lethargy or delirium can signal the onset of myxedema coma, which requires immediate medical attention. |
| Reorient the patient frequently. Have a clock and calendar visible and use radio or television for orientation. | This ensures that the patient has the information necessary to answer neurologic assessment questions appropriately. |
| Clearly explain all procedures to the patient before performing them. Provide adequate time for the patient to ask questions. | This promotes a better understanding of procedures for a patient who may have memory impairment. |
| If necessary, remind the patient to complete activities of daily living such as bathing and brushing hair. | As above. |
| Encourage visitors to discuss topics of special interest to the patient. | This will enhance the patient's alertness. |
| Administer the thyroid replacement hormones as prescribed. | Thyroid replacement increases metabolic rate, which in turn promotes cerebral blood flow. Patients are started on low doses that are increased gradually, based on serial laboratory tests (TSH and $T_4$), and adjusted until the TSH is in a normal range. Dose titration prevents hyperthyroidism caused by too much exogenous hormone. Therapy is continued for the patient's lifetime. |
| For patients with secondary hypothyroidism, avoid administering thyroid supplements. | Thyroid supplements can promote acute symptoms in patients with secondary hypothyroidism and therefore are contraindicated. |

## Patient Problem/Analyze Cues/Prioritize Hypotheses

# Risk for Disease (Myxedema Coma)

*due to* inadequate response to treatment of hypothyroidism or stressors such as infection

**Desired Outcomes/Generate Solutions:** The patient is free of symptoms of myxedema coma, as evidenced by HR of 60 bpm or greater; BP of 90/60 mm Hg or greater (or within the patient's normal range); RR of 12 breaths/minute or more with normal depth and pattern; and orientation to person, place, and time. Alternatively, if myxedema coma occurs, it is detected, reported, and treated promptly.

| ASSESSMENT—RECOGNIZE CUES/ INTERVENTIONS—TAKE ACTION | RATIONALES |
|---|---|
| Assess the patient for hypoxia. Immediately report significant findings to health care providers. | Circumoral or peripheral cyanosis, pulse oximetry less than 88%, and a decrease in the level of consciousness are signs of hypoxia, which may signal that the patient is in heart failure and/or about to experience cardiac arrest. |
| Check the medication doses carefully before administration, especially sedatives. | Because of decreased metabolism, drug action times are prolonged. Patients with hypothyroidism do not tolerate sedatives, and therefore central nervous system depressants are contraindicated unless absolutely necessary to manage the patient during a crisis. |
| Monitor for signs of toxicity if sedatives or barbiturates are administered. | Signs of toxicity include altered mental status, decreased BP, decreased RR, and shallow breathing. |
| Monitor the laboratory work, including complete metabolic panel, complete blood count, lipids, and glucose. | If in a coma, the patient should be evaluated for the following abnormalities, which are associated with myxedema coma: anemia, elevated creatine phosphokinase, elevated creatinine, elevated transaminases, hypercapnia, hyperlipidemia, hypoglycemia, hyponatremia, hypoxia, leukopenia, and respiratory acidosis. |

Continued

| ASSESSMENT—RECOGNIZE CUES/ INTERVENTIONS—TAKE ACTION | RATIONALES |
|---|---|
| In the presence of myxedema coma, implement the following: | |
| • Restrict fluids or administer hypertonic saline as prescribed. | This will correct hyponatremia. A too-rapid correction could cause central pontine myelinolysis, which is brain cell dysfunction caused by the destruction of the myelin sheath covering nerve cells in the brainstem (pons). |
| • As prescribed, administer and carefully monitor IV thyroid replacement hormones with IV hydrocortisone and IV glucose. | In the treatment of hypoglycemia, rapid IV administration of thyroid hormone can precipitate hyperadrenalism. This can be avoided by concomitant administration of IV hydrocortisone. Although concomitant administration of IV hydrocortisone helps prevent adrenal problems, it may cause hypoadrenalism if not carefully monitored. |
| • Monitor for signs of heart failure. Notify the health care provider of any significant findings. | Jugular vein distention, crackles, shortness of breath, peripheral edema, weakening peripheral pulses, and hypotension are signs of heart failure, which can occur secondary to hypothyroidism and lead to myxedema coma. |
| • Prepare to transfer the patient to the ICU. Keep oral airway and manual resuscitator at the bedside in the event of seizure, coma, or the need for ventilatory assistance | This enables emergency treatment for a decreased ventilatory drive. |

## ✔ PATIENT–FAMILY TEACHING AND DISCHARGE PLANNING

When providing patient–family teaching, focus on sensory information, avoid giving excessive information, and initiate a visiting nurse referral for necessary follow-up teaching. Part of the initial assessment should include asking about existing knowledge of the disease, ability for self-management, and psychologic acceptance. Include verbal and written information about the following:

✔ Thyroid replacement drugs should be taken in the morning to avoid insomnia 1–2 hours before breakfast for best absorption.

✔ Medications, including drug name, purpose, dosage, schedule, precautions, and potential side effects. Also discuss drug–drug, food–drug, and herb–drug interactions.

✔ When managing hypothyroidism while pregnant, dosage adjustments must be made every 4 weeks to avoid fetal growth retardation related to untreated maternal hypothyroidism.

✔ Reminder that thioamides, iodides, and lithium are contraindicated because they decrease thyroid activity. Be sure the patient is aware that thyroid replacement medications are to be taken for life.

✔ Dietary requirements and restrictions, which may change as hormone replacement therapy takes effect.

✔ Expected changes that can occur with hormone replacement therapy: increased energy level, weight loss, and decreased peripheral edema. Neuromuscular problems should improve as well.

✔ Importance of continued, frequent medical follow-up; confirm date and time of next medical appointment.

✔ Importance of avoiding physical and emotional stress, and ways for the patient to maximize coping mechanisms for dealing with stress.

✔ Signs and symptoms that necessitate medical attention, including fever or other symptoms of upper respiratory, urinary, or oral infections and signs and symptoms of hyperthyroidism, which may result from excessive hormone replacement.

✔ Available resources:
  • American Thyroid Association: www.thyroid.org
  • Hormone Foundation: www.hormone.org

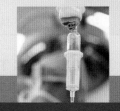

# Syndrome of Inappropriate Antidiuretic Hormone 52

## OVERVIEW/PATHOPHYSIOLOGY

Syndrome of inappropriate antidiuretic hormone (SIADH) is a potentially lethal condition involving an alteration in sodium and water balance resulting from excessive production or release of ADH. It is a condition in which there is serum hypoosmolality and undiluted urine production in patients with normal adrenal, thyroid, renal, hepatic, and cardiac function who do not have hypotension, volume depletion, or other physiologic causes of ADH (vasopressin). Increased ADH levels increase the permeability of the renal distal tubule and collecting duct, leading to the reabsorption of water into the circulation. This causes increased extracellular fluid, decreased plasma osmolality, increased glomerular filtration, and decreased sodium levels. ADH stimulates the nephron to produce aquaporin (AQP), a specific water channel protein, on the surface of the interstitial cells lining the collecting duct. The presence of AQP in the wall of the distal nephron allows the resorption of water from the duct lumen according to the osmotic gradient and excretion of concentrated urine.

Secretion of ADH results in urine concentration and reduced urine output. SIADH is considered a paraneoplastic syndrome that can result from immune system dysfunction due to the presence of tumor cells.

SIADH is the most frequent cause of hyponatremia, which is the most common electrolyte imbalance in hospitalized patients. Mild hyponatremia (serum sodium less than 135 mEq/L) occurs in 15%–22% of hospitalized patients and 7% of ambulatory patients, whereas moderate hyponatremia (serum sodium less than 130 mEq/L) occurs in 1%–7% of hospitalized patients. Hyponatremia is often caused by extracellular fluid volume depletion associated with many diuretics that cause a significant loss of sodium along with water. Hyponatremia is important to manage because of its potential morbidity and should be recognized as an indicator of underlying disease.

ADH is produced in the hypothalamus, is stored in the posterior pituitary, and regulates free water volume in the kidney. Hyponatremia resulting from chronic SIADH is not always caused by reduced water excretion or volume overload. Plasma ADH level may not be high, and measurement is often not helpful in establishing the diagnosis. Findings may reflect dilute (hypoosmolar) plasma and hyponatremia with a normal circulating blood volume. Morbidity and mortality of hyponatremia associated with SIADH stem from cerebral edema and abnormal nerve function. Values of serum sodium less than 100 mEq/L are life threatening.

ADH is a key component in the regulation of fluid and electrolyte balance through direct effects on renal water regulation. Water is reabsorbed in the distal nephron, where the kidney both concentrates and dilutes urine in response to the ADH level. ADH stimulates the nephron to produce AQP, a specific water channel protein, on the surface of the interstitial cells lining the collecting duct. The presence of AQP in the wall of the distal nephron allows the resorption of water from the duct lumen according to the osmotic gradient and excretion of concentrated urine.

## HEALTH CARE SETTING

Acute care

## ASSESSMENT

**Signs and symptoms.** Decreased urine output with concentrated urine. Signs of water intoxication may appear, including the altered level of consciousness (LOC), muscle cramps, fatigue, headache, diarrhea, anorexia, nausea, vomiting, and seizures. Symptoms related to hyponatremia will vary depending on the degree of hyponatremia. As serum sodium level falls, symptoms become more severe. **Note:** Because of loss of $Na^+$, edema will not accompany the fluid volume excess.

**Physical assessment.** Weight gain without edema, elevated blood pressure (BP), altered mental status. Laboratory values must be correlated with physical findings. The goal of assessment is to differentiate between SIADH and a compensatory response of ADH release in patients with chronic, mild volume depletion/dehydration.

**History.** Cancers of the lung, pancreas, duodenum, and prostate, which can secrete a biologically active form of ADH. Other common causes include pulmonary disease (e.g., tuberculosis, pneumonia, chronic obstructive pulmonary disease, empyema), acquired immunodeficiency syndrome, head trauma, brain tumor, intracerebral hemorrhage, meningitis, and encephalitis. Positive-pressure ventilation, physiologic stress, chronic metabolic illness, and a wide variety of medications (chlorpropamide, acetaminophen, oxytocin, narcotics, general anesthetic, carbamazepine, thiazide diuretics, tricyclic antidepressants, neuroleptics, angiotensin-converting enzyme inhibitors, cancer chemotherapy agents) all have been linked to SIADH.

## DIAGNOSTIC TESTS

**Serum Na⁺ level.** Decreased to less than 135 mEq/L.

**Serum osmolality.** Decreased to less than 280 mOsm/kg.

**Urine osmolality.** Elevated disproportionately relative to plasma osmolality.

**Urine Na⁺ level.** Increased to more than 20 mEq/L. Increases to more than 60 mEq/L are common. Urine Na⁺ level (e.g., increased) is best evaluated in comparison with serum Na⁺ level (e.g., decreased).

**Urine specific gravity.** More than 1.030.

**Serum arginine vasopressin (antidiuretic hormone) level.** May be normal to elevated, depending on the type of SIADH present.

**Water load test.** Excretion of water or urine output may be reduced to 30%–40% of the ingested load in the presence of VP production. Normal urine output is 78%–82% of the ingested water load during the 4-hour test. In SIADH, low plasma osmolality is present with highly concentrated urine, with decreased plasma sodium indicating abnormal secretion of ADH/VP.

**Urinary aquaporin-2.** May be useful in the differentiation of SIADH from other causes of hyponatremia.

## Patient Problems/Analyze Cues/Prioritize Hypotheses

# Fluid Imbalance/Electrolyte Imbalance

*due to* SIADH or its management

**Desired Outcomes/Generate Hypotheses:** Within 72 hours of initiating treatment, the patient verbalizes orientation to time, place, and person; has stable weight; BP is 90–140/60–85 mm Hg or within the patient's baseline range, urine output is at least 30 mL/hour; and heart rate is 60–100 bpm. Na⁺ levels are within or return to normal limits.

| ASSESSMENT—RECOGNIZE CUES/ INTERVENTIONS—TAKE ACTION | RATIONALES |
| --- | --- |
| **!** Assess for clinical signs of hyponatremia and fluid overload. Promptly report significant findings or changes to the health care provider. | Hyponatremia causes changes in neurologic/neuromuscular symptoms including lethargy, coma, seizures, headache, confusion, and weakness. Sodium levels of less than 120 mEq/L can cause life-threatening symptoms. Decreasing LOC, elevated BP and central venous pressure, urine output less than 30 mL/hour, and weight gain are signs of fluid overload that may occur with SIADH. |
| Monitor the laboratory results for hyponatremia and indicators of water intoxication. Report significant findings to the health care provider. | Decreased serum Na⁺ and plasma osmolality, urine osmolality elevated disproportionately in relation to plasma osmolality, and increased urine Na⁺ are values that may be seen with SIADH. Water retention may occur secondary to increased ADH secretion that dilutes the blood and results in reduced amounts of more concentrated urine. |
| Initiate fluid restriction (800–1000 mL/day), if needed and prescribed, to prevent fluid overload. Explain the necessity of this treatment to the patient and significant other. Do not keep water or ice chips at the bedside. | Restricting fluids to the amount manageable by the kidneys will allow the restoration of normal serum Na⁺ levels and osmolality without complications from pharmacotherapy. |
| Elevate the head of bed (HOB) 10–20 degrees, especially if fluid overload is present. | A slightly elevated HOB promotes venous return and thus reduces ADH release. Fluid overload can sometimes result in cerebral edema, which may add to problems with neural regulation of ADH secretion. |
| Monitor the daily weight during the same time and conditions each day. | Daily weight will help monitor changes in fluid balance. |
| Administer the vasomotor receptor antagonists as prescribed; carefully observe and document the patient's response. | These medications promote the normalization of hyponatremia. |
| **!** Administer the hypertonic (3%) saline slowly as prescribed. | This may be given if the patient has severe hyponatremia. Rate of administration is slow so that it only increases sodium levels to no more than 8–12 mEq/L in the first 24 hours. The administration rate is based on serial serum Na⁺ levels to decrease the risk for neurologic damage (osmotic demyelination), particularly if the hyponatremia is chronic rather than acute. |

## ASSESSMENT—RECOGNIZE CUES/ INTERVENTIONS—TAKE ACTION / RATIONALES

| ASSESSMENT—RECOGNIZE CUES/ INTERVENTIONS—TAKE ACTION | RATIONALES |
|---|---|
| Make sure that specimens for laboratory tests are drawn on time and results are reported to the health care provider promptly. | Serum blood levels of Na⁺ are assessed to determine whether the patient has hypernatremia as a result of aggressive treatment. |
| Institute seizure precautions as indicated and per agency policy. For more information, see "Seizures and Epilepsy," Chapter 42. | Seizures can occur in the presence of hyponatremia associated with SIADH. |

## Problems for Patients Undergoing Intracranial Surgery

### Patient Problems/Analyze Cues/Prioritize Hypotheses

# Risk for Increased Intracranial Pressure

*due to* complications that can occur as a result of intracranial surgery

**Desired Outcomes/Generate Solutions:** Optimally, the patient demonstrates the baseline level of mental acuity and verbalizes orientation to person, place, and time. The patient and significant other verbalize an accurate understanding of the importance of avoiding Valsalva-type maneuvers and describe signs and symptoms of increased intracranial pressure (ICP).

| ASSESSMENT—RECOGNIZE CUES/ INTERVENTIONS—TAKE ACTION | RATIONALES |
|---|---|
| Assess for changes in mental status or LOC, sluggish or unequal pupils, and changes in respiratory rate or pattern. | These are indicators of increased intracranial pressure (ICP). Neurologic deterioration may necessitate computed tomography scan. |
| Monitor for decreased vision, eye muscle weakness, abnormal extraocular eye movements, double vision, and airway obstruction. Report significant findings to the health care provider. | The surgery may interfere with cranial nerves governing eye movements and visual acuity—II, III, IV, and VI. |
| Measure the intake and output hourly for 24 hours, and monitor urine specific gravity every 1–2 hours. Monitor weight daily for evidence of weight gain or loss. | Intracranial surgical procedures may prompt either SIADH or diabetes insipidus caused by swelling or tissue integrity disturbances in the area of the pituitary gland or hypothalamus. |
| In the presence of suspected cerebrospinal fluid (CSF), elevate HOB and immediately report any suspicious drainage. | Raising the HOB decreases the potential for bacteria entering the brain. The presence of CSF represents a serious breach in cranial integrity. |
| Elevate the HOB 30 degrees. | This elevation will help decrease ICP and swelling. Dexamethasone may be prescribed to reduce cerebral swelling. |
| Explain that coughing, sneezing, and other Valsalva-type maneuvers must be avoided. | These actions can stress the operative site and increase ICP. |
| As indicated, obtain the prescription for a mild cathartic or stool softener. | This will help prevent straining with bowel movements. |

## ADDITIONAL PROBLEMS:

| | |
|---|---|
| *Risk for Impaired Cognition*, due to altered cerebral function | Chapter 48 |
| *Risk for Infection* | Chapter 37 |

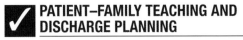

## ✓ PATIENT–FAMILY TEACHING AND DISCHARGE PLANNING

When providing patient–family teaching, speak slowly and simply, avoid giving excessive information, and initiate a visiting nurse referral for necessary follow-up teaching. Include verbal and written information about the following:
- ✓ Signs and symptoms of infection, which necessitate medical attention: fever, nuchal rigidity, moderate to severe headache, and photophobia.
- ✓ Importance of fluid restriction for the prescribed period if the patient was hypervolemic. Assist the patient with planning permitted fluid intake (e.g., by saving liquids for social and recreational situations as indicated).
- ✓ How to safely enrich diet with Na⁺ and K⁺ salts, particularly if ongoing diuretic use is prescribed.
- ✓ How to use daily weight measurements to assess hydration status.

✓ Signs of hyponatremia and hypervolemia: altered LOC, fatigue, headache, nausea, vomiting, and anorexia, any of which should be reported promptly to the health care provider.

✓ Medications, including drug name, dosage, route, purpose, precautions, and potential side effects. Also discuss drug–drug, food–drug, and herb–drug interactions. Encourage the patient to report to the health care provider all alternative and complementary health strategies being used.

✓ Importance of continued medical follow-up; confirm date and time of next medical appointment.

✓ How to obtain a medical alert bracelet and identification card outlining diagnosis and emergency treatment by contacting MedicAlert Foundation at www.medicalert.org.

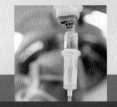

# Abdominal Trauma 53

## OVERVIEW/PATHOPHYSIOLOGY

Abdominal trauma accounts millions of emergency department visits in the United States annually and often causes serious injury to major organs and blood vessels. It is essential to understand the mechanism of the injury (blunt, penetrating, or combination) and the abdominal organs and blood vessels affected to avoid complications in the recovery period. Astute serial assessments in the posttraumatic period may prevent serious consequences and avoid life-threatening situations. Abdominal injuries often are associated with multisystem trauma. See also discussions in "Pneumothorax/Hemothorax," Chapter 14; "Spinal Cord Injury," Chapter 43; and "Traumatic Brain Injury," Chapter 45.

Knowledge of the injury mechanism and location assists the nurse in anticipating specific injuries to abdominal organs and vessels. Abdominal trauma, along with thoracic and musculoskeletal trauma, especially below the fourth rib, is an indicator that specific abdominal organs are at risk for injury. Solid organs (liver, kidneys, and spleen) may bleed profusely with trauma and may result in hypovolemic shock; hollow organs (stomach and intestines) may collapse or rupture, releasing caustic substances into the peritoneum, which may lead to peritonitis. Injury also may result from the movement of organs within the body, particularly at the transition between rigidly fixed and mobile organs. Injury to the urinary bladder is not common but may be associated with pelvic fractures. Rectal and vaginal examinations are necessary to assess for injury and bleeding.

Blunt trauma may be caused by falls, assaults, motor vehicle collisions, or sports injuries and involve direct transmission of energy to solid or hollow organs, most commonly affecting the spleen and liver. Splenic injury should be suspected in the presence of left lower rib fractures. Rupture may not be immediately obvious, reinforcing the need for ongoing assessments. Pain radiating to the left shoulder (Kehr sign) may indicate blood beneath the diaphragm from splenic bleeding. Pain radiating to the right shoulder may indicate injury to the liver. Other organs that may be affected by blunt trauma include the kidneys and, occasionally, the pancreas and small and large intestines. Bleeding is the most common complication, resulting in increased morbidity and mortality. Abdominal vessels are sometimes injured when blunt abdominal trauma occurs, and this may lead to shock and death if not recognized early. Signs of blood loss may not be evident initially; therefore, continual assessment is essential.

Gunshot, stabbing, or impalement may cause penetrating trauma, and the external appearance of the wound often does not accurately represent internal damage. If the lower esophagus, stomach, or intestines are injured by penetration, complications from the release of irritating gastric and intestinal fluids into the peritoneum and free air below the diaphragm may occur. Penetrating injuries to the solid organs may cause fatal damage if not identified early.

## HEALTH CARE SETTING

Emergency care, trauma center, acute care surgical unit, rehabilitation center

## ASSESSMENT

As with all trauma patients, immediate life-threatening problems must be identified, and treatment initiated before the more detailed secondary assessments are completed.

**Caution:** Recently injured patients should be evaluated frequently for peritoneal signs (generalized abdominal pain or tenderness, guarding and splinting of the abdominal wall, abdominal wall rigidity, rebound tenderness, abdominal pain with movement or coughing, abdominal distention, and decreased or absent bowel sounds). Umbilical and flank areas must also be assessed for bruising, which may indicate retroperitoneal hemorrhage. The health care provider must be notified immediately of these signs of bleeding as well as evidence of shock, gastric or rectal bleeding, or gross hematuria.

***Vital signs and hemodynamic measurements.*** Vital signs (VS) should be assessed continually to detect changes early. Gradual or sudden changes may signal hemorrhage after trauma, with tachycardia, impaired capillary refill, and hypotension, key indicators of bleeding or shock. Respiratory assessment is also essential because ventilatory excursion may be diminished because of pain, thoracic injury, or limited diaphragmatic movement caused by abdominal distention, which may impede oxygenation.

***Pain.*** Mild tenderness to severe abdominal pain may be present, with pain either localized to the site of injury or diffuse. Blood or fluid collection within the peritoneum causes irritation and may cause guarding, distention, rigidity, and rebound tenderness.

***Gastrointestinal symptoms.*** Nausea and vomiting may be present after blunt or penetrating trauma secondary to bleeding or obstruction.

**Note:** *Absence of signs and symptoms, especially in patients who have sustained head or spinal cord injury, does not exclude the presence of major abdominal injury.*

**Inspection.** Abrasions and ecchymoses are suggestive of underlying injury. For example, ecchymosis over the left upper quadrant (LUQ) suggests possible splenic injury. Ecchymotic areas around the umbilicus or flanks are suggestive of retroperitoneal bleeding. Erythema and ecchymosis across the lower abdomen suggest intestinal or bladder injury caused by lap belts. Ecchymoses may take hours to days to develop, depending on the rate of blood loss. Abdominal distention may signal bleeding, free air, or inflammation.

**Auscultation.** Bowel sounds should be auscultated frequently, especially in the first 24–48 hours after injury. Auscultate before percussion and palpation to avoid stimulating the bowel and confounding assessment findings. Bowel sounds may be decreased or absent with abdominal organ injury and intraperitoneal bleeding. However, the presence of bowel sounds does not exclude significant abdominal injury. Bowel sounds in the chest could indicate a ruptured diaphragm with small bowel herniation into the thorax. Absence of bowel sounds is suggestive of ileus or other complications, such as bleeding, peritonitis, or bowel infarction. Presence of an abdominal bruit (turbulent blood flow through vessels) could indicate arterial injury.

**Note:** *Percuss and palpate painful areas last. If the patient's pain is severe, do not percuss or palpate because more advanced studies are indicated for evaluation.*

**Percussion.** Tympany suggests the presence of gas. Percussion may reveal unusually large areas of dullness over ruptured blood-filled organs (e.g., a fixed area of dullness in the LUQ suggests a ruptured spleen).

**Palpation.** Tenderness or pain to palpation suggests abdominal injury. Blood or fluid in the abdomen can result in signs and symptoms of peritoneal irritation.

## DIAGNOSTIC TESTS

**Hemoglobin and hematocrit.** This is done to determine baseline values because hemoglobin (Hgb) and hematocrit (Hct) will not change until fluid resuscitation begins.

**Urinalysis.** Blood in the urine may be a sign of kidney or bladder damage.

**White blood cell count.** Leukocytosis is expected immediately after injury. Splenic injuries in particular result in the rapid development of a moderate to high white blood cell (WBC) count. A later increase in WBCs or a shift to the left reflects an increase in the number of neutrophils, which signals an inflammatory response and possible intraabdominal infection.

**Platelet count.** Mild thrombocytosis is seen immediately after traumatic injury. Thrombocytopenia may be present after a massive hemorrhage.

**Glucose.** Glucose is initially elevated because of catecholamine release and insulin resistance associated with major trauma. Glucose metabolism is abnormal after major hepatic resection, and patients should be monitored to prevent hypoglycemic episodes.

**Amylase.** Elevations reflect pancreatic or upper small bowel injury.

**Liver function tests.** Elevations reflect hepatic injury.

**Arterial blood gases.** To determine the presence of hypoxemia, hypercapnia, and respiratory or metabolic acidosis or alkalosis.

**Type and crossmatch.** To prepare for blood replacement if required.

**Radiographic examination.** Initially, flat and upright chest radiographic examinations exclude chest injuries (commonly associated with abdominal trauma) and establish a baseline. Subsequent chest radiographic examinations aid in detecting complications, such as atelectasis and pneumonia. In addition, chest and pelvic radiographic examinations may reveal fractures, missiles, foreign bodies, free intraperitoneal air, hematoma, or hemorrhage. Plain abdominal films are not useful in blunt trauma because they cannot define blood in the peritoneum.

**Ultrasound.** A rapid, noninvasive assessment tool for detecting intraabdominal hemorrhage may be done in the emergency department. The focused assessment sonogram for trauma (FAST) is a rapid bedside examination that has a sensitivity, specificity, and accuracy rate of more than 90% in detecting 100 mL or more of intraabdominal blood or fluid. Four areas are evaluated: the perihepatic and hepatorenal space, the perisplenic area, the pelvis, and the pericardium. A single negative FAST cannot absolutely exclude intraabdominal bleeding. FAST is used in conjunction with the full trauma evaluation.

**Computed tomography.** Reveals organ-specific blunt abdominal injury and quantifies the amount of blood and source of hemorrhage in the abdomen. Computed tomography (CT) images the ureters and can detect the extravasation of urine. Disadvantages are the expense and time required to perform the examination. Patients with positive CT scan require diagnostic laparotomy. **Caution:** A nurse always must accompany a patient in an unstable condition during the CT scan.

**Peritoneal lavage.** May be done to detect blood, bile, intestinal contents, and urine in the peritoneal cavity.

**Occult blood.** Gastric contents, urine, and stool must be tested for occult blood because bleeding can occur as a result of direct injury, causing significant complications.

**Angiography.** Performed to evaluate the injury to spleen, liver, pancreas, duodenum, and retroperitoneal vessels. **Caution:** Ensure adequate hydration and monitor urine output closely for 24–48 hours after angiography because the large amount of contrast used may cause renal failure, especially in older adults or in patients with preexisting cardiovascular or renal disease. Decreased urinary output and increased blood urea nitrogen and creatinine may indicate contrast-associated acute tubular necrosis.

## Patient Problem/Analyze Cues/Prioritize Hypotheses

# Impaired Gas Exchange

*due to* shallow respirations caused by pain from injury or surgical incision, chemical irritation of blood or bile on pleural tissue, and diaphragmatic elevation caused by abdominal distention

**Desired Outcome/Generate Solutions:** Within 24 hours of admission or surgery, the patient becomes eupneic with a respiratory rate (RR) of 12–20 breaths/minute and clear breath sounds; $O_2$ saturation is greater than 92%.

| ASSESSMENT—RECOGNIZE CUES/ INTERVENTIONS—TAKE ACTION | RATIONALES |
|---|---|
| Assess the quality of breath sounds, RR, presence/absence of cough, and sputum characteristics. | Individuals sustaining abdominal trauma are likely to be tachypneic, with poor ventilatory effort. |
| Monitor the oximetry readings every 2–4 hours. | $O_2$ saturation 92% or less usually signals the need for supplemental oxygen. |
| Report significant findings to health care provider. | Poor ventilatory effort may result in atelectasis or pneumonia. |
| Administer the supplemental oxygen as prescribed. Monitor and document effectiveness. | Supplemental $O_2$ is delivered until the patient's arterial blood gas or oximetry values while breathing room air are acceptable. Oxygen is essential to recovery. |
| Encourage and assist the patient with coughing, deep breathing, incentive spirometry, and turning every 2–4 hours. | These measures help prevent pneumonia and atelectasis. |
| Administer the analgesics at dose and frequency that relieves pain and associated impaired chest excursion. | Reducing pain will enable full chest excursion for better oxygenation. |
| Instruct the patient on methods to splint the abdomen. | This information will help reduce pain on movement, coughing, and deep breathing, which in turn will aid the respiratory effort. |
| For additional interventions, see "Perioperative Care," Chapter 4, for *Impaired Gas Exchange*. | |

## Patient Problems/Analyze Cues/Prioritize Hypotheses

# Risk for Hemorrhage

*due to* abdominal trauma

**Desired Outcome/Generate Solutions:** Within 4 hours of admission or on definitive repair (e.g., surgery), the patient is normovolemic, as evidenced by systolic blood pressure (SBP) of 90 mm Hg or higher (or within the patient's baseline range), heart rate (HR) of 60–100 bpm, urinary output at least 30 mL/hour, warm extremities, brisk capillary refill (2 seconds or less), distal pulses at least 2+ on a 0–4+ scale, and absence of orthostasis.

| ASSESSMENT—RECOGNIZE CUES/ INTERVENTIONS—TAKE ACTION | RATIONALES |
|---|---|
| In *recently injured* patients, assess BP continually in the presence of obvious bleeding or unstable VS. | Health care providers must be notified for even a small drop in blood pressure that is sudden, especially in a trauma patient in whom extent of injury is unknown. In the young trauma patient, excellent neurovascular compensation results in a near-normal BP until there is large intravascular volume depletion. |

Continued

## ASSESSMENT—RECOGNIZE CUES/ INTERVENTIONS—TAKE ACTION

## RATIONALES

| ASSESSMENT—RECOGNIZE CUES/ INTERVENTIONS—TAKE ACTION | RATIONALES |
|---|---|
| Be alert to and report increasing diastolic BP (DBP) and decreasing SBP. | Increasing diastolic pressure with decreasing systolic pressure is a sign of hypovolemic shock. The difference between the SBP and the DBP is termed *pulse pressure.* When the pulse pressure is narrowed (less than 25% of SBP), this signals decreasing cardiac output and increasing peripheral vascular resistance in the presence of hypovolemic shock. |
| Assess the extremities for temperature, color, capillary refill, and strength of distal pulses. Report significant findings. | Pallor, coolness, delayed capillary refill (2 seconds or more), and decreased or absent peripheral pulses are physical indicators of bleeding/hemorrhage/shock. |
| Assess the HR, RR, and anxiety level (early) and confusion, lethargy, and coma (later). Immediately report significant findings. | Tachycardia (HR more than 100 bpm) and tachypnea (RR more than 20 breaths/minute) are clinical indicators of bleeding/hemorrhage/shock as are anxiety, confusion, lethargy, and coma. |
| | Early detection and treatment of shock are essential to prevent irreversible cardiovascular collapse and death. |
| Monitor the HR and cardiovascular status continually until the patient's condition is stable. Report dramatic changes to the health care provider. | Tachycardia and hypotension occur with bleeding. VS should be assessed continually to detect changes early for prompt intervention. |
| Administer the prescribed fluids rapidly through large-caliber (18-gauge or larger) intravenous (IV) catheters in patients with evidence of active blood loss. | Massive blood loss is frequently associated with abdominal injuries. Restoration and maintenance of adequate intravascular volume are essential. Ringers lactate or an isotonic solution is administered. Packed red blood cells are administered to replace blood loss, especially with Hgb less than 8 g/dL. Patients with abdominal trauma must have two large-bore IV lines inserted peripherally or centrally for rapid replacement of volume. |
| Evaluate the IV flow rate frequently during rapid volume resuscitation and monitor the patient closely. | These assessments will help prevent fluid volume overload and complications such as heart failure. |
| Titrate IV fluid therapy to maintain SBP greater than 90 mm Hg. | Maintaining SBP greater than 90 mm Hg is essential for adequate peripheral perfusion. |
| Ensure that large volumes of fluid are warmed before they are infused. | Warming is necessary to prevent hypothermia. |
| Measure the urinary output hourly if a catheter is in place or when the patient voids. | Low urine output reflects inadequate intravascular volume and decreased renal perfusion. |
| Be alert to decreasing urinary output and to infrequent voiding. Report significant findings. | Deficient fluid volume is an indicator that renal perfusion may be severely compromised. |
| Note and report the significant increases in the amount of drainage, especially if it is sanguineous. | An increase in sanguineous drainage signifies bleeding, and immediate intervention may be required to maintain hemodynamic stability. |
| Measure all output from drainage tubes and catheters, noting color, consistency, and odor (e.g., "coffee grounds," burgundy, bright red). Monitor and measure the quantity of bloody stools. | These measurements provide an estimate of ongoing blood loss. |
| Note the frequency/number of dressings used in performing dressing changes due to saturation with blood. | This assessment estimates the amount of blood lost via the wound site. |

## Patient Problem/Analyze Cues/Prioritize Hypotheses

# Acute Pain

*due to* the irritation caused by intraperitoneal blood or secretions, trauma or surgical incision, or manipulation of organs during surgery

*Desired Outcomes/Generate Solutions:* Within 4 hours of admission, the patient's subjective perception of pain decreases, as documented by pain scale. Nonverbal indicators, such as grimacing, are absent or diminished. The patient's pain is controlled without sedation.

| ASSESSMENT—RECOGNIZE CUES/ INTERVENTIONS—TAKE ACTION | RATIONALES |
|---|---|
| Assess for the presence and location of traumatic, preoperative, and postoperative pain. Use a pain scale, rating discomfort from 0 (no pain) to 10 (worst pain). | Pain related to trauma is an indicator of the extent of injury. Preoperative pain is anticipated and is a vital diagnostic aid. Location and character of postoperative pain also can be important. For example, incisional and some visceral pain can be anticipated, but intense or prolonged pain, especially when accompanied by other peritoneal signs, can signal bleeding, bowel infarction, infection, or other complications. Autonomic nervous system response to pain can complicate the assessment of abdominal injury and hypovolemia. A pain scale helps quantify pain and determine subsequent relief obtained. |
| Administer the analgesics as prescribed and indicated. | An alert patient should not suffer severe pain while awaiting surgical evaluation. Postoperatively prescribed analgesics should be administered on a continual or regular schedule promptly with additional analgesia as needed, or patient-controlled analgesia (PCA) provided. Analgesics are helpful in relieving pain and in aiding the recovery process by promoting greater ventilatory excursion. As the severity of pain lessens, alternative analgesics such as nonsteroidal antiinflammatory drugs (e.g., ketorolac, ibuprofen) may be prescribed if not contraindicated by patient history of gastric bleeding. |
| Encourage the patient to request analgesic before the pain becomes severe. | Prolonged stimulation of pain receptors results in increased sensitivity to painful stimuli and will increase the amount of drug required to relieve pain. |
| If possible, obtain an accurate drug and alcohol use history. | Intoxication often is involved in traumatic events. Patients may be drug or alcohol users, with a higher-than-average tolerance for opioids, requiring adjusted dosage for adequate pain relief. (Opioids can decrease gastrointestinal [GI] motility and may delay the return to normal bowel function.) These individuals may suffer symptoms of alcohol withdrawal (tremors, weakness, tachycardia, elevated BP, delusions, agitation, hallucinations) or opioid withdrawal (lacrimation, rhinorrhea, anxiety, tremors, muscle twitching, mydriasis, nausea, abdominal cramps, vomiting), and this will necessitate prompt recognition and treatment. |
| Use withdrawal scales if needed. | Withdrawal scales enable standardized assessment and treatment. |
| Monitor the PCA, if prescribed, and document effectiveness, using pain scale. Monitor RR and sedation when patient is using a PCA. | For this and other interventions/rationales, see discussions in "Pain," Chapter 5. |
| Incorporate nonmedication pain relief measures such as positioning, massage, music, and distraction to aid in pain reduction. Provide these instructions to the patient and family members. | Nonpharmacologic maneuvers support analgesia therapy in reducing pain. |

## Patient Problem/Analyze Cues/Prioritize Hypotheses

# Risk for Infection

*due to* inadequate primary defenses occurring with disruption of the internal organs (particularly of the GI tract) and traumatically inflicted open wound, multiple indwelling catheters and drainage tubes, and compromised immune state caused by blood loss and metabolic response to trauma

*Desired Outcome/Generate Solutions:* The patient is free of infection, as evidenced by temperature less than 100°F (37.7°C); HR of 100 bpm or less; no significant changes in mental status; orientation to person, place, and time; and absence of unusual erythema, edema, tenderness, warmth, or drainage at surgical incisions or wound sites.

| ASSESSMENT—RECOGNIZE CUES/ INTERVENTIONS—TAKE ACTION | RATIONALES |
|---|---|
| Wash your hands before and after all patient encounters. | Hand washing is the number one defense against infection. |
| Assess the VS for temperature increases and associated increases in heart and RRs. Notify the health care provider of sudden temperature elevations. | These signs are indicators of infection. |
| Assess mental status, orientation, and level of consciousness (LOC) as frequently as needed. | Mental status changes, confusion, or deterioration from baseline LOC can signal infection. |
| Evaluate the incisions and wound sites for unusual erythema, warmth, tenderness, edema, delayed healing, and purulent or unusual drainage. | These signs are evidence of localized infection. |
| Assess the amount, color, character, and odor of all drainage, and report significant findings. | Foul-smelling or abnormal drainage can occur with infection and should be reported for prompt intervention. |
| Ensure the patency of all surgically placed tubes or drains. Irrigate or attach to low-pressure suction as prescribed. Maintain continuity of closed drainage systems; use sterile technique when emptying drainage and recharging suction containers. Promptly report loss of tube patency. | Blocked drainage systems may promote infection and abscess formation. Maintaining a closed drainage system, and using the sterile technique, decrease the risk of infection. |
| Administer the antibiotics as prescribed on time. Reschedule parenteral antibiotics if a dose is delayed more than 1 hour. Check blood levels as indicated (e.g., with vancomycin and gentamicin). | Failure to administer antibiotics on schedule may result in inadequate blood levels and treatment failure. |
| Administer the pneumococcal vaccine to patients with total splenectomy, as prescribed. | This measure minimizes the risk for postsplenectomy sepsis. |
| Administer the tetanus immune globulin and tetanus toxoid as prescribed. | Risk for tetanus after trauma increases if the patient has not been immunized within the past 10 years. |
| Change dressings as prescribed, using the sterile technique; change one dressing at a time. | These interventions prevent infection and cross-contamination from various wounds. |
| Use drains, closed drainage systems, or drainage bags to remove and collect GI secretions. | These measures prevent contamination of the surgical incision site. |
| ⚠ If the patient has or develops an evisceration, do not reinsert tissue or organs. Place sterile, saline-soaked gauze over the evisceration, and cover it with a sterile towel until the surgeon can evaluate the evisceration. | Evisceration is an emergent, life-threatening situation. Preventing infection and maintaining homeostasis are essential until a surgical intervention can be made. |
| If evisceration is present, notify surgeon and keep the patient on bedrest in semi-Fowler position with knees bent. | This position reduces strain on eviscerated organs. Bedrest minimizes disruption to the abdominal organs, preventing further tissue damage and risk for infection. |
| Maintain nothing by mouth (NPO) status for the patient when evisceration is present. | The patient may need emergency surgery. |

## Patient Problem/Analyze Cues/Prioritize Hypotheses

# Risk for Ineffective Tissue Perfusion

*due to* interrupted blood flow to the abdominal viscera occurring with vascular disruption or occlusion, or *due to* moderate-to-severe hypovolemia caused by hemorrhage

***Desired Outcomes/Generate Solutions:*** The patient has adequate GI tissue perfusion, as evidenced by normoactive bowel sounds; soft, nondistended abdomen; and return of bowel elimination. Gastric secretions, drainage, and excretions are negative for occult blood.

| ASSESSMENT—RECOGNIZE CUES/ INTERVENTIONS—TAKE ACTION | RATIONALES |
|---|---|
| Auscultate for bowel sounds hourly in recently injured patients and at least every 8 hours during the recovery phase. Report significant findings. | Absent or diminished bowel sounds may be anticipated for up to 72 hours after trauma or surgery. Prolonged or sudden absence of bowel sounds may signal bowel ischemia or infarction and must be reported promptly for intervention. |
| Assess the patient for signs of peritonitis and report significant findings. | Signs of peritoneal irritation (generalized abdominal pain or tenderness, guarding, abdominal wall rigidity, rebound tenderness, abdominal pain with movement or coughing, abdominal distention, and decreased or absent bowel sounds) may occur acutely secondary to injury or may not develop until days or weeks later if complications caused by slow bleeding or other mechanisms occur. |
| Evaluate the laboratory data for evidence of bleeding (e.g., serial Hct and Hgb); elevated liver or pancreatic enzymes; and report significant findings. | Decreases in Hgb and Hct signify bleeding. Increases in liver or pancreatic enzymes indicate hepatic or pancreatic inflammation or injury. |
| Document the amount and character of GI secretions, drainage, and excretions and report significant findings. | Changes suggestive of bleeding (presence of frank or occult blood), infection (e.g., increased or purulent drainage), or obstruction (e.g., failure to eliminate flatus or stool within 72 hours after surgery) may signal the presence of a complication that necessitates timely intervention. |
| Assess the patency of gastric or intestinal tube. | Gastric decompression requires a patent tube to prevent the accumulation of gas or fluid in the stomach. |
| Ensure adequate intravascular volume (see discussion in *Risk for Hemorrhage*, earlier). | Adequate intravascular volume optimizes organ perfusion. |

## Patient Problem/Analyze Cues

# Impaired Skin Tissue Integrity

*due to* direct trauma and surgery, drain or tube insertion, catabolic posttraumatic state, and altered circulation

***Desired Outcome/Generate Solutions:*** Ongoing, the patient exhibits wound healing, and/or the skin remains nonerythemic and intact.

| ASSESSMENT—RECOGNIZE CUES/ INTERVENTIONS—TAKE ACTION | RATIONALES |
|---|---|
| Assess the wounds, fistulas, and drain sites at routine intervals and report significant findings. | These measures identify signs of irritation, infection, and ischemia (i.e., erythema, edema, purulent drainage) for prompt intervention. |
| Identify the infected and devitalized tissue. Aid in their removal by irrigation, wound packing, or preparing the patient for surgical debridement. | Removal of devitalized tissue is essential for wound healing to progress. |
| Promptly change all dressings that become soiled with drainage or blood. Protect skin surrounding tubes, drains, or fistulas, keeping the areas clean and free from drainage. | Gastric and intestinal secretions and drainage are irritating and can lead to skin excoriation. |

Continued

| ASSESSMENT—RECOGNIZE CUES/ INTERVENTIONS—TAKE ACTION | RATIONALES |
|---|---|
| If necessary, apply ointments, skin barriers, or drainage bags. Apply reusable dressing supports such as an abdominal binder or tubular mesh gauze. | These measures aid in preventing skin excoriation. <br><br> Dressing supports aid in keeping dressings in place and prevent excessive injury to surrounding skin by frequent tape removal. |
| Consult a wound, ostomy, continence/enterostomal therapy nurse for complex or involved cases and follow evidence-based recommendations. | Consulting with experts and following evidence-based recommendations can substantially aid in preventing skin damage. |
| Consult a nutritionist to ensure adequate protein and calorie intake (see *Risk for Impaired Nutrition*, following). | Adequate nutrition is necessary for tissue healing to occur. |
| For more information, see "Managing Wound Care," Chapter 75. | |

## Patient Problem/Analyze Cues/Prioritize Hypotheses

# Risk for Impaired Nutrition

*due to* decreased intake secondary to trauma and disruption of GI tract integrity (traumatic or surgical) and increased caloric need due to hypermetabolic posttraumatic state

*Desired Outcome/Generate Solutions:* By at least 24 hours before hospital discharge, the patient has adequate nutrition, as evidenced by maintenance of baseline body weight and positive or balanced nitrogen (N) state.

| ASSESSMENT—RECOGNIZE CUES/ INTERVENTIONS—TAKE ACTION | RATIONALES |
|---|---|
| Collaborate with the health care provider, nutritionist, and pharmacist to assess the patient's metabolic needs based on the type of injury, activity level, and nutritional status before injury. <br><br> Parenteral feedings are administered if enteral feedings cannot be tolerated. If patients are fed enterally, the feeding tube must be placed distal to the injury. | Patients with abdominal trauma have complex nutritional needs because of the hypermetabolic state associated with major trauma and traumatic or surgical disruption of normal GI function. Infection and sepsis often contribute to a negative nitrogen (N) state and increased metabolic needs. Prompt initiation of enteric feedings and administration of supplemental calories, proteins, vitamins, and minerals are essential for healing. |
| Monitor laboratory values, including prealbumin, albumin, total protein, and blood glucose. | Prealbumin, albumin, and total protein are indicators of nutritional stores and guide nutritional replacement. Patients with hepatic or pancreatic injury may be unable to regulate blood sugar levels. |
| Confirm the placement of the feeding tube before each tube feeding. After initial insertion, check the radiograph for position of the tube. Mark to determine tube migration, secure the tubing in place, and reassess every 4 hours and before each feeding. | Determining the correct placement of the feeding tube before instilling medications or feedings is essential to prevent aspiration or instillation of liquids or medications into the lungs. |
| Use caution and consult the surgeon before irrigating nasogastric (NG) or other tubes that have been placed in or near recently sutured organs. | Some NG tubes are sutured in place; irrigation or movement of the tube could disrupt sutures and cause bleeding. |
| Assess the pH of gastric aspirate. | A pH of less than 5 usually signals gastric placement. However, acid blockade medications may alter pH. |
| Avoid opioid analgesics if possible; administer prescribed nonnarcotic analgesics (e.g., ketorolac). | Opioid analgesics decrease GI motility and may contribute to nausea, vomiting, abdominal distention, and ileus. |
| For more information, see "Providing Nutritional Support," Chapter 76. | |

## Patient Problem/Analyze Cues/Prioritize Hypotheses

# Risk for Post Trauma Response

*due to* life-threatening event or severe trauma

***Desired Outcomes/Generate Solutions:*** By at least 24 hours before hospital discharge, the patient verbalizes aspects of the psychosocial impact of the event and does not exhibit signs of severe stress reaction, such as display of inconsistent affect, suicidal or homicidal behavior, or extreme agitation or depression. The patient cooperates with the treatment plan.

| ASSESSMENT—RECOGNIZE CUES/ INTERVENTIONS—TAKE ACTION | RATIONALES |
|---|---|
| Assess the patient's mental status at regular intervals. Be alert to indicators of severe stress reaction, such as display of affect inconsistent with statements or behavior, suicidal or homicidal statements or actions, extreme agitation or depression, and failure to cooperate with instructions related to care. | Many victims of major abdominal trauma sustain life-threatening injury. The patient is often aware of the situation and fears death. Even after the physical condition stabilizes, the patient may have a prolonged or severe reaction triggered by the recollection of the trauma. |
| Assess for organic causes that may contribute to the posttraumatic response. | Severe pain, alcohol intoxication or withdrawal, electrolyte imbalance, metabolic encephalopathy, and impaired cerebral perfusion are potential contributors to the posttraumatic response and should be treated accordingly. |
|  Consult specialists such as a psychiatrist, psychologist, psychiatric nurse practitioner, or pastoral counselor if the patient displays signs of severe stress reaction described previously. | Specialized intervention supports the patient and may prevent long-term suffering or suicide. |
| For other interventions, see "Psychosocial Support for the Patient" Chapter 8. | |

---

### ADDITIONAL PROBLEMS:

### ✓ PATIENT–FAMILY TEACHING AND DISCHARGE PLANNING

Anticipate extended physical and emotional rehabilitation for the patient and significant other. When providing patient–family teaching, focus on sensory information, avoid giving excessive information, and initiate a visiting nurse referral for necessary follow-up teaching. Include verbal and written information about the following:

- ✓ Self-management. Assessment of the patient's ability to manage own care should be completed before hospital discharge. Identification of support persons to assist with care should be initiated early.
- ✓ Probable need for emotional care, even for patients who have not required extensive physical rehabilitation. Provide referrals to support groups for trauma patients and family members.
- ✓ Availability of rehabilitation programs, extended care facilities, and home health agencies for patients unable to accomplish self-care on hospital discharge.
- ✓ Availability of rehabilitation programs for substance abuse, as indicated. Immediately after the traumatic event, patient and family members are very impressionable, making this period an ideal time for patients with substance abuse issues to begin to resolve the problem.
- ✓ Medications, including drug name, purpose, dosage, schedule, precautions, and potential side effects. Also discuss drug–drug, herb–drug, and food–drug interactions. Encourage patients taking antibiotics to take medications for prescribed length of time, even though they may not have symptoms. If the patient received a tetanus immunization, ensure that he or she receives documentation of the immunization.
- ✓ Wound and catheter care and dressing changes. Have the patient or caregiver describe and demonstrate proper technique before hospital discharge. Reinforce the importance of hand washing before and after all care activities to prevent infection.
- ✓ Activity. Restrictions and recommendations should be reviewed thoroughly with the patient and caregivers. An at-home assessment may be necessary if activity is severely limited or adaptations are necessary. Consider referral to an occupational therapist or physical therapist.

✓ Diet/nutrition. Review diet recommendations with the patient/family. If enteral or parenteral feeding is necessary, have the patient or caregiver describe and demonstrate the correct technique before hospital discharge. Home health care services may be warranted for support and evaluation.

✓ Importance of seeking medical attention if indicators of infection or bowel obstruction occur (e.g., fever, severe or unusual abdominal pain, nausea and vomiting, unusual drainage from wounds or incisions, a change in bowel habits).

✓ Injury prevention. After traumatic injury, the patient and family members are especially likely to respond to injury prevention education. Provide instructions on proper seat-belt applications (across pelvic girdle rather than across soft tissue of lower abdomen), safety for infants and children, and other factors suitable for individuals involved.

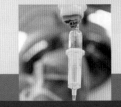

# Appendicitis 54

## OVERVIEW/PATHOPHYSIOLOGY

Appendicitis is the most commonly occurring inflammatory lesion of the bowel and one of the most common reasons for abdominal surgery. Appendicitis occurs most often in adolescents and young adults and is more common in males than females. The appendix is a blind, narrow tube that extends from the inferior portion of the cecum and generally is believed to serve no known useful function. However, it has been postulated that the appendix may be associated with the immune system and that it also may act as a repository for beneficial bacteria. Appendicitis can be caused by obstruction of the appendiceal lumen by a fecalith (hardened bit of fecal material), inflammation, a foreign body, or a neoplasm. Obstruction prevents drainage of secretions that are produced by epithelial cells in the lumen, thereby increasing intraluminal pressure and compressing mucosal blood vessels. This tension eventually impairs local blood flow, which can lead to necrosis, perforation, and peritonitis. Inflammation and infection result from normal bacteria invading the devitalized wall. Severe inflammation can lead to a ruptured appendix, which can cause local or generalized peritonitis and therefore surgery should be done as soon as the diagnosis is made. Patients are treated with fluids and antibiotics before surgery.

## HEALTH CARE SETTING

Acute care surgical unit. Inpatient status for ruptured appendix with peritonitis; 1-day length of stay for uncomplicated laparoscopic appendectomy without complications.

## ASSESSMENT

Signs and symptoms vary because of differences in anatomy, size, and age. The sequence of symptoms can be significant in the differential diagnosis. Abdominal discomfort, indigestion, and bowel irregularity occur first.

***Early stage.*** Pain usually occurs in either the epigastric or umbilical area and may be vague and diffuse or associated with mild cramping. Nausea and vomiting are not always present, but if they occur, they follow the onset of pain. Fever and leukocytosis occur later.

***Intermediate (acute) stage.*** Over a period of a few hours, pain shifts from the midabdomen or epigastrium to the right lower quadrant (RLQ) at McBurney's point (approximately 2 inches from the anterior superior iliac spine on a line drawn from the umbilicus) and is aggravated by walking, coughing, and movement. Pain may be accompanied by a sensation of constipation (gas-stoppage sensation). Anorexia, malaise, occasionally diarrhea, and diminished peristalsis also can occur.

On physical assessment, the patient may experience pain in the RLQ elicited by light palpation of the abdomen; presence of rebound tenderness; RLQ guarding, rigidity, and muscle spasms; tachycardia; low-grade fever; and pain elicited with rectal examination. A palpable, tender mass may be felt in the peritoneal pouch if the appendix lies within the pelvis.

> **Note:** *Physical assessment is performed in four steps—inspection, auscultation, percussion, and palpation—in that order, to avoid stimulating the abdomen by palpation and percussion, which can affect bowel sounds.*

***Acute appendicitis with perforation.*** Increasing, generalized pain, and may exhibit a positive psoas (pain with right thigh extension), obturator (pain with passive internal rotation of the flexed thigh), and Rovsing signs (RLQ pain when left lower quadrant is palpated); recurrence of vomiting. On physical assessment, the patient usually exhibits temperature increases to more than 101.4°F (38.5°C) and generalized abdominal rigidity. Typically, the patient remains rigid with flexed knees. Presence of abscess can result in a tender, palpable mass. The abdomen may be distended.

## DIAGNOSTIC TESTS

***Abdominal computed tomography scan.*** Has an accuracy rate of 95% overall and should be performed before a laparotomy.

***White blood cell count with differential.*** Reveals the presence of leukocytosis and an increase in neutrophils. A shift to the left with more than 75% neutrophils is a consistent finding in the later stages of appendicitis.

***C-reactive protein assay.*** Blood test that detects the presence of an inflammatory process. Elevated levels are seen with appendicitis.

***Abdominal ultrasound.*** May be done to rule out appendicitis or conditions that mimic it, such as Crohn's disease, diverticulitis, or gastroenteritis. Higher success rate for diagnosis is found in children.

***Abdominal radiographic examination.*** May reveal the presence of a fecalith. About half of these patients may have radiographic findings of localized air-fluid levels, increased soft tissue density

411

in the RLQ, and indications of localized ileus. If perforation has occurred, the presence of free air is noted.

**Urinalysis.** To rule out genitourinary conditions mimicking appendicitis; may reveal microscopic hematuria and pyuria. This test result usually is normal.

**Stool test for calprotectin.** A protein that is a biomarker for identifying acute appendicitis.

**Intravenous pyelogram.** May be performed to rule out ureteral stone or pyelitis.

## Patient Problem/Analyze Cues/Prioritize Hypotheses

# Risk for Infection

*due to* inadequate primary defenses (danger of rupture, peritonitis, abscess formation) occurring with the inflammatory process

**Desired Outcome/Generate Solutions:** The patient is free of infection/sepsis, as evidenced by normothermia, heart rate of 100 bpm or less, blood pressure of at least 90/60 mm Hg, respiratory rate of 12–20 breaths/minute with normal depth and pattern (eupnea), absence of chills, soft and nondistended abdomen, and bowel sounds 5–34/minute in each abdominal quadrant.

| ASSESSMENT—RECOGNIZE CUES/ INTERVENTIONS—TAKE ACTION | RATIONALES |
| --- | --- |
| ⚠ Assess and document the quality, location, and duration of the pain; presence of nausea; and the patient's positioning. | Signs of worsening appendicitis that can lead to rupture include pain that becomes accentuated; recurrent vomiting; and the patient assuming a side-lying or supine position with flexed knees. Pain that worsens and then disappears is a signal that rupture may have occurred. |
| ⚠ Assess the vital signs for elevated temperature, increased pulse rate, hypotension, and shallow/rapid respirations. Assess the abdomen for rigidity, distention, and decreased or absent bowel sounds. Report significant findings to the health care provider. | Any of these indicators can occur with rupture. |
| Administer the antibiotics as prescribed. | Antibiotics are indicated to prevent systemic infection and to treat intraabdominal infection. |
| Assess the patient's mobility for ambulation with a limp or pain with hip extension. | Retrocecal abscess may irritate the psoas muscle as it traverses the area of posterior RLQ of the abdomen and results in pain with hip extension. |
| Teach the postoperative incisional care as well as care of drains if the patient is to be discharged with them. | Maintaining a clean incision and avoiding contamination of drains help prevent infection in areas in which the skin is no longer intact. |
| | An incisional drain may be inserted in the presence of abscess, rupture, or peritonitis to facilitate drainage of exudate and peritoneal fluid and avoid complications of infection. |
| Provide instructions for the prescribed antibiotics if the patient is to be discharged with them. | Antibiotics prevent or treat systemic infection from a ruptured appendix. See "Peritonitis," Chapter 62, for more information. |

## Patient Problem/Analyze Cues/Prioritize Hypotheses

# Acute Pain

*due to* the inflammatory process

**Desired Outcomes/Generate Solutions:** Within 1–2 hours of pain-relieving interventions, the patient's subjective perception of pain decreases, as documented by pain scale. Objective indicators, such as grimacing, are absent or diminished.

| ASSESSMENT—RECOGNIZE CUES/ INTERVENTIONS—TAKE ACTION | RATIONALES |
|---|---|
| Assess and document the quality, location, and duration of the pain. Devise a pain scale with the patient, rating discomfort from 0 (no pain) to 10 (worst pain). | These characteristics of discomfort may be seen during the following stages of appendicitis: <br><br> *Early stage:* Abdominal pain (either epigastric or umbilical) that may be vague and diffuse, nausea and vomiting, fever, and sensitivity over appendix area. <br><br> *Intermediate (acute) stage:* Pain that shifts from the epigastrium to the RLQ at McBurney's point (approximately 2 inches from the anterior superior iliac spine on a line drawn from the umbilicus) and is aggravated by walking or coughing. The pain may be accompanied by a sensation of constipation (gas-stoppage sensation). Anorexia, malaise, occasional diarrhea, and diminished peristalsis also can occur. <br><br> *Acute appendicitis with perforation:* Increasing, generalized pain; recurrence of vomiting; increasing abdominal rigidity. |
| Medicate with antiemetics, sedatives, and analgesics as prescribed; evaluate and document the patient's response, using the pain scale. | These agents reduce nausea and pain. Opioids are avoided until diagnosis is certain because they mask clinical signs and symptoms. |
| Encourage the patient to request medication *before* symptoms become severe. | Prolonged stimulation of pain receptors results in increased sensitivity to painful stimuli and will increase the amount of drug required to relieve the discomfort. |
| Teach the technique for slow, diaphragmatic breathing. | This technique reduces stress and helps promote comfort by relaxing tense muscles. |
| Help position the patient for optimal comfort. | Many patients find comfort from a side-lying position with knees bent, whereas others find relief when supine with pillows under the knees (avoiding pressure on popliteal area). These positions help to reduce pain by decreasing traction on the abdomen. |

## Patient Problem/Analyze Cues/Prioritize Hypotheses

# Risk for Health Care–Associated Complication (Reaction to Iodinated Contrast Medium)

*due to* allergy to contrast dye administration during computed tomography (CT) scan procedure

***Desired Outcome/Generate Solutions:*** After completion of the CT scan procedure, the patient has no significant changes in vital signs, has no adverse reactions, and is able to tolerate increased fluid intake and void at least 30 mL/hour to excrete contrast dye.

| ASSESSMENT—RECOGNIZE CUES/ INTERVENTIONS—TAKE ACTION | RATIONALES |
|---|---|
| • Before the procedure, assess the patient for allergies to iodine, shellfish, and previous allergic reaction to iodinated or other contrast media. If these allergies exist, notify the health care provider. | An iodine-based contrast medium may cause an anaphylactic response in patients allergic to these substances. |
| • If patient taking Metformin, notify health care provider and do not administer before and after the procedure as per provider orders. | Intravascular administration of iodinated contrast media to patients who are receiving metformin, an oral antidiabetic agent, can result in lactic acidosis. |

Continued

## ASSESSMENT—RECOGNIZE CUES/ INTERVENTIONS—TAKE ACTION

## RATIONALES

| ASSESSMENT—RECOGNIZE CUES/ INTERVENTIONS—TAKE ACTION | RATIONALES |
| --- | --- |
| Obtain prescribed laboratory tests, such as blood urea nitrogen and creatinine levels. Notify the health care provider if levels are elevated. | If levels are elevated, the patient is at increased risk for renal failure secondary to the contrast medium. |
| Administer the preprocedure medication as prescribed. | Premedication with prednisone and diphenhydramine may be prescribed to decrease or prevent contrast media reaction. A nonionic, hypoallergenic contrast dye may be used instead. |
| Instruct the patient to increase fluids and report any decrease in urinary output from his or her normal range. | Increased fluid intake promotes contrast dye excretion and prevents dye-induced renal failure. |
| Instruct the patient to contact the health care provider immediately if rash, hives, tachycardia, or dyspnea occurs. | Reactions to contrast media can occur starting from 2 to 6 hours after the procedure and to within 7 days after contrast dye injection. |

### ADDITIONAL PROBLEM:

| | |
| --- | --- |
| "Perioperative Care" | Chapter 4 |

### ✓ PATIENT–FAMILY TEACHING AND DISCHARGE PLANNING

When providing patient–family teaching, focus on sensory information, and avoid giving excessive information. Include verbal and written information about the following:

- ✓ Medications, including drug name, dosage, purpose, schedule, precautions, and potential side effects. Also discuss drug–drug, food–drug, and herb–drug interactions.
- ✓ Care of incision, including dressing changes and bathing restrictions if appropriate.
- ✓ Indicators of infection: fever, chills, incisional pain, redness, swelling, and purulent drainage.
- ✓ Postsurgical activity precautions: avoid lifting heavy objects (more than 10 lb) for the first 6 weeks or as directed, be alert to and rest after symptoms of fatigue, get maximum rest, and gradually increase activities to tolerance.
- ✓ Importance of avoiding enemas for the first few postoperative weeks. Caution the patient about the need to check with the health care provider before having an enema.

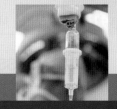

# Cholelithiasis, Cholecystitis, and Cholangitis 55

## OVERVIEW/PATHOPHYSIOLOGY

Cholelithiasis, or gallstones, is the most common disorder of the biliary system in the United States, affecting up to 10% of the adult population, with women affected at a rate double that of men. Gallstones may be found anywhere in the biliary system and may lodge in the gallbladder or in the cystic duct, and cause pain, nausea, and vomiting. Many people with gallstones have no symptoms; however, these individuals are at risk for developing cholecystitis, cholangitis, or pancreatitis. Gallstones are classified as cholesterol or pigment stones. Cholesterol stones, which originate in the gallbladder, are more common in the United States and represent most cases. Factors contributing to the formation of cholesterol stones include obesity, rapid weight loss (e.g., due to bariatric surgery), multiparity, hyperlipidemia, diets high in cholesterol, diabetes mellitus, and medications. Pigment stones account for 30% of gallstones and are divided into two types: black pigment stones and calcium bilirubinate stones. Black pigment stones are shiny, hard, and tar-like and consist of inorganic material. Calcium bilirubinate stones are soft and brown and have a foul odor. Factors leading to the formation of pigment stones include cirrhosis, ileal disease, hemolytic anemia, truncal vagotomy, hyperparathyroidism, and infections of the bile duct. Patients with mixed stones have both cholesterol and pigment stones.

The incidence of gallstones is predominant in adult females and increases after age 40 years. Cholelithiasis is commonly seen in patients with diseases such as diabetes mellitus, regional enteritis, and certain blood dyscrasias. Usually, cholelithiasis is asymptomatic until a stone becomes lodged in the cystic duct or bile duct. If the obstruction is unrelieved, biliary colic causes an acute, sharp pain when the gallbladder contracts while a stone is lodged in the cystic duct. Biliary colic eventually leads to acute cholecystitis.

*Choledocholithiasis* is the term used to describe gallstones that have migrated to the common bile duct. *Acute cholecystitis* results from bile stasis, bacterial infection, or ischemia of the gallbladder. When the cystic tract becomes obstructed, the gallbladder becomes distended. Structural changes such as swelling and thickening of the gallbladder walls can occur. Additionally, serosal edema, mucosal sloughing, and congestion within the venous and lymphatic systems occur. Ultimately, ischemia can occur, resulting in gangrene or perforation. With chronic cholecystitis, stones almost always are present, and the gallbladder walls are thickened and fibrosed.

*Ascending cholangitis or acute cholangitis* (inflammation of the biliary ducts) is the most serious complication of gallstones and is more difficult to diagnose than either cholelithiasis or cholecystitis. It is caused by an impacted stone in the common bile duct, resulting in bile stasis, bacteremia, and septicemia if left untreated. Cholangitis is most likely to occur when an already infected bile duct becomes obstructed. Bacteria enter the duct from the adjacent duodenum. It is believed that chronic bacteremia within the bile duct can eventually cause *primary sclerosing cholangitis* with the hallmarks, including biliary duct fibrosis (intrahepatic and extrahepatic) and inflammatory changes. Mortality rate is high if not recognized and treated early.

## HEALTH CARE SETTING

Primary care; acute care

## ASSESSMENT

**Cholelithiasis.** Patients report a history of occasional discomfort after eating. As the stone moves through the duct or becomes lodged, a sudden onset of mild, aching pain occurs in the mid-epigastrium after eating (especially after a high-fat meal) and increases in intensity during a colic attack, potentially radiating to the right upper quadrant (RUQ), right subscapular region, right shoulder, or back and can last 1–4 hours. Nausea, vomiting, tachycardia, mild fever, and diaphoresis also can occur. Patients who develop gallstone pancreatitis may be completely symptom free until they develop the symptoms of pancreatitis.

**Acute cholecystitis.** When acute cholecystitis develops, patients experience RUQ pain, fever, and leukocytosis. There may be a history of discomfort after eating, including regurgitation, flatulence, belching, epigastric heaviness, indigestion, heartburn, chronic upper abdominal pain, and nausea. Amber-colored urine, clay-colored stools, pruritus, jaundice, steatorrhea, fever, and bleeding tendencies can be present if there is biliary obstruction. Symptoms may be vague. An acute attack may last 7–10 days, but it usually resolves in several hours.

**Cholangitis.** Fever is present in nearly all the patients with bacterial cholangitis. Jaundice, chills, abdominal pain, mental confusion, and lethargy are part of the presenting symptoms. Leukocytosis and elevated bilirubin are present in 80% of cases.

# PHYSICAL ASSESSMENT

*Cholelithiasis.* Palpation of the RUQ reveals a tender abdomen during episodes of biliary colic. Otherwise, between episodes of pain, the examination is usually normal.

*Acute cholecystitis.* Palpation elicits tenderness localized behind the inferior margin of the liver. With progressive symptoms, a tender, globular mass may be palpated behind the lower border of the liver. Rebound tenderness and guarding also may be present. With the patient taking a deep breath, palpation over the RUQ elicits Murphy sign (pain and inability to inspire when the examiner's hand comes in contact with the gallbladder).

*Cholangitis.* Hypotension and mental confusion are present in severe cases.

> **Note:** *Cholangitis is a surgical emergency requiring prompt decompression of the biliary tract.*

# DIAGNOSTIC TESTS

*Ultrasonography.* Ultrasonography is the preferred test for confirming the presence of gallstones, as well as their number, size, and location. Ultrasound can also identify gallbladder wall changes such as thickening and edema, as well as the presence of sludge and fluid collection. Ultrasonography is readily available, does not expose the patient to radiation, and is noninvasive and inexpensive.

*Percutaneous transhepatic cholangiography.* Percutaneous transhepatic cholangiography is a procedure performed during which contrast is injected into one or more bile ducts. It is often done after bile duct blockage is noted on the ultrasound.

*Endoscopic retrograde cholangiopancreatography.* Visualization and evaluation of the biliary tree or pancreatic duct. Endoscopic retrograde cholangiopancreatography (ERCP) is useful to both diagnose and remove common bile duct stones and can also help with the evaluation of anatomic structures.

ERCP does have its risks because complications such as ERCP-induced pancreatitis, hemorrhage, perforation, and cholangitis are possible.

*Magnetic resonance imaging and magnetic resonance cholangiopancreatography.* Magnetic resonance imaging (MRI) and magnetic resonance cholangiopancreatography (MRCP) also can be used to diagnose common bile duct stones; however, unlike ERCP, common bile duct stones cannot be removed with MRCP. MRI is not available at every institution and requires patient cooperation. Because MRCP is a more expensive test, its use is limited, although it can be a helpful study to assess RUQ pain in pregnancy and biliary tree abnormalities.

*Computed tomography scan.* Although ultrasonography is preferred over computed tomography (CT) for suspected gallbladder disease, CT of the abdomen is used in cases of uncertain diagnosis, presence of complications, or suspicion of additional pathologies. A drawback of CT is its low sensitivity in the detection of gallstones.

*Complete blood count with differential.* To assess for the presence of infection or blood loss. Infection and inflammation cause leukocytosis. White blood cell counts greater than 18,000 suggest possible gangrene or gallbladder perforation.

*Bilirubin tests (serum and urine) and urobilinogen tests (urine and fecal).* May be performed to differentiate among hemolytic disorders, hepatocellular disease, and obstructive disease. Usually, there is an increase of bilirubin in the plasma and urine with biliary disease.

*Serum liver enzyme test.* Usually normal in cholecystitis but often becomes abnormal in the presence of prolonged cholecystitis or common duct stones. If elevated in cholecystitis, it is usually associated with worse outcomes.

*Prothrombin time and International Ionized Ratio (INR).* To assess for prolonged clotting time secondary to faulty vitamin K absorption.

*Electrocardiogram.* To rule out cardiac disease. Pain that may present as cholelithiasis or cholecystitis may actually be cardiac pain.

## Patient Problem/Analyze Cues/Prioritize Hypotheses

# Acute Pain

*due to* the obstructive or inflammatory process

**Desired Outcomes/Generate Solutions:** The patient's subjective perception of pain decreases within 1 hour of intervention, as documented by a pain scale. Nonverbal indicators, such as grimacing, are absent or diminished.

| ASSESSMENT—RECOGNIZE CUES/ INTERVENTIONS—TAKE ACTION | RATIONALES |
|---|---|
| Monitor the patient for pain, including spasms. Devise a pain scale with the patient, rating discomfort on a scale of 0 (no pain) to 10 (worst pain). Assess the patient before and after interventions for the effectiveness of discomfort relief. | Using a pain scale enables a more objective measurement of discomfort and subsequent relief obtained. |

| ASSESSMENT—RECOGNIZE CUES/ INTERVENTIONS—TAKE ACTION | RATIONALES |
|---|---|
| Explain that a low-Fowler position will minimize discomfort. | This position decreases tension on abdominal contents to promote comfort. |
| Provide instructions to the patient about the prescribed diet. | The prescribed diet will prevent spasms and varies according to the patient's condition. |
| During an acute attack, nothing by mouth (NPO) status with intravenous (IV) fluids may be instituted in preparation for possible surgery. The diet advances to the patient's tolerance, and small, frequent feedings of a low-fat diet are recommended for both acute and chronic conditions. | This diet minimizes the secretion of bile salts and subsequent gallbladder spasms. |
| After cholecystectomy, a low-fat diet is used initially, and fatty foods may be introduced gradually to the patient's level of tolerance. | Fats are introduced gradually to decrease the risk of gastrointestinal symptoms. |
| Administer a bile salt–binding agent as prescribed. | These drugs bind with bile salts in the intestine to facilitate their excretion and may also provide relief from pruritus caused by prolonged obstructive jaundice. |
| Administer the analgesics as prescribed and report significant side effects. | Nonsteroidal antiinflammatory drugs or opioid analgesics may be indicated, depending on pain severity. For postoperative patients, epidural, continuous IV, and patient-controlled infusions of opioid analgesics are used with increasing frequency and superior efficacy (see "Pain," Chapter 5, for more information). |
| | IV ketorolac every 6 hours for 4–8 doses has shown benefit in controlling postoperative pain with these patients, reducing the need for opioid analgesics. It should not be used for more than 5 days because of its toxic effects. respiratory depression associated with its cumulative effects. |
| Administer the acid suppression therapy if prescribed. | This therapy neutralizes gastric hyperacidity and reduces associated pain. $H_2$ blockers and antacids should be used as the first-line therapy. |

## Patient Problem/Analyze Cues/Prioritize Hypotheses

# Nausea

*due to* the obstructive or inflammatory process

***Desired Outcomes/Generate Solutions:*** The patient reports that nausea and associated vomiting have decreased within 1 hour of interventions. Nonverbal indicators, such as retching, are absent or diminished.

| ASSESSMENT—RECOGNIZE CUES/ INTERVENTIONS—TAKE ACTION | RATIONALES |
|---|---|
| Monitor the patient for nausea using a scale from 1 to 10. Assess the patient before and after interventions for the effectiveness of relief. | Using a scale enables a more objective measurement of nausea and subsequent relief obtained. |
| Instruct the patient and significant other about the prescribed diet. | The prescribed diet will prevent nausea and varies according to the patient's condition. This diet minimizes the secretion of bile salts and subsequent gallbladder spasms. |
| During an acute attack, NPO status with IV fluids may be instituted in preparation for possible surgery. With severe nausea and vomiting, a gastric tube is inserted and attached to low, intermittent suction. The diet advances to the patient's tolerance, and small, frequent feedings of a low-fat diet are recommended for both acute and chronic conditions. | |
| After cholecystectomy, a low-fat diet is used initially, and fatty foods may be introduced gradually to the patient's level of tolerance. | |
| Administer the acid suppression therapy if prescribed. | This therapy neutralizes gastric hyperacidity and reduces associated nausea and digestive upset. |
| Administer the antiemetics as prescribed. | Antiemetics are given to control nausea and vomiting. |

## Patient Problem/Analyze Cues/Prioritize Hypotheses

# Risk for Disease (Recurring Bile Obstruction)

*due to* postsurgical drainage issues

**Desired Outcome/Generate Solutions:** The patient exhibits diminishing dark-brown drainage of less than 1000 mL/day and the presence of a soft and nondistended abdomen, normal skin color, brown stools, and straw-colored urine.

| ASSESSMENT—RECOGNIZE CUES/ INTERVENTIONS—TAKE ACTION | RATIONALES |
|---|---|
| Monitor the color of the skin, sclera, urine, and stool. | If obstruction recurs and bile is forced back into the bloodstream, the skin becomes jaundiced (yellow), urine is amber colored, and stools are clay colored (clay color is normal if bile is drained through a T-tube). Brown color should return to the stools after the bile begins to drain normally into the duodenum. |
| If a T-tube is present, note and record color, amount, odor, and consistency of drainage from T-tube or wound drain every 2 hours on the day of surgery and at least every shift thereafter. | Initially, drainage will be dark brown with small amounts of blood and can amount to 500–1000 mL/day. Greater amounts of blood or drainage should be reported to the health care provider. The amount should subside gradually as swelling diminishes in the common duct and drainage into the duodenum normalizes. |
| | **Note:** Laparoscopic surgery for common bile duct exploration often does not necessitate the insertion of a T-tube. |
| Ensure that drainage collection devices are positioned lower than the level of the common bile duct. | This will prevent reflux of drainage when the patient is ambulating. |
| Be alert to abdominal distention, rigidity, and complaints of diaphragmatic irritation (caused by inflammation or bleeding and, in this case, is pain referred to the right shoulder) along with cessation or significant decrease in the amount of drainage. If these signs occur, notify the health care provider immediately and anticipate tube replacement with a 14-French catheter. | These are indicators of a dislodged or clogged drainage tube causing bile leakage into the abdomen or backup of bile, necessitating timely intervention. |

### ADDITIONAL PROBLEMS:

| | |
|---|---|
| *Risk for Infection* | Chapter 4 |
| *Risk for Impaired Skin Integrity*, due to pruritus | Chapter 59 |
| *Risk for Hemorrhage* | Chapter 4 |

### PATIENT–FAMILY TEACHING AND DISCHARGE PLANNING

When providing patient–family teaching, focus on sensory information, avoid giving excessive information, and initiate a visiting nurse referral for necessary follow-up monitoring of postoperative patients. Include verbal and written information about the following:

- ✓ Notifying health care provider if the following indicators of recurrent biliary obstruction occur: dark urine, pruritus, jaundice, clay-colored stools. Inform the patient that loose stools may occur for several months as the body adjusts to the continuous flow of bile.
- ✓ Medications, including drug name, dosage, schedule, purpose, precautions, and potential side effects. Also discuss drug–drug, food–drug, and herb–drug interactions.
- ✓ Care of dressings and tubes if applicable at hospital discharge, and monitoring of incision and drain sites for signs of infection (e.g., fever, persistent redness, pain, purulent discharge, swelling, increased local warmth). The patient should not submerge the abdomen in the bathtub with incisions and drain sites present.
- ✓ Importance of maintaining a diet low in fat and eating frequent, small meals for medically managed patients.
- ✓ Importance of follow-up appointments with the health care provider; reconfirm the time and date of the next appointment.
- ✓ Avoiding alcoholic beverages during first 2 postoperative months to minimize the risk for pancreatic involvement.
- ✓ Necessity of postsurgical activity precautions: avoid lifting heavy objects (more than 10 lb) for the first 4–6 weeks or as directed, rest after periods of fatigue, get maximum amounts of rest, and gradually increase activities to tolerance. Postsurgical patients may experience fatty food intolerance (e.g., flatulence, cramps, diarrhea) for several months after surgery until the body recovers.

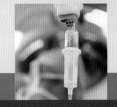

# Cirrhosis 56

## OVERVIEW/PATHOPHYSIOLOGY

Cirrhosis is a chronic and irreversible end-stage liver disease, resulting in liver cell death. As cells die, they are replaced with nonfunctioning fibrous tissue. Hepatomegaly, or liver enlargement, results from fibrous tissue, nodules, and fat build-up. Hepatomegaly leads to abdominal distention and shortness of breath due to pressure on the diaphragm. Eventually, blood flow to the liver is impaired as the portal vein becomes obstructed. As a result of impaired blood flow, essential functions of the liver become disrupted, including digestion, metabolism, glycogen storage, protein synthesis, blood coagulation, hormone metabolism, fluid and electrolyte balances, and detoxification of chemicals. The liver holds approximately 13% of the body's total blood supply, and as the portal vein becomes obstructed, blood flow backs up into the spleen and gastrointestinal (GI) tract. Patients with cirrhosis are at high risk for serious bleeding.

Alcohol abuse is one of the major causes of liver disease, which often appears after 10–20 years of heavy drinking. Often other liver insults, such as malnutrition, chronic viral hepatitis or nonalcoholic fatty liver disease, increase the risk factors for liver disease in alcohol users. The spectrum of the disease starts with fatty liver and progresses to alcoholic hepatitis and ultimately to chronic hepatitis with fibrosis or cirrhosis. In most cases, simple, uncomplicated fatty liver can be reversed within weeks by abstaining from alcohol. Within 6 months of abstinence, even scarring and nodules can show reversal. However, with continued alcohol abuse, liver cell regeneration does not occur in an organized way and results in abnormal blood vessel and bile duct structure. This leads to poor blood flow to the liver causing decreased liver cell nutrition and oxygenation. Eventually decreased liver function occurs.

Cirrhosis also can be caused by any chronic liver disease such as chronic hepatitis B, hepatitis C virus, hereditary hemochromatosis, nonalcoholic liver steatohepatitis, autoimmune hepatitis, Wilson disease, or alpha-1 antitrypsin deficiency.

Cardiac cirrhosis is caused by chronic and severe right-sided heart failure. Venous congestion, parenchymal damage, liver cell necrosis, and fibrosis all occur from poor right-sided cardiac output.

## HEALTH CARE SETTING

Primary care, acute care

## ASSESSMENT

**Signs and symptoms.** Many patients with early cirrhosis have no symptoms or just complain of fatigue. Later symptoms vary, depending on the degree of impaired hepatocellular function. Manifestations are related to the degree of liver failure and the severity of portal hypertension. Late signs and symptoms may include jaundice, weakness, fatigability, weight loss, pruritus, fever, anorexia, nausea, occasional vomiting, abdominal pain, diarrhea, peripheral edema, loss of libido, endocrine problems, skin lesions, and hematologic problems. Urine may be dark (brownish) because of the presence of urobilinogen, and stools may be pale and clay colored because of the absence of bilirubin.

**Physical assessment.** Jaundice, hepatomegaly, ascites, peripheral edema, pleural effusion, and fetor hepaticus (a musty, sweetish odor on the breath). There may be slight changes in personality and behavior, which can progress to coma (a result of hepatic encephalopathy); spider angiomas, testicular atrophy, gynecomastia, pectoral and axillary alopecia (a result of hormonal changes); splenomegaly; hemorrhoids (a result of portal hypertension complications); spider nevi; purpuric lesions; and palmar erythema.

**History.** Excessive alcohol ingestion, chronic hepatitis B or C infection, exposure to hepatotoxic drugs or chemicals, biliary or metabolic disease.

## DIAGNOSTIC TESTS

**Complete blood count.** Red blood cells may be decreased in hypersplenism and decreased with hemorrhage. White blood cells and platelet counts may be decreased with hypersplenism and increased with infection.

*Bilirubin levels.* Elevated because of failure in hepatocyte metabolism and obstruction in some instances. Very high or persistently elevated levels are considered a poor prognostic sign, reflective of the poor excretory function of the liver.

*Alkaline phosphatase levels.* Normal to mildly elevated in most cases. In primary biliary cholangitis, it is 2–3 times more than normal levels, reflective of biliary tract dysfunction.

*Aspartate aminotransferase and alanine aminotransferase levels.* Usually elevated to more than 300 U with acute liver failure and normal or mildly elevated with chronic liver failure. Alanine aminotransferase is more specific than aspartate aminotransferase for hepatocellular damage.

*Albumin levels.* Reduced, especially with ascites. Persistently low levels suggest a poor prognosis. This test is not a perfect indicator of liver function because it is affected by poor nutrition and fluid status.

*Gamma-glutamyl transpeptidase.* Levels likely will be elevated, especially in patients who use alcohol or other substances toxic to the liver.

*Globulins.* Important in forming antibodies, proteins, and clotting factors. There are three types of globulins: alpha, beta, and gamma. Elevated gamma globulin levels occur in advanced cirrhosis.

*Sodium level.* Normal to low sodium is retained but is associated with water retention, which results in normal serum sodium levels or even a dilutional hyponatremia. Severe hyponatremia is often present in the terminal stage and is associated with tense ascites and hepatorenal syndrome.

*Potassium level.* Slightly reduced unless the patient has renal insufficiency, which would result in hyperkalemia. Chronic hypokalemic acidosis is common in patients with chronic alcoholic liver disease.

*Glucose level.* Hypoglycemia is possible because of impaired gluconeogenesis and glycogen depletion in patients with severe or terminal liver disease.

*Ammonia level.* May be elevated because of the inability of the failing liver to convert ammonia to urea and shunting of intestinal blood via collateral vessels. GI hemorrhage, infection, or an increase in intestinal protein from dietary intake can increase ammonia levels.

**Note:** *Serum ammonia sample must be transported to the laboratory immediately for processing.*

*Coagulation.* Prothrombin time (PT)/international normalized ratio (INR) is elevated and, in severe liver disease, unresponsive to vitamin K therapy. The failing liver is unable to synthesize clotting factors. Coagulation abnormalities usually include not only factor V but also factors II, VII, IX, and X. These tests are more sensitive in reflecting the synthesis function of the liver.

**Urine tests.** Urine bilirubin is increased; urobilinogen is normal or increased; and proteinuria may be present.

**Ascitic fluid analysis.** Straw-colored or clear fluid is present in liver cirrhosis. Fluid should be cultured if spontaneous bacterial peritonitis is suspected.

**Liver biopsy.** Performed for three reasons: to establish a diagnosis, to assess disease prognosis, and as a tool to assist in disease management. Liver biopsy produces a tissue specimen for histologic analysis. It is considered the definitive test for determining the extent of disease in cirrhosis.

**Radiologic studies.** Ultrasound may be used to assess the size of the liver and spleen, screen for liver tumors (particularly hepatocellular carcinoma), and assess for signs of biliary obstruction. A Doppler study can also be performed to assess blood flow through the portal vessels. Computed tomography of the abdomen and magnetic resonance imaging (MRI) can show great detail related to the assessment of hepatic vasculature and any thrombus. With MRI, a cholangiogram can be performed, eliminating the need for endoscopic retrograde cholangiopancreatography.

**Angiographic studies.** Establish portal vein patency and visualize portosystemic collateral vessels to determine the cause of and the effective treatment for variceal bleeding. Portal venous anatomy must be established before such operations as portal systemic shunt or hepatic transplantation. In patients with previously constructed surgical shunts, loss of patency may be confirmed as a factor leading to the present bleeding episode. The most common procedure is portal venography by indirect angiography. The femoral artery is catheterized, and contrast material is injected into the splenic artery. Contrast material flows through the spleen into the splenic and portal veins.

**Esophagogastroduodenoscopy (or upper endoscopy).** Visualizes the esophagus and stomach directly through a fiberoptic endoscope. Varices in the esophagus and upper portion of the stomach are identified, and attempts are made to identify the exact source of bleeding.

**Paracentesis.** Performed in the following circumstances: new-onset ascites, ascites present at the time of hospital admission, and signs and symptoms of infection (fever, leukocytosis) in patients with ascites. Paracentesis is considered safe, even in patients with coagulopathies. It is important not to delay paracentesis if spontaneous bacterial peritonitis is suspected.

## Patient Problem/Analyze Cues/Prioritize Hypotheses

# Impaired Gas Exchange

*due to* alveolar hypoventilation resulting from shallow breathing occurring with ascites or hepatic hydrothorax; altered oxygen-carrying capacity of the blood occurring with anemia; and possible ventilation/perfusion mismatching

**Desired Outcome/Generate Solutions:** Within 24 hours of admission, the patient has adequate gas exchange, as evidenced by $PaCO_2$ of 35–45 mm Hg, $PaO_2$ of 80 mm Hg or more, $O_2$ saturation greater than 92%, and respiratory rate (RR) of 12–20 breaths/minute with normal depth and pattern (eupnea).

| ASSESSMENT—RECOGNIZE CUES/ INTERVENTIONS—TAKE ACTION | RATIONALES |
|---|---|
| Monitor the arterial blood gas values and pulse oximetry; notify the health care provider of $PaO_2$ less than 80 mm Hg or $O_2$ saturation 92% or less. Administer the oxygen as prescribed. | These lower-than-normal values usually signal the need for supplemental oxygen. |
| Obtain baseline abdominal girth measurement, and measure girth either daily or every shift. Measure around the same circumferential area each time, marking the site with indelible ink. Report significant findings to the health care provider. | An increase in abdominal girth indicates increased ascitic fluid accumulation, which can cause pressure on the diaphragm with subsequent dyspnea. |
| During complaints of dyspnea or orthopnea, assist the patient into semi-Fowler or high-Fowler position. | These positions promote gas exchange, which is likely to be altered by the pressure of ascitic fluid on the diaphragm. |
| Encourage position changes and deep breathing at frequent intervals. Teach the use of incentive spirometry. | Deep breathing expands the alveoli and aids in mobilizing secretions to the airway. |
| Include ambulation and movement from bed to chair as a part of position changes and deep breathing exercises. | Getting the patient out of bed will prevent deconditioning of the muscles and enable the patient to better perform incentive spirometry. |
| If secretions are present, ensure that the patient coughs frequently. | Coughing further promotes mobilization and clearing of secretions. |
| ! Notify the health care provider if the patient has fever, chills, diaphoresis, and adventitious breath sounds. | These are indicators of respiratory infection, which can lead to complications such as pneumonia and respiratory distress. Patients with severe cirrhosis are weak and, with poor maintenance of secretions, are more susceptible to infections. |
| ! Position the patient in a side-lying position during episodes of vomiting. | This position decreases the risk for aspiration, which could result in respiratory complications such as pneumonia. |

## Patient Problem/Analyze Cues/Prioritize Hypotheses

# Risk for Hemorrhage

*due to* decreased coagulation factors and portal hypertension

***Desired Outcomes/Generate Solutions:*** The patient is free of bleeding/hemorrhage, as evidenced by blood pressure (BP) of at least 90/60 mm Hg; heart rate (HR) of 100 bpm or less; warm extremities; distal pulses greater than 2 on a 0–4 scale; brisk capillary refill (less than 2 seconds); and orientation to person, place, and time. Bruising, melena, and hematemesis are absent.

| ASSESSMENT—RECOGNIZE CUES/ INTERVENTIONS—TAKE ACTION | RATIONALES |
|---|---|
| ! Assess the vital signs (VS) every 4 hours (or more frequently if VS are outside of the patient's baseline values). | Upper GI hemorrhage is common in patients with chronic liver disease and can result from esophageal varices, portal hypertensive gastropathy, duodenal or gastric ulcers, or Mallory–Weiss tear (mucosal laceration at the juncture of the distal esophagus and proximal stomach). Early diagnosis is essential to enable appropriate intervention. Hypotension and increased HR, as well as cool extremities, delayed capillary refill, decreased amplitude of distal pulses, mental status changes, and decreasing level of consciousness (LOC), are indicators of hypovolemia and hemorrhage. |
| • Assess for signs of bleeding such as bruising, melena, and hematemesis are signs of bleeding. <br><br> Assess for signs of significant bleeding such as altered VS, irritability, air hunger, pallor, and weakness. Notify the health care provider of significant findings. | These signs of bleeding and significant bleeding necessitate prompt intervention. |

Continued

| ASSESSMENT—RECOGNIZE CUES/ INTERVENTIONS—TAKE ACTION | RATIONALES |
|---|---|
| Inspect stools for the presence of blood; perform stool occult blood test as indicated. | This is an assessment for bleeding within the GI tract. |
| Monitor the PT and INR for abnormality. | INR: Normal range is less than 2 seconds for patients not receiving anticoagulant therapy.<br><br>PT: Normal range is 10.5–13.5 seconds. A PT that is prolonged signals the patient is at risk for bleeding. |
| Instruct the patient to avoid swallowing foods that are chemically or mechanically irritating. | Rough or spicy foods, hot foods, hot liquids, and alcohol may be injurious to the esophagus and result in bleeding. |
| Provide instructions on the importance of avoiding actions such as sneezing, lifting, or vomiting. | These actions increase intra-abdominothoracic pressure, which can result in bleeding. |
| Administer stool softeners as prescribed. | Stool softeners help prevent straining with defecation, which puts patients at risk for bleeding. |
| As appropriate, encourage the intake of foods rich in vitamin K (e.g., spinach, cabbage, cauliflower, liver). | These foods may help decrease PT/INR and reduce bleeding risk. |
| ⚠ As often as possible, avoid invasive procedures such as giving injections and taking rectal temperatures. | If clotting is altered, invasive procedures could result in prolonged bleeding. |
| ⚠ Monitor the patient undergoing band ligation or injection sclerotherapy of varices for increased HR, decreased BP, pallor, weakness, and air hunger. | These are signs of esophageal perforation caused by the treatment of varices, whether by injection, cautery, or the scope itself. |
| ⚠ If signs of perforation occur, notify the health care provider immediately, keep the patient nothing by mouth (NPO), and prepare for gastric suction. Administer antibiotics as prescribed to prevent infection. | NPO status and gastric suction prevent leakage of fluid, secretions, and food through the perforation into the mediastinum. This emergency situation necessities immediate intervention. |

## Patient Problem/Analyze Cues/Prioritize Hypotheses

# Fluid Imbalance

*due to* compromised regulatory mechanism with the sequestration of fluids occurring with portal hypertension and hepatocellular failure

***Desired Outcome/Generate Solutions:***  By at least 24 hours before hospital discharge, the patient is normovolemic, as evidenced by stable or decreasing abdominal girth, RR of 12–20 breaths/minute with normal depth and pattern (eupnea), HR of 100 bpm or less, edema of 1 or less on a 0–4 scale, and absence of crackles (rales).

| ASSESSMENT—RECOGNIZE CUES/ INTERVENTIONS—TAKE ACTION | RATIONALES |
|---|---|
| Obtain the baseline abdominal girth measurement. | A baseline assessment enables comparison for subsequent assessments. Girth measurements indicate the amount of ascitic fluid in the abdomen and provide information regarding the effectiveness of medical treatment. |
| Place the patient in a supine position and mark the abdomen with indelible ink. Measure girth daily or every shift as appropriate. | These measures ensure accurate serial measurements from the same circumferential site. |
| Monitor and record weight and intake and output (I&O). | The output should be equal to or exceed intake. Weight loss should not exceed 0.5 kg/day (1.1 lb/day) except in the presence of massive edema or ascites, which would permit a greater loss. Rapid diuresis from diuretics can lead to loss or shifts in electrolytes, particularly sodium, leading to encephalopathy and elevated creatinine. |

| ASSESSMENT—RECOGNIZE CUES/ INTERVENTIONS—TAKE ACTION | RATIONALES |
|---|---|
| ⚠ Assess the degree of edema from 1 (barely detectable) to 4 (deep, persistent pitting) and document accordingly. | The presence of edema signals excess sodium intake or low serum albumin. Low albumin levels are associated with ascites; persistently low levels suggest a poor prognosis. |
| ⚠ Monitor serum sodium and potassium values and report abnormalities to the health care provider. | Optimal values are serum sodium of 135–145 mEq/L and serum potassium of 3.5–5 mEq/L. Sodium is retained but is associated with water retention, which results in normal serum sodium levels or even a dilutional hyponatremia. Severe hyponatremia is present in the terminal stage and is associated with tense ascites and hepatorenal syndrome. Potassium may be slightly reduced unless the patient has renal insufficiency, which would result in hyperkalemia. Chronic hypokalemic acidosis is common in patients with chronic alcoholic liver disease. |
| ⚠ Be alert to dyspnea, basilar crackles that do not clear with coughing, orthopnea, and tachypnea. Report significant findings to the health care provider. | These are clinical indicators of pulmonary edema, which occurs from excess fluid volume in the circulatory system. Symptoms also may be present with pleural effusion caused by a small defect in the right hemidiaphragm, which develops with acute, rapid shortness of breath as the abdomen decompresses. |
| Administer frequent mouth care and provide ice chips to help minimize thirst. | These measures help minimize thirst while not compounding problems with fluid volume excess. |
| As indicated, remind the patient to avoid food and nonfood items that contain sodium, such as antacids, baking soda, and some mouthwashes. | Sodium may be restricted because of retention by the kidneys. |
| Elevate the lower extremities. | This will decrease peripheral edema. |
| Apply antiembolism hose or support stockings, sequential compression devices, or pneumatic foot compression devices as prescribed. | These garments/devices decrease peripheral edema by external compression of the extremities. |
| ⚠ Monitor for signs of variceal hemorrhage (see *Risk for Hemorrhage*, earlier). | Rapid increases in intravascular volume can precipitate variceal hemorrhage in susceptible individuals. |

## Patient Problem/Analyze Cues/Prioritize Hypotheses

# Body Weight Problem (Weight Loss)

*due to* anorexia, nausea, or malabsorption

**Desired Outcome/Generate Solutions:**  By at least 24 hours before hospital discharge, the patient demonstrates progress toward adequate nutritional status as evidenced by stable weight, balanced I&O, stable blood glucose levels, and normal electrolyte values.

| ASSESSMENT—RECOGNIZE CUES/ INTERVENTIONS—TAKE ACTION | RATIONALES |
|---|---|
| Assess and record I&O; weigh the patient daily. | These measures help assess the adequacy of diet/nutritional intake and measure the effectiveness of diuretic therapy for ascites. |
| Explain dietary restrictions. Encourage the patient to eat foods that are permitted within dietary restrictions. | With fluid retention and ascites, sodium and fluids are restricted. |
| | Sodium intake should be less than 2000 mg daily in the presence of ascites/edema. |
| | Fluid restriction of 1.5 L/day may be required in the presence of ascites/edema. |
| | 20%–30% of calories should be from fat. |
| | Malnourished patients may need 30–40 kcal/kg/day of protein. |

Continued

| ASSESSMENT—RECOGNIZE CUES/ INTERVENTIONS—TAKE ACTION | RATIONALES |
|---|---|
| Monitor the glucose levels. | Patients with cirrhosis may have glucose intolerance or diabetes. No more than 5–6 g/kg/day of glucose should be given. |
| Encourage small, frequent meals, including a bedtime snack or late evening meal, and caution the patient to avoid missing meals. | This helps ensure adequate nutrition without causing bloating from large meals. |
| Administer the parenteral or enteral nutrition if prescribed (see "Providing Nutritional Support," Chapter 76). | Parenteral nutrition is administered only if nutritional needs cannot be met through oral or enteral routes. Enteral nutrition may be used in patients with a functional gut who cannot meet their protein energy needs by the oral route. |
| Encourage significant others to bring desirable foods as permitted. | Patients are more likely to consume foods they like. |
| Administer the following prescribed medications: acid suppression agents, antiemetics, and cathartics. | These agents decrease gastric distress, which may facilitate intake. |
| Manage the prescribed therapies such as diuresis, colloid replacement, and paracentesis. | These therapies relieve/mobilize ascites and decrease pressure on intraabdominal structures, which may decrease a sense of early satiety caused by severe ascites. |
| ⚠ Encourage the abstinence of alcohol in patients with alcoholic cirrhosis. | This remains the primary intervention in patients with alcohol-induced cirrhosis. Abstinence can result in healing of reversible factors of alcoholic liver disease over a period of months. Continued use of alcohol will further damage the liver to the point of irreversibility. |

### Patient Problem/Analyze Cues/Prioritize Hypotheses

# Risk for Impaired Cognition

*due to* neurosensory changes occurring with cerebral accumulation of ammonia or GI bleeding

**Desired Outcome/Generate Solutions:** The patient verbalizes orientation to person, place, and time; exhibits intact signature; and is free of signs of injury caused by neurosensory changes.

| ASSESSMENT—RECOGNIZE CUES/ INTERVENTIONS—TAKE ACTION | RATIONALES |
|---|---|
| Perform a baseline assessment of the patient's personality characteristics, LOC, and orientation. Enlist aid of the patient's significant others to help determine slight changes in personality or behavior. | Having a baseline assessment will help determine subsequent changes in personality or behavior, which could progress to hepatic coma if left unchecked. |
| ⚠ Be alert to generalized muscle twitching and asterixis (flapping tremor induced by dorsiflexion of wrist and extension of fingers). Report significant findings to the health care provider. | Asterixis may be present in advanced cirrhosis. |
| ⚠ Monitor for indicators of GI bleeding, including melena or hematemesis. Report bleeding promptly to the health care provider. | GI bleeding can precipitate hepatic encephalopathy. |
| ⚠ Keep side rails up and the bed in its lowest position and assist with ambulation when need is determined. | These measures protect the patient from injury that could be precipitated by a confused state. Because of the patient's encephalopathy and resulting neurosensory changes, reminders and reorientation are necessary to help ensure the patient's safety. Additionally, the patient may be experiencing alcohol withdrawal (in cases of alcohol cirrhosis), which would place the patient at risk for seizures. |
| ⚠ Avoid opioid analgesics and phenothiazines. Use caution when administering sedatives, antihistamines, and other agents affecting the central nervous system. | Opioids and sedatives are metabolized by the liver and therefore are contraindicated. Small doses of benzodiazepines with a short half-life may be administered if absolutely necessary. |

## ADDITIONAL PROBLEMS:

| | |
|---|---|
| *Deficient Knowledge* (causes of hepatitis and modes of transmission) | Chapter 59 |
| *Fatigue* | Chapter 59 |

## ✓ PATIENT–FAMILY TEACHING AND DISCHARGE PLANNING

When providing patient–family teaching, focus on sensory information, avoid giving excessive information, and initiate a visiting nurse referral for necessary follow-up teaching of any skilled care needed after discharge. Include verbal and written information about the following:

- ✓ Medications, including drug name, purpose, dosage, schedule, precautions, and potential side effects. Also discuss drug–drug, food–drug, and herb–drug interactions.
- ✓ Dietary restrictions, in particular those of sodium, protein, and ammonia.
- ✓ Refer patient to dietician.
- ✓ Potential need for lifestyle changes, including avoiding alcoholic beverages. Stress that alcohol cessation is a major factor in the survival of this disease. Include appropriate referrals (e.g., to Alcoholics Anonymous, Al-Anon, and Alateen). As appropriate, provide referrals to community nursing support agencies.
- ✓ Awareness of hepatotoxic agents, especially over-the-counter drugs, including acetaminophen, aspirin, and many popular complementary and alternative use medications, such as herbals, dietary supplements, and vitamins.
- ✓ Importance of deep breathing exercises when ascites is present.
- ✓ Indicators of variceal bleeding/hemorrhage (i.e., vomiting blood, change in LOC) and need to inform the health care provider if they occur.
- ✓ Telephone numbers to call in case questions or concerns arise about therapy or disease after discharge. Additional general information can be obtained by contacting the National Institute of Diabetes and Digestive and Kidney Diseases at www.niddk.nih.gov.
- ✓ For patients awaiting transplantation, provide the following information: United Network for Organ Sharing at www.unos.org.
- ✓ As an additional information source, refer patients to American Liver Foundation at www.liverfoundation.org.

# Crohn's Disease 57

## OVERVIEW/PATHOPHYSIOLOGY

Crohn's disease (CD) is a chronic inflammatory disease that can involve any part of the gastrointestinal (GI) tract from the mouth to the anus. Usually, the disease occurs segmentally, demonstrating discontinuous areas of disease with segments of healthy bowel in between. In 45%–50% of cases, the end of the ileum and cecum/ascending colon are involved (ileocolitis); in 35% of cases, the terminal ileum is affected (ileitis); and in 20% of cases, the colon alone is affected (Crohn's colitis). A small number of patients have involvement of the jejunum, duodenum, stomach, esophagus, and mouth; in these cases, the ileum, colon, or both are also involved. Approximately 30%–35% of patients have perianal fistulas, fissures, or abscesses. The disease affects all layers of the bowel: the mucosa, submucosa, circular and longitudinal muscles, and serosa, predisposing to intestinal strictures and fistulas. A family history of this disease or ulcerative colitis occurs in 15%–20% of affected patients.

The cause of CD is unknown, but theories include infection, immunologic factors, environmental factors, and genetic predisposition. In a genetically susceptible subject, an outside agent or substance, such as a bacterium, virus, or other antigens, interacts with the body's immune system to trigger the disease or may cause damage to the intestinal wall, initiating or accelerating the disease process. The resulting inflammatory response continues unregulated by the immune system. As a result, inflammation continues to damage the intestinal wall, causing the symptoms of CD. It is a chronic disease that has no cure. However, there are effective treatments to aid in controlling the disease. Initial treatment is nonoperative, individualized, and based on symptomatic relief. Surgery is reserved for complications rather than used as a primary form of therapy.

CD is generally diagnosed between the ages of 15 and 35 years, but it also can occur in young children and in people 70 years of age or older. The prevalence is essentially equal in women and in men. CD is seen more frequently in the Caucasian population and in Ashkenazi Jews than in non-Caucasian populations and in people of non-Jewish descent. It is more prevalent in urban, developed countries with temperate climates than in rural, more southern countries. However, the increasing incidence is being observed in African American populations and in Japan and South America. Cigarette smoking has been shown to increase the risk for developing CD and is associated with resistance to medical therapy and recurrence of disease after surgery.

## HEALTH CARE SETTING

Primary care, with possible hospitalization due to complications

## ASSESSMENT

*Signs and symptoms.* Clinical presentation varies as a direct reflection of the location of the inflammatory process and its extent, severity, and relationship to contiguous structures. Sometimes, onset is abrupt, and the patient can appear to have appendicitis, ulcerative colitis, intestinal obstruction, or a fever of obscure origin. Acute symptoms include right lower quadrant (RLQ) pain, tenderness, spasm, flatulence, nausea, fever, and diarrhea. A more typical picture is insidious onset with more persistent but less severe symptoms, such as vague abdominal pain, unexplained anemia, and fever. Diarrhea—liquid, soft, or mushy stools—is the most common symptom. The presence of gross blood is rare. Abdominal pain is a common symptom, and it may be colicky or crampy, initiated by meals, centered in the lower abdomen, and relieved by defecation because of chronic partial obstruction of the small intestine, colon, or both. As the disease progresses, anorexia, malnutrition, weight loss, anemia, lassitude, malaise, and fever can occur in addition to fluid, electrolyte, and metabolic disturbances.

*Physical assessment.* In early stages, the examination is often normal but may demonstrate mild tenderness in the abdomen over the affected bowel. In more advanced disease, a palpable mass may be present, especially in the RLQ with terminal ileum involvement. Persistent rectal fissure, large ulcers, perirectal abscess, or rectal fistula is the first indication of disease in 15%–25% of patients with small bowel involvement and in 50%–75% of patients with colonic involvement. Rectovaginal, abdominal, and enterovesical fistulas also can occur. Extraintestinal manifestations characteristic of UC do occur, but less commonly (10%–20%).

## DIAGNOSTIC TESTS

*Stool examination.* Usually, reveals occult blood; frank blood may be noted in the stools of patients with colonic involvement or with ulcerations and fistulas of the rectum. A few patients have a presenting symptom of bloody diarrhea. Stool cultures and smears rule out bacterial and parasitic disorders. Specimens are also examined for fecal fat. Stool also is examined for the presence of white blood cells (WBCs) and certain proteins, the presence of which suggests inflammation.

**Sigmoidoscopy.** Evaluates possible colonic involvement and obtains rectal biopsy. The finding of granulomas on mucosal biopsy argues strongly for the diagnosis of CD. However, because granulomas are more numerous in the submucosa, suction biopsy of the rectum provides deeper, larger, and less traumatized specimens for a better diagnostic yield than mucosal biopsy obtained through an endoscope.

**Colonoscopy.** May help differentiate CD from UC. Characteristic patchy inflammation (skip lesions) rules out UC. However, colonoscopy usually does not add useful diagnostic information in the presence of positive findings from sigmoidoscopy or radiologic examination. When diagnosis is unclear and there is a question of malignancy, colonoscopy provides the means of directly visualizing mucosal changes and obtaining biopsies, brushings, and washings for cytologic examination. Colonoscopy also may assist in planning for surgery by documenting the extent of colonic disease. The evolving techniques of high-resolution and high-magnification endoscopy have the potential for detecting subtle mucosal changes.

**Note:** *Because of the risk for perforation, this procedure may be contraindicated in patients with acute phases of Crohn's colitis or when deep ulcerations or fistulas are known to be present.*

**Endoscopic ultrasonography.** Aids in the diagnosis of perirectal fistula and abscesses and in detecting transmural depth of inflammation in the bowel or esophagus, using an endoscopically placed ultrasound probe.

**Small bowel enteroscopy.** Permits visualization of the upper GI tract to identify areas of inflammation and bleeding to the level of the midjejunum.

**Wireless capsule.** Permits visualization of the small intestine to identify abnormalities. The patient swallows a large capsule that contains a small disposable camera; images are transmitted to a receiver on the patient's waist. New capsules that contain light filters to enhance mucosal abnormalities are under development and study.

**Note:** *Use is contraindicated if strictures exist because strictures can prevent the capsule from progressing through the intestine; surgical removal of the capsule may be required.*

**Barium enema and upper GI series with small bowel follow-through.** Contribute to diagnosis of CD. Involvement of only the terminal ileum or segmental involvement of the colon or small intestine almost always indicates CD. Thickened bowel wall with stricture (string sign) separated by segments of normal bowel, cobblestone appearance, and presence of fistulas and skip lesions are common findings. A double-contrast barium enema technique may increase sensitivity in detecting early or subtle changes.

**Note:** *Barium enema may be contraindicated in patients with acute phases of Crohn's colitis because of the risk for perforation. Upper GI barium series is contraindicated in patients in whom intestinal obstruction is suspected.*

**Computed tomography.** Complements information gathered through endoscopy and conventional radiography. In advanced disease, computed tomography (CT) clearly delineates extraluminal complications (e.g., abscess, phlegmon, bowel wall thickening, mesenteric inflammation). CT has been used also to percutaneously drain fistulas (colovesicular, enterovesicular, colovaginal, enterocolonic) and to evaluate perirectal disease, enterocutaneous fistula, and sinus tracts.

**Computed tomography enterography.** An emerging modality for specialized visualization of the small intestine and lumen and for depicting inflammatory changes.

**Magnetic resonance imaging and magnetic resonance enterography.** Imaging techniques used to evaluate extraluminal complications (e.g., perirectal fistula, sinus tracts, and abscesses) and the small intestine. Because they use a magnetic field and radio waves, their advantage is not exposing predominantly young patients to x-ray radiation as would occur with CT and computed tomography enterography.

**Serum antibody testing.** In difficult-to-diagnose cases, may be helpful in differentiating CD from UC.

**Radionuclide imaging.** Intravenous (IV) indium-111– or technetium-99m–labeled leukocytes migrate to areas of active inflammation and are then identified by scans performed after 4 and 24 hours. This procedure aids in differentiating CD from UC and evaluating abscess and fistula formation.

**Blood tests.** Are nonspecific for diagnosis of CD but help determine whether the inflammatory process is active and evaluate the patient's overall condition. Anemia may be present and may be microcytic because of iron deficiency from chronic blood loss and bone marrow depression secondary to chronic inflammatory process or megaloblastic because of folic acid or vitamin $B_{12}$ deficiency (usually seen only in patients with extensive ileitis causing malabsorption). Increased WBC count, sedimentation rate, and C-reactive protein reflect disease activity and inflammation. Hypoalbuminemia corresponds with disease activity and results from decreased protein intake, extensive malabsorption, and significant enteric loss of protein. Hypokalemia is seen in patients with chronic diarrhea; hypophosphatemia and hypocalcemia are seen in patients with significant malabsorption. Liver function studies may be abnormal secondary to pericholangitis.

**Urinalysis and urine culture.** May reveal urinary tract infection secondary to enterovesicular fistula.

**Tests for malabsorption.** Because patients with active, extensive disease (especially when it involves the small intestine) may develop malabsorption and malnutrition, the following tests are clinically significant: D-xylose tolerance test (for upper jejunal involvement); Schilling test (for ileal involvement); serum albumin, carotene, calcium, and phosphorus levels; and fecal fat (steatorrhea).

## Patient Problem/Analyze Cues/Prioritize Hypotheses

# Dehydration

*due to* the active loss of GI fluids occurring with diarrhea or the presence of a GI fistula

*Desired Outcomes/Generate Solutions:* The patient is normovolemic within 24 hours of admission, as evidenced by balanced intake and output (I&O), urinary output of 30 mL/hour or more, specific gravity of 1.010–1.030, blood pressure (BP) of 90/60–120/70 mm Hg (or within the patient's normal range), respiratory rate (RR) of 12–20 breaths/minute, stable weight, elastic skin turgor, and moist mucous membranes. The patient reports that diarrhea is controlled. Serum electrolytes potassium, sodium, and chloride are all within optimal values.

| ASSESSMENT—RECOGNIZE CUES/ INTERVENTIONS—TAKE ACTION | RATIONALES |
|---|---|
| Assess the I&O and urinary specific gravity, weigh the patient daily, and monitor laboratory values to evaluate fluid and electrolyte status. | These assessments monitor for fluid loss and electrolyte imbalance. GI fluid losses (nasogastric suction, vomiting, diarrhea, fistula) can lead to hyponatremia, hypokalemia, and hypochloremia. Optimal values are serum potassium 3.5–5.0 mEq/L, serum sodium 135–145 mEq/L, and serum chloride 96–106 mEq/L. Critical values: potassium less than 2.5 or more than 6.5 mEq/L, sodium less than 120 or more than 160 mEq/L, chloride less than 80 or more than 115 mEq/L. |
| Assess the frequency and consistency of stools. | This assessment monitors for the presence and amount of blood, mucus, fat, and undigested food, which occur secondary to the underlying inflammatory process. |
| Assess for the presence of thirst, poor skin turgor, dryness of mucous membranes, fever, and concentrated (specific gravity greater than 1.030) and decreased urinary output. | These are indicators of dehydration. |
| Maintain the patient on parenteral replacement of fluids and electrolytes as prescribed. | This will promote anabolism and healing. |
| When the patient is taking food orally, provide the prescribed diet. Assess tolerance to the diet by determining the incidence of cramping, diarrhea, and flatulence. Modify the diet plan accordingly. | Bland diets low in residue, roughage, and fat but high in protein, calories, carbohydrates, and vitamins provide good nutrition and reduce excessive stimulation of the bowel. A diet free of milk, milk products, gas-forming foods, alcohol, and iced beverages reduces cramping and diarrhea. |

## Patient Problem/Analyze Cues/Prioritize Hypotheses

# Risk for Disease (Intraabdominal Complications)

*due to* decreased immune response and defense mobilization to combat the intestinal inflammatory process

*Desired Outcome/Generate Solutions:* The patient is free from indicators of infection and intraabdominal injury/dysfunction, as evidenced by normothermia; heart rate (HR) of 60–100 bpm; RR of 12–20 breaths/minute; normoactive bowel sounds; absence of abdominal distention, rigidity, and localized pain and tenderness; absence of nausea and vomiting; negative culture results; no significant change in mental status; and orientation to person, place, and time.

| ASSESSMENT—RECOGNIZE CUES/ INTERVENTIONS—TAKE ACTION | RATIONALES |
|---|---|
| Assess for abdominal distention, abdominal rigidity, and increased episodes of nausea and vomiting. | These are indicators of intestinal obstruction. Contributing factors to the development of intestinal obstruction include use of opioids and prolonged use of antidiarrheal medication. |
| Assess for fever, increased RR and HR, chills, diaphoresis, and increased abdominal discomfort. | These indicators can occur with intestinal perforation, abscess or fistula formation, or generalized fecal peritonitis and septicemia. **Note:** Systemic therapy with corticosteroids and antibiotics can mask the development of these complications. |
| Evaluate mental status, orientation, and level of consciousness every 2–4 hours. | Mental cloudiness, lethargy, and increased restlessness can occur with peritonitis and septicemia. |
| Obtain cultures of blood, urine, fistulas, or other possible sources of infection, as prescribed, if the patient has a sudden temperature elevation. | Abscesses or fistulas to the abdominal wall, bladder, or vagina are common in CD and are potential sources of infection, as are abscesses or fistulas to other loops of the small bowel and colon. |
| Monitor culture reports and notify the health care provider promptly of any positive results. | Prompt the recognition of abnormal results enables early and appropriate interventions. |
| If draining fistulas or abscesses are present, change dressings and pouching system or irrigate tubes or drains as prescribed. Note the color, character, and odor of all drainage. | Foul-smelling or abnormal drainage, which can signal infection, or loss of tube/drain patency should be reported to the health care provider promptly for intervention. |
| Refer to wound, ostomy, continence (WOC)/enterostomal therapy (ET) nurse for fistula management as needed. | This referral provides expert assistance in the management of complex draining wounds and/or fistulas. |
| Administer the antibiotics as prescribed and on the prescribed schedule. | Maintaining the therapeutic serum level of antibiotics will help control suppurative complications (e.g., bacterial overgrowth) and perianal fistulas in patients with mild-to-moderate colonic or ileocolonic CD. |
| Administer the immunomodulators and biologic agents as prescribed. | These agents aid in healing, especially with refractory disease or active disease unresponsive to conventional therapy. |
| Use good hand hygiene before and after caring for the patient and dispose of dressings and drainage using proper infection control techniques. | These measures prevent the transmission of potentially infectious organisms. Because immunomodulators, steroids, and biologic agents can reduce the response of the immune system, the patient can be at increased risk for infection and therefore should be monitored closely. |

Patient Problem/Analyze Cues/Prioritize Hypotheses

# Acute Pain

*due to* the intestinal inflammatory process

***Desired Outcomes/Generate Solutions:*** The patient's subjective perception of discomfort decreases within 1 hour of intervention, as documented by a pain scale. Objective indicators, such as grimacing, are absent or diminished.

| ASSESSMENT—RECOGNIZE CUES/ INTERVENTIONS—TAKE ACTION | RATIONALES |
|---|---|
| Assess and document the characteristics of discomfort and assess whether it is associated with the ingestion of certain foods or with emotional stress. | The discomfort of pain, nausea, and abdominal cramping may be associated with certain foods or emotional stress. |
| Devise a pain scale with the patient, rating discomfort from 0 (no pain) to 10 (worst pain). Teach the patient to eliminate foods that cause cramping and discomfort. | A pain scale will help determine the degree of relief obtained after interventions have been implemented. |

Continued

| ASSESSMENT—RECOGNIZE CUES/ INTERVENTIONS—TAKE ACTION | RATIONALES |
|---|---|
| As prescribed, keep the patient nothing by mouth (NPO) and provide parenteral nutrition. | These measures allow bowel rest, which will help alleviate discomfort. |
| Administer antidiarrheal medications and analgesics as prescribed. | These medications are given to reduce abdominal discomfort, often with a concomitant decrease in abdominal cramping. |
| • **Evaluate outcomes**<br><br>Assess the patient's response to these medications. Report significant findings to the health care provider. | • If the patient does not respond appropriately to standard antidiarrheal medications and mild sedation, the presence of obstruction, bowel perforation, or abscess formation is suspected. |
| Instruct the patient to request analgesia before pain becomes severe. | Prolonged stimulation of pain receptors results in increased sensitivity to painful stimuli and increases the amount of medication required to relieve discomfort. |
| Instruct the patient in the use of nonpharmacologic methods of pain relief, such as guided imagery, relaxation, massage, heat or cold therapy, and distraction. | These methods provide comfort, can decrease anxiety, and may result in more effective response to analgesics. |
| Administer antiemetic medications before meals. | These agents enhance appetite when nausea is a problem. |
| For additional information, see "Pain," Chapter 5. | |

## Patient Problem/Analyze Cues/Prioritize Hypotheses

# Diarrhea

*due to* the intestinal inflammatory process

***Desired Outcome/Generate Solutions:*** The patient reports a reduction in the frequency of stools and a return to soft, formed stool consistency within 3 days of hospital admission.

| ASSESSMENT—RECOGNIZE CUES/ INTERVENTIONS—TAKE ACTION | RATIONALES |
|---|---|
| Assess the patient's bowel pattern. If the patient is experiencing frequent and urgent passage of loose stools, provide a covered bedpan or commode or be sure the bathroom is easily accessible and ready to use at all times. | Providing easy access to a bedpan, commode, or bathroom promotes patient safety, reduces stress, and enables patients to cope with diarrhea more effectively. |
| Administer antidiarrheal medications as prescribed. | These agents decrease fluidity and the number of stools, inhibit GI peristaltic activity, and increase transit time and stool consistency. |
| Administer cholestyramine as prescribed. | This agent controls diarrhea if bile salt deficiency (because of ileal disease or resection) is contributing to this problem. |
| Instruct the patient to eliminate or decrease the fat content in the diet. | Fat can increase diarrhea in individuals with malabsorption syndromes. |
| Instruct the patient to follow a bland diet low in residue, roughage, and fat but high in protein, calories, carbohydrates, and vitamins. | This diet provides good nutrition and reduces the stimulation of the intestine. |
| Instruct the patient to restrict raw vegetables and fruits; whole-grain cereals; condiments; gas-forming foods; alcohol; iced and carbonated beverages; and, in lactose-intolerant patients, milk and milk products. | These foods and beverages also can precipitate diarrhea and cramping. When remission occurs, a less restricted diet can be tailored to the individual patient, excluding foods known to precipitate symptoms. |
| Provide instructions to the patient about vitamin and mineral supplementation and, if indicated, cholestyramine. | Patients with involvement of the small intestine often require supplementation of vitamins and minerals, especially calcium, iron, folate, and magnesium secondary to malabsorption or to compensate for foods excluded from the diet. Patients with extensive ileal disease or resection often require vitamin $B_{12}$ replacement, and if bile salt deficiency exists, cholestyramine and medium-chain triglycerides may be needed to control diarrhea and reduce fat malabsorption and steatorrhea. Vitamin D deficiency is common in these patients and may require replacement with cholecalciferol. |

## Patient Problem/Analyze Cues

# Fatigue

*due to* the generalized weakness and the prescribed rest occurring with the intestinal inflammatory process

**Desired Outcome/Generate Solutions:** The patient adheres to the prescribed rest regimen and sets appropriate goals for self-care as the condition improves (optimally within 3–7 days of admission).

| ASSESSMENT—RECOGNIZE CUES/ INTERVENTIONS—TAKE ACTION | RATIONALES |
|---|---|
| Keep the patient's environment quiet. | This will facilitate needed rest. |
| Assist with activities of daily living (ADLs) and plan nursing care to provide maximum rest periods. | Adequate rest is necessary to sustain remission. |
| Facilitate coordination of health care providers. Provide 90 minutes for undisturbed rest. | This enables rest periods between care activities. |
| As prescribed, administer anxiolytics. | These agents promote rest and reduce anxiety. |
| As the patient's physical condition improves, encourage self-care to the greatest extent possible and assist the patient with setting realistic, attainable goals. | These measures enable the patient to increase endurance incrementally to his or her tolerance and prevent problems associated with prolonged bedrest. |

## Patient Problem

# Deficient Knowledge (Medications)

*due to* the unfamiliarity with medications used for the treatment of CD

**Desired Outcome/Generate Solutions:** Immediately after teaching, the patient verbalizes accurate information about the medications used during exacerbations of CD.

| ASSESSMENT—RECOGNIZE CUES/ INTERVENTIONS—TAKE ACTION | RATIONALES |
|---|---|
| Provide instructions to the patient about the following, referring to the therapeutic agent or combination of agents prescribed: | Treatment is customized based on the type and severity of symptoms. |
| **Aminosalicylates: Sulfasalazine and 5-Aminosalicylic Acid (5-ASA) Preparations** | |
| | These medications work on the intestinal lining to decrease inflammation. |
| **Sulfasalazine** | |
| | This medication is given to treat acute exacerbations of colonic and ileocolonic disease. Although sulfasalazine does not prevent the recurrence of CD, patients who respond tend to benefit from long-term therapy and relapse when the agent is discontinued. It appears to be more effective in patients with mild-to-moderate disease limited to the colon than in those with disease limited to the small bowel. |
| • Folic acid supplements are necessary during treatment. | Sulfasalazine impairs folate absorption. |
| • A complete blood count must be done within the first 4 months of treatment. | WBCs may be lowered with this medication, and anemia can occur (uncommon). |
| • Liver enzymes must be checked within the first year of treatment. | Hepatitis, though uncommon, has occurred. |

Continued

| ASSESSMENT—RECOGNIZE CUES/ INTERVENTIONS—TAKE ACTION | RATIONALES |
|---|---|
| • Notify the health care provider immediately if discoloration of the skin or urine occurs. | Sulfasalazine may produce orange-yellow discoloration of the skin and urine and could cause contact lenses to turn yellow. |
| • Men may want to check for infertility by sperm analysis. | Infertility has occurred in some men, although it reverses when patients stop taking the medication. |
| • Be alert to the following side effects: fever, skin rash, joint pain, nausea, headache, or fatigue when the dose exceeds 4 tablets/day. | Most side effects are sulfa related and caused by the sulfa component of the drug. |

**5-ASA Preparations**

| | |
|---|---|
| | 5-ASA is used in patients unable to tolerate sulfasalazine. Extended-release mesalamine (Pentasa) and delayed-released mesalamine (Asacol) are used for mildly to moderately active ileocolonic and ileal disease and for maintenance therapy in selected patients. They may delay or prevent postoperative recurrence when initiated soon after ileal and colonic resection. |
| • Kidney profile and urine examination, including blood urea nitrogen and creatinine must be done annually. | There is a risk for kidney damage with high doses (above 4000 mg/day). |

**Corticosteroids**

| | |
|---|---|
| | These agents reduce the active inflammatory response by depressing the immune system, decreasing edema in moderate-to-severe forms, and controlling exacerbations in chronic disease. The oral route is most effective for the disease limited to the small intestine. |
| • Blood pressure will be checked during each clinic/office visit. | Secondary hypertension is a potential side effect. |
| • Blood glucose must be measured after 1 month of therapy, and then every 3 months. | Increased blood glucose levels may occur with the use of these drugs. |
| • Schedule an eye examination annually. However, notify the health care provider immediately if experiencing eye pain or vision changes because some complications may result in permanent vision loss. | There is potential for cataract formation, glaucoma, and temporary vision changes during treatment with steroids. Also, extraintestinal manifestations of CD can involve the eye. |
| • Schedule bone mineral density scanning if on corticosteroids for more than 3 consecutive months or if on recurrent courses of corticosteroids. | Bone loss can occur with prolonged use of steroids and as a result of chronic inflammation. |
| • Be alert to rounding of face (moon face), acne, increased appetite and weight gain, red marks/blotches on skin, facial hair, severe mood swings, weakness, and leg cramps. | These are typical side effects with corticosteroids. |
| • As active disease subsides, corticosteroid doses are tapered but never discontinued abruptly. | The goal is eventual elimination of the medication to prevent complications from long-term use. Abrupt discontinuation of corticosteroids may cause adrenal insufficiency. |
| • In some cases of chronic disease, continuous corticosteroid therapy may be necessary. | Many patients with CD become steroid dependent, meaning they are symptomatic with low-dose therapy (5–15 mg/day) or with total discontinuation of the drug. |
| • A nonsystemic steroidal agent, budesonide, is approved for the treatment of mild-to-moderate disease involving the ileum and cecum or ascending colon. | It provides benefits of traditional therapy with reduced side effects because it is nonsystemic and therefore primarily released in the GI tract. It is used for flare-ups but not commonly for maintenance therapy. |
| • Avoid grapefruit and grapefruit juice when taking budesonide. | They may increase drug effects. |
| • Topical therapy is an effective route. | Topical therapy with hydrocortisone has controlled inflammation through retention enemas for patients with proctosigmoiditis (involvement to 40 cm); suppositories have been used for patients with Crohn's proctitis. |

| ASSESSMENT—RECOGNIZE CUES/ INTERVENTIONS—TAKE ACTION | RATIONALES |
|---|---|
| **Immunomodulators** Azathioprine 6-Mercaptopurine (6-MP) Methotrexate | These agents modify the immune system in order to decrease inflammation. They may take several months to be effective. After they take effect, they allow dosage reduction or withdrawal of corticosteroids in steroid-dependent patients, are used for maintenance therapy with a lower relapse rate, and aid in healing and reducing drainage of perianal fistulas. |
| • If taking azathioprine or 6-MP, complete blood counts must be done every other week until dose has been stable for 6 months and then monitored every month for 3 months, then once every 3 months. | Lowered WBC count, anemia, low platelet levels, low hemoglobin levels, and abnormal liver enzyme levels can occur. |
| • Be alert to and report the following when taking azathioprine or 6-MP: allergic reaction (fever, skin rash, joint aches), pancreatitis (severe abdominal pain typically radiating through the back), and infection. | These are possible side effects/allergic reactions. |
| • Methotrexate is used with extreme caution in people with preexisting liver disease or who consume significant quantities of alcohol. Blood cell counts and liver enzymes are checked monthly for the first 3 months, then at 3-months intervals. | This drug can affect liver function. |
| • Methotrexate is contraindicated during pregnancy. In women anticipating pregnancy, methotrexate should be discontinued for at least 3 months before planned conception. | It may cause fetal death and congenital abnormalities and can be transferred through breast milk. |
| • There is a risk for malignancy with immunomodulators. | Lymphoma has occurred, but the risk is considered to be low. |
| **Biologic Agents** Anti–tumor necrosis factor (anti-TNF) agents  Adalimumab  Certolizumab pegol  Infliximab Integrin receptor antagonists  Natalizumab  Vedolizumab | These anti-TNF agents block a protein called TNF-alpha that promotes inflammation in the intestine. These agents inhibit the migration of cells that cause inflammation from moving out of the blood vessels into GI tissues. All these genetically engineered agents listed are designed to block inflammation or to stimulate anti-inflammatory processes in the body. They are used intravenously (infliximab, natalizumab, and vedolizumab) or subcutaneously (adalimumab and certolizumab pegol) to treat and maintain remission of moderate-to-severe active disease unresponsive to conventional therapy. Infliximab also is used to treat and maintain remission in fistulizing disease. Vedolizumab is used to treat and maintain steroid-free remission in patients who are unresponsive or intolerant to an anti-TNF agent or to an immunomodulator. |
| • Report sore throat, upper respiratory infection, abscesses, sinusitis, and bronchitis. | There is a risk for altered immune response with these medications; therefore, the risk for infection is increased. |
| • There is a risk for malignancy. | Lymphoma has occurred in some patients. |
| • Infusion- and injection-site–related reactions that occur during or shortly after administration include fever, chills, headache, low BP, rash, muscle and joint pain, chest pain, itching, and shortness of breath. A reaction may occur during and up to 2 hours after infusion. | These reactions usually are of short duration and almost always respond to treatment with acetaminophen, antihistamines, corticosteroids, or epinephrine as prescribed. |
| • A tuberculosis skin test should be performed before therapy is initiated. | Treatment of latent tuberculosis infection is needed before starting infliximab therapy. |
| • Inform all health care providers of the use of biologic agents and also the use of immunomodulatory agents and corticosteroids, before receiving vaccines. | Live-virus vaccines should not be administered until therapy stops because these agents may affect normal immune response. However, the immune status of the individual should be assessed on a case-by-case basis to determine risks versus benefits. |

Continued

| ASSESSMENT—RECOGNIZE CUES/ INTERVENTIONS—TAKE ACTION | RATIONALES |
| --- | --- |
| • Before considering treatment with natalizumab, testing must be done for the John Cunningham (JC) virus. | The patient is at increased risk for a severe brain condition, progressive multifocal leukoencephalopathy, that occurs from infection with the JC virus. |
| **Combination Therapy** | |
| • Immunomodulators and biologic agents | Both may be more effective in combination to maintain remission. However, there may be an increased risk for side effects. |
| • Ensure that the patient verbalizes accurate knowledge about the purpose, precautions, and potential side effects of any prescribed medication he or she will be taking. Refer to the previous sections that describe the potential side effects/allergic reactions that can occur with both types of medications. | A knowledgeable individual is more likely to adhere to the therapeutic regimen and promptly report untoward side effects to the health care provider. |

## ADDITIONAL PROBLEMS:

| | |
| --- | --- |
| *Risk for Infection* | Chapter 4 |
| *Risk for Injury* | Chapter 4 |
| *Risk for Spiritual Distress* | Chapter 8 |
| *Impaired Gastrointestinal Function* | Chapter 58 |
| *Risk for Impaired Tissue Perfusion (Stomal Tissue)* | Chapter 58 |
| *Risk for Impaired Skin Integrity (Peristomal Skin)* | Chapter 58 |

## ✔ PATIENT–FAMILY TEACHING AND DISCHARGE PLANNING

When providing patient–family teaching, focus on sensory information, avoid giving excessive information, and initiate a visiting nurse referral for necessary follow-up teaching. Include verbal and written information about the following:

✓ Medications, including drug name, rationale, dosage, schedule, route of administration, precautions, and potential side effects. Also discuss drug–drug and food–drug interactions.

✓ Discuss herbal/alternative therapies, such as vitamins, herbs, dietary supplements, minerals, homeopathy, and probiotics, in order to minimize interactions with prescribed medications and adverse effects.

✓ Importance of taking medications as prescribed in order to maintain remission and prevent flares.

✓ Importance of tobacco cessation because smoking is associated with resistance to medical therapy, recurrence of disease after surgery, and shortened duration of remission.

✓ Signs and symptoms that necessitate medical attention, including fever, nausea and vomiting, abdominal discomfort, any significant change in appearance and frequency of stools, or passage of stool through the vagina or stool mixed with urine, any of which can signal recurrence or complications of CD.

✓ Importance of dietary management to promote nutritional and fluid maintenance and prevent abdominal cramping, discomfort, and diarrhea.

✓ Importance of perineal/perianal skin care after bowel movements.

✓ Importance of balancing activities with rest periods, even during remission, because adequate rest is necessary to sustain remission.

✓ Referral to community resources: Crohn's & Colitis Foundation of America at www.ccfa.org

✓ Teens with IBD at www.justlikemeibd.org;

✓ Online community at www.ccfacommunity.org,

✓ Facebook at https://www.facebook.com/ccfafb

✓ Twitter at www.twitter.com/crohnscolitisfn.

✓ Importance of follow-up medical care, including supportive psychotherapy, because of the chronic and progressive nature of CD.

In addition, if the patient has a fecal diversion (colostomy or ileostomy):

✓ Care of the incision, dressing changes, and bathing.

✓ Care of the stoma and peristomal skin, use of ostomy equipment, and method for obtaining supplies.

✓ Gradual resumption of ADLs, excluding heavy lifting (more than 10 lb), pushing, or pulling for 6–8 weeks to prevent incisional herniation.

✓ Referral to community resources, including home health care agency, WOC/ET nurse, local ostomy association, the United Ostomy Association of America (UOAA) main website at www.ostomy.org, and the UOAA Discussion Board at www.uoaa.org/forum.

✓ Importance of reporting signs and symptoms that require medical attention, such as change in stoma color from the normal bright and shiny red; lesions of stomal mucosa that may indicate recurrence of disease; peristomal skin irritation; diarrhea or constipation, fever, chills, abdominal pain, distention, nausea, and vomiting; and incisional pain, local increased temperature, drainage, swelling, or redness.

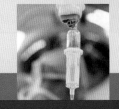

# Fecal Diversions: Colostomy, Ileostomy, and Ileal Pouch-Anal Anastomoses

## OVERVIEW/PATHOPHYSIOLOGY

See Chapter 63 for information on Ulcerative Colitis. See Chapter 57 for information on Crohn's Disease.

## HEALTH CARE SETTING

Acute care on surgical unit, primary care, home care after hospital discharge

## SURGICAL INTERVENTIONS

It is sometimes necessary to interrupt the continuity of the bowel because of intestinal disease or its complications. A fecal diversion may be necessary to divert stool around a diseased portion of the bowel or, more commonly, out of the body. A fecal diversion can be located anywhere along the bowel, depending on the location of the diseased or injured portion, and it can be permanent or temporary. The most common sites for fecal diversion are the colon and ileum.

**Colostomy.** Created when the surgeon brings a portion of the colon to the surface of the abdomen. An opening in the exteriorized colon permits the elimination of flatus and stool through the stoma. Any part of the colon may be diverted into a colostomy. The ostomy is further described by its anatomic site such as ascending, transverse, descending, and sigmoid colostomies. The more distal the ostomy, the more likely that the drainage will resemble feces that would have been eliminated from an intact colon and rectum.

*Transverse colostomy.* Most commonly created stoma to divert feces on a temporary basis. Surgical indications include relief of bowel obstruction before definitive surgery for tumors, inflammation, diverticulitis, or colon perforation secondary to trauma. Stool can be liquid to paste-like or soft and unformed, and bowel elimination is unpredictable. A temporary colostomy may be double barreled, with a proximal stoma through which stool is eliminated and a distal stoma, called a *mucus fistula*, adjacent to the proximal stoma. More commonly, a loop colostomy is created with a supporting rod placed beneath it until the exteriorized loop of colon heals to the skin.

*Descending or sigmoid colostomy.* Usually a permanent fecal diversion. Rectal cancer is the most common cause for surgical intervention. Stool is usually formed, and some individuals

may have stool elimination at predictable times. In a permanent colostomy, the surgeon brings the severed end of the colon to the abdominal skin surface. The severed end becomes the stoma from which stool is excreted. The diseased or injured portion of the colon and/or rectum is resected and removed. To create the stoma, the colon above the skin surface is rolled back on itself to expose the mucosal surface of the intestine. The end of the cuff is sutured to the subcutaneous tissues with absorbable sutures to hold it in place as it heals.

*Temporary colostomy.* Typically created when there is significant inflammation in the diseased portion of the bowel (e.g., perforated diverticulum or ulcerative colitis [UC]) or when rectum-sparing surgery is performed for colorectal cancer. When a temporary colostomy is created, the severed end of the colon is brought through the abdominal wall as for a permanent colostomy. The diseased or injured portion of the colon is resected and removed. The remaining rectum or rectosigmoid is oversewn and left in the peritoneal cavity; it is referred to as a *Hartmann pouch*. After the inflammatory process has resolved (e.g., 3–6 months), the colostomy is reversed and reattached to the bowel of the Hartmann pouch, thus reconstructing the continuity of the bowel and normal bowel elimination.

**Permanent ileostomy.** Created by bringing a distal portion of the resected ileum through the abdominal wall. Surgical indications include UC, CD, and familial adenomatous polyposis (FAP) requiring excision of the entire colon and rectum. For any ileostomy, the output is usually liquid (or, more rarely, paste-like) and is eliminated continually. The more proximal the ileostomy, the more active are digestive enzymes within the effluent (stool) and the greater their potential for irritation to exposed skin around the stoma. A collection pouch is worn over the stoma on the abdomen to collect gas and fecal discharge.

*Temporary ileostomy.* Usually a loop stoma with or without a supporting rod in place beneath the loop of the ileum until the exteriorized loop of ileum heals to the skin. The purpose is to divert the fecal stream away from a more distal anastomotic site or fistula repair until healing has occurred.

*Continent (Koch pouch) ileostomy.* An intraabdominal pouch constructed from approximately 40 to 45 cm of distal ileum. Intussusception of a 10-cm portion of ileum is performed to form an outlet nipple valve from the pouch to the skin of the abdomen, where a stoma is constructed flush with the skin. The intraabdominal pouch can hold approximately 500 mL of fecal material and is therefore continent for gas and fecal discharge. It must be emptied approximately four times daily by inserting a catheter through the stoma. No external pouch is needed, and a Band-Aid or small dressing is worn over the stoma to collect mucus. Surgical indications include UC and FAP requiring removal of the colon and rectum. CD is generally a contraindication for this procedure because the disease can recur in the pouch, necessitating its removal. A long-term complication of the Kock pouch is pouchitis. See under "ileal pouch-anal anastomosis" (IPAA) next, with the exception that tenesmus is not a symptom for a patient with a Kock pouch.

***Ileal pouch-anal anastomosis.*** A two-stage surgical procedure developed to preserve fecal continence and prevent the need for a permanent ileostomy. During the first stage after total colectomy and removal of the rectal mucosa, an ileal reservoir or pouch is constructed and lowered into position in the pelvis just above the rectal cuff. Then the ileal outlet from the pouch is brought down through the cuff of the rectal muscle and anastomosed to the anal canal. The anal sphincter is preserved, and the resulting ileal pouch provides a storage place for feces. A temporary diverting ileostomy is required for 2–3 months to allow healing of the anastomosis. The second stage

occurs when the diverting ileostomy is taken down and fecal continuity is restored. Initially, the patient experiences fecal incontinence and 10 or more bowel movements per day. After 3–6 months, the patient experiences decreased urgency and frequency with 4–8 bowel movements per day. This procedure is an option for patients requiring colectomy for UC or FAP. Its use is controversial in patients with CD. It is contraindicated with incontinence problems. Pouchitis is a long-term complication of IPAA. Its cause is unknown but may be the stasis of bacteria in the ileal pouch. However, *Clostridium difficile* infection is now being increasingly recognized as a potential cause of pouchitis.

About 40% of patients who undergo IPAA surgery for UC develop pouchitis at least once (Barnes et al., 2020). Symptoms of pouchitis include increased stool frequency, cramping, tenesmus, and bleeding. Pouchitis has been effectively treated with metronidazole or ciprofloxacin. Probiotics also may be effective in preventing and maintaining remission in patients with recurrent pouchitis.

> **Note:** *Consult a wound, ostomy, continence (WOC)/ enterostomal therapy (ET) nurse, if available, because he or she has expertise in all aspects of fecal diversion management and the related patient care.*

## Patient Problem/Analyze Cues/Prioritize Hypotheses

# Risk for Impaired Tissue Perfusion (Stomal Tissue)

*due to* improperly fitted appliance resulting in damage to stomal tissue and/or impaired circulation

***Desired Outcome/Generate Solutions:*** The patient's stoma remains red, moist, viable, and intact.

| ASSESSMENT—RECOGNIZE CUES/ INTERVENTIONS—TAKE ACTION | RATIONALES |
|---|---|
| **After Colostomy or Conventional Ileostomy (Permanent or Temporary)** | |
|  Assess the stoma for viability every 8 hours. | The stoma should be red, moist, and shiny with mucus. A stoma that is pale, dark purple to black, or dull in appearance may indicate circulatory impairment and should be documented and reported to the health care provider immediately. |
| | If necrosis (tissue death) of the stoma occurs, it will most likely occur within 24 hours to 5 days after surgery. The necrosis can be superficial or deep. |
| Recalibrate the skin barrier opening to the size of the stoma with each pouch change. | Stomas become less edematous over a period of 6–8 weeks after surgery, necessitating changes in the size of the skin barrier opening. The skin barrier opening should be the exact circumference of the stoma, or as recommended by the manufacturer, to prevent stomal constriction, which can result in increased edema of and decreased blood flow to the stoma as well as to prevent laceration of the stoma. Commercial templates are available to aid in estimating the size of the opening needed for the skin barrier. |

## ASSESSMENT—RECOGNIZE CUES/ INTERVENTIONS—TAKE ACTION

### After Continent Ileostomy (Kock Pouch)

Change the 4×4 dressing around the stoma every 2 hours or as often as it becomes wet.

Assess the stoma for viability with each dressing change.

## RATIONALES

The stoma should be red, moist, and shiny with mucus. A stoma that is pale, dark purple to black, or dull in appearance may indicate circulatory impairment and should be documented and reported to the health care provider immediately.

If necrosis of the stoma occurs, it will most likely occur within 24 hours to 5 days after surgery. Necrosis can be superficial or deep.

## Patient Problem/Analyze Cues/Prioritize Hypotheses

# Risk for Impaired Skin Integrity (Peristomal Skin)

*due to* exposure to stool/small bowel effluent, soaps, solvents, or appliance material

***Desired Outcome/Generate Solutions:*** The patient's peristomal skin has no erythema and remains intact.

## ASSESSMENT—RECOGNIZE CUES/ INTERVENTIONS—TAKE ACTION

With each pouch change, apply a pectin, gelatin, methylcellulose-based, or synthetic solid-form skin barrier around the stoma.

When cutting the skin barrier to fit over the stoma, measure the circumference of the stoma and ensure the opening has the same circumference as the stoma, or is cut as recommended by the manufacturer. Remove the release paper and apply the sticky surface directly to the peristomal skin.

For some pouching systems, the skin barrier may be a separate barrier to be used with an adhesive-backed pouch, part of a two-piece system, or an integral part of a one-piece pouch system. Pectin-based paste also may be used to "caulk" around the barrier and compensate for irregular surfaces on the peristomal skin.

Remove the skin barrier and inspect the skin every 3–4 days. Monitor the peristomal skin for erythema, erosion, serous drainage, bleeding, and induration. Carefully document abnormal findings and report them to the health care provider.

Discontinue the use of irritating materials and substitute other materials.

Patch-test the patient's abdominal skin.

Recalibrate the skin barrier opening to the size of the stoma with each change.

## RATIONALES

This barrier will protect peristomal skin from irritation caused by contact with stool or small bowel effluent.

The skin barrier should cover the peristomal skin to prevent contact with stool.

A pectin-based paste may prevent undermining of the barrier with effluent and protect the skin immediately adjacent to the stoma.

These indicators may signal infection, irritation, or sensitivity to the materials placed on the skin.

Accurate documentation and health care provider notification will promote early interventions to prevent skin breakdown or inflammation. With irritant dermatitis, erythema, erosion, and skin damage are confined to areas of stool or irritant contact. In allergic dermatitis, margins of contact are more blurred, may extend beyond the area of contact as inflammation progresses, and are pruritic.

This will help heal and protect irritated and/or denuded skin.

This will determine sensitivity to suspected materials. A dermatology consult may be required.

Stomas become less edematous over a period of 6–8 weeks after surgery, necessitating changes in the size of the skin barrier opening. The skin barrier opening should be the exact circumference of the stoma, or as recommended by the manufacturer, to prevent contact of stool with the skin. Commercial templates are available to aid in estimating the size of the opening needed for the skin barrier.

Continued

| ASSESSMENT—RECOGNIZE CUES/ INTERVENTIONS—TAKE ACTION | RATIONALES |
|---|---|
| Instruct the patient to immediately report any burning or itching under the skin barrier or any fecal odor. | Burning, itching, and odor are signs that stool or effluent may have contacted the skin. To prevent skin irritation or breakdown, the skin barrier should be changed immediately. |
| Empty the pouch when it is one-third to one-half full of stool and/or gas. | This helps ensure the maintenance of a secure pouch seal. A pouch with a larger amount of stool and/or gas could break the seal. |

### After Continent Ileostomy (Kock Pouch)

| | |
|---|---|
| Assess the site for erythema, induration, drainage, or erosion around the stoma. Report significant findings to the health care provider. | These are signs of infection, irritation, or sensitivity to materials placed on the skin. |
| Assess the catheter every 2 hours for patency and irrigate with sterile as prescribed. Notify the health care provider if solution cannot be instilled, if there are no returns from the catheter, or if leakage of irrigating solution or pouch contents appears around the catheter. | These measures check for and help prevent catheter obstruction. Instilling 30 mL of saline will clear the catheter and liquefy the secretions/effluent without adding unnecessary pressure on the pouch walls and areas of anastomosis. |
| Avoid stress on the ileostomy catheter and its securing suture. | This will prevent tissue destruction and catheter dislodgment. |
| As prescribed, maintain the catheter on low, continuous suction or gravity drainage. | The catheter was inserted through the stoma into the continent ileostomy pouch during surgery to prevent stress on the nipple valve and maintain pouch decompression so that suture lines are allowed to heal without stress or tension. |
| Change the 4×4 dressing around the stoma every 2 hours or as often as it becomes wet. | This will help prevent peristomal skin irritation. |
| Report frank bleeding to the health care provider. | Ostomy drainage will be serosanguineous at first and mixed with mucus. Bloody drainage may indicate a GI bleed and must be treated immediately. |

### After IPAA

| | |
|---|---|
| After the first stage of the operation, perform routine care for the temporary diverting ileostomy. | See earlier discussion for "After colostomy or conventional ileostomy (permanent or temporary)." |
| Maintain perineal/perianal skin integrity by gently cleansing the area with water and cotton balls or soft tissues. | After the first stage of the operation, the patient may have incontinence of mucus. |
| Avoid soap. | Soap can cause itching and irritation. |
| Place an absorbent pad over the rectal area at night. | This will absorb oozing mucus from the anus. |
| After the second stage of the operation (when the temporary diverting ileostomy is taken down), assess the patient's defecation pattern. | The patient likely will experience frequency and urgency of defecation. |
| Assess the perineal/perianal skin for erythema and denuded areas. | Proteolytic enzymes present in effluent can cause skin breakdown. |
| Wash the perineal/perianal area with warm water or commercial perineal/perianal cleansing solution, using a squeeze bottle, cotton balls, or soft tissues. | This will promote comfort and cleanse the perineal/perianal area to ensure skin integrity. |
| Do not use toilet paper. If desired, dry the area with hair dryer on a cool setting. | Toilet paper can cause skin irritation. A hair dryer on a cool setting will prevent skin irritation potentially caused by other materials. |
| Provide sitz baths. | These will promote comfort and help clean the perineal/perianal area. |
| Apply the protective skin sealants or ointments. | This will help maintain skin integrity. |
| | **Note:** Skin sealants containing alcohol should not be used on irritated or denuded skin because the high alcohol content would cause a painful burning sensation; apply only to intact skin. |

## Patient Problems/Analyze Cues/Prioritize Hypotheses

# Impaired Gastrointestinal Function

*due to* the disruption of normal function with a fecal diversion

**Desired Outcomes/Generate Solutions:** Within 2–4 days after surgery, the patient has bowel sounds and eliminates gas and stool through the fecal diversion. Within 3 days after teaching has been initiated, the patient verbalizes understanding of measures that will maintain a normal elimination pattern and demonstrates care techniques specific to the fecal diversion.

| ASSESSMENT—RECOGNIZE CUES/ INTERVENTIONS—TAKE ACTION | RATIONALES |
|---|---|
| **After Colostomy and Conventional Ileostomy (Permanent and Temporary)** | |
| Assess the intake and output (I&O). Empty stool from the bottom opening of the pouch and assess the quality and quantity of stool. Record the volume of liquid stool and its color and consistency. | This assessment documents the return of normal bowel function and its quality and quantity. Expect serosanguineous to serous liquid drainage and flatus initially. Colostomy output of clear brown, liquid stool usually begins within 3–4 days. Ileostomy output of liquid, bilious effluent usually begins within 24–48 hours. Output consistency thickens as solid food is ingested and varies with the type of ostomy. |
| **After Continent Ileostomy (Kock Pouch)** | |
| Assess the I&O and record the amount, color, and consistency of output. | The patient likely will have bright-red blood or serosanguineous liquid drainage from the Kock pouch during the early postoperative period. |
| As gastrointestinal (GI) function returns after 3–4 days, assess and document the color and character of output. | Usually, drainage changes from blood-tinged to greenish-brown liquid. When ileal output appears, suction (if used) is discontinued, and the pouch catheter is connected to or maintained on gravity drainage. |
| Check and irrigate the catheter every 2 hours and as needed. | This will maintain catheter patency. As the patient's diet progresses from clear liquids to solid food, ileal output thickens. |
| If the patient reports abdominal fullness in the area of the pouch along with decreased fecal output, catheter placement and patency should be assessed. | Decreased fecal output along with GI symptoms may indicate an output blockage. |
| When the patient is alert and taking food by mouth, teach the catheter irrigation procedure, which should be performed every 2 hours; demonstrate how to empty pouch contents through the catheter into the toilet. | The pouch effluent begins to thicken in consistency when the patient is taking food by mouth. Irrigation liquefies effluent for easier flow through the catheter. Frequent irrigations prevent overdistention of the pouch. |
| Before hospital discharge, provide instructions to the patient on how to remove and reinsert the catheter. | Teaching, followed by a return demonstration, helps ensure that learning has occurred and facilitates the retention of that information. |
| **After IPAA** | |
| Assess the patient for temperature elevation accompanied by perianal pain and discharge of purulent, bloody mucus from drains and anal orifice. Report significant findings to the health care provider. | These are signs of infection or anastomotic leak, which should be reported for prompt intervention. |
| If drains are present, irrigate them as prescribed. | Irrigation helps maintain patency, decrease stress on suture lines, and decrease the incidence of infection. |
| Assess the output from IPAA. | This assessment monitors the quantity, quality, and consistency of output. Also see the earlier discussion, "After colostomy or conventional ileostomy (permanent or temporary)," for the monitoring of output from a temporary diverting ileostomy. |
| After the first stage of the operation, advise the patient to wear a small pad in the perianal area to absorb mucus drainage. | This will prevent soiling of outer garments. After the first stage of the operation, the patient may experience oozing of mucus from the anus. |

Continued

| ASSESSMENT—RECOGNIZE CUES/ INTERVENTIONS—TAKE ACTION | RATIONALES |
|---|---|
| After the second stage of the operation (when the temporary diverting ileostomy is taken down), assess the patient's output. | The patient likely will have incontinence and 15–20 bowel movements per day with urgency when on a clear-liquid diet. The number of bowel movements decreases to 6–12/day and the consistency thickens when the patient is eating solid foods. |
| Assist with perianal care and apply protective skin care products. | This helps maintain perineal/perianal skin integrity. If nocturnal incontinence is especially troublesome, the catheter can be placed in the reservoir and connected to a gravity drainage bag overnight. |
| Administer the hydrophilic colloids and antidiarrheal medications as prescribed. | These agents decrease the frequency and fluidity of stools. |
| Provide a diet consultation. | The patient can learn about foods that cause liquid stools (spinach, raw fruits, highly seasoned foods, green beans, broccoli, prune and grape juices, alcohol) and increase intake of foods that cause thick stools (cheese, ripe bananas, applesauce, creamy peanut butter, gelatin, pasta). |
| Reassure the patient that frequency and urgency are temporary and that as the reservoir expands and absorbs fluid, bowel movements should become thicker and less frequent. | This reassurance may decrease anxiety about the disruption of the patient's usual bowel pattern. |

## Patient Problem/Analyze Cues/Prioritize Hypotheses

# Risk for Negative Self-Image

*due to* the presence of a fecal diversion

***Desired Outcome/Generate Solutions:*** Within 5–7 days after surgery, the patient demonstrates actions that reflect beginning acceptance of the fecal diversion and improvements in his or her self-image, as evidenced by acknowledging body changes, viewing the stoma, and participating in care of the fecal diversion.

| ASSESSMENT—RECOGNIZE CUES/ INTERVENTIONS—TAKE ACTION | RATIONALES |
|---|---|
| Assess the patient for expressed concerns about the fecal diversion. | Many concerns may be expressed by patients experiencing a fecal diversion. Some patients view incontinence as a return to infancy. The following concerns may be expected: physical, social, and work activities will be curtailed significantly; rejection, isolation, and feelings of uncleanliness will occur; everyone will know about the altered pattern of fecal elimination; and loss of voluntary control may occur. |
| Assess carefully for and listen closely to expressed or nonverbalized needs. | Each patient will react differently to the surgical procedure. |
| Encourage the patient to discuss feelings and concerns; clarify any misconceptions. Involve family members in discussions because they too may have concerns and misconceptions. | Concerns about body image may be reduced by talking about them. Such discussions also enable clarification about misconceptions. |
| Provide a calm and quiet environment for the patient and significant other to discuss the surgery. Initiate an open, honest discussion. | An open discussion enables understanding of the patient's perspective of the impact the diversion will have and assists in the development of an individualized plan of care that will help the patient. |
| Encourage the patient to participate in care. | Optimally, this will promote acceptance of the fecal diversion and enhance a sense of control. |

| ASSESSMENT—RECOGNIZE CUES/ INTERVENTIONS—TAKE ACTION | RATIONALES |
|---|---|
| Assure the patient that physical, social, and work activities will not be affected by the presence of a fecal diversion. | Resuming the previous lifestyle with minimal disruption is an essential component of the rehabilitation. It helps rebuild a sense of independence and self-esteem. |
| Expect the patient to have concerns about sexual acceptance. If you are uncomfortable talking about sexuality with patients, be aware of these potential concerns and arrange for a consultation with someone who can speak openly and honestly about these problems. | Although these concerns usually are not expressed overtly, anxieties center on change in body image; fears about odor and the ostomy appliance interfering with intercourse; conception, pregnancy, and discomfort from the perianal wound and scar in women; and impotence and failure to ejaculate in men, especially after more radical dissection of the pelvis in patients with cancer. Discussing these concerns will help patients cope with their feelings and provide accurate information about perceived sexual difficulties. |
| Consult the patient's health care provider about a visit by another person with an ostomy. | Patients gain reassurance and build positive attitudes and body image by seeing a healthy, active person who has undergone the same type of surgery, and it expands their support systems as well. |

## Patient Problem/Analyze Cues/Prioritize Hypotheses

# Deficient Knowledge (colostomy irrigation)

*due to* the unfamiliarity with the colostomy irrigation procedure

*Desired Outcome/Generate Solutions:* Within 3 days after initiation of teaching, the patient demonstrates proficiency with the procedure for colostomy irrigation.

**Note:** *Provide instructions to the patient on how to irrigate the colostomy per facility policy and procedures. If this protocol is not available, teach the patient how to perform the irrigation procedure as outlined next.*

| ASSESSMENT—RECOGNIZE CUES/ INTERVENTIONS—TAKE ACTION | RATIONALES |
|---|---|
| Provide instructions on the following steps and have the patient return the demonstration: | An appropriate candidate is a patient who has one or two formed stools each day at predictable times. |
| The prescribed colostomy irrigation is taught to patients with permanent descending or sigmoid colostomy. Colostomy irrigation is performed daily or every other day so that wearing a pouch becomes unnecessary. | The patient must be able to manipulate the equipment, remember the technique, and be willing to spend approximately 1 hour/day performing the procedure. |
| | It may take 4–6 weeks for the patient to have stool elimination regulated with irrigation. |
| | Instructions are provided so that the patient can correctly manage their ostomy care after discharge. |
| | A return demonstration with an explanation for each step will enable the nurse to determine the patient's knowledge level and facilitate learning retention for the patient. |
| Position the irrigating sleeve over the colostomy, centering the stoma in the opening. Secure the sleeve in place with an adhesive disk on the sleeve or with a sleeve belt. | The irrigation sleeve provides controlled diversion of stool and irrigation solution into the toilet. |
| Fill the enema/irrigation container with 500–1000 mL (1–2 pints) of warm water. With the patient in a sitting position on the toilet or on a chair facing the toilet, position the sleeve so that it empties into the toilet. Hang the enema/irrigation container so that the bottom surface is at the patient's shoulder level. | The volume of water must be titrated for each patient to produce colon distention without causing cramping or excessive stretching of the colon wall. |

Continued

PART I: Medical-Surgical Nursing Care Plans

| ASSESSMENT—RECOGNIZE CUES/ INTERVENTIONS—TAKE ACTION | RATIONALES |
| --- | --- |
| Open the slide or roller clamp and flush the tubing; re-clamp the tubing. | This removes air from the tubing. |
| Gently dilate the stoma with a gloved finger lubricated with water-soluble lubricant. | This enables the patient to identify the direction of the intestinal lumen and the presence or absence of obstructing stool or stomal stenosis. |
| Lubricate the cone, with or without the attached catheter, and slowly insert into the stoma. | This prevents bowel perforation. If the cone has an attached catheter, the catheter should be inserted no more than 3 inches. |
| Hold the cone gently, but firmly, in place against the stoma. | This prevents the backflow of irrigant. |
| Let water slowly enter the stoma from the container through the tubing; allow 15 minutes for fluid to enter the colon. | This prevents cramping caused by too rapid an infusion. |
| **Note:** If cramping occurs while water is flowing, stop the flow and leave the cone in place until the cramping passes. Then the flow of water may be resumed. | This likely will stop the cramping. If cramping does not resolve, the colon is probably ready to evacuate and should be allowed to do so. |
| After water has entered the colon, advise the patient to hold the cone in place for a few seconds and then gently remove it. | This ensures a complete infusion of the water. |
| Leave the sleeve in place for 30–40 minutes. | This enables water and stool to be eliminated. |
| When elimination is complete, remove the irrigation sleeve and cleanse and dry the peristomal area. | Cleaning and drying the skin help prevent skin irritation. |
| Apply a small dressing or security pouch over the colostomy between irrigations. | This collects mucus drainage from the stoma. **Note:** During the initial adaptation period, a drainable pouch is worn between irrigations to collect the expected spillage of stool. |

## ADDITIONAL PROBLEMS:

| | |
| --- | --- |
| Risk for Injury (Perioperative) | Chapter 4 |
| Risk for Infection | Chapter 4 |
| Difficulty Coping | Chapter 8 |
| Risk for Spiritual Distress | Chapter 8 |

 **PATIENT–FAMILY TEACHING AND DISCHARGE PLANNING**

When providing patient–family teaching, focus on sensory information, avoid giving excessive information, and initiate a visiting nurse referral for necessary follow-up teaching. Include verbal and written information about the following:

- ✓ Medications, including drug name, rationale, dosage, schedule, route of administration, precautions, and potential side effects. Also discuss drug–drug, herb–drug, and food–drug interactions.
- ✓ Importance of dietary management to promote nutritional and fluid maintenance.
- ✓ Care of incision, dressing changes, and permission to take baths or showers after sutures and drains are removed.
- ✓ Care of stoma, care of peristomal and perianal skin, use of ostomy equipment, and method for obtaining supplies.
- ✓ Gradual resumption of activities of daily living, excluding heavy lifting (more than 10 lb), pushing, or pulling for 6–8 weeks to prevent the development of incisional herniation.

- ✓ Referral to community resources including home health care agency, WOC/ET nurse, local ostomy association, and the United Ostomy Association of America (UOAA) main website at www.ostomy.org and the UOAA Discussion Board at www.uoaa.org/forum; or provide additional resources: Wound, Ostomy and Continence Nurses Society at www.wocn.org; Osto Group (a donation-based non-profit organization that provides ostomy supplies to the uninsured free of charge except for shipping and handling) at www.ostogroup.org; Crohn's and Colitis Foundation of America at www.ccfa.org.
- ✓ Refer to the Hollister website for Do's and Don'ts regarding sex after ostomy surgery. https://www.hollister.com/en/ostomycare/ostomylearningcenter/livingwithanostomy/sexafterostomysurgerydosanddonts.
- ✓ Importance of follow-up care with the health care provider and WOC/ET nurse; confirm date and time of next appointment.
- ✓ Importance of reporting signs and symptoms that necessitate medical attention, such as change in stoma color from normal bright and shiny red; peristomal or perianal skin irritation; any significant changes in appearance, frequency, and consistency of stools; fever, chills, abdominal pain, or distention; and incisional pain, increased local warmth, drainage, swelling, or redness; and signs and symptoms of pouchitis, including diarrhea, cramping, tenesmus, and bleeding.

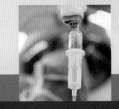

# Hepatitis 59

## OVERVIEW/PATHOPHYSIOLOGY

Viral hepatitis is the most common form of hepatitis and may be caused by one of five viruses that are capable of infecting the liver: hepatitis A (HAV), B (HBV), C (HCV), D, (HDV), or E. HDV is not a stand-alone hepatitis. HDV does not exist outside the presence of HBV. Although the various types have similar signs and symptoms, the mode of transmission and the course of the disease varies with each type. When hepatocytes are damaged, necrosis and autolysis can occur, which in turn lead to abnormal liver functioning. Generally, these changes are completely reversible after the acute phase. In some cases, however, massive necrosis can lead to acute liver failure and death.

Patients with *acute hepatitis* may not have symptoms, but others may have gastrointestinal symptoms such as nausea, vomiting, diarrhea, or constipations. Patients may also complain of right upper quadrant tenderness from liver inflammation. Jaundice, dark urine, and clay-colored stool are caused by decreased bilirubin metabolism. The acute phase lasts from 1 to 6 months. Most patients have a complete recovery from acute hepatitis.

*Chronic hepatitis* is inflammation of the liver for more than 6 months. Patients with chronic hepatitis may be asymptomatic, and without medical intervention, continual destruction of the infected hepatocytes occurs. Scar tissue eventually develops, leading to irreversible cirrhosis and decreased liver function. Forms of chronic hepatitis are associated with infection from HBV, HCV, and HDV; viral infections such as cytomegalovirus; excessive alcohol consumption; inflammatory bowel disease; and autoimmunity (chronic active lupoid hepatitis).

*Alcoholic hepatitis* occurs as a result of tissue necrosis caused by alcohol abuse; it is nonviral and noninfectious. Generally, it is a precursor to cirrhosis (see Chapter 56), but it may occur simultaneously with cirrhosis.

Jaundice is a condition in which the skin, sclera, and mucous membranes become yellow from increased serum levels of bilirubin (total serum bilirubin more than 2.5 mg/dL) and can occur with any hepatitis. Jaundice may be seen in any patient with impaired hepatic function and occurs as bilirubin begins to be excreted through the skin. Pruritis (itchy skin) may accompany jaundice, which may cause intense discomfort. There is also an increased excretion of urobilinogen and bilirubin by the kidneys, resulting in darker, almost brownish, urine. Jaundice is classified as follows.

*Prehepatic (hemolytic).* Caused by increased production of bilirubin following erythrocyte destruction. Prehepatic jaundice is implicated when the indirect (unconjugated) serum bilirubin is more than 0.8 mg/dL.

*Hepatic (hepatocellular).* Caused by the dysfunction of the liver cells (hepatocytes), which reduces their ability to remove bilirubin from the blood and form it into bile. Hepatic jaundice is also implicated with indirect serum bilirubin and is associated with acute hepatitis.

*Posthepatic (obstructive).* Caused by the obstruction of the flow of bile out of the liver and resulting in backed-up bile through the hepatocytes to the blood. Posthepatic jaundice is implicated when direct serum bilirubin is more than 0.3 mg/dL.

## HEALTH CARE SETTING

Primary care, with possible brief hospitalization resulting from complications

## ASSESSMENT

*Signs and symptoms.* Nausea, vomiting, malaise, anorexia, epigastric discomfort, aversion to smoking, muscle or joint aches, fatigue, irritability, pruritus, slight to moderate temperature increases, dark urine, clay-colored stools, and jaundice.

*Physical assessment.* Presence of jaundice; palpation of lymph nodes and abdomen may reveal lymphadenopathy, ascites (excess fluid in the peritoneal cavity), hepatomegaly, and splenomegaly. Liver size is usually small with acute hepatic failure.

*History and risk factors.* Clotting disorders, multiple blood transfusions, excessive alcohol ingestion, parenteral drug use, exposure to hepatotoxic chemicals or medications (including over-the-counter [OTC] medications or herbal supplements), travel to developing countries, men who engage in sexual activities with other men, prostitutes/heterosexuals with multiple sexual partners, injection drug users.

## DIAGNOSTIC TESTS

*Immunoglobulins.* Chronic infection markers are present for HBV, HCV, and HDV. They are HBsAg, anti-HBc IgG for hepatitis B; anti-HCV (enzyme-linked immunosorbent assay) and HCV RNA quantitation for hepatitis C; and anti-HDV IgG for hepatitis D.

*Serum enzymes.* Aspartate aminotransferase and alanine aminotransferase are initially elevated and then drop.

Gamma-glutamyl transpeptidase is elevated early in liver disease and persists as long as cellular damage continues.

*Other hematologic tests.* Total bilirubin may be elevated, and prothrombin time (PT) and INR may be prolonged. Differential white blood cell count reveals leukocytosis, monocytosis, and atypical lymphocytes.

*Urine tests.* Reveal elevation of urobilinogen, mild proteinuria, and mild bilirubinuria.

*Liver elastography.* Mostly done in place of a liver biopsy. Use of an ultrasound for patients with chronic liver disease to detect the extent of tissue damage and scar tissue formation, by measuring the fibrosis stage (stiffness) of the liver tissue (Kennedy et al., 2018).

*Liver biopsy.* Although this procedure is performed to obtain a definitive diagnosis of hepatitis, clinically it is not always advisable because of the high risk for bleeding. When performed, a biopsy is obtained percutaneously or by laparoscopy to collect a specimen for histologic examination to confirm differential diagnosis.

## Patient Problem/Analyze Cues/Prioritize Hypotheses

# Fatigue

*due to* the decreased metabolic energy production occurring with faulty absorption, metabolism, and storage of nutrients

***Desired Outcome/Generate Solutions:*** By at least 24 hours before hospital discharge, the patient relates decreasing fatigue and increasing energy.

| ASSESSMENT—RECOGNIZE CUES/ INTERVENTIONS—TAKE ACTION | RATIONALES |
|---|---|
| Conduct a diet history. Consult the dietitian regarding increased intake of carbohydrates or other high-energy food sources within prescribed dietary limitations. Encourage significant others to bring in desirable foods if permitted. Monitor and record the intake. | The patient's diet history is done to determine food preferences. A dietician will help ensure that the patient is provided with the appropriate diet.<br><br>The patient will be more willing to eat those foods that they enjoy.<br><br>Intake documentation will provide the health care team with a record on the patient's daily fluid and caloric consumption.<br><br>In general, dietary management consists of giving palatable meals as tolerated without overfeeding. If oral intake is substantially decreased, parenteral or enteral nutrition may be initiated. Sodium restrictions may be indicated in the presence of fluid retention. Protein is moderately restricted, or eliminated, depending on the degree of mental status changes (i.e., encephalopathy). If no mental status changes are noted, normal amounts of high biologic-value protein are indicated to facilitate tissue healing, promote energy, and decrease fatigue. All alcoholic beverages are strictly forbidden. When appetite and food selection are poor, vitamins may be given to supplement dietary intake. |
| Encourage small, frequent feedings, and provide emotional support during meals. | Smaller and more frequent meals are usually better tolerated in patients who are fatigued, nauseated, and anorexic. |
| Provide rest periods of at least 90 minutes before and after activities and treatments. | Rest facilitates recovery after the body has experienced stress and may be indicated when symptoms are severe, with a gradual return to normal activity as symptoms subside. |
| Advise the patient to avoid exercise immediately after meals. | Exercise after meals increases the potential for nausea and vomiting, which could cause loss of nutrients and exacerbate fatigue. |
| Keep frequently used objects within easy reach. | This will help conserve the patient's energy. |
| Decrease environmental stimuli; place patient in a room away from the nurses' station; offer relaxing music; and speak with the patient in short, simple terms. | These measures promote rest and sleep and decrease sensory overload. |
| Administer acid suppression therapy, antiemetics, antidiarrheal medications, and cathartics as prescribed. | These agents minimize gastric distress and promote the absorption of nutrients, which will help provide energy and reverse feelings of fatigue. |

## Patient Problem/Analyze Cues/Prioritize Hypotheses

# Deficient Knowledge (Disease Process)

*due to* unfamiliarity with the causes of hepatitis and modes of transmission

***Desired Outcome/Generate Solutions:*** Within the 24-hour period before hospital discharge, the patient verbalizes accurate knowledge about the causes of hepatitis and measures that help prevent transmission.

| ASSESSMENT—RECOGNIZE CUES/ INTERVENTIONS—TAKE ACTION | RATIONALES |
|---|---|
| Assess the patient's health care literacy (language, reading, comprehension). Assess the culture and culturally specific information needs. | This assessment helps ensure that information is selected and presented in a manner that is culturally and educationally appropriate. |
| Assess the patient's knowledge about the disease process and educate as necessary. | Determining a patient's level of knowledge will facilitate the development of an individualized teaching plan. |
| Speak to patient in an objective tone to ensure that no moral judgments about alcohol/drug use or sexual behavior are conveyed. | This will promote the patient's confidence in you. |
| Instruct the patient and significant others about the importance of wearing gloves and using good hand hygiene if contact with body fluids such as urine, blood, wound exudate, or feces is possible. | These measures help prevent the spread of infection. |
| If appropriate, advise patients with HAV that crowded living conditions with poor sanitation should be avoided if possible. If needed, refer patient to Social Services to aid them in securing an appropriate living arrangement. | This information may prevent recurrence. |
| Remind patients with HBV and HCV that they should modify sexual behavior as directed by the health care provider. Explain that blood donation is no longer possible. | For patients with HBV and HCV, contact with blood is a likely mode of transmission, and blood contact can occur with some types of sexual activities. For patients with HBV, sexual contact is a likely mode. |
| ⚠ Advise patients with HBV that their sexual partners should receive HBV vaccine. | For patients with HBV, sexual contact is a likely mode of transmission. |
| ⚠ Refer the patient to drug treatment programs as necessary. | Drug use not only is a causative factor but also can further damage the liver. |

## Patient Problem/Analyze Cues/Prioritize Hypotheses

# Risk for Impaired Skin Integrity

*due to* scratching caused by pruritus

***Desired Outcome/Generate Solutions:*** The patient reports reduced pruritus, as evidenced by intact skin and verbalized reduction in itching.

| ASSESSMENT—RECOGNIZE CUES/ INTERVENTIONS—TAKE ACTION | RATIONALES |
|---|---|
| Keep the patient's skin moist by using tepid water or emollient baths, avoiding alkaline soap (which is a stronger soap; use transparent soaps such as a glycerin soap), and applying emollient lotions at frequent intervals. | Hot water and alkaline soaps can dry the skin and may cause irritation in patients with sensitive skin. Emollients and lipid creams (i.e., Eucerin) are used to keep skin moist and supple. |
| Encourage the patient not to scratch skin and to keep nails short and smooth. | These measures help prevent skin breakdown and infection. |

Continued

| ASSESSMENT—RECOGNIZE CUES/ INTERVENTIONS—TAKE ACTION | RATIONALES |
|---|---|
| Suggest the use of knuckles if the patient must scratch. Wrap or place gloves on the patient's hands (especially comatose patients). | Knuckles and gloved hands are less traumatic to the skin and tissue than fingernails. |
| Assess the skin for scratches and lesions and treat any skin breakdown promptly as per facility policy and/or as prescribed. | This will help prevent infection. Pathogens can enter the body through nonintact skin. |
| • Administer antihistamines as prescribed; observe closely for excessive sedation. | Antihistamines may be used for symptomatic relief of pruritus. However, if used, they are administered with caution and in low doses because they are metabolized by the liver. |
| | Some antihistamines may cause sedation, which may increase the patient's fall risk. |
| Encourage the patient to wear loose, soft clothing; provide soft linens (cotton is best). | These measures help prevent abrasions caused by tight clothing or rough material on skin that is already compromised. |
| Keep the environment cool. | Cool temperatures help prevent further skin irritation caused by perspiration. |
| Change soiled linen as soon as possible. | This measure helps prevent further irritation caused by waste products or fluids having constant skin contact. |

## Patient Problem/Analyze Cues/Prioritize Hypotheses

# Risk for Hemorrhage

*due to* the decreased vitamin K absorption and decreased coagulation factors

***Desired Outcome/Generate Solutions:*** The patient is free of bleeding, as evidenced by negative tests for occult blood in the feces and urine and absence of ecchymotic areas and bleeding at the gums and injection sites.

| ASSESSMENT—RECOGNIZE CUES/ INTERVENTIONS—TAKE ACTION | RATIONALES |
|---|---|
| Monitor the PT and International Normalized Ratio (INR) levels daily. | These assessments measure coagulation associated with vitamin K synthesis. Optimal range for PT is 10.5–13.5 seconds and INR 1.1 or below. In hepatitis, PT is prolonged and INR is elevated because of the inability of the liver to produce coagulation factors. |
| Monitor the platelet count daily. | These assessments detect thrombocytopenia. Optimal range is 150,000–400,000/mm$^3$. In hepatitis, platelet count is decreased because of the decrease in the production of thrombopoietin or platelet pooling caused by splenomegaly and portal hypertension. |
| Monitor the hematocrit (Hct) and hemoglobin (Hgb) daily. | These assessments detect decreases that may indicate occult bleeding. Optimal ranges are Hct 40%–54% (male) and 37%–47% (female) and Hgb 14–18 g/dL (male) and 12–16 g/dL (female). |
| Handle the patient gently (e.g., when turning or transferring). | This measure helps minimize the risk for bleeding within the tissues. |
| Minimize intramuscular injections. Rotate sites and use small-gauge needles. Administer medications orally or intravenously when possible. | Bleeding may result from the use of large-bore needles. Rotating sites help prevent tissue damage caused by frequent injections in the same tissue. |
| Apply moderate pressure after an injection, but do not massage the site. | These measures minimize bleeding at the injection site while preventing excessive pressure on the tissue. |
| Observe for ecchymotic areas. Inspect gums and test urine and feces for bleeding. Report significant findings to the health care provider. | These assessments detect early signs of bleeding potential and abnormal bleeding sources. |

## ASSESSMENT—RECOGNIZE CUES/INTERVENTIONS—TAKE ACTION

## RATIONALES

| ASSESSMENT—RECOGNIZE CUES/INTERVENTIONS—TAKE ACTION | RATIONALES |
|---|---|
| Instruct the patient to use an electric razor and soft-bristle toothbrush. | These measures minimize the risk for bleeding from cuts or abrasions caused by a razor or hard bristles. |
| Administer vitamin K as prescribed. | For patients with prolonged PT and elevated INR, vitamin K is a cofactor that modifies clotting factors to provide a site for calcium binding—an essential part of the clotting function. Patients with severe hepatic failure may not respond to vitamin K and may require transfusions of fresh frozen plasma before invasive procedures. |

## ADDITIONAL PROBLEM:

| | |
|---|---|
| *Risk for Hemorrhage*, if the patient develops encephalopathy | Chapter 56 |

## PATIENT–FAMILY TEACHING AND DISCHARGE PLANNING

When providing patient–family teaching, focus on sensory information, avoid giving excessive information, and initiate a visiting nurse referral for necessary follow-up teaching. Include verbal and written information about the following:

✓ Importance of rest and getting adequate nutrition. When appropriate, provide a list of high biologic-value protein food sources or protein foods to avoid and sample menus to demonstrate how these foods may be incorporated into or excluded from the diet. Instruct the patient to eat frequent, small meals; to eat slowly; and to chew all food thoroughly.

✓ Instruct the patient to rest for 30–60 minutes after meals. Initiate a dietitian consult as needed for diet instruction.

✓ Importance of avoiding hepatotoxic agents, including OTC drugs and herbal supplements. Examples of OTC drugs include aspirin and other salicylates, nonsteroidal antiinflammatory drugs, acetaminophen, alcohol, and vitamin A.

✓ Prescribed medications (e.g., multivitamins), including drug name, purpose, dosage, schedule, potential side effects, and precautions. Also discuss drug–drug, food–drug, and herb–drug interactions.

✓ Importance of informing health care providers, dentists, and other health care workers of the hepatitis diagnosis.

✓ Potential complications, including delayed healing, skin injury, and bleeding tendencies.

✓ Importance of avoiding alcohol during recovery.

✓ Referral to alcohol/drug treatment programs as appropriate.

✓ Provide information about organizations available for education:
  • Centers for Disease Control and Prevention: www.cdc.gov/ncidod/diseases/hepatitis/index.htm
  • Hepatitis B Foundation: https://www.hepb.org/

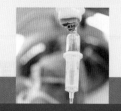

# Pancreatitis 60

## OVERVIEW/PATHOPHYSIOLOGY

The pancreas serves both endocrine (hormonal) and exocrine (nonhormonal) functions. (Pancreatic endocrine function is discussed in "Diabetes Mellitus," Chapter 47.) The exocrine portion constitutes 98% of its tissue mass. Exocrine secretions, which are produced by the acini cells, empty through a series of lobular ducts into the main pancreatic duct, where they are released into the duodenum. Exocrine function is the secretion of potent enzymes, proteases, lipases, and amylases that act to reduce proteins, fats, and carbohydrates, respectively, into simpler chemical substances. Pancreatic proteases (trypsin, chymotrypsin, carboxypeptidases A and B, elastase, and phospholipase A) aid in protein digestion. Pancreatic lipase acts on fats to produce glycerides, fatty acids, and glycerol; pancreatic amylase acts on starch to produce disaccharides. The pancreas also secretes sodium bicarbonate to neutralize the strongly acidic gastric content as it enters the duodenum. The resultant mixture of acids and bases provides an optimal pH of 8.3 for the activation of pancreatic enzymes.

Pancreatitis, which can be acute or chronic, is an inflammation of the pancreas with varying degrees of edema, hemorrhage, and necrosis. The damage can lead to fibrosis, stricture, and calcifications. Acute pancreatitis occurs when pancreatic ductal flow becomes obstructed and digestive enzymes escape from the pancreatic duct into surrounding tissue. Self-destruction of the pancreas produces edema, hemorrhage, and necrosis of pancreatic and surrounding tissue, causing severe pain. Biochemical abnormalities and disruption of cardiopulmonary, renal, metabolic, and gastrointestinal (GI) function are likely. Pancreatitis has been associated with gallstones (most common cause), alcoholism (second most common cause), surgical manipulation, abdominal trauma, abdominal vascular disease, heavy metal poisoning, infectious agents (viral, bacterial, mycoplasmal, parasitic), medications, and some allergic reactions. Pancreatitis also is associated with familial hyperlipidemia and can be induced by endoscopic retrograde cholangiopancreatography (ERCP). Most acute pancreatitis cases are mild, require a short hospitalization, and leave no long-term adverse effects. Complications of acute pancreatitis include pancreatic abscess, hemorrhage, pancreatic pseudocyst, fistula formation, and transient hypoglycemia. Acute, life-threatening complications include renal failure, hemorrhagic pancreatitis, septicemia, adult respiratory distress syndrome (ARDS), shock, and disseminated intravascular coagulation.

Chronic pancreatitis is characterized by varying degrees of pancreatic insufficiency, which results in decreased production of enzymes and bicarbonate and malabsorption of fats and proteins. The digestion of fat is affected most severely. As a result, a high-fat content in the bowel stimulates water and electrolyte secretion, which produces diarrhea. The action of bacteria on fecal fat produces flatus, fatty stools (steatorrhea), and abdominal cramps. Often diabetes mellitus (DM) occurs as a result of chronic pancreatitis because of damage to the insulin-producing beta cells and resultant deficient insulin production. Chronic pancreatitis is also associated with complications of DM, chronic pain, maldigestion, pseudocysts, and bleeding.

## HEALTH CARE SETTING

Primary care with hospitalization for acute pancreatitis and complications of chronic pancreatitis

## ASSESSMENT

**Acute pancreatitis.** Symptoms vary according to the severity of the attack. Sudden onset of constant, severe mid-epigastric or left upper quadrant abdominal pain often occurs after a large meal or alcohol intake. Pain frequently radiates to the back or left shoulder and is somewhat relieved by a sitting position with the spine flexed. It is caused by biliary tree obstruction, enzymes irritating pancreatic and surrounding tissue, and the resulting edema. Nausea and vomiting, sometimes with persistent retching, usually occur and are caused by bowel hypermotility or ileus. Pain may be increased after vomiting because of increased pressure on the ducts, leading to further obstruction of secretions and tissue damage. Fever is usually present as well as hypotension and tachycardia. Jaundice suggests biliary tree obstruction. Extreme malaise, restlessness, respiratory distress, and diminished urinary output may be present. Hypovolemic shock may be present from bleeding into the pancreas, or distributive shock may occur secondary to systemic inflammatory response syndrome (SIRS).

**Physical assessment.** Diminished or absent bowel sounds, suggesting the presence of ileus; mild to moderate ascites; generalized abdominal tenderness; tachypnea, crackles (rales) at lung bases related to atelectasis, and interstitial fluid accumulation; diminished ventilatory excursion related to splinting and guarding with pain; low-grade fever (100°F–102°F [37.7°C–38.8°C]) or pronounced fever with abscess or sepsis; and agitation, confusion, and altered mental status may occur because of electrolyte/metabolic abnormalities or acute alcohol withdrawal. Gray-blue discoloration of the flank (Grey Turner sign) or blue-red discoloration around the umbilicus (Cullen sign) sometimes is present with pancreatic hemorrhage.

**Chronic pancreatitis.** Constant, dull epigastric pain; steatorrhea resulting from malabsorption of fats and protein; weight loss; and onset of symptoms of DM (polydipsia, polyuria, polyphagia).

**History.** Biliary tract disease; chronic excessive alcohol consumption; physical trauma to the abdomen (especially in young people); peptic ulcer disease; viral infection; ERCP; cystic fibrosis; neoplasms; shock; and use of certain medications, such as estrogen-containing oral contraceptives, glucocorticoids, sulfonamides, chlorothiazides, and azathioprine.

## DIAGNOSTIC TESTS

**Serum amylase.** When significantly elevated (more than 500 units/dL), rules out acute abdomen conditions, such as cholecystitis, appendicitis, bowel infarction/obstruction, and perforated peptic ulcer and confirms the presence of pancreatitis. These levels return to normal 48–72 hours after the onset of acute symptoms, even though clinical indicators may continue. Sensitivity is limited in patients with alcoholic pancreatitis and hypertriglyceridemia.

**Serum lipase.** Has higher specificity and sensitivity than serum amylase. It rises more slowly than serum amylase and persists longer. Both lipase and amylase levels reflect the degree of necrotic pancreatic tissue.

**Blood glucose.** Hyperglycemia occurs because of interference with beta cell function. It is transient with acute pancreatitis

but common with chronic pancreatitis, during which DM is likely to develop.

**Ultrasound, magnetic resonance imaging, computed tomography.** May reveal an enlarged and edematous pancreatic head or abscess, pseudocyst, or calcification.

**Magnetic resonance cholangiopancreatography.** Used to visualize pancreatic and common bile ducts and may be used if an ERCP is not feasible.

**Endoscopic retrograde cholangiopancreatography.** A combined endoscopic-radiographic tool that is used to study the degree of pancreatic disease through assessment of biliary-pancreatic ductal systems. It allows direct visualization of the ampulla of Vater, diagnoses biliary stones and duct stenosis, and distinguishes cancer of the pancreas from pancreatic calculi. ERCP is not performed until the acute episode has subsided.

**Potassium.** Hyperkalemia will occur in the presence of tissue damage, metabolic acidosis, and renal failure in severe cases.

**Serum calcium and magnesium.** May be lower than normal. On electrocardiogram, hypocalcemia is evidenced by prolonged QT segment with a normal T wave.

**Complete blood count.** Elevated white blood cell (WBC) count caused by inflammatory process. Polymorphonuclear bodies may increase if bacterial peritonitis is present secondary to duodenal rupture. Hematocrit (Hct) may be elevated or decreased.

**Abdominal radiographic examination.** May show the dilation of the small or large bowel and the presence of pancreatic calcification in chronic pancreatitis.

## Patient Problem/Analyze Cues/Prioritize Hypotheses

# Acute Pain

*due to* the inflammatory process of the pancreas

**Desired Outcomes/Generate Solutions:** Within 6 hours of intervention, the patient's subjective perception of discomfort decreases, and it is controlled within 24 hours, as documented by pain scale. Nonverbal indicators, such as grimacing and splinting of abdominal muscles, are absent or diminished.

| ASSESSMENT—RECOGNIZE CUES/ INTERVENTIONS—TAKE ACTION | RATIONALES |
|---|---|
| Assess for and document the degree and character of the patient's discomfort. Devise a pain scale with the patient, rating discomfort on a scale of 0 (no pain) to 10 (worst pain). | Pain characteristics may signal varying problems (see the "Assessment" section). Baseline and subsequent use of a pain scale help determine effectiveness of pain relief. |
| Assess the patient's previous responses to pain and previously effective pain relief measures. | The patient's previous history of pain and how well it was managed influence perceptions and trust in present pain relief measures. |
| Consider possible cultural and spiritual influences that may affect the patient's beliefs regarding pain. | Some cultures allow less outward show of pain, whereas others do not prohibit expressions of pain. |
| Ensure that the patient maintains limited activity or bedrest. | Rest helps minimize pancreatic secretions and pain. |

Continued

| ASSESSMENT—RECOGNIZE CUES/ INTERVENTIONS—TAKE ACTION | RATIONALES |
|---|---|
| Maintain nothing by mouth (NPO) status and monitor nasogastric (NG) tube function if it is used. | NPO status is initiated early in the course of illness to decrease the stimulus for pancreatic secretions and reduce stress in the GI tract. NG suction is generally used only in more severely ill patients who have unrelieved vomiting. After acute pain and ileus have resolved, the patient is given clear liquids and the diet is advanced as tolerated. |
| Administer the analgesics, antispasmodic agents, steroids, histamine-2 ($H_2$)-receptor blockers, antiemetics, and other medications as prescribed. Be alert to the patient's response to medications, using the pain scale. | Analgesics and antispasmodic agents reduce discomfort associated with pancreatitis. Steroids may be given to reduce inflammation in certain types of pancreatitis when infection is not a problem. |
| | $H_2$-receptor blockers are given to reduce gastric acid secretion, which stimulates pancreatic enzymes. Antiemetics are given for nausea and vomiting. Antacids are given to neutralize gastric acid and reduce associated pain. |
| Instruct the patient to request an analgesic before pain becomes severe. | Pain is more easily managed when it is treated before it becomes severe. If the analgesic is ineffective, the health care provider should be notified because the patient may require another intervention. Optimally, analgesics are administered by patient-controlled pumps. |
| Avoid intramuscular (IM) injections in individuals with clotting or bleeding complications. | Transdermal analgesics or small, frequent doses of intravenous opioids usually are more effective than IM injections, which also increase the risk for bleeding in individuals with bleeding/clotting complications. |
| Assist the patient in attaining a position of comfort. | A sitting or supine position with the knees flexed often helps relax abdominal muscles. |
| Emphasize nonpharmacologic pain interventions (e.g., relaxation techniques, distraction, guided imagery, massage). | These interventions are especially important for patients in whom chronic pancreatitis develops and who are prone to chemical dependence. |
| Prepare significant others for personality changes and behavioral alterations associated with extreme pain and opioid analgesic. Reassure them that these are normal responses. | Pancreatitis can be very painful. Family members sometimes misinterpret the patient's lethargic or unpleasant disposition and may even blame themselves. |
| Monitor the patient's respiratory pattern and level of consciousness (LOC) closely. | Both may be depressed by the large amount of opioids usually required to control pain. |
| Report $O_2$ saturation of 92% or less and respiratory rate (RR) under 10 bpm. | Continuous pulse oximetry identifies decreasing oxygen saturation associated with hypoventilation. Values of 92% or less often signal need for supplemental oxygen. Decreased $O_2$ saturation and RR indicate opioid-induced respiratory depression and must be treated with an opioid antagonist and reported to the provider. |
| Consider referral to a pain management team. | A pain management team can help with conventional pain control measures during acute pain situations in patients with chronic or frequent bouts of pancreatitis or with low pain tolerance. Less conventional measures, such as nerve blocks that interfere with transmission of pain sensations along visceral nerve fibers, are effective in the relief of pancreatic pain. Bilateral splanchnic nerve or left celiac ganglion blocks may be performed as well. |

For additional pain interventions, see "Pain," Chapter 5.

## Patient Problem/Analyze Cues/Prioritize Hypotheses

# Risk for Infection

*due to* the tissue destruction with resulting necrosis occurring with the release of pancreatic enzymes

*Desired Outcome/Generate Solutions:* The patient remains free of infection, as evidenced by body temperature of less than 100°F (less than 37.7°C); negative culture results; heart rate (HR) of 60–100 bpm; RR of 12–20 breaths/minute; blood pressure (BP) within the patient's baseline range; and orientation to person, place, and time.

| ASSESSMENT—RECOGNIZE CUES/ INTERVENTIONS—TAKE ACTION | RATIONALES |
|---|---|
| Assess the patient's temperature every 4 hours. | An increase may signal infection. **Note:** Hypothermia may precede hyperthermia in some individuals, particularly older adults. |
| ! If there is a sudden elevation in temperature, obtain specimens for culture of blood, sputum, urine, wound, drains, and other sites as indicated. Monitor culture reports, and report findings promptly to the health care provider. | Cultures enable the detection of a developing necrotic pancreas or presence of an abscess. The body may be developing SIRS, which is a precursor to sepsis. SIRS is manifested by two or more of the following: body temperature higher than 100.4°F (38°C) or lower than 98.6°F (36°C), RR more than 20 breaths/minute or $CO_2$ less than 32 mm Hg, HR greater than 90 bpm, WBC count greater than 12,000 $mm^3$ or less than 4000 $mm^3$, or presence of more than 10% immature neutrophils ("bands"). |
| ! Assess BP, HR, and RR every 4 hours. | Increases in HR (up to 100–140 bpm) and RR are associated with infection of the necrotic pancreatic tissue and SIRS. BP may be either transiently high or low with significant orthostatic hypotension. |
| Monitor all secretions and drainage for changes in appearance or odor that may signal infection. | Sputum, for example, can become more copious and change in color from clear to white to yellow to green in the presence of infection. |
| ! Assess the mental status, orientation, and LOC every 4–8 hours. Document and report significant deviations from baseline. | Impairments may occur with alcohol withdrawal, hypotension, electrolyte imbalance, or hypoxia and from the sepsis associated with the necrotic, infected pancreas. |
| Administer the parenteral antibiotics as prescribed. | This measure helps maintain bacteriacidal serum levels. |
| Reschedule antibiotics if a dose is delayed for more than 1 hour. | Failure to administer antibiotics on schedule can result in inadequate blood levels and treatment failure. |
| Use good hand hygiene before and after caring for the patient and dispose of dressings and drainage carefully. | These measures help prevent the transmission of potentially infectious agents. |

## Patient Problems/Analyze Cues

# Fluid and Electrolyte Imbalance

*due to* the active loss occurring with NG suctioning, vomiting, diaphoresis, or pooling of fluids in the abdomen and retroperitoneum

*Desired Outcomes/Generate Solutions:* The patient is normovolemic within 8 hours of hospital admission, as evidenced by HR of 60–100 bpm, central venous pressure (CVP) of 2–6 mm Hg (5–12 cm $H_2O$), brisk capillary refill (less than 2 seconds), peripheral pulse amplitude greater than 2+ on a 0–4+ scale, urinary output at least 30 mL/hour, or 0.5 mL/kg/hour and stable weight and abdominal girth measurements. Electrolytes, sodium and calcium, are within normal limits.

| ASSESSMENT—RECOGNIZE CUES/ INTERVENTIONS—TAKE ACTION | RATIONALES |
|---|---|
| Assess the vital signs (VS) every 2–4 hours. | This assessment enables the detection of a falling BP and increasing HR (100–140 bpm), which can occur with moderate to severe fluid loss. |

Continued

| ASSESSMENT—RECOGNIZE CUES/ INTERVENTIONS—TAKE ACTION | RATIONALES |
|---|---|
| Assess the intake and output (I&O) and monitor CVP, if available, every 2–4 hours. Weigh the patient daily and note trends. | CVP less than 2 mm Hg can occur with volume-related hypotension, and output greater than intake signals fluid loss. Weight decreases when fluid is lost, or intake is insufficient. |
| Correlate weight measurements with I&O ratios. | Fluid loss requires immediate replacement to prevent shock and acute renal failure. Approximately 1 kg weight=1 L fluid. |
| Measure the orthostatic VS initially and every 8 hours. | This enables the detection of decreasing BP and increasing HR on standing, which suggests the need for crystalloid and/or colloid volume expansion. |
| Administer the parenteral solutions (lactated Ringer solution is preferred) and plasma volume expanders as prescribed. | These measures help maintain adequate circulating blood volume. Fluid resuscitation reduces morbidity among patients with acute pancreatitis. |
| Monitor closely for adventitious breath sounds, increased weight, and drop in Hct without concomitant blood loss. | These are signs of fluid overload and potentially of pulmonary edema associated with overly aggressive fluid resuscitation. In cases of severe acute pancreatitis, patients develop a profound loss of circulating blood volume and need adequate fluid resuscitation quickly, sometimes as much as 5–6 L/day. This increases the risk for fluid overload, especially if the patient has been hypotensive and the kidneys are not functioning well enough to handle the large amounts of fluid. The fluid overload can lead to pulmonary edema and respiratory failure. Respiratory dysfunction is the most frequent complication of severe, acute pancreatitis and one of the main causes of early death. |
| Monitor the values of the following for irregularities: Hct, hemoglobin (Hgb), WBC count, calcium, glucose, blood urea nitrogen (BUN), creatinine, and potassium. | Irregularities can occur in patients with infection, inflammatory response, and bleeding caused by necrotic pancreas and would be outside the following normal values: Hct 40%–54% (male) and 37%–47% (female), Hgb 14–18 g/dL (male) and 12–16 g/dL (female), calcium 8.5–10.5 mg/dL (4.3–5.3 mEq/L), glucose 140 mg/dL (2-hour postprandial if no history of diabetes) and 65–110 mg/dL (fasting), BUN 6–20 mg/dL, potassium 3.5–5 mEq/L, and WBC count 4500–11,000 mm$^3$. |
| Be alert to positive Chvostek sign (facial muscle spasm) and Trousseau sign (carpopedal spasm), muscle twitching, tetany, or irritability. | These signs are indicators of hypocalcemia, which can occur with electrolyte loss. |
| Administer the electrolytes (calcium and potassium) as prescribed. | Replacement of these electrolytes helps prevent cardiac dysrhythmias, tetany, and other problems caused by their specific decreases. |

## Patient Problem/Analyze Cues

# Impaired Gas Exchange

*due to* ventilation–perfusion mismatching occurring with atelectasis or accumulating pulmonary fluid (pleural effusion)

***Desired Outcome/Generate Solutions:*** After interventions, the patient has adequate gas exchange, as evidenced by RR of 12–20 breaths/minute with eupnea, oxygen saturation greater than 92%; no significant changes in mental status; orientation to person, place, and time; and breath sounds that are clear and audible throughout the lung fields.

## ASSESSMENT—RECOGNIZE CUES/ INTERVENTIONS—TAKE ACTION

## RATIONALES

 Assess and document the RR every 2–4 hours as indicated by the patient's condition. Note the pattern, degree of excursion, and whether the patient uses accessory muscles of respiration. Report significant deviations from baseline to the health care provider.

Irregular pattern, decreased chest excursion, and use of accessory muscles of respiration occur with impending respiratory compromise (can occur with ARDS and respiratory failure) and may be a sign of inadequate pain control or worsening pancreatitis.

Auscultate both lung fields every 4–8 hours.

Presence of abnormal (crackles, wheezes) or diminished breath sounds can occur with fluid overload.

Assess the sputum production and promptly report to the health care provider an increase or color change (from clear to white to yellow to green) in respiratory secretions.

Copious secretions that change color can indicate respiratory tract infection; copious secretions without color changes can occur with pulmonary edema.

Assess for changes in mental status, restlessness, agitation, and alterations in mentation.

These are early signs of hypoxia.

Monitor the pulse oximetry every 8 hours or as indicated (report oxygen saturation 92% or less). Monitor arterial blood gas results as available (report $Pao_2$ less than 80 mm Hg).

These decreased values usually signal the need for supplementary oxygen.

Administer the oxygen as prescribed. Monitor the oxygen delivery system at regular intervals.

Hypoxia is an early sign of impending respiratory failure and necessitates oxygen delivery.

Elevate the head of bed 30 degrees or higher, depending on the patient's comfort level.

This position optimizes ventilation and oxygenation.

If pleural effusion or another defect is present on one side, position the patient with the unaffected lung dependent.

This position maximizes ventilation–perfusion relationship, which optimizes oxygenation.

 Avoid overaggressive fluid resuscitation.

This could lead to hypoxia, heart failure, pleural effusions, and respiratory failure.

Explain to the patient and significant others that the patient is at risk for hypostatic pneumonia.

Pancreatitis results in decreased production of surfactant, and pain limits adequate respiratory excursion, increasing the potential for hypostatic pneumonia.

Provide instructions on the use of a hyperinflation device (e.g., incentive spirometer) followed by coughing exercises. Explain that emphasis of this therapy is on inhalation to expand the lungs maximally. Ensure that the patient inhales slowly and deeply 2 times normal tidal volume and holds the breath for at least 5 seconds at the end of inspiration. Monitor the patient's progress and document in nurses' notes.

Deep breathing expands alveoli and helps mobilize secretions to the airways, while coughing further mobilizes and clears secretions. Ten deep breaths each hour are recommended to maintain adequate alveolar inflation.

When appropriate, provide instructions to the patient on splinting wounds or upper abdomen.

Splinting helps reduce pain and enable effective cough.

Instruct the patient on the cascade cough (i.e., a succession of more short and forceful exhalations) to patients who cannot cough effectively.

A cascade cough helps keep lungs expanded when abdominal pain would not otherwise enable deep cough.

Encourage activity as prescribed.

Activity helps mobilize secretions and promote effective airway clearance.

## Patient Problem/Analyze Cues

# Risk for Disease (Paralytic Ileus)

*due to* bowel dysfunction occurring with electrolyte disturbance

***Desired Outcome/Generate Solutions:*** After interventions, GI motility normalizes, as evidenced by the presence of bowel sounds and flatus and absence of nausea, vomiting, and abdominal distention.

| ASSESSMENT—RECOGNIZE CUES/ INTERVENTIONS—TAKE ACTION | RATIONALES |
| --- | --- |
| Assess for the absence of flatus/bowel sounds or change in bowel sounds and the presence of abdominal cramping or pain. | These findings may be present with bowel dysfunction, which can occur with an electrolyte imbalance (particularly hypokalemia) resulting directly from severe pancreatitis. |
| Assess for bowel sounds in all four abdominal quadrants. | Bowel dysfunction may occur at any point along the GI tract. Diminished or absent bowel sounds suggest the presence of ileus and therefore must be auscultated in all four quadrants before NPO can be rescinded. Hypoactive sounds (3–5/minute) indicate decreased motility; hyperactive sounds (more than 34/minute) can be caused by anxiety, infectious diarrhea, irritation of intestinal mucosa from blood, or gastroenteritis. High-pitched tinkling sounds (hyperperistalsis) occur during intestinal obstruction, usually accompanied by cramping pain. |
| In the absence of bowel sounds, keep the patient NPO. | Fluids and food are not tolerated until the bowel returns to normal function, as evidenced by bowel sounds. |
| After recommencement of fluids and food, monitor for bowel movements and emesis. | Absence of emesis and the presence of bowel movements indicate return of normal GI function. |

## Patient Problem/Analyze Cues/Prioritize Hypotheses

# Body Weight Problem (Weight Loss)

*due to* anorexia, dietary restrictions, poor nutrition, and digestive dysfunction

**Desired Outcome/Generate Solutions:** The patient attains baseline body weight and exhibits a positive or balanced nitrogen state on nitrogen studies by the 24-hour period before hospital discharge.

| ASSESSMENT—RECOGNIZE CUES/ INTERVENTIONS—TAKE ACTION | RATIONALES |
| --- | --- |
| Assess for polyphagia, polydipsia, and polyuria. | These indicators of a hyperglycemic state reflect the need for health care provider evaluation and intervention to ensure proper metabolism of carbohydrates if the endocrine function is impaired. Hyperglycemia occurs because of interference with beta cell function. It is transient with acute pancreatitis but common with chronic pancreatitis, during which diabetes is likely to develop. |
| Monitor the blood glucose levels for the presence of hyperglycemia. Adjust insulin amounts according to capillary blood glucose levels, as prescribed. | Laboratory values of fasting blood sugar and bedside monitoring of blood glucose may reveal abnormalities in blood glucose levels and direct the appropriate insulin therapy (see "Diabetes Mellitus," Chapter 47, for more information). |
| Note the amount and degree of steatorrhea (foamy, foul-smelling stools high in fat content). | This is an indicator of fat malabsorption, which is common with chronic pancreatitis. Steatorrhea can indicate the recurrence of the disease process or ineffectiveness of drug therapy and should be reported to the health care provider. |
| Weigh the patient at the same time and same setting daily. | Progressive weight loss may signal the need to change the diet or provide enzyme replacement therapy. |

## ASSESSMENT—RECOGNIZE CUES/ INTERVENTIONS—TAKE ACTION | RATIONALES

| ASSESSMENT—RECOGNIZE CUES/ INTERVENTIONS—TAKE ACTION | RATIONALES |
|---|---|
| Deliver enteral or parenteral nutrition as prescribed. | Enteral feedings are being used with increasing frequency but should be infused past the ligament of Treitz (the ligament that transitions the duodenum to the jejunum) to avoid pancreatic stimulation. Parenteral nutrition likely is instituted if distal enteral feedings are unobtainable or unsuccessful within 5–7 days. |
| Monitor the blood glucose level every 4 hours if administering parenteral nutrition. | Blood glucose needs to be monitored with parenteral nutrition because of the high glucose level in the fluids. |
| Provide oral hygiene at frequent intervals. | This measure enhances appetite and minimizes nausea. |
| When the gastric tube is removed, provide the diet as prescribed. | Small, high-carbohydrate, low-fat meals at frequent intervals (six per day) with protein added according to tolerance is the usual diet for patients with pancreatitis. |
| Instruct the patient to avoid coffee, tea, alcohol, and nicotine or other gastric irritants. | These are stimulants that increase pancreatic enzyme secretion. |
| As prescribed, administer the pancreatic enzyme supplements. | Pancreatic enzyme supplements are given before introducing fat into the diet to enable its digestion. |
| If prescribed, administer other dietary supplements that support nutrition and caloric intake. | These supplements, which may include products that consist of medium-chain triglycerides (MCTs) such as MCT oil, do not require pancreatic enzymes for absorption. |
| Avoid administering pancreatic enzymes with hot foods or drinks. | Heat deactivates its enzyme activity. |
| Provide meals in small feedings throughout the day. | Smaller, more frequent meals may help alleviate bloating, nausea, and cramps experienced by some patients. |

## ✔ PATIENT–FAMILY TEACHING AND DISCHARGE PLANNING

When providing patient–family teaching, focus on sensory information, avoid giving excessive information, and initiate a visiting nurse referral for necessary follow-up teaching. Include verbal and written information about the following:

✔ Cause for the current episode of pancreatitis, if known, so that recurrence may be avoided.

✔ Alcohol consumption, which can cause or exacerbate acute or chronic pancreatitis.

✔ Diet: frequent, small meals that are high in carbohydrates and protein. Food should be bland until gradual return to a normal diet is prescribed. Remind the patient to avoid enzyme stimulants, such as coffee, tea, nicotine, and alcohol.

✔ Medications, including drug name, purpose, dosage, schedule, precautions, and potential side effects. Also discuss drug–drug, food–drug, and herb–drug interactions.

✔ Signs and symptoms of DM, including fatigue, weight loss, polydipsia, polyuria, and polyphagia.

✔ Necessity of medical follow-up; confirm time and date of next medical appointment.

✔ Potential for recurrence of steatorrhea as evidenced by foamy, foul-smelling stools that are high in fat content.

✔ Weighing daily at home; importance of reporting weight loss to the health care provider.

✔ If surgery was performed, instruct the patient on how to prevent infection and on the indicators of wound infection: redness, swelling, discharge, fever, pain, or increased local warmth.

✔ Availability of chemical dependency programs to prevent/treat drug dependence, which is a common occurrence with chronic pancreatitis; or to treat alcoholism. Discuss the availability of community support groups, such as the following:

- Alcoholics Anonymous: www.aa.org
- Narcotics Anonymous: www.na.org

✔ For more information, contact the National Institute of Diabetes and Digestive and Kidney Diseases at www.niddk.nih.gov

# Peptic Ulcer Disease 61

## OVERVIEW/PATHOPHYSIOLOGY

Peptic ulcers are erosions of the upper gastrointestinal (GI) tract mucosa, extending through the muscularis mucosa and potentially into the muscularis propria. They may occur anywhere the mucosa is exposed to the erosive action of gastric acid and pepsin. Commonly, ulcers are gastric or duodenal, but the lower esophagus, surgically created stomas, and other areas of the upper GI tract may be affected. Autodigestion of mucosal tissue and ulceration are associated with increased acidity of the stomach juices or increased sensitivity of the mucosal surfaces to damage. Ulcers can penetrate deeply into the mucosal layers and become a chronic problem, or they can be more superficial and manifest as an acute problem resulting from severe physiologic or psychologic trauma, infection, or shock (stress ulceration of the stomach or duodenum). The most common causes of peptic ulcer disease are the use of nonsteroidal antiinflammatory drugs (NSAIDs) and infection with *Helicobacter pylori*. Duodenal and gastric ulcers may be complications of other diseases but also can occur in association with high-stress lifestyle, smoking, and the use of irritating drugs. Ulceration may occur as a part of Zollinger–Ellison syndrome, in which gastrinomas (gastrin-secreting tumors) of the pancreas or other organs develop. Gastric acid hypersecretion and ulceration subsequently occur.

> **Note:** *Ulcers are differentiated from erosions by the depth of penetration. Erosions, such as with gastritis, are small superficial mucosal lesions that do not penetrate the muscularis mucosa.*

*H. pylori* infection is a major risk factor for peptic ulcer disease. *H. pylori* can reside below the mucosa of the stomach because it produces the enzyme *urease*, which hydrolyzes urea to ammonia and carbon dioxide, providing a buffering alkaline halo. Infection can begin in childhood and go undetected for years because there may be no symptoms until gastric or duodenal ulceration or gastritis occurs. Transmission of *H. pylori* has been determined to be by fecal–oral and oral–oral routes. A high duodenal acid load is one of the characteristics of duodenal ulcer disease inasmuch as it reduces the concentration of bile acids that normally inhibit the growth of *H. pylori*. Gastric ulcers tend to occur on the lesser curvature of the stomach. Ulcers in both locations are characterized by slow healing leading to metaplasia. In turn, a greater colonization with *H. pylori* causes slow healing and results in a vicious cycle.

Serious and disabling complications, such as hemorrhage, GI obstruction, perforation, peritonitis, or intractable ulcer pain are common. With treatment, ulcer healing usually occurs within 4–6 weeks (gastric ulcers can take as long as 12–16 weeks to heal), but there is potential for recurrence in the same or another site.

## HEALTH CARE SETTING

Primary care; acute care for complications

## ASSESSMENT

***Signs and symptoms.*** In gastric ulcers, burning, gnawing, dull epigastric pain typically 1–2 hours after eating. Discomfort occurs more often between meals and at night. In duodenal ulcers, eating usually alleviates discomfort; with gastric ulcer, pain often worsens after meals. Patients may also experience bloating, nausea, and vomiting. Older adults have less sensory perception in the stomach and may not experience pain as a symptom. In addition, some patients with active ulcers are asymptomatic. However, on evaluation, there may be findings of ulcers, gastritis, and other conditions. Even so, pain symptoms warrant further investigation.

Hematemesis, melena, dizziness, and syncope are associated with an actively bleeding ulcer. Sudden, severe epigastric pain, often radiating to the right shoulder, suggests perforation of an ulcer. Pain described as piercing through to the back suggests penetration of the ulcer into adjacent posterior structures in the abdomen.

***Physical assessment.*** Tenderness over the involved area of the abdomen. With perforation, there is severe pain (see "Peritonitis," Chapter 62, for more information) and rebound tenderness. With penetration, the pain is usually altered by changes in back position (extension or flexion).

***History and risk factors.*** NSAID use; smoking; use of irritating agents such as caffeine, alcohol, corticosteroids, salicylates, reserpine, indomethacin, or phenylbutazone; disorders of the endocrine glands, pancreas, or liver; and hypersecretory conditions, such as Zollinger–Ellison syndrome.

## DIAGNOSTIC TESTS

***Endoscopy.*** Allows visualization of the stomach (gastroscopy), duodenum (duodenoscopy), both stomach and duodenum (gastroduodenoscopy), or the esophagus, stomach, and duodenum (esophagogastroduodenoscopy) by the passage of a lighted, fiberoptic, flexible endoscope. It is the most accurate procedure to determine the presence and location of an ulcer. A biopsy may be performed as part of the endoscopy procedure. Biopsied tissue can be obtained for a rapid urease testing (CLO test) and also may be sent for histologic examination and for culture and sensitivity to identify *H. pylori* infection.

***Helicobacter pylori testing.*** Serum antigen testing identifies exposure to *H. pylori* bacteria; this is the least expensive means of identifying *H. pylori* infection. However, antibody tests remain positive many months after successful therapy and are not reliable for assessing therapy effectiveness. A breath test is available to identify *H. pylori* infection by detecting carbon dioxide and ammonia as by-products of the action of the bacterium's urease in the patient's expired air. Rapid urease testing,

histologic identification of the microorganism, and culture are other direct tests for *H. pylori*. Direct tests and stool antigen testing require discontinuation of all drugs that suppress *H. pylori* for 2 weeks before testing.

***Barium swallow.*** An imaging test that uses a contrast agent (e.g., barium) to detect abnormalities.

Postprocedure care involves the administration of prescribed laxatives and enemas to facilitate passage of the barium and prevent constipation and fecal impaction.

***Complete blood count.*** Reveals a decrease in hemoglobin (Hgb), hematocrit (Hct), and red blood cells when acute or chronic blood loss accompanies ulceration.

***Stool for occult blood.*** Positive if bleeding is present.

## Patient Problem/Analyze Cues/Prioritize Hypotheses

# Risk for Disease (Gastrointestinal Hemorrhage, Perforation, Obstruction)

*due to* the ulcerative process

***Desired Outcome/Generate Solutions:*** The patient is free of signs and symptoms of bleeding, obstruction, perforation, and peritonitis as evidenced by negative results for occult blood testing, passage of stool and flatus, soft and nondistended abdomen, good appetite, and normothermia.

| ASSESSMENT—RECOGNIZE CUES/INTERVENTIONS—TAKE ACTION | RATIONALES |
|---|---|
| Assess for hematemesis and melena. Check all nasogastric (NG) aspirate, emesis, and stools for occult blood. Report positive findings. | Bleeding can occur with an ulcerative process. |
| Monitor the results of complete blood count and coagulation studies. | Hct less than 40% (male) or less than 37% (female) and Hgb less than 14 g/dL (male) or less than 12 g/dL (female) are indicators of bleeding and should be reported promptly. |
| | Partial thromboplastin time greater than 70 seconds, prothrombin time greater than 12.5 seconds, or International normalized ratio more than 1.1 are longer than normal clotting times. |
| If prescribed, insert an NG tube. | An NG tube will enable the evacuation of blood from the stomach, monitoring of bleeding, and gastric lavage as prescribed. |
| NG tubes are contraindicated in patients who have or are suspected of having esophageal varices. | Trauma from tube insertion could result in hemorrhage. |
| Monitor the O₂ saturation by oximetry and report O₂ saturation 92% or less. | Usually, patients with O₂ saturation 92% or less require oxygen supplementation. |
| If the patient is actively bleeding or if Hct and Hgb are low, administer the prescribed O₂. | A low Hct and Hgb indicate an anemic state, which means there is less available Hgb for oxygen transport. |
| Assess for and note abdominal pain, abnormal (increased peristalsis, "rushes," or "tinkles") or absent bowel sounds, distention, anorexia, nausea, vomiting, and inability to pass stool or flatus. | These are indicators of obstruction, a serious complication of peptic ulcers, which necessitates prompt notification of the health care provider for rapid intervention. |
| Be alert to sudden or severe abdominal pain, distention, and rigidity; fever; nausea; and vomiting. Notify the health care provider immediately of significant findings. | These are indicators of perforation and peritonitis, serious complications of peptic ulcers that necessitate prompt notification of health care provider for rapid intervention. |
| | See "Peritonitis," Chapter 62, for more information. |
| Describe to the patient signs and symptoms of GI complications and the importance of reporting them promptly to the staff or the health care provider if they occur. | A knowledgeable patient likely will report these signs promptly, which will enable rapid treatment. |

Patient Problem/Analyze Cues/Prioritize Hypotheses

# Impaired Tissue Integrity (Gastric Mucosal Tissue)

*due to* GI exposure to chemical irritants (gastric acid, pepsin)

**Desired Outcome/Generate Solutions:** Gastric and duodenal mucosal tissues heal and remain intact as evidenced by reduced or absent abdominal pain.

## ASSESSMENT—RECOGNIZE CUES/ INTERVENTIONS—TAKE ACTION

## RATIONALES

| ASSESSMENT—RECOGNIZE CUES/ INTERVENTIONS—TAKE ACTION | RATIONALES |
|---|---|
| Administer the antibiotics as prescribed, usually as part of combination therapy (e.g., amoxicillin, clarithromycin, metronidazole, tetracycline, levofloxacin). | Antibiotics function to kill the *H. pylori* bacterium. A combination of two antibiotics may be more effective and less likely to fail because of antibiotic resistance. A history of past antibiotic use by the patient is important to assess potential resistance. Also, known resistance rates in the area where the patient lives may assist in determining which antibiotics are used for treatment. |
| | Antibiotics are administered in combination with a proton pump inhibitor (PPI), and possibly bismuth subsalicylate, as eradication therapy for *H. pylori*. (See the next two interventions.) |
| Administer the *H. pylori* eradication therapy for *H. pylori*–associated ulceration. | The highest eradication rates are obtained with a triple-drug regimen of PPI, clarithromycin, and amoxicillin. Metronidazole is substituted for amoxicillin in those patients who are allergic to penicillin. Treatment is given for 7–14 days. Some patients may receive a four-drug regimen, with the addition of bismuth subsalicylate. |
| Administer the acid suppression therapy as prescribed: | This therapy is given for acute episodes of ulceration. |
| • PPIs (e.g., omeprazole, esomeprazole, lansoprazole, pantoprazole, rabeprazole, dexlansoprazole) | PPIs deactivate the enzyme system that pumps hydrogen ions ($H^+$) from the parietal cells, thus inhibiting gastric acid secretion. They are used for short-term treatment of active duodenal and gastric ulcers and for long-term treatment of gastroesophageal reflux disease and hypersecretory conditions. Omeprazole and lansoprazole are now available over the counter (OTC). |
| • Histamine-2 ($H_2$)-receptor blockers (e.g., cimetidine, nizatidine, famotidine) | These agents are administered by mouth (PO) or intravenous route to suppress the secretion of gastric acid and facilitate ulcer healing. They also can be used prophylactically for limited periods of time, especially in patients susceptible to stress ulceration. They are administered with meals at least 1 hour apart from antacids because antacids can reduce their absorption. They are available both through prescription and OTC, and although time to relief obtained is longer than with antacids, their effects last longer. |
| • Sucralfate | This is an antiulcer agent that coats the ulcer with a protective barrier so that healing can occur. It must be taken before meals and at bedtime. It should not be taken within 30 minutes of antacids because acid facilitates adherence of sucralfate to the ulcer. |
| • Antacids | Antacids are administered orally or through an NG tube to provide quick, symptomatic relief, facilitate ulcer healing, and prevent further ulceration. They can be administered prophylactically in patients who are especially susceptible to ulceration. Antacids are administered after meals and at bedtime or given periodically by NG tube for patients who are intubated. |

| ASSESSMENT—RECOGNIZE CUES/ INTERVENTIONS—TAKE ACTION | RATIONALES |
|---|---|
| • Misoprostol<br>Avoid or use the misoprostol cautiously in women of childbearing age. | This is a synthetic prostaglandin $E_1$ analog that enhances the body's normal mucosal protective mechanisms and decreases acid secretion. The drug may be used in the healing and prevention of NSAID-induced ulcers for people requiring high doses of NSAIDs for the treatment of arthritis and other chronic pain conditions.<br><br>Because it can cause spontaneous abortions, this medication is used with caution in women of childbearing years who could be pregnant. |
| Stress the importance of taking medications at prescribed intervals, not just for symptomatic relief of pain. | Initial pain relief does not mean the ulcer is completely healed. |
| Refer the patient to community resources and support groups for assistance in smoking cessation or abstinence from drinking. | Smoking increases acid secretions and decreases mucosal blood flow, thereby inhibiting ulcer healing. Alcohol also slows the healing process. |

## ADDITIONAL PROBLEM:

*Acute Pain*                                      Chapter 57

## ✓ PATIENT–FAMILY TEACHING AND DISCHARGE PLANNING

When providing patient–family teaching, focus on sensory information, avoid giving excessive information, and initiate a visiting nurse referral for necessary follow-up teaching of skilled needs. Include verbal and written information about the following:

✓ Importance of following a prescribed diet to facilitate ulcer healing, prevent exacerbation or recurrence, or control postsurgical dumping syndrome. If appropriate, arrange a consultation with a dietitian.

✓ Medications, including drug name, rationale, dosage, schedule, precautions, and potential side effects. Also discuss drug–drug, food–drug, and herb–drug interactions.

✓ Signs and symptoms of exacerbation and recurrence, as well as potential complications.

✓ Care of incision line and dressing change technique, as necessary.

✓ Signs of wound infection, including persistent redness, swelling, purulent drainage, local warmth, fever, and foul odor.

✓ Role of lifestyle alterations in preventing exacerbation or recurrence of ulcer, including smoking cessation (smoking impairs ulcer healing and has been associated with a higher incidence of complications and the need for surgical repair of the ulcer), stress reduction, decreasing or eliminating consumption of alcohol, and avoidance of irritating foods and drugs (alcohol, caffeine, coffee, NSAIDs, and aspirin are associated with increased acidity and GI erosions and ulcerations). Note that $H_2$-receptor blockers are more effective in individuals who are nonsmokers.

✓ Referral to a health care specialist for assistance with stress reduction as necessary.

✓ Referrals to community support groups, such as Alcoholics Anonymous at www.aa.org

✓ Referrals to other reliable websites:
  • American Gastroenterologic Association: www.gastro.org (use Patient Center link)
  • Cleveland Clinic Peptic Ulcer Disease: https://my.clevelandclinic.org/health/diseases/10350-peptic-ulcer-disease

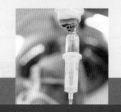

# Peritonitis 62

## OVERVIEW/PATHOPHYSIOLOGY

Peritonitis is the inflammatory response of the peritoneum to offending chemical and/or bacterial agents invading the peritoneal cavity. The inflammatory process can be local or generalized and may be classified as primary, secondary, or tertiary, depending on the pathogenesis of the inflammation. Primary peritonitis, such as spontaneous bacterial peritonitis, occurs when blood-borne organisms enter the peritoneal cavity without intraabdominal pathology. Secondary peritonitis is caused by the rupture or perforation of abdominal organs. Common events include abdominal trauma, postoperative leakage of gastrointestinal (GI) content or blood into the peritoneal cavity, intestinal ischemia, ruptured or inflamed abdominal organs, poor sterile techniques (e.g., with peritoneal dialysis), and direct contamination of the bloodstream. Tertiary peritonitis is a persistent abdominal sepsis without a focus on infection, and it may follow treatment of a previous episode of peritonitis. The peritoneum responds to invasive agents by attempting to localize the infection with a shift of the omentum (the "guardian of the abdominal cavity") to wall off the inflamed area. Inflammation of the peritoneum results in tissue edema, the development of fibrinous exudate, and hypermotility of the intestinal tract. As the disease progresses, paralytic ileus occurs, and intestinal fluid, which then cannot be reabsorbed, leaks into the peritoneal cavity. As a result of the fluid shift, cardiac output and tissue perfusion are reduced, leading to impaired cardiac and renal function. If infection or inflammation continues, respiratory failure and shock can ensue. Peritonitis often is progressive and can be fatal. It is the most common cause of death after abdominal surgery, and mortality is dictated by the patient's overall health, including nutritional and immune status and organ function.

## HEALTH CARE SETTING

Acute care surgical unit, critical care unit

## ASSESSMENT

### Signs and symptoms.

*Early findings.* Acute abdominal pain with movement, tenderness over involved area, anorexia, nausea, vomiting, chills, fever, rigor, malaise, weakness, hiccoughs, diaphoresis, absence of bowel sounds, and abdominal distention and rigidity (often described as board-like).

*Later findings.* Dehydration (e.g., thirst, dry mucous membranes, oliguria, concentrated urine, poor skin turgor).

**Physical assessment.** Presence of tachycardia, hypotension, and shallow and rapid respirations caused by abdominal distention and discomfort. Often the patient assumes a supine position with knees flexed or side-lying with knees drawn up toward the chest. Palpation usually reveals peritoneal irritation as shown by distention, abdominal rigidity with general or localized tenderness, guarding, and rebound or cough tenderness. However, as many as one-fourth of these patients will have minimal or no indications of peritoneal irritation. Auscultation findings include hyperactive bowel sounds during the gradual development of peritonitis and the absence of bowel sounds or infrequent high-pitched sounds ("tinkling" or "squeaky") during later stages if paralytic ileus occurs. Ascites may be present as demonstrated by shifting areas of dullness on percussion.

**History.** Abdominal surgery, cirrhosis, peptic ulcer disease, cholecystitis, acute necrotizing pancreatitis, other GI disorders, acute salpingitis, ruptured appendix or diverticulum, trauma, peritoneal dialysis.

## DIAGNOSTIC TESTS

**Serum tests.** May reveal the presence of leukocytosis, usually with a shift to the left (may be the only sign of tertiary peritonitis); hemoconcentration; elevated blood urea nitrogen; and electrolyte imbalance, particularly hypokalemia. Hypoalbuminemia and prolonged prothrombin time, in combination with leukocytosis, are especially characteristic.

**Urinalysis.** Often performed to rule out genitourinary involvement (e.g., pyelonephritis).

**Paracentesis for peritoneal aspiration with culture and sensitivity and cell count.** May be performed to determine the presence of blood, bacteria, bile, pus, and amylase content and identify the causative organism. Gram stain of ascitic fluid is positive in only about 25% of these patients. Diagnosis of bacterial peritonitis is confirmed by positive culture of ascitic fluid and cell count and differential of the ascitic fluid notable for elevated polymorphonuclear count of 250 cells/mm$^3$ or greater. Ascitic fluid also may be tested for total protein, glucose concentration, and lactate dehydrogenase to differentiate spontaneous bacterial peritonitis from secondary bacterial peritonitis.

**Abdominal radiographic examination.** To determine the presence of distended loops of bowel and abnormal levels of

PART I: Medical-Surgical Nursing Care Plans

fluid and gas, which usually collect in the large and small bowel in the presence of a perforation or obstruction. "Free air" under the diaphragm also may be visualized, which indicates a perforated viscus.

**Computed tomography, ultrasound, and magnetic resonance imaging.** May be used to evaluate abdominal pain and more clearly delineate nondistinct areas found by plain abdominal radiographic examination. May be done to identify ascites and abscesses.

**Chest radiographic examination.** Abdominal distention may elevate the diaphragm. Pain from peritonitis may limit respiratory

excursion and lead to associated infiltrates in the lower lobes. In later stages, changes in serum osmolality allow for pleural effusions to occur.

**Contrast radiographic examination.** May be used to identify specific intestinal pathologic conditions. Water-soluble contrast (e.g., meglumine diatrizoate) may be used to evaluate suspected upper GI perforation.

**Radionuclide scans.** Gallium, Hepatobiliary Iminodiacetic Acid (lidofenin), and liver-spleen scans may be used to identify intraabdominal abscess.

## Patient Problem/Analyze Cues/Prioritize Hypotheses

# Risk for Disease (Septic Shock)

*due to* worsening/recurring peritonitis

**Desired Outcome/Generate Solutions:** The patient is free of symptoms of worsening/recurring peritonitis or septic shock, as evidenced by normothermia, blood pressure (BP) 90/60–120/70 mm Hg (or within the patient's baseline range), heart rate (HR) of 60–100 bpm, absence of chills, presence of eupnea, urinary output at least 30 mL/hour, central venous pressure (CVP) of 2–6 mm Hg (5–12 cm $H_2O$), decreasing abdominal girth measurements, and minimal tenderness to palpation.

| ASSESSMENT—RECOGNIZE CUES/ INTERVENTIONS—TAKE ACTION | RATIONALES |
| --- | --- |
| Assess the abdomen every 1–2 hours during the acute phase and every 4 hours after the patient is stabilized. | To determine the presence, pitch, and frequency of bowel sounds. Bowel sounds initially may be frequent but later are absent as peritonitis advances. The patient may have decreased/absent bowel sounds with an ileus; intermittent loud, rushing bowel sounds with an obstruction; abdominal rigidity, distention, rebound tenderness; hyperresonance/tympany with an ileus or free air in the abdomen; and loss of dullness over the liver (free air in the abdomen). |
| *Lightly* palpate the abdomen for evidence of increasing rigidity or tenderness. | This would signal disease progression. If the patient experiences increased pain on removal of your hand, rebound tenderness is present. |
| Measure the abdominal girth. Notify the health care provider of significant findings. | Girth measurements monitor for increasing distention, which would signal the development of ascites. |
| Assess the vital signs (VS) and skin at least every 2 hours and more frequently if the patient's condition is unstable. Be alert to signs of septic shock: increased temperature, hypotension, tachycardia, shallow and rapid respirations, urine output less than 30 mL/hour, and CVP less than 2 mm Hg (less than 5 cm $H_2O$). | In the early stage of shock (preshock or warm shock), skin usually is warm, pink, and dry secondary to peripheral venous pooling, and BP and CVP begin to drop. In the late stage of shock, extremities become pale and cool because of decreasing tissue perfusion. |
| If prescribed, insert a nasogastric tube and connect it to low suction. | Suction prevents or decreases distention. |
| Administer the antibiotics as prescribed; ensure close adherence to schedules for maintenance of bactericidal serum levels. Antibiotics are commonly administered intravenously and may also be directly instilled into the peritoneal cavity by surgically placed catheters. | Combination broad-spectrum antibiotic therapy is rapidly begun to ensure the treatment of Gram-negative bacilli and anaerobic bacteria. Common agents include cephalosporins (cefotaxime, cefepime), aminoglycosides (gentamicin), ampicillin, ofloxacin, and metronidazole |
| If administering aminoglycosides, collect blood samples for renal function and therapeutic blood monitoring. Collaborate with the pharmacist who will be determining the drug dose after assessing the patient's renal function and drug's therapeutic blood level. | Aminoglycoside therapeutic levels are monitored because nephrotoxicity and ototoxicity are associated with these drugs. To be effective, these drugs must be eight times higher than the lowest concentration of the drug needed to kill a standard amount of the targeted bacteria. |

Continued

| ASSESSMENT—RECOGNIZE CUES/ INTERVENTIONS—TAKE ACTION | RATIONALES |
|---|---|
| Monitor the complete blood count (CBC), especially white blood cells (WBCs), hematocrit, and hemoglobin. | With peritonitis, WBC count is elevated due to infection and hematocrit and hemoglobin are elevated due to hemoconcentration with decreased plasma volume. |
| Maintain the sterile technique with dressing changes and all invasive procedures. | This prevents/reduces the spread of infection. |
| Instruct the patient on signs and symptoms of recurring peritonitis and the importance of reporting them promptly if they occur: fever, chills, abdominal pain, vomiting, and abdominal distention. | An informed individual likely will report these signs promptly for rapid treatment. |

## Patient Problem/Analyze Cues

# Acute Pain

*due to* the inflammatory process, fever, and tissue damage

**Desired Outcomes/Generate Solutions:** The patient's subjective perception of pain decreases within 1 hour of intervention, as documented by a pain scale. Nonverbal indicators, such as grimacing and abdominal guarding, are absent or diminished.

| ASSESSMENT—RECOGNIZE CUES/ INTERVENTIONS—TAKE ACTION | RATIONALES |
|---|---|
| Assess and document the character and severity of discomfort every 1–2 hours. Devise a pain scale with the patient, rating discomfort on a scale of 0 (no pain) to 10 (worst pain). | This assessment will not only define the type of pain but also will monitor the relief of discomfort obtained to determine the effectiveness of the treatment. |
| After diagnosis has been made, administer the opioids, other analgesics, and sedatives as prescribed. | These medications relieve severe pain and discomfort after the diagnosis has been confirmed. Because potent analgesics can mask diagnostic symptoms, opioids should not be administered until surgical evaluation has been completed. |
| Encourage the patient to request analgesic *before* pain becomes severe. Document the relief obtained, using the pain scale. | Pain management is more effective when analgesia is given before pain becomes too severe. Prolonged stimulation of pain receptors results in increased sensitivity to painful stimuli and will increase the amount of analgesia required to relieve pain. |
| Keep the patient on bedrest. Provide a restful and quiet environment. | Rest minimizes pain, which can be aggravated by activity and stress. |
| Instruct the patient in methods to splint the abdomen. | Splinting reduces pain on movement, coughing, and deep breathing. |
| Keep the patient in a position of comfort, usually semi-Fowler position with the knees bent. | This position promotes a fluid shift to the lower abdomen, which will reduce pressure on the diaphragm and enable deeper and easier respirations. Raising the knees will decrease stress on the abdominal wall. |
| See "Pain," Chapter 5, for other pain interventions. | |

## Patient Problem/Analyze Cues/Prioritize Hypotheses

# Nausea

*due to* the inflammatory process, fever, and tissue damage

**Desired Outcome/Generate Solutions:** Within 1–2 hours of interventions, the patient verbalizes decreased nausea, and there is a reduction in the number of episodes of vomiting.

| ASSESSMENT—RECOGNIZE CUES/ INTERVENTIONS—TAKE ACTION | RATIONALES |
|---|---|
| Assess the patient for nausea and vomiting. Administer antiemetics (e.g., hydroxyzine, ondansetron, prochlorperazine, promethazine) as prescribed; instruct the patient to request medication *before* nausea becomes severe. | These medications, when given early, combat nausea and vomiting before they become more difficult to control. |
| Provide instructions to the patient on the technique of slow, diaphragmatic breathing. | This technique reduces stress and promotes comfort and relaxation by increasing the oxygenation of tissues and relaxing tense muscles. |
| Offer mouth care and lip moisturizers frequently. | Oral care helps relieve discomfort from continuous or intermittent suction, poor mouth hygiene, dehydration, and nothing by mouth (NPO) status. |

## Patient Problem/Analyze Cues/Prioritize Hypotheses

# Impaired Gas Exchange

*due to* alveolar hypoventilation and decreased depth of respirations that may occur with guarding, opioid administration, fatigue, and/or other causes of decreased respiratory effort in the patient critically ill with peritonitis

***Desired Outcomes/Generate Solutions:*** The patient has an effective breathing pattern and optimal gas exchange, as evidenced by $PaO_2$ at least 80 mm Hg; oxygen saturation greater than 92%; BP 90/60–120/70 mm Hg (or within the patient's baseline range); HR of 100 bpm or less; and orientation to person, place, and time. Eupnea occurs within 1 hour after pain-relieving intervention.

| ASSESSMENT—RECOGNIZE CUES/ INTERVENTIONS—TAKE ACTION | RATIONALES |
|---|---|
| ⚠ Monitor the VS, ABG, and oximetry results for evidence of hypoxemia. | The following are indicators of hypoxemia and usually signal the need for supplemental oxygen: $PaO_2$ less than 80 mm Hg, low oxygen saturation (92% or less), and the following clinical signs: hypotension, tachycardia, tachypnea, restlessness, confusion or altered mental status, central nervous system depression, and possibly cyanosis. |
| ⚠ Auscultate the lung fields. Note and document the presence of adventitious breath sounds. | This assessment monitors ventilation and detects pulmonary complications, such as pleural effusion. Pleural effusion, an accumulation of fluid in the pleural space, can develop in later stages of peritonitis because of changes in serum osmolality. Decreased breath sounds and pleural friction rub are diagnostic of pleural effusion. |
| Keep the patient in semi-Fowler or high-Fowler position; encourage deep breathing and coughing, and use of the incentive spirometer. Assist with and monitor the effects of incentive spirometry. | These positions and exercises aid respiratory effort and promote deep breathing to enhance oxygenation and coughing to clear pulmonary secretions. |
| Instruct the patient in splinting the abdomen. | Splinting enables better chest excursion to facilitate respiratory hygiene. |
| Administer the oxygen as prescribed. | Oxygen supports increased metabolic needs and treats hypoxia. |

## Patient Problem/Analyze Cues/Prioritize Hypotheses

# Body Weight Problem (Weight Loss)

*due to* NPO status, vomiting, and intestinal suctioning

***Desired Outcome/Generate Solutions:*** By at least 24 hours before hospital discharge, the patient demonstrates optimal progress toward adequate nutritional status as evidenced by stable weight/weight gain and balanced or positive nitrogen (N) state.

| ASSESSMENT—RECOGNIZE CUES/INTERVENTIONS—TAKE ACTION | RATIONALES |
|---|---|
| Keep the patient NPO as prescribed during the acute phase. | Oral fluids are not resumed until the patient has passed flatus and the gastric/intestinal tube has been removed. If the patient has an ileus, a nasogastric tube will be inserted to decompress the abdomen. |
| Reintroduce the oral fluids as ordered gradually after motility has returned, as evidenced by bowel sounds, decreased distention, and passage of flatus. | This ensures that the patient will tolerate fluids through the intestines, which may have become irritated from the inflammatory process. |
| Support the patient with peripheral parenteral nutrition or total parenteral nutrition (TPN), as prescribed, depending on the duration of the acute phase (usually by day 5). | If the GI tract is nonfunctioning, TPN usually is initiated in the early stages to promote nutrition and protein replacement. |
| Assess the serum electrolytes and intake and output daily. | Daily measurements of serum electrolytes and calculations of fluid volume are performed to determine the necessary types of fluid and electrolyte replacement to correct hypovolemia, hypoproteinemia, and anemia. |
| Administer the replacement electrolytes and fluids such as crystalloids, colloids (albumin, Plasmanate), blood, and blood products as prescribed. | Fluid and electrolyte replacement maintains hydration and restores electrolytes and nutrients lost in gastric/intestinal tube output and fluid shifts. |
| Describe to the patient the rationale for tube placement and NPO status; underlying pathologic condition (as appropriate); need for close monitoring of fluid intake and output; and, eventually, diet advancement. | A knowledgeable patient likely will adhere to the treatment regimen and report symptoms that would necessitate timely intervention. |

## ADDITIONAL PROBLEMS:

| | |
|---|---|
| *Risk for Infection* | Chapter 4 |
| *Activity Intolerance* | Chapter 1 |
| *Risk for Impaired Musculoskeletal System Function* | Chapter 1 |
| *Risk for Fluid Imbalance (Fluid Overload or Dehydration)* | Chapter 76 |

 **PATIENT–FAMILY TEACHING AND DISCHARGE PLANNING**

When providing patient–family teaching, focus on sensory information, avoid giving excessive information, and initiate a visiting nurse referral for necessary monitoring of wound care and follow-up teaching. Include verbal and written information about the following:

✓ Medications, including drug name, dosage, schedule, purpose, precautions, and potential side effects. Also discuss drug–drug, food–drug, and herb–drug interactions.
✓ Activity alterations as prescribed by the health care provider, such as avoiding heavy lifting (more than 10 lb), resting after periods of fatigue, getting maximum amounts of rest, and gradually increasing activities to tolerance.
✓ Notifying the health care provider of the following indicators of recurrence: fever, chills, abdominal pain, vomiting, abdominal distention.
✓ If the patient has undergone surgery, note indicators of wound infection: fever, pain, chills, incisional swelling, persistent erythema, purulent drainage.
✓ Importance of follow-up medical care; confirm date and time of next medical appointment.

# Ulcerative Colitis 63

## OVERVIEW/PATHOPHYSIOLOGY

Ulcerative colitis (UC) is a nonspecific, chronic inflammatory bowel disease (IBD) that causes inflammation and ulcers in the digestive tract. UC is a disease of the mucosa and submucosa of the colon and rectum. Generally, the disease begins in the rectum and sigmoid colon, but it can extend proximally and uninterrupted as far as the cecum. In 30%–50% of cases, the rectum (proctitis) or rectosigmoid (proctosigmoiditis) is affected; in 30%–40% of cases, the disease extends to the splenic flexure (left-sided or distal colitis); and in 20%–30% of cases, the disease extends proximally to involve the entire colon (pancolitis). In some instances, a few centimeters of distal ileum are affected. This is sometimes referred to as *backwash ileitis*, and it occurs in only about 10% of patients with UC involving the entire colon. In most patients, the extent of colonic involvement is maintained from onset through the disease course, with the patient experiencing flare-ups and remissions. UC initially affects the mucosal layer. Eventually, small mucosal layer abscesses form that ultimately penetrate the submucosa, spread horizontally, and allow sloughing of the mucosa, creating ulcerative lesions. The muscular layer (muscularis) generally is not affected, but the serosal layer may have congested and dilated blood vessels.

The cause of UC is unknown, but theories posit an interaction of external agents, host responses, and genetic immunologic factors creating the pathogenic responses. In a genetically susceptible subject, an outside agent or substance, such as a bacterium, virus, or other antigens, interacts with the body's immune system to trigger the disease or may cause damage to the intestinal wall, initiating or accelerating the disease process. The resulting inflammatory response continues unregulated by the immune system. As a result, inflammation continues to damage the intestinal wall, causing symptoms of UC. Medical therapy is based on symptomatic relief. The goals are to terminate the acute attack, induce and maintain remission, maintain quality of life, and prevent complications. Surgical intervention is indicated only when the disease is unresponsive to medical management or when the patient develops a disabling complication. Total proctocolectomy cures UC and results in the construction of a permanent fecal diversion.

The most firmly established risk factor for developing IBD is a positive family history. There is a 10-fold increase in risk for IBD in first-degree relatives of patients with UC. Individuals with UC develop colonic adenocarcinomas at 10 times the rate of the general population. UC can occur at any age but is generally diagnosed in the third decade of life with a second peak in the fifth and sixth decades. There is no difference in gender distribution; however, men are more likely than women to be diagnosed in the fifth and sixth decades of life. Incidence is higher in the Caucasian population and in Ashkenazi Jews than in non-Caucasian populations and in people of non-Jewish descent. UC is more prevalent in urban, developed countries with temperate climates than in rural, more southern countries. It is more common in nonsmokers and former smokers, suggesting that smoking has a protective effect and may decrease the severity of symptoms. Appendectomy before age 20 may reduce risk.

## HEALTH CARE SETTING

Primary care; acute care for complications

## ASSESSMENT

### Signs and symptoms.

Bloody diarrhea is the most common sign of ulcerative colitis. The clinical picture can vary from acute episodes with a frequent discharge of watery stools mixed with blood, pus, and mucus, accompanied by fever, abdominal pain, fatigue, and tenesmus (urge to defecate when bowel is empty), to loose or frequent stools, to formed stools coated with a little blood. However, nearly two-thirds of patients have crampy abdominal pain and varying degrees of fever, vomiting, anorexia, weight loss, and dehydration. Remissions and exacerbations are common. Extracolonic manifestations also can occur, including polyarthritis, skin lesions (erythema nodosum, pyoderma gangrenosum), liver impairment, and ophthalmic complications (iritis, uveitis). Extracolonic manifestations may precede overt bowel disease, and their clinical activity may be related or unrelated to the clinical activity of the bowel disease.

### Physical assessment.
With mild disease, there is no significant abdominal tenderness; left lower quadrant (LLQ) cramps are commonly relieved by defecation. With moderate disease, abdominal pain and tenderness may be present; mild fever (temperature 99°F–100°F [37.2°C–37.7°C]), anemia (hematocrit [Hct] 30%–40%), and hypoalbuminemia (3–3.5 g/dL) may be present. With severe disease, abdominal pain and tenderness are present, especially in the LLQ; distention and a tender, spastic anus also may be present; fever (temperature greater than 100.4°F [38°C]), severe anemia (Hct less than 30%), and impaired nutrition with hypoalbuminemia (less than 3 g/dL)

and weight loss are present. With rectal examination, the mucosa may feel gritty and the examining gloved finger may be covered with blood, mucus, or pus.

*Risk factors.* Duration of active disease more than 10 years, pancolitis, and family history of colon cancer.

## DIAGNOSTIC TESTS

*Stool examination.* Reveals the presence of frank or occult blood. Stool cultures and smears rule out bacterial and parasitic disorders. Stool is examined also for white blood cells (WBCs) and certain proteins such as calprotectin, the presence of which suggests inflammation.

*Sigmoidoscopy.* Reveals red, granular, hyperemic, and extremely friable mucosa; strips of inflamed mucosa undermined by surrounding ulcerations, which form pseudopolyps; and thick exudate composed of blood, pus, and mucus.

> **Note:** *Enemas should not be given before the examination because they can produce hyperemia and edema and may cause exacerbation of the disease. A limited prep may be given to facilitate visualization during examination.*

*Colonoscopy.* Will help determine the extent of the disease and differentiate UC from Crohn's disease through both endoscopic appearance and histologic examination of biopsy tissues. Serial colonoscopy is also performed to monitor patients with chronic UC at risk for colon carcinoma. The evolving techniques of high-resolution and high-magnification endoscopy have the potential for detecting subtle mucosal changes. *Chromoendoscopy* is a staining technique used during surveillance colonoscopy in which a blue dye is used to improve the detection of flat neoplastic lesions or polyps.

> **Note:** *Colonoscopy may be contraindicated in patients with acute disease because of the risk for perforation or hemorrhage.*

*Barium enema.* Reveals mucosal irregularity from fine serrations to ragged ulcerations, narrowing and shortening of the colon, presence of pseudopolyps, loss of haustral markings, and presence of spasms and irritability. Double-contrast technique may facilitate the detection of superficial mucosal lesions. With a double-contrast technique, barium is instilled into the colon as with a conventional barium enema, but most of the barium is then withdrawn and the colon is inflated with air, which causes a thin coating of barium to line the intestinal wall. The double-contrast technique has become the gold standard for evaluating patients for colitis.

> **Note:** *Collect specimens before barium enema is performed.*

> **Note:** *Because they produce hyperemia and edema and may cause exacerbation of the disease, irritant cathartics and enemas should not be given before the examination.*

*Abdominal plain films (flat plate).* An important tool for screening severely ill patients when colonoscopy and barium enema are contraindicated. An abdominal flat plate may reveal fecal residue, appearance of mucosal margins, widening or thickening of visible haustra, and colonic wall diameter. In patients with suspected ileus, obstruction, or perforation, the flat plate film reveals abnormal gas and fluid levels or the presence of free air in the peritoneal cavity.

*Computed tomography.* Used to identify suspected complications of UC (e.g., toxic megacolon, pneumatosis coli).

*Radionuclide imaging.* To identify the extent of disease activity, especially when colonoscopy and barium enema are contraindicated. Injections of indium-111–labeled autologous leukocytes are used to identify areas of active inflammation.

**Blood tests**
Complete blood count (CBC)
- Typically shows iron-deficiency anemia from blood loss.
- Elevated WBC—this may indicate toxic megacolon or perforation.
- Low levels of sodium, potassium, chloride, bicarbonate, and magnesium may occur due to fluid and electrolyte loss.
- Decreased albumin may be present due to poor nutrition.
- Increase erythrocyte sedimentation rate and C-reactive protein may indicate inflammation.

## Patient Problem/Analyze Cues/Prioritize Hypotheses

# Dehydration

*due to* the active loss occurring with gastrointestinal (GI) bleeding/hemorrhage and diarrhea

*Desired Outcomes/Generate Solutions:* The patient is normovolemic within 24 hours of admission, as evidenced by balanced intake and output, elastic turgor, moist mucous membranes, stable weight, blood pressure (BP) of 90/60–120/70 mm Hg (or within the patient's baseline range), and respiratory rate (RR) of 12–20 breaths/minute. Serum electrolytes, Hct, hemoglobin (Hgb), and red blood cells (RBCs) are all within optimal values as outlined in the following third rationale.

| ASSESSMENT—RECOGNIZE CUES/ INTERVENTIONS—TAKE ACTION | RATIONALES |
|---|---|
| Assess for hypotension, increased heart rate (HR) and RR, pallor, diaphoresis, and restlessness. Assess stool for quality (e.g., is it grossly bloody and liquid?) and quantity (e.g., is it mostly blood or mostly stool?). Report significant findings to the health care provider. | These are signs of bleeding/hemorrhage. |
| Assess for thirst, poor skin turgor (may not be a reliable indicator of hydration in the older adult), dryness of mucous membranes, fever, and concentrated (specific gravity greater than 1.030) and decreased urinary output. | These are indicators of dehydration. |
| Assess the intake and output and urine specific gravity; weigh the patient daily; and assess the laboratory values to evaluate fluid, electrolyte, and hematologic status. | These assessments evaluate fluid, electrolyte, and hematologic status. Optimal values are serum $K^+$ 3.5–5.0 mEq/L, Hct 40%–54% (male) and 37%–47% (female), Hgb 14–18 g/dL (male) and 12–16 g/dL (female), and RBCs 4.5–6 million/$mm^3$ (male) and 4–5.5 million/$mm^3$ (female). Hypokalemia is common because of the prolonged diarrhea. Prolonged anemia may result in decreased Hct, Hgb, and RBCs. |
| Assess the frequency and consistency of stool. For frequent bowel movements, keep a stool count and measure liquid stools. Assess and record the presence of blood, mucus, fat, and undigested food. | Although bloody diarrhea is most commonly seen, the patient may experience acute episodes with a frequent discharge of watery stools mixed with blood, pus, and mucus, accompanied by fever, abdominal pain, rectal urgency, and tenesmus; loose or frequent stools; or formed stools coated with a little blood. |
| Provide a parenteral replacement of fluids, electrolytes, and vitamins as prescribed. | These measures maintain the acutely ill patient and are guided by laboratory test results. |
| Administer the blood products and iron as prescribed. | This will help correct existing anemia and losses caused by hemorrhage. |
| Provide a bland, high-protein, high-calorie, low-residue diet as prescribed, when the patient is taking food by mouth (PO). | Nutritional management varies with the patient's condition. A low-residue elemental diet provides good nutrition with low fecal volume to allow bowel rest. A bland, high-protein, high-calorie, low-residue diet with vitamin and mineral supplements and excluding raw fruits and vegetables provides good nutrition and decreases diarrhea. Milk and wheat products are restricted to reduce cramping and diarrhea in patients with lactose and gluten intolerance. |
| Assess the tolerance to the diet. | Cramping, diarrhea, and flatulence are signs the patient is not tolerating the diet. |

## Patient Problem/Analyze Cues/Prioritize Hypotheses

# Risk for Disease (Septicemia)

*due to* the perforation of deeply inflamed colonic mucosa

**Desired Outcome/Generate Solutions:** The patient is free of signs of perforation, toxic mega-colon, septicemia, and septic shock, as evidenced by normothermia; HR of 60–100 bpm; RR of 12–20 breaths/minute with normal depth and pattern (eupnea); normoactive bowel sounds; absence of abdominal distention, tympany, or rebound tenderness; negative culture results; no mental status changes; and orientation to person, place, and time.

| ASSESSMENT—RECOGNIZE CUES/ INTERVENTIONS—TAKE ACTION | RATIONALES |
|---|---|
| Assess for fever, chills, increased respiratory and HRs, diaphoresis, and increased abdominal discomfort. | These indicators can occur with perforation of the colon and potentially result in localized abscess or generalized fecal peritonitis and septicemia. **Note:** Systemic therapy with corticosteroids and antibiotics can mask the development of this complication. |

Continued

| ASSESSMENT—RECOGNIZE CUES/ INTERVENTIONS—TAKE ACTION | RATIONALES |
|---|---|
| Report any evidence of sudden abdominal distention associated with the preceding symptoms. | Together these indicators can signal toxic megacolon. Factors contributing to the development of this complication include hypokalemia, barium enema examinations, and use of opioids and anticholinergics. Surgery to prevent perforation is indicated in patients with fulminant disease or toxic megacolon whose condition worsens or does not improve in 48–72 hours. |
| Assess the mental status, orientation, and level of consciousness every 2–4 hours. | Mental cloudiness, lethargy, and increased restlessness can signal impending or actual septic shock. |
| If the patient has a sudden temperature elevation, culture blood and other sites as prescribed. Assess the culture reports, notifying the health care provider promptly of any positive cultures. | A temperature spike can signal septicemia; a culture will identify causative organism if present. |
| Assess the WBC counts, lactate levels. | Patients with severe UC can have markedly elevated WBC counts—greater than 20,000/mm$^3$ and occasionally as high as 50,000/mm$^3$. Critical values are less than 2500/mm$^3$ and greater than 30,000/mm$^3$.<br><br>Elevated lactate levels are done to determine the development of sepsis. |
| Administer the antibiotics as prescribed and in a timely fashion. | This measure ensures optimal blood levels of the effective therapeutic dose in order to kill the bacteria and control infection in the patient with acute pancolitis or toxic megacolon because secondary bacterial infection of deeply inflamed mucosa is likely. |

## Patient Problem/Analyze Cues/Prioritize Hypotheses

# Acute Pain

*due to* the intestinal inflammatory process

***Desired Outcomes/Generate Solutions:*** Within 1 hour of intervention, the patient's subjective perception of discomfort decreases as documented by pain scale. Objective indicators, such as grimacing, are absent or diminished.

| ASSESSMENT—RECOGNIZE CUES/ INTERVENTIONS—TAKE ACTION | RATIONALES |
|---|---|
| Assess and document the characteristics of the discomfort and assess whether it is associated with the ingestion of certain foods or medications or with emotional stress. Devise a pain scale with the patient, rating discomfort from 0 (no pain) to 10 (worst pain). Eliminate foods that cause cramping and discomfort. | These assessments help determine the discomfort trigger and degree to which discomfort is alleviated after intervention. |
| Assess for intensification of symptoms. Notify the health care provider of significant findings. | This can indicate the presence of complications, which should be treated promptly. |
| As prescribed, maintain the patient nothing by mouth (NPO) or on Total parenteral nutrition (TPN) to provide bowel rest. | These measures provide bowel rest, which should help alleviate symptoms. |
| Keep the patient's environment quiet. Facilitate coordination of health care providers to provide rest periods between care activities. Allow 90 minutes for undisturbed rest. | Rest promotes healing. |
| Administer the anxiolytics as prescribed. | These agents promote rest and reduce anxiety, which optimally will lessen symptoms. |

PART I: Medical-Surgical Nursing Care Plans

## ASSESSMENT—RECOGNIZE CUES/ INTERVENTIONS—TAKE ACTION

- Administer the hydrophilic colloids, anticholinergics, and antidiarrheal medications as prescribed.
- Opioids and anticholinergics should be administered with extreme caution.

Instruct the patient to request medication before discomfort becomes severe.

Instruct the patient in the use of nonpharmacologic methods of pain relief, such as guided imagery, relaxation, massage, heat or cold therapy, and distraction.

## RATIONALES

These agents relieve cramping and diarrhea.

Opioids and anticholinergics may contribute to the development of toxic megacolon.

Cramping and diarrhea are more easily controlled if they are treated before they become severe.

These methods provide comfort and can decrease anxiety and may result in a more effective response to analgesics.

### Patient Problem/Analyze Cues/Prioritize Hypotheses

# Diarrhea

*due to* the inflammatory process of the intestines

**Desired Outcomes/Generate Solutions:** The patient's stools become soft and formed, and frequency is lessened within 3 days of admission. Potassium level is within normal limits.

## ASSESSMENT—RECOGNIZE CUES/ INTERVENTIONS—TAKE ACTION

Assess and record the amount, frequency, and character of stools. When possible, measure liquid stools.

Assess serum electrolytes, particularly Potassium, for abnormalities. Alert the health care provider to Potassium less than 3.5 mEq/L. (Critical value: Potassium less than 2.5 mEq/L.)

Provide a covered bedpan, commode, or bathroom that is easily accessible and ready to use at all times.

Empty the bedpan and commode promptly.

- Administer the hydrophilic colloids, anticholinergics, and antidiarrheal medications as prescribed.
- Opioids and anticholinergics should be administered with extreme caution

Administer the topical corticosteroid or aminosalicylate preparations and antibiotics by retention enema, as prescribed.

If the patient has difficulty retaining the enema for the prescribed amount of time, consult the health care provider about the use of corticosteroid foam.

## RATIONALES

Although bloody diarrhea is the cardinal symptom, the clinical picture can vary from acute episodes with a frequent discharge of watery stools mixed with blood, pus, and mucus, accompanied by fever, abdominal pain, rectal urgency, and tenesmus, to loose or frequent stools, to formed stools coated with a little blood.

Hypokalemia is often present because of colonic losses (diarrhea) and renal losses in patients taking high doses of corticosteroids.

This will control odor and decrease the patient's anxiety and self-consciousness. Easy access promotes patient safety and enables the patient to cope with diarrhea more effectively.

This will remove the source of odor and decrease the patient's anxiety about incontinence.

These agents decrease fluidity and number of stools as well as inhibit GI peristaltic activity.

Opiods and anticholinergics may contribute to the development of toxic megacolon.

These agents reduce mucosal inflammation in patients with mild disease limited to the rectum and sigmoid colon. In patients with acute moderate to severe disease and with more extensive (pancolonic) disease, oral or intravenous corticosteroid therapy is initiated. In patients not responding to steroids or aminosalicylates, immunosuppressive immunomodulatory therapy may be initiated to reduce inflammation.

Corticosteroid foam is easier to retain and administer.

Continued

| ASSESSMENT—RECOGNIZE CUES/ INTERVENTIONS—TAKE ACTION | RATIONALES |
|---|---|
| Administer the probiotics or fish oil, as prescribed. | Probiotics are beneficial bacteria that restore balance to the intestinal environment, with resulting reduction in inflammation. Omega-3 fatty acids found in fish oil appear to benefit patients with active UC by decreasing inflammation; they must be taken in large quantity. |

## Patient Problem/Analyze Cues/Prioritize Hypotheses

# Risk for Impaired Skin Integrity (Perineal/Perianal Skin)

*due to* the persistent diarrhea

**Desired Outcome/Generate Solutions:**  The patient's perineal/perianal skin remains intact with no erythema.

| ASSESSMENT—RECOGNIZE CUES/ INTERVENTIONS—TAKE ACTION | RATIONALES |
|---|---|
| Assess the perineal/perianal skin for erythema and denuded areas. | Frequent liquid stools, particularly if bloody, can cause skin breakdown. |
| Provide the materials or assist the patient with cleansing and drying the perineal area after each bowel movement. | These measures help keep skin clean and intact. |
| Instruct the patient to wash and dry perineal/perianal area with warm water and nonirritating cleansing agent, using a squeeze bottle, cotton balls, or soft tissues. | These measures help keep the skin clean and intact and promote comfort. Sitting on the toilet may make this procedure easier. |
| Instruct the patient to clean perineal area with soft wipes and not to use toilet paper. | Toilet paper can cause skin irritation. |
| Teach the patient to avoid scrubbing during cleansing. | Friction can cause mechanical skin injury. |
| After the skin has been cleansed and dried, provide protective skin care products (skin preparations, gels, or barrier films). | These products prevent irritation caused by frequent liquid stools and maintain perianal skin integrity. Skin care products containing alcohol should not be used on broken or denuded skin because the alcohol content causes a painful burning sensation. |
| • Administer the hydrophilic colloids, anticholinergics, and antidiarrheal medications as prescribed.<br>• Opioids and anticholinergics should be administered with extreme caution | These agents decrease fluidity and number of stools and inhibit GI peristaltic activity. **Opioids and anticholinergics may** contribute to the development of toxic megacolon. |

## Patient Problem/Analyze Cues

# Deficient Knowledge (Medications)

*due to* unfamiliarity with the purpose and precautions of medications used with UC

**Desired Outcome/Generate Solutions:**  Immediately after teaching interventions (if the patient is not hospitalized) or within the 24-hour period before hospital discharge, the patient verbalizes accurate information about medications used with UC, including their purpose and necessary precautions.

PART I: Medical-Surgical Nursing Care Plans

## ASSESSMENT—RECOGNIZE CUES/ INTERVENTIONS—TAKE ACTION

Provide the following medication information to patients:

- Drug action
- Drug administration—dosage, route, time
- Drug-to-drug interactions
- Drug interactions with food
- Side effects

- If a patient is prescribed oral corticosteroids, instruct the patient to taper medication as prescribed and never stop suddenly stop taking medication.

For additional information on side effects and precautions, see "Crohn's Disease," Chapter 57, *Deficient Knowledge (Medications).*

Instruct patient to never crush extended (delayed) release tablets or open extended (delayed) release capsules.

If prescribed, combination therapy that includes oral and rectal administration of mesalamine may be needed.

Advise patient that medications do not cure UC but are a treatment option that also includes diet and possibly surgery.

## RATIONALES

Patient education regarding prescribed drugs will increase patient's knowledge and promote safe self-administration of drugs and compliance with therapeutic health care regimen.

Sudden discontinuation of corticosteroids may cause adrenal crisis, which can be life threatening.

Extended or delayed-release drugs release small amounts of medication into a person's system over a long period of time. Crushing an extended-release tablet or opening an extended-release capsule may cause rapid absorption of a large dose that was intended to be released slowly over time and may cause drug toxicity.

Combination therapy may be more effective in treating than using the oral form alone.

Medications are used to prevent signs and symptoms such as diarrhea and bleeding. Foods and drinks that include caffeine, dairy, carbonation, and high amounts of fiber may cause UC flare-ups. Surgery may cure UC when the affected bowel is removed.

### ADDITIONAL PROBLEMS:

| | |
|---|---|
| *Risk for Infection* | Chapter 4 |
| *Risk for Hemorrhaging* | Chapter 4 |
| *Difficulty Coping* | Chapter 8 |
| *"Fecal Diversions: Colostomy, Ileostomy, and Ileal Pouch-Anal Anastomoses,"* for relevant problems if bowel diversion surgery is performed. | Chapter 58 |

## PATIENT–FAMILY TEACHING AND DISCHARGE PLANNING

When providing patient–family teaching, focus on sensory information, avoid giving excessive information, and initiate a visiting nurse referral for necessary follow-up teaching. Include verbal and written information about the following:

✓ Medications, including drug name, rationale, dosage, schedule, route of administration, precautions, and potential side effects. Also discuss drug–drug and food–drug interactions. **Note:** Caution patients receiving high-dose steroid therapy to avoid abrupt discontinuation of steroids to prevent precipitation of adrenal crisis. Withdrawal symptoms include weakness, lethargy, restlessness, anorexia, nausea, and muscle tenderness. Instruct the patient to notify the health care provider if these symptoms occur.

✓ Herbal/alternative therapies, such as vitamins, herbs, dietary supplements, minerals, and homeopathy in order to minimize interactions with prescribed medications and adverse effects. Discuss with the patient that even though a probiotic is indicated for the dietary management of UC, it should be used under the supervision of the prescribing health care provider.

✓ Importance of taking medications as prescribed in order to maintain remission and prevent flares.

✓ Signs and symptoms that necessitate medical attention, including fever, nausea and vomiting, diarrhea or constipation, and any significant change in appearance and frequency of stools, any of which can signal exacerbation of the disease.

✓ Dietary management to promote nutritional and fluid maintenance and prevent abdominal cramping, discomfort, and diarrhea.

✓ Importance of perineal care after bowel movements.

✓ Enteral or parenteral feeding instructions if the patient is to supplement diet or is NPO.

✓ Referral to community resources, including the Crohn's & Colitis Foundation of America, Inc., at www.ccfa.org; the Teens with IBD website at www.justlikemeibd.org; and the following social media: Online Community at www.ccfa-community.org, Facebook at https://www.facebook.com/ccfafb, and Twitter at www.twitter.com/crohnscolitisfn.

✓ Importance of follow-up medical care, particularly for patients with long-standing disease because so many of them develop colonic adenocarcinoma.

✓ Referral to a mental health specialist if recommended by the health care provider.

In addition, if the patient has a fecal diversion (colostomy, ileostomy, or ileal pouch-anal anastomosis):

✓ Care of incision, dressing changes, and permission to take baths or showers after sutures and drains are removed.

✓ Care of stoma, peristomal/perianal skin, or perineal wound; use of ostomy equipment; and method for obtaining supplies. Sitz baths may be indicated for perineal wound.

✓ Medications that are contraindicated (e.g., laxatives) or that may not be well tolerated or absorbed (e.g., antibiotics, enteric-coated tablets, long-acting tablets).

✓ Gradual resumption of activities of daily living, excluding heavy lifting (more than 10 lb), pushing, or pulling for 6–8 weeks to prevent incisional herniation.

✓ Referral to community resources, including home health care agency, wound, ostomy, continence/enterostomal therapy nurse, the local ostomy association, and the United Ostomy Association of America (UOAA) main website at www.ostomy.org and the UOAA Discussion Board at www.uoaa.org/forum.

✓ Importance of reporting signs and symptoms that require medical attention, such as change in stoma color from the normal bright and shiny red; peristomal or perianal skin irritation; diarrhea; incisional pain, local increased temperature, drainage, swelling, or redness; signs and symptoms of fluid and electrolyte imbalance; and signs and symptoms of mechanical or functional obstruction.

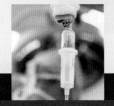

# Anemias of Chronic Disease 64

## OVERVIEW/PATHOPHYSIOLOGY

Erythropoietin (EPO) is a naturally occurring protein hormone produced and released by the kidneys (90%) and liver (10%). The kidneys are stimulated to release EPO in response to low blood oxygenation. EPO then stimulates stem cells in the bone marrow to develop and produce red blood cells (RBCs). Individuals with decreased renal function (e.g., chronic kidney disease [CKD]) often become anemic because their kidneys cannot produce EPO. In other chronic conditions (cancer, heart failure, human immunodeficiency virus [HIV], rheumatologic disorders, inflammatory bowel disease, Castleman disease), elevated cytokines (such as interleukin-6) may reduce bone marrow erythrocyte production, reduce erythropoietic response in the bone marrow, restrict iron recycling from the liver due to hepcidin blocking intestinal iron absorption and its release from macrophages and hepatocytes, reduce iron absorption from the gut, and shorten erythrocyte survival. Recombinant human EPO (epoetin alpha) has provided some benefits for patients with CKD, for some patients receiving chemotherapy for cancer, and for patients undergoing treatment for infection with HIV, but it may pose risks for life-threatening cardiovascular events. Because anemia may be caused by other conditions, including blood loss, hemolysis, and inadequate dietary intake of iron, vitamin $B_{12}$ (cobalamine), or folate, these conditions must be ruled out before the ultimate cause of anemia can be identified.

## HEALTH CARE SETTING

Primary care; acute care for blood transfusion or treatment for sequelae of chronic diseases

## ASSESSMENT

**Chronic indicators.** The patient may have no symptoms or may have brittle hair and nails and pallor. In the presence of severe and chronic disease, shortness of breath, dizziness, and fatigue may be present even at rest. The patient may have a history of CKD, dialysis therapy, cancer within the bone marrow (e.g., leukemia), cancer chemotherapy, or other chronic conditions (e.g., HIV, heart failure, diabetes).

**Acute indicators.** Fatigue, decreased ability to concentrate, cold sensitivity, menstrual irregularities, and loss of libido.

**Physical assessment.** Tachycardia, palpitations, tachypnea, exertional dyspnea, pale mucous membranes, pale nail beds, and vertigo.

## DIAGNOSTIC TESTS

**Blood count.** RBCs, hemoglobin (Hgb), and hematocrit (Hct) are low because the percentage of RBCs in the total blood volume is decreased.

**Mean corpuscular volume.** May be within normal limits or slightly decreased. In iron deficiency anemia, the mean corpuscular volume (MCV) will be decreased; in cobalamin and folic acid deficiencies, the MCV will be increased.

**Ferritin.** May be within normal limits or increased. If it is less than 30 mcg/L, there is a coexisting iron deficiency.

**Total iron-binding capacity.** Decreased.

**Reticulocyte count.** Within normal limits to slightly decreased.

**Serum iron levels.** Within normal limits to decreased.

**Transferrin.** Within normal limits to decreased.

**Cobalamin (vitamin B12) folate.** Within normal limits.

**C-reactive protein.** Elevated.

**Erythrocyte sedimentation rate.** Elevated.

## Patient Problem/Analyze Cues/Prioritize Hypotheses

# Activity Intolerance

*due to* anemia and the decreased oxygen-carrying capacity of the blood occurring with decreased RBCs

***Desired Outcomes/Generate Solutions:*** After treatment, Hgb and Hct levels are within medical goals and the patient reports an absence of fatigue, dizziness, and headaches. The patient perceives exertion at 3 or less on a 0–10 scale and tolerates exercise/activity, as evidenced by the respiratory rate of 12–20 breaths/min, eupnea, and heart rate of 100 bpm or less.

| ASSESSMENT—RECOGNIZE CUES/ INTERVENTIONS—TAKE ACTION | RATIONALES |
|---|---|
| Assess for signs of activity intolerance. Ask the patient to rate perceived exertion on a 0–10 scale (see "Immobility," Chapter 1, for *Activity Intolerance*). | Fatigue, dyspnea on exertion, dizziness, palpitations, headaches, and verbalization of increased exertion level (rated perceived exertion more than 3) are signs of activity intolerance and decreased tissue oxygenation, and the patient should stop or modify the activity until signs of increased exertion are no longer present with the activity. |
| [!] Assess the risk for falling and implement appropriate strategies. | Because of the potentially slow, progressive nature of this anemia, patients may not be aware of weaknesses and limitations leading to reductions in strength and balance. Patient falls can result in severe injury, prolonged hospitalization, and even death. |
| Monitor the oximetry; report the O$_2$ saturation 92% or less. | O$_2$ saturation 92% or less may signal the need for supplementary oxygen. |
| Administer the oxygen as prescribed; encourage deep breathing. | Both measures augment oxygen delivery to the tissues. |
| Facilitate the coordination of care providers, allowing time for at least 90 minutes of undisturbed rest. | Fewer interruptions in rest enable patients to benefit from the undisturbed rest/sleep they need until the anemia is resolved. |
| Encourage gradually increasing activities to tolerance as the patient's condition improves. | This promotes endurance while preventing problems caused by prolonged bedrest. |
| Consider this effective measure: Setting mutually agreed-on goals with the patient (e.g., "Let's plan this morning's activity goals. Could you walk up and down the hall once, or twice?" or appropriate amount, depending on the patient's tolerance). | |
| Administer the intravenous blood components (usually packed RBCs) as prescribed. | This will increase the number of circulating RBCs, which in turn will increase the blood's oxygen-carrying capacity. |
| [!] Double-check the type and crossmatching and the patient identifiers as per facility policy and monitor for and report signs of transfusion reaction. | These measures reduce the risk for delivering the wrong type of blood to the patient and enable rapid treatment if a transfusion reaction occurs. |
| Reassure the patient that fatigue symptoms usually are relieved and tolerance for exercise/activity increased with the treatment plan. | RBC production is improved through additional EPO (RBCs are not responsive to normal EPO levels in chronic conditions). |
| Treatment may include | Iron and B12, and folate replenish Hgb and depleted iron and other deficiencies if needed. |
| • packed RBCs or EPO replacement (recombinant EPO [epoetin alpha or darbepoetin alfa]), | People with chronic diseases, especially older individuals, may not have a normal dietary intake of these substances. Supplements will maximize normal erythropoiesis. |
| • administration of iron and other supplements (cobalamine, folate) as prescribed, and | |
| • a diet high in iron and vitamins. | Improvements in dietary intake and strength also may help reduce symptoms. |

## ADDITIONAL PROBLEM:

*Risk for Infection*, due to myelosuppression          Chapter 6

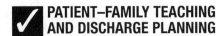

## PATIENT–FAMILY TEACHING AND DISCHARGE PLANNING

When providing patient–family teaching, focus on sensory information, avoid giving excessive information, and initiate a visiting nurse referral for necessary follow-up teaching. Include verbal and written information about the following:

✓ Importance of a well-balanced diet, especially iron intake, if appropriate, which is found in foods such as red meat, dark green vegetables, legumes, and certain fruits (apricots, figs, raisins). Refer to a clinical dietitian as prescribed.

✓ Importance of safety during mobility when experiencing weakness and fatigue. Instruct the patient and family/caregivers on safety strategies; recommend referral to physical therapy as appropriate.

✓ Special instructions for taking iron (and its concomitant risk for constipation), if appropriate, depending on the type prescribed. Therapy may need to be continued for 4–6 months to replace iron stores adequately.

✓ Necessity and consent for EPO replacement therapy to be continued for the duration of the underlying condition.

✓ When self-administering EPO, importance of *not* shaking medication vial before taking it. Shaking the vial may denature glycoprotein in the solution and render it biologically inactive. Any discolored solution or solution with particulate matter should not be used.

✓ Other medications, including drug name, dosage, purpose, schedule, precautions, and potential side effects. Also, discuss drug–drug, herb–drug, and food–drug interactions.

✓ Risks and benefits for RBC transfusion (as explained by the health care provider) and a necessity for signed consent to the transfusion.

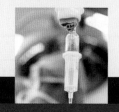

# Disseminated Intravascular Coagulation 65

## OVERVIEW/PATHOPHYSIOLOGY

Disseminated intravascular coagulation (DIC) is an acute and serious coagulation disorder characterized by paradoxical clotting and hemorrhage. The sequence usually progresses from massive clot formation, depletion of clotting factors, and activation of diffuse fibrinolysis to hemorrhage. DIC occurs secondary to widespread coagulation factors in the bloodstream caused by extensive surgery, burns, shock, sepsis, neoplastic diseases, or abruptio placentae; extensive destruction of blood vessel walls caused by eclampsia, anoxia, or heat stroke; or damage to blood cells caused by hemolysis, sickle cell disease, or transfusion reactions. Although clotting and bleeding occur simultaneously, organ failure related to thromboses of vital organs (e.g., kidneys, lungs, central nervous system, liver) is usually the primary life-threatening concern. Prompt assessment of the disorder can result in a good prognosis. Usually, affected patients are transferred to the intensive care unit (ICU) for careful monitoring and aggressive therapy.

## HEALTH CARE SETTING

Acute care/critical care unit

## ASSESSMENT

*Clinical indicators.* Bleeding of abrupt onset; oozing from venipuncture sites or mucosal surfaces; bleeding from surgical sites; and presence of hematuria, blood in stool (melena or hematochezia), hemoptysis, spontaneous ecchymosis (bruising), petechiae, purpura fulminans (extensive skin hemorrhagic necrosis), pallor, or mottled skin. The patient also may bleed from the vagina (menometrorrhagia), nose (epistaxis), and oral mucous membranes. Joint pain and swelling may signal bleeding into joints. The complaint of headache or mental status changes may indicate intracranial hemorrhage and/or stroke. Symptoms of hypoperfusion can occur, including decreased urine output and abnormal behavior.

*Physical assessment.* Abdominal assessment may reveal signs of gastrointestinal (GI) bleeding, such as guarding; distention (increasing abdominal girth measurements);

hyperactive, hypoactive, or absent bowel sounds; and a rigid, board-like abdomen. With significant hemorrhage, patients may exhibit the following: systolic blood pressure (SBP) less than 90 mm Hg and diastolic BP less than 60 mm Hg; heart rate (HR) greater than 100 bpm; peripheral pulse amplitude 2+ or less on a 0–4+ scale; respiratory rate (RR) greater than 22 breaths/minute; shortness of breath; urinary output less than 30 mL/hour; secretions and excretions positive for blood; cool, pale, clammy skin; lack of orientation to person, place, and time; or changes in mental status. Jaundice from excessive hemolysis also may be present.

*Risk factors.* Infection, burns, trauma, hepatic disease, hypovolemic shock, severe hemolytic reaction, malignancy, obstetric complications, and hypoxias.

## DIAGNOSTIC TESTS

*Oxygen saturation (SpO$_2$).* Low (less than 92%), indicating a tissue perfusion problem.

*Serum fibrinogen.* Low because of abnormal consumption of clotting factors in the formation of fibrin clots.

*Platelet count.* Less than 100,000/mm$^3$, indicating increased utilization by bleeding and/or sequestration in large clots

*Fibrin split products.* Increased, indicating the widespread dissolution of clots. Fibrinolysis produces fibrin split products, also known as *fibrin degradation products* (FDPs), as an end product.

*D-Dimers.* The by-products of fibrinolysis, D-dimers are increased in DIC and, along with increased FDPs, are considered diagnostic of DIC.

*Prothrombin time.* Normal, low, or possibly increased because of depletion of clotting factors.

*Partial thromboplastin time.* Normal, low, or possibly high because of depletion of clotting factors.

*Protein C.* Low because normal anticoagulation is impaired. Protein C is a coagulation inhibitor.

*Peripheral blood smear.* Shows fragmented red blood cells (RBCs; schistocytes).

## Patient Problem/Analyze Cues/Prioritize Hypotheses

# Risk for Disease (Excessive Clotting)

*due to* the widespread coagulation factors in the bloodstream with DIC

***Desired Outcome/Generate Solutions:*** After treatment, the patient is free of the signs of excessive clotting as evidenced by BP of 90/60 mm Hg or greater and HR of 100 bpm or less (or within the patient's baseline range); $SpO_2$ greater than 92%; peripheral pulse amplitude 2+ or greater on a 0–4+ scale; urinary output 30 mL/hour or more; equal and normoreactive pupils; normal/baseline motor function; orientation to person, place, and time; and no mental status changes.

| ASSESSMENT—RECOGNIZE CUES/ INTERVENTIONS—TAKE ACTION | RATIONALES |
|---|---|
| Assess for coagulation/thrombus formation as follows: | DIC is an acute coagulation disorder characterized by paradoxical clotting and hemorrhage. |
| • Monitor the vital signs (VS), particularly BP, HR, and peripheral pulses. | Decreased BP, increased HR, and decreased amplitude of peripheral pulses may signal that coagulation and thrombus formation are occurring. This in turn can lead to digital ischemia and gangrene. |
| • Perform the neurologic checks, including orientation, mental status assessments, pupillary reaction to light, level of consciousness (LOC), and motor response. | Deficits may signal that cerebral perfusion is ineffective and should be reported promptly. Signs may be general, such as increased confusion, agitation, or seizures, and become more focal, such as a unilateral widened pupil. |
| • If signs of decreased cerebral perfusion occur, implement fall precautions as appropriate | It is important to protect the patient from injury caused by cerebral impairment |
| • Monitor the intake and output; report the significant findings. | Urine output less than 5 mL/kg/hour in the presence of adequate intake may indicate renal vessel thrombosis. |
| • Monitor for hemorrhage from intravenous (IV) catheters, surgical wounds, GI and genitourinary (GU) tracts, and mucous membranes. | Hemorrhage is a potential risk after fibrinolysis. See *Risk for Hemorrhaging*, which follows. |
| • Monitor oxygen saturation by pulse oximetry every 4 hours or as indicated; report oxygen saturation 92% or less. | Oxygen perfusion may be compromised by pulmonary emboli and/or pulmonary hemorrhage. Oxygen saturation 92% or less often signals the need for supplement oxygen. |
| Monitor the laboratory work for values suggestive of DIC. | Increased D-dimer values, low serum fibrinogen (less than 200 mg/dL), low platelet count (less than 100,000/mm³), increased Fibrin Split Products (FSPs) (9 mcg/mL or greater), possible increased prothrombin time (PT) (greater than 11–15 seconds), and possible increased partial thromboplastin time (greater than 40–100 seconds) are common with DIC. Monitoring these values will promote timely interventions. |
| Report the significant findings to the patient's health care provider; prepare for emergent blood product transfusion, medical support, and transfer to ICU if the condition worsens. | The patient may require careful monitoring and aggressive therapy. |
| Administer the anticoagulant agents as prescribed and assess frequently for signs and symptoms of bleeding. | Heparin may be of value in some cases to prevent or treat clotting-related ischemia. so that excessive bleeding does not occur. |
| Administer the blood products as prescribed. | Packed RBCs replace blood volume; platelets may be needed to restore hemostasis for severe bleeding; fresh frozen plasma (FFP) and/or cryoprecipitate also may be used for severe bleeding and low fibrinogen levels. |
| Double-check the blood product and type as per facility policy, and monitor for and report the signs of transfusion reaction, including chills, back pain, dyspnea, hives, and wheezing. | These precautions help ensure the patient receives the correct blood product and type, which otherwise could result in transfusion reaction. |

## Patient Problem/Analyze Cues/Prioritize Hypotheses

# Risk for Hemorrhaging

*due to* the depletion of clotting factors and the fibrinolysis component of DIC

***Desired Outcome/Generate Solutions:*** After treatment, the patient is free of signs of bleeding/hemorrhage, as evidenced by SBP of 90 mm Hg or greater; HR of 100 bpm or less (or within the patient's normal range); RR of 12–20 breaths/minute and demonstrates eupnea; urinary output of 30 mL/hour or 5 mL/kg/hour or more; secretions and excretions negative for blood; stable abdominal girth measurements; orientation to person, place, and time; and no changes in mental status.

| ASSESSMENT—RECOGNIZE CUES/ INTERVENTIONS—TAKE ACTION | RATIONALES |
|---|---|
| Assess the LOC and monitor the VS at frequent intervals; report significant changes. | Hypotension, tachycardia, dyspnea, disorientation, and changes in mental status can signal hemorrhage. |
| Inflate cuff only as high as needed to obtain reading. Alternate arms with each BP check. | Frequent BP readings may cause bleeding under the cuff. Alternating arms reduces repeated tissue trauma. |
| Assess for abdominal pain, abdominal distention, changes in bowel sounds, and a board-like abdomen. | These are signs of GI bleeding. |
| Check the stool, urine, emesis, and nasogastric drainage for blood using point-of-care testing or send it to the laboratory immediately. | A positive test signals the presence of blood in the GI/GU tracts and should be reported to the health care provider promptly for rapid intervention. |
| Assess the puncture sites regularly. | This assessment will detect external bleeding or oozing. |
| When possible, treat bleeding sites with ice, pressure, rest, and elevation. Administer the thrombin-soaked gauze, such as Gelfoam, or topical thrombin powder if prescribed. | These interventions will slow bleeding by vasoconstriction, gravity, and coagulation. |
| Be alert to visual changes, headache, and joint pain. | Visual changes may signal retinal hemorrhage. Joint pain and headache are other signs that bleeding may be occurring and could be life threatening. |
| Monitor the coagulation and other hematologic laboratory values. | Increased PT and INR are signs that clotting factors are depleted and the patient is at risk for hemorrhage. |
| Prevent or promptly control vomiting, coughing, and straining with bowel movements. Avoid giving intramuscular injections and minimize venipunctures as appropriate. | These measures minimize the potential for bleeding. |
| Administer the blood products (packed RBCs, platelets, FFP), and IV fluids as prescribed. See the precautions listed with the previous nursing diagnosis. | These products help counteract deficiencies causing the bleeding and support blood volume. Cryoprecipitate or FFP may be used if fibrinogen is low; platelets may be given if they are less than 10,000/mm³ or if there is bleeding. |
| Instruct patients to use electric shaver and soft-bristle toothbrush and to avoid forceful nose blowing (dab instead), bending down (head lower than the heart), and potentially traumatic procedures (e.g., enemas, rectal temperatures). | These precautions reduce the risk for bleeding. Razors, hard bristles, rectal thermometers, and enema nozzles, for example, could break the skin and mucous membranes, causing bleeding. |
| Report significant findings to the patient's health care provider. Prepare for emergent blood product transfusion, medical support, and transfer to the ICU if the condition worsens. | The patient may require aggressive therapy and careful monitoring. |

Patient Problem/Analyze Cues/Prioritize Hypotheses

# Risk for Impaired Skin/Tissue Integrity

*due to* the altered circulation occurring with hemorrhage or thrombosis

**Desired Outcome/Generate Solutions:** The patient's skin and tissue remain non erythemic and intact.

| ASSESSMENT—RECOGNIZE CUES/ INTERVENTIONS—TAKE ACTION | RATIONALES |
|---|---|
| Assess the patient's skin, noting changes in color, temperature, and sensation. | Erythema that does not clear after removal of pressure or changes in color, sensation, and temperature may signal decreased perfusion that can lead to tissue damage. |
| Ensure that the patient turns every 2 hours and consider the use of protective measures on elbows and heels and enhanced pressure-distribution mattress padding. Do not pull on patient's extremities when assisting patient to change positions. | These measures eliminate or minimize pressure points that could damage the skin/tissue. |
| As prescribed, encourage the active range of motion (ROM) of all extremities every 2 hours. | ROM exercise reduces tissue pressure and promotes circulation. |
| Ensure that the patient's extremities are warm. | Warmth helps prevent tissue hypoxia, which would increase the risk for tissue damage/necrosis. |
| Use alternatives to tape to hold dressings in place, such as gauze wraps or net gauze if tape causes injury. If tape is necessary, use paper tape. | Tape removal could damage fragile skin and tissue. Paper tape is the least damaging to skin. |
| If the patient has areas of breakdown, see "Managing Wound Care," Chapter 75. | |

## ADDITIONAL PROBLEM:

| | |
|---|---|
| *Risk for Hemorrhaging*, due to anticoagulation therapy | Chapter 15 |

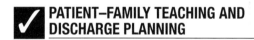

## PATIENT–FAMILY TEACHING AND DISCHARGE PLANNING

See the patient's primary diagnosis.

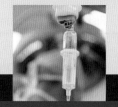

## OVERVIEW/PATHOPHYSIOLOGY

Polycythemia is a chronic disorder characterized by excessive production of red blood cells (RBCs). As RBCs increase, blood volume, blood viscosity, and hemoglobin (Hgb) concentration increase, causing excessive workload for the heart and congestion of organs (e.g., liver, kidney), hemorrhage, and vascular events (venous thromboembolism, stroke, heart failure, and myocardial infarction).

Primary polycythemia (*Polycythemia vera* [PV]) arises from a chromosomal mutation (a *JAK2* V617F mutation) most often affecting men of Jewish descent, with onset in late midlife. PV results in increased RBC mass, leukocytosis, and thrombocytosis. The *JAK2* V617F is a point mutation change that causes continuous activation of intracellular pathways responsible for the activation of erythropoietin (Lichtman et al., 2017).

Because of increased viscosity and decreased microcirculation, mortality is high if the condition is left untreated. In addition, there is potential for this disorder to evolve into other hematopoietic disorders, such as myelofibrosis and acute leukemia.

*Secondary polycythemia* results from an abnormal increase in erythropoietin production and caused by hypoxia that occurs with chronic lung or cardiovascular disease, defective oxygen transport, prolonged living in high altitudes, or by other conditions. Other conditions that may cause polycythemia include cancers or benign tumors that produce erythropoietin (EPO).

## HEALTH CARE SETTING

Primary care; acute care for complications

## ASSESSMENT

***Signs and symptoms.*** Fatigue, fevers, muscle pain, headache, dizziness, tinnitus, paresthesias, visual disturbances, dyspnea, thrombophlebitis, joint pain, bone pain, painful pruritus, night sweats, chest pain, palpitations, abdominal discomfort, weight loss, dull foot pain at night, and a feeling of "fullness," especially in the head.

***Physical assessment.*** Hypertension, engorgement of retinal blood veins, crackles, weight loss, cyanosis, changes in mentation or mood (delirium, psychotic depression, mania), ruddy complexion (especially palmar aspects of hands and plantar surfaces of feet), splenomegaly, hepatomegaly, gastrointestinal (GI) disturbances (ulcers, GI bleed), nosebleeds.

## DIAGNOSTIC TESTS

***Complete blood count.*** Increased RBC mass (8–12 million/mm$^3$), Hgb (more than 18.5 g/dL in women and 16.5 g/dL in men), hematocrit ([Hct] more than 48% in women and 52% in men), and leukocytes (more than 10,000/mcL); and overproduction of thrombocytes (more than 400,000/mcL) are diagnostic of polycythemia.

***Platelet count.*** Elevated as a result of increased production.

***Liver function studies.*** Increased direct and indirect bilirubin is possible due to red cell hemolysis and liver vascular congestion.

***Bone marrow aspiration.*** Reveals RBC proliferation, and 95% of patients demonstrate a *JAK2* V617F mutation.

***Uric acid levels.*** May be increased because of increased nucleoprotein, an end product of RBC breakdown.

***Erythropoietin levels.*** Elevated in secondary polycythemia and decreased in PV.

***$O_2$ saturation.*** Normal (greater than 92%); should be measured both at rest and after exercise.

---

## Patient Problem/Analyze Cues/Prioritize Hypotheses

# Acute Pain

*due to* the discomfort of headache, angina, pruritus, and abdominal and joint pain occurring with altered circulation caused by blood hyperviscosity

***Desired Outcomes/Generate Solutions:*** Within 1 hour of intervention, the patient's subjective perception of discomfort decreases, as documented by a pain scale. Objective indicators, such as grimacing, are absent or diminished. The patient states that lifestyle behaviors are not compromised because of discomfort.

| ASSESSMENT—RECOGNIZE CUES/ INTERVENTIONS—TAKE ACTION | RATIONALES |
|---|---|
| Assess for the presence of headache, angina, abdominal pain, and joint pain. Devise a pain scale with the patient, rating discomfort from 0 (no pain) to 10 (worst pain). | The patient provides a personal baseline report, enabling the nurse to more effectively monitor subsequent increases and decreases in pain. The use of a pain intensity scale allows more accurate documentation of discomfort and subsequent relief obtained after analgesia has been administered. |
| Monitor for complaints of calf pain and tenderness. | These are indicators of peripheral thrombosis, which can lead to pulmonary embolus or stroke and therefore should be reported promptly for immediate intervention. |
| In the presence of joint or skin discomfort, rest the joint and elevate the extremity. Use gentle range of motion (ROM) exercises as tolerated. Caution patients to avoid crossing legs and wearing restrictive clothing. Apply the cool compresses or ice. | Elevation may help increase circulation and prevent the pooling of hyperviscous blood in the joints. ROM helps improve circulation. Ice is used (short term) to decrease severe joint pain. **Note:** In the presence of pruritus, skin may become painful and swollen, exacerbated by heat or exposure to water. Topical antihistamines or lotions generally are not helpful. |
| Administer the analgesics as prescribed. | Analgesics reduce pain. |
| Avoid the analgesics containing aspirin or nonsteroidal antiinflammatory drugs unless prescribed by the health care provider. | These medications may exacerbate bleeding associated with thrombocytosis (high number of ineffective platelets) but may be helpful in alleviating microvascular symptoms. |
| Instruct the patient to request analgesia before pain becomes too intense. | Pain is easier to control before it becomes severe. Prolonged stimulation of pain receptors results in increased sensitivity to painful stimuli and will increase the amount of medication required to relieve pain. |
| Provide instructions on measures that reduce pruritus, such as avoiding hot baths and taking medications as prescribed. | Hot baths exacerbate pruritus. Medications that may be prescribed include paroxetine, antihistamines, and steroids. In PV, there is potentially an increased number of mast cells in the skin and elevated histamine levels. Paroxetine (a selective serotonin reuptake inhibitor and antidepressant) potentially works by its vasomotor effects. Antihistamines and steroids reduce the inflammatory manifestations of the vascular congestion. |
| Encourage the use of nonpharmacologic pain control, such as relaxation and distraction. | These are pain measures that potentiate analgesics and do not have side effects. |
| For more information, see "Pain," Chapter 5. | |

## Patient Problem/Analyze Cues/Prioritize Hypotheses

# Risk for Inadequate Tissue Perfusion (Multisystem)

*due to* blood hyperviscosity

***Desired Outcome/Generate Solutions:*** The patient has adequate renal, peripheral, cardiac, and cerebral perfusion as evidenced by urinary output 30 mL/hour or 0.5 mL/kg/hour or more; peripheral pulses 2+ or more on a scale of 0–4+; distal extremity warmth; adequate (baseline) muscle strength; no mental status changes; and orientation to person, place, and time.

| ASSESSMENT—RECOGNIZE CUES/ INTERVENTIONS—TAKE ACTION | RATIONALES |
|---|---|
| Assess the intake and output; report significant findings. | Urine output less than 30 mL/hour or 0.5 mL/hour in the presence of adequate intake can signal renal congestion and decreased perfusion. |

Continued

| ASSESSMENT—RECOGNIZE CUES/ INTERVENTIONS—TAKE ACTION | RATIONALES |
|---|---|
| Assess the circulation by palpating peripheral pulses; assess distal extremities. | Pulse amplitude 2+ or less on a scale of 0–4+ and coolness in distal extremities can signal disruption of peripheral tissue perfusion secondary to hyperviscosity of the blood. |
| Assess for muscle weakness and decreases in sensation and level of consciousness (LOC). | These are indicators of thrombosis. Any new signs or symptoms could indicate a medical emergency. |
| If patient has muscle weakness, decreased sensation and LOC, assist with ambulation or initiate fall prevention measures, depending on the degree of deficit. | These measures reduce the risk for further thrombosis as well as protect patients from injury caused by declining neurologic status. |
| In the absence of signs of cardiac and renal failure, provide prescribed intravenous (IV) hydration and encourage fluid intake to decrease blood viscosity. | Inadequate hydration can increase blood viscosity and contribute adversely to polycythemia. |
| Perform or coordinate the phlebotomy as prescribed. | Phlebotomy to maintain a Hct of less than 43% in women and 45% in men has been shown to improve survival. |
| Encourage the patient to change position every hour when in bed or to exercise and ambulate to tolerance. | These measures promote circulation and reduce the risk for thrombosis. |
| Instruct the patient to avoid tight or restrictive clothing and provide instructions on signs and symptoms of venous thromboembolism. | Tight clothing could impede blood flow/circulation, increasing the risk for thromboses. |
| Administer the antiplatelet and myelosuppressive agents, as prescribed. | Anticoagulants (low-dose aspirin or anagrelide) and/or chemotherapy agents are given to inhibit bone marrow function and reduce the overproduction of blood cells and the potential for thrombosis. |
| Monitor the complete blood count (CBC). | Antiplatelet and myelosuppressive agents can affect bone marrow function and place the patient at risk for myelosuppression, blood counts should be monitored. |
| If the patient smokes, encourage enrollment in a smoking cessation program. | Smoking significantly increases the potential of a thromboembolic event. |

## Patient Problem

# Body Weight Problem (Weight Loss)

*due to* anorexia occurring with feelings of fullness resulting from organ system congestion

***Desired Outcome/Generate Solutions:*** By at least 24 hours before hospital discharge, the patient exhibits adequate nutrition as evidenced by maintenance of or return to baseline body weight or a 1- to 2-lb weight gain.

| ASSESSMENT—RECOGNIZE CUES/ INTERVENTIONS—TAKE ACTION | RATIONALES |
|---|---|
| Assess the fluid and nutrition balance by weighing the patient daily. | This will help identify the trend of the patient's nutritional status. |
| Assess the fluid volume intake; encourage the intake if indicated. | These measures will maximize hydration and vascular blood flow. |
| Encourage the patient to eat small, frequent meals. Document intake. | Smaller, more frequent meals usually are better tolerated than larger, less frequent meals. |
| Request that significant others bring in the patient's favorite foods if they are unavailable in the hospital. | This promotes the likelihood the patient will eat. |
| Advise the patient to avoid spicy foods and to eat mild foods. | Mild foods are better tolerated. |

| ASSESSMENT—RECOGNIZE CUES/ INTERVENTIONS—TAKE ACTION | RATIONALES |
| --- | --- |
| Instruct the patient to avoid intake of iron and citrus with meals. | These restrictions help minimize abnormal RBC proliferation and iron overload. Citrus increases the absorption of iron. |
| As indicated, obtain a dietary consultation. | Such a referral will enable more detailed instruction/discussion about foods to eat and those to avoid. |
| Provide instructions to the patient or significant other on how to record and maintain fluid and food intake diary. | This will help them monitor trends in food intake and ensure monitoring of hydration status. |

### Patient Problem/Analyze Cues/Prioritize Hypotheses

# Risk for Inadequate Tissue Perfusion (Cerebral and Cardiac)

*due to* hypovolemia occurring with phlebotomy

**Desired Outcome/Generate Solutions:** The patient has adequate cerebral and cardiopulmonary perfusion as evidenced by no mental status changes; orientation to person, place, and time; heart rate of 100 bpm or less; blood pressure of 90/60 mm Hg or greater (or within the patient's baseline range); absence of chest pain; and respiratory rate of 20 breaths/minute or less.

| ASSESSMENT—RECOGNIZE CUES/ INTERVENTIONS—TAKE ACTION | RATIONALES |
| --- | --- |
| Before the procedure, review the patient's Hgb, Hct, and platelet counts. | This is to assess the appropriateness of therapy and goal of treatment. |
| During the procedure, assess for tachycardia, hypotension, chest pain, or dizziness; notify the patient's health care provider of significant findings. | These are signs of ineffective perfusion as a result of phlebotomy. |
| During the phlebotomy procedure, keep the patient recumbent. | This position helps prevent dizziness or hypotension as a result of phlebotomy. |
| After the procedure, assist the patient in a sitting position for 5–10 minutes before ambulation and assess for headache and weakness. | This will help prevent orthostatic hypotension. For more information about orthostatic hypotension, see "Immobility," Chapter 1, for *Risk for Altered Blood Pressure (Orthostatic Hypotension)*. |
| Provide instructions to the patient about the potential for orthostatic hypotension and the need for caution when standing for at least 2–3 days after phlebotomy. | This information will help protect against injury caused by falling as a result of orthostatic hypotension. |
| Provide the IV hydration as prescribed. | Adequate hydration improves blood flow to the tissues. |
| Explain that vigorous exercise should be avoided within 24 hours after phlebotomy and that adequate hydration should be maintained. | Vigorous exercise and lack of hydration could cause further fluid loss, hypotension, and red cell vascular congestion, whereas maximizing fluids improves blood flow. |

## ✓ PATIENT–FAMILY TEACHING AND DISCHARGE PLANNING

When providing patient–family teaching, focus on sensory information, avoid giving excessive information, and initiate a visiting nurse referral for necessary follow-up teaching. Include verbal and written information about the following:

✓ Need for continued medical follow-up, including laboratory studies and the potential for phlebotomy.

✓ Medications, including drug name, purpose, dosage, schedule, precautions, and potential side effects. Also discuss drug–drug, herb–drug, and food–drug interactions.

✓ Importance of augmenting fluid intake (e.g., greater than 2.5 L/day) to decrease blood viscosity and of avoiding smoking; provide smoking cessation information as appropriate.

✓ Signs and symptoms that necessitate medical attention: angina, muscle weakness, numbness and tingling of extremities, decreased tolerance to activity, mental status changes, joint pain, and bleeding.

✓ Nutrition: Importance of maintaining a balanced diet to increase resistance to infection and of limiting the dietary or supplemental intake of iron to help minimize abnormal RBC proliferation and iron overload.

# Thrombocytopenia 67

## OVERVIEW/PATHOPHYSIOLOGY

Thrombocytopenia is a relatively common coagulation disorder that results from a decreased number of platelets. It can be congenital or acquired, and it is classified according to cause. Causes include deficient production of thrombocytes, as occurs with bone marrow disease (e.g., leukemia, aplastic anemia), or accelerated platelet destruction occurring from loss or increased use, as in hemolytic anemia, thrombotic thrombocytopenic purpura (TTP), idiopathic (immune) thrombocytopenic purpura (ITP), disseminated intravascular coagulation (DIC), or damage by dialysis and devices such as prosthetic heart valves, as well as hypersplenism and hypothermia. Potential triggers include an autoimmune disorder, severe vascular injury, and spleen malfunction. In addition, thrombocytopenia can occur as a side effect of certain medications, such as chemotherapy. Regardless of cause or trigger, the disorder affects coagulation and hemostasis. With chemical-induced thrombocytopenia, prognosis is good after withdrawal of the offending drug. Prognosis for other types depends on the form of thrombocytopenia and the individual's baseline health status and response to treatment.

> **Note:** *Thrombocytopenia may be the first sign of systemic lupus erythematosus (SLE) or infection.*

*TTP* is an uncommon syndrome that is characterized by thrombocytopenia, hemolytic anemia, neurologic abnormalities, fever (in the absence of infection), and renal abnormalities, although all features may not be present. TTP is often associated with hemolytic uremic syndrome (HUS) and is thus referred to as TTP-HUS. It is often caused by a deficiency of a plasma enzyme (ADAMTS13), which is responsible for regulating von Willebrand factor (vWF) and platelet adhesion. Without the enzyme, large vWFs attach to activated platelets, thereby promoting platelet aggregation and loss of circulating platelets. This syndrome may be triggered by certain medications (e.g., cyclosporine, clopidogrel), infections (shigella), pregnancy, or autoimmune disorders, such as SLE.

*ITP*, the most common acquired thrombocytopenia, is caused by proteins on the platelet cell membrane that stimulate the production of antiplatelet immunoglobulin G (IgG) antibodies. These platelets travel to the spleen, where they are recognized as foreign and destroyed by macrophages. Additionally, platelet production from megakaryocytes is impaired. The acute form is most often seen in children (2–6 years of age) and may be related to a previous viral infection. The chronic form is seen more often in adults (18–50 years of age) and may be of unknown origin.

*Heparin-induced thrombocytopenia (HIT)* is a disorder in which heparin triggers an antibody response. Another name is *heparin-induced thrombocytopenia and thrombosis syndrome or HITTS*. The heparin-antibody complexes bind to platelet surfaces, causing activated platelets to aggregate, leading to further thrombosis and, because of increased utilization, thrombocytopenia. Because the platelets are activated (although low in number), HIT is also associated with both arterial and venous thrombosis rather than bleeding.

## HEALTH CARE SETTING

Primary care; hospitalization for complications

## ASSESSMENT

***Chronic indicators.*** Long history of mild bleeding or hemorrhagic episodes from the mouth, nose, gastrointestinal (GI) tract, or genitourinary (GU) tract. Increased bruising (ecchymosis) and petechiae also have been noted.

***Acute indicators.*** Fever, splenomegaly, acute and severe bleeding episodes, weakness, lethargy, malaise, hemorrhage into mucous membranes, gum bleeding, and GU or GI bleeding. Prolonged bleeding can lead to a shock state with tachycardia, shortness of breath, and decreased level of consciousness (LOC). Optic fundal hemorrhage decreases vision and may preclude potentially fatal intracranial hemorrhage.

> **Note:** *With TTP and HIT, the individual may exhibit signs associated with platelet thrombus formation (such as skin necrosis) and ischemic organ failure (decreased renal function or neurologic changes).*

## DIAGNOSTIC TESTS

***Platelet count.*** Can vary from only slightly decreased to nearly absent. Less than 100,000/mm³ is significantly decreased; less than 20,000/μL (20×10⁹/L) results in a serious risk for hemorrhage.

***Peripheral blood smear.*** May reveal megathrombocytes (large platelets), which are present during premature destruction of platelets, as well as reticulocytosis and fragmented red cells.

***Lactate dehydrogenase.*** May be elevated.

**Bilirubin.** Increased.

**Complete blood count.** Low hemoglobin and hematocrit levels because of blood loss or aggregates with clotting; white blood cell count usually within normal range.

**Coagulation studies.**

*Bleeding time:* Increased because of decreased platelets.

*Partial thromboplastin time:* May be increased or within normal range.

*Prothrombin time:* May be increased or within normal range.

*International normalized ratio:* Increased.

*International sensitivity index:* Increased.

**Bone marrow aspiration.** Reveals an increased number of megakaryocytes (platelet precursors) in the presence of ITP and HIT but may be decreased in other causes of thrombocytopenia.

**Antibody screen.** May be positive because of the presence of IgG platelet antibodies, positive HIT or drug-dependent antibodies, and ADAMTS13 deficiency.

**Doppler ultrasound.** Identifies changes in blood flow secondary to the presence of a thrombus. See "Venous Thrombosis/Thrombophlebitis," Chapter 26, for more information about venous thrombosis.

## Patient Problem/Analyze Cues/Prioritize Hypotheses

# Risk for Hemorrhaging

*due to* the deficient production of thrombocytes, as occurs with bone marrow disease (e.g., leukemia, aplastic anemia) or accelerated platelet destruction

**Desired Outcome/Generate Solutions:** The patient is free of the signs of bleeding, as evidenced by secretions and excretions negative for blood, blood pressure (BP) of 90/60–120/70 mm Hg or within the patient's baseline range, heart rate of 100 bpm or less, respiratory rate of 12–20 breaths/minute with normal depth and pattern (eupnea), and absence of bruising or active bleeding.

| ASSESSMENT—RECOGNIZE CUES/ INTERVENTIONS—TAKE ACTION | RATIONALES |
|---|---|
| Assess for hematuria, melena, epistaxis, hematemesis, hemoptysis, menorrhagia, bleeding gums, petechiae, severe ecchymosis, or decreased BP and increased pulse. | These are signs of bleeding that could occur as a result of thrombocytopenia. |
| Teach the patient to be alert to and report the above indicators promptly as well as any headache or changes in vision. | Prompt patient-reported outcomes may improve treatment decisions and control of the disorder. |
| Monitor the platelet count daily and coagulation studies at least weekly or as prescribed. | Optimal range is 150,000–400,000/mm³. Less than 100,000/mm³ is significantly decreased; less than 20,000/mm³ results in a serious risk for hemorrhage. |
| Ensure that there is a current type and crossmatch in the blood bank for red blood cells (RBCs). | RBC transfusions would be necessary to help maintain intravascular volume in the event acute bleeding occurs. |
| Prevent or promptly control symptoms that can trigger bleeding, such as retching, vomiting, coughing, and straining with bowel movements. | Straining and similar actions increase intracranial pressure and can result in intracranial hemorrhage. |
| When possible, avoid venipuncture. If performed, apply pressure on site for 5–10 minutes or until bleeding stops. Do not give intramuscular injections. If injections are necessary, use the subcutaneous route with a small-gauge needle. | The patient is at risk for prolonged bleeding because of the decreased platelet count. |
| Advise the patient to avoid straining at stool and other strenuous activities. | Straining increases intracranial pressure and can result in intracranial hemorrhage. |
| Obtain a prescription for stool softeners, if indicated. Provide instructions to the patient on constipation prevention as described in "Immobility," Chapter 1, for *Constipation*. | These measures help prevent constipation, thereby minimizing the need to strain at stool and risk for bleeding. |
| Instruct the patient to use an electric razor and soft-bristle toothbrush and to avoid cutting nails, walking in bare feet, and wearing tight clothing. | These items minimize the risk for injury and hence bleeding. |

Continued

PART I: Medical-Surgical Nursing Care Plans

| ASSESSMENT—RECOGNIZE CUES/<br>INTERVENTIONS—TAKE ACTION | RATIONALES |
|---|---|
| Instruct the patient about the association of alcohol consumption, smoking, and use of aspirin or nonsteroidal antiinflammatory drugs (NSAIDs) with increased risk for bleeding. | Alcohol may suppress bone marrow production of blood cells, smoking affects circulation, and aspirin and NSAIDs reduce platelet adhesion. |
| As prescribed, administer the following treatments:<br><br>Corticosteroids<br><br>Argatroban<br><br>Intravenous immunoglobulin<br><br>IV anti-D immune globulin<br><br>Rituximab<br><br>Thrombopoietin receptor agonists<br><br>Eculizumab<br><br>Monitor the patient appropriately and provide the patient and family education regarding these treatments. | *Corticosteroids* enhance vascular integrity and diminish platelet destruction.<br><br>*Argatroban* directly inhibits thrombin and is used in the treatment of HIT.<br><br>*Intravenous immunoglobulin (IV IgG)* increases platelet count by impeding the antibody production that destroys platelets.<br><br>*IV anti-D immune globulin* increases platelet count by impeding antibodies that destroy platelets because the antibodies are bound to red cells versus the platelets.<br><br>*Rituximab* increases platelet count by its immunosuppressive properties in ITP.<br><br>*Thrombopoietin receptor agonists* (e.g., Romiplostim, Eltrombopag) may be indicated for ITP for patients who fail other therapies.<br><br>*Eculizumab* may be prescribed for complement-associated TTP-HUS syndrome by inhibiting complement.<br><br>Careful patient monitoring will aid the nurse to evaluate treatment outcomes.<br><br>Patient/family education will aid patient and family to understand treatment needs and side effects. |
| Administer the platelets as prescribed. | Platelet transfusion is used if platelet destruction or deficient formation is the primary cause of the disorder or if the risk for increased microthrombi and organ ischemia is not of primary concern. It provides only temporary relief because the half-life of platelets is only 3–4 days and may be even shorter with ITP (i.e., minutes to hours).<br><br>If used, human leukocyte antigens (HLA)-matched or crossmatched platelets may improve clinical response. |
| Double-check the blood product and type as per facility policy and monitor for and report signs of transfusion reaction, including chills, back pain, dyspnea, hives, and wheezing. | These precautions help ensure that the patient receives the correct blood product and type, which otherwise could result in transfusion reaction. |
| Ensure the patient has been informed of the risks and benefits of all blood product transfusions by the health care provider and that the patient signs consent to the transfusion. | Although the risk for life-threatening reactions and infections is low, patients must be informed as to the risks and benefits by the health care provider. |
| Ensure that if thrombocytopenia was caused by a medication, the medication is noted in the patient's chart as an allergen. | Removal of the offending agent (e.g., medication-induced TTP) is the first step in resolving the disorder. |
| Monitor for infection and bleeding postoperatively after splenectomy. | Splenectomy may be indicated for ITP that is not responsive to medical therapies, such as steroids, IV IgG, and others. Surgical procedures may pose risk for infection and bleeding. |

## Patient Problem/Analyze Cues/Prioritize Hypotheses

# Risk for Inadequate Tissue Perfusion (Multisystem)

*due to* the thrombotic component in TTP and HIT, which results in sensitization and clumping of platelets in the blood vessels

***Desired Outcome/Generate Solutions:*** The patient's perfusion is adequate, as evidenced by no mental status changes; orientation to person, place, and time; normoreactive pupillary responses; absence of headaches, dizziness, and visual disturbances; peripheral pulses greater than 2+ on a 0–4+ scale; and urine output 30 mL/hour or more.

| ASSESSMENT—RECOGNIZE CUES/ INTERVENTIONS—TAKE ACTION | RATIONALES |
|---|---|
| Assess for changes in mental status, LOC, and pupillary response. Monitor for headaches, dizziness, or visual disturbances. | These changes and findings are indicators of ineffective cerebral tissue perfusion and may indicate a medical emergency. |
| Palpate peripheral pulses on all extremities. Compare distal extremities for color, warmth, and character of pulses. | Pulse amplitude 2+ or less on a 0–4+ scale is a signal of ineffective peripheral tissue perfusion (thrombosis), as are differences in color, warmth, and pulse character when comparing one extremity to the other. |
| Assess the urine output. | Adequate renal perfusion is reflected by urine output 30 mL/hour (0.5 mL/kg/hour) or more for consecutive 2 hours. Amounts less than that may signal decreased renal perfusion as a result of thrombosis. |
| Monitor the fluid intake. | The patient should be well hydrated (2–3 L/day if not medically contraindicated) to increase perfusion to the small vessels. |
| Coordinate care for plasma exchange, which may entail physician placement of a large-bore apheresis catheter. | Plasma exchange may be performed in TTP and HIT to remove large platelet complexes from the patient's plasma and replace normal plasma. |

## Patient Problem/Analyze Cues/Prioritize Hypotheses

# Acute Pain

*due to* the discomfort occurring with hemorrhagic episodes or blood extravasation into the tissues

*Desired Outcomes/Generate Solutions:* Within 1 hour of intervention, the patient's subjective perception of discomfort decreases, as documented by pain scale. Objective indicators, such as grimacing, are absent or diminished.

| ASSESSMENT—RECOGNIZE CUES/ INTERVENTIONS—TAKE ACTION | RATIONALES |
|---|---|
| Assess for fatigue, malaise, and joint pain. Devise a pain scale with the patient, rating discomfort on a scale of 0 (no pain) to 10 (worst pain). | This assessment will help determine the degree and type of discomfort. The pain scale also will help assess the degree of relief obtained after treatment/intervention. |
| Maintain a calm, quiet environment. Facilitate the coordination of care providers, allowing time for periods of undisturbed rest. | These measures promote rest, which will help decrease discomfort and fatigue. |
| Elevate the patient's legs. Support the legs with pillows. | These measures help minimize joint discomfort in the lower extremities. |
| Avoid raising the bed at the knee. Choose chairs with padding or provide padding on the seats. | These measures help prevent the occlusion of popliteal vessels. |
| Use a bed cradle; provide socks, as needed, for warmth. | A bed cradle will decrease pressure on tissues of the lower extremities. Decreased circulation results in extremity coolness. |
| Administer the analgesics as prescribed. Reassess pain and document relief obtained, using the pain scale. | Analgesics reduce pain. The pain scale will help assess the degree of relief obtained after treatment/intervention. |
| Avoid the use of aspirin and NSAIDs. | These agents are contraindicated because of their antiplatelet action, which would increase the risk for bleeding. |
| Instruct the patient to request analgesic before the pain becomes severe. | Pain is more readily controlled when it is treated before it gets severe. Prolonged stimulation of pain receptors results in increased sensitivity to painful stimuli and will increase the amount of drug required to relieve pain. |

See "Pain," Chapter 5, for more information.

---

### ADDITIONAL PROBLEM:

"Perioperative Care" for *Risk for Hemorrhaging,*    Chapter 4
    due to invasive procedure

---

 **PATIENT–FAMILY TEACHING AND DISCHARGE PLANNING**

When providing patient–family teaching, focus on sensory information, avoid giving excessive information, and initiate a visiting nurse referral for necessary follow-up teaching. Include verbal and written information about the following:

✓ Importance of preventing trauma, which can cause bleeding.

✓ Seeking medical attention for any signs of bleeding, infection, or clotting. Review signs and symptoms of common infections, such as upper respiratory, urinary tract, and wound infections. Signs and symptoms of common infections are described in "Care of the Kidney Transplant Recipient," Chapter 31, *Risk for Infection.* Also teach the patient to assess for hematuria, melena, hematemesis, hemoptysis, menometrorrhagia, oozing from mucous membranes, and petechiae.

✓ Importance of regular medical follow-up for laboratory studies and vaccinations.

✓ If the patient is discharged with a corticosteroid prescription, provide an explanation of side effects of steroids, including weight gain, headache, capillary fragility, hypertension, moon facies, thinning of arms and legs, mood changes, acne, buffalo hump, edema formation, risk for GI hemorrhage, delayed wound healing, and increased appetite. Review the need to take medication with food, immediately take missed doses, and not precipitously discontinue medication.

✓ Other medications, including drug name, dosage, purpose, schedule, precautions, and potential side effects. Also discuss drug–drug, herb–drug, and food–drug interactions.

✓ Importance of obtaining a medical alert bracelet and identification card outlining diagnosis and emergency treatment. Contact MedicAlert Foundation at www.medicalert.org.

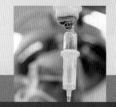

# Amputation 68

## OVERVIEW/PATHOPHYSIOLOGY

Amputation, the removal of part or all of a limb through bone, is now less commonly performed as an orthopedic surgical intervention than it was before advances in antibiotic therapy, treatment for musculoskeletal neoplasms, and microsurgery/limb salvage techniques. Lower extremity amputation may still be the treatment of choice for complications of diabetes mellitus such as peripheral vascular disease (PVD), for severe trauma, or for osteomyelitis or other infections that are refractory to antibiotic treatment. Persons with PVD account for approximately 55% of lower extremity amputations in the Western world. Amputation may be necessary on rare occasions because of tumors or due to congenital limb deficiencies in infants and children.

Although most lower extremity amputations are performed because of disease, most upper extremity amputations are the result of trauma. Amputation and prosthesis use may offer the patient improved functional ability.

## HEALTH CARE SETTING

Critical care unit, acute care surgical unit, orthopedic rehabilitation unit

## ASSESSMENT

***Chronic disease.*** Patients with advanced PVD often complain of extremity pain in a definable muscle group (usually calf muscles) precipitated by exercise and promptly relieved by rest. This pain is distinguished from that of diabetic neuropathy, which is distributed along dermatomes rather than confined to a specific muscle group; neuropathy is also constant and unrelated to exercise. Signs of PVD on the lower extremities include cool skin temperature, thin, brittle, shiny skin on legs and feet, hair loss on legs, weak pulses in legs and feet, and wounds that won't heal over pressure points like the heels and ankles. The affected limb is often a dark-red color (rubor) when it is dependent, but pale when leg is elevated. Amputation also may be needed because of metabolic bone disorders (e.g., osteosarcoma of Paget disease) or massive muscle necrosis that results from an acute thromboembolic event or untreated compartment syndrome. Amputation in the event of a bone or soft tissue tumor is much less common than in the past because of the advent of sophisticated limb salvage procedures.

***Trauma.*** A mangled extremity is common with high-energy injuries. The patient may have multiple injuries, and surgical priority must be given to injuries that may be life threatening. Trauma may result in a complete amputation, a near or partial amputation, or a segmental amputation of an extremity.

## DIAGNOSTIC TESTS

WBC with differential—done to determine the presence of infection

***Ankle–arm (ankle–brachial) index.*** The most widely used noninvasive test for evaluating PVD. Blood pressure is measured at both ankles and arms after the patient has been supine, with the arms and legs at the same level as the heart, for at least 10 minutes. The ankle cuff should be placed on the leg between the malleolus and the calf and should completely encircle the leg. Anterior tibial and posterior tibial systolic pressures will be obtained on each leg, and the higher of the two values will be used as the ankle pressure measurement. Ankle–brachial index (ABI) is calculated by dividing the highest ankle blood pressure by the highest recorded brachial pressure in the arms. A normal resting ABI of 1–1.4 indicates the pressure in the ankle is equal to or greater than the pressure in the arm, suggesting no significant narrowing or blockage of blood flow. A decrease in the ABI (0.9 or lower) is a sensitive indicator that significant PAD is present.

***Doppler ultrasound.*** Evaluates blood flow to the extremities. It can reliably distinguish exercise-related effects from severe ischemia.

***Transcutaneous $O_2$ pressure.*** Measured after oxygen sensors are applied to the skin. By determining oxygen tension (desired value is 30–50 mm Hg, depending on the site of assessment and current patient health), the provider can identify areas of lesser perfusion in the affected extremity. This test offers the most accurate indirect measure of blood flow and the best prediction of residual limb healing potential.

***Angiography.*** Confirms circulatory impairment to determine the appropriate level for amputation. This invasive study involves radiographic imaging after the injection of a contrast dye into a blood vessel. It is most useful if the patient is a candidate for angioplasty or arterial reconstruction.

Patient Problem/Analyze Cues/Prioritize Hypotheses
# Acute Pain
*due to* phantom limb sensation

***Desired Outcome/Generate Solutions:*** Within 1 hour of intervention, the patient's subjective perception of pain decreases, as documented by pain intensity rating scale.

| ASSESSMENT—RECOGNIZE CUES/ INTERVENTIONS—TAKE ACTION | RATIONALES |
|---|---|
| Assess the patient's pain using an appropriate pain intensity rating scale, such as the visual analog scale, Wong-Baker FACES Pain Rating Scale, Faces Pain Scale—Revised, or FLACC (face, legs, activity, crying, consolability) scale. | The patient provides a personal baseline report, enabling the nurse to more effectively assess subsequent increases and decreases in pain. For the patient who is too young or unable to comprehend the quantitative scales, the nurse will use the FLACC scale based on observations. |
| Administer the simple (nonopioid) analgesics (i.e., acetaminophen), nonsteroidal antiinflammatory drugs, opioid analgesics, and adjuncts as prescribed and reassess their effectiveness in approximately 1 hour using the pain intensity rating scale. Document the preintervention and postintervention pain intensity scores. | Although opioids provide effective treatment of incisional pain, they may be ineffective for phantom limb sensation because they do not alter the response of afferent nerves to noxious stimuli. Higher opioid doses are often required to treat phantom limb sensation. |
| | Anticonvulsants such as gabapentin, pregabalin, and topiramate may be effective for neuropathic pain, and the muscle relaxer baclofen may be used to control spasms and cramps in the phantom limb. Tricyclic antidepressants not only offer analgesia but also may be used to elevate mood. **N-methyl-D-aspartate (NMDA)** receptor antagonists affect the body's ability to relay nerve signals and have been effective in relieving phantom limb pain. A lidocaine patch also may be helpful when applied near the surgical wound. |
| Ensure adequate pain management before elective amputation surgery. | This measure decreases the likelihood that phantom limb sensation will develop. Patients with unmanaged preoperative pain are more likely to experience phantom limb sensation. |
| Explain that continued sensations often arise postoperatively from the amputated part and may be painful, irritating, or simply disconcerting. Instruct the patient to report any of these sensations if experienced. | This information prepares patients for the potential experience of phantom limb sensation. |
| Provide instructions to the patient about the use of counterirritation to manage painful sensations. | Counterirritation is based on the gate control theory of pain. It may manage painful sensations by providing a new stimulus to compete with the patient's pain. The simplest form of counterirritation involves systematic rubbing of the painful part. |
| Apply and maintain an elastic dressing over the residual limb. | Use of an elastic dressing will decrease swelling and thus pain. Its use also facilitates measurement for and use of a prosthetic. |
| As indicated, use transcutaneous electrical nerve stimulation (TENS) on the contralateral limb. | TENS may provide effective short-term management of phantom limb sensation. Use on the residual limb has been associated with exacerbation of pain and should be avoided. |
|  Consider pain management interventions such as distraction, guided imagery, relaxation, and biofeedback. | These nonpharmacologic methods augment pharmacologic pain management. |
| Instruct the patient to begin to massage the residual limb 3 weeks postoperatively. After surgical wound healing is complete, vigorous stimulation of the end of the residual limb may be prescribed. This can be accomplished by hitting the end of the limb with a rolled towel. | Massage will desensitize the area in preparation for the prosthesis. Early prosthesis use may reduce the incidence of phantom limb sensation. |
| Encourage the patient to consider the use of sympathetic blocking agents, acupuncture, ultrasound, and injection with local anesthetics if standard treatment is ineffective. | Additional modalities may be used to decrease phantom limb sensation. |

| ASSESSMENT—RECOGNIZE CUES/ INTERVENTIONS—TAKE ACTION | RATIONALES |
|---|---|
| Refer the patient to a pain clinic. | Pain clinics enable a comprehensive interprofessional program to manage chronic phantom limb sensation. |
| Explore the possible impact of phantom limb pain on the patient's ability to function on the job or in interpersonal relationships. | Attempts to cope with chronic pain can cause fatigue and deplete the patient's resources, leaving little energy for work and relationships. |
| For more information, including the use of patient-controlled analgesia, see "Pain," Chapter 5. | |

## Patient Problem/Analyze Cues/Prioritize Hypotheses

# Impaired Mobility

*due to* severe pain, and potential contracture occurring with lower extremity amputation

***Desired Outcomes/Generate Solutions:*** Within 24 hours of instruction, the patient verbalizes understanding of the prescribed exercise regimen and performs exercises independently. The patient is free of symptoms of contracture, as evidenced by optimal range of motion (ROM) of joints and maintenance of muscle mass.

| ASSESSMENT—RECOGNIZE CUES/ INTERVENTIONS—TAKE ACTION | RATIONALES |
|---|---|
| Assess the ROM of the affected extremity and the patient's ability to perform prescribed exercises. | Accurate assessment ensures the creation of an individualized exercise program that will enable the appropriate progression of the patient's activity. |
| Collaborate with the patient to establish a goal for pain management, using both pharmacologic and nonpharmacologic measures. | Effective pain management promotes early movement and ambulation, which in turn aid in the prevention of flexion contractures. An early return to activity also prevents loss of muscle strength and increases local circulation to improve wound healing. |
| If prescribed, elevate the affected extremity for the first 24 hours postoperatively. | During the first 24 hours after surgery, elevation decreases swelling and thus aids in pain management and mobility. Elevation is discontinued after 24 hours to prevent hip flexion contracture. |
| Assist in the performance of ROM exercises daily for the mobility of proximal joints. | Performance of ROM exercises contributes to optimal joint function and decreases the risk for the development of flexion contractures. |
| Perform extremity elevation and ROM exercises *only* if prescribed by the health care provider. | A residual limb with deficient vascular supply must not be elevated to avoid further compromise of circulation. |
| On the second postoperative day, ensure that the patient keeps the residual lower limb flat when at rest. | This position will decrease the risk for hip flexion contracture. Other strategies to prevent contracture include assisting the patient to lie prone for 1 hour 4 times daily. |
| Provide instructions to the patient on the following prescribed exercises, which may include:<br><br>• Above-knee amputation (AKA): The patient attempts to straighten the hip from a flexed position against resistance or perform gluteal-setting exercises.<br><br>• Below-knee amputation: The patient attempts to straighten the knee against resistance or perform quadriceps exercises. The patient also should perform exercises for AKA. | These prescribed exercises increase the strength of muscle extensors. |

## Patient Problem/Analyze Cues/Prioritize Hypotheses

# Difficulty Coping

*due to* traumatic loss of limb

*Desired Outcome/Generate Solutions:* Within 72 hours after surgery, the patient begins to show adaptation to the loss of the limb and demonstrates interest in resuming role-related responsibilities.

| ASSESSMENT—RECOGNIZE CUES/ INTERVENTIONS—TAKE ACTION | RATIONALES |
|---|---|
| Assess the patient's current perception and acceptance of the amputation and residual limb. | The patient's current response to the residual limb will guide the nurse's interventions. |
| Assist the patient with coping and adapting to the loss of the limb while maintaining a sense of what is perceived as the normal self. | Strategies include introducing the patient to others who have successfully adapted to a similar amputation (e.g., through local or national support, such as Amputees in Motion). Teaching aids such as books, pamphlets, audiovisuals, and videotapes can be used to demonstrate how others have adapted to amputation. |
| Encourage the patient to look at and touch the residual limb and verbalize feelings about the amputation. Provide privacy for the patient and significant others to express feelings regarding the amputation. Show an accepting attitude and encourage significant others to accept the patient's new appearance. | The patient may have a stereotyped image of disability and unattractiveness after amputation. These emotions may be suppressed during rehabilitation but reemerge later. Addressing stereotypical thinking early in recovery and actively involving the patient in education will help provide a sense of participation and control. |
| Discuss ways the patient may alter task performance to continue to function in vocational and interpersonal roles. Assistive devices may be needed for continued functioning in the current vocational role. If the patient's health precludes continued performance in the current vocational role, referral and counseling for retraining may be needed. | This promotes independence. |
| Encourage the use of a prosthesis (if prescribed) as soon as possible after surgery. | Whether the amputation is the result of trauma, chronic illness, or cancer, the patient is likely to experience a period of grieving. Disbelief and anger often mark the initial response. The patient may believe attainment of independence and future goals is impossible. The early use of a prosthesis helps patients promptly return to mobility and resume typical activities. |
| For patients who continue to have difficulty coping with the amputation, provide a referral to a mental health professional such as an advanced practice psychiatric nurse or a psychologist. | Trained professionals can help explore the impact of amputation on the patient's life and review strategies for adaptation. |

## Patient Problem/Analyze Cues/Prioritize Hypotheses

# Deficient Knowledge (post op care of residual limb)

*due to* unfamiliarity with the care of the residual limb and prosthesis and signs and symptoms of skin irritation or pressure necrosis

*Desired Outcomes/Generate Solutions:* Within 24 hours of hospital discharge, the patient verbalizes knowledge about the care of the residual limb and prosthesis and correctly demonstrates how to wrap the residual limb. The patient verbalizes knowledge about indicators of pressure necrosis and irritation from the shrinkage device or prosthesis.

| ASSESSMENT—RECOGNIZE CUES/ INTERVENTIONS—TAKE ACTION | RATIONALES |
|---|---|
| Assess the patient's health literacy (language, reading, comprehension). Assess culturally specific information needs and current knowledge level. | This assessment helps ensure that educational materials are selected and presented in a manner that is culturally and educationally appropriate. |

**Instruct the Patient About the Following:**

| | |
|---|---|
| • For the first 24 hours after surgery, elevate the residual limb as prescribed. | Elevation reduces edema and pain. |
| • After this period, keep the residual lower limb flat when at rest in bed. | A flat position reduces the risk for hip flexion contracture. |
| • When seated, elevate the residual lower limb. | Elevating the residual lower limb reduces dependent edema when the patient is seated. |
| • Apply the prescribed shrinkage device such as an elastic wrap or sock. | A shrinkage device molds and prepares the residual limb for possible prosthesis fitting. Application of the elastic wrap is begun with a recurrent turn over the distal end of the residual limb; then diagonal circumferential turns are made, overlapping to two-thirds the width of the wrap. Wrapping in a circular pattern may compromise the blood supply to the residual limb. The shrinkage device should be wrapped snugly but not too tightly to avoid impeding circulation and healing. It should remain smooth and free of wrinkles to avoid causing skin breakdown or uneven shrinkage of the residual limb. |
| • Ensure that all tissue is contained by the elastic wrap. | The goal of wrapping is to form a cone-shaped residual limb. If any tissue is allowed to bulge, proper fitting of the prosthesis will be difficult. |
| • Perform rewrapping and careful inspection of the residual limb at least every 4–6 hours or as determined by the surgeon or agency protocol. Rewrapping may need to be done more often if the elastic wrap becomes loose. | Assessment of the limb at regular intervals will detect early skin impairment and allow intervention. |
| | Rewrapping also ensures that the elastic wrap remains snug enough to effectively mold the residual limb for the prosthesis. |
| • Use extra padding with moleskin or lamb's wool. | Extra padding prevents irritation to areas susceptible to pressure. |
| Teach the patient to monitor the residual limb for skin abrasions, blisters, hair follicle infection, or other impairments. | These findings indicate skin irritations or pressure necrosis caused by the shrinkage device or prosthesis. |
| Explain that if erythema persists after massage, the patient should notify the health care provider. | Persistent erythema may be an early sign of pressure ulcer development. |
| If prescribed, instruct the patient to leave any open areas on the residual limb exposed to air for 1-hour periods 4 times daily. Verify wound care preferences with the patient's surgeon. | Prolonged dressing of wounds can trap moisture that can contribute to wound maceration. Exposure to air allows the wound surface to dry naturally to facilitate healing. |
| Teach the daily routine of skin cleansing with soap and water. | Soap and water have adequate antibacterial effects. Washing also helps toughen skin on the residual limb in preparation for prosthesis use. Patients should be taught to avoid applying lotions, alcohol, powder, or oils unless prescribed because they can cause excessive wound dryness. |
| Instruct the patient to dry the residual limb thoroughly before any shrinkage device is applied. | Retained moisture can cause skin maceration, which would contribute to fungal growth. |
| Instruct the patient to change the shrinkage device daily, washing it with mild soap and water and drying it thoroughly before reapplication. | Use of a soiled shrinkage device can contribute to wound infection. |
| Instruct the patient to begin to massage the residual limb 3 weeks postoperatively. | Massage will break up adherent scar tissue and prepare the skin for the stress of prosthesis wear. |
| Ensure that the patient receives complete instructions in the care of the prosthesis by a nurse expert or certified prosthetist-orthotist. | Patients need to be encouraged to accept the residual limb and become adept at self-care in order to be independent as quickly as possible. |

## ADDITIONAL PROBLEMS:

| | |
|---|---|
| *Constipation*, due to decreased mobility and use of opioid analgesics | Chapter 69 |
| *Impaired Mobility*, due to musculoskeletal pain and unfamiliarity with the use of immobilization devices | Chapter 69 |

## PATIENT–FAMILY TEACHING AND DISCHARGE PLANNING

When providing patient–family teaching, focus on sensory information, avoid giving excessive information, and make appropriate referrals (e.g., visiting or home health nurse, community health resources) for follow-up teaching. Include verbal and written information about the following:

- ✓ Medications and supplements, including name, dosage, purpose, schedule, precautions, and potential side effects. Also discuss drug–drug, herb–drug, and food–drug interactions.
- ✓ How and where to purchase necessary supplies and equipment for self-care.
- ✓ Care of residual limb and prosthesis.
- ✓ Indicators of wound infection that require medical attention such as swelling, persistent redness, purulent discharge, local warmth, systemic fever, and pain. Suggest the use of a small hand mirror if needed to examine incision and residual limb.
- ✓ Prescribed exercise regimen, including rationale for each exercise, number of repetitions for each, and frequency of exercise periods.
- ✓ Ambulation with assistive devices and prosthesis on level and uneven surfaces and on stairs. The patient should demonstrate independence and achievement of physical therapy goals before hospital discharge. For the patient with upper extremity amputation, independence with the performance of activities of daily living should be demonstrated before discharge.
- ✓ Importance of follow-up care, date of next appointment, and a telephone number to call if questions arise.
- ✓ Referral to visiting, public health, or home health nurses as necessary for ongoing care after hospital discharge. Also consider referral to an appropriate resource person if the patient has continued difficulty with grief or body image disturbance.
- ✓ Referral to community resources, including local amputation support activities, and to Amputees in Motion at www.amputeesinmotion.org or Amputee Coalition at www.amputee-coalition.org.

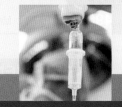

# Fractures 69

## OVERVIEW/PATHOPHYSIOLOGY

A fracture is a break in the continuity of a bone. It occurs when stress is placed on the bone that exceeds its biologic loading capacity. Most commonly, the stress is the result of trauma. Pathologic fractures can occur when the bone's decreased loading capacity cannot tolerate even normal stress, as with osteoporosis.

## HEALTH CARE SETTING

Emergency care, acute care, primary care

## ASSESSMENT

**Physical findings.** Include loss of normal bony or limb contours, edema, ecchymosis, limb shortening, decreased range of motion (ROM) of involved and adjacent joints, and false motion (occurs outside a joint). The patient may describe crepitus, but this should not be elicited by the health care provider because of the risk for injury to surrounding soft tissues. Complicated or complex fractures can present with signs and symptoms of perforated internal organs, neurovascular dysfunction, joint effusion, or excessive joint laxity. Open fractures involve a break in the skin and will exhibit a wound in the area of suspected fracture; bone may be exposed in the wound.

**Acute indicators.** Fractures cause either insidious and progressive pain or sudden onset of severe pain. They are usually associated with trauma or physical stress, such as jogging, strenuous exercise, or a fall. In the event of pathologic fracture, the patient typically describes signs and symptoms associated with the underlying pathology.

**Complications.** *Delayed union* is the failure of bone fragments to unite within the expected time frame based on factors such as the patient's age. Lack of any bony union is known as *nonunion*, which is demonstrated by nonalignment and lost function secondary to lost bony rigidity. *Pseudoarthrosis* is a state in which the fracture fails to heal, and a false joint develops at the fracture site. *Avascular necrosis* occurs when the fracture interrupts the blood supply to a segment of bone, causing eventual bone death. *Myositis ossificans* involves heterotrophic bone formation (abnormal, out of the normal area). It occurs most commonly in the arms, thighs, and hips. *Complex regional pain syndrome* (or reflex sympathetic dystrophy) is an incompletely understood process that results in pain out of proportion to the injury, with reduced function, joint stiffness, and trophic changes in soft tissue and skin following a traumatic event such as a fracture. Other fracture complications include altered sensation, limb-length discrepancies, and chronic lymphatic or venous stasis.

> **Note:** *Any patient with a suspected fracture should be treated as though a fracture is present until diagnosis is made. Interventions should include immobilization of the affected area and careful monitoring of neurovascular function distal to the injury. Any restrictions to swelling (e.g., rings, wristwatches, bracelets) should be removed before they can contribute to neurovascular dysfunction. Ice and elevation, if tolerated and appropriate based on the type of injury, can be used to decrease swelling.*

## DIAGNOSTIC TESTS

Most fractures are identified easily with standard anteroposterior and lateral radiographic examination. Occasionally special radiographic views are needed, such as the mortise view with bimalleolar ankle fractures (showing joint spaces between the fibula, tibia, and talus) or radiographic examination through the open mouth to identify fractures of the odontoid process. Magnetic resonance imaging may be useful in evaluating complicated fractures, but its ability to identify different bone densities is limited. Intraarticular fractures may be diagnosed with arthroscopy. Bone scans, computed tomography scans, tomograms, stereoscopic films, and arthrograms also can be used.

## Patient Problem/Analyze Cues/Prioritize Hypotheses

# Acute Pain

*due to* injury, surgical repair, and/or rehabilitation therapy

**Desired Outcomes/Generate Solutions:** Within 1–2 hours of intervention, the patient's subjective perception of pain decreases as indicated by a lower pain intensity rating. The patient demonstrates the ability to perform activities of daily living (ADLs) with minimal complaints of discomfort.

| ASSESSMENT—RECOGNIZE CUES/ INTERVENTIONS—TAKE ACTION | RATIONALES |
|---|---|
| Assess the patient's pain using an appropriate pain intensity rating scale, such as the visual analog scale, Wong–Baker FACES Pain Rating Scale, Faces Pain Scale—Revised, or FLACC (face, legs, activity, crying, consolability) scale. | The patient provides a personal baseline report, enabling the nurse to more effectively assess subsequent increases and decreases in pain. For the patient who is too young or unable to comprehend the quantitative scales, the nurse will use the FLACC scale based on observations. |
| If appropriate, instruct hospitalized surgical patients in the use of patient-controlled analgesia (PCA) or epidural analgesia. | Understanding the principles of PCA or epidural analgesia will help patients obtain better pain management. |
| If PCA or epidural analgesia is used, verify with another nurse per facility policy that the PCA or epidural pump contains the prescribed medication and concentration with prescribed settings for patient dosing, continuous infusion, and/or clinician-activated bolus. | Verification of the prescribed medication and pump settings is critical to the safe delivery of the analgesia. |
| Instruct the family/significant other that only the patient may administer a dose of analgesia from the PCA pump. | If the family administers medication by the PCA pump, the patient may experience negative effects from overmedication (e.g., excessive sedation). |
| If PCA or epidural analgesia is used, frequently assess patient's respirations and sedation scale as per the facility's policy.  Administer an opioid antagonist such as Naloxone to reverse respiratory depression as per facility policy. | Intravenous (IV) opioids may cause oversedation and respiratory depression, which may be life threatening. If respiratory depression occurs, an administration of an opioid antagonist will reverse the opioid effects. |
| Assist the patient with coordinating the time of peak effectiveness of analgesics with periods of exercise or ambulation. | Careful timing of analgesics enables the patient to achieve optimal pain management before exercise or ambulation. Participation in the exercise regimen (e.g., physical therapy) contributes to the expediency of recovery. |
| As prescribed, administer the nonsteroidal antiinflammatory drugs (NSAIDs) and assess the effectiveness of the patient's pain management as well as adverse effects. | Because of the potential for excessive bleeding after NSAID administration, it is important to monitor for hemorrhage at the surgical site. |
| • Do not administer low-molecular-weight heparin (LMWH) to a patient who has an indwelling epidural catheter | Although anticoagulants are commonly prescribed after orthopedic surgery, LMWH must not be administered if the patient has an indwelling epidural catheter as it can cause an epidural hematoma. LMWH can be given 2 hours after the epidural catheter has been removed. |
| Use the nonpharmacologic pain management methods, such as guided imagery, relaxation, massage, distraction, biofeedback, cold therapy, and music therapy. Traditional nursing interventions such as back rubs and repositioning also should be included in the pain management plan of care. | Nonpharmacologic methods can augment pharmacologic pain management strategies. These methods may be indicated for a patient who avoids the use of analgesics or experiences minimal pain management with prescribed analgesics. |
| If an intraarticular anesthetic or opioid was administered intraoperatively, advise the patient that lack of pain in the immediate postoperative period should *not* be mistaken for the ability to move the joint excessively. | Patients with minimal postoperative pain may be tempted to increase activity, putting unnecessary stress on the fracture site. Prescribed activity and weight-bearing status must be carefully followed to avoid additional injury to the affected extremity. |

## Patient Problem/Analyze Cues/Prioritize Hypotheses

# Risk for Injury (Compartment Syndrome)

*due to* the interruption of capillary blood flow occurring with increased pressure within the myofascial compartment

***Desired Outcomes/Generate Solutions:*** The patient has an adequate peripheral neurovascular function in the involved extremity, as evidenced by normal muscle tone, brisk capillary refill (less than 2 seconds or consistent with the contralateral extremity), normal tissue pressures (15 mm Hg or less, as determined by the invasive diagnostic procedure), minimal edema or tautness, and absence of paresthesia. The patient verbalizes the understanding of the importance of reporting symptoms indicative of impaired neurovascular function.

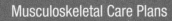

| ASSESSMENT—RECOGNIZE CUES/ INTERVENTIONS—TAKE ACTION | RATIONALES |
|---|---|
| ⚠ Assess the patient's pain at regular intervals as defined by the health care provider or agency policy, immediately informing the provider of increased pain or pain not managed by analgesia. | Increased or unrelenting pain, or pain out of proportion to the injury, often is the first sign of developing compartment syndrome. |
| ⚠ Assess the tissue pressures in all compartments as prescribed if an intracompartmental pressure device is available. | Continued assessment of high-risk patients (e.g., adolescents or young adults with traumatic injury; confused or developmentally disabled patients who cannot accurately report symptoms) should be done to avoid possible complications. The site of fracture or repair (e.g., high tibial osteotomy) also can increase the risk for developing compartment syndrome. |
| ⚠ Alert the health care provider to pressures higher than 10 mm Hg. | Sustained high pressures may indicate developing compartment syndrome; if pressures exceed systolic blood pressure, perfusion to the extremity is threatened. |
| ⚠ Assess the neurovascular status at regular intervals by checking temperature (circulation), movement, and sensation in the affected extremity. | Paresthesia (second "P"), pallor (third "P"), and poikilothermia (coolness due to diminished blood flow to distal tissues) (fourth "P") are additional signs of a developing compartment syndrome. True paralysis or pulselessness (fifth "P") is a late sign of compartment syndrome, which indicates significant ischemia/limb impairment. |
| Apply ice and elevate the affected extremity when prescribed. | A fractured limb is typically elevated for the first 24 hours to decrease swelling. Ice is applied to cause vasoconstriction in the area of injury, which decreases edema and aids in pain management. Because edema can contribute to the development of compartment syndrome, these early interventions may be critical. |
| ⚠ When acute compartment syndrome is suspected, avoid the use of ice and elevation. | Ice and elevation may further compromise vascular supply in an extremity that is already experiencing ischemia secondary to developing compartment syndrome. |
| ⚠ In response to changes in the neurovascular condition, contact the health care provider promptly. Adjust the constricting device as prescribed (e.g., loosen elastic wrap around a splint or bivalved cast). Wrap dressing around a split cast. | When swelling places, patients at risk for compartment syndrome, the constricting device (e.g., cast, splint, circumferential dressing) must be loosened down to skin level to prevent further swelling and compromise to the affected extremity. Wrapping a dressing around a split cast aids in the continued immobilization of fracture fragments. |
| Instruct the patient and significant others about symptoms of neurovascular compromise that should be reported immediately (e.g., changes in temperature, sensation, color, or ability to move digits of the affected extremity). | Awareness of the risk for compartment syndrome will enable the patient to respond more quickly to possible symptoms and reduce a delay in treatment. |

## Patient Problem/Analyze Cues/Prioritize Hypotheses

# Impaired Mobility

*due to* musculoskeletal pain and unfamiliarity with the use of immobilization devices

***Desired Outcomes/Generate Solutions:*** By at least 24 hours before hospital discharge, the patient maintains appropriate body alignment with external fixation devices in place or demonstrates appropriate use of a home traction device. The patient uses mobility aids safely. The patient verbalizes the understanding of the use of analgesics and adjunctive methods to decrease pain.

| ASSESSMENT—RECOGNIZE CUES/ INTERVENTIONS—TAKE ACTION | RATIONALES |
|---|---|
| Assess the patient's health literacy (language, reading, comprehension). Assess the culturally specific information needs. | This assessment helps ensure that materials are selected and presented in a manner that is culturally and educationally appropriate. |
| Provide instructions on proper body alignment, most commonly with joints in neutral position if an external fixation device has been applied. | Maintenance of a neutral position decreases the risk for contracture formation, which would affect the patient's mobility. |
| If orthotic devices are used to maintain position, teach exercises and ROM to do when the device is removed. | Prolonged use of the orthotic can cause impaired joint mobility. Exercise at regular intervals will help maintain joint flexibility. |
| Instruct the patient and significant others to perform active and/or passive ROM exercises of adjacent joints every 8 hours as appropriate. | ROM exercises help preserve joint mobility and decrease the risk for contracture formation. |
| When appropriate, instruct the patient and significant others in care of an extremity in traction, including signs and symptoms of complications (e.g., skin impairment from unrelieved pressure, impaired neurovascular function, and pin site infection for skeletal traction). | Knowledge will help ensure optimal healing and prompt treatment in case of complications. |
| Instruct the patient and significant others in care of an extremity in external fixator, performance of prescribed exercises while in the fixator, and signs and symptoms of complications (see the previous intervention). | Knowledge will help ensure optimal healing and prompt treatment in case of complications. |
| Instruct the patient and significant others in care of the casted extremity and in signs and symptoms of complications (e.g., skin maceration, impaired neurovascular function). | A knowledgeable patient should be able to demonstrate cast care, describe the neurovascular assessment of the distal extremity, describe the assessment of the evidence of unrelieved pressure beneath the cast, demonstrate the performance of prescribed exercises, and describe the prevention of skin maceration to ensure optimal healing and prompt treatment in case of problems. |
| Instruct the patient in use of crutches, walker, cane, or other mobility aids. | Safe use enables early mobilization and decreases risk for additional injury. |
| Instruct the patient and significant others in use of analgesics and nonpharmacologic pain management methods. | Effective pain management will increase the patient's ability to participate in appropriate exercise and activity. |

## Patient Problem/Analyze Cues/Prioritize Hypotheses

# Risk for Impaired Skin and Tissue Integrity

*due to* irritation and pressure with an immobilization device (e.g., cast, splint)

**Desired Outcomes/Generate Solutions:** Within 8 hours of immobilization device application, the patient verbalizes knowledge about indicators of unrelieved pressure. The patient relates the absence of discomfort under the immobilization device and exhibits intact skin when the device is removed.

| ASSESSMENT—RECOGNIZE CUES/ INTERVENTIONS—TAKE ACTION | RATIONALES |
|---|---|
| When assisting with the application of a cast or other immobilization device, ensure adequate padding is applied over bony prominences of the affected extremity. | Bony prominences are at risk for skin breakdown. Padding decreases pressure over these areas. |
| Handle a drying cast only with palms of the hands. | Handling a wet cast with fingers can cause indentations that create pressure points on underlying skin. Using palms of the hands ensures a smooth surface as the cast dries and decreases the likelihood of underlying pressure points. |

| ASSESSMENT—RECOGNIZE CUES/ INTERVENTIONS—TAKE ACTION | RATIONALES |
|---|---|
| Ensure that all cast surfaces are alternately exposed to air. | Exposure to air facilitates drying of the cast. |
| Petal edges of plaster casts with tape or moleskin if a cast liner was not applied. | Petaling prevents rough cast edges from causing skin irritation/impairment. It also prevents cast crumbs from falling into the cast and causing pressure areas with additional skin irritation/impairment. |
| Pad surfaces of other immobilization devices as well. | Padding decreases pressure on skin underneath the devices. |
| Instruct the patient never to insert anything between the immobilization device and skin. | Foreign objects inserted into the cast may cause skin irritation that leads to infection. It also may cause bunching of the cotton material placed between the cast and skin, which would result in pressure points under the cast. |
| Advise the patient to notify the health care provider of severe itching. | The health care provider may prescribe a medication to relieve itching. Scratching the unaffected side in a similar location also may provide relief. |
| Instruct the patient and significant others about indicators of unrelieved pressure under the immobilization device, such as pain, burning sensation, foul odor from the opening, or drainage on the device. | An informed individual is more likely to report these findings quickly, which will enable prompt treatment to avoid further impairment. |

## Patient Problem/Analyze Cues/Prioritize Hypotheses

# Constipation

*due to* decreased mobility and the use of opioid analgesic

**Desired Outcomes/Generate Solutions:** Within 8 hours of immobilization device application, the patient verbalizes understanding of strategies to maintain normal bowel elimination. The patient maintains bowel elimination in his or her baseline pattern.

| ASSESSMENT—RECOGNIZE CUES/ INTERVENTIONS—TAKE ACTION | RATIONALES |
|---|---|
| Assess the patient's usual bowel pattern and habits to ensure regular elimination. | Use of proven strategies will help the patient more quickly regain the usual bowel elimination pattern. |
| Encourage the choice of diet items that will facilitate normal bowel elimination. | High-fiber foods (e.g., bran, whole grains, nuts, raw and coarse vegetables, fruits with skins) add bulk to stool to promote bowel elimination. |
| If not contraindicated, encourage the patient to drink adequate fluids. | Fluid intake helps promote soft stool for easier elimination. |
| If the patient desires, request a prescription for stool softener and/or laxative. Reassess the bowel elimination for response to medication and initiate additional treatment as needed to return normal bowel function. | Pharmacologic intervention may be needed to maintain normal bowel elimination. |
| If a stool softener or laxative is ineffective, the patient may require a rectal suppository or enema administration to facilitate elimination. | |
| Encourage the mobility to the extent of the prescribed activity parameters. | Mobility promotes peristalsis and hence improves bowel elimination. The patient thus should not be left in bed or allowed to use a bedside commode if additional mobility can be tolerated. |
| As indicated, identify with patient their current risks for constipation. | Decreased mobility, use of opioid analgesics, and inconsistent food intake can adversely influence bowel elimination. |

Patient Problem/Analyze Cues/Prioritize Hypotheses

# Impaired Functional Ability

*due to* physical limitations present with a cast, immobilizer, or orthotic devices that affect self-care

**Desired Outcome/Generate Solutions:** Within 48 hours of initiation of immobilization, the patient demonstrates the optimal performance of ADLs.

| ASSESSMENT—RECOGNIZE CUES/ INTERVENTIONS—TAKE ACTION | RATIONALES |
|---|---|
| Assess the patient's self-care limitations. | Thorough assessment enables the implementation of appropriate self-care strategies. |
| Ensure that the patient receives the prescribed treatment for pain. | Unmanaged pain can severely limit attempts to mobilize, making performance of self-care tasks difficult or impossible. |
| Incorporate a structured exercise regimen that will increase strength and endurance. Direct the regimen toward the development of muscle groups needed for the patient's specific activity deficit. | A patient with insufficient strength to manipulate immobilized extremities needs planned exercise to assist in managing self-care while in a cast or immobilizer. Increased strength and endurance contribute to independence in self-care. |
| As indicated, refer the patient to occupational therapy and reinforce the correct use of assistive devices and dressing/grooming aids as needed. | Use of appropriate assistive devices maximizes self-care ability. Sock donners, long-handled reachers and brushes, raised toilet seats, and other devices minimize stress on joints. Clothing also can be adapted for greater ease in dressing (e.g., zipper pulls, Velcro closures); adaptive clothing also accommodates a cast or external fixator. |
| When needed, instruct significant others on how to assist the patient with self-care activities. | Although independence with self-care is the goal, the involvement of the significant other can minimize the need for skilled home services. A knowledgeable significant other also can reinforce professional health instructions given to the patient. |
| If indicated, refer patient to care management/social services department of the hospital. | The patient may require assistance with funding for assistive equipment or home help. Care management/social services staff also can identify community agencies that loan equipment or have other volunteer services. |

Patient Problem/Analyze Cues/Prioritize Hypotheses

# Deficient Knowledge

*due to* unfamiliarity with the function of the external fixation, the performance of pin care, and the signs and symptoms of pin site infection

**Desired Outcomes/Generate Solutions:** By at least 24 hours before hospital discharge, the patient verbalizes knowledge of the rationale for the external fixator and indicators of pin site infection. The patient or significant other demonstrates the performance of pin care.

| ASSESSMENT—RECOGNIZE CUES/ INTERVENTIONS—TAKE ACTION | RATIONALES |
|---|---|
| Assess the patient's health care literacy (language, reading, comprehension). Assess culturally specific information needs and the current knowledge level. | This assessment helps ensure educational materials are selected and presented in a manner that is culturally and educationally appropriate. |

| ASSESSMENT—RECOGNIZE CUES/ INTERVENTIONS—TAKE ACTION | RATIONALES |
|---|---|
| Describe to the patient the rationale for use of the fixator with the type of fracture or injury, emphasizing patient benefits: external fixation consists of skeletal pins that penetrate the fracture fragments and are attached to universal joints. These joints are in turn attached to rods, which provide stabilization and form a frame around the fractured limb for immobilization. | A patient who is knowledgeable about the device and its purpose is more likely to care for the device judiciously to ensure bone fragment immobilization. |
| Provide instructions to the patient and significant others for appropriate handling and care of the external fixator. | Although some fixation devices can be used safely as a handle to lift the limb, this activity is contraindicated with other devices because it may lead to loosening of skeletal pins and loss of bone fragment immobilization. Awareness of care requirements for the patient's specific type of fixation device is critical. |
| Instruct the patient and significant others to support the extremity with pillows, two hands, slings, and other devices as necessary. | Adequate support of the extremity prevents stress on skeletal pins. Stress on pins can contribute to loosening and loss of bone fragment immobilization. |
| Instruct the patient and significant others in pin care as prescribed by the health care provider. | A knowledgeable patient and significant other will more likely be able to properly care for their injury. |
| For external fixator pins, some health care providers require daily cleansing; chlorhexidine is the most commonly used skin preparation solution, although some health care providers may recommend dilute hydrogen peroxide. Iodine-based mixtures may cause corrosion of some fixation devices and interfere with pin site assessment. Antibacterial ointments and small dressings also may be prescribed for pin sites. | |
| Instruct the patient and significant others to identify possible indicators of infection at pin sites, including persistent redness, swelling, drainage, increasing pain, local warmth, and body temperature greater than 100.4°F (38°C). Instruct the patient to report abnormal findings immediately to the health care provider. | The patient and significant others must recognize signs of infection and report them to the health care provider for prompt assessment and treatment. |
| If an orthotic device is used, ensure that the patient and significant others are aware of its purpose and able to identify areas of excessive pressure and follow the prescribed schedule for adjunctive/ROM exercises. | Devices should be kept clean and dry to decrease the risk for infection at pin sites. |
| Orthotics may be added to the external fixator to prevent wristdrop, footdrop, contracture, or other joint dysfunction. | |
| Advise the patient of the need for maintaining adequate fracture immobilization and scheduling follow-up care. | Failure to immobilize the fracture adequately may lead to delayed union, malunion, or nonunion. Adherence to the weight-bearing prescription for lower extremities and follow-up assessment of the device will ensure fracture immobilization is maintained. |

## ✔ PATIENT–FAMILY TEACHING AND DISCHARGE PLANNING

When providing patient–family teaching, focus on sensory information, avoid giving excessive information, and make appropriate referrals (e.g., visiting or home health nurse, community health resources) for follow-up teaching. Include verbal and written information about the following:

✓ Medications and supplements, including name, dosage, purpose, schedule, precautions, and potential side effects. Also discuss drug–drug, herb–drug, and food–drug interactions.

✓ Use of nonpharmacologic methods of pain management.

✓ Appropriate use of elevation and thermotherapy.

✓ Importance of performing prescribed exercises.

✓ Rationale for therapy (i.e., casting, external fixation, internal fixation).

✓ Precautions of therapy.

✓ *Casts:* Caring for the cast, monitoring neurovascular function of distal extremity, identifying evidence of unrelieved pressure beneath cast, signs of infection, and preventing skin maceration.

✓ *Internal fixation devices:* Caring for the wound, noting signs of wound infection, following appropriate weight-bearing prescription for lower extremity fracture.

✓ *External fixator:* Demonstrating pin care, identifying evidence of pin site infection, knowing when to notify the health care provider of problems with the fixator, using prescribed orthotics, monitoring neurovascular function of the distal extremity.

✓ Use of assistive devices/ambulatory aids. Ensure the patient can perform return demonstration and is independent with devices/aids before hospital discharge.

✓ Materials necessary for wound care at home, with names of agencies that can provide additional supplies.

✓ Importance of follow-up care, date of next appointment, and telephone number to call if questions arise.

✓ For all patients who receive allograft bone for bone graft and who have questions about these grafts, resources for information include the following organizations:

- American Red Cross: www.redcross.org
- AlloSource: www.allosource.org

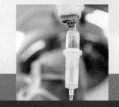

# Joint Replacement Surgery 70

## OVERVIEW/PATHOPHYSIOLOGY

### Total hip arthroplasty

Surgery to repair a hip fracture is the standard of care. The type of surgical intervention depends on the location and severity of the fracture and the patient's age. There are four types of hip fracture repair surgeries: (1) closed reduction with percutaneous pinning, this type of surgery is minimally invasive and is done to stabilize the femoral neck and head with screws; (2) repair with internal fixation devices (screws or other hardware); (3) replacement of the femoral head with a prosthesis; and (4) total hip arthroplasty (THA). THA involves surgical resection of the hip joint and its replacement with an endoprosthesis. THA may be necessary for conditions such as osteoarthritis, rheumatoid arthritis, Legg–Calvé–Perthes disease, avascular necrosis, hip fracture, developmental hip dysplasia, and benign or malignant bone tumors. Because conservative treatments usually fail to decrease the impact of disease on the patient's functional ability, surgery becomes the next intervention. Arthroscopy, osteotomy, excision, hip-resurfacing arthroplasty, or arthrodesis (joint fusion) may be considered before the patient and surgeon choose THA.

Historically, THA has been restricted to older patients because the life of the implant has been traditionally estimated at 20 years. However, younger patients with severe disease are now undergoing this procedure. Advanced age is not an absolute contraindication for THA because poor surgical outcomes appear to be related more to comorbidities than to aging alone. Contraindications to surgery include recent or active joint sepsis, arterial impairment, deficit to the extremity, or neuropathic joint. The individual's inability to cooperate in postoperative interventions and rehabilitation may also be a relative contraindication.

With THA, both femoral and acetabular components will be replaced. A typical prosthesis design includes a polyethylene-lined metal cup that fits over a metal femoral component. Metal-on-metal, ceramic-on-polyethylene, and ceramic-on-ceramic components are also used. The ceramic-on-ceramic components show very little wear and have minimal particle debris, thus extending the life of the hip arthroplasty. Components may be secured in place with cement (polymethylmethacrylate), or noncemented components with porous or roughened surfaces may be chosen to enable bony ingrowth. Because cemented components typically allow early weight bearing, they may be ideal for the patient whose activities do not place great demand on the joint but who would benefit from early mobility. The noncemented arthroplasty requires early weight-bearing restriction but accepts more strenuous activity after bony ingrowth is complete.

Early complications of infection, breakage, and loosening now occur less commonly because of improved surgical techniques and prosthetics. Infection risk has been substantially decreased with the administration of prophylactic antibiotics and improved perioperative protocols. However, potential complications still include dislocation and aseptic loosening of components. The patient is also at risk for venous thromboembolism (VTE).

### Total knee arthroplasty

When there is severe deterioration and instability of the knee joint, a total knee arthroplasty (TKA) may be done. TKA involves surgical resection of the knee joint and its replacement with an endoprosthesis. TKA may be necessary for conditions such as osteoarthritis, rheumatoid arthritis, gouty arthritis, hemophilic arthritis, osteochondritis dissecans, and severe knee trauma. Because conservative treatments have failed to decrease the impact of disease on functional ability in most patients, surgery is the next intervention. Viscosupplementation treatment injections, arthroscopy, osteotomy, unicompartmental arthroplasty, arthrodesis (joint fusion), or use of a joint spacer may be considered before the patient and surgeon choose TKA.

Contraindications to surgery include recent or active sepsis in the joint, arterial impairment or deficit in the extremity, and neuropathic joint. The individual's inability to cooperate in postoperative interventions and rehabilitation may also be a relative contraindication. Postoperative risk for VTE is addressed by hydration, early ambulation, and anticoagulant medications. The risk for dislocation is minimal, but component loosening is a long-term complication that may necessitate revision arthroplasty.

## HEALTH CARE SETTING

Acute care surgical unit; rehabilitation unit

## DIAGNOSTIC TESTS

Various tests are combined with patient history and physical findings to confirm the presence of conditions that necessitate joint replacement. Radiographic examination is commonly required.

Patient Problem/Analyze Cues/Prioritize Hypotheses

# Risk for Injury

*due to* interrupted arterial blood flow occurring with compression from the abduction pillow after THA and edema or use of a bulky postoperative dressing after TKA

**Desired Outcomes/Generate Solutions:** The patient maintains adequate peripheral neurovascular function distal to the operative site, as evidenced by warmth, appropriate color for race, capillary refill less than 2 seconds, and ability to dorsiflex/plantar flex the foot and feel sensations. The patient verbalizes the understanding of the potential peripheral neurovascular complications and the importance of promptly reporting signs of impairment.

| ASSESSMENT—RECOGNIZE CUES/ INTERVENTIONS—TAKE ACTION | RATIONALES |
|---|---|
| Assess the neurovascular function of the operative leg at regular intervals as prescribed by the surgeon or in accordance with hospital policy. Compare to the contralateral (nonoperative) leg and preoperative baseline assessment. Notify the health care provider of abnormal findings. | Pressure from the abductor pillow (THA) or a bulky knee dressing (TKA) can interrupt arterial blood flow and compress the peroneal and tibial nerves. These nerves provide movement and sensation to the calf and foot muscles. Loss of sensation or movement signals impaired nerve function and must be reported promptly to the health care provider. |
| Apply cold therapy as prescribed at the operative site. | Swelling increases intracompartmental pressure in the lower leg, potentially interrupting arterial blood flow and compromising nerve function. Ice application is an important early intervention to decrease swelling. |
| Provide the patient with information about the risk for neurovascular impairment and the importance of promptly reporting alterations in sensation, strength, movement, temperature, and color of the operative extremity. | These findings indicate impaired nerve function. Nerve damage can lead to severe disability with footdrop and paresthesia. The patient's knowledge of signs of impairment leads to prompt reporting, enabling health care providers to initiate appropriate, timely treatment. |
| Instruct the patient to perform the prescribed exercises (e.g., ankle pumps, heel slides) at regular intervals (e.g., 4 times an hour while awake). | Exercises stimulate circulation to the distal extremity and decrease the risk for neurovascular dysfunction. |

Patient Problem/Analyze Cues/Prioritize Hypotheses

# Risk for Inadequate Tissue Perfusion

*due to* the development of VTE

**Desired Outcome/Generate Solutions:** The patient exhibits adequate tissue perfusion in the lower extremities, as evidenced by maintenance of normal skin temperature and absence of calf pain and/or swelling.

| ASSESSMENT—RECOGNIZE CUES/ INTERVENTIONS—TAKE ACTION | RATIONALES |
|---|---|
| Assess for and promptly report to the health care provider the patient's complaints of swelling, warmth, or pain/tenderness along the vein tracts in the lower extremities. | Close monitoring for these signs of thrombosis is imperative to ensure timely treatment. The patient's awareness of indicators also contributes to the early identification and treatment of potential thrombotic complications. |
| Encourage the patient to perform ankle pumps/heel slides at regular intervals. | These exercises cause calf muscle contraction. Muscle contraction increases blood return to the heart and decreases the risk for thrombus development. |

| ASSESSMENT—RECOGNIZE CUES/ INTERVENTIONS—TAKE ACTION | RATIONALES |
|---|---|
| Maintain antiembolic stockings, intermittent pneumatic compression devices, or venous foot pump compression devices whenever the patient is in bed or chair. | These devices compress leg muscles and promote blood return to the heart, decreasing the risk for thrombus development. |
| Remove compression devices when the patient ambulates. | Attempting to ambulate without removing compression devices increases the risk for the patient falling. |
| Encourage the patient to perform other prescribed exercises and participate fully in the physical therapy (PT) program. | Early mobilization decreases the risk for thrombus formation. |
| Unless contraindicated, encourage the fluid intake to maintain adequate hydration. Maintain intravenous fluids as prescribed. | Dehydration contributes to the development of sluggish blood flow and blood clots. Adequate hydration will decrease VTE risk. |
| Instruct the patient regarding the use of anticoagulants and other VTE prevention modalities. | Because of the increased risk for VTE with joint replacement surgery, the surgeon will prescribe anticoagulant therapy. In addition, passive prevention strategies (e.g., sequential compression device) may be implemented. |
| Administer the anticoagulants as prescribed and review results of relevant blood tests, ensuring that the health care provider has been informed of laboratory results. | Anticoagulants will increase coagulation times and may alter other blood levels such as platelet counts. It is important to assess coagulation times to ensure therapeutic levels in those patients who are receiving meds that affect blood levels. Since some anticoagulants lower platelet counts, it is important to monitor levels so that the provider is notified if levels become abnormal. |
| | Review *Risk for Hemorrhaging* in "Pulmonary Embolus," Chapter 15. |

## Patient Problem/Analyze Cues/Prioritize Hypotheses

# Risk for Hemorrhaging

*due to* joint arthroplasty surgery

***Desired Outcome/Generate Solutions:*** Within 24 hours of surgery, the patient is free of symptoms of excessive bleeding or hematoma formation, as evidenced by maintenance of heart rate, respiratory rate, and blood pressure (BP) within the patient's baseline range; balanced intake and output; output from wound drain of 10 mL/hour or less; brisk capillary refill (less than 2 seconds or consistent with preoperative assessment); peripheral pulses 2+ or more on 0–4+ scale; and warmth and normal color in the operative extremity distal to the surgical site.

| ASSESSMENT—RECOGNIZE CUES/ INTERVENTIONS—TAKE ACTION | RATIONALES |
|---|---|
| When assessing vital signs (VS), also assess drainage from the wound drainage system and/or on the surgical dressing. Promptly report to the health care provider output from the drainage system that exceeds 50 mL/hour or a dressing that is more than 50% saturated. | During wound closure, it is possible that a bleeding vessel may be overlooked or that bleeding will begin later during the patient's recovery. Careful assessment of wound drainage will detect excessive output. |
| Assess the patient's VS, subjective complaints, and neurovascular function. Report abnormal findings. | Patient complaints of warmth beneath the dressing, sensation of "things crawling" under the dressing, increasing pressure or pain, or coolness distal to the area of surgery can occur with hemorrhage or hematoma formation. |
| Reassess the VS at regular intervals as determined by the surgeon's directive or agency policy for hypotension and increasing pulse rate. | These signs suggest shock or hemorrhage. |
| Assess for pallor, decreased peripheral pulses, slowed capillary refill, or coolness of the distal extremity. | These signs can occur with hemorrhage or hematoma formation. |

Continued

| ASSESSMENT—RECOGNIZE CUES/ INTERVENTIONS—TAKE ACTION | RATIONALES |
|---|---|
| • If hemorrhage or hematoma formation is suspected, notify the health care provider promptly for intervention. | These interventions are done to control bleeding. |
| • Interventions may include limb elevation or application of an elastic wrap or compression dressing to provide direct pressure on the site of bleeding | |
| If the patient's VS suggest shock related to suspected hemorrhage or hematoma formation and the health care provider is unavailable, expose the surgical area by loosening the dressing. | This allows direct inspection of and pressure application to the area. Compression will usually control hemorrhage; if not, a thigh-high BP cuff over sheet wadding will serve as a tourniquet until the health care provider arrives for definitive therapy. |

## Patient Problem/Analyze Cues/Prioritize Hypotheses

# Impaired Mobility

*due to* postoperative musculoskeletal pain and immobilization devices

**Desired Outcomes/Generate Solutions:** By at least 24 hours before hospital discharge, the patient demonstrates appropriate use of ambulatory aids. The patient verbalizes understanding of the use of analgesics and adjunctive methods to decrease pain when performing prescribed exercises or activities.

| ASSESSMENT—RECOGNIZE CUES/ INTERVENTIONS—TAKE ACTION | RATIONALES |
|---|---|
| Assess the patient's health literacy (language, reading, comprehension). Assess the culturally specific information needs and current knowledge level. | This assessment helps ensure materials are selected and presented in a manner that is culturally and educationally appropriate. |
| Reinforce the instructions by the physical therapist on the use and care of ambulatory aids such as a walker or crutches. Include the use of the ambulatory aid on stairs or in other situations the patient may experience at home after discharge. | Patients need to be aware of equipment maintenance and techniques for safe use to avoid injury. |
| Reinforce the instructions by the physical therapist on exercises that improve muscle strength and increase joint flexibility. | Improved muscle strength and joint flexibility contribute to earlier mobilization and safe use of ambulatory aids. Exercises for both lower extremities and upper extremities should be included in the prescribed regimen. |
| Instruct the patient and significant others in the use of analgesics and nonpharmacologic pain management methods. | Effective pain management will enable patients to become mobile more quickly, decreasing the risk for complications associated with impaired physical mobility. |

## Patient Problem/Analyze Cues/Prioritize Hypotheses

# Deficient Knowledge (patients undergoing the posterolateral approach to THA)

*due to* unfamiliarity with appropriate activity precautions to decrease the risk for dislocation of the operative hip

**Desired Outcome/Generate Solutions:** At least 24 hours before hospital discharge, the patient verbalizes knowledge about the potential for dislocation of the operative hip and activity precautions that decrease the risk for dislocation.

| ASSESSMENT—RECOGNIZE CUES/ INTERVENTIONS—TAKE ACTION | RATIONALES |
|---|---|
| Assess the patient's health literacy (language, reading, comprehension). Assess culturally specific information needs and current knowledge level. | This assessment helps ensure materials are selected and presented in a manner that is culturally and educationally appropriate. |
| During preoperative instruction, advise the patient of the potential for postoperative dislocation. | Risk for dislocation remains high until the periarticular tissues heal around the endoprosthesis (approximately 6 weeks). If dislocation occurs once, the potential for recurrence is increased because of stretching of periarticular tissues. A confirmed dislocation is initially treated with closed reduction using conscious sedation (procedural sedation). Recurrent dislocations may require revision arthroplasty or surgery to tighten periarticular tissues. A knowledgeable patient is more likely to understand the rationale for and adhere to activity and positional restrictions. |
| Show the patient an endoprosthesis and describe how it can be dislocated when positional restrictions are not followed (i.e., flexion of the hip past 90 degrees, internal rotation, or adduction). | Seeing how certain positions result in dislocation will help patients understand the need for and to adhere to positional restrictions. |
| During preoperative instruction, explain and demonstrate the use of ambulatory aids and assistive devices for activities of daily living (ADLs) that enable independence without violating positional restrictions. | Preoperative introduction to ambulatory aids and ADL assistive devices enables patients to become familiar with the devices and techniques for use. This instruction is critical if outpatient (ambulatory) surgery is expected. |
| After surgery, reinforce positional restrictions and discuss activities that may violate restrictions, including pivoting on the operative leg, sitting on a toilet seat of regular height, bending over to tie shoelaces, or crossing legs. | After THA using the posterolateral approach, the patient may use an abduction wedge to prevent internal rotation and keep the hip from crossing the midline (i.e., maintain abducted position). Avoidance of flexion past 90 degrees also is required to decrease risk for dislocation. |
| Reinforce the need to get out of bed on the affected side. | Getting out of bed on the affected side decreases the risk for dislocation by keeping the patient from crossing the legs. |
| Confirm the patient's need for assistive devices for use at home after discharge. Refer patient to occupational therapy for assistive device access and instructions to perform activities of daily living. Refer the patient to the case manager or provide contact information for medical equipment suppliers that sell these items. Ensure the patient verbalizes understanding of the use of these devices, demonstrates positional restrictions and muscle-strengthening exercises, and can perform ADLs independently using appropriate assistive devices. | Self-care tasks such as dressing, bathing, and toileting may require the use of assistive devices such as a long-handled reacher and sock donner. Patients with posterior precautions may need bathroom equipment such as an elevated toilet seat. PT generally includes a program of muscle-strengthening exercises and gait training with a walker or crutches to maximize mobility. Exercises also target the upper extremities because their weakness can make it difficult to use a walker or crutches. |
| Instruct the patient to report pain in the hip, buttock, or thigh, or prolonged limp. | These symptoms may indicate prosthesis loosening. |

### Problem/Analyze Cues/Prioritize Hypotheses

# Deficient Knowledge (TKA postoperative care)

*due to* unfamiliarity with prescribed exercises for the involved extremity following TKA

***Desired Outcome/Generate Solutions:*** Within 30 minutes of instruction, the patient demonstrates and verbalizes understanding of prescribed exercises.

| ASSESSMENT—RECOGNIZE CUES/ INTERVENTIONS—TAKE ACTION | RATIONALES |
|---|---|
| Assess the patient's health literacy (language, reading, comprehension). Assess the culturally specific information needs. | This assessment helps ensure materials are selected and presented in a manner that is culturally and educationally appropriate. |
| Reinforce the instructions for the muscle-strengthening and joint range-of-motion exercise regimen. Reinforce the written instructions that describe the exercises, listing frequency and number of repetitions for each one. | Prescribed exercises will facilitate the return of normal joint function and reinforce gains in joint mobility. An effective method is to teach the appropriate exercise, demonstrate it, and then have patients return the demonstration. |
| Maintain a compression dressing or knee immobilizer if prescribed. | These devices are used to immobilize the knee in extension at rest and can also be used during ambulation. |
| Administer the analgesia before exercise. | Effective pain control is key for patient mobility. |

## ADDITIONAL PROBLEMS:

| | |
|---|---|
| *Acute Pain*, due to injury, surgical repair, and/or rehabilitation therapy | Chapter 69 |
| *Low Self-Esteem*, due to pain, decreased joint function, or body image changes that interfere with sexual performance | Chapter 71 |

 **PATIENT–FAMILY TEACHING AND DISCHARGE PLANNING**

When providing patient–family teaching, focus on sensory information, avoid giving excessive information, and make appropriate referrals (e.g., visiting or home health nurse, community health resources, case manager) for follow-up teaching. Include verbal and written information about the following:
- ✓ Medications and supplements, including name, dosage, purpose, schedule, precautions, and potential side effects. Also discuss drug–drug, herb–drug, and food–drug interactions.
- ✓ Any precautions related to wound care and signs of infection (e.g., persistent redness or pain, swelling or localized warmth, fever, purulent drainage) or other complications of surgery.

- ✓ Need to avoid placing objects such as a pillow or towel roll under the knee for patients with TKA.
- ✓ Need to maintain appropriate oral hygiene to decrease the risk for periprosthetic infection; discuss possible prophylactic antibiotics with the health care provider before any minor surgical procedure (e.g., dental surgery) based on risk stratification (e.g., immunocompromise from treatment for inflammatory arthropathy).
- ✓ Activity restrictions related to surgical approach and weight-bearing restrictions related to prosthesis type.
- ✓ Use of prescribed immobilization device such as abductor wedge for patients with THA.
- ✓ Frequency of exercise and rationale for exercise performance. Ensure the patient independently demonstrates each exercise.
- ✓ For ADL and ambulation, ensure the patient demonstrates independence in the use of walker/crutches and other assistive devices before discharge from hospital or ambulatory surgery center.
- ✓ Assessment of neurovascular condition at least four times daily, including need to immediately report to the provider symptoms such as numbness and tingling or coolness in extremity.
- ✓ Importance of follow-up care, date of next appointment, and a telephone number to call if questions arise.

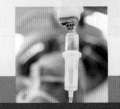

## OVERVIEW/PATHOPHYSIOLOGY

Osteoarthritis (OA) is the most prevalent articular disease in adults 65 years of age and older. It is a disorder that slowly progresses with manifestations in the synovial joints as a gradual loss of articular cartilage occurs. In OA, chondrocytes within the joint fail to synthesize a good-quality matrix in terms of both resistance and elasticity; this makes the cartilage more prone to deterioration. OA is recognized as a process in which all joint structures produce new tissue in response to joint injury or cartilage destruction. This chronic, progressive disease is characterized by gradual loss of articular cartilage combined with thickening of the subchondral bone and formation of bony outgrowths (osteophytes or spurs) at the joint margins. Affected individuals experience increasing pain and loss of function, with possible joint deformity. The prevalence of OA varies among different populations, but it is a universal human problem that actually may begin by 20–30 years of age. Most people are affected by 40 years of age, but few experience symptoms until after 50 or 60 years of age. OA affects women more than men.

OA may be classified as either *idiopathic* or *secondary*. Idiopathic OA occurs in individuals with no history of joint injury or disease or of systemic illness that might contribute to the development of arthritis. Aging may be one influence on the deterioration of cartilage in arthritic joints, but additional evidence suggests the existence of an autosomal recessive trait for gene defects that causes premature cartilage destruction. The prevalence of OA in postmenopausal women also suggests estrogen loss increases the risk of the disease. In contrast, secondary OA has an identifiable cause. Any condition or event that directly damages or overloads articular cartilage or causes joint instability can result in arthritic changes. Secondary OA typically occurs in younger individuals because of congenital processes (e.g., Legg–Calvé–Perthes disease), trauma, repetitive occupational stress, hemophilic joint hemorrhage, or infection.

OA is characterized by *site specificity*, with certain synovial joints showing higher disease prevalence. These include the weight-bearing joints (hips, knees); cervical and lumbar spine; distal interphalangeal (DIP), proximal interphalangeal (PIP), and metacarpophalangeal joints in the hands; and metatarsophalangeal joints in the feet (bunion deformity, or hallux valgus). The hips are most often affected in men and the hands in women, especially after menopause.

## HEALTH CARE SETTING

Primary care

## ASSESSMENT

**Signs and symptoms.** Joint pain and stiffness are the dominant symptoms and the most common reason for seeking medical evaluation. However, because the onset of pain is typically insidious, the patient may not be able to recall exactly when it began. The patient often describes an "aching" asymmetric pain that increases with joint use and is relieved by rest, especially in the early stages of OA. Pain often is worse with using stairs, standing, and walking; less pain is experienced at night and when sitting. As the disease progresses, however, night pain or pain at rest is likely to occur. The patient also may state that pain increases with cool, damp, and rainy weather. This has been attributed to changes in intraarticular pressure associated with the fall in barometric pressure that precedes inclement weather. Joint stiffness ranges from slowness to pain with initial movement. Early morning stiffness is common but typically lasts less than 30 minutes. Stiffness after periods of rest or inactivity (articular gelling or gel phenomenon) is also characteristic of OA but resolves within several minutes. The patient may describe a squeaking, creaking, or grating with movement (crepitus) caused by loose cartilage particles in the joint capsule.

**Physical assessment.** Contralateral joints should be compared for symmetry, size, shape, color, appearance, temperature, and pain. Bony enlargement is common, and affected joints are likely to be tender to palpation. Reduced range of motion (ROM) is extremely common in osteoarthritic joints and contributes greatly to disability. Generally, it is related to osteophyte formation, joint surface incongruity from severe loss of cartilage, or spasm and contracture of surrounding muscle. Locking during movement may be accentuated by mild effusion and soft tissue swelling. Large effusions are uncommon in OA and could suggest other processes such as septic arthritis or gout. Crepitation during passive movement is present in more than 90% of patients with knee OA and indicates loss of cartilage integrity. Deformities may include Heberden nodes on DIP joints and Bouchard nodes on PIP joints of the hands. Almost 50% of patients with knee OA have a joint malalignment, typically a varus (an excessive inward angulation) deformity due to cartilage loss in the medial compartment. Leg-length discrepancy may be noted due to loss of joint space in advanced hip OA. In addition, muscular atrophy may be seen in advanced disease secondary to joint splinting for pain relief.

## DIAGNOSTIC TESTS

OA almost always can be diagnosed by history and physical examination.

**Laboratory tests.** To rule out other arthropathic conditions (e.g., rheumatoid arthritis, septic arthritis) and to establish baselines before starting therapy.

**Complete blood count.** Suggested for patients who will be taking nonsteroidal antiinflammatory drugs (NSAIDs) for arthritis symptom management, with an additional complete blood count prescribed periodically to screen for anemia caused by occult gastrointestinal (GI) bleeding.

**Renal and liver function tests.** For patients starting aspirin or NSAID therapy, with further testing done every 6 months to assess for side effects such as electrolyte imbalance, hepatitis, or renal insufficiency.

**Rheumatoid factor, erythrocyte sedimentation rate, and C-reactive protein.** None excludes a diagnosis of OA in the older patient. About 20% of healthy older adults have positive rheumatoid factor, and measures of inflammation tend to rise with age. The evaluation of inflammation is useful to rule out chronic conditions such as polymyalgia rheumatica. Synovial fluid analysis is another reliable method for differentiating OA from inflammatory arthritic disorders.

**Radiographic examination.** Radiographic findings do not always correlate with the severity of the patient's clinical symptoms. As disease progresses, radiographic examination will reveal joint space narrowing, osteophytes at joint margins, subchondral cysts, and altered shape of bone ends that suggests bone remodeling.

**Magnetic resonance imaging.** Much more sensitive than radiographic examination in marking the progression of joint destruction.

## Patient Problem/Analyze Cues/Prioritize Hypotheses

# Pain

*due to* arthritic joint changes and associated therapy

**Desired Outcome/Generate Solutions:** Within 1–2 hours of intervention, the patient's perception of pain decreases, as documented by scoring on a pain intensity scale. The patient demonstrates the ability to perform activities of daily living with minimal discomfort.

| ASSESSMENT—RECOGNIZE CUES/ INTERVENTIONS—TAKE ACTION | RATIONALES |
|---|---|
| Assess the patient's pain using an appropriate pain intensity rating scale, such as the visual analog scale, Wong–Baker FACES Pain Rating Scale, Faces Pain Scale—Revised, or FLACC (face, legs, activity, crying, consolability) scale. | The patient provides a personal baseline report, enabling the nurse to more effectively assess subsequent increases and decreases in pain. For the patient who is too young or unable to comprehend the quantitative scales, the nurse will use the FLACC scale based on observations. |
| Administer the simple (nonopioid) analgesics (i.e., acetaminophen), NSAIDs, opioid analgesics, and adjuncts as prescribed and reassess their effectiveness in approximately 1 hour using pain intensity rating scale. Document the preintervention and postintervention pain intensity scores. | Pain management is a treatment priority for OA. Mobility is enhanced when pain level is manageable. |
| Acetaminophen is recommended by the American College of Rheumatology as the initial treatment for OA pain. If acetaminophen is ineffective, low-dose over-the-counter NSAIDs or salicylates are recommended for patients with normal renal function and no prior history of GI problems. Prescriptive NSAID doses are indicated if pain persists or worsens. | |
| Observe for adverse effects of NSAIDs, such as GI bleeding or renal failure. | Traditional NSAIDs, such as ibuprofen or naproxen sodium, may increase the risk for gastric ulceration or renal impairment because they inhibit cyclooxygenase-1, which reduces prostaglandin levels in the stomach and kidneys. They also reduce renal circulation by decreasing the synthesis of renal prostaglandins. |

| ASSESSMENT—RECOGNIZE CUES/ INTERVENTIONS—TAKE ACTION | RATIONALES |
|---|---|
| Provide instructions to the patient about the risk for cardiovascular events such as myocardial infarction (MI) and stroke with high doses of NSAIDs. | Patients should know the risk of long-term NSAID use. Except for aspirin, NSAID use has been associated with an increased risk of heart disease. In particular, the risk of MI from NSAID use rises in proportion to the individual's underlying risk. |
| Advise the patient to coordinate time of peak effectiveness of the analgesic or NSAID with periods of exercise or other use of arthritic joints. | Careful timing of analgesics enables patients to achieve optimal pain management before exercise or ambulation. Participation in the exercise regimen helps maintain joint function. |
| Apply the topical analgesics as prescribed. | Topical application may help with localized pain management for the OA patient. Capsaicin cream in particular has been shown to reduce knee pain significantly when used with other prescribed arthritis medications. |
| • Use nonpharmacologic methods of pain management, such as guided imagery, relaxation, massage, distraction, biofeedback, heat or cold therapy, and music therapy. Include traditional nursing interventions such as back rubs and repositioning in the pain management plan of care. | Nonpharmacologic methods can augment pharmacologic pain management strategies. These methods may be critical for patients who avoid the use of analgesics or experience minimal pain management with prescribed analgesics. |
| • Thermal therapy in particular may lessen pain and stiffness. Ice can be helpful during occasional episodes of acute inflammation, whereas heat therapy may be beneficial for stiffness. Heat therapy is delivered through numerous modalities, including hot packs, ultrasound, whirlpool, paraffin wax, and massage. | |
|  Instruct the patient about the purpose and use of glucosamine and chondroitin. | Efficacy of these agents is not conclusively supported by scientific literature. However, anecdotal reports do indicate that some patients experience positive effects. Because patients with OA continue to try these therapies, the nurse must be prepared to discuss their use. |
| Caution the patient to avoid joint immobilization for more than a week. | Additional stiffness and discomfort can result from prolonged joint rest. |
| Refer the patient to occupational therapy as indicated and encourage the use of assistive devices and dressing/grooming aids as needed based on the assessment of the patient's pain-related self-care limitations. | Use of appropriate assistive devices decreases pain during attempts at self-care. Sock donners, long-handled reachers and brushes, raised toilet seats, and other devices may help minimize stress on joints. Clothing also can be adapted for greater ease in dressing (e.g., zipper pulls, Velcro closures). |

## Patient Problem/Analyze Cues/Prioritize Hypotheses

# Impaired Mobility

*due to* musculoskeletal impairment and the need for adjustment to a new walking gait with assistive device

***Desired Outcomes/Generate Solutions:*** Within 1 week of instruction, the patient demonstrates adequate upper body strength for use of an assistive device. The patient demonstrates appropriate use of the assistive device on flat and uneven surfaces.

| ASSESSMENT—RECOGNIZE CUES/ INTERVENTIONS—TAKE ACTION | RATIONALES |
|---|---|
| Assess to ensure the patient has necessary strength of the upper extremities to use the prescribed assistive device. | Many older adults have impaired upper body strength. Upper extremities must be strong enough to support body weight and allow safe use of prescribed assistive devices such as crutches or walker. |

Continued

| ASSESSMENT—RECOGNIZE CUES/ INTERVENTIONS—TAKE ACTION | RATIONALES |
|---|---|
| As indicated, teach the armchair push-ups to attain and maintain triceps muscle strength. | Armchair push-ups target the triceps muscles, which are critically important for safe ambulation with crutches or walker. |
| Patients should be encouraged to perform 10 repetitions several times daily if possible. | Repetition of armchair push-ups will improve triceps muscle strength. |
| Ensure that height of the walker, crutches, or cane allows the patient to have approximately 15 degrees of elbow flexion when ambulating. | The assistive device must be appropriately sized to enable the patient's safe use. |
| Ensure that crutch tops rest 1–1.5 inches (width of two fingers) below the patient's axillae. | This position avoids upper extremity paresthesia caused by pressure of the crutch tops on the brachial plexus. |
| Supervise the use of the prescribed assistive device. Ensure that the patient can use the assistive device to get in and out of a motor vehicle safely. | Supervised practice helps ensure that the patient will be able to use the device safely on different surfaces and in multiple settings. Ambulation should begin in small increments on a flat surface and progress to all surfaces that the patient is expected to encounter. |

## Patient Problem/Analyze Cues/Prioritize Hypotheses

# Deficient Knowledge (Medications)

*due to* unfamiliarity with the potential interactions between NSAIDs, anticoagulants, and herbal products

***Desired Outcome/Generate Solutions:*** Within 1–2 hours of instruction, the patient verbalizes understanding of potential interactions between NSAIDs, anticoagulants, and herbal products that potentiate bleeding.

| ASSESSMENT—RECOGNIZE CUES/ INTERVENTIONS—TAKE ACTION | RATIONALES |
|---|---|
| Assess the patient's health care literacy (language, reading, comprehension). Assess the culturally specific information needs and current knowledge level. | This assessment helps ensure that materials are selected and presented in a manner that is culturally and educationally appropriate. |
|  Determine the patient's use of NSAIDs, anticoagulants, and herbal products that potentiate bleeding (e.g., ginkgo, ginger, turmeric, chamomile, kelp, horse chestnut, garlic, dong quai). | Herbal supplements, particularly ginger and turmeric, have been shown to reduce the pain and inflammation of arthritis. However, patients need to be aware that these herbs can potentiate bleeding. Concurrent use of anticoagulants and NSAIDs increases the risk of bleeding. |
|  Advise the patient to discuss with the health care provider of concurrent use of herbal products or anticoagulants while taking NSAIDs for arthritis symptom management. | The provider should be aware of any products that increase the patient's bleeding risk. |
| Provide patient education on signs of occult bleeding such as black or tarry stools, hematuria, bleeding gums, and coughing up or vomiting blood. | A knowledgeable patient is more likely to recognize and immediately report signs of occult bleeding. |

## Patient Problem/Analyze Cues/Prioritize Hypotheses

# Low Self-Esteem

*due to* pain, decreased joint function, or body image changes that interfere with sexual performance

***Desired Outcome/Generate Solutions:*** Within 1 week of intervention, the patient describes increased self-esteem related to improved physical and psychological comfort during sexual intimacy.

| ASSESSMENT—RECOGNIZE CUES/ INTERVENTIONS—TAKE ACTION | RATIONALES |
|---|---|
| Discuss and assess the possible problems with sexual performance related to decreased joint function, pain, or body image. | This discussion encourages patients to verbalize feelings related to body image changes, pain experience, and mobility that may affect interest in and ability to have sexual intercourse. |
| Encourage the patient to use relaxation strategies (e.g., warm bath if medically permissible) to alleviate pain and stiffness before sexual intercourse. | Relaxation strategies decrease muscle tension, which contributes to joint pain, and allow increased flexibility of connective tissues that support the joints. |
| Encourage the use of analgesics before sexual intercourse to enable easier movement. | Careful timing of analgesics enables patients to achieve optimal pain management before sexual intercourse. |
| Discuss the other ways to preserve intimacy (e.g., caressing and holding) in a relationship if intercourse is difficult. | Exploration of additional ways to demonstrate intimacy will reinforce the patient's ability to maintain/strengthen the relationship despite the effects of OA. |
| Instruct the patient about the disease process and alternative positions that promote comfort during sexual intercourse. | Understanding the impact of OA on mobility will allow patients to choose positions that decrease stress on joints during sexual intercourse. |

## ADDITIONAL PROBLEMS:

| | |
|---|---|
| *Impaired Functional Ability*, due to pain and limitations in joint ROM affecting self-care | Chapter 69 |
| *Fatigue*, due to persistent discomfort, effects of prolonged immobility, and psychoemotional demands of chronic illness | Chapter 73 |

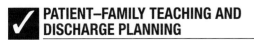

## PATIENT–FAMILY TEACHING AND DISCHARGE PLANNING

When providing patient–family teaching, focus on sensory information, avoid giving excessive information, and initiate a visiting nurse/home health or community services referral for necessary follow-up teaching whenever possible. Include verbal and written information about the following:

- ✓ Medications and supplements, including name, dosage, purpose, schedule, precautions, and potential side effects. Also discuss drug–drug, herb–drug, and food–drug interactions.
- ✓ Importance of laboratory follow-up (e.g., blood or urine testing) for needed monitoring while the patient is taking selected medications.
- ✓ Proper use of heat or cold therapy, as appropriate to joint condition.
- ✓ Importance of joint protection, with balance of rest and activity.
- ✓ Use, care, and replacement of orthotics and assistive devices.
- ✓ Weight reduction, if indicated.
- ✓ Importance of follow-up care, date of next appointment, and a telephone number to call if questions arise.
- ✓ Referral to community resources, including local arthritis support activities, such as Arthritis Foundation at www.arthritis.org.
- ✓ Additional information on arthritis may be available through the National Institute of Arthritis and Musculoskeletal and Skin Diseases (NIAMS) Information Clearinghouse at http://www.niams.nih.gov/health_info/.

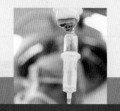

# Osteoporosis 72

## OVERVIEW/PATHOPHYSIOLOGY

Osteoporosis ("porous bone") is the most common metabolic bone disease. It is characterized by a reduction in both bone mass and bone strength, while bone size remains constant. These changes make bone more brittle and susceptible to fractures. It is eight times more common in women than in men for several reasons: bone resorption begins earlier in women and becomes more rapid at menopause; pregnancy and breastfeeding deplete a woman's skeletal reserve; and women have longer life expectancies, Osteoporosis affects more than 54 million people in the United States (National Osteoporosis Foundation, n.d.) and is responsible for more than 2 million fractures annually. Three types of osteoporosis have been identified: postmenopausal, senile, and secondary.

***Postmenopausal osteoporosis (type I).*** Affects females; clinical symptoms appear 10–15 years after menopause due to lack of estrogen.

***Senile (age-associated) osteoporosis (type II).*** Affects both males and females, more commonly after 70 years of age; related to calcium deficiency, an aging skeleton, and decreased physical activity.

***Secondary osteoporosis.*** Affects both males and females; results from another disease process (e.g., chronic kidney failure/liver disease, rheumatoid arthritis, celiac disease, and other malabsorption syndromes), hormonal conditions (e.g., diabetes mellitus, hyperparathyroidism), medications and therapies (e.g., glucocorticoids, anticoagulants, anticonvulsants, cyclosporines, radiation therapy), malnutrition/protein deficiency, and disuse (e.g., spinal cord injury/loss of biomechanical function, long-term bedrest).

## HEALTH CARE SETTING

Primary care; acute care for complications. Individuals with osteoporosis are seen in all health care settings for primary diagnoses other than osteoporosis.

## ASSESSMENT

***Signs and symptoms.*** Because of the insidious onset of osteoporosis, many individuals are not diagnosed until they experience an acute fracture or receive evidence from radiographic examinations obtained for other conditions (e.g., chest radiographic examination to confirm pneumonia). Vertebral compression fractures can develop gradually, resulting in back discomfort and loss of height. Severe chronic flexion of the vertebral spine (kyphosis or "dowager's hump") may inhibit the function of multiple organ systems (e.g., gastrointestinal, respiratory). With severe spinal deformities, the patient often describes the difficulty in obtaining clothes that fit well.

### Risk factors

***Unchangeable factors.*** Female biologic gender, age, family history, body size (small frame, slight build), ethnicity (Caucasian, Asian).

***Changeable factors.*** Serum hormones (surgical or physiologic menopause, hypogonadism), diet (lifelong low-calcium intake, decreased protein intake, increased caffeine intake).

***Lifestyle factors.*** Smoking, alcohol use, sedentary activity level.

***Other influences.*** Medications, hyperthyroidism, hyperparathyroidism, multiple myeloma, transplantation, chronic diseases.

## DIAGNOSTIC TESTS

Use of one or more tests is common.

***Laboratory tests.*** Serum and urinary markers of bone remodeling can help to determine disease cause but they cannot accurately determine bone density or fracture risk. Cannot accurately determine bone density or fracture risk, but serum and urinary markers of bone remodeling can help in determining disease cause. Serum calcium is usually within normal levels in osteoporosis, but urinary calcium may be elevated. In addition, 25-hydroxyvitamin D can be used to assess vitamin D deficiency, which can affect calcium absorption and bone health.

***Standard anteroposterior and lateral radiographic examinations of the spine.*** Provide diagnosis for osteoporotic fractures or kyphosis. They have limited use in diagnosing disease before a fracture, however, because changes are not evident on plain films until at least 30% of bone mineral density has been lost.

***Bone mineral density tests.*** Can measure the amount of bone in specific areas of the skeleton to predict the risk for fracture. Dual-energy x-ray absorptiometry (DEXA, also called DXA) is the gold standard for measuring bone density by testing bone mass in the spine, femoral neck, and wrist. This method is precise and economical; short procedure times mean minimal radiation exposure. The National Osteoporosis Foundation and the World Health Organization recommend bone density testing using central DEXA.

Peripheral screening tests may be useful when central DEXA is not available; they can help identify people who may benefit from additional testing. For example, quantitative computed tomography measures bone density at sites throughout the body but is most often used in the spine. It is accurate but costly and delivers a considerable amount of radiation. In the heel, quantitative ultrasound compares favorably with density measurements obtained by DEXA. It is also an easy, low-cost, radiation-free diagnostic aid.

*Bone biopsy.* Useful in differential diagnosis of metabolic bone diseases such as osteoporosis and osteomalacia. It also can be useful for diagnosis in individuals with early onset of osteoporosis (age younger than 50 years) or those with severe demineralization.

## Patient Problem/Analyze Cues/Prioritize Hypotheses

# Deficient Knowledge: Disease Management

*due to* unfamiliarity with the prevention of osteoporosis, its treatment, and importance of adequate dietary calcium intake/supplementation

*Desired Outcome/Generate Solutions:* Within 48 hours of instruction, the patient verbalizes knowledge of the disease process, possible treatments, and importance of adequate calcium intake.

| ASSESSMENT—RECOGNIZE CUES/ INTERVENTIONS—TAKE ACTION | RATIONALES |
|---|---|
| Assess the patient's health care literacy (language, reading, comprehension). Assess culturally specific information needs and current knowledge level. | This assessment helps ensure that materials are selected and presented in a manner that is culturally and educationally appropriate. |
| Assess the patient's understanding of the nature of osteoporosis and the potential diminished response to treatment if not initiated until symptoms appear. | Because of the insidious onset of osteoporosis, many individuals are not diagnosed until they experience an acute fracture or receive radiographic evidence from x-ray films obtained for other conditions (e.g., chest radiograph to confirm pneumonia). |
| Include instruction on osteoporosis prevention as a routine part of health teaching for children, adolescents, and adults. | Adults need to recognize factors that increase their risk for osteoporosis (e.g., female, increasing age, small frame, Caucasian or Asian race). As children and adolescents experience bone growth, their bone quality can be improved through awareness of osteoporosis prevention strategies. |
| Instruct the patient about proper nutrition in relation to calcium and vitamin D intake. | Appropriate nutrition is the foundation of osteoporosis prevention and treatment, and consistent calcium intake is especially important. A knowledgeable patient is more likely to adhere to prevention and treatment strategies. Vitamin D is needed for adequate intestinal absorption of calcium; see discussion of vitamin D later in this patient problem. |
| Ensure that the health care provider has recommended or approves the use of calcium supplements for the patient. | Although calcium is important to bone health, supplementation should be done on the advice of the health care provider. Excessive calcium intake can lead to nephrolithiasis in susceptible individuals. |
| Inform the patient that, although calcium supplements come in numerous forms, calcium carbonate is inexpensive and commonly available. | This information may promote adherence to health care regimen. |
| Calcium carbonate is best absorbed when taken with food because of its dependence on stomach acid for absorption. | |
| Inform patients taking a proton pump inhibitor (PPI) that they will need to take calcium citrate, an alternate form of the supplement. | Use of PPIs for gastric reflux or other conditions alters the acidic environment of the stomach and decreases the absorption of calcium carbonate. Thus the use of calcium citrate, which can be absorbed, is indicated for persons taking PPIs. |

Continued

## ASSESSMENT—RECOGNIZE CUES/ INTERVENTIONS—TAKE ACTION

## RATIONALES

| ASSESSMENT—RECOGNIZE CUES/ INTERVENTIONS—TAKE ACTION | RATIONALES |
|---|---|
| Instruct the patient read the label on calcium supplement to determine the amount of *elemental calcium* available in supplements and verbalize the recommended calcium dosage. | *Elemental calcium* refers to the amount of calcium in a supplement that is available for the body to absorb.<br><br>There is no added benefit in taking more calcium than is required, and supplementation is unnecessary if dietary intake is adequate. |
| Instruct the patient not to take calcium and iron supplements at the same time. | The two elements bind with each other, and absorption of both will be impaired. |
| Review the patient's medication profile. | Because calcium may reduce the absorption of other medications, the nurse should carefully time administration of all medications to ensure maximal absorption. |
| Caution the patient to avoid taking more than 500–600 mg of calcium at one time and to spread doses over the entire day. | Excessive intake can lead to hypercalcemia, which may cause muscle weakness, constipation, and heart block. In addition, a dose in excess of 600 mg will not be fully absorbed. |
| Remind the patient to drink a full glass of water with each supplement. | Adequate hydration minimizes the risk for developing renal calculi. |
| Remind the patient of the need for sunlight to enable vitamin D activation. | Vitamin D is required for calcium absorption. Without enough vitamin D, one can't form enough of the hormone calcitriol. This in turn leads to insufficient calcium absorption from the diet. |
| Instruct patient that sunscreen or sunblock should be used for all exposure but sun protection factor 8 can reduce the production of vitamin D by 95%. | Exposure to sunlight is needed for cutaneous synthesis of vitamin D. An average of 15 minutes of exposure to the hands, face, arms, and legs typically meets the vitamin D requirement for most people. |
| Provide education on nutritional sources of vitamin D (e.g., milk, fortified products such as orange juice, fatty fish such as tuna). | |
| Instruct the patient to avoid vitamin D supplementation if dietary intake is adequate unless prescribed. | Supplements may be needed by institutionalized persons, those living in extreme northern or southern latitudes, and people with limited sun exposure. However, excessive intake is discouraged because of risk for toxicity. |
| Remind patient that vitamin D is often included in calcium supplements, so the patient should read supplement labels before selecting a separate vitamin D product. | |
| • If hormone replacement therapy (HRT) has been prescribed, explain its purpose, action, and precautions.<br>• Encourage your female patient to discuss with health care providers about personal risks and benefits. | HRT risks may include heart disease, blood clots, stroke, and breast cancer. Education about the risks and benefits of HRT will enable the patient to make informed decisions. |
| Provide instructions to the patient about the possible medications prescribed for the treatment of osteoporosis, indications for use, possible side effects, administration time and method, and need for follow-up laboratory tests. | A knowledgeable patient is likely to adhere to the drug therapy and report necessary signs and symptoms to ensure prompt treatment of untoward side effects. |
| Encourage patients needing invasive dental treatment, such as tooth extractions, root canals, or dental implantations, to have dental work completed before starting treatment with a bisphosphonate. | Bisphosphonate-related osteonecrosis of the jaw is a condition found in patients who are taking bisphosphonates during invasive dental treatments. |
| If dental extraction is unavoidable, instruct the patient to consult with the bisphosphonate prescriber about the possible interruption of treatment. | |
| Provide the patient with instructions about the importance of weight-bearing exercise and associated activity restrictions. | Weight-bearing exercise contributes to increased bone density and prevents bone loss. |
| Remind patients with established osteoporosis that they should avoid vigorous unsupervised exercise, and their exercise regimen should not include spinal flexion through activities such as toe touches and sit-ups. Caution patients that rotational exercises such as golf and bowling may lead to vertebral injury by creating excessive compressive forces. Instruct patients that walking is generally considered a safe weight-bearing exercise. | Knowledge about activities that could cause injury will decrease patients' participation in risky behaviors. |

<u>Patient Problem/Analyze Cues/Prioritize Hypotheses</u>

# Risk for Injury

*due to* fall risk, spontaneous fracture, comorbidities, and unsafe environment

**Desired Outcome/Generate Solutions:** Within 24 hours of instruction, the patient describes strategies to decrease the risk for fall or fracture.

| ASSESSMENT—RECOGNIZE CUES/ INTERVENTIONS—TAKE ACTION | RATIONALES |
|---|---|
| Assess the patient's fall risk using a recognized fall risk assessment tool. Refer to the health care provider as necessary for additional evaluation of any identified deficits. | Delirium/dementia, cardiovascular disorders, decreased mobility, generalized weakness, abnormal elimination needs, impaired vision or hearing, and use of medications that affect blood pressure, balance, or level of consciousness can lead to falls and possible fracture in a patient with decreased bone density. |
| | Often the spontaneous fracture of a weakened bone causes the fall. The person with osteoporosis is also more at risk for injury (i.e., fragility fractures) if he or she falls. |
| Assist the patient and significant others in assessing the presence of and eliminating environmental hazards that may increase the risk for falls in the home. | Poor lighting, scatter rugs, electrical cords or oxygen tubes that cross floors or halls, and narrow stairs without adequate railing and lighting can increase fall risk. |
| Encourage the patient to avoid unnecessary inactivity because of fear of falling. | Inactivity can place an individual at greater risk for fractures by further decreasing bone density, increasing muscle atrophy, and contributing to orthostasis. |
| Encourage adequate intake of calcium and vitamin D, as well as appropriate use of prescribed osteoporosis medications. | Calcium and vitamin D contribute to bone health. Their adequate intake may decrease risk for injury if a fall occurs. Other prescribed medications such as bisphosphonates or Selective Estrogen Receptor Modulators (SERMs) must be taken as prescribed for optimal bone health. |
| Instruct the patient to avoid lifting heavy objects, with weight limits stipulated by the health care provider. | Lifting puts patients with osteoporosis at risk for vertebral compression fractures. |
| Discuss with patient to develop strategies to maintain routine activities without an increase in risk for vertebral injury. | |
| Collaborate with physical therapy to educate and encourage patient to participate in exercise regimens that improve balance. | Aerobic walking and strength training by upper and lower body exercises have been shown to improve standing balance, which will help decrease risk for falls. |

<u>Patient Problem/Analyze Cues/Prioritize Hypotheses</u>

# Deficient Knowledge: Diet

*due to* inadequate intake of foods/supplements containing calcium and vitamin D

**Desired Outcomes/Generate Solutions:** Within 24 hours of instruction, the patient demonstrates adequate intake of calcium and vitamin D. The patient plans a 3-day menu that provides sufficient intake of both.

| ASSESSMENT—RECOGNIZE CUES/ INTERVENTIONS—TAKE ACTION | RATIONALES |
|---|---|
| Assess the patient's health care literacy (language, reading, comprehension). Assess culturally specific information needs and current knowledge level. | This assessment helps ensure that materials are selected and presented in a manner that is culturally and educationally appropriate. |

Continued

| ASSESSMENT—RECOGNIZE CUES/ INTERVENTIONS—TAKE ACTION | RATIONALES |
|---|---|
| Assess the patient's knowledge of and ability to select foods high in calcium, including cheese and milk. | This information will aid the nurse to identify patient teaching needs. Food is a better source of calcium than supplements. |
| If the patient is unable to tolerate dairy products, explore other food choices that can ensure adequate calcium intake (e.g., broccoli, sardines). | |
| Assessment should include any limitations on food selection imposed by lower financial income. | |
| Instruct the patient about the purpose and recommended daily intake of calcium and vitamin D. | An informed patient will have the knowledge to make appropriate food choices. |
| | Proper nutrition is the foundation of osteoporosis prevention and treatment. Consistent calcium intake alone cannot prevent or cure osteoporosis, but it is an important part of an overall prevention or treatment program. |
| Provide sample menus that include adequate daily amounts of calcium and vitamin D. Guide the patient in developing a 3-day menu that includes appropriate intake of foods containing calcium and vitamin D. | Sample menus demonstrate easy ways in which adequate calcium and vitamin D can be incorporated into the daily diet. |
| Provide instructions on the necessity for adequate exposure to sunlight to prevent vitamin D deficiency. | See *Deficient Knowledge* earlier in this chapter for a discussion of vitamin D. |
| If the patient has limited exposure to sunlight (e.g., resident of a long-term care facility), instruct the patient regarding vitamin D supplementation to ensure adequate calcium absorption as prescribed. | See *Deficient Knowledge* earlier in this chapter for a discussion of vitamin D. |

## ADDITIONAL PROBLEMS:

| | |
|---|---|
| *Constipation*, due to decreased mobility and use of opioid analgesics and calcium supplements | Chapter 69 |
| *Pain*, due to arthritic joint changes and associated therapy | Chapter 71 |
| *Impaired Mobility*, due to musculoskeletal impairment and adjustment to new walking gait with an assistive device | Chapter 71 |
| *Self Care Deficit*, due to pain and limitations in joint range of motion affecting self-care | Chapter 73 |
| *Risk for Disturbed Body Image*, due to joint deformities | Chapter 73 |

 ## PATIENT–FAMILY TEACHING AND DISCHARGE PLANNING

When providing patient–family teaching, focus on sensory information, avoid giving excessive information, and make appropriate referrals (e.g., visiting or home health nurse, community health resources, case manager) for follow-up teaching. Include verbal and written information about the following:

✓ Description of disease process and recommended treatment.

✓ Medications and supplements, including name, dosage, purpose, schedule, precautions, and potential side effects. Also discuss drug–drug, herb–drug, and food–drug interactions.

✓ Prescribed dietary regimen, including rationale for food choices.

✓ Prescribed exercise regimen, including need to avoid movements that twist or compress the spine (e.g., situps) as well as high-impact activities.

✓ Importance of establishing fall prevention measures in the home (e.g., placing handrail in tub or shower, installing nightlights, avoiding use of throw rugs). Arrange for a home visit from a nurse or physical therapist as necessary.

✓ Importance of reporting to the health care provider any indicators of pathologic fracture (i.e., deformity, pain, edema, ecchymosis, limb shortening, false motion, decreased range of motion, or crepitus). Stress the need to promptly report any indicators of vertebral fractures (e.g., paresthesia, weakness, paralysis, radicular pain, or change in bowel or bladder function) because of risk for possible spinal cord or nerve compression.

✓ Importance of follow-up care, date of next appointment, and telephone number to call if questions arise.

✓ Referral to community resources, including local osteo-porosis support activities:

- National Osteoporosis Foundation: www.nof.org
- National Institute of Arthritis and Musculoskeletal and Skin Diseases Information Clearinghouse, Information Specialist: www.niams.nih.gov

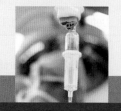

# Rheumatoid Arthritis 73

## OVERVIEW/PATHOPHYSIOLOGY

Rheumatoid arthritis (RA) is a chronic systemic autoimmune disease associated with severe morbidity and functional decline caused by inflammation of connective tissue, primarily in the synovial joints. The mortality rate of persons with RA is double that of the general population, particularly if the disease is not well managed. Individuals with RA are at increased risk for cardiovascular events. Women are affected two to three times more often than men. Although no single known cause exists for RA, theory suggests that it occurs in a susceptible host who initially experiences an immune response to an antigen. Because complex genetic factors appear to be involved, the antigen is probably not the same in all patients. Autoimmunity has been suggested as a cause because of the association of RA with the occurrence of rheumatoid factor (RF), the antibody against abnormal immunoglobulin G. Support for a genetic predisposition has come from studies of disease clusters in families, and formal genetic studies have confirmed this familial aggregation. No microorganism has been cultured from blood and synovial tissue or fluid with enough reproducibility to determine an infectious etiology for RA. In addition, no environmental factors have been identified as disease precipitators.

The immune response appears to center on synovial tissue, where disease changes are first seen. Synovitis develops when immune complexes are deposited onto the synovial membrane or superficial articular cartilage. As hypertrophied synovium invades surrounding tissues, highly vascularized fibrous exudate (*pannus*) forms to cover the entire articular cartilage. Pannus also scars and shortens adjacent tendons and ligaments to create the laxity, subluxation, and contractures characteristic of RA.

## HEALTH CARE SETTING

Primary care; acute care for complications

## ASSESSMENT

**Signs and symptoms.** Nonspecific symptoms such as fatigue, anorexia, weight loss, and generalized stiffness may precede the onset of joint complaints. Stiffness typically becomes more localized as time progresses. Morning joint stiffness lasting at least 1 hour is common, but it may last for hours. The patient often complains of joint pain and swelling, especially in the hands and wrists. Knees, ankles, and metatarsophalangeal joints also may be affected. The patient describes increasing difficulty with mobility and performance of activities of daily living (ADLs).

**Physical assessment.** During early disease, examination may reveal spindle-shaped fingers, with swan-neck and boutonnière deformities due to flexion contractures that occur with disease progression. Ulnar deviation, a "zigzag" wrist deformity, is also likely. Metatarsal-head subluxation and hallux valgus (bunion) in the feet may lead to walking disability and pain. Affected symmetric (bilateral) joints are typically swollen, red, warm, and tender with decreased range of motion (ROM). Patients also may exhibit guarded movement and gait abnormalities due to joint changes. Subcutaneous nodules may be noted over bony prominences, extensor surfaces, or juxtaarticular areas; hoarseness may be evident if nodules have invaded the vocal chords.

## DIAGNOSTIC TESTS

Diagnosis of RA is based primarily on physical findings and patient history. Radiographic studies are not usually needed to make a diagnosis. Laboratory results are helpful in confirming diagnosis and monitoring disease progression.

**Rheumatoid factor.** Higher titers appear to be correlated with severe and unremitting disease. However, the RF titer has little prognostic value, and serial titers have no usefulness in following disease process.

**Anti–cyclic citrullinated protein antibody test.** Tests for an antibody associated with RA. The test is useful for early diagnosis and can identify people who are more likely to develop severe RA.

**Antinuclear antibodies.** Positive antinuclear antibody (ANA) means autoantibodies are present but does not confirm the presence of an autoimmune disease or need for treatment. Many people have low positive ANA without clinical evidence of RA.

**Erythrocyte sedimentation rate and C-reactive protein.** Elevation is a general indicator of active inflammation. C-reactive protein (CRP) values change more quickly than erythrocyte sedimentation rate, making CRP useful in assessing the effectiveness of RA medications.

**Synovial fluid analysis.** Fluid is opaque and cloudy yellow, with elevated white blood cell count and polymorphonuclear leukocytes in the presence of RA. Glucose level will be lower than serum glucose.

**Radiographic examination of affected joints.** Radiographs may be inconclusive in early disease, but baseline films, especially of the hands, aid in monitoring disease progression. Presence of erosions also helps determine prognosis. With advanced disease, loss of articular cartilage leads to narrowed joint space. Subluxation and joint malalignment can be identified on radiographs, reflecting changes noted on physical examination.

Osteopenia or osteoporosis may be evident in the patient with RA who has been treated with corticosteroids.

> **Bone scan.** Detects early synovial changes.
>
> **Arthroscopy.** Reveals pale, hypertrophic synovium with destruction of cartilage and formation of fibrous scar tissue.

## Patient Problem/Analyze Cues/Prioritize Hypotheses

# Deficient Knowledge (Medications)

*due to* unfamiliarity with medications used in RA treatment

**Desired Outcome/Generate Solutions:** Immediately after a teaching intervention, the patient verbalizes accurate information about the prescribed RA medications.

| ASSESSMENT—RECOGNIZE CUES/ INTERVENTIONS—TAKE ACTION | RATIONALES |
|---|---|
| Assess the patient's health care literacy (language, reading, comprehension). Assess culturally specific information needs and current knowledge level. | This assessment helps ensure that materials are selected and presented in a manner that is culturally and educationally appropriate. |
| Provide instruction to the patient about medications prescribed for the treatment of arthritis: indications for use, possible side effects, administration time and method, and need for follow-up laboratory tests. | Drug therapy remains the cornerstone of an interdisciplinary approach to care for patients with RA. A knowledgeable patient is likely to adhere to drug therapy and report necessary signs and symptoms to ensure prompt treatment of untoward side effects. |
| [!] Instruct the patient to minimize exposure to ill individuals and immediately report personal illness to the physician. | Several RA drugs cause immunosuppression and can increase a patient's risk for illness. Illness, particularly if resistant to conventional treatment (e.g., common cold), should be reported immediately to the health care provider for more aggressive treatment. |
| [!] Remind the patient that laboratory monitoring of renal and liver function is necessary when taking disease-modifying antirheumatic drugs (DMARDs) and biologic response modifiers (BRMs), both of which are commonly used medications for people with RA. | Patients should be instructed to complete all follow-up laboratory tests as prescribed because the potential is great for renal and hepatic toxicity with DMARDs and BRMs, |
| [!] Instruct the patient who is taking nonsteroidal antiinflammatory drugs (NSAIDs) about the signs and symptoms of acute kidney injury (AKI) and adverse gastrointestinal (GI) effects. | NSAIDs are linked to increased risk for AKI and GI adverse effects. AKI symptoms may include flank pain, malaise, oliguria. GI adverse effects may include abdominal pain, nausea, diarrhea, and internal bleeding. Patients must be able to seek prompt medical attention for any suspected kidney injury or serious GI effects. |
| [!] Explain that caution is necessary for long-term use of oral corticosteroids. Patients who take corticosteroids should receive additional instruction on risks associated with long-term use. | Corticosteroids may be used to address the inflammation related to RA. Long-term use of these drugs is associated with the development of avascular necrosis or osteoporosis and therefore should not be a mainstay of treatment for the patient with RA. |
| [!] Instruct patient who is taking corticosteroids to never abruptly stop taking them. Instruct the patient to taper corricosteroid withdrawal as prescribed. | Abrupt withdrawal from corticosteroids causes adrenal insufficiency, which may be a life-threatening condition. Tapering the withdrawal of corticosteroids provides the adrenal glands time to resume their normal function. |

# Patient Problem/Analyze Cues/Prioritize Hypotheses
# Self-Care Deficit

*due to* pain and limitations in joint ROM affecting self-care

**Desired Outcome/Generate Solutions:** Within 1 week of instruction, the patient verbalizes/exhibits increased independence in dressing/grooming.

| ASSESSMENT—RECOGNIZE CUES/ INTERVENTIONS—TAKE ACTION | RATIONALES |
| --- | --- |
| Assess the impact of pain and limitations in joint ROM on performance of ADLs (e.g., dressing/bathing activities). | Recognition of the extent to which the disease has affected the patient's ability to perform ADLs independently enables the nurse and the patient to develop an individualized care/teaching plan for dressing/grooming. |
| Assess pain and ROM in joints used in dressing/grooming (e.g., small joints in hands; elbows, shoulders, knees). | Independence in dressing/grooming can be quickly lost as small joints become affected by the disease. Strategies for self-care must take into consideration any limitations in the small joints. |
| Refer the patient to an occupational therapist as indicated. | The occupational therapist is able to evaluate the need for dressing/bathing/toileting aids. Sock donners, buttoners, long-handled reachers and brushes, raised toilet seats, and other devices may help minimize stress on joints. Clothing also can be adapted to promote independence in dressing (e.g., zipper pulls, elastic shoelaces, Velcro closures). |
| Instruct the patient to coordinate the time of peak effectiveness of the prescribed analgesics and antiinflammatory medications with periods of joint use for self-care activities. | Careful timing of analgesics enables patients to achieve optimal pain management before performing ADLs that can stress small joints. |
| Collaborate with physical therapy to provide instructions to the patient about exercises that increase joint flexibility and decrease pain during joint use for self-care. | Joint flexibility is critical to a patient's ability to perform ADLs independently. Pain should be minimized to facilitate joint use as well. |
| Refer the patient to the Arthritis Foundation (AF) Exercise Program for local programs as well as online exercise guides and programs. | The AF Exercise Program is available "live" in many locations, with a search function on the AF website. The community-based program includes ROM exercises to promote flexibility and decrease pain. AF also offers information to help the patient create an effective home exercise program: http://www.arthritis.org/living-with-arthritis/exercise/. |

# Patient Problem/Analyze Cues/Prioritize Hypotheses
# Fatigue

*due to* the state of persistent discomfort, effects of prolonged mobility, and psychoemotional demands of chronic illness

**Desired Outcome/Generate Solutions:** Within 24 hours of instruction and interventions, the patient verbalizes a reduction in fatigue.

| ASSESSMENT—RECOGNIZE CUES/ INTERVENTIONS—TAKE ACTION | RATIONALES |
| --- | --- |
| Assess the patient's sleep pattern and suggest strategies that facilitate adequate rest (e.g., warm bath at bedtime). | Adequate rest helps patients maintain a more normal routine and decreases the risk for disease exacerbation. |
| Assess the patient's ability to manage pain and encourage the use of interventions to maximize the quality of rest periods. | Effective use of pain management interventions contributes to improved quality of rest periods. |

| ASSESSMENT—RECOGNIZE CUES/ INTERVENTIONS—TAKE ACTION | RATIONALES |
|---|---|
| Assess the patient's stress or emotional distress. Suggest coping strategies or refer the patient to an appropriate clinical specialist in psychiatric nursing. | Stress and emotional distress may increase fatigue and exacerbate disease symptoms. By understanding the patient's response to chronic illness, significant others may support efforts to maintain routine activities. If the patient is unable to develop and use effective coping strategies independently, referral may be warranted. |
| Help the patient identify the time that fatigue occurs, its relationship to necessary activities, and activities that relieve or aggravate symptoms. | With planning, patients should be able to optimize their ability to participate in routine and recreational activities. Patients also can anticipate fatigue-producing activities and plan rest periods accordingly. |
| Help the patient evaluate food preparation methods that may contribute to fatigue.  For example, the patient might set the table for the next day's breakfast before going to bed at night, use convenience foods whenever possible, or prepare food while seated on a stool at the kitchen counter. | This allows the patient to conserve energy by positional changes and during times of the day when fatigue occurs. |
| Encourage the patient to pace activities and allow adequate rest periods during the day. | Balance of rest and activity decreases the patient's risk for becoming fatigued. Fatigue contributes to stress and possible disease exacerbations. |
| Discuss the rationale for a stepped approach to exercise that increases endurance and strength without fatiguing the patient. Encourage the patient to set realistic exercise goals and share them with associated health care providers. | Endurance and strength should be increased gradually. An aggressive exercise program may cause fatigue and exacerbate disease symptoms. |
| Collaborate with physical therapy to instruct the patient in use of assistive devices used for ambulation. | A variety of devices are available to support small joints during routine activities and to assist with ambulation, thus minimizing stress and fatigue. The patient who uses appropriate assistive devices is also generally able to continue with routine activities and avoid social isolation. |

## Patient Problem/Analyze Cues/Prioritize Hypotheses

# Risk for Disturbed Body Image

*due to* joint deformities and the effects of corticosteroid use (e.g., weight gain due to fluid retention and increased appetite)

*Desired Outcome/Generate Solutions:* Within 1 month of intervention, the patient verbalizes positive adjustment to body changes.

| ASSESSMENT—RECOGNIZE CUES/ INTERVENTIONS—TAKE ACTION | RATIONALES |
|---|---|
| Assess the patient for negative body image. | Manifestations of negative body image may be different in each patient. Examples may include refusal to discuss or participate in care, withdrawal from social contacts, and avoidance of intimate relationships. Early identification of a changing body image provides an opportunity for overcoming isolating effects of the disease. |
| Assess the patient for negative feelings about body image linked specifically to the use of assistive devices/mobility aids. | The nurse can help select the least obtrusive aids, which will help patients maintain a more normal body image. |

Continued

| ASSESSMENT—RECOGNIZE CUES/ INTERVENTIONS—TAKE ACTION | RATIONALES |
|---|---|
| Provide anticipatory counseling about possible joint deformities/body image changes as the disease progresses, including ways for the patient to prepare for the reaction of others. | Awareness of the likelihood of deformity will enable patients to develop strategies that make routine encounters and regular activities easier. Patients also can anticipate times when RA deformities may be especially apparent and respond in ways that will minimize potential embarrassment or inconvenience. |
| Encourage participation in support groups for patients with RA. | Support group members can be good role models for successful coping. |
| Demonstrate positive regard for the patient and acceptance of any physical changes associated with chronic illness. | The nurse's consistent positive regard will help the patient avoid equating self with the disease process. It is critical that the patient recognize the disease as a separate entity rather than the defining element of his or her life. |

## ADDITIONAL PROBLEMS:

| | |
|---|---|
| *Pain*, due to arthritic joint changes and associated therapy | Chapter 71 |
| *Impaired Mobility*, due to musculoskeletal impairment and adjustment to new walking gait with an assistive device | Chapter 71 |

## PATIENT–FAMILY TEACHING AND DISCHARGE PLANNING

When providing patient–family teaching, focus on sensory information, avoid giving excessive information, and make appropriate referrals (e.g., visiting or home health nurse, community health resources) for follow-up teaching. Include verbal and written information about the following:

✓ Treatment regimen, including physical therapy and exercises, systemic rest/principles of joint protection, and cryotherapy.

✓ Importance of laboratory follow-up (e.g., blood or urine testing) for needed monitoring while the patient is taking selected medications.

✓ Medications and supplements, including name, dosage, schedule, precautions, and potential side effects. Also discuss drug–drug, herb–drug, and food–drug interactions.

✓ Nutrition: Research has shown several positive connections between food or nutritional supplements (e.g., omega-3 fatty acids as in fish and fish oil) and some types of arthritis, including RA. Increased fiber intake from grains, fruits, and vegetables may also reduce inflammation. However, omega-6 fatty acids (e.g., found in some plant oils, many snack foods, margarine, egg yolks, and meats) may increase the risk for inflammation and obesity. Some specific diets that are known to have harmful side effects include those that rely on large doses of alfalfa, copper salts, or zinc, or the so-called immune power diet or the low-calorie/low-fat/low-protein diet.

✓ Risk for folic acid deficiency that requires supplementation when taking methotrexate.

✓ Potential complications of disease and therapy, as well as the need to recognize and seek medical attention promptly if they occur.

✓ Potential concurrent pathologic conditions, such as pericarditis and ocular lesions, and need to report them promptly to the health care provider.

✓ Use, care, and replacement of splints, orthotics, and assistive devices.

✓ Use of adjunctive aids as appropriate, including long-handled reacher, long-handled shoehorn, elastic shoelaces, Velcro fasteners, crutches, walker, and cane.

✓ Referral to visiting/public health or home health nurses as necessary for ongoing care after discharge.

✓ Importance of follow-up care, date of next appointment, and telephone number to call if questions arise.

✓ Referral to community resources, including local arthritis support activities, and to the following:
  - AF: www.arthritis.org
  - National Institute of Arthritis and Musculoskeletal and Skin Diseases Information Clearinghouse, Information Specialist: www.niams.nih.gov

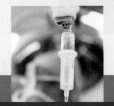

# HIV/AIDS 74

## OVERVIEW/PATHOPHYSIOLOGY

Human immunodeficiency virus (HIV) causes a life-threatening illness called *acquired immunodeficiency syndrome* (*AIDS*). AIDS is characterized by the disruption of cell-mediated immunity. This breakdown of the immune system is manifested by opportunistic infections such as *Pneumocystis jirovecii* pneumonia ([PJP], previously *Pneumocystis carinii* pneumonia) or tumors such as Kaposi sarcoma (KS). It is estimated that the total number of people living with HIV is 1.2 million. According to the Centers for Disease Control and Prevention (CDC) (2019), 36,801 people were diagnosed in the United States with HIV. From 2015 to 2019 the estimated annual number of new HIV infections decreased by 9% (CDC, HIV in the United States: At a Glance, 2019).

Confirmed routes of HIV transmission include the following:

- *Blood*: Exposure to HIV-infected blood by sharing contaminated needles or other drug paraphernalia, unsterile invasive instruments, exposure to needlesticks or sharps, transfusion with contaminated blood, and mucocutaneous exposure to blood or other infected body fluids, which includes the oral route.
- *Genital secretions*: Exposure to HIV-infected genital secretions during sexual activity. Anal-receptive sex with an HIV-infected person is the greatest sexual risk for exposure to HIV, followed by vaginal sex.
- *Breast milk*: Infant exposure to HIV-infected breast milk from an HIV-infected woman.
- *Perinatal*: Fetal exposure to HIV during all stages of pregnancy with the highest rates of transmission during labor and delivery.

HIV infection has transcended all racial, social, sexual, and economic barriers, and all persons who engage in risk behaviors are at risk for transmission. Health care workers who come into contact with infectious body fluids are also at risk. Understanding and practicing universal precautions are essential for all health care workers. Prophylaxis of HIV drugs after an exposure is available for the prevention of HIV infection in case an occupational or high-risk nonoccupational exposure occurs. It must be initiated within 72 hours of exposure.

The CDC recommends that all persons aged 13–64 years be screened for HIV at least once in their lifetime as part of routine testing. Individuals with certain risk factors should be tested more frequently, including people who exchange money for sex or men who have sex with men. In cases in which a screening is necessary in a more time-efficient manner, HIV testing can be conducted by a rapid test, which yields results within as little as 20 minutes. Anyone with a positive HIV antigen/antibody test result must be considered infectious and capable of transmitting the virus and should be started on HIV medications as soon as possible.

HIV targets CD4+ T cells, weakening the immune system. When CD4+ T cell count reaches 200 or below, the body becomes increasingly vulnerable to various infections such as PCP pneumonia or thrush. This phase of HIV infection is called AIDS. Thus HIV is a chronic viral disease that covers a wide spectrum of illnesses and symptoms over a variable course of time.

Since the introduction of highly active antiretroviral therapy (HAART), there has been a dramatic reduction in HIV-related morbidity and mortality. Strict adherence to a combination of antiretroviral agents blocks viral replication at different points in the life cycle of HIV. The use of antiretroviral agents reduces the amount of virus circulating in the blood. Reduction of this viral load allows the immune system to recover and slow progression of the disease, resulting in reduction in symptoms, opportunistic diseases, and inflammatory complications. This prolongs survival time and improves the quality of life. Additionally, consistent use of HAART has been found to reduce the risk of HIV transmission to others (CDC, 2017). Recent advances in HAART have led to once-daily combinations that improve adherence and have reduced side effects. These combination pills contain either two or three different medications since treatment with a single agent is never sufficient. As a result, HAART is currently recommended for all persons living with HIV (US Department of Health and Human Services [DHHS] Panel on Antiretroviral Guidelines for Adults and Adolescents, 2018), compared with the previous recommendation of starting at a CD4+ T cell count of 500. Plans for individuals with HIV must include the discussion of adherence to medications and risk for resistance, the importance of ongoing follow-up, and the prevention of HIV transmission to others.

## HEALTH CARE SETTING

Primary care, hospice, and home care with possible acute care hospitalization resulting from complications or occurrence of opportunistic infections

## ASSESSMENT

**HIV risk assessment.** With continued transmission of HIV infection and the incidence of new infections, which is independent of race, gender, sexual preference, or age, continuous HIV risk assessment and prevention education within all clinical settings are essential. Health care providers have a responsibility to assess each patient's risk for HIV infection and to be sensitive to issues of sexual preferences and practices as well as cultural values, norms, and traditions. A risk assessment should be used not only for the purpose of recommending testing but also for the development of a "patient-centered" risk reduction plan.

**Stages of HIV disease (for untreated individuals).** The four stages of HIV infection can be categorized as acute infection, asymptomatic, symptomatic, and AIDS.

*Acute or primary infection.* The acute or primary infection stage is a period of rapid viral replication during which the person may experience flu-like symptoms at the time of seroconversion, although not everyone will experience these symptoms. If this stage develops, it is generally within 2–4 weeks after becoming infected with the HIV virus. The viral load is frequently greater than 1 million. It is now believed that starting HIV medications during this phase preserves immune system architecture (US DHHS, AIDS Info, 2017).

*Asymptomatic stage.* The asymptomatic stage is a period when the immune system continues to mount a massive response to HIV, causing a drop in viral load, but viral replication continues. Patients achieve a viral load plateau, typically in the thousands, and continue to be infectious during this time. This stage may last 10 years or more, and the patient may remain free of symptoms or opportunistic infections.

*Early symptomatic stage.* The early symptomatic stage consists of a rate of viral replication that remains relatively constant. The gradual failure of the immune system results in the inability to control the virus, causing increased viral load. The CD4+ T cell count falls during this stage, and symptoms such as night sweats and weight loss may present.

*Advanced stage, acquired immunodeficiency syndrome.* AIDS, the advanced stage, is characterized by a depletion of CD4+ T cells. This results in the CD4+ T cell count falling below 200 or the development of an AIDS-defining illness, such as PCP pneumonia or chronic intestinal cryptosporidiosis. Clinical manifestations include wasting and opportunistic diseases such as viral, bacterial, and fungal infections, as well as neoplasms. Dementia also can occur, characterized by cognitive impairment and mood changes.

**Physical assessment.** The following indicators are commonly seen with HIV infection.

*General.* Fever, night sweats, weight loss.

*Cutaneous.* Herpes zoster or simplex lesions, seborrheic or other dermatitis, fungal infections of the skin (candidiasis) and nail beds (onychomycosis), KS lesions, and warts.

*Head/neck.* "Cotton-wool" spots visualized on funduscopic examination; oral KS; candidiasis (thrush); hairy leukoplakia; aphthous ulcers; enlarged, hard, and occasionally tender lymph nodes.

*Respiratory.* Tachypnea, dyspnea, diminished or adventitious breath sounds (crackles or wheezing).

*Gastrointestinal.* Enlargement of the liver or spleen, nausea, vomiting, persistent diarrhea, constipation, hyperactive bowel sounds, abdominal distention, inguinal lymphadenopathy.

*Genital/rectal.* KS lesions, herpetic lesions, candidiasis, balanitis, warts, syphilitic chancres, rectal or cervical dysplasia, fistulas, human papillomavirus–related neoplasms.

*Neuromuscular.* Neuropathy, flattened affect, apathy, withdrawal, memory deficits, headache, muscle atrophy, speech deficits, gait disorders, generalized weakness, incontinence.

## DIAGNOSTIC TESTS

A variety of diagnostic tests are used for specific reasons in the course of HIV infection. First-generation testing methods could require up to 6 months for the person to develop enough antibodies to trigger a reactive result. The period when a person is infectious but the HIV antibody is not yet detectable is referred to as the "window period." Individuals who test negative should be retested in 10 days to 3 months, depending on the sensitivity of the HIV test used to confirm seronegativity. The CDC currently recommends routine HIV screening for all individuals 13–64 years old, regardless of risk factors. The following tests are used to determine HIV infection.

**Western blot.** A confirmatory test used to separate specific viral proteins of HIV. A reactive Western blot is defined by a specific pattern of protein bands separated by electrophoresis on a strip of nitrocellulose paper. Three of the following bands must be present for reactivity: p24, p41, p65, or p120. While this is no longer the standard of care, this test still provides valuable information.

**Enzyme-linked immunosorbent assay.** A laboratory technique in which chemically modified antibodies attach to a sample. These modified antibodies can change color such as with an at-home pregnancy test or can radioactively imprint photographic film. In HIV, the patient's antibody from his or her blood bridges the gap between the test antigen and the modified antibody of the test.

**Rapid test.** Indicates the presence of the HIV antibody in oral fluid, serum, and/or whole blood within minutes. It is used in clinics and as a home test kit using a finger prick or saliva. This test is not as accurate as laboratory tests using a drawn blood sample.

**HIV RNA test.** Used to monitor the viral load clinically. It may be used as a test method and can detect infection in as early as 1 week. However, it may not be sufficiently sensitive for screening tests.

**CD4+ T cell count.** A measure of the amount of CD4+ T cells per milliliter in the blood. It is a marker for the impact of HIV infection on the immune system and the individual's susceptibility to infections. With increased viral load, there is a reduction in CD4+ T cell counts because of the destruction of these lymphocytes by HIV. A CD4+ T cell count of less than 200 is diagnostic of AIDS. Frequency of CD4+ T cell count testing is determined by clinical presentation and laboratory results.

***Viral load testing.*** Only 3%–4% of the virus is located in the plasma. The remaining amount exceeding 90% is located in lymphoid and other tissues. The viral load test measures the free virus in the plasma but not in these other areas. It is used to determine the response of antiretroviral treatment, monitor the development of drug resistance, and determine the need to change antiretroviral treatment. When a patient is on HAART, the goal is an undetectable viral load.

***Viral resistance testing.*** Testing for viral resistance to specific antiretroviral drugs is routine clinical practice. Before initiating treatment, this test is used to determine whether the virus is already resistant to a specific agent. It is also used to assess treatment failure and help determine appropriate changes in antiretroviral agents. The different types of resistance testing include genotypic assays, phenotypic assays, and virtual phenotype.

## Patient Problem/Analyze Cues/Prioritize Hypotheses
# Nonadherence

*due to* impaired judgment, socioeconomic status, antiretroviral side effects, or lack of information regarding the antiretroviral regimen

***Desired Outcome/Generate Solutions:*** After intervention, the patient states and exhibits improved adherence to the antiretroviral medication regimen.

| ASSESSMENT—RECOGNIZE CUES/ INTERVENTIONS—TAKE ACTION | RATIONALES |
|---|---|
| Assess for missed doses of antiretrovirals. Note and record any missed doses. | Antiretroviral medications will help decrease the viral load and increase the CD4+ T cell count, thus decreasing the risk for infection and other HIV-related complications. **Note:** Adherence is the most common issue related to individuals with HIV. |
| Assess for adherence to the entire antiretroviral regimen. | Antiretroviral regimens need to be taken in their entirety in order to optimize effect and decrease the risk for resistance. |
| Assess for side effects to antiretrovirals and provide nonpharmacologic and pharmacologic interventions (as prescribed) to decrease side effects. | Side effects may be one reason for nonadherence. Interventions may help improve adherence. |
| Assess for the rationale behind poor adherence and help the patient develop a strategy for improving adherence. | Assessing for specific reasons behind poor adherence can assist in providing patient-specific adherence counseling. |
| Instruct the patient on the role of antiretrovirals in improving the immune system, aiding in healing infections, preventing additional opportunistic infections and HIV-related complications, and reducing HIV transmission. | Knowledge regarding the role of antiretrovirals in improving immune system response to infections and other HIV-related complications may improve adherence. |
| Explain the need for 100% adherence in order to prevent viral resistance to antiretrovirals. | Resistance to antiretrovirals can develop with even just a few missed doses, thereby decreasing the number of treatment options and potentially increasing the pill burden. |

## Patient Problem/Analyze Cues/Prioritize Hypotheses
# Impaired Gas Exchange

*due to* altered oxygen exchange occurring with pulmonary infiltrates, hyperventilation, and sepsis

***Desired Outcomes/Generate Solutions:*** After treatment or intervention, the patient has adequate gas exchange, as evidenced by a respiratory rate (RR) of 12–20 breaths/minute with eupnea and absence of adventitious sounds such as wheezes, crackles, or rubs. There is no nasal flaring or other clinical indicators of respiratory dysfunction. By hospital discharge, the patient's oximetry demonstrates $O_2$ saturation greater than 92%–95%, depending on age, underlying cause, acute illness, or fluid overload. Arterial blood gas (ABG) results are as follows: $PaO_2$ 80 mm Hg or higher, $PaCO_2$ 35–45 mm Hg, and pH 7.35–7.45.

| ASSESSMENT—RECOGNIZE CUES/ INTERVENTIONS—TAKE ACTION | RATIONALES |
| --- | --- |
| Assess the respiratory status as often as indicated by the patient's condition. Assess the rate, rhythm, quality, cough, and sputum production. | With respiratory dysfunction, respiratory distress can be exhibited with accessory muscles use, flaring of nares, presence of adventitious sounds, cough, changes in color or character of sputum, or cyanosis. |
| Maintain the continuous or frequent monitoring of $O_2$ saturation by pulse oximetry. Report findings of less than 92%. | $O_2$ saturation 92% or less may signal the need for supplementary oxygen and should be reported to the health care provider. |
| Assess the ABG results for changes and report abnormal findings. | Decreased $PaCO_2$ (less than 35 mm Hg) and increased pH (greater than 7.45) can occur with hyperventilation. Increased $PaCO_2$ (higher than 45 mm Hg) and decreased pH (less than 7.35) can occur with respiratory failure. |
| As prescribed, initiate or adjust the oxygen therapy. | This measure helps ensure optimal oxygenation. |
| Administer the oxygen with humidity. | Humidity alleviates convective losses of moisture and relieves mucous membrane irritation, which can predispose to coughing spells. |
| Instruct the patient to report changes in cough dyspnea that increases with exertion. | These indicators may be seen with opportunistic respiratory disease. |
| Provide chest physiotherapy as prescribed. Encourage the use of incentive spirometry at frequent intervals. | These measures help loosen secretions, prevent atelectasis, and improve the expectoration of secretions. |
| Reposition the patient every 2 hours and assist with ambulation and sitting up as tolerated. | Repositioning and walking help prevent stasis of lung fluids. |
| Assess for changes in color or character of sputum; obtain sputum for culture and sensitivity if indicated and as prescribed. | Changes in color and character of sputum may signal infection; a culture confirms infection type. |
| Group nursing activities to provide the patient with uninterrupted periods of rest, optimally 90–120 minutes at a time. | Rest promotes optimal chest excursion. |
| If administering corticosteroids, be alert for additional infections or other potential side effects. | Corticosteroids may be given to improve breathing in persons with PCP pneumonia. Side effects of corticosteroids include masking of symptoms and increased susceptibility to infection. |

**Patient Problems/Analyze Cues/Prioritize Hypotheses**

# Risk for Infection

*due to* inadequate immune system function and malnutrition

**Desired Outcome/Generate Solutions:** The patient is free of additional infections, as evidenced by clinical observations and appropriate cultures or biopsies.

| ASSESSMENT—RECOGNIZE CUES/ INTERVENTIONS—TAKE ACTION | RATIONALES |
| --- | --- |
| Assess for persistent fevers, night sweats, fatigue, involuntary weight loss, persistent and dry cough, persistent diarrhea, and headache. | These are indicators of opportunistic infections that can occur as a result of breakdown of the patient's immune system. |
| Monitor the laboratory data, especially complete blood count, differential, and cultures, to evaluate the course of infection. Be alert to abnormal results and notify the health care provider of significant findings. | Increased/positive values may signal the presence/type of infection. |

## ASSESSMENT—RECOGNIZE CUES/INTERVENTIONS—TAKE ACTION / RATIONALES

| ASSESSMENT—RECOGNIZE CUES/INTERVENTIONS—TAKE ACTION | RATIONALES |
|---|---|
| Assess the temperature and vital signs at frequent intervals. Perform a complete physical assessment at least every 8 hours. | These assessments identify changes from baseline assessment that signal fever or sepsis. In addition to increased temperature, other signs include diaphoresis, confusion or mental status changes, decrease in the level of consciousness, increased heart rate (HR), and decreased blood pressure (BP) secondary to the vasodilator effect of the increased body temperature. |
| Assess for changes in breath sounds. | Diminished breath sounds or adventitious sounds may indicate opportunistic disease and/or an increasing level of pulmonary infiltrates. PJP may be seen in HIV disease when the immune system is extremely compromised (CD4+ T cell counts below 200). Other opportunistic infections that can manifest with pulmonary signs and symptoms include *Mycobacterium tuberculosis* and bacterial pneumonia. |
| Maintain strict sterile technique for all invasive procedures. | This helps prevent the introduction of new pathogens. |
| Assist the patient in maintaining meticulous body hygiene. | This measure helps prevent spread of organisms from body secretions into skin breaks, especially if the patient has diarrhea. |
| Encourage the patient to engage in frequent deep breathing, coughing, and incentive spirometry exercises. | These exercises promote pulmonary health, which will help prevent respiratory infections. |
| Assess the sites of invasive procedures for erythema, swelling, local warmth, tenderness, and purulent exudate. | These are signs of localized infection. |
| Enforce good hand hygiene practices before and after contact with the patient. | Hand washing minimizes the risk for transmitting infectious organisms from (and to) the staff and other patients. |
| Provide instructions on home care considerations for infection prevention after hospital discharge (see "Patient–Family Teaching and Discharge Planning" below). | This reinforces the importance of infection protection and promotes adherence after hospital discharge. |
| When providing care to patients with active tuberculosis (TB) or unknown TB status, wear respiratory protection consistent with current recommendations from the CDC and Occupational Safety and Health Administration. | This helps prevent the spread of disease. See "Pulmonary Tuberculosis," Chapter 16, for more information. |

## Potential Problem/Analyze Cues

# Diarrhea

*due to* opportunistic infections; medication side effects, including chemotherapy; HIV-related gastrointestinal (GI) changes; or food intolerance

**Desired Outcome/Generate Solutions:** By the time of hospital discharge, the patient has formed stools and a bowel elimination pattern that is normal for him or her.

| ASSESSMENT—RECOGNIZE CUES/INTERVENTIONS—TAKE ACTION | RATIONALES |
|---|---|
| Be alert to cool and clammy skin, increased HR (greater than 100 bpm), increased RR (greater than 20 breaths/minute), and decreased urinary output (less than 30 mL/hour or 0.5 mL/kg/hour). | These are signs of hypovolemia that could result from prolonged diarrhea. |
| Assess for anxiety, confusion, muscle weakness, cramps, dysrhythmias, weak pulse, and decreased BP. | These are indicators of electrolyte imbalance that could occur because of fluid loss. |

Continued

| ASSESSMENT—RECOGNIZE CUES/ INTERVENTIONS—TAKE ACTION | RATIONALES |
|---|---|
| Maintain accurate intake and output. | This measure monitors for changes in fluid volume status. |
| Monitor the stool cultures. | Cultures identify causative organisms. |
| Perform hand hygiene with soap and water after handling stool. | Hand hygiene is recommended by the CDC when contact with blood or body fluids is possible. Using soap and water is the best method for infection control, particularly when spores (i.e., *Clostridium difficile*) are found in stool cultures. In these cases, hand gels are considered ineffective. |
| Encourage the patient to increase fluid intake as long as there are no fluid restrictions. | Increased fluid intake helps prevent dehydration. |
| Protect anorectal area by keeping it cleansed and using compounds such as zinc oxide or sitz baths. | This measure prevents or slows skin excoriation caused by diarrhea. |
| Instruct the patient to avoid large amounts (greater than 300 mg/day) of caffeine. | Caffeine increases peristalsis and can promote diarrhea. |

## Patient Problem

# Body Weight Problem (Weight Loss)

*due to* diarrhea and nausea associated with side effects of medications, malabsorption, anorexia, dysphagia, and fatigue

***Desired Outcomes/Generate Solutions:*** By hospital discharge, the patient has adequate nutrition, as evidenced by stable or increased weight. The patient states that nausea and other GI side effects associated with HAART are controlled.

| ASSESSMENT—RECOGNIZE CUES/ INTERVENTIONS—TAKE ACTION | RATIONALES |
|---|---|
| Assess the nutritional status daily, noting weight, caloric intake, and protein values. | Progressive weight loss, wasting of muscle tissue, loss of skin tone, and decreases in total protein can adversely affect wound healing and impair the patient's ability to fight infection. |
| Provide small, frequent, high-calorie, high-protein meals, allowing sufficient time for the patient to eat. Offer supplements between feedings. | Smaller, more frequent meals may be more easily tolerated. Higher calorie/protein meals will provide the adequate nutrition necessary to promote healing. |
| Provide the supplemental vitamins and minerals as prescribed. | These supplements replace deficiencies. |
| Assess and provide the oral hygiene before and after meals. | Oral hygiene minimizes anorexia and helps treat stomatitis. |
| If the patient feels isolated socially, encourage significant others to visit at mealtimes and bring the patient's favorite high-calorie, high-protein foods from home. | Patients likely will benefit from socialization at mealtime, which also may promote intake of these high-calorie, high-protein foods. |
| If the patient is nauseated, provide instructions for deep breathing and voluntary swallowing. | These measures help decrease stimulation of the vomiting center. |
| Administer the antiemetics as prescribed. | Antiemetics helps prevent or minimize nausea. |
| Encourage the patient to request medication as early as possible. | Nausea/vomiting is easier to control when it is treated before it gets too severe or is prolonged. |

| ASSESSMENT—RECOGNIZE CUES/ INTERVENTIONS—TAKE ACTION | RATIONALES |
|---|---|
| If the patient is dysphagic, encourage intake of fluids that are high in calories and protein; provide different flavors and textures for variation. | Fluids may be better tolerated than foods when the patient has dysphagia because they are less irritating; fluids that contain supplemental nutrients will help ensure optimal intake. |
| Collaborate with speech therapy to assist persons with swallowing difficulties. | Speech therapists are integral members of the interprofessional team to diagnose and manage oral and pharyngeal dysphagia |
| Discuss the potential need for total parenteral nutrition (TPN) with the health care provider. | TPN is the administration of liquid nutrition through a peripheral venous access. It promotes caloric intake in patients whose ability for oral intake is impaired. |

## Patient Problem/Analyze Cues/Prioritize Hypotheses

# Impaired Cognition

*due to* altered sensory integration, reception, and transmission occurring with infection, space-occupying lesions in the central nervous system (CNS), or HIV dementia

***Desired Outcomes/Generate Solutions:*** After intervention, the patient verbalizes orientation to person, place, and time. Optimally, by hospital discharge, the patient correctly completes exercises in logical reasoning, memory, perception, concentration, attention, and sequencing of activities.

| ASSESSMENT—RECOGNIZE CUES/ INTERVENTIONS—TAKE ACTION | RATIONALES |
|---|---|
| Assess for minor alterations in personality traits that cannot be attributed to other causes, such as stress or medication. Interview family/friends regarding personality changes. | This assessment may help rule out medication side effects versus opportunistic diseases. |
| Assess for slowing of all cognitive functioning, with problems in the areas of attention, concentration, memory, perception, logical reasoning, and sequencing of activities. | These are signs of dementia. |
| Encourage the patient to report persistent headaches, dizziness, or seizures. | These indicators may signal CNS involvement. |
| Note any cranial nerve involvement that differs from the patient's past medical history. | Most commonly the fifth (trigeminal), seventh (facial), and eighth (acoustic) nerves are involved in infectious processes of the CNS. |
| Assess for signs of mental aberration, blindness, aphasia, hemiparesis, or ataxia. | These indicators may signal the presence of opportunistic infections. |
| Divide the activities into small, easily accomplished tasks. | Pacing activities decreases frustration and increases the likelihood of completion. |
| Maintain a stable environment (e.g., do not change the location of furniture in the room). | A stable environment helps the patient remain familiarized with the immediate surroundings. |
| Write the notes as reminders; maintain a calendar of appointments. Provide some mechanism (e.g., pillbox) to ensure medication adherence. | Patients will require these reminders to complete tasks, take medications, and make appointments as independently as possible. |
| Remind patient of the importance of reporting increasing severity of headaches, blurred vision, gait disturbances, or blackouts. Notify the health care provider of all significant findings. | These indicators identify neurologic changes that necessitate treatment intervention. |

## Patient Problem/Analyze Cues/Prioritize Hypotheses
# Pain

*due to* physical and chemical factors associated with prolonged immobility, infections, and peripheral neuropathy

***Desired Outcomes/Generate Solutions:*** Within 1–2 hours of intervention, the patient's subjective perception of pain decreases, as documented by pain scale. Nonverbal indicators of discomfort, such as grimacing, are absent or diminished.

| ASSESSMENT—RECOGNIZE CUES/ INTERVENTIONS—TAKE ACTION | RATIONALES |
| --- | --- |
| Assess and record the following: location, onset, duration, and factors that precipitate and alleviate the patient's pain. With the patient, establish a pain scale, rating pain from 0 (no pain) to 10 (worst pain). | Competent pain management requires a frequent and thorough assessment of these factors. Using a pain scale provides an objective measurement that enables the assessment of pain management strategies. |
| Administer the analgesics as prescribed. Encourage the patient to request medication before the pain becomes severe. | Pain that is allowed to become severe is more difficult to control. Prolonged stimulation of pain receptors results in increased sensitivity to painful stimuli and will increase the amount of medication required to relieve pain. |
| Provide heat or cold applications to affected areas (e.g., apply heat to painful joints and cold packs to reduce swelling associated with infections or multiple venipunctures). | Heat and cold applications are effective nonpharmacologic measures that reduce pain and augment the effects of analgesics. |
| Encourage diversional activities (e.g., soothing music; quiet conversation; reading; slow, rhythmic breathing). | Diversion is a means of increasing pain tolerance and decreasing its intensity. |
| Instruct patient about techniques such as deep breathing, biofeedback, and relaxation exercises. | These techniques reduce pain intensity by decreasing skeletal muscle tension. |
| Discuss with the health care provider the desirability of a capped venous catheter for long-term blood withdrawal. | This measure will help reduce pain in patients in whom frequent venipunctures cause discomfort. |
| Administer back rubs and massage. | These measures promote relaxation and comfort. |

## Patient Problem/Analyze Cues/Prioritize Hypotheses
# Activity Intolerance

*due to* generalized weakness and decreased muscle tone occurring with prolonged inactivity

***Desired Outcome/Generate Solutions:*** Before hospital discharge, the patient rates perceived exertion and/or pain on exertion at 3 or less on a 0–10 scale and exhibits tolerance to exercise/activity, as evidenced by HR of 20 bpm or less over resting HR, RR of 20 breaths/minute or less, and systolic BP (SBP) of 20 mm Hg or less over or under resting SBP.

| ASSESSMENT—RECOGNIZE CUES/ INTERVENTIONS—TAKE ACTION | RATIONALES |
| --- | --- |
| Assess the HR, RR, and BP before and immediately after activity, and ask the patient to rate his or her perceived exertion. See "Immobility," Chapter 1, for *Activity Intolerance* for details about rating perceived exertion. | This assessment monitors tolerance to activity. If the patient's rating of perceived exertion is more than 3, or if he or she exhibits signs of exercise/activity intolerance, the activity should be stopped or modified. |

| ASSESSMENT—RECOGNIZE CUES/ INTERVENTIONS—TAKE ACTION | RATIONALES |
|---|---|
| Assess the oximetry or ABG values to ensure that the patient is oxygenated adequately; adjust the oxygen delivery accordingly. | Oxygen saturation 92% or less may signal the need for supplemental oxygen or an increase in oxygen delivery. |
| Monitor the electrolyte levels. | This helps determine whether muscle weakness is caused by hypokalemia. |
| Plan adequate (90- to 120-minute) rest periods between scheduled activities. Adjust activities as appropriate. | This will help reduce the patient's energy expenditure. |
| As much as possible, encourage the regular periods of exercise. | Exercise helps prevent cardiac intolerance to activities, which can occur quickly after periods of prolonged inactivity. |
| Advise the patient to keep anecdotal notes (perhaps in journal format) on exacerbation and remission of signs and symptoms. | Anecdotal notes are useful tools for self-examination as well as for reporting to the health care provider, who may use this information to alter or modify treatment or develop new strategies. |

## Patient Problem/Analyze Cues/Prioritize Hypotheses

# Deficient Knowledge (Disease)

*due to* unfamiliarity with the disease process, prognosis, lifestyle changes, and treatment plan

***Desired Outcome/Generate Solutions:*** Before hospital discharge, the patient verbalizes accurate information about the disease process, prognosis, behaviors that increase the risk for transmitting the virus to others, and the treatment plan.

| ASSESSMENT—RECOGNIZE CUES/ INTERVENTIONS—TAKE ACTION | RATIONALES |
|---|---|
| Assess the patient's health care literacy (language, reading, comprehension). Assess the culture and culturally specific information needs. | This assessment helps ensure that information is selected and presented in a manner that is culturally and educationally appropriate. |
| Assess the patient's knowledge about HIV disease, including pathophysiologic changes that may occur, ways the disease is transmitted, and how to prevent other infections. Correct misinformation and misconceptions as necessary. | This assessment enables the formulation of an individualized teaching plan to improve the patient's health and quality of life. |
| Assess the patient's knowledge about HAART and viral resistance. Correct misinformation and misconceptions as necessary. | This information enables nurses to formulate individualized teaching plans to improve adherence and help prevent viral resistance to HAART. |
| Provide information about private and community agencies that are available to help with tasks such as handling legal affairs, cooking, housecleaning, and nursing care. Provide telephone numbers and addresses for HIV support groups and self-help groups. | Lack of knowledge about these services and groups may add unnecessary stress to the patient's illness. A social worker may be able to provide more resources. |
| Provide literature that explores myths and realities of the HIV disease process. | This information helps patients engage in activities that will improve, rather than harm, their health. |
| Remind the patient of the importance of informing sexual partners of the patient's HIV condition and avoiding high-risk behaviors known to transmit the virus, such as not adhering to strict condom usage. | These measures reduce the risk of transmitting the virus to others. |
| Involve the significant other in the teaching and learning process. | Involving the significant other in the teaching process not only provides information to him or her but also enables the significant other to reinforce teaching for the patient. |
| Provide the patient and significant other with names and addresses or phone numbers of HIV resources (see "Patient–Family Teaching and Discharge Planning" below). | These resources provide information about current therapies, support services, and funding for medications. |

Special Needs Care Plans

## Patient Problems/Analyze Cues/Prioritize Hypotheses

# Anxiety

*due to* significant life, physical, or emotional changes and social isolation

**Desired Outcome/Generate Solutions:** After intervention, the patient expresses feelings and is free of harmful anxiety, as evidenced by HR of 100 bpm or less, RR of 20 breaths/minute or less with normal depth and pattern (eupnea), and BP within the patient's baseline range.

| ASSESSMENT—RECOGNIZE CUES/ INTERVENTIONS—TAKE ACTION | RATIONALES |
|---|---|
| Assess for verbal or nonverbal expressions of problems coping. | Subtle cues such as guilt for past actions, uncertainty, concerns about rejection, isolation, and suicidal ideation may signal problems with coping. |
| Spend time with the patient and encourage expressions of anxieties, feelings, and concerns. Support effective coping patterns (e.g., by allowing the patient to cry or talk rather than denying his or her legitimate concerns). | Before patients can learn effective coping strategies, they must first clarify their feelings. Verbalizing feelings in a nonthreatening, nonjudgmental environment can help them deal with unresolved/ unrecognized issues that may be contributing to the current stressor. |
| Provide accurate information about HIV disease, related diagnostic procedures, and emerging treatments. | Some anxieties may be realistic, whereas others may necessitate clarification based on current treatment information. |
| If the patient hyperventilates, teach them to mimic your normal respiratory pattern (eupnea). | This is an effective calming technique. |

## Patient Problem/Analyze Cues/Prioritize Hypotheses

# Risk for Disturbed Body Image

*due to* biophysical changes resulting from KS lesions, wasting, lipodystrophy, and lipoatrophy

**Desired Outcome/Generate Solutions:** Before hospital discharge, the patient expresses positive feelings about themselves to the family, significant other, and primary nurse.

| ASSESSMENT—RECOGNIZE CUES/ INTERVENTIONS—TAKE ACTION | RATIONALES |
|---|---|
| Encourage the patient to express feelings, especially the way they view or feel about self. Provide positive feedback; help the patient focus on facts rather than myths or exaggerations. | These measures provide an environment conducive to free expression and promote understanding of health status, which may clarify misconceptions that may be contributing to the disturbed body image. |
| Provide a referral to a nutritionist if appropriate. | A nutrition expert will assist in establishing a healthy diet that will minimize body changes. |
| Provide access to clergy, psychiatric nurse, social worker, psychologist, or HIV counselor as appropriate. | The patient may require specialized counseling, especially if he or she is at risk for self-harm. |
| Encourage the patient to join and share feelings with an HIV support group. | Many people benefit from support groups and sharing experiences with others who are having similar experiences. |

## ADDITIONAL PROBLEMS:

| Impaired Mobility | Chapter 6 |
| Risk for Spiritual Distress | Chapter 8 |
| Difficulty Coping (Family) | Chapter 9 |
| Impaired Skin Integrity | Chapter 75 |

## ✓ PATIENT–FAMILY TEACHING AND DISCHARGE PLANNING

When providing patient–family teaching, focus on sensory information, avoid giving excessive information, and initiate a visiting nurse referral for necessary follow-up teaching. Include verbal and written information about the following:

✓ Importance of reporting any new symptoms of infection or changes in neurologic status (e.g., increasing severity of headaches, blurred vision, gait disturbances, blackouts) immediately to the health care provider.

✓ Necessity of modifying high-risk sexual behaviors.

✓ Prescribed medications, including drug name, dosage, purpose, and potential side effects. Also discuss drug–drug, herb–drug, and food–drug interactions. Instruct the patient and significant other in the necessity of taking antiretroviral medications as prescribed to avoid viral resistance.

✓ Importance of the patient's adherence to HAART regimens, which is critical to patients and the clinicians providing and monitoring their care. Interruptions in drug treatment can lead to the development of virus resistant to specific antiretroviral drugs, which can result in treatment failure and limiting of future treatment options. Health care providers and patient partnerships characterized by shared decision-making have been identified as a key component in successful HIV treatment.

✓ Strategies for promoting HIV treatment adherence. These must be customized to meet the needs of each patient. The approach must be patient centered and include ongoing education, psychosocial and community support, and resources that involve both patient-directed and provider-directed strategies.

✓ Because of decreased resistance to infection, particularly in persons with CD4+ T cell counts below 200, the importance of limiting contact with individuals known to have active infections. In addition, pets may harbor various fungal, protozoal, and bacterial organisms in their excrement. Therefore contact with birdcages, cat litter, and tropical fish tanks should be avoided.

✓ Necessity for meticulous hygiene to prevent the spread of any extant or new infectious organisms. To avoid exposure to fungi, damp areas in bathrooms (e.g., shower) should be cleaned with solutions of bleach, refrigerators should be cleaned thoroughly with soap and water, and leftover food should be disposed of within 2–3 days.

✓ Techniques for self-assessment of early signs of infection (e.g., erythema, tenderness, local warmth, swelling, purulent exudate) in all cuts, abrasions, lesions, or open wounds.

✓ Importance of avoiding the use of recreational drugs, which are believed to potentiate immunosuppressive processes, lower resistance to infection, and can be linked to transmission.

✓ Significance and importance of refraining from donating blood.

✓ Principles and importance of maintaining a balanced diet; ways to supplement diet with multivitamins and other food sources, such as high-calorie substances (e.g., Isocal, Ensure).

✓ Because of increased susceptibility to foodborne opportunistic organisms, fruits and vegetables should be washed thoroughly; meats should be cooked thoroughly at appropriate temperatures; and raw eggs, raw fish (sushi), and unpasteurized milk should be avoided.

✓ Care of the venous access device, including technique for self-administration of TPN or medications; and care of gastric tube and administration of enteral tube feedings if appropriate (see "Providing Nutritional Support," Chapter 76).

✓ Importance of avoiding fatigue by limiting participation in social activities, getting maximum amounts of rest, and minimizing physical exertion.

✓ Importance of maintaining medical follow-up appointments.

✓ Advisability of sharing feelings with significant other or within a support group.

✓ With discharge planning, discuss immunization status with the treating provider.

✓ Educate partner about pre-exposure prophylaxis (if not HIV+); encourage testing.

✓ In addition, provide the following information regarding HIV resources:
- Public Health Service AIDS Hotline: (800) CDC-INFO or (800) 232-4636
- National Sexually Transmitted Diseases Hotline/American Social Health Association: (800) 227-8922
- CDC HIV/AIDS information: www.cdc.gov/hiv/
- Association of Nurses in AIDS Care: www.anacnet.org
- National Institutes of Health, National Institute of Allergy and Infectious Diseases: www.niaid.nih.gov
- HRSA, Bureau of HIV/AIDS: www.hab.hrsa.gov
- AIDS Education and Training Centers National Resource Center: http://aidsetc.org
- National HIV/AIDS Clinician Consultation Center, Clinician Post-Exposure Prophylaxis Hotline (PEPline): (800) 933-3413 and www.ucsf.edu/hivcntr

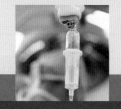

# Managing Wound Care 75

A wound is a disruption of tissue integrity caused by trauma, surgery, or an underlying medical disorder. Wound management is directed at promoting healing and preventing infection and deterioration in wound status.

## WOUNDS CLOSED BY PRIMARY INTENTION: OVERVIEW/PATHOPHYSIOLOGY

Clean, surgical, or traumatic wounds whose edges are closed with sutures, clips, tissue glue, or sterile tape strips are referred to as *wounds closed by primary intention*. Individuals at high risk for disruption of healing by primary intention are those who are elderly and/or have diabetes, malnutrition, fluid and electrolyte imbalance, prior radiation, chronic obstructive pulmonary disease (COPD), peripheral vascular disease (PVD), surgery lasting longer than 2 hours, intraoperative blood loss greater than 500 mL, or receiving medical therapy (chemotherapy, corticosteroid, or immunosuppressive drug administration).

## HEALTH CARE SETTING

Primary care, acute care, critical care

## ASSESSMENT

**Healing by primary intention.** Warm, reddened, indurated, tender incision line is seen immediately after surgery. After 1 or 2 days, epithelial cells migrate across the incision line and seal the wound. Over time, a scar is visible. Healing is complete when structural and functional integrity is reestablished, which may take up to 2 years.

**Impaired healing.** Impaired healing is seen as surgical site infection (SSI), dehiscence (opening of incision after surgery) with or without evisceration (incision opens, and organs are visible), and delayed healing. SSI includes three categories: superficial incisional SSI, deep incisional SSI, and organ/space SSI. SSI occurs within 30 days of surgery or up to 1 year if the incision involves an implant. SSI symptoms include purulent drainage; signs of inflammation (warmth, redness, pain, or tenderness); localized swelling; abscess; fever greater than 100.4°F (38°C); positive culture; and dehiscence. Evisceration also may occur. Risk for dehiscence is characterized by lack of an adequate inflammatory response and manifested by the reduction in initial redness, warmth, and induration or inflammation that persists or occurs after the fifth postinjury day; continued drainage from the incision line 2 days after injury (when no drain is present). Patients who are elderly may not exhibit classic signs of impaired healing but only changes in cognition or functional status that lead to the search for the site of infection.

## DIAGNOSTIC TESTS

***Culture and sensitivity of tissue by biopsy or swab.*** To determine organism and optimal antibiotic treatment. Sample is obtained from clean tissue, not from exudate, pus, or necrotic tissue. Infection is present when there are greater than $10^5$ organisms/g.

***White blood cell count with differential.*** Increased white blood cell (WBC) with a shift to the left seen with SSI.

***Radiographic evaluation.*** To identify abscess.

***Computed tomography/magnetic resonance imaging.*** To identify osteomyelitis (bone infection).

## Patient Problem/Analyze Cues/Prioritize Hypotheses

# Risk for Infection

*due to* contamination

***Desired Outcomes/Generate Solutions:*** The patient exhibits abatement of signs and symptoms of SSI. The incision has well-approximated wound edges, no inflammatory response past the fifth day after the injury, and no drainage.

| ASSESSMENT—RECOGNIZE CUES/ INTERVENTIONS—TAKE ACTION | RATIONALES |
|---|---|
| Assess the incision for drainage, purulent exudate, excessive inflammatory response, localized swelling, and abscess. | These signs and symptoms indicate SSI. |
| Assess vital signs for fever greater than 100.4°F (38°C) and increased heart rate (HR). Check blood pressure (BP). Document findings. | Elevated temperature and HR are possible signs of infection. BP and HR within the patient's usual range indicate the adequacy of perfusion to support healing. |
| Assess for hyperglycemia with serial capillary glucose measures and maintain blood glucose less than 200 mg/dL or the level set by the health care provider using insulin as prescribed. | Hyperglycemia increases the risk for infection. |
| Assess the pulse oximetry. Report $O_2$ saturation 92% or less and consult the health care provider about the administration of $O_2$. | Oxygen saturation 92% or less often signals the need for supplemental oxygen to support tissue healing and prevent/treat infection. |
| Anticipate the need for antibiotics. | Systemic antibiotics are used to treat SSI. |
| Assess the hydration status by monitoring peripheral pulses, moisture of mucous membranes, skin turgor, volume and specific gravity of urine, and intake and output. | Hypovolemia inhibits adequate perfusion and prevents antibiotics from reaching the wound site. |
| Assess the nutritional status (see "Providing Nutritional Support," Chapter 76, for details). | Nutrients are needed for repair. |
| Assess the wound pain using a numeric rating scale. | Pain causes vasoconstriction and may impair healing. |
| Treat pain with pharmacologic and nonpharmacologic interventions, including homeopathic/naturopathic agents. Anticipate pain associated with dressing change and premedicate as needed. | |
| Wash hands and use universal precautions in wound care. | Hand washing and universal precautions prevent cross-contamination. Intact skin is kept clean and free from drainage to maintain skin integrity, the body's first line of defense. |
| Cleanse the intact skin around the incision daily with soap and water and keep it dry. | |
| Keep the incision dry. Maintain the dressing that was applied in the operating room (OR) until changed by surgeon or as per surgeon's postoperative orders. | To maintains sterile wound environment. |
| If drainage saturates the dressing, notify surgeon, change the dressing, and clean the incision with sterile saline as prescribed by surgeon; apply a dry sterile dressing. | Moisture supports the growth of microorganisms. A dry environment inhibits microorganism growth. Most surgical dressings are changed after 48–72 hours by the health care provider or as prescribed. Saturated dressings may cause the incision to become macerated and increase the risk for infection. Sterile technique eliminates the introduction of nosocomial organisms and helps prevent infection. Drains remove excess fluid and exudate from the surgical site. |
| Follow agency policy in using sterile/clean technique when changing dressings. If a drain is present, maintain its sterility and patency (e.g., empty drainage reservoir and recharge suction on closed drainage systems if needed), and handle it gently to prevent it from becoming dislodged. | |
| Encourage deep breathing every 2 hours while the patient is awake. Provide incentive spirometry. Splint the incision with a pillow/binder as needed. | Deep breathing promotes oxygenation, which enhances wound healing. Splinting reduces tension on the incision. |
| Stress the importance of position changes at least every 2 hours and activity as tolerated. | Movement, exercise, and activity promote ventilation and circulation, and hence oxygenation to the tissues. |
| For nonrestricted patients, ensure a fluid intake of at least 30 mL/kg body weight/day. | Adequate hydration is critical to wound healing, perfusion, and antibiotics reaching the operative site. |
| Provide a diet with adequate protein, vitamin C, and calories. If the patient complains of feeling full when eating three meals per day, give more frequent small feedings. Encourage between-meal high-protein supplements (e.g., yogurt, milkshakes). | Positive nitrogen balance and nutrients support wound healing. Smaller, more frequent meals are often more easily tolerated. |
| If wound care is necessary after hospital discharge, provide instructions on clean dressing change procedure to the patient and significant other. Immunosuppressed patients require sterile technique. | Clean technique is used at home because most people have antibodies to familiar organisms. Immunosuppressed patients have an increased risk for infection. |

Special Needs Care Plans

Patient Problem/Analyze Cues/Prioritize Hypotheses

# Risk for Health Care–Associated Complication (Wound Dehiscence With or Without Evisceration)

*due to* obesity, diabetes, or tension on the suture line

**Desired Outcomes/Generate Solutions:** The patient exhibits a well-approximated incision, no drainage after 48 hours (except where a drain in present), and an appropriate inflammatory response (erythema, induration, warmth, and pain) that lasts up to 5 days.

| ASSESSMENT—RECOGNIZE CUES/ INTERVENTIONS—TAKE ACTION | RATIONALES |
|---|---|
| Assess the incision for drainage, separation of edges, and decreased or excess inflammation (redness, pain/tenderness, warmth, swelling). | The incision line usually is sealed after 48 hours; continued drainage indicates potential for disruption. Decreased inflammation may indicate an inadequate immune response and result in the inhibition of collagen deposition. Increased inflammation may indicate increased bioburden and the possibility of infection. |
| Splint the incision with a pillow or a binder. | Support reduces tension on the incision line during mobility and coughing. |
| If dehiscence/evisceration occurs when the patient is out of bed, return the patient to bed and position at a 45-degree angle unless the patient is hemodynamically unstable, and if so, position flat. | Treatment and stabilization necessitate being in bed. |
| In the presence of dehiscence (with or without evisceration), immediate treatment involves keeping subcutaneous tissues moist using sterile saline and sterile dressings. Notify the health care provider. | Moisture maintains tissue viability. Sterility prohibits the introduction of microorganisms. |
| If dehiscence is present, anticipate that the patient will need an ongoing dressing that keeps the tissue moist. | With dehiscence, moisture will help maintain tissue viability as the wound heals by secondary intention. |
| If evisceration occurs, anticipate that the patient will return to the OR for surgery. | Organs need to be maintained within a body cavity, and muscle and fascia need to be repaired; this is performed surgically in the OR. |

## ADDITIONAL PROBLEMS:

## ✓ PATIENT–FAMILY TEACHING AND DISCHARGE PLANNING

When providing patient–family teaching, focus on sensory information, avoid giving excessive information, and initiate a home health referral for necessary follow-up teaching. Include verbal and written information about the following:

- ✓ Local wound care, including type of equipment necessary, wound care procedure, and therapeutic and potential side effects of topical agents used. Have the patient or significant other demonstrate dressing change procedure before hospital discharge.
- ✓ How/where to obtain wound care supplies.

- ✓ Signs and symptoms of infection and improvement or deterioration in wound status, highlighting those that necessitate notification of the health care provider or clinic (e.g., fever, thicker exudate).
- ✓ Diet that promotes wound healing. Discuss the importance of adequate protein and calorie intake. Involve dietitian, the patient, and significant other as necessary.
- ✓ Activities that maximize ventilatory status: a planned regimen for ambulatory patients and deep breathing and turning (at least every 2 hours) for those on bedrest.
- ✓ Importance of taking pain medication, antibiotics, multivitamins, and supplements of iron and zinc as prescribed. For all medications to be taken at home, provide the following: drug name, purpose, dosage, schedule, precautions, and potential side effects. Also discuss drug–drug, herb–drug, and food–drug interactions.
- ✓ Importance of follow-up care with the health care provider; confirm time and date of next appointment, if known. If not known, ensure that the patient/family knows how to and is able to get this information.
- ✓ If needed, arrange for a visit by a home health nurse before hospital discharge.

## WOUND HEALING BY SECONDARY INTENTION: OVERVIEW/ PATHOPHYSIOLOGY

Wounds healing by secondary intention are those with tissue loss or heavy contamination that form granulation tissue and contract (get smaller in size) in order to heal. Most often, impairment of healing is caused by contamination and inadequate blood flow, hypoxemia, and malnutrition. These wounds may occur secondary to surgery or be associated with an underlying medical condition, for example, PVD or diabetes. Individuals at high risk for disruption of healing by secondary intention have similar risk factors as those healing by primary intention; that is, they are elderly/or have diabetes, malnutrition, fluid and electrolyte imbalance, prior radiation, COPD, PVD, surgery lasting longer than 2 hours, intraoperative blood loss greater than 500 mL, or receiving medical therapy (chemotherapy, steroid, or immunosuppressive drug administration).

## HEALTH CARE SETTING

Acute care, critical care, primary care, long-term care, home care

## ASSESSMENT

**Healing by secondary intention.** Initially, the wound edges are inflamed, indurated, and tender. At first, granulation tissue is pink, progressing to a deeper pink and then to a beefy red; wound tissues should be moist. Epithelial cells from the tissue surrounding the wound gradually migrate across the granulation tissue. As healing occurs, the wound edges become pink, the angle between surrounding tissue and the wound becomes less acute, wound contraction occurs, and the wound gets smaller. Occasionally, a wound has a tract or sinus that gradually decreases in size as healing occurs. When a drain is in place, volume, color, and odor of the drainage are evaluated. Time frame for healing depends on wound size and location and on the patient's physical and psychologic status. Healing is complete when structure and function have been reestablished.

**Impaired healing.** Exudate/slough/necrotic tissue is present on the floor and walls of the wound. Note distribution, color, odor, volume, and adherence of the exudates/slough/dead tissue and damage to skin surrounding the wound, including disruption, discoloration, swelling, local increased warmth, and increasing pain. Elderly patients may not exhibit classic signs of impaired healing but may only exhibit changes in cognition or functional status that would lead the provider to assess for infection.

## DIAGNOSTIC TESTS

**Culture with tissue biopsy or swab.** To determine the presence of infection and optimal antibiotic.

**Complete blood count with white blood cell differential.** Complete blood count to assess hematocrit level and for the presence of severe anemia (less than 25 g/dL). Increased WBC count signals infection, whereas a decrease occurs with immunosuppression. Monitor the lymphocyte count (1800/mm³ or less) as a sign of malnutrition.

**Radiographic evaluation/magnetic resonance imaging/ computed tomography/bone scan.** To determine the presence of osteomyelitis.

**Diagnostic work to identify the underlying cause of pathology with chronic wounds.** Invasive/noninvasive studies to diagnose such disorders as venous disease, arterial disease, and diabetic foot ulcer.

---

### Patient Problem/Analyze Cues/Prioritize Hypotheses

# Risk for Disease (Delayed Wound Healing)

*due to* the presence of contaminants, metabolic disorders (e.g., diabetes), perfusion defect (e.g., arterial/venous disease), medical therapy (e.g., chemotherapy, radiation therapy), or malnutrition

**Desired Outcomes/Generate Solutions:** The patient's wound exhibits the following signs of healing: wound edges are inflamed, indurated, and tender; with epithelialization, edges become pink; granulation tissue develops over time (identified by pink tissue that becomes beefy red); and there is no odor, exudate, or necrotic tissue. The patient or significant other successfully demonstrates wound care procedure before hospital discharge, if appropriate.

| ASSESSMENT—RECOGNIZE CUES/ INTERVENTIONS—TAKE ACTION | RATIONALES |
|---|---|
| Assess for decreased or excessive inflammatory response; epithelialization that is slowed or mechanically disrupted or noncontiguous around the wound; granulation tissue that remains pale, excessively dry, or excessively moist; and the presence of odor, exudate, slough, and/or necrotic tissue. | These are signs of impaired healing. |

Continued

| ASSESSMENT—RECOGNIZE CUES/ INTERVENTIONS—TAKE ACTION | RATIONALES |
|---|---|
| Ensure good hand hygiene and use universal precautions with wound care. | This prevents cross-contamination. |
| Cleanse the drainage or secretions from intact skin surrounding the wound with a mild disinfectant (e.g., soap and water). Do not use friction with cleansing if tissue is friable. | Cleansing removes chemical irritants and bacterial contaminants. |
| Cleanse the wound with each dressing change using 100–150 mL solution (e.g., saline, water, 0.5%–1.0% acetic acid) and a 35-mL syringe with an 18-gauge angiocatheter, following prescriber's orders and infection prevention procedures outlined in agency policy. | Use of an angiocatheter facilitates dislodging and removal of bacteria and loosens necrotic tissue, foreign bodies, and exudates. |
| When topical enzymes are prescribed, use them on necrotic tissue only and follow package directions carefully. | Enzymes remove necrotic tissue and spare healthy tissue. |
| Apply the prescribed dressings following meticulous infection prevention procedures. | Depending on the patient's individual needs, these dressings keep healthy wound tissue moist. |
| When prescribed, apply antimicrobial dressings for infection. | Silver dressings, honey dressings, cadexomer carbohydrate or polyethylene glycol slow-release, and polyhexamethylene biguanide reduce bacteria counts over a 2- to 4-week period. |
| Insert dressing gently into all tracts. Do not overfill. | This promotes the gradual closure of those areas. |
| When a drain is used, maintain its patency, prevent its kinking, and secure the tubing to prevent the drain from becoming dislodged. | Drains remove excess tissue fluid or purulent drainage. |
| Use the sterile technique when caring for drains. | Organisms may move into tissue by way of the drain. Sterile technique reduces the risk for contamination and ingress of organisms. |
| With closed drainage systems, empty the drainage reservoir and document the volume removed. Maintain suction as needed. | Suction aids in the removal of excess fluid. |
| With negative pressure therapy, maintain pressure and change the dressing as prescribed. | This therapy reduces bacterial load and enhances blood flow to support healing. |
| Provide care consistent with the underlying pathology, for example, venous ulcer (compression) or arterial ulcer (support for arterial flow) as prescribed. | Healing requires implementation of local and systemic care that supports the overall plan for treating the patient's pathology. Failure to provide care consistent with the overall plan of care may undermine positive patient outcomes. |
| Provide instructions to the patient or significant other on the prescribed wound care procedure, if indicated. | Wound care may be required after the patient is discharged. |

## ADDITIONAL PROBLEMS:

| | |
|---|---|
| *Risk for Impaired Skin Integrity* | Chapter 3 |
| *Acute Pain* | Chapter 5 |
| *Ineffective Tissue Perfusion* | Chapter 18 |
| *Risk for Impaired Skin Integrity* | Chapter 47 |

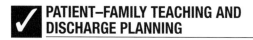 PATIENT–FAMILY TEACHING AND DISCHARGE PLANNING

See teaching and discharge planning interventions in "Wounds Closed by Primary Intention," earlier.

## WOUND HEALING BY TERTIARY INTENTION: OVERVIEW/ PATHOPHYSIOLOGY

Tertiary healing (delayed primary intention) occurs when a wound is initially left open after surgical removal (debridement) of all nonviable tissue. The wound may also be left open to allow for drainage of wounds with high bacterial content. Eventually, the wound edges are sutured closed after a period of time and when the infection is controlled, the wound appears clean, and there is evidence of good tissue perfusion.

## See Patient Problem/Analyze Cues/ Prioritize Hypotheses: (Risk for Infection)

*due to* contamination

## See Patient Problem/Analyze Cues/ Prioritize Hypotheses: *Risk for Disease (Delayed Wound Healing) under Wound Healing by Secondary Intention*

### PATIENT–FAMILY TEACHING AND DISCHARGE PLANNING

See teaching and discharge planning interventions in "Wounds Closed by Primary Intention," earlier.

### Pressure Injury: Overview/Pathophysiology

Pressure injury (PI) is localized damage to the skin and/or underlying soft tissue, usually over a bony prominence, or related to a medical or other devices. The injury can present as intact skin or an open ulcer and may be painful. Injury results from intense and/or prolonged pressure or pressure in combination with shear. Tissue tolerance for pressure and shear is influenced by microclimate, nutrition, perfusion, comorbidities, and condition of the soft tissue.

High-risk patients include elderly persons and those with decreased mobility, decreased level of consciousness (LOC), impaired sensation, debilitation, incontinence, sepsis/elevated temperature, malnutrition, or a previous PI.

## HEALTH CARE SETTING

Primary care, acute care, critical care, long-term care, assisted care, home care

## ASSESSMENT

Risk assessment and skin assessment together identify high-risk individuals on admission and with daily assessments during hospitalization using a standard assessment schema. PI severity is staged on a scale of 1–4 or classified as unstageable or having deep tissue injury. Other categories of PI are medical device–related PI (MDRPI) and mucosal membrane PI (MMPI).

- *Stage 1 PI:* Nonblanchable erythema of intact skin. The skin is intact skin with a localized area of nonblanchable erythema, which may appear differently in darkly pigmented skin. Blanchable erythema or changes in sensation, temperature, or firmness may precede visual changes. Color changes do not include purple or maroon discoloration, which may indicate deep tissue PI.
- *Stage 2 PI:* Partial-thickness skin loss with exposed dermis. The wound bed is viable, pink or red, and moist and also may present as an intact or ruptured serum-filled blister. Adipose (fat) and deeper tissues are not visible. Granulation tissue, slough, and eschar are not present. These injuries commonly result from adverse microclimate and shear in the skin over the pelvis and shear in the heel. **Note:** This stage should not be used to describe moisture-associated skin damage, including incontinence-associated dermatitis, intertriginous dermatitis, medical adhesive–related skin injury, or traumatic wounds (skin tears, burns, abrasions).
- *Stage 3 PI:* Full-thickness skin loss. There is full-thickness loss of skin in which adipose (fat) is visible in the ulcer, and granulation tissue and epibole (rolled wound edges) are often present. Slough and/or eschar may be visible. The depth of tissue damage varies by anatomic location; areas of significant adiposity can develop deep wounds. Undermining and tunneling may occur. Fascia, muscle, tendon, ligament, cartilage, and/or bone are not exposed. If slough or eschar obscures the extent of tissue loss, this is an unstageable PI.
- *Stage 4 PI:* Full-thickness skin and tissue loss. There is full-thickness skin and tissue loss with exposed or directly palpable fascia, muscle, tendon, ligament, cartilage, or bone in the ulcer. Slough and/or eschar may be visible. Epibole (rolled edges), undermining, and/or tunneling often occur. Depth varies by anatomical location. If slough or eschar obscures the extent of tissue loss, this is an unstageable PI.
- *Unstageable PI:* Obscured full-thickness skin and tissue loss. There is full-thickness skin and tissue loss in which the extent of tissue damage within the injury cannot be confirmed because it is obscured by slough or eschar. If slough or eschar is removed, a stage 3 or stage 4 PI will be revealed. Stable eschar (i.e., dry, adherent, intact without erythema or fluctuance) on an ischemic limb or the heel(s) should not be removed.
- *Deep Tissue PI (DTPI):* Persistent nonblanchable deep-red, maroon, or purple discoloration. Intact or nonintact skin with localized area of persistent nonblanchable deep-red, maroon, or purple discoloration or epidermal separation revealing a dark wound bed or blood-filled blister. Pain and temperature change often precede skin color changes. Discoloration may appear differently in darkly pigmented skin. DTPI results from intense and/or prolonged pressure and shear forces at the bone-muscle interface. It may evolve rapidly to reveal the actual extent of tissue injury or may resolve without tissue loss. If necrotic tissue, subcutaneous tissue, granulation tissue, fascia, muscle, or other underlying structure is visible, this indicates a full-thickness PI (unstageable, stage 3, or stage 4). Do not use DTPI to describe vascular, traumatic, neuropathic, or dermatologic conditions.

### ADDITIONAL PRESSURE INJURY DEFINITIONS:

#### Medical Device–Related Pressure Injury

This category describes the etiology of the injury. MDRPIs result from the use of diagnostic or therapeutic devices. The resultant PI generally conforms to the pattern or shape of the device. The injury is staged using the staging system.

#### Mucosal Membrane Pressure Injury

MMPI is found on mucous membranes with a history of a medical device in use at the injury site. Because of the anatomy of the tissue, MMPI cannot be staged. High-risk patients include elderly persons and those who have decreased mobility, decreased LOC, impaired sensation, debilitation, incontinence, sepsis/elevated temperature, malnutrition, or previous PI.

*Do not downstage during PI assessment. The injury is always described at its greatest depth (e.g., healing stage 4 injury) because tissue lost in a PI is not replaced; rather the hole is filled with scar tissue.*

## DIAGNOSTIC TESTS

See Diagnostic Tests in "Wound Healing by Secondary Intention."

## Patient Problem/Analyze Cues/Prioritize Hypotheses

# Risk for Impaired Skin/Tissue Integrity

*due to* excessive tissue pressure and shear

***Desired Outcomes/Generate Solutions:*** The patient's tissue remains intact. The patient or significant other participates in preventive measures and verbalizes an accurate understanding of the rationale for these interventions.

| ASSESSMENT—RECOGNIZE CUES/ INTERVENTIONS—TAKE ACTION | RATIONALES |
|---|---|
| Assess the PI risk and skin status daily. Focus on tissue over bony prominences and inspect mucous membranes when a medical device is present. Use a standard risk assessment scale such as the Braden Scale. Document the findings. | Early identification of risk and injury enables timely prevention and treatment. |
| Establish and post a position-changing schedule. | This communicates established turning and position-changing schedule for the staff and the patient/family and reinforces its importance. |
| **[!]** Ensure the following position changes: | Turning removes pressure from tissues and prevents ischemia. There is an inverse relationship between pressure and time in PI formation. Heavier patients need to change position more frequently because fat tissue is poorly perfused. |
| • Turn immobile patients every 2 hours using appropriate assistive devices (e.g., turning sheet, sliding board). Assist those able to turn themselves. | |
| • Use pillows, foam wedges, or gel pads to maintain lateral positioning as needed | Proper body alignment is maintained with assistive devices. |
| • Assist/remind wheelchair-bound patients to perform chair push-ups/ change position every 1–2 hours. | Position changes ensure periodic relief from pressure. |
| • For high-risk patients and those with a history of previous PI, provide pressure-relief measures more frequently. | Healed PIs have a lower pressure tolerance than uninjured skin. |
| • Keep the head of bed at or below 30 degrees and position the bed flat when not contraindicated. Alternate the supine position with prone when possible and 30-degree or less elevated side-lying positions. | Greater head elevation increases shearing when patients slide down in bed. A side-lying position at 30 degrees or less prevents high pressure on the trochanter. |
| **[!]** • For immobile patients, raise their heels off the bed surface ("float heels"). | This totally relieves pressure on heels, an area of increased PI risk due to little subcutaneous tissue. |
| **[!]** • Lift rather than drag patients during position changes and transferring; use a transfer board/draw sheet to facilitate the patient's movement. | Lifting minimizes friction and shear on tissue during activity. |
| **[!]** • Use sufficient staff and assistive devices to move or position the patient. Consider using a trapeze for those able to help position self. | This prevents friction and shear and promotes staff safety. |
| • Apply heel and elbow protection as needed. | These protectors prevent shearing when the patient moves. |
| • Consider the need for a mattress such as foam, low air loss, alternating air, gel, or water. | These mattresses reduce pressure on body tissues. Facility policy dictates the appropriate mattress. |
| • Encourage the patient to maintain or increase the current level of activity. Mobilize early and progressively. | Activity promotes blood flow, which helps prevent impaired skin/tissue integrity. |
| • Do not massage over bony prominences. | Massage can result in skin/tissue damage. |
| • Cleanse the skin daily and at the time of soiling. Use moisture barriers, diapers (for pediatrics), and disposable adult briefs as needed. | These measures minimize skin exposure to moisture and chemical irritants. |

| ASSESSMENT—RECOGNIZE CUES/ INTERVENTIONS—TAKE ACTION | RATIONALES |
|---|---|
| • For patients with excessive perspiration, ensure frequent bathing and bedding changes. | Perspiration reduces tissue tolerance. |
| • Maximize protein, calorie, and fluid intake, taking into consideration the patient's overall condition. | Adequate nutrition and fluid are critical to maintaining tissue integrity. |

## Patient Problem/Analyze Cues/Prioritize Hypotheses

# Impaired Skin Integrity

*due to* excessive pressure and shear, altered circulation, and the presence of contaminants or irritants (chemical, thermal, or mechanical)

***Desired Outcomes/Generate Solutions:*** Stages 1 and 2 show progressive healing over days to weeks; stages 3 and 4 may require months to heal. For injuries that can be healed, a 30% reduction in wound size occurs in 4 weeks. After intervention and instruction, the patient or significant other verbalizes causes and preventive measures for PI and successfully participates in the plan of care to promote healing and prevent further breakdown.

| ASSESSMENT—RECOGNIZE CUES/ INTERVENTIONS—TAKE ACTION | RATIONALES |
|---|---|
| Assess the PI and stage (see Assessment, earlier). | Assessment provides data on ulcer status. |
| | Frequency of assessment is determined by agency policy or instructions for home care. |
| Apply the preventive interventions to all patients with a PI. | Those who have a PI are at risk for additional injury due to pressure and shear. |
| Avoid positioning on the PI. | External pressure reduces blood flow and increases the risk for ischemia and further tissue injury. |
| Anticipate and treat wound pain before dressing change. | Pain causes vasoconstriction and may reduce blood flow to the injury. Adequate perfusion is needed for healing. |
| Ensure good hand hygiene and use universal precautions with wound care. | This measure prevents cross-contamination. |
| Cleanse the PI using a dressing that is consistent with the status of the injury (described under "Wound Healing by Secondary Intention," earlier). Maintain a moist physiologic environment. Change dressings as indicated, using meticulous infection prevention procedure. Clean technique with standard precautions is used for most dressing changes. | Dressings provide a physiological environment to aid with healing. Moisture is needed for cells to migrate to close the injury. Dressings minimize contaminants. |
| Avoid using dressing/tape on damaged skin. If tape must be used, apply paper tape. | Removal of adherent tape/dressing may further disrupt friable tissue. Paper tape is the least offensive to fragile skin. |
| Keep the patient's skin clean with regular bathing and be especially conscientious about washing urine and feces from the skin. | Incontinence causes chemical irritation to the skin and reduces tissue tolerance to external pressure. Soap should be used and then thoroughly rinsed from the skin. |
| Apply heel and elbow protection as needed. | These protectors absorb moisture and prevent shearing when the patient moves. |
| For patients with excessive perspiration, ensure frequent bathing and bedding changes. | Perspiration reduces tissue tolerance. |
| Instruct the patient and significant other about the importance of and measures to prevent excess pressure. | Knowledgeable individuals are more likely to adhere to prevention measures. |

## ADDITIONAL PROBLEMS:

| | |
|---|---|
| *Risk for Impaired Skin Integrity* | Chapter 3 |
| *Acute Pain* | Chapter 5 |

 **PATIENT–FAMILY TEACHING AND DISCHARGE PLANNING**

When providing patient–family teaching, focus on sensory information, avoid giving excessive information, and initiate a home health referral for necessary follow-up teaching. Consider including verbal and written information about the following:

✓ Location of local medical supply stores that have pressure-reducing mattresses and wound care supplies.

✓ Planning a schedule for changing the patient's positions.

See "Wounds Closed by Primary Intention," earlier, for other teaching and discharge planning interventions.

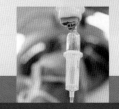

# Providing Nutritional Support 76

Adequate nutrition is necessary to meet the body's demands in order to maintain normal body composition and function. A patient's nutritional status may be affected by disease or injury state (i.e., cancer or trauma), physical factors (e.g., poor dentition or mobility), social factors (e.g., isolation, lack of financial resources), or psychologic factors (e.g., mental illness). In addition, cultural beliefs (e.g., vegetarian diet) and age (e.g., older adults with cognitive impairment causing them to forget to eat) may influence overall nutrition intake.

Poor nutrition is associated with impaired wound healing, pressure injuries, infections, increased hospital stays, and associated costs. All individuals should be assessed for imbalanced nutrition risk. Nutrition support should be considered when individuals are unable or expected to be unable to meet nutritional needs through oral intake. Nutrition support should be initiated within 24–28 hours in critically ill adult individuals unable to meet needs orally.

## HEALTH CARE SETTING

Acute care

## ASSESSMENT

### Food and nutrition history

A dietary history is compiled to reveal the adequacy of usual and recent food intake. Based on the information obtained, the nurse may identify the need to consult with a Registered Dietitian Nutritionist (RDN) for additional interventions. Nutritional assessment should include excesses or deficiencies of nutrients and any special eating patterns such as vegetarian or prescribed diets, fad diets, and excessive supplementation. The patient's perception of and actual intake may differ from what they actually ingest, and therefore family, significant others, or caregivers should be included when obtaining a dietary history. The nursing care plan should identify anything that impairs adequate selection, preparation, ingestion, digestion, absorption, or excretion of nutrients, as follows:

- Food allergies, food aversions, and use of prescribed or over-the-counter nutritional supplements.
Alternative therapies such as use of herbs or other "natural" supplements.
- Over-the-counter medications.
- Recent unplanned weight loss or gain.

- Chewing or swallowing difficulties, dental health problems, dentures (and their fit), missing teeth, no teeth, and/or loose teeth.
- Nausea, vomiting, or pain with eating.
- Altered pattern of elimination (e.g., constipation, diarrhea).
- Chronic disease affecting utilization of nutrients (e.g., malabsorption, pancreatitis, diabetes mellitus).
- Surgical resection; disease of the gut or accessory organs of digestion (i.e., pancreas, liver, gallbladder).
- Pregnancy or lactating.
- Use of medications that affect gastrointestinal (GI) function (e.g., laxatives, antacids, antibiotics, antineoplastic drugs)
- Use of alcohol and/or illegal drugs that may affect appetite, digestion, or utilization or excretion of nutrients.

## PHYSICAL ASSESSMENT

The current assessment findings should be compared with past assessments, especially related to the following:
- Loss of muscle and adipose tissue.
- Clothing that does not fit.
- Work and muscle endurance.
- Ability to maintain activities of daily living.
- Changes in mobility and/or activities.
- Changes in hair, skin, or neuromuscular function.
- Excessive bruising or bleeding (may reflect vitamin K deficiency).
- Alopecia or seborrheic dermatitis (may reflect biotin deficiency).
- Scaly dermatitis (may reflect essential fatty acid deficiency).
- Sores at the edges of the mouth, facial rash, peeling of the skin on the palms of the hands and soles of the feet, and brittle nails (may reflect zinc deficiency.)
Dry, scaling skin; brittle nails; and/or dry hair (may reflect calcium deficiency).

***Height.*** Used to determine the ideal weight and body mass index (BMI). If the patient's height is unavailable or impossible to measure, obtain an estimate from the family or significant other.

***Weight.*** Used by many to determine nutritional status, but fluctuations may be a result of amputation, dehydration, diuresis, fluid retention (renal failure, edema, third spacing), fluid resuscitation, wound dressings, or clothing. One liter of fluid equals approximately 2 lb or 1 kg. The patient should be asked to recall usual weight, weight changes (gains and losses), and the time frame in which these occurred. Unintentional loss in weight of greater than 10% over a 6-month period is considered significant and may be associated with severe malnutrition. The greater the unintentional weight loss, the more predictive this weight loss may be of mortality.

**Body mass index.** Used to evaluate the weight of adults. One calculation and one set of standards are applicable to both men and women:

$$BMI\ (kg/m^2) = Weight/Height\ (m^2)$$

You may also refer to the following Centers for Disease Control and Prevention (CDC) online BMI calculator: https://www.cdc.gov/healthyweight/assessing/bmi/adult_bmi/english_bmi_calculator/bmi_calculator.html.

BMI is interpreted using standard weight categories for adults 20 years and older. BMI values between 18.5 and 24.9 are considered normal or healthy weight. Overweight is defined as a BMI between 25 and 29.9, obesity is a BMI greater than 30, and extreme obesity a BMI greater than 40. A BMI below 18.5 is considered underweight. A BMI of less than 18.5 and greater than 40 is associated with high nutrition risk and mortality. However, BMI alone is not an adequate measure of nutritional status. Referral to an RDN for underweight and obese individuals should be considered. Height, weight, and BMI should be documented in the medical record.

**Nutritional support modalities.** Specialized nutritional support refers to the provision of an artificial formulation of nutrients by enteral (via mouth or tube directly to the stomach or small intestine) or parenteral route for the treatment or prevention of malnutrition. Oral supplements are the preferred route because they are less invasive, more natural, and less costly, whereas tube feeding is preferred over parenteral nutrition (PN).

### Types of feeding tubes

*Small-bore nasal tubes.* Defined as 12 French or smaller. Composition may be polyurethane, silicone, or polyvinyl chloride, and the usual length is 36–55 inches. It may or may not require a stylet for insertion. Location cannot be verified in the GI tract when using auscultation after injecting an air bolus, asking the patient to speak, or submerging the tube's proximal tip into a glass of water. Standard of practice dictates that an abdominal radiographic examination is needed for confirmation of placement. The US Food and Drug Administration (FDA) has approved the use of an electromagnetically guided placement device to confirm tube placement. There continues to be a risk for misplacement regardless of the technique used for placement. The physician determines whether the distal tip ends in the stomach or small intestine. It also may be inserted using endoscopy- or fluoroscopy-guided placement. Because of their diameter and composition, these tubes are easily dislocated proximally in the GI tract without any resultant external signs.

*Large-bore nasal tubes.* Defined as larger than 12 French with a composition of either polyurethane or polyvinyl chloride. Usual length of the tube is 36 inches. A stylet is not required for insertion. Insertion may be by a nurse. Placement is confirmed by withdrawal of gastric fluid or radiographic examination.

*Gastrostomy tubes.* Enter the stomach directly through the abdominal wall and usually are anchored with either a balloon or disk on the inside of the stomach. Usually, they are 12 French or larger. Composition may be polyurethane, silicone, or rubber, and they may contain multiple ports, in addition to the main lumen, for the insertion of air into the balloon and delivery of medications. Initially, a physician in radiology, endoscopy, or surgery performs the insertion. If not placed during surgery (i.e., open laparotomy), the common term used to describe the tube is *percutaneous endoscopically inserted gastrostomy.* Reinsertion by a nurse is determined by agency policy. Inadvertent removal of a tube in position for less than 6 weeks should be considered a medical emergency, and the health care provider should be contacted immediately.

*Gastrostomy button.* Placed into a mature gastrostomy stoma. It fits into the stoma tract flush with the outer abdominal wall. The button contains an anti-reflux valve to prevent leakage, but gastric samples or residuals usually cannot be obtained via the button.

*Jejunostomy tubes.* Placed by a physician either surgically or percutaneously (*percutaneous endoscopically inserted jejunostomy*). The diameter is usually about 12–18 French. Confirmation of position requires radiographic examination with contrast. No residuals should be obtained from this tube. If the tube becomes displaced, the entry site into the jejunum will close down rapidly (approximately 20–30 minutes). Reinsertion by a nurse is determined by agency policy but is not recommended without special training.

*Gastrostomy-jejunostomy tubes.* Enters the stomach directly through the abdominal wall with a small-bore jejunostomy tube placed through the main lumen of the gastrostomy and the distal tip positioned in the jejunum.

### Feeding sites

*Stomach.* Simulates normal GI functions; may be used for bolus, intermittent, or continuous feedings; indicated for patients who have intact gag or cough reflexes.

*Duodenum, jejunum.* Must be used for continuous feedings only to prevent dumping syndrome and diarrhea. Small-bore diameter tube is recommended.

## Parenteral Nutrition

PN provides some or all nutrients by the intravenous (IV) route. PN is used to provide complete nutrition for patients who cannot receive enteral nutrition or to supplement the nutritional needs of patients who are unable to absorb sufficient calories through the GI tract. PN is more expensive than enteral nutrition and can potentially lead to the development of severe complications more rapidly.

## Parenteral nutrition administration site

**Central venous catheter and peripherally inserted central catheter.** Used for all IV solutions whose final concentration is greater than 12.5% dextrose or a solution with an osmolarity of 800 mOsm/L or greater. (If unsure or information is unavailable on the infusion container related to infusion route, consult with a pharmacist or refer to hospital policy.) Use of central venous catheter (CVC) requires a large central vein with the distal tip of the catheter in the superior vena cava. A peripherally inserted central catheter (PICC) line is inserted into a large peripheral vein such as the basilic, brachial, cephalic, or medial cubital veins of the arm. The flow of blood through the large vessels rapidly dilutes hypertonic solutions and decreases the potential for thrombophlebitis.

## Transitional feeding

Patients who have received PN for more than 2–3 weeks may have some mucosal atrophy of the bowel and will need a period of adjustment before the bowel can fully resume its usual functions of digestion and absorption. The best diet advancement includes starting with clear liquids, then advancing to a regular diet. Also, because these individuals have been ill, the lactase in their stomachs has decreased, placing them at higher risk for lactose deficiency. Therefore, they should limit or avoid a full liquid diet because of the increased incidence of bloating, nausea, and diarrhea associated with lactose deficiency.

## Patient Problem/Analyze Cues/Prioritize Hypotheses

# Body Weight Problem (Weight Loss)

*due to* the inability to ingest, digest, or absorb carbohydrates, protein, and/or fat

*Desired Outcome/Generate Solutions:* The patient has stabilization of weight at the desired level or steady weight gain of ½–1 lb/week; presence of wound granulation (i.e., pinkish-white tissue around wound edges; wound edges approximating together), and absence of infection (see *Risk for Infection*, later).

| ASSESSMENT—RECOGNIZE CUES/ INTERVENTIONS—TAKE ACTION | RATIONALES |
|---|---|
| **For Oral Nutrition:** | |
| Collaborate with an RDN to assess for nutritional deficiencies within 24 hours of admission with a nutritional screening tool. | Hospitalized patients are at risk for developing protein-energy malnutrition. Baseline assessment enables comparison with subsequent assessments, which may reveal problems that may require interventions. |
| Assess for food allergies/intolerances and avoid these foods. | Individuals with celiac disease, for example, will have severe GI reactions (i.e., bloating, abdominal cramping, diarrhea) when exposed to even small amounts of wheat and other gluten-containing products. |
| Obtain weight weekly. | Stabilizing weight or a weight gain of 1/2–1 lb/week is the usual goal if weight gain is desired. |
| Position the patient in high-Fowler position for eating. | This promotes a normal position for eating and decreases the risk for aspiration. |
| Provide small, frequent feedings of diet compatible with the disease state and the patient's ability to ingest foods. | After an illness, early satiety may be a problem. Small, frequent meals are likely to increase intake. |
| Respect food aversions, religious guidelines, and food preferences. | Individuals will eat more readily and frequently when consuming preferred foods that are within dietary allowances. |
| Provide liquid nutritional supplements as prescribed. | Supplements increase calories consumed and help meet recommended daily allowances (RDAs) for vitamins and minerals needed for recovery. |
| Serve the nutrition supplements cold or over ice according to patient preference. | Serving cold will help enhance palatability. |
| Provide a psychologic support to patient. | Emotional health influences appetite. |

Continued

| ASSESSMENT—RECOGNIZE CUES/ INTERVENTIONS—TAKE ACTION | RATIONALES |
|---|---|
| Involve significant other in meal rituals for companionship. | Patients who eat alone tend to eat less. |
| **For Enteral or PN in the Acute Care Setting:** | |
| Collaborate with an RDN to assess for nutritional deficiencies within 24 hours of admission with a nutritional screening tool; document and reassess weekly. | Hospitalized patients are at risk for developing protein-calorie malnutrition. Baseline assessment enables comparison with subsequent assessments, which may reveal problems that may require intervention. |
| Assess initial and at least weekly values of electrolytes, blood urea nitrogen (BUN), creatinine, phosphorus, and magnesium. | Values outside the normal range may signal changing metabolic status, decreased renal function, or refeeding syndrome. |
| Assess daily for refeeding syndrome in patients with risk factors. | Risk for refeeding syndrome occurs after a large carbohydrate infusion in a patient with previous inadequate food intake and may result in fluid retention, hypophosphatemia, hypokalemia, hypomagnesium, increased diarrhea, and cardiac dysrhythmias. |
| Assess the other laboratory data initially and then at least weekly; liver function tests, including albumin, alkaline phosphatase, total bilirubin. | These laboratory values provide data about tolerance, clearance, and metabolism by organs and stabilization of the disease process. |
| Assess for fluid imbalance, especially fluid overload.<br><br>Fluid excess may be manifested by peripheral edema, adventitious breath sounds (especially crackles), and weight gain (1 kg = 1000 mL). | Patients may be especially susceptible to fluid excess because low protein levels in the blood cause a decrease in oncotic pressure in the vessels, resulting in fluid retention. |
| Assess the patient's weight initially and daily during an acute illness, then advance to weekly. | Stabilized weight or weight gain of 1/2–1 lb/week is the usual goal if weight gain is an intended goal. Weight trend also assesses the fluid status and disease process. |
| Administer continuous enteral feedings using a feeding pump at the prescribed rate. | A steady infusion rate decreases feelings of fullness and avoids peaks in blood glucose levels. Postoperative patients may experience gastric ileus and benefit from feedings delivered into the small bowel. |
| Check the infused volume and rate every 4 hours. | This helps ensure the accuracy of the prescribed delivery. |
| If prescribed, administer the intermittent bolus feeding over 30–40 minutes by gravity infusion. Do not use plunger to force feeding into stomach. | Intermittent bolus feeding is similar to the natural pattern of eating, and infusion through gravity prevents overfeeding and mucosal damage that may occur with plunging/forcing feeding directly into stomach. |
| Administer the PN using a volumetric pump at the prescribed rate. | There is potential for complications if dextrose or electrolytes are infused too quickly, such as hyperglycemia and hyperkalemia. An approved continuous rate for volume is better tolerated. |
| Check the infused volume and rate every hour or as per facility policy. | Checking volume and rate prevents volume overload and other complications that could occur when using the pump. |

**Note:** If fluid in PN infuses before a new bag is available, replace the empty bag with 10% Dextrose until the PN replacement is available to prevent hypoglycemia.

## Patient Problem/Analyze Cues/Prioritize Hypotheses

# Risk for Aspiration

*due to* GI feeding or delayed gastric emptying

***Desired Outcome/Generate Solutions:*** The patient is free of aspiration problems as evidenced by auscultation of clear lung sounds, vital signs (VS) remain within patient's baseline, and no signs of respiratory distress.

| ASSESSMENT—RECOGNIZE CUES/ INTERVENTIONS—TAKE ACTION | RATIONALES |
|---|---|
| Mark the nasogastric (NG) tube at the time of placement to determine the length exiting from the body. Check this mark to determine tube migration. Secure tubing in place per agency policy. | The NG tube can easily slide out of the nose because of nasal discharge, sweat, and loosening of the tape or tube holder. The tube also may migrate beyond the pylorus over time. |
| ⚠ Reassess the tube position as per agency policy every 4 hours and before each feeding. | If tube migration is suspected or the tube is reinserted, obtain x-ray to confirm placement. |
| ⚠ Assess the respiratory status every 4 hours, including respiratory rate, effort, and adventitious breath sounds.<br>• Regurgitation or vomiting of gastric contents.<br>• Aspiration from the oropharynx of saliva and upper airway secretions. | Lung sounds should be clear, and there should be no signs of respiratory distress before infusing a feeding.<br>Aspiration of gastric contents is a risk factor for ventilator-associated pneumonia, which is the leading cause of hospital-associated death.<br>Aspiration of bacteria from the oral and pharyngeal areas may cause bacterial pneumonia. |
| Monitor the temperature every 4 hours; report any parameters as defined by the health care provider. | Temperature outside of parameters as defined by the health care provider should be reported. An increased temperature occurs with aspiration pneumonia. |
| Auscultate the bowel sounds every 8 hours. | High-pitched or absent bowel sounds, abdominal distention, or nausea can occur with ileus, decreased tolerance to the feeding, and small bowel obstruction. These problems can lead to vomiting and aspiration and therefore should be reported promptly. |
| ⚠ Depending on the patient's medical condition, raise the head of bed 30 degrees or higher or place the patient in a right side-lying position during and for 1 hour after administration of a bolus or intermittent feeding. | These positions promote gravity flow from the greater stomach curvature through the pylorus into the duodenum and decrease the risk for aspiration. |
| Stop the tube feeding 1/2–1 hour before chest physical therapy or placing the patient supine. | This measure enables complete emptying of the stomach and decreases the potential for aspiration. |
| Check residuals per agency policy. | High-volume residuals may be a sign of intolerance because of ileus or small bowel obstruction, either of which can lead to vomiting and aspiration. |
| Recognize that no residuals or minimal volume should be obtained from a tube placed into the small intestine. | Unlike the stomach, the small intestine does not function as a reservoir and therefore normally will not hold volume because of forward peristalsis. |
| ⚠ Avoid the use of formulas that have been tinted with coloring to assess for aspiration. | Published case reports describe fatal metabolic acidosis secondary to the excessive use of food coloring in enteral feedings. This practice has received a warning from the FDA and should not be used under any circumstance. |

## Patient Problem/Analyze Cues/Prioritize Hypotheses

# Diarrhea

*due to* medications, dumping syndrome, bacterial contamination, or formula intolerance

**Desired Outcome/Generate Solutions:** The patient has formed stools within 2–3 days of intervention.

| ASSESSMENT—RECOGNIZE CUES/ INTERVENTIONS—TAKE ACTION | RATIONALES |
|---|---|
| Assess the abdomen and GI status: bowel sounds, distention, cramping, nausea, and frequency of bowel movements. | These assessments establish a baseline and reference point from which the current trend can be compared. Hyperactive bowel sounds may occur with increased stooling, along with signs and symptoms of distention, cramping, and nausea. |
| Ask the patient to define diarrhea. Determine the patient's normal stool pattern. | One loose stool does not mean a patient has diarrhea. Liquid intake normally produces a pasty stool, and patients may misinterpret this as diarrhea. Enteral feedings may produce several soft-formed stools per day. |
| Assess the hydration status by recording and evaluating intake and output every shift and checking weight daily. Obtain the parameter from the health care provider for notification. | An example of a parameter established by the health care provider for dehydration would be a decrease in urinary output to less than 30 mL/hour × 4 hours or 0.5 mL/kg/hour or increased stool output greater than a specific volume in an 8-hour period. Daily weight measurement is used to assess fluid status. For example, a loss of 1 kg/day could signal a loss of 1000 mL of fluid. |
| Review patient's medication record for medications that may cause diarrhea, especially in those patients with a history of multiple bowel surgeries, GI hypersecretion, or intestinal failure.  Refer to the pharmacist for guidance. | Pharmacists are knowledgeable about medications that cause diarrhea as well as those that are used to treat diarrhea associated with GI abnormalities. Some of these medications include prokinetic agents and stool softeners. |
| Contact the pharmacy about elixirs being administered. Discuss with the health care provider and pharmacist changing the form of medication or switching to another medication within the same class. | Most elixirs contain sorbitol, which will increase transit time in the intestines and cause diarrhea. |
| Consult with the health care provider regarding the collection of a stool sample for bacterial culture and sensitivity, ova and parasites, or *Clostridioides difficile*. | Diarrhea may be caused by bacteria or parasites. If *C. diff* is present, the volume of the daily stool output may exceed 500 mL and will occur whether or not the individual consumes food or enteral products. This type of diarrhea is considered secretory because the fluid is secreted from the intestinal wall and can lead to imbalances in fluid status. |
| Do not administer an antidiarrheal medication until the stool culture (if prescribed) is confirmed as negative. | Giving this medication when the stool culture is positive increases the risk for toxic megacolon and bowel perforation. |
| If the patient is receiving a bolus feeding, consult with provider to switch to intermittent or continuous feedings. | Bolus feedings may contribute to dumping syndrome, which would result in increased diarrhea. |
| Follow agency guidelines for handling of enteral products, feeding tube, and feeding sets. Change all equipment per agency policy. | Bacteria can grow in feeding sets and on hands of the caregiver and could cause diarrhea if allowed to be transported to the patient. |
| Store and discard all production according to manufacturer's instructions. | Products must be discarded 24 hours after they are opened as per manufacturer's instructions. These products are a potential growth media for bacteria and could cause diarrhea if the product that has been opened more than 24 hours is given to the patient. Unopened products should be stored at room temperature to prevent clumping of proteins in the container. |
| Follow agency and manufacturer guidelines for length of time that enteral solution products can be used. | This reduces the risk for bacterial contamination. Closed systems reduce the risk for touch contamination. |
| ! Identify the tube as enteral access before attaching the closed system. | This measure reduces the risk for inadvertent infusion of enteral feeding into an IV port. |

## Patient Problem/Analyze Cues/Prioritize Hypotheses

# Nausea

*due to* the underlying medical condition, too rapid infusion of enteral product, food intolerance, or medication administration

***Desired Outcome/Generate Solutions:*** After interventions, the patient has no nausea with food intake.

| ASSESSMENT—RECOGNIZE CUES/ INTERVENTIONS—TAKE ACTION | RATIONALES |
|---|---|
| Assess the abdomen for distention and auscultate bowel sounds. | Absence of or high-pitched bowel sounds may signal ileus or obstruction. Decreased bowel sounds may indicate the need to decrease the feeding and check stool output. Distention may appear either with ileus or with decreased motility. These signs would necessitate notifying the health care provider for intervention. |
| Assess for and record flatus and bowel movements. | Decreased bowel movements and flatus may indicate ileus or partial obstruction. |
| Assess the electrolyte values, especially potassium. | Hypokalemia is associated with ileus and nausea. |
| Administer an antiemetic as prescribed. | An antiemetic decreases/eliminates nausea. |
| Administer the medication on an empty stomach only when indicated. | Medications such as analgesics may cause nausea if given without food. |
| Offer food in small portions, 6 times per day. | Smaller meals are better tolerated than larger meals. |
| Give chewing gum or hard candies as needed, if permitted. | Providing some sugar to the system may stimulate the GI tract and decrease nausea. |
| Suggest the patient brush teeth and tongue every 8 hours and as needed. | A bad taste in the mouth may increase nausea in some individuals. |
| If the odor of food induces nausea, remove the food immediately. | This will help eliminate nausea caused by odor. |
| Consult with provider to reduce the rate/minute of enteral formula infusion. | Nausea may be caused by an increased infusion rate, which may result in delayed gastric emptying, overdistention, or constipation. |
| If the patient is receiving a bolus infusion, consult with the provider to change to intermittent or continuous. | Overdistention with a bolus infusion may cause or increase nausea, whereas a slower infusion rate with an intermittent or continuous infusion may be better tolerated. |
| If medically indicated, consult with the provider to order a bowel suppository. | This will stimulate the intestinal tract. Nausea may occur secondary to constipation or decreased motility. |

## Patient Problem/Analyze Cues/Prioritize Hypotheses

# Constipation

*due to* inadequate fluid and fiber in the diet

***Desired Outcome/Generate Solutions:*** The patient states that he or she has had a soft bowel movement within 3–4 days of this patient problem (or within the patient's usual pattern).

| ASSESSMENT—RECOGNIZE CUES/ INTERVENTIONS—TAKE ACTION | RATIONALES |
|---|---|
| Assess the abdomen for distention and auscultate bowel sounds. | A distended abdomen may signal a backup of stool and gas in the colon. |

Continued

Special Needs Care Plans

| ASSESSMENT—RECOGNIZE CUES/ INTERVENTIONS—TAKE ACTION | RATIONALES |
|---|---|
| If the patient is receiving a formula that contains fiber, assess the intake of free water. | Fiber pulls more fluid into the intestines. When a patient is "dry" from medical therapy, there is no extra water to pull, and if no extra water is available, constipation will occur. Optimally, water intake should be 1 mL/calorie of intake or 30–50 mL/kg body weight to compensate for losses that occur normally through respirations, urination, fever, and so on. |
| Give free water every 4 hours or as prescribed and after each medication for enterally fed patients. Encourage adequate oral fluid intake for patients on an oral diet. | Free water helps maintain fluid balance and patency of the feeding tube, as well as promote soft stools and prevent constipation. |
| Discuss with the health care provider and pharmacist the possibility of a reduction in the amount of opioids being administered. | Opioid medications are constipating. The patient may need a stool softener or motility enhancer. |
| Consider a stool softener, especially if the patient regularly uses a laxative at home. | If the patient is unable to increase water needs effectively, a stool softener will prevent straining and decrease the risk for constipation. |

## Patient Problem

# Impaired Swallowing

*due to* decreased or absent gag reflex, facial paralysis, mechanical obstruction, fatigue, weight loss, or decreased strength or excursion of muscles involved in mastication

***Desired Outcome/Generate Solutions:*** Before food or fluids are initiated, the patient demonstrates adequate cough and gag reflexes and the ability to ingest foods by the phases of swallowing as instructed.

| ASSESSMENT—RECOGNIZE CUES/ INTERVENTIONS—TAKE ACTION | RATIONALES |
|---|---|
| Consult with speech pathologist to assess oral motor function within 24 hours of admission or on a change in a medical condition. | If the patient has adequate oral motor functioning, oral intake can be increased with dietary texture restrictions. Otherwise, texture restrictions (e.g., puree), liquid restrictions (e.g., thickened liquids), or tube feedings should be considered to prevent aspiration. |
| Assess cough and gag reflexes before the first feeding. | Patients who develop gastric reflux or vomit can aspirate if their cough and gag reflexes are not intact. |
| Offer semisolid foods and progress to thicker textures as tolerated if prescribed by provider in collaboration with speech pathologist. | If the patient is likely to have difficulty with swallowing, liquids will be the most difficult and most likely to be aspirated. |
| Coach the patient through the phases of ingesting food: opening the mouth, inserting food, closing the lips, chewing, transferring food from side to side in the mouth and then to the back of the oral cavity, elevating the tongue to the roof of the mouth (hard palate), and swallowing between breaths. | With illness, muscles may become weaker, and this may result in bad habits of rushing swallowing and moving food into the trachea rather than into the esophagus, where it is less likely to be aspirated. |
| Order extra sauces, gravies, or liquids if dryness of the oral cavity impairs swallowing ability. | This moistens each bite of food for patients in whom dryness of the oral cavity impairs swallowing ability. |
| If tolerated, keep the patient in high-Fowler position for 1/2 hour after eating. | This position minimizes the risk for aspiration by promoting gravity flow through the stomach and into the duodenum. |
| Provide mouth care before and after meals and dietary supplements. | This measure ensures that all traces of food are removed, preventing subsequent aspiration. |

| ASSESSMENT—RECOGNIZE CUES/ INTERVENTIONS—TAKE ACTION | RATIONALES |
|---|---|
| Provide small, frequent meals. | Six smaller feedings per day may increase muscle strength needed for swallowing and be less likely to result in rushing, which could cause aspiration. |
| Provide foods at temperatures acceptable to the patient. | Foods that are too hot or too cold could rush swallowing and lead to aspiration. |
| As indicated, obtain services of a speech, or occupational therapist. | These specialists assist in retraining or facilitating the patient's swallowing. |

## Patient Problem/Analyze Cues/Prioritize Hypotheses

# Risk for Infection

*due to* invasive procedures, nasoenteric or nasogastric tube, PN, decreased nutritional intake, malnutrition, and suppression of the immune system

*Desired Outcome/Generate Solutions:* The patient is free of infection as evidenced by temperature, pulse, and respirations within the patient's normal range and absence of the following clinical signs of sepsis: erythema, swelling at the catheter insertion site, chills, fever, and glucose intolerance.

| ASSESSMENT—RECOGNIZE CUES/ INTERVENTIONS—TAKE ACTION | RATIONALES |
|---|---|
| Assess the patient routinely for signs and symptoms of infection, including white blood cell (WBC) count with differential for values outside normal range and increased temperature. | A higher value signals infection. Infection requires extra calories. Fever increases fluid requirements. |
| Assess bedside glucose for values outside the normal range. If the individual is glucose intolerant, begin glucose checks as prescribed and administer insulin as prescribed by the health care provider. | Glucose intolerance is a sign of sepsis. An increase in glucose also promotes bacterial growth and increases the risk for infection. Insulin is given to maintain blood glucose within normal limits. |
| Assess the IV catheter insertion site every 12 hours for erythema, swelling, or purulent discharge. | These are signs of local infection. |
| Change gauze dressings over IV sites routinely every 48 hours or immediately if the integrity is breached. Change transparent semipermeable membrane dressing at least every 7 days. | Gauze dressings prevent visualization of the insertion site. Blood on the gauze is considered a break in the dressing's integrity |
| Use meticulous sterile technique when changing CVC and PICC dressings, IV fluid bags, or administration lines. Follow agency policy for central line dressing changes. | These measures reduce the possibility of infection. |
| Consult the health care provider to obtain a prescription for blood cultures at two sites as outlined by the CDC in patients with a central line who are febrile with a rising WBC count. | Two positive cultures may indicate a bloodstream infection requiring antibiotic treatment. |
| Restrict the use of the lumen used for the administration of PN, if possible. Avoid drawing blood specimens or other fluids, pressure monitoring, or medication administration, if possible. | When PN is being administered, most infections of catheters and blood are related to the insertion site or tubing sets. |
| Change all administration sets, as per agency guidelines. | This is a standard infection prevention protocol. |

Patient Problem/Analyze Cues/Prioritize Hypotheses
# Risk for Fluid Imbalance (Fluid Overload or Dehydration)
*due to* the failure of regulatory mechanisms, hyperglycemia, medications, fever, infection, fluid administration, or immobility

***Desired Outcome/Generate Solutions:*** The patient's hydration status is balanced and adequate, as evidenced by baseline VS, serum glucose 70–140 mg/dL, balanced I&O, no more than 1–2 lb weight gain per week, and serum electrolytes and WBC count within normal limits.

| ASSESSMENT—RECOGNIZE CUES/ INTERVENTIONS—TAKE ACTION | RATIONALES |
|---|---|
| Assess the rate and volume of nutritional support every 4 hours. | This assessment helps ensure the prescribed rate and volume are delivered, thereby preventing volume overload or deficiency. |
| Assess the patient's weight daily | Daily weight measurement is used to assess fluid status. For example, a loss of 1 kg/day could signal a loss of 1000 mL of fluid. |
| Assess the I&O every 8 hours or more frequently if medically indicated. | This measure assesses for imbalances and trends toward fluid overload or dehydration. |
| Assess the electrolytes daily or as frequently as prescribed. | Changes in sodium, chloride, and BUN levels may indicate changes in fluid status. |
| Assess for signs of circulatory overload during fluid replacement. | Signs of circulatory overload may occur during fluid replacement, including peripheral edema, bounding pulse, jugular distention, and adventitious lung sounds (especially crackles). Circulatory overload is more likely to occur in older adults or individuals with heart failure or other chronic medical conditions such as renal insufficiency in which output is decreased, even if fluids are delivered properly. |

### ADDITIONAL PROBLEM:

*Risk for Health Care–Associated Complication (Wound Dehiscence With or Without Evisceration)*    Chapter 75

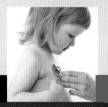

# Asthma 77

## OVERVIEW/PATHOPHYSIOLOGY

Asthma is a chronic, reversible (in most cases) obstructive airway disease characterized by a pathophysiologic triad consisting of inflammation, mucosal edema, and bronchospasm. The inflammatory response causes increased sensitivity of the airways and is the most common feature of asthma.

Asthma is one of the leading causes of chronic illness in children, but the prevalence and associated morbidity rates are decreasing. An estimated 6.2 million children younger than 18 years had asthma in 2015, while 4.2 million (5.8%) had asthma in 2020. About 50% of the children with asthma experienced an asthma attack or episode in 2020. There is an increased incidence in boys, children of low-income families with inadequate health care, as well as Blacks, American Indians/Alaskan Natives, and Puerto Ricans. Asthma is one of the leading causes of school absences, and it is the third leading cause of hospitalizations, resulting in 790,478 emergency department visits and about 64,500 hospitalizations in 2019 in children less than 18 years (CDC, 2022a). About 44% of children with current asthma had uncontrolled asthma in 2018–2020. The incidence was higher in boys than in girls (CDC, 2022b). If not properly managed, asthma can be a life-threatening disease, with more boys than girls dying from asthma. The rate of asthma-related ED visits is significantly higher in Black children as are the death rates (CDC, 2022a; National Institute of Health, 2022).

The National Asthma Education and Prevention Program published updated guidelines for diagnosis and management in 2007. The Expert Panel Report 3 focused on guidelines for deciding treatment based on individual needs (looking at age and severity) and level of asthma control and determined that regular monitoring is essential so that treatment can be adjusted as needed. Guidelines for children were expanded to include three age ranges with a stepwise approach for severity and control. Severity classification included intermittent or persistent (mild, moderate, or severe). Each step included patient/family education, environmental control, and management of comorbidities. It noted that assessing asthma control and adjusting therapy depend on the classification of control (well controlled, not well controlled, and very poorly controlled). The National Heart, Lung, and Blood Institute (NHLBI) 2020 Focused Updates to the Asthma Management Guidelines cover six priority topics based on age and severity of symptoms:

- Intermittent inhaled corticosteroids help control inflammation.
- Long-Acting Muscarinic Antagonists (LAMA) or Long-Acting Beta-2 Agonists (LABA) as added on to inhaled corticosteroids—relax the airway muscles. **Note**: LABA are preferred for children under 12 and most people over 12 with asthma that is not controlled with inhaled corticosteroids (ICS) alone.
- Indoor allergen reduction
- Immunotherapy (e.g., allergy shots)
- Fractional exhaled nitric oxide (FeNO) testing for children 5 and over
- Bronchial thermoplasty (not generally recommended).

These changes are designed to improve the care of people with asthma and to help their doctors make informed decisions about the management of their asthma. There is a continued emphasis that all treatment plans need to include an assessment of environmental factors, provide child and/or parent education, and manage comorbidities (NHLBI, 2020).

## HEALTH CARE SETTING

Primary care for chronic care management, with possible hospitalization resulting from severe acute attacks.

## ASSESSMENT

It is important to obtain a detailed history of current problems as well as past episodes, including frequency and severity of asthma attacks, ED visits, any hospitalizations, and/or intubations due to respiratory distress.

***Common early warning signs.*** Breathing changes (different from child's norm), sneezing, moodiness, headache, itchy/watery eyes, dark circles under eyes, easy fatigue, sore throat, trouble sleeping, trouble eating (e.g., an infant having difficulty sucking on a bottle), chest or throat itchiness, the downward trend in peak flow values, cough—especially at night or early morning (a common symptom of asthma), slight tightness in the chest.

***Symptoms of acute episode.*** Coughing, shortness of breath, anxiety, apprehension, tightness in chest, and wheezing (primarily on expiration).

***Severe asthma symptoms.*** Severe coughing (e.g., hacking, paroxysmal) progressing shortness of breath, tightness in the chest and/or wheezing, apprehension, and difficulty talking, eating, or concentrating.

**Symptoms of severe respiratory distress and impending respiratory failure.** Profuse diaphoresis, sitting upright and refusing to lie down, suddenly becoming agitated or becoming quiet when previously agitated, decrease in or absence of wheezing.

**Physical assessment.** The chest has hyperresonance on percussion. Breath sounds are loud and coarse, with sonorous crackles throughout the lung fields. Prolonged expiration is noted. Coarse rhonchi may be heard, as well as generalized inspiratory and expiratory wheezing. As obstruction increases, wheezing becomes higher pitched. With minimal obstruction, wheezing may be mild, heard only on end expiration with auscultation, or absent. Breath sounds and crackles may become inaudible with a severe obstruction or bronchospasm. Posturing occurs to facilitate breathing. Pulsus paradoxus (an abnormally large decrease in systolic blood pressure and pulse wave amplitude during inspiration) also may be noted because of lung hyperinflation. Children with chronic asthma may develop a barrel chest with depressed diaphragm, elevated shoulders, and increased use of accessory muscles of respiration.

**Caution:** If symptoms are untreated or treated unsuccessfully, an acute asthma attack may progress to *status asthmaticus*, a severe unrelenting attack. Status asthmaticus is an acute, severe, and prolonged asthma attack in which respiratory distress continues despite vigorous therapeutic measures and may result in death.

## DIAGNOSTIC TESTS

**Arterial blood gas values.** Reveal status of oxygenation and acid–base balance. In severe asthma exacerbation with $PaO_2$ less than 60 mm Hg (on room air) and $PaCO_2$ of 42 mm Hg or greater, the child may have cyanosis and initially may show signs of alkalosis due to hyperinflation. The alkalosis might progress to acidosis as exacerbation or attack worsens. While arterial blood gas (ABG) values are not usually checked in children, they may be obtained while in an intensive care unit and with an initial assessment to provide atraumatic care. When possible, topical anesthetics are used to decrease pain and anxiety with blood draws needed to obtain an ABG.

**Pulse oximetry.** A noninvasive method that reveals decreased $O_2$ saturation (usually less than 93%–95%, depending on the facility's protocol) and helps provide atraumatic care.

**Pulmonary function tests (spirometry).** Provide an objective method of evaluating the presence and degree of lung disease, as well as response to treatment, and usually can be performed reliably on children by 5 or 6 years of age. These tests typically show diminished expiratory flows, such as the forced expiratory volume in the first second ($FEV_1$).

**Fractional exhaled nitrous oxide (FeNO) testing.** Measures the amount of nitrous oxide, a by-product of inflammation, exhaled. This can be used for children 5 and older if diagnosis or approach to treatment is uncertain.

**Note**: Not usually done for acute episode.

**Chest radiographic examination.** To rule out pneumonia and assess for air trapping. It is also used to evaluate possible cardiomegaly secondary to pulmonary hypertension resulting from chronic obstruction. Typical findings in a child with significant asthma symptoms are hyperinflation, atelectasis, and flattened diaphragm.

**Complete blood count.** May show slight elevation during acute asthma, but white blood cell elevations greater than $12,000/mm^3$ or an increased percentage of band cells may indicate a respiratory infection. Eosinophils greater than $500/mm^3$ tend to suggest an allergic or inflammatory disorder.

**Peak expiratory flow rate.** Assesses the severity of asthma by measuring the maximum flow of air that can be forcefully exhaled in 1 second using a peak flow meter (PFM). Each child's peak expiratory flow rate (PEFR) varies according to age, height, gender, and race. After the personal best value is established, it is recommended that it be done 1–2 times/day in children with moderate to severe persistent asthma. The child needs to measure the PEFR three times with at least 30 seconds between each measurement and then record the highest reading. Maintaining a diary or log book is beneficial and helps direct the plan of care. Although this test is used for monitoring control, it is not used for the initial diagnosis. Most children 5 years of age and older can use the PFM effectively.

**Sputum.** Gross examination may reveal increased viscosity or "mucus plugs." Culture and sensitivity may reveal microorganisms if infection was the precipitating event. Cytologic examination will reveal elevated eosinophils, which is commonly associated with asthma. It is rarely done in children.

**Serum theophylline level.** Important baseline indicator for patients who are receiving this oral medication, although it is used infrequently. The current guidelines call for a serum concentration of 5–15 mcg/mL. Theophylline toxicity can occur with serum levels greater than 20 mcg/mL. Side effects include nausea, vomiting, headache, irritability, and insomnia. Early signs of toxicity are nausea, tachycardia, irritability, and seizures. Dysrhythmias occur at serum levels greater than 30 mcg/mL.

Oral theophylline is not recommended for acute asthma exacerbations (American Pharmacists Association, 2021).

**Skin testing.** The 2020 Focused Updates to the Asthma Management Guidelines recommended changing the consideration of subcutaneous allergen immunotherapy (allergy shots) to a recommendation for people who have allergic asthma and whose symptoms worsen after being exposed to certain allergens.

## Patient Problems/Analyze Cues/Prioritize Hypotheses

# Dyspnea/Risk for Impaired Respiratory System Function

*due to* bronchospasm, mucosal edema, and increased mucus production

***Desired Outcomes/Generate Solutions:*** *Child with a significant asthma attack:* Within 48 hours of interventions/treatment, adventitious breath sounds, cough, and increased work of breathing (WOB) are decreased. Within 72 hours, the respiratory rate (RR) returns to the child's baseline range, and retractions and nasal flaring disappear. *Child with a mild asthma attack:* Within 3 hours after interventions/treatment, adventitious breath sounds and cough are decreased, and retractions and nasal flaring are absent.

> **Note:** *WOB means ease or effort of breathing. Signs of increased WOB include nasal flaring, retractions, and use of accessory muscles.*

| ASSESSMENT—RECOGNIZE CUES/ INTERVENTIONS—TAKE ACTION | RATIONALES |
| --- | --- |
| Assess respiratory status with the initial assessment, with each vital sign check, and as needed. | After establishing the baseline, changes can be detected quickly with subsequent assessments, enabling rapid intervention. |
| Assess RR, heart rate (HR), $O_2$ saturation, and breath sounds before and 5–10 minutes or per unit policy/after each nebulizer treatment or metered-dose inhaler (MDI) administration. | These assessments help determine the child's status and the effectiveness of medication in decreasing bronchospasm or mucosal edema and enabling more effective airway clearance. |
| Position the child in high-Fowler position and encourage deep breathing. | This will ensure the child has maximum lung expansion and that medication will be dispersed more effectively, thereby improving airway clearance. |
| Administer nebulizer treatment or MDI, usually albuterol, as prescribed. | These therapies decrease bronchospasm or mucosal edema, thereby opening the airway and enabling more effective airway clearance. |
| Use a spacer or holding chamber when administering MDI unless contraindicated (e.g., Serevant Diskus). | This is the most effective method of getting the maximum amount of medication delivered to a child. A mask may be required with a spacer in children younger than 5 years or children who are unable to seal their lips effectively around the mouthpiece. |
| Hold the albuterol treatment if the HR is:<br>• Greater than 180 bpm (children 2–3 years)<br>• Greater than 160 bpm (children 3–6 years)<br>• Greater than 140 bpm (children 6–12 years)<br>• Greater than 120 bpm (children older than 12 years)<br>• Or per health care provider's parameters<br>Notify the health care provider as directed. | Tachycardia is a major side effect of albuterol. When it is present, the health care provider needs to assess the patient to ensure that the side effects of medication do not outweigh the benefit of decreasing bronchospasm. |
| Check PEFR in children 5 years and older before and after each albuterol treatment using PFM, if possible. | These assessments monitor the effectiveness of the medication in decreasing bronchospasm and increasing effective airway clearance. For more information about PEFR, see the "Diagnostic Tests" section. |
| Encourage deep breathing and effective cough and expectoration every 2 hours while awake. Have young children blow on a pinwheel or blow bubbles to facilitate deep breathing. | This loosens and expectorates secretions (many young children cough up secretions and swallow them) and will lead to more effective airway clearance. |
| Teach children 7 years and older breathing exercises and controlled breathing. | Children younger than 7 years are diaphragmatic breathers normally. Proper diaphragmatic breathing decreases WOB and improves chest wall mobility and airway clearance. |

Continued

| ASSESSMENT—RECOGNIZE CUES/ INTERVENTIONS—TAKE ACTION | RATIONALES |
|---|---|
| Administer other medications (inhaled, intravenous [IV], or by mouth [PO]) as prescribed (usually corticosteroids). | Corticosteroids decrease inflammation, thereby improving airway clearance. Antibiotics are given only if a bacterial infection is present. |
| Assess and document the intake and output (I&O) every 4 hours or as ordered. Ensure that a minimum urine output (UO) of 1 mL/kg/hour is met (the amount may vary based on the age of child and/or guidelines from health care provider). | Assessing I&O on a regular basis alerts one to inadequate intake or output before the child shows signs of dehydration. Dehydration thickens secretions and decreases airway clearance. |
| Assess the hydration status every 4 hours or more often as indicated, including the level of consciousness (LOC), anterior fontanel (if the child is younger than 2 years), abdominal skin turgor, and UO. | Because of increased insensible water loss (owing to increased RR, metabolic rate, and secretions), the child may still become dehydrated *even if* receiving maintenance fluids and having appropriate I&O. Ongoing assessments detect early changes and provide a more prompt resolution of the problem. Dehydration thickens secretions and decreases airway clearance. Signs of dehydration include decreasing LOC, sunken fontanel/eyes, tented abdominal skin, and decreasing UO. |
| Encourage maintenance fluids, preferably orally, that are appropriate for the child's weight. | Fluids thin mucus and improve the ability to expectorate it, which promotes airway clearance. Some children may need IV fluids because of increased WOB. |
| Provide specific guidelines for hydration (maintenance fluids). | For example, a 2-year-old child who needs 1200 mL/day and drinks from a 4-oz "sippy" cup, needs to drink 10 "sippy" cupfuls/day. Understanding appropriate care improves adherence to the treatment regimen and decreases symptoms. |
| Avoid iced fluids and limit caffeinated fluids. | Iced fluids may trigger bronchospasm. Excessive intake of caffeinated fluids may increase the risk for cardiovascular and central nervous system side effects of many medications. |

## Patient Problem/Analyze Cues/Prioritize Hypotheses

# Fatigue

*due to* disease state (hypoxia and increased work of breathing [WOB])

***Desired Outcome/Generate Solutions:*** Within 48 hours after treatment/interventions, the child exhibits decreased fatigue as evidenced by less irritability and restlessness, improved sleeping pattern, and ability to perform usual activities.

| ASSESSMENT—RECOGNIZE CUES/ INTERVENTIONS—TAKE ACTION | RATIONALES |
|---|---|
| Assess the HR, RR, and WOB every 4 hours or more frequently for increases from the child's norm. Report significant findings. | Recognizing and reporting changes promptly facilitates appropriate actions that resolve the problem and decrease the likelihood of fatigue. |
| Assess for signs of hypoxia (restlessness, fatigue, irritability, tachycardia, dyspnea, and change of LOC). | Recognizing the symptoms of hypoxia promptly enables timely treatment and decreases fatigue. |
| Provide a calm and restful environment. Ensure the child's physical comfort. Consolidate care; organize nursing care to provide periods of uninterrupted rest and sleep. | These measures promote rest and decrease stress, oxygen demand, and fatigue. |
| Encourage the parents' presence, especially with younger children. | The parents' presence decreases fear and anxiety, thereby decreasing $O_2$ consumption and fatigue. |
| Encourage quiet, age-appropriate play activities as the child's condition improves. | Emotional and physical comfort increases a sense of well-being, promotes rest, and decreases oxygen expenditure and fatigue. |

## Patient Problem/Analyze Cues/Prioritize Hypotheses

# Anxiety

*due to* illness (e.g., trouble breathing and/or respiratory distress), loss of control, and medical/nursing management of illness

***Desired Outcome/Generate Solutions:*** After interventions/treatments, the child/parents verbalize and/or exhibit decreased anxiety.

| ASSESSMENT—RECOGNIZE CUES/ INTERVENTIONS—TAKE ACTION | RATIONALES |
|---|---|
| Assess the child's/parents' understanding of the child's anxiety. | This enables support and teaching to be more appropriate and effective. |
| Explain all procedures/interventions performed on the child (e.g., blood drawing, starting IVs) to the child in a developmentally appropriate manner and/or parents. | Knowledge often helps decrease anxiety and promotes family-centered care. |
| Explain the purpose of equipment used on the child (HR monitor, $O_2$ and pulse oximeter, blood pressure [BP] monitor). | Increased understanding of equipment decreases fear of pain, which in turn will decrease anxiety. |
| Use therapeutic play by providing child with equipment (e.g., oral syringe, stethoscope, blood pressure cuff) in children older than 3 years. | Playing with items that will be used in the care of the child also helps decrease anxiety. For example, put a BP cuff on a doll or teddy bear or let the child put the cuff on you. |
| Provide a quiet room where the child can be closely observed. | Increased stimuli increases anxiety. |
| Encourage the parents to stay with the child if possible. | This promotes a sense of security, which will decrease the child's anxiety. |
| Avoid making the parents feel guilty if they are unable to stay. | Parents are already anxious about the child being ill and in a hospital. |
| Keep the parents informed of the child's progress, including what is being done and why. | This decreases their anxiety. The child easily perceives parental anxiety. |
| Talk quietly and calmly to the child in age-appropriate language. Reassure the child that you are available and will be there to help. | Establishing rapport increases trust and decreases anxiety. |
| Encourage transitional objects (items from the child's home, such as a blanket or teddy bear). | Such items increase a feeling of security and decrease anxiety. |
| Facilitate coordination of care. | This avoids disturbing the child any more than necessary, which would otherwise increase the anxiety level. |

## Family Problem/Analyze Cues/Prioritize Hypotheses

# Difficulty Coping

*due to* the child having a chronic illness and/or emergent hospitalization

***Desired Outcome/Generate Solutions:*** Within 1 month of diagnosis, the family provides a normal environment for the child and copes effectively with the symptoms, management, and effects of asthma.

| ASSESSMENT—RECOGNIZE CUES/ INTERVENTIONS—TAKE ACTION | RATIONALES |
|---|---|
| Assess for and use every opportunity to reinforce the family's understanding of asthma and its therapies. | Accurate knowledge enables the family to cope more effectively with the child's chronic illness. |
| Instruct the parents to have realistic expectations about the child's asthma. | Knowing what to expect enables families to cope more effectively. Expectations will vary, depending on the child's developmental age and severity of the asthma. |
| Encourage the parents and siblings to focus on the child as a normal child who needs some lifestyle modifications. | The child needs to be the focus, not the disease. Normalizing the environment as much as possible promotes the child as the focus. |
| Reinforce the importance of helping the siblings cope with/adapt to having a sibling with a chronic illness. | This supports family-centered care and increases the likelihood of more normal family processes. |
| Reinforce to the parents the importance of setting consistent behavior limits and not enabling secondary gain for an asthma attack. | Discipline and guidelines are essential for all children to develop appropriate behavior. |
| Reinforce the need to use PFM at least 1–2 times/day and/or implement the child's asthma action plan. | Understanding the importance of monitoring the child's status enables the family to cope more effectively and incorporate monitoring into the daily routine, thereby promoting normalization and the child's optimal health status. |
| Teach the child/parents how to give respiratory treatments (nebulizer, MDI) correctly, using the prescribed medication and administering it with proper technique. | This information eliminates confusion about the correct administration of medications and method of delivery, thereby improving the ability to cope with managing a chronic illness. |
| Include parents in the care of their child as much as possible while the child is hospitalized. | This increases having a more normal environment for the child and parent and improving their ability to cope with the new care needs of the child. |
| Encourage the family to contact the school (nurse, teachers, coaches) to develop a 504 plan for the child. | This promotes the family's coping while facilitating the child's improvement. A 504 plan makes accommodations in the school environment so that the child can function better and thereby learn more effectively. For example, a child who is allergic to grass will not be assigned to a classroom with windows that open near a field of grass when the grass is being mowed. |
| Refer the family to appropriate support groups and community agencies. | These groups/agencies help children and families function and deal with chronic illness more effectively. |

<u>**Patient/Parent Problem/Analyze Cues/Prioritize Hypotheses**</u>

# Deficient Knowledge

*due to* unfamiliarity with the purpose, precautions, and potential side effects of prescribed medications

***Desired Outcome/Generate Solutions:*** After interventions/instructions, the child and/or parents verbalize accurate information about the prescribed medications.

| ASSESSMENT—RECOGNIZE CUES/ INTERVENTIONS—TAKE ACTION | RATIONALES |
|---|---|
| **Teach the Parents and Child (Depending on the Child's Age and Severity of Disease) the Following:** | |
| **Long-Term Control Medications** | |
| These are taken daily to achieve and maintain control of persistent asthma. Intermittent use may be indicated for children 0–4 years with recurrent wheezing for a short course per the 2020 Focused Update to Asthma Management Guidelines (NHLBI, 2020). | |
| **Corticosteroids** | |
| These are the most potent antiinflammatory medications. | |
| *Inhaled oral corticosteroid (ICS) medications, such as fluticasone (Flovent HFA), beclomethasone (Qvar), and flunisolide (Aerospan)* | |
| • Rinse the mouth and gargle with water after oral inhalation. Do not swallow. | This helps prevent thrush (oral candidiasis). |
| • Administer some corticosteroids using a spacer or holding chamber (e.g., Flovent HFA). | These devices may enhance drug delivery and efficiency of the inhaled form and help decrease the incidence of thrush.<br><br>Some MDIs have built-in spacers, for example, Aerospan. |
| • Monitor for and report fatigue, headache, oral thrush, sinus infection or sinusitis, hoarseness, throat irritation, nasal congestion. | These are potential side effects; dosage may need to be changed.<br><br>**Warning/Precautions**: May cause growth suppression especially in younger children or in patients receiving high doses for prolonged periods of time.<br><br>Paradoxical bronchospasm that may be life-threatening may occur with the use of inhaled bronchodilating agents |
| • Do not decrease dose or discontinue without the consent of the health care provider. | This is a maintenance medication, and the child may have exacerbation of symptoms if it is decreased or discontinued inappropriately. |
| *Oral corticosteroids, such as prednisolone and prednisone* | |
| • Monitor for and report headaches, sore throat, mood changes, sleep disturbances, seizures, increased blood sugar, diarrhea, nausea, gastrointestinal (GI) bleeding (seen in emesis, stools), weight gain, increased appetite, and tissue swelling. | These are potential side effects; dosage may need to be changed.<br><br>**Warning/Precautions**: May cause growth suppression especially in younger children or in patients receiving high doses for prolonged periods of time.<br><br>May cause osteoporosis (at any age) or inhibition of bone growth in pediatric patients. |
| • Take cautiously with barbiturates, carbamazepine, phenytoin, rifampin, or isoniazid. | These medications may reduce the effects of prednisone and increase risk for GI ulcer. |
| • Observe carefully if taking salicylates, toxoids, nonsteroidal antiinflammatory drugs, or diuretics that are potassium depleting. | These drugs may increase the risk for GI ulcer when taken with corticosteroids. |
| • Limit the use of caffeine and alcohol.<br><br>Take after meals or with food or milk | They may increase risk for GI ulcer or cause stomach irritation. |

Continued

| ASSESSMENT—RECOGNIZE CUES/INTERVENTIONS—TAKE ACTION | RATIONALES |
|---|---|
| • **Caution:** Inform all health care providers about steroid use. | It may be necessary to avoid vaccinations while taking prednisone. Live virus vaccines may increase the risk for viral infection. Vaccines, in general, may have decreased effect. |
| • Do not change or discontinue dose without the consent of the health care provider. | Long-term steroid dosage needs to be decreased carefully to allow for gradual return of pituitary–adrenal axis functioning. Failure to do so can result in adrenal insufficiency. |

### Cromolyn (oral inhalation)

This antiasthmatic agent prevents the release of mast cells (e.g., histamine) after exposure to an allergen. It is not recommended as an initial treatment of persistent asthma or routine use but may be considered for exercise or allergen-induced bronchospasm (American Pharmacists Association, 2021).

**Note**: Not addressed in 2020 Focused Updates to the Asthma Management Guidelines (NHLBI, 2020).

| ASSESSMENT—RECOGNIZE CUES/INTERVENTIONS—TAKE ACTION | RATIONALES |
|---|---|
| • Administer this medicine only in a power-operated nebulizer that has an adequate flow rate and is equipped with a face mask or mouthpiece per health care provider. | Utilizing the most appropriate delivery device increases the effectiveness of the inhaled medication. Hand-squeezed bulb nebulizers should not be used as they will not deliver the medication effectively. |
| • Assess for and report drowsiness, burning or pruritis of the nose, nausea, stomach pain, rash, transient cough, sneezing, and/or nasal congestion | These are potential side effects. |
| • Explain that a decrease in asthma symptoms should occur after the medication has been taken for 2–4 weeks on a regular basis. | Therapeutic response should occur within 2–4 weeks if used on a regular basis. |

### Leukotriene modifiers such as montelukast (Singulair)

These antiasthmatic agents decrease inflammation and bronchoconstriction.
**Note**: Not addressed in the 2020 Focused Update to Asthma Management Guidelines

| ASSESSMENT—RECOGNIZE CUES/INTERVENTIONS—TAKE ACTION | RATIONALES |
|---|---|
| • Assess for and report a variety of potential dermatological issues, for example, eczema and urticaria: headache, changes in behavior/mood, abdominal pain, fatigue, dizziness, cough, diarrhea, laryngitis, pharyngitis, nausea, earache, sinus discomfort, and viral infections. | These are potential side effects. |

**Note:** Side effects vary depending on the age of the child.

| ASSESSMENT—RECOGNIZE CUES/INTERVENTIONS—TAKE ACTION | RATIONALES |
|---|---|
| • Assess for agitation, aggression, depression, sleep disturbances, hallucinations, stuttering, suicidal thoughts, and behavior. Stop medication and report immediately to health care provider | **Warnings/Precautions**: Neuropsychiatric events have been reported in patients with and without a previous history of psychiatric disorder. Risks and benefits need to be discussed with child/parent. (American Pharmacists Association, 2021). |
| • For granules: Give directly into the mouth, dissolved with 5 mL of cold or room-temperature baby formula or breast-milk, or mixed with a spoonful cold or room-temperature foods (using only applesauce, mashed carrots, rice, or ice cream). Do not dissolve in other liquids or foods. Administer within 15 minutes of opening the packet. | Following these guidelines ensures the stability of the granules and a better therapeutic response. |
| • Check with the health care provider or pharmacist before taking any other medications. | These medications may interact with numerous other medications. |

### Immunomodulators such as omalizumab (Xolair)

These medications are used to treat moderate to severe persistent immunoglobulin E–mediated allergic asthma not controlled with ICS. This medication is administered subcutaneously monthly. It is used in children 6 years old and older (American Pharmacists Association, 2021).

| ASSESSMENT—RECOGNIZE CUES/INTERVENTIONS—TAKE ACTION | RATIONALES |
|---|---|
| • Assess for and report headache, dizziness; fatigue; urticaria, pruritus; local injection site reactions (bruising and pain occur within 1 hour and may last up to 8 days); pain in joints, arms, or legs; fracture; and otitis media, earache. | These are potential side effects. |

| ASSESSMENT—RECOGNIZE CUES/ INTERVENTIONS—TAKE ACTION | RATIONALES |
|---|---|
| • Assess for and report any signs of allergic reactions such as difficulty breathing, swelling of the throat or tongue, cough, chest tightness, and generalized itching to the health care provider immediately. | Anaphylaxis reactions usually occur within 2 hours but may be delayed up to 24 hours or longer. The patient must have this medication administered by a health care professional and be observed a minimum of 2 hours after the first three injections. Observation should be for at least 30 minutes after subsequent injections or per institution policy.<br><br>**Note**: As of April 2020, FDA temporarily allowed self-administration of prefilled syringes for selected patients due to COVID-19 pandemic (American Pharmacists Association, 2021). |
| • Do not alter medications without consulting the health care provider. | This is a maintenance medication. The child may have exacerbation of symptoms if medications are decreased or discontinued inappropriately. |
| **LAMAs such as salmeterol (Serevent Diskus) and Formoterol (Perforomist)**<br><br>LABAs relax bronchial smooth muscles to relieve bronchospasm but should be used in patients whose asthma is not adequately controlled with long-term controller medications such as ICS and never as a monotherapy. **(United States Boxed Warning):** Monotherapy with LABAs is contraindicated to treat asthma. LABAs increase the risk for asthma-related deaths as well as asthma-related hospitalizations in pediatric and adolescent patients. (American Pharmacists Association, 2021).<br><br>**Note**: 2020 Focused Updates to the Asthma Management Guidelines state that in children 4 years and older with moderate to severe asthma, the preferred treatment is an ICS with formoterol that can be used as a daily controller and quick-relief therapy in a single inhaler (NHLBI, 2020). | |
| • Assess for and report increased blood pressure, dizziness, headache, rash, increased blood sugar, nausea, pain in joints, cough, nasal congestion, throat irritation, or respiratory/sinus infections. | These are potential side effects. |
| • Before inhaling med, breathe out fully but do not exhale into Serevent Diskus device. Activate and use only holding it in a level, horizontal position. Inhale quickly and deeply through the Diskus, take the device out of your mouth, try to hold your breath for 5–10 seconds, and then exhale slowly. | This increases drug delivery and efficiency. |
| • Do not use with a spacer or wash the mouthpiece. You can wipe the mouthpiece with a dry cloth. Keep the Diskus dry. | The powder would coat the inside of the spacer and not be delivered to the patient. |
| • Rinse mouth after using Serevent as directed by the health care provider. | To prevent thrush |
| • Use Serevent Diskus powder up to 6 weeks after removing the protective foil or when the counter reads "0." | Serevent powder for inhalation is stable for 6 weeks after removal from the foil packet. |
| **LAMAs such as tiotropium (Spiriva Respimat)**<br><br>LAMAs block the parasympathetic nerve reflexes that cause airways to constrict, thereby inhibiting bronchospasm. Recommended for use in children 6 years old and older if LABA cannot be used but only with ICS or if the child using ICS+LABA is still not controlled (American Pharmacists Association, 2021; NHLBI, 2020). | |
| • Assess for and report dry mouth, sore throat, upper respiratory infections (URIs), and sinusitis. | These are the most common side effects. |
| • Assess for and report chest pain, indigestion, dizziness and blurred vision, headache, abdominal pain, constipation, and rhinitis. | These are potential side effects. **Warning/Precautions:** Paradoxical bronchospasm may occur with inhaled agents. |

Continued

## ASSESSMENT—RECOGNIZE CUES/ INTERVENTIONS—TAKE ACTION

## RATIONALES

| ASSESSMENT—RECOGNIZE CUES/ INTERVENTIONS—TAKE ACTION | RATIONALES |
|---|---|
| • Before using the first time, Spiriva Respimat cartridge is inserted into Spiriva Respimat inhaler and the unit is primed. Prime by actuating the inhaler to the ground until an aerosol cloud is visible and repeat three times and then the unit is ready for use. **Note**: If not used for 3 days or longer, actuate the unit once to prepare it for use. If not used for more than 21 days, repeat the initial priming sequence again. | Priming before use enhances the correct delivery of medication. |
| • Keep the cap closed. Turn the base until it clicks, then open the cap, inhale and exhale deeply and slowly facing away from the inhaler. Place the inhaler in your mouth with lips surrounding the mouthpiece, point the inhaler to the back of your throat, press the button while inhaling slowly and deeply, try to hold your breath for 10 seconds or as long as possible, turn your head away from the inhaler and exhale slowly. Close lid. | This increases drug delivery and efficiency. |
| • Rinse mouth after using Spiriva Respimat. | To prevent thrush. |
| • Explain that a decrease in asthma symptoms should occur after the medication has been taken for up to 4–8 weeks on a regular basis. | Maximum benefits may take up to 4–8 weeks of receiving medication on a regular basis as prescribed. Intermittent use will not provide the desired relief of symptoms. |
| • Check with the health care provider or pharmacist before taking any other medications. | Multiple medications may interact with tiotropium. |

**Methylxanthines such as theophylline (rarely used now)**

These are weak bronchodilators.

| | |
|---|---|
| • Assess for and report GI upset, GI reflux, vomiting, nausea, abdominal pain/ulcer, hyperactivity, headache, insomnia, restlessness, seizures, tremors, and increased pulse rate. | These are the most common side effects. |
| • Limit caffeine (e.g., caffeinated beverages and chocolate). | Excessive intake may increase the risk for cardiovascular and central nervous system side effects. |
| • Limit intake of charcoal-broiled foods. | Excessive intake may increase elimination or decrease the effectiveness of medication. |
| • Check with the health care provider or pharmacist before taking any other medications. | Numerous medications increase or decrease theophylline level. |

**Quick-Relief Medications**

These medications decrease bronchospasm, thereby opening the airway and enabling more effective airway clearance. They are used to treat acute signs and symptoms and pretreat exercise-induced asthma.

**Short-acting inhaled beta-2 agonists (SABAs) such as albuterol (ProAir HFAI or Ventolin HFA)**

SABAs are bronchodilators.

| | |
|---|---|
| • Assess for and report excitement, nervousness, pharyngitis, bronchospasm, exacerbation of asthma, shakiness, increased HR, palpitations, tremor, insomnia, nausea, and headache. | These are potential side effects and vary with different age groups, for example, tremor frequency increases with age, excitement occurs in children 2–14 years, and shakiness in children 6–14 years. Central nervous system stimulation, hyperactivity, and insomnia occur more often in younger children than in adults. Side effects also vary with dosage and route of administration (American Pharmacists Association, 2021). |
| • Use with caution in patients with cardiovascular disease. | Side effects from these medications are more significant in patients with cardiovascular disease, high blood pressure, or heart failure. |
| • If using an MDI, use with a spacer or holding chamber. Children younger than 4 years need a face mask along with the spacer or holding chamber. | These devices increase drug delivery and efficiency. |
| • Limit caffeinated beverages if taking albuterol. | Caffeine may increase the side effects of albuterol. |

| ASSESSMENT—RECOGNIZE CUES/ INTERVENTIONS—TAKE ACTION | RATIONALES |
|---|---|
| • Check with the health care provider or pharmacist before taking other medications. | Numerous medications increase or decrease the effects/toxicity of albuterol. |
| *Anticholinergics such as ipratropium (Atrovent HFA) oral inhalation* | |
| These bronchodilator/antiasthmatic agents may be used for acute moderate to severe asthma exacerbations if poor response to initial SABA therapy during first treatment in acute care setting (e.g., ED). Questionable benefit for maintenance therapy (American Pharmacists Association, 2021). | |
| • Assess for and report bronchitis, sinusitis, headache, tachycardia, nervousness, cough, hoarseness, dry mouth, and drying of respiratory secretions. | These are potential side effects, but systemic effects are rare. **Warning/Precautions**: Hypersensitivity reactions (urticaria, angioedema, rash bronchospasm, oropharyngeal edema), including anaphylaxis, have been reported. Stop medication immediately. Paradoxical bronchospasm that may be life-threatening may occur with inhaled bronchodilators. If occurs, discontinue and seek alternative therapy (American Pharmacists Association, 2021). |
| • If using an MDI, use with a spacer or holding chamber. Children younger than 4 years need a face mask along with the spacer or holding chamber. | These devices increase drug delivery and efficiency. |
| • Shake the inhaler well before use with a spacer. | Shaking the inhaler before use ensures the consistency of the dose delivered. |
| *Oral and IV corticosteroids (also see under long-term control medication) such as methylprednisolone or prednisolone.* | |
| These antiinflammatory agents are usually given for a short time. | |
| • Assess for and report dizziness, headache, anxiety, GI discomfort, and cough. | These are potential side effects. |
| • Give oral medication with food or milk. | Food/milk decreases GI upset. |

## ADDITIONAL PROBLEMS:

"Bronchiolitis" for *Dehydration*      Chapter 79
"Cystic Fibrosis" for *Impaired Gas Exchange.*      Chapter 82
     However, with asthma, be aware that
     oxygen saturation needs to be greater than
     93%–95%, depending on agency protocol.

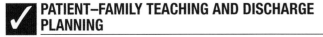

## ✔ PATIENT–FAMILY TEACHING AND DISCHARGE PLANNING

When providing child/family teaching, focus on sensory information, avoid giving excessive information, and initiate a visiting nurse referral for necessary follow-up teaching and assessment as needed. Utilize a variety of teaching methods (e.g., videos, iPads/tablets, and webinars as well as verbal and written) depending on learning style and resources of child/family. Stress the importance of family-centered care, which is viewing the family as a unit that is the "constant" in the child's life and maintaining or improving the health of the family and its members in a holistic manner. Include information about the following, ensuring that it is written at a level understandable to child/family:

✓ What is asthma? Discuss the definition, signs and symptoms, and pathophysiology.

✓ Identification of specific triggers for the child that can precipitate an attack and removal of as many of them as possible from the environment. Asthma triggers vary for each child. The most common triggers of asthma are URI, cigarette smoke, exercise, stress, anxiety, and weather changes. Other triggers unique to the environment are important (e.g., humid weather, frequent rainy days, local industry). Additional common triggers include pollens, dust mites, mold, cockroaches, rodents, and pet dander. Indoor allergen reduction is one of the six areas in NHLBI 2020 Focused Updates. Strong odors also may be a trigger.

✓ Importance of personal asthma action plan with green, yellow, and red zone values specific for the child. This plan is set up by the health care provider based on the child's best score/PEFR except for younger children unable to use PFM. Zone values will be based on symptoms infant/child exhibits. Zones are established similar to a stoplight. The green zone is a score 80%–100%

of the child's best score and with no symptoms present. The yellow zone is a score 50%–80% of the child's best score and signals caution: the child may need extra asthma medicine. Follow guidelines in the child's personal asthma action plan. The red zone is a score that is below 50% of the child's best score and signals an emergency situation. Follow the asthma action plan and call the health care provider. A sample asthma action plan is available at https://www.nhlbi.nih.gov/health/asthma/treatment-action-plan (also includes "How to Control Things That Make Your Asthma Worse"), or https://www.nationaljewish.org/NJH/media/pdf/pdf-asthma-action-plan_v2.pdf (includes early warning signs and worsening symptoms for babies as well as children and adults).

✓ Correct PFM technique. Most children between 5 and 6 years old can use PFM. Document return demonstration before discharge. The child needs to check this rate at least daily and more often if the rate is decreased. The child needs to keep a log to document PEFR.

✓ Maintaining asthma symptom diary, especially for a child with frequent symptoms.

✓ Medications, including drug name, route, purpose, and type (controller: long-term management or short-acting immediate relief), dosage, precautions, and potential side effects. Also discuss drug–drug, food–drug, and herb–drug interactions.

✓ Proper technique for using MDIs with spacer (holding chamber) or spacer with a mask (usually for a child younger than 5 years), as directed by health care provider. Document adequate return demonstration. Remind the family that over-the-counter (OTC) inhalers contain medications that can interfere with the prescribed therapy. Instruct the child/parent to contact the health care provider before trying any OTC medications. Instruct the child/parent in sequencing of inhalers; bronchodilator inhalers are used 15 minutes before administration of the steroid inhaler. The preferred treatment is one inhaler with both meds.

✓ Cleaning and care of equipment—nebulizer, MDI, or other medication delivery systems, including assessment of when the canister is low or empty.

✓ If the child is taking oral corticosteroids while at home, instructions to ensure that he or she receives the correct amount each day, especially if the medication is going to be tapered. Missing a dose may decrease the effectiveness. Also, discuss side effects and the importance of taking with food to prevent stomach irritation.

✓ Importance of taking medication at home and at school as directed. Medication in the original bottle/canister (with prescribing label) and a written prescription from the health care provider are needed for the child to be able to take any medication at school.

✓ Importance of knowing early warning signs before an acute attack (e.g., fatigue, sneezing, sore throat, itchy/watery eyes, headache, slight tightness in chest, drop in PFM values). These differ for each child.

✓ Signs and symptoms of increased respiratory distress in children related to age (e.g., an infant may have increased RR when sleeping, decreased interest in eating/drinking, nasal flaring, grunting, retractions). Other signs and symptoms include difficulty speaking in sentences, inability to walk short distances, hunched posture, and PFM values in the red zone.

✓ Importance of avoiding contact with infectious individuals, especially those with respiratory infection.

✓ Recommendation that the child receives annual influenza if over 6 months old and all age-appropriate vaccinations.

✓ Importance of follow-up care on a regular basis (not just emergency department). Confirm the date and time of the next appointment.

✓ Phone numbers to call if questions or concerns arise about therapy or disease.

✓ When to call the health care provider:
  • To refill medications.
  • PEFR in yellow zone 24 hours or child has an event such as coughing, wheezing, chest tightness, or shortness of breath.
  • PEFR in red zone or the child is in increased respiratory distress.
  • Immediate reliever/quick-relief medication (albuterol) needed more often than every 4 hours.
  • Reliever medication not helping.

✓ When to call emergency medical services:
  • The child is in severe respiratory distress.
  • The child is gray/blue.
  • The child is unable to answer questions or seems confused.

✓ Importance of communication with the child's school or group child care regarding the child's condition, need for medication, and activity level.

✓ Legal rights of the child—Section 504 of Rehabilitation Act of 1973: Each student with a disability is entitled to accommodation needed to attend school and participate as fully as possible in school activities. This accommodation may be related to a medical condition or an educational issue. More details are at https://www.verywellfamily.com and search for 504 Plan.

✓ Guidelines for attendance, activity level, and exercise at school or group child care.

✓ Referral to community resources, such as the local and national American Lung Associations, for educational programs for children with asthma. Additional general information can be obtained by contacting:
  • American Lung Association: https://www.lung.org/
  • Allergy & Asthma Network: https://allergyasthmanetwork.org/
  • Asthma and Allergy Foundation of America: https://aafa.org/asthma/ National Heart, Lung, and Blood Institute: Asthma resources for patients and caregivers https://www.nhlbi.nih.gov/LMBBasthma/asthma-publications-patients-and-caregivers

- Centers for Disease Control and Prevention: Learn how to control asthma. https://www.cdc.gov/asthma/ (http://www.cdc.gov/asthma-DELETE)
✓ Several links for children and adolescents include:
  - *Dusty the Asthma Goldfish and His Asthma Triggers Funbook*, and *Why Is Coco Orange?*: https://www. epa.gov/asthma/publications-about-asthma#1tab-1. Dusty's funbook is an educational activity book that helps children learn more about asthma triggers. Coco and his friends learn about air quality and how to stay healthy when air quality is bad.
  - *Huff & Puff: An Asthma Tale:* https://vimeopro.com/ healthnutsmedia/huff-and-puff-an-asthma-tale/ page/1. Seven videos where the Big Bad Wolf huffs and puffs and has an asthma attack!
  - *Allie and Andy's Awesome Asthma and Allergy Activity Booklet:* https://community.aafa.org/blog/9-ways-to-teach-children-about-asthma "How Asthma makes Me Feel" https://allergyasthmanetwork.org/what-is-asthma/asthma-in-babies-and-children (2nd video on page). Heartrending 6-minute YouTube video with children telling with their pictures and in their own words how they felt during and after an attack.

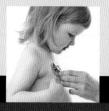

# Attention-Deficit Hyperactivity Disorder 78

## OVERVIEW/PATHOPHYSIOLOGY

Attention-deficit hyperactivity disorder (ADHD) is a neuro-developmental/neurobehavioral disorder involving developmentally inappropriate behavior. ADHD is one of the most common chronic illnesses diagnosed in children and adolescents in the United States. The statistics for the number of children affected vary depending on source and population but currently occurred in 8.7% of children between 3 and 17 years old in 2016–2019 data (Bitsko et al., 2022). Although the exact etiology is unknown, it probably involves a combination of genetics, environment, and development. ADHD is seen more often in children who have a family member with ADHD, particularly a parent or sibling with ADHD or another mental disorder. Some other risk factors include exposure to environmental toxins (e.g., lead and pesticides) or medications; prematurity; and brain injury (CHADD, n.d.a.; Hockenberry et al., 2019). Gray et al. in 2020 noted that about 50% of children with ADHD had insomnia which can exacerbate their symptoms leading to problems with school performance, family relationships, mood, and quality of life. ADHD most commonly occurs in association with language and learning disorders per the American Academy of Pediatrics (AAP) Clinical Practice Guidelines (2019). ADHD is more common in males than females, and most children affected continue to demonstrate symptoms into adolescence and adulthood. There is some belief that ADHD is not "outgrown" but that people learn to compensate. Wesemann and Cleve (2018) and the American Academy of Pediatrics (2019) note that Black and Hispanic children are less likely to be diagnosed and treated for ADHD. Studies note that children and adolescents with ADHD have lower grades and higher rates of retention in grade level and dropping out of school than their peers. Studies also show higher rates of unintentional injury and emergency department visits. Interpersonal relationships and social developments can also be affected. Thus ADHD may affect all realms of the child's and adolescent's world, including home, school, and friends. There is also a significant economic burden that affects the child, family, health care resources, educational services, and society. Zhao et al. (2019) noted that families with a child with ADHD incurred a total economic burden over the course of the child's development that was more than five times greater compared to children without ADHD.

## HEALTH CARE SETTING

Primary care.

## ASSESSMENT

Includes comprehensive history and physical examination with a thorough cardiovascular examination, detailed neurologic examination, family assessment, and school assessment.

**Signs and symptoms.** The behaviors exhibited are not unusual aspects of any child's behavior. The difference lies in the quality of motor activity and developmentally inappropriate inattention, impulsivity, and hyperactivity displayed. The symptoms vary with developmental age and may range from a few to numerous different symptoms. The core symptoms include inattention, hyperactivity, and impulsivity. Children may experience significant functional problems such as school difficulties, academic underachievement, troublesome interpersonal relationships with family members and peers, and low self-esteem.

**Physical assessment.** A complete physical examination including vision and hearing screening and a thorough cardiovascular examination is needed. To rule out any severe neurologic disorders, a detailed neurologic examination is also required.

The Guidelines for the Diagnosis of ADHD were revised by the AAP in October 2011, expanded slightly by the American Psychiatric Association in 2013, and updated in 2019. The current guidelines change the focus on the evaluation, diagnosis, and treatment of ADHD in children 4–18 years old, highlighting the importance of identifying comorbid conditions (Zimlich, 2019). Without any significant change in the guidelines, they include the following:

1. The age range to include any child 4–18 years of age presenting with academic or behavioral problems and symptoms of inattention, hyperactivity, or impulsivity.
2. Use of specific criteria for the diagnosis using the *Diagnostic and Statistical Manual of Mental Health Disorders* (DSM-5) criteria.
3. Importance of obtaining information concerning the child's symptoms/behavior in more than one setting (especially from school). Obtain information from multiple sources (e.g., from parents or guardians, other family members, teachers, and mental health workers).

4. Evaluation for comorbid conditions that may make the diagnosis more difficult or complicate treatment planning including emotional or behavioral disorders (e.g., anxiety and behavior problems), developmental disorders (e.g., learning and language disorders), and physical conditions (e.g., tics or apnea). The primary care provider should refer child to a specialist if they find co-occurring conditions that the child is not experienced in diagnosing or treating. **Note:** Studies have shown that 75% of children/adolescents with ADHD have another DSM-5 condition, for example, specific learning disorder, anxiety and/or depression, and oppositional defiant disorder. "ADHD Complex" is now being used for these children/adolescents (Gephart, 2020).

5. Primary care clinicians should consider this a chronic condition; thus children and youth with ADHD have special health care needs and should follow the principles of the chronic care model and medical home. The medical home model originated by the AAP refers to the delivery of quality coordinated care integrating health promotion, acute care, and chronic care in a planned family-centered manner.

6. Specific guidance per treatment of preschool-aged children (4–6 years), school-aged children, and adolescents (6–18 years).

> **Note:** *The 2019 AAP Clinical Practice guidelines included two attachments—a process of care algorithm and an article "Systems barriers to the care of children and adolescents with ADHD."*

***Multidisciplinary evaluation.*** Includes the primary pediatrician (and possibly a developmental pediatrician, pediatric neurologist, or pediatric psychiatrist), psychologist, pediatric/school nurse, classroom teacher, specialty teachers as appropriate, and the child's parents/caregivers to obtain all perspectives of the child's behavior.

***Detailed history.*** Both medical and developmental history and descriptions of the child's behavior need to be obtained from as many observers as possible. Traumatic experiences, psychiatric, and other disorders (lead poisoning, seizures, partial hearing loss, psychosis, and witnessing sexual activity and/or violence) need to be ruled out.

It is important to focus on school-based skills including fine and gross motor skills.

***Psychologic testing.*** Valuable in determining a variety of deficits and helpful in identifying the child's intelligence and achievement levels.

***Behavioral checklists and adaptive scales.*** Helpful in measuring social adaptive functioning in children with ADHD. Examples include Conners' Rating Scales and Vanderbilt ADHD Scales, both include several specific versions (e.g., parents or teachers).

## DIAGNOSTIC TESTS

ADHD is a diagnosis of exclusion. There is no definitive test for ADHD.

### Patient Problem/Analyze Cues/Prioritize Hypotheses

# Risk for Impaired Psychological Status (Decreased Impulse Control)

*due to* excessive environmental stimuli resulting in an inability to concentrate, control impulses, and organize thoughts in a manner appropriate for age and development

***Desired Outcomes/Generate Solutions:*** Within 1 month of this diagnosis, the child completes activities of daily living and shows behavioral improvement in the school setting. Within one semester, the child shows improvement in academic activities.

| ASSESSMENT—RECOGNIZE CUES/ INTERVENTIONS—TAKE ACTION | RATIONALES |
|---|---|
| Encourage parents/teachers to provide a structured environment and consistency. | Structure and consistency offer opportunities for children to focus on areas that need improvement. |
| Promote ongoing communication between parents and teachers. | Consistency among family and teachers in reinforcing the same guidelines improves the child's ability to concentrate. |
| Encourage parents/teachers to decrease stimuli when concentration is important. | Children with ADHD are easily distracted by extraneous stimuli. Removing those stimuli should improve concentration. For example, parents/teachers should have the child do homework in a quiet area without TV or radio or sit in a quiet section of the classroom, not near an open door or window. |

## Patient Problem/Analyze Cues/Prioritize Hypotheses

# Low Self-Esteem

*due to* negative responses and lack of approval from others regarding behavior

**Desired Outcome/Generate Solutions:** Within 1 month of this diagnosis, the child achieves at least one goal, lists strengths, and elicits fewer negative responses from others.

| ASSESSMENT—RECOGNIZE CUES/ INTERVENTIONS—TAKE ACTION | RATIONALES |
| --- | --- |
| Assess the child's interactions with others. | This assessment helps determine the existence/degree of negative responses from other people. |
| Reward positive behavior and provide limit setting as needed. Avoid negative comments and giving attention for negative behavior. | Positive reinforcement is an effective way to improve behavior and self-esteem. |
| Help the child set goals that are age appropriate, realistic, and achievable. Set a timetable to achieve step-by-step progress until he or she accomplishes the overall goal. | Achieving goals increases self-esteem. If the child has difficulty completing assignments, divide the assignment into manageable tasks. For example, for an essay assignment: day 1, make an outline; day 2, begin literature search; day 3, begin writing the paper; day 4, finish the paper and have someone review it; day 5, finalize the paper. |
| Encourage the child to make a list of his or her strengths. Teach self-questioning techniques (e.g., "What am I doing?" and "How is that going to affect others?"). Encourage positive self-talk (e.g., "I did a good job with that!"). Provide feedback accordingly. | These activities encourage positive self-thought and build self-esteem. |

## Patient Problem/Analyze Cues/Prioritize Hypotheses

# Risk for Injury

*due to* increased activity level, limited judgment skills, and impulsivity

**Desired Outcome/Generate Solutions:** The child remains free from signs of trauma.

| ASSESSMENT—RECOGNIZE CUES/ INTERVENTIONS—TAKE ACTION | RATIONALES |
| --- | --- |
| Reinforce to the parents the importance of the child using appropriate safety equipment/protective device (e.g., seat belt and bicycle helmet). | Using this equipment/device decreases likelihood of trauma. |
| Encourage the parents to model the use of appropriate safety equipment/protective devices. | Children are more likely to wear a seat belt or bicycle helmet if their parents wear them also. |
| Encourage the parents to set clear limits on where the child may ride a bike or play and to offer choices from several safe areas the child can go. | Clear, simple guidelines are easier for a child with ADHD to focus on and follow. Allowing the child some choice improves compliance, which decreases the likelihood of injury. |
| Encourage the child's participation in active play rather than in passive activities (e.g., playing softball rather than playing video games). | Active play helps children grow physically and cognitively. It also helps the child with ADHD to redirect energy in a safe and effective manner, thus decreasing the risk for injury/trauma. |
| Reinforce the importance of the parents monitoring the child's activities on a regular basis. | Adequate supervision decreases likelihood of injury/trauma. |
| Instruct the parents to reinforce positive behavior with feedback and intermittent rewards. | This encourages appropriate behavior and activity, thereby decreasing the risk for injury/trauma. |

## Patient/Parent Problem/Analyze Cues/Prioritize Hypotheses

# Deficient Knowledge

*due to* unfamiliarity with chronicity of ADHD and its treatment

***Desired Outcome/Generate Solutions:*** Within 1 month of this diagnosis, the child and/or parents verbalize an accurate understanding of the chronic condition of ADHD and possible treatments.

| ASSESSMENT—RECOGNIZE CUES/ INTERVENTIONS—TAKE ACTION | RATIONALES |
|---|---|
| Assess the parents' and child's understanding (depending on the child's age) of ADHD. As indicated, teach them about the disorder, including the fact that it is chronic. | This assessment enables the development of an individualized teaching plan. Accurate knowledge about the condition facilitates understanding of the need for ongoing treatment and ways to manage it realistically. |
| Encourage parents/teachers to provide a calm, structured environment and consistency. | Structure and consistency offer opportunities for the child to focus on areas that need improvement. |
| Promote ongoing communication between the teacher and family. | Frequent communication between the parents and teacher/school, especially when the child is first diagnosed, facilitates everyone working together to maximize the child's ability to function more appropriately. |
| Discuss different treatment strategies, based on the age of child and any comorbidities. | This information promotes the understanding that no single treatment strategy is *the* answer and that there are multiple strategies that may help the child, such as medication, behavioral/psychosocial interventions (parent training in behavior management and education, behavior modification, teacher training in behavioral classroom interventions/proper classroom placement and management, counseling, and psychotherapy), combined or multimodal treatment, and biofeedback. |

## Patient/Parent Problem/Analyze Cues/Prioritize Hypotheses

# Deficient Knowledge

*due to* unfamiliarity with the purpose, precautions, and potential side effects of prescribed medications

***Desired Outcome/Generate Solutions:*** Within 1 week of starting medication, the child and/or parents verbalize accurate information about the prescribed medications.

| ASSESSMENT—RECOGNIZE CUES/ INTERVENTIONS—TAKE ACTION | RATIONALES |
|---|---|
| **Teach the Following to the Parents/Child:** | |
| **Stimulant Medications** | This is the first-line treatment for children and adolescents but generally not for preschoolers (PTBM – parent training in behavior management, is the recommended primary intervention, if available) (AAP, 2021). |
| *Short, intermediate, and long-acting methylphenidate (e.g., Ritalin); short, intermediate, and long-acting dextroamphetamine (e.g., Dexedrine); mixed dextroamphetamine/amphetamine (e.g., Adderall); and dexmethylphenidate (e.g., Focalin)* | Stimulants are given to promote attentiveness and decrease restlessness by increasing dopamine and norepinephrine levels, which leads to stimulation of the inhibitory system of the central nervous system (CNS). |
| • Medications can be titrated up every 3–7 days per clinician's directive until a decrease in symptoms occurs or the maximum dose is reached. | A slow increase allows time to determine whether medication is effective. This requires close monitoring with the clinician to evaluate the child's physical condition and symptom relief. The goal is to have maximum benefit with minimal side effects. |

## ASSESSMENT—RECOGNIZE CUES/ INTERVENTIONS—TAKE ACTION

## RATIONALES

| ASSESSMENT—RECOGNIZE CUES/ INTERVENTIONS—TAKE ACTION | RATIONALES |
|---|---|
| • Assess for and report decreased appetite, stomachache or headache, and trouble sleeping (AAP, 2019; CHADD, n.d.b.). | The most common side effects are usually short term but may require either dosage adjustment or change in schedule. |
| • Assess for and notify the health care provider if the child develops or has increased aggression or hostility, depression, delusional thinking, hallucinations, or mania. | These are serious side effects and will require a change in dosage or medication. |
| • Assess for and report circulation problems in fingers and toes. | Side effect/concern that may require a change in dosage or medication |
| • Assess for and report tics (involuntary movements of a small group of muscles such as of the face). | Tics occur in 15%–30% of children and are usually transient. This medication is contraindicated if the child/family member has motor tics or Tourette syndrome. |
| • Assess for and report the child becoming overfocused while on medication or appearing dull or overly restricted. | These changes are seen in children receiving too high a dose or who are overly sensitive. Decreasing the dose usually resolves these problems. |
| • Assess height, weight, and blood pressure (BP) at regular follow-up visits with the prescribing clinician. | Suppression of growth may occur with long-term use, and it can also increase BP. |
| • Assess for and report decreased impulsiveness, improved social interaction, and increased academic productivity and accuracy. | This will indicate the effectiveness of medication. |
| • Take the medication on an empty stomach 30–45 minutes before meals, if possible, for most forms. | Absorption of methylphenidate is increased when taken with meals, with the exception of extended/sustained-release forms (may be taken with or without meals but must be taken with water, milk, or juice). It must be taken daily in the morning, and the tablet must not be crushed, chewed, or divided. |
| | Taking all forms of the medication at a consistent time is most important. Dosage can be adjusted to counteract the effects of any decreased absorption as long as the medication is taken consistently with or without food. |
| • Avoid taking amphetamines with acidic foods, juices, or vitamin C. | When taken with these foods and drinks, the amphetamine blood level may be reduced and, therefore, not be as effective as desired. |
| • Do not crush, chew, or break sustained-release forms. | Action of the medication will change and probably not be as effective. |
| • Take the last daily dose several hours before bedtime. | This reduces the potential for insomnia. |
| • Apply transdermal patch (e.g., Daytrana) to the hip 2 hours before needed and remove 9 hours later. It may be removed earlier if shorter duration of effect is needed or if late-day undesired effects occur. Apply to clean, dry skin; alternate site of application daily; apply immediately after opening protective foil; do not cut the patch; apply at the same time each day; and press the patch firmly for 30 seconds. | This patch is approved for children 6–17 years of age. Applying the patch in the appropriate site, manner, and time improves the effectiveness of this form of the medication. |
| • Monitor the application site for local adverse reactions (e.g., skin lightened under or around patch) and allergic contact sensitization. | These side effects may require a dosage adjustment or change in the form of medication. |
| • Get all prescriptions filled at the same pharmacy or give a list of all current medications to every pharmacy used. | There are many drug interactions with these medications. An informed pharmacist can identify all potential interactions among medications. For example, methylphenidate may increase serum levels of tricyclic antidepressants, phenytoin, phenobarbital, and warfarin. Monoamine oxidase inhibitors (MAOIs) or general anesthetics potentiate methylphenidate. |
| • Limit caffeine and decongestants. | They are stimulants and can potentiate medications the child is receiving. |
| • Avoid the use of the previously listed CNS stimulants in patients with serious cardiac problems. | They could place the patient at increased risk for sympathomimetic effects of CNS stimulants, including sudden death in children. American Heart Association recommends that all children with ADHD being treated with stimulants have thorough cardiovascular assessments before initiation of therapy. |
| | **United States Boxed Warning**: Serious cardiovascular events, including sudden death in children with preexisting structural cardiac abnormalities or serious heart problems. |

| ASSESSMENT—RECOGNIZE CUES/ INTERVENTIONS—TAKE ACTION | RATIONALES |
|---|---|
| • Avoid the use in patients with marked agitation, tension, or anxiety. | These medications may exacerbate symptoms of behavior disturbance and thought disorders. |
| • Prolonged use may lead to drug dependency. Abrupt withdrawal after taking high doses or after a prolonged time may cause withdrawal. Therefore patients might need to be weaned off these medications rather than abruptly stopped if possible. | **United States Boxed Warning:** There is also the potential for drug dependency with these medications. |
| • The child needs to be carefully screened for any abuse history, and the family must ensure the medication is secured. | **United States Boxed Warning:** There is a high potential for abuse with these medications by the child or others. |
| • Avoid the use of the previously listed CNS stimulants in children who have taken an MAOI within the past 14 days. | These drugs could precipitate a hypertensive crisis. |
| • Caution is necessary when taken by children with seizures. | These medications may lower the seizure threshold. |
| • Children should have a periodic drug holiday (e.g., no medication during the summer) or periodic discontinuation. | This assesses the child's requirement for medication, decreases tolerance, and limits suppression of linear growth and weight. |
| • Reevaluate the child at appropriate intervals while receiving these medications. | This assesses the effectiveness and whether the child still needs to be on the medication at all. Some studies have shown children to have improved behavior even after going off the medication. |
| • Use with caution in preschool-aged children and only if behavior therapy is not effective. | Young children are more sensitive to adverse effects. Methylphenidate may be used if behavioral interventions do not relieve symptoms and child continues to have serious problems. Several medications are now approved by the United States Food and Drug Administration (FDA) for use in children 3–5 years (all are forms of dextroamphetamine and dextroamphetamine and amphetamine that are short-acting/immediate release drugs such as Adderall). Although FDA approved, they are still not recommended for use in children per current guidelines (AAP, 2019; American Pharmacists Association, 2021). |

**Norepinephrine Reuptake Inhibitor (Nonstimulant)**

| | |
|---|---|
| *Atomoxetine (e.g., Strattera)* | This medication is given to improve attentiveness, enhance the ability to follow through on tasks with less distraction and forgetfulness, and diminish hyperactivity. The exact mechanism of action is unknown, but it is believed to be related to the selective inhibitor of presynaptic norepinephrine transporter, resulting in norepinephrine reuptake inhibition. |
| • Assess for and report headache, dizziness, insomnia, upper abdominal pain, vomiting, decreased appetite, dry mouth, or cough. | These are the most common side effects and may require either dosage adjustment or change in schedule. |
| • Assess for and report chest pain or palpitations, urinary retention or difficulty voiding, appetite loss and weight loss, mood swings, or insomnia. | These are significant side effects and will require some changes either in dosage or medication. |
| • Assess weight on a regular basis and ensure the dose prescribed is appropriate for weight before administering. | The dose is based on weight. An accurate weight is needed to get optimal effects of the medication with minimal side effects. It is also important to note whether the child is losing weight. If so, it may be necessary to interrupt therapy. |
| • Assess baseline heart rate (HR) and BP with dose increases and periodically while on therapy. | This medication may cause significantly increased HR, significantly increased BP, and palpitations; if so, the dose needs to be adjusted. This is especially important for a child with preexisting hypertension. |
| • Observe closely for and report behavioral changes (e.g., emergence of irritability or agitation), including increased aggression and hostility, which may be a precursor to emerging suicidal ideation. | **United States Boxed Warning:** There is an increased risk for suicidal ideation in children and adolescents with this medication, especially for the first few months and after dose changes. |
| • Avoid the use of atomoxetine in patients with serious cardiac problems. | This medication could put patients at increased risk for serious cardiovascular events, including sudden death in children. American Heart Association recommends that all children with ADHD who are treated with atomoxetine have a thorough cardiovascular assessment before initiation of therapy. |

Continued

| ASSESSMENT—RECOGNIZE CUES/ INTERVENTIONS—TAKE ACTION | RATIONALES |
|---|---|
| • Use cautiously with Albuterol or other beta-2 agonists, vasopressor drugs, or CYP2D6 inhibitors (e.g., paroxetine, fluoxetine, and quinidine). | Beta-2 agonists potentiate cardiovascular effects of this medication; CYP2D6 inhibitors may increase blood levels and toxicity. |
| • Do not use within 2 weeks of taking MAOIs. | This may precipitate a hypertensive crisis. |
| • Get all prescriptions filled at the same pharmacy or give a list of all current medications to every pharmacy used. | This drug interacts with many medications. An informed pharmacist can identify all potential interactions among medications. |
| • Assess for a decrease in ADHD symptoms within the first 4–6 weeks of starting the medication. | It may take up to 4–6 weeks to get the maximum response. If adequate response has not been achieved, it may be necessary to titrate dosing or try another medication. |
| • Reevaluate the patient's physical condition and ADHD symptoms at appropriate intervals. | Ongoing, regular assessments will detect problems before they become severe as well as assess the effectiveness and whether the medication needs to be continued. |

**Other Approved Nonstimulant Medications**

| | |
|---|---|
| *Clonidine extended-release form only*—one of three medications approved by AAP other than stimulants to treat ADHD | An alpha-2–adrenergic agonist, this medication regulates levels of neurotransmitters and norepinephrine. It may be effective in decreasing ADHD symptoms alone or in combination with stimulant medications. |
| • Avoid the use of clonidine in patients with serious cardiac problems. | This medication could put the patient at increased risk for serious cardiovascular events, including sudden death in children. American Heart Association recommends that all children with ADHD who are treated with clonidine have a thorough cardiovascular assessment before initiation of therapy. |
| • Assess for and report dry mouth, dizziness, drowsiness, irritability, fatigue, constipation, anorexia, palpitations, and local skin reactions with patch. | These are side effects that may necessitate a change in dosage. |
| • Assess for and report immediately: palpitations, bradycardia, hypotension, edema, rapid weight gain, confusion, and hallucinations. | These are serious side effects that require prompt attention. |
| • Do not stop the medication abruptly. It is necessary to slowly wean off the medication. | The patient will go through withdrawal symptoms. |
| • Watch the child closely if clonidine is given with CNS depressants. | Additive sedation would occur if given with CNS depressants, including alcohol, antihistamines, opioid analgesics, and sedative/hypnotics. |
| • Assess for a decrease in symptoms of ADHD, especially after 2–4 weeks on the medication. | It may take an extended period of time to get maximum response from the medication. If there is no decrease in ADHD symptoms, it may be necessary to have the dose increased or the medication changed. |
| • Get all prescriptions filled at the same pharmacy or give a list of all current medications to every pharmacy used. | This medication interacts with many others, such as cardiac, antihypertensive, tricyclic antidepressants, and psychiatric medications. An informed pharmacist can identify all potential interactions among medications. |
| *Guanfacine extended-release form only* | This medication, an alpha-2–adrenergic agonist, regulates levels of neurotransmitters and norepinephrine and may be effective in decreasing ADHD symptoms alone or in combination with stimulant medications. It is very similar to clonidine. |
| • Assess for and report immediately: bradycardia, hypotension, orthostatic hypotension, and syncope, especially during the first month of taking the medication. | These are significant side effects that may be more apparent during the first month of therapy. If severe, it may be necessary to change the dose of medication or change the medication. |
| • Assess for and report immediately: rash; hives; itching; difficulty breathing; tightness in the chest; swelling in the mouth, face, lips, or tongue; rapid HR; or palpitations. | These are significant side effects that may require immediate action. |
| • Assess for constipation, dizziness, drowsiness, dry mouth, or tiredness. | These are side effects that may necessitate dose change if significant. This medication causes less drowsiness than clonidine. |

See "Clonidine," earlier, for the last two assessments/interventions.

Family Problem/Analyze Cues/Prioritize Hypotheses

# Difficulty Coping

*due to* the need for constant and close supervision of the child, hyperactivity of the child, or the stigma associated with a child with impulsive or aggressive behavior

***Desired Outcome/Generate Solutions:*** Within 1 week of diagnosis, family members (including siblings, depending on their developmental age) discuss the child's needs and develop a plan to provide the necessary support.

| ASSESSMENT—RECOGNIZE CUES/ INTERVENTIONS—TAKE ACTION | RATIONALES |
|---|---|
| Assess the family's knowledge/understanding of current coping status. | This assessment will help ensure that support and assistance will be more effective. |
| Assist the family with problem-solving ways of managing the child's behavior and needs. | Positive reinforcement, time-out, response cost, or token rewards are examples of effective behavioral techniques for children with ADHD. |
| Provide handouts for caregivers explaining behavioral management techniques. | Verbal and written guidelines promote understanding. Handouts increase consistency among caregivers and improve their ability to meet the child's needs. |
| Enable the family (including siblings) to vent concerns and problems. | Discussing concerns increases their ability to cope with the situation. |
| Help identify community resources for support (e.g., many school systems have ADHD support groups, local Children and Adults With ADHD [CHADD] chapter). | Support groups often help families function and cope more effectively. |
| Encourage the family to advocate for their child within the school system (Individualized Education Program [IEP] or 504 accommodation plan as appropriate). | Many parents are unaware of the rights of disabled children. Environmental accommodation and appropriate classroom placement help children with ADHD reach their maximum potential by concentrating better, controlling impulses, and improving organizational ability. For example, for a child with ADHD, the desk may be placed in the front and on the quieter side of the classroom, and the child may be given extra time to complete tests. This involvement/support by the family increases the potential for the child to function well/succeed. |

### ADDITIONAL PROBLEM:

| | |
|---|---|
| "Psychosocial Support for the Patient's Family and Significant Others," for relevant psychosocial care plans that would help family members cope with ADHD, such as *Anxiety* and *Difficulty Coping*. | Chapter 9 |

 PATIENT–FAMILY TEACHING

The child with ADHD may have a wide variety of symptoms and treatment modalities. Providing support and information about the disease is essential because of the stigma associated with ADHD. When providing child/family teaching, focus on sensory information and avoid giving excessive information and initiate visiting nurse referral follow-up assessment and teaching as needed. Utilize a variety of teaching methods (e.g., videos, iPads/tablets, and webinars as well as verbal and written) depending on learning style and resources of child/family. Stress family-centered care, which is viewing the family as a unit that is the "constant" in the child's life and maintaining or improving the health of the family and its members). Include information about the following (ensure that written information is at a level the reader can understand):

✓ Clarification of myths and realities concerning ADHD: The child is not "bad," "lazy," or "stupid."

✓ Safety measures relative to developmental age, impulsivity, inattentiveness, and hyperactivity. These stresses will change as the child gets older.

✓ Importance of multiple approaches necessary to treat ADHD, not just medications.

✓ Medications, including drug name; purpose; dosage; frequency; precautions; drug–drug, food–drug, and herb–drug interactions; and potential side effects.

✓ Suggestions to help with side effect of decreased appetite:
  • Give stimulant medication with or after meals rather than before.
  • Encourage nutritious snacks in the evening when medication effects are decreasing.
  • Offer small meals often with healthy "on-the-go" snacks.
✓ Importance of taking medication as directed at home and school. Medication in the original pharmacy bottle and written prescription from the health care provider are needed for the child to be able to take medication at school.
✓ Importance of monitoring pill count and prescription drug monitoring as appropriate since most ADHD medications are controlled substances.
✓ Importance of consistency, structure, and routine for the child with ADHD.
✓ Importance of collaboration of family, the health care provider, and school for optimal outcome.
✓ Importance of supporting siblings and including them in the "plan." Help them cope with/adapt to having a brother/sister with a chronic illness.
✓ Environmental manipulation and appropriate classroom placement, which increase the child's ability to function optimally.
✓ Suggestions regarding house rules:
  • Give clear, specific directions.
  • Use positive rewards; do not punish.
  • Implement a contingency plan.
✓ Suggestions to help children with ADHD:
  • Daily picture with schedule of activities and events.
  • Index cards with written steps or pictures.
  • Organized backpack and notebook.
  • Physical relaxation techniques.
  • Standing when needing to work at his or her desk.
  • Two chairs (can move back and forth between them).
  • Boundaries in the classroom.
  • Provide *only* needed materials.
  • Include short, fast-paced tasks.
  • Soothing music, carpet, earplugs.
  • One step at a time—the student verbalizes the step, performs the step, and then moves on to the next step.
  • Positive self-talk and reinforcement practices.
✓ Suggestions to facilitate communication between the family and school, including daily written communication with the teacher per behavior (gives a better overall evaluation of the effectiveness of medication/behavioral modification).
✓ Legal rights of the child.
✓ Individuals With Disabilities Education Act: Requires states to identify, diagnose, educate, and provide related services for children 3–21 years old.
✓ IEP: Multidisciplinary team designs this plan to facilitate special education and therapeutic strategies and goals for

each eligible child. Parents need to be involved in this process.
✓ Section 504 of Rehabilitation Act of 1973: Each student with a disability is entitled to the accommodation needed to attend school and participate as fully as possible in school activities.
✓ Signs that indicate when to contact the health care provider:
  • Child seems very drowsy.
  • Child is unable to concentrate after being on medication for several weeks.
  • Child physically harms self or others.
  • No improvement is seen in school performance over 1–2 months.
✓ Importance of follow-up care, including the primary pediatrician and multidisciplinary team.
✓ Referral to community resources such as support groups, pediatricians who are comfortable dealing with ADHD, child psychologists, and local community services boards, including:
  • CHADD: http://www.chadd.org.
  • National Resource Center for ADHD (program of CHADD)—Educational/legal rights for children with ADHD in public schools (http://www.chadd.org/for-parents/education/) or Centers for Disease Control and Prevention: ADHD. My child has been diagnosed with ADHD, now what? Detailed information per treatment for parents, including extensive information on behavioral therapy and training for parents as well as medications, is found at https://www.cdc.gov/ncbddd/adhd/treatment.html.
  • Center for Parent Information and Resources: Central "hub" of networks and products created for the Parent Centers serving families of children with disabilities. Some examples include a resource library, newsletters, and webinars, which is found at https://parentcenterhub.org/ptacs.
  • HealthyChildren.org (supported by AAP): https://www.healthychildren.org/English/health-issues/conditions/adhd.
  • *Hi, It's Me! I Have ADHD by Katelyn Mabry (2020).* With colorful pictures and kid-friendly language and based on the author's personal experiences growing up, she shares the thoughts, feelings, emotions, and experiences of a child dealing with the many challenges of ADHD. It offers insight into the world of ADHD, presenting a list of tips and printable coloring/journal pages. This rhyming picture book helps children struggling with ADHD feel empowered. It is available on Amazon.com.
  • *Marvin's Monster Diary 2 (+Lyssa): ADHD Emotion Explosion (But I Triumph, Big Time): An ST4 Mindfulness Book for Kids* (4) (Monster Diaries) by Raun Melmed and Caroline Bliss Larsen with illustrator Arief Kriembonga, 2019. Marvin is a lovable

monster with a 12-stringed baby fang guitar, a rambunctious case of ADHD, and a diary to record it all. Marvin got it together in Marvin's Monster Diary: ADHD Attacks, but his lab partner Lyssa's emotional roller coaster is a little out of control. His diary

teaches kids how to be mindful, observe their surroundings, and take time to think about their actions in a funny, relatable way. It is available on Amazon.com.

## OVERVIEW/PATHOPHYSIOLOGY

Bronchiolitis is an acute infection that causes inflammation and obstruction of the bronchioles, the smallest, most distal sections of the lower respiratory tract. Severe bronchiolitis rarely occurs in children older than 2 years and has a peak incidence at less than 6 months of age (Centers for Disease Control and Prevention [CDC], 2022). Bronchiolitis is one of the major causes of hospitalization in children younger than 2 years (Freeman & Bajaj, 2022). Before 2020 seasonal patterns were consistent with the greatest incidence in the fall, winter, and early spring in most of the United States. Florida had an earlier respiratory syncytial virus (RSV) season with a longer duration. The incidence of RSV in the traditional 2020–2021 season was low but started rising in the spring 2021 and continued through the spring, summer, and fall. This "interseasonal" activity was very different from the usual seasonal pattern and was not followed by a second wave of increased RSV activity in the winter of 2021–2022 (American Academy of Pediatrics [AAP], 2022).

Acute bronchiolitis is most often a viral infection and is most often caused by the RSV, with almost all young children being infected by the age of 2 years. Other common causes are adenoviruses, human metapneumovirus, parainfluenza, and, occasionally, *Mycoplasma pneumoniae* (Hockenberry et al., 2019). RSV is highly contagious and transmitted by droplets and direct contact with secretions or indirectly on contaminated surfaces. Infants/children infected with RSV are usually contagious for 3–8 days but may become contagious 1 or 2 days before showing symptoms. Some infants and immunocompromised children may be infectious for up to 4 weeks (CDC, n.d.a). RSV is the leading cause of lower respiratory tract disease (e.g., bronchiolitis and pneumonia) in infants, causing more than 58,000–80,000 hospitalizations and 2.1 million outpatient visits in children younger than 5 years annually (CDC, n.d.b). Most infants and young children can be cared for at home, but approximately 1%–2% of those younger than 6 months who are infected may need to be hospitalized (CDC, 2022).

## HEALTH CARE SETTING

Primary care with possible hospitalization for respiratory distress

## ASSESSMENT

Initially upper respiratory infection symptoms for 2–3 days: fever, rhinorrhea, and cough. In children less than 6 months, the only symptoms may be irritability, decreased activity and appetite, and/or apnea.

***Acute respiratory distress.*** Expiratory wheezing, tachypnea with respiratory rate (RR) of 60–80 breaths/minutes or more, nasal flaring, paroxysmal nonproductive cough, increased respiratory effort or work of breathing (WOB), cyanosis, retractions, difficulty feeding because of increased RR, posttussive (after coughing) emesis, irritability, lethargy.

***Physical assessment.*** Auscultation of expiratory wheezing and crackles or rhonchi. Symptoms of dehydration may be present: decreased level of consciousness (LOC), sunken anterior fontanel (if younger than 2 years), dry or sticky oral mucosa, decreased abdominal skin turgor, and decreased urine output (UO).

### Risk factors for severe respiratory syncytial virus bronchiolitis

- Infants, especially 6 months or younger
- Premature infants
- Chronic lung disease (CLD)/bronchopulmonary dysplasia and less than 2 years old
- Congenital heart disease (CHD) and less than 2 years old
- Immunodeficiency
- Neuromuscular disorders, especially those who have difficulty swallowing or clearing secretions (risk factor)

**Note:** *Management and medications for children with the previously listed congenital/chronic conditions may vary from the general recommendations in the AAP 2014 guidelines for children from 1 month to 23 months. Updated guidance per prophylaxis during the 2022–2023 RSV Season from AAP in November 2022.*

## DIAGNOSTIC TESTS

Diagnosis is made based on history and physical examination. Neither the AAP Clinical Practice Guideline: The Diagnosis, Management, and Prevention of Bronchiolitis (2014) nor Hockenberry et al. (2019) recommend routinely prescribing laboratory and radiologic studies.

**Arterial blood gases.** May be done initially to determine the degree of hypoxemia and acid-base imbalance in infants/children in severe distress. Topical anesthetics are used if possible to decrease pain and anxiety (atraumatic care).

**Pulse oximetry.** Noninvasive method of monitoring oxygen saturation. It facilitates atraumatic care of the infant.

**Chest radiographic examination.** Usually shows hyperinflation with mild interstitial infiltrates, but segmental atelectasis occurs infrequently. Not usually done unless health care provider suspects pneumonia.

**Respiratory syncytial virus washing on nasal or nasopharyngeal secretions.** To identify the cause of respiratory distress; detects RSV antigen.

## Patient Problems/Analyze Cues/Prioritize Hypotheses

# Dyspnea/Risk for Impaired Respiratory System Function

*due to* airway obstruction caused by bronchiolar edema and increased mucus production occurring with a respiratory infection

**Desired Outcomes/Generate Solutions:** Within 24–48 hours of treatment/intervention, the child exhibits decreased RR and decreased WOB. By discharge the child is able to manage respiratory secretions as evidenced by more normal RR and minimal WOB.

| ASSESSMENT—RECOGNIZE CUES/ INTERVENTIONS—TAKE ACTION | RATIONALES |
|---|---|
| Assess the respiratory status every 2 hours: LOC, RR, breath sounds, signs of increased WOB (nasal flaring, retractions, use of accessory muscles), cough, and skin and mucous membrane color. | Early identification of changes that might indicate increasing respiratory distress (decreased LOC, increased RR, adventitious or decreasing breath sounds, increased WOB, and pallor or cyanosis) ensures prompt intervention, which results in decreased severity of respiratory symptoms. |
| Assess the heart rate (HR), RR, O₂ saturation, and breath sounds before and after nebulizer treatment, if administered. | These assessments monitor the effectiveness of treatment and for its side effects. **Note:** The use of albuterol or epinephrine-like racemic epinephrine is no longer recommended by the AAP (2014). |
| Hold the nebulizer treatment if the child's HR is greater than parameters set by the health care provider. | Tachycardia is one of the main side effects of racemic epinephrine. (Side effects should not outweigh the benefit of improving airway clearance.) |
| Administer hypertonic saline with handheld nebulizer if it is prescribed. | Nebulized hypertonic saline may be used for hospitalized children, but it is not recommended for use in the emergency department. |
| Instill saline nose drops, wait 1–2 minutes, and suction the nares before feedings and as needed. | Instilling saline drops before suctioning is helpful if the secretions are not loose or if the child sounds congested. Suctioning before feedings to clear the nares will improve intake because infants are obligate nose breathers. Suctioning often causes nasal edema if using a bulb syringe. |

Patient Problem/Analyze Cues/Prioritize Hypotheses

# Impaired Gas Exchange

*due to* airway obstruction caused by bronchiolar edema and increased mucus production

***Desired Outcomes/Generate Solutions:*** Immediately after treatment/intervention, the child attains $O_2$ saturation greater than 90% (Justice & Le, 2022). By discharge the child maintains $O_2$ saturation greater than 90% on room air (unless child was $O_2$ dependent before the illness).

| ASSESSMENT—RECOGNIZE CUES/ INTERVENTIONS—TAKE ACTION | RATIONALES |
|---|---|
| Assess for signs and symptoms of hypoxia (restlessness, change in LOC, and dyspnea). Remember that cyanosis is a late sign of hypoxia in children. | Ongoing observation results in early detection of problems and early intervention, thereby decreasing the severity of the hypoxia if it occurs. |
| Assess the respiratory status every 2 hours: LOC, RR, breath sounds, signs of increased WOB (nasal flaring, retractions, and use of accessory muscles), cough, and skin and mucous membrane color. | This ensures early identification of changes that might indicate increasing respiratory distress. See details in the previous patient problem. |
| Assess the vital signs every 2–4 hours and as needed. | Hypoxia causes an increase in HR, RR, and blood pressure (BP). A drop in BP and decreasing RR may be signs of impending respiratory arrest. |
| Maintain continuous oximetry initially and document at least every 2 hours if the child is receiving $O_2$ and/or has moderate to severe respiratory distress or per health care providers' orders. | Oximetry provides continuous monitoring of $O_2$ saturation and alerts nurses to changes. |
| Spot-check $O_2$ saturation every 4–8 hours when the child is clinically improving (feeding well with minimal respiratory distress and maintaining $O_2$ saturation greater than 90%). | Feeding well and minimal respiratory distress while maintaining $O_2$ saturation greater than 90% are good indicators of improvement in a child, and therefore less frequent monitoring is appropriate. |
| Provide humidified $O_2$ by nasal cannula to maintain $O_2$ saturation greater than 90%. | Delivering oxygen increases oxygen to the tissues. Oxygen is drying to the nasal mucosa as well as to mucus in the airway, so proper humidification to liquify secretions is important. |
| Report to the health care provider if $O_2$ saturation is 90% or less. | $O_2$ saturation of 90% or less may indicate deteriorating condition. |
| Position the child for maximum ventilation (e.g., head elevated but without compression on the diaphragm). | Children are diaphragmatic breathers until 7 years of age. Preventing the compression of the diaphragm enables optimal breathing effort. |
| Use an apnea monitor for an infant or young child at high risk for or with a history of apnea. | This monitor ensures quick detection of deterioration in status or apneic episode. |
| Consolidate care to provide maximum rest. | Oxygen needs to decrease with decreased energy expenditure. |
| Provide a neutral thermal environment. | An environment in which the child does not need to use any energy to cool or warm self reduces $O_2$ demand. |

Patient Problem/Analyze Cues/Prioritize Hypotheses

# Dehydration

*due to* increased insensible loss (owing to increased RR, fever, and increased metabolic rate) and decreased intake

***Desired Outcome/Generate Solutions:*** Within 4–8 hours after treatment the child has adequate fluid volume as evidenced by alertness and responsiveness, soft anterior fontanel (in child younger than 2 years), moist oral mucous membrane, elastic skin turgor, and normal UO (e.g., infant UO more than 2–3 mL/kg/hour, toddler and preschooler UO 2 mL/kg/hour, school-age UO 1–2 mL/kg/hour, and adolescent UO 0.5–1 mL/kg/hour).

| ASSESSMENT—RECOGNIZE CUES/ INTERVENTIONS—TAKE ACTION | RATIONALES |
|---|---|
| Assess the hydration status: LOC, anterior fontanel (in child younger than 2 years), oral mucous membrane, abdominal skin turgor, and UO every 4 hours. | The child may be receiving maintenance fluids but still be dehydrated because of increased insensible losses. Frequent assessment leads to early recognition of problems and quicker treatment. Deficient fluid volume may be evidenced by decreased LOC, sunken anterior fontanel, dry or sticky oral mucous membrane (if not a mouth breather), tented abdominal skin, and decreased UO. |
| Assess the intake and output every 2–4 hours. Weigh all diapers. Ensure minimum UO of 1 mL/kg/hour is met or per health care provider's directive. | These assessments enable earlier intervention if a deficit is noted. |
| Assess the daily weights, using the same scale at the same time of day and without any clothing (including diaper) for infants or the same clothing for a child. | Short-term weight changes are the most reliable measurement of fluid loss or gain. Consistency in the time weighed, clothing, and scale improves the accuracy of weight. |
| Assess the temperature every 4 hours and treat per the health care provider's directive. | Increased body temperature increases insensible fluid loss. |
| Ensure that the child is receiving at least daily maintenance fluids based on his or her weight or per health care provider order. | Daily maintenance fluid requirements need to be met in order for the child to have adequate hydration. The smaller the child, the greater the percentage of body weight is water. To meet minimal fluid requirements, the necessary volume is calculated based on the child's weight in the following way: Up to 10 kg: 100 mL/kg/24 hours=_____ 10–20 kg: 50 mL/kg/24 hours=_____ Greater than 20 kg: 20 mL/kg/24 hours=_____ Total amount=maintenance fluid requirement *For example, a child weighs 23 kg:* 10 kg×100 mL/kg/24 hour=1000 mL/24 hours 10 kg×50 mL/kg/24 hours=500 mL/24 hours 3 kg×20 mL/kg/24 hours=60 mL/24 hours 23 kg=1560 mL/24 hours Maintenance fluid requirement for a child weighing 23 kg is 1560 mL/24 hours. |
| Offer a variety of liquids frequently that the child likes (e.g., frozen juices, popsicles, Pedialyte, Rice-Lyte, breast milk, and formula). | This replaces measurable and insensible fluid losses and helps liquefy secretions. A child is more likely to cooperate if offered preferred fluids. |
| Do not offer by mouth (PO) fluids if the child's RR is more than 60–80 breaths/minutes (depending on child's age and baseline RR) while awake. | There is an increased chance of aspiration when a child is tachypneic. |
| Administer the nasogastric tube (NGT) feedings as prescribed if the child is unable to take oral fluids. If the child is unable to tolerate NGT feedings, intravenous (IV) fluids may be prescribed. | The child may not be able to take adequate oral fluid because of respiratory distress. Administering NGT fluids ensures that the child receives maintenance fluids and usually is easier to insert than an IV access. |

## ADDITIONAL PROBLEMS:

"Asthma" for *Fatigue* due to hypoxia and        Chapter 77
increased work of breathing, and
*Anxiety* due to illness, loss of control, and
medical/nursing interventions.

### PATIENT–FAMILY TEACHING AND DISCHARGE PLANNING

When providing child/family teaching, focus on sensory information, avoid giving excessive information, and initiate a visiting nurse referral for necessary follow-up teaching and assessment as needed. Utilize a variety of teaching methods, including videos, tablets, and webinars, depending on learning style and resources of child/family. Stress the importance of family-centered which is viewing as a unit that is the "constant" in the child's life and maintaining or improving the health of the family and its members in a holistic manner. Include verbal and written information about the following (ensure that written information is at a level the reader can understand):

✓ Bronchiolitis: definition, signs and symptoms, basic pathophysiology, length/progression of illness, and routes of transmission.

✓ If the child is on medications: drug name, route, purpose, type, dosage, precautions, and potential side effects. Also discuss drug–drug, food–drug, and herb–drug interactions.

✓ Despite having RSV bronchiolitis, the child can develop another RSV infection.

✓ Risk factors for developing RSV infection/bronchiolitis:
  • Exposure to tobacco smoke
  • Group child care attendance
  • School-aged siblings
  • Crowded living conditions (two or more children in the same bedroom)
  • Multiple births and/or premature infant
  • CLD, CHD, or immunocompromised state
  • Born within 12 weeks of RSV season (usually November to April)
  • Formula-fed (resulting in decreased maternal antibodies) rather than breastfed
  • Low socioeconomic status

✓ Guidelines for preventing RSV infection/bronchiolitis:
  • Good hand hygiene
  • Keeping anyone with a fever or cold away from the child
  • Avoiding secondhand smoke
  • Avoiding crowds and group child care

✓ Importance of checking hydration status at least several times a day when the child is ill. (The younger the child is and the less he or she weighs, the greater the percentage of body weight is water. Therefore dehydration occurs much more quickly than it would in an older child or adult.)

  • Is the child alert and interactive? The child would not be as alert and interactive as usual if dehydrated.
  • Check the anterior fontanel (soft spot) on top of the head (in children younger than 2 years). If it is sunken, the child may be dehydrated.
  • Check inside the mouth, not the lips. If dry or sticky and the child is not a mouth breather, the child is dehydrated.
  • Pinch skin on the abdomen. If it sits up like a tent instead of falling down right away, the child is dehydrated.
  • How many wet diapers does the child usually have a day? If the number of diapers is decreased or they are not as wet as usual, the child may be dehydrated.

✓ How much should the child drink per day? Give parents the information they can understand, such as an infant who weighs 9 kg needs 900 mL/day for maintenance fluids, which is 30 oz. If the infant drinks from 4-oz bottles, he or she needs to take about eight 4-oz bottles of fluid/day to get maintenance fluids. Infant may need more if increased fluid loss (e.g., fever or diarrhea.)

✓ Use of normal saline nose drops and bulb syringe to clear nares before feedings. An infant breathes primarily through the nose until 5–6 months old, so if the nose is congested, he or she cannot breathe and, therefore, cannot drink or eat. Suction before feedings/meals and before bedtime. Do not suction too often because it can lead to increased nasal congestion resulting from nasal edema when using a bulb syringe.

✓ Continued prophylaxis against RSV with palivizumab (Synagis) if already receiving prophylaxis or per prescription (e.g., monthly intramuscular medication that gives passive immunity against RSV during RSV season, usually November through April but has been occurring "intraseasonally" in different areas of the country since the spring of 2021). This is generally recommended for infants born before 29 weeks of gestation, those with hemodynamically significant CHD or CLD of prematurity that are less than 12 months old at the start of RSV season. This medication may be given more than 5 months in a row depending on a local surge of RSV (AAP, 2022).

✓ The child may still have some signs and symptoms of RSV/bronchiolitis but may return to babysitter/group child care if he or she does not have a fever, is eating well, has had a follow-up visit to the health care provider, and is believed to be no longer contagious. Most healthy infants recover in 7–10 days.

✓ Importance of follow-up care; typically follow-up appointment is made within 24–48 hours after discharge.

✓ Phone number to call in case questions or concerns arise about treatment or disease after discharge.

✓ When to call the health care provider:
  • Fever increases.
  • Rate of breathing increases (more than 60 breaths/minute [varies depending on the age of the infant/child]).

- Nostrils flare out with each breath when the child is resting (crying will cause this to happen when the child is not having breathing problems).
- The chest sinks in with each breath.
- The child looks like he or she is working harder to breathe.
- The lips turn gray or blue (cold can make lips look very pale and almost blue).
- The child exhibits signs of dehydration.

✓ Importance of infant/child receiving all routine childhood immunizations and rationale for giving immunizations.

✓ Importance of cardiopulmonary resuscitation and safety training.

✓ Refer to community resources such as local and national American Lung Associations. Additional information can be obtained by contacting:

- American Lung Association: https://www.lung.org/lung-health-diseases/lung-disease-lookup/rsv.

- HealthyChildren.org (from AAP): https://www.healthychildren.org/English/health-issues/conditions/chest-lungs/Pages/RSV-When-Its-More-Than-Just-a-Cold.aspx Updated 2022.
- KidsHealth Resource Center for Nemours Associates: https://www.kidshealth.org/CareSource/en/parents/bronchiolitis.html?ref=search Detailed information sheet and short video "Does My Child Need Antibiotics?"
- RSVProtection: Information about the disease, treatment, and prevention of RSV. https://www.rsvprotection.com/what-is-rsv-disease.html.
- Centers for Disease Control and Prevention (CDC): Information about the disease, treatment, and prevention, as well as other information about RSV: https://www.cdc.gov/rsv/.

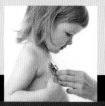

# Burns 80

## OVERVIEW/PATHOPHYSIOLOGY

Burn injuries represent one of the most painful and devastating traumas a person can experience. Although most burns in children are relatively minor and do not require hospitalization, fire- and burn-related injuries are a leading cause of death from injury in children aged 1–14 years. Thermal burns result from contact with a thermal agent such as a flame, hot surface, or hot liquid (e.g., hair curlers/curling irons, radiators, kerosene heaters, wood burning stoves, ovens and ranges, irons, gasoline, and fireworks) and are the leading causes of fire/burn injuries in children 19 years and younger. Scald burns are the most common type of thermal burns.

The causative agent for burns varies depending on the child's developmental age. For instance, in children 4 years and younger hospitalized with burn-related injuries, most are treated for scald burns caused by hot liquids, steam, hot foods (e.g., coffee or soup), or grease, with the highest incidence in children younger than 2 years. Scald injuries often occur in everyday activities such as bathing, cooking, and eating.

The most common type of burn-related injury in older children is flame burn. In 2020, approximately 61,526 children aged 0–19 years were seen in the ED and released, with 9361 hospitalizations and 228 deaths from fire and burn injuries. About 93% of deaths were residential, which was 5% more than in 2018. Boys were at a higher risk for death from fires than girls, as were African American children (Safe Kids Worldwide, 2022). In 2021, an estimated 2465 children of 15 years and younger, with the highest incidence in children 5–9 years, were treated in emergency departments for injuries involving fireworks, with about 30% of the estimated firework-related injuries occurring in children of less than 15 years (Consumer Product Safety Commission, 2022). Although the rate of deaths in children 0–19 years old has decreased 53% from 2006 to 2008, the cost is still overwhelming. The estimated medical- and work-related costs for fatal and nonfatal fire and burn injuries in 2020 were $1.12 billion, with an additional estimated quality-of-life loss cost of $1.17 billion (Safe Kids Worldwide, 2022).

The least common types of burn injuries are chemical (usually touching or ingesting a caustic agent such as cleaning solution), electrical (possibly due to household electrical and extension cords in younger children), and radiation (caused by prolonged exposure to ultraviolet rays of the sun or to other sources of radiation such as x-rays) (Safe Kids Worldwide, 2022).

It is estimated that 9.7% of cases of burns annually are the result of nonaccidental trauma (Loos et al., 2020). These cases involve a history inconsistent with the distribution of the burn, the burn injury inconsistent with the child's developmental age, or unusual burns such as immersion (glove-and-stocking) burns or contact burns from cigarettes or irons, and/or there was a delay in seeking treatment. This type of injury occurs most often in children of less than 3 years, with scald burns being the most common cause (Hockenberry et al., 2019).

### Factors affecting severity of the burn and seriousness of the injury

1. Percentage of total body surface area (TBSA) burned: One formula that is often used is the modified rule of nine for children (i.e., the percentage of TBSA of head varies with the age of child; at 1 year old, it is 17%; at 10 years old, it is 11%; and in an adult, it is 7%) (Hockenberry et al., 2019). Another formula used is Lund–Browder chart for children (Merk & Co., 2023).

2. Burn depth:
   a. Superficial (first-degree) burn involves epidermis and heals within 5–7 days without scarring.
   b. Partial-thickness (second-degree) injury involves epidermis and varying degrees of the dermis. It may be superficial (usually heals in about 14 days with variable scarring) or deep dermal, which is similar to full-thickness burns but hair follicles and sweat glands remain intact (usually heals in about 21 days if no infection occurs, with extensive scarring). The wound blanches with pressure.
   c. Full-thickness (third-degree) burn involves the epidermis and dermis and extends into the subcutaneous tissue. Nerve endings, sweat glands, and hair follicles are destroyed. It cannot reepithelialize and requires surgical excision and wound grafting. This tissue does not blanch. Frequently, there are superficial and partial-thickness burns to the surrounding tissue with both intact and exposed nerve endings.
   d. Fourth-degree is a full-thickness burn that involves underlying structures—muscles, fascia, and bones and may necessitate amputation if on an extremity or autografting (Hockenberry et al., 2019).

3. Wound location: Certain body areas carry a higher risk for complications and require specialized care (e.g., burns of the hands and feet and across joints can interfere with growth and development because of scar formation).

4. Age of the child: For example, the very thin skin of a premature infant would take longer to heal and be damaged more easily than that of a healthy 3-year-old.
5. Causative agent.
6. Presence of respiratory involvement.
7. General health of the child.
8. Presence of concomitant injuries.

### Children most at risk

- Children 4 years and younger because of their natural curiosity and lack of awareness of danger are especially at risk for scald and contact burns and for sparkler injury.
- Children with disabilities related to developmental level or physical inability to get out of harm's way are especially at risk for scald and contact burns.
- Boys are at greater risk than girls.
- Children in homes without smoke detectors are at greatest risk for fires and fire-related death and injury.
- Children 5–14 years old are at highest risk for fireworks-related injuries.

### Differences in the effects of burn injury in children

- There is a higher mortality rate in children less than 2 years old who have been burned compared with older children and adults with comparable burns.
- Lower temperatures and shorter exposure time can cause more severe burns in children than in adults because of the child's thinner skin.
- Larger body surface area compared with adults puts severely burned children at increased risk for fluid and heat loss.
- The greater proportion of body fluid to mass in children increases the risk for dehydration and cardiovascular problems because of less effective cardiovascular response to changing intravascular volume. The younger the child, the greater the percentage of water is total body weight, and the greater his or her percentage of extracellular fluid (i.e., interstitial fluid surrounds the cell; intravascular fluid is within the blood vessels or plasma; and transcellular fluid such as spinal fluid and sweat).
- Because of smaller muscle mass and less body fat than adults, children are at increased risk for protein and calorie deficiency.
- The younger the child, the less mature the immune system, and the greater the risk for infection.
- Extensive burns may result in delayed growth.
- Hypertrophic scarring is increased, and scar maturation is prolonged.

## HEALTH CARE SETTING

Emergency department, with possible hospitalization and/or referral to specialized burn center for significant burns or burns at high risk for complications; some burns are treated in primary care, and others at home.

## ASSESSMENT

Varies significantly depending on the classification of the degree of burning and seriousness of the injury.

### Superficial burn (e.g., mild sunburn)

Erythema, moderate discomfort/pain, blanches with pressure, and good capillary refill.

### Partial-thickness burn

- *Superficial:* Fluid-filled blisters, skin red to ivory with moist surfaces, considerable pain, blanches with pressure, and refills.
- *Deep:* May or may not have fluid-filled blisters; blisters are often flat and dehydrated, making skin feel like tissue paper; color is mottled, waxy white, and with a dry surface. Nerve endings are intact, so pain is severe on exposure to air or water.

### Full-thickness burn

Varies in color from red to tan, waxy white, brown, or black. It does not blanch with pressure. Edema is present. It has a dry, leathery appearance and lacks sensation because of destruction of nerve endings. However, because it is usually surrounded by superficial and partial-thickness burns that have intact nerve endings, adjacent areas will likely be painful.

### Respiratory compromise

Upper airway edema related to injury starts within a few minutes, and the airway may occlude in minutes to a few hours, although it may be delayed up to 24–48 hours. The presence of singed nasal hairs may suggest thermal injury to the upper airway; therefore airway mucosa must be monitored closely.

### Respiratory distress

Abdominal breathing in a child older than 7 years (children are primarily abdominal breathers until that age), head bobbing with respiratory effort, nasal flaring, coughing, stridor, wheezing.

### Burn shock

With severe burns (greater than 15%), a type of hypovolemic shock may occur with increased heart rate (HR), increased respiratory rate (RR), low blood pressure (BP), hypothermia, pallor, cyanosis, decreased level of consciousness (LOC), and poor muscle tone. May occur with smaller burns in younger children.

> **Note:** *Blood pressure in children can remain normotensive initially even in a state of hypovolemia.*

### Physical assessment

It is also important to assess for other injuries such as fractures and internal injuries.

### Complications

- *Pulmonary complications are the leading cause of death in thermal trauma:* Inhalation injury, aspiration of gastric contents, bacterial pneumonia, pulmonary edema/insufficiency, and emboli. Pneumonia is the leading cause of infection and death. Indications of respiratory tract compromise include wheezing, increased secretions, wet rales, carbonaceous secretions, and hoarseness.
- *Wound sepsis:* Disorientation is one of the first signs of overwhelming sepsis.
- *Gastrointestinal complications:* Feeding intolerance, mucosal ulceration, and bleeding, especially in the stomach and duodenum.

## DIAGNOSTIC TESTS

> **Note:** *Topical anesthetics are used with blood draws, if possible, to decrease pain and anxiety and to provide atraumatic care.*

### Arterial blood gas level

To determine acid–base balance; variations from baseline may signal respiratory compromise with respiratory acidosis as well as lactic/metabolic acidosis.

### Chemistries

- *Fluid and electrolytes:* Deficits of fluid and sodium occur with burn shock.
- *Blood urea nitrogen and creatinine:* Elevations occur because of tissue destruction, oliguria, and decreased circulating volume.
- *Glucose:* May be elevated in young infants. Stress may cause either hypoglycemia or pseudodiabetes, resulting in elevated glucose levels.

---

## Patient Problem/Analyze Cues/Prioritize Hypotheses

# Dehydration

*due to* fluid shift from the intravascular to interstitial compartment, increased metabolic demands, and decreased intake

**Desired Outcomes/Generate Solutions:** Within 4 hours after intervention/treatment, the child has adequate fluid volume as evidenced by normal LOC for the child, soft anterior fontanel (in a child younger than 2 years), moist oral mucous membranes, good/elastic abdominal skin turgor (on unaffected areas), capillary refill less than 2 seconds, and normal urine output (UO). For example, infant UO more than 2–3 mL/kg/hour; toddler and preschooler UO 2 mL/kg/hour; school-aged child UO 1–2 mL/kg/hour; and adolescent UO 0.5–1 mL/kg/hour.

| ASSESSMENT—RECOGNIZE CUES/ INTERVENTIONS—TAKE ACTION | RATIONALES |
| --- | --- |
| Assess the hydration status every 4 hours: LOC, anterior fontanel (in a child younger than 2 years), oral mucous membrane, abdominal skin turgor, capillary refill, and UO. **Note:** Edema may occur around the burn or from fluid shifts. | The child may be receiving maintenance fluids after initial fluid resuscitation but still be dehydrated because of significantly increased insensible water losses, especially in a child with burns. Frequent assessment leads to early detection of problems and quicker treatment. Signs of impaired hydration include decreasing LOC, sunken fontanel, dry and sticky oral mucous membrane, tenting of abdominal skin, capillary refill more than 2 seconds, and decreased UO. |
| Assess the intake and output every 2 hours. Weigh all diapers, 1 mL=1 g. Ensure that the minimum UO of 1 mL/kg/hour is met, depending on the age of child. | This assessment determines whether the child is receiving appropriate intake and has adequate output. |
| Assess the vital signs (VS), capillary refill, and LOC every 4 hours for changes related to hypovolemia. | Hypovolemia may be present because of reduced circulating blood volume that occurs with plasma loss in burns. Tachycardia, changes in tissue perfusion (e.g., capillary refill more than 2 seconds), and alteration in LOC are early signs of hypovolemic shock. BP will be normal initially because increased systemic vascular resistance helps to maintain it. However, perfusion with a normal BP may be inadequate to meet the body's demands. Therefore decreased BP can be a late sign of hypovolemia in children. |

Continued

| ASSESSMENT—RECOGNIZE CUES/ INTERVENTIONS—TAKE ACTION | RATIONALES |
|---|---|
| Assess the daily weights, using the same scale at the same time of day and with the same amount of clothing (no clothes, including diaper in infants). | Short-term weight changes are the most reliable measurement of fluid loss or gain. Excessive weight gain could indicate fluid retention; weight loss could signal dehydration or excessive fluid loss. Either would interfere with wound healing. Consistency in weighing increases accuracy. |
| Administer the intravenous (IV) fluids as prescribed. | Fluid resuscitation is required in children with burns greater than 10% TBSA. Fluids help maintain general circulation to vital organs and capillary circulation to viable skin. |
| Assess the IV site hourly. | Peripheral IV lines in children can infiltrate and cause tissue damage in a short period of time, especially in younger children. Thus the patient would not be receiving the needed fluid systemically as well as having additional tissue damage. |
| When stabilized, ensure that the child receives *at least* maintenance fluids based on their weight and health care providers' guidelines. | The smaller the child, the greater the percentage of body weight that is water and the larger the percentage of extracellular fluid. Because of fluid loss from the burn injury, increased metabolic demands related to the child's age, and increased catecholamine release caused by burn stress, the child probably will need more than maintenance fluids. First, use this formula to determine maintenance fluids:<br><br>Up to 10 kg: 100 mL/kg/24 hours=_____<br><br>10–20 kg: 50 mL/kg/24 hours=_____<br><br>More than 20 kg: 20 mL/kg/24 hours=_____<br><br>= maintenance fluid requirement<br><br>*For example, a child weighs 33 kg:*<br><br>10 kg×100 mL/kg/24 hours=1000 mL/24 hours<br><br>10 kg×50 mL/kg/24 hours=500 mL/24 hours<br><br>13 kg×20 mL/kg/24 hours=260 mL/24 hours<br><br>33 kg=1760 mL/24 hours<br><br>Maintenance fluid requirement for a child weighing 33 kg is 1760 mL/24 hours. Remember that the child probably will need *more* than maintenance fluids. |
| Alert the health care provider promptly to significant findings or changes. | This helps ensure timely treatment. |

<u>Patient Problem/Analyze Cues/Prioritize Hypotheses</u>

# Acute Pain

*due to* thermal injuries and medical-surgical interventions

**Desired Outcome/Generate Solutions:** Within 30 minutes to 1 hour after treatment/intervention, the child's pain level is decreased (to 4 or less on the developmentally appropriate scale with 0–10 rating; FLACC [face, legs, activity, cry, and consolability]; Wong–Baker Faces; or numeric) or at a level acceptable to the child.

| ASSESSMENT—RECOGNIZE CUES/ INTERVENTIONS—TAKE ACTION | RATIONALES |
|---|---|
| Assess the child's developmental level, previous use of pain scales, and establish the appropriate pain scale (e.g., FLACC, Wong–Baker Faces, or numeric). | A pain scale increases the ability to accurately assess pain and the degree of relief obtained. |
| Assess the level of pain every 2–4 hours, as well as before and after pain medication administration (e.g., 1 hour after by mouth [PO] medications, 10–20 minutes after IV medications). | These assessments detect early changes in pain level and assess the effectiveness of pain medications. |
| • Provide pain medications/nonpharmacologic pain relief measures around the clock on a regular basis, not as needed.<br><br>Utilize Child Life if available to help with nonpharmacological pain relief. | Scheduled rather than as-needed pain relief provides better and more reliable pain control. Prolonged stimulation of pain receptors results in increased sensitivity to painful stimuli and will increase the amount of analgesia needed to relieve pain. Pain relief measures such as distraction; relaxation; repositioning; guided imagery; cutaneous stimulation such as massage, heat, or cold; and positive self-talk increase the effectiveness of medications.<br><br>Child Life Specialists work with children to help them cope with their medical experience—frequently using age-appropriate methods of distraction, relaxation, guided imagery, etc. |
| Explain how patient-controlled analgesia (PCA) works and that the child cannot give self too much medication. Encourage the child/parent to use PCA when needed if it is available. | Most experts believe that when a child is capable of pushing the button on the pump, usually by 5–6 years of age, he or she can self-administer pain medication. Some facilities allow PCA by proxy—the parent or nurse can administer the medication if the child is too ill or cannot understand the concept of pushing the button to relieve the pain. |
| Reassure the parent that addiction rarely occurs when medication is used to relieve pain. | Fear of addiction may decrease the use of pain medication. |
| Premedicate the child before painful procedures. Use a topical anesthetic to decrease the trauma of blood draws/IV insertion, if possible (atraumatic care). Some anesthetics, such as ketamine, may also be used to prevent/control procedural pain. | Pain medications given before painful procedures will help control pain. The time frame before the procedure depends on the route (e.g., 10–20 minutes IV and 1 hour PO). |
| Explain all procedures at the developmental level appropriate for the child. | Anxiety increases pain; knowing what to expect may decrease anxiety. |

## Patient Problem/Analyze Cues/Prioritize Hypotheses

# Injury (Skin/Tissue)

*due to* burns

***Desired Outcomes/Generate Solutions:*** The skin/graft site heals without signs of infection (e.g., drainage, erythema, edema, or pain). Superficial burns heal within 7 days without scarring; deep partial-thickness burns heal within 30 days with varying degrees of scarring.

| ASSESSMENT—RECOGNIZE CUES/ INTERVENTIONS—TAKE ACTION | RATIONALES |
|---|---|
| Assess both the child and wound/graft/donor site(s) at least every 4 hours for signs and symptoms of infection. | These assessments ensure prompt recognition of problems, more rapid treatment, and maximum healing. Infection indicators include change in LOC, hypothermia or hyperthermia, odor, drainage, increased edema, increased erythema, and increased pain. |
| Assess the graft at least every 4 hours for evidence of hematoma, edema, or sloughing of graft; notify the health care provider promptly if noted. | Early recognition of the problem and prompt treatment increase the chance of saving the graft. |
| Carefully clean the wound and tissue immediately surrounding the wound as prescribed. | Cautious cleansing is necessary to avoid damaging the epithelialization of granulating skin and decrease the risk for infection. Infection would further damage the already traumatized tissue, disrupt epithelialization, and delay healing. |
| Provide appropriate pain control measures before removing the dressing and beginning wound care. | A relaxed, more comfortable patient facilitates careful wound cleansing. |
| Débride the wound as prescribed. | Débridement promotes healing by removing dead or injured tissue so that the wound has an environment conducive to healing. |
| Apply ointment and/or dressings as prescribed using clean/sterile technique. | These measures protect the wound, decrease the risk for infection, and promote healing. |
| Minimize the child scratching and picking at the wound, using methods appropriate for his or her developmental age. | This promotes better wound healing and decreases scarring. Methods for developmental age include: <br>• Young child: distraction and supervision. <br>• Older child: explanations of the importance of not scratching, picking, or hitting the wound. |
| Perform active (or ensure passive) range-of-motion (ROM) exercises to affected joints as prescribed. | These exercises promote reabsorption of edema, prevent contracture formation, and improve healing. |
| Position for minimal stress/pressure on the wound/graft. | Proper positioning promotes healing and protects the wound/graft. For example, do not allow the child to lie on the wound; use a cradle to keep sheets/blankets off the graft site. |
| Offer high-calorie, high-protein meals and snacks, providing foods the child likes. | The child has increased metabolism and catabolism because of the burn injury and therefore needs increased calories and protein to promote positive nitrogen balance, which facilitates healing. Offering foods the child likes increases the likelihood of increased intake. |
| Administer vitamins and minerals (e.g., vitamins A, B, C, zinc, and iron) as prescribed. | These supplements facilitate wound healing and epithelialization. |
| For more detailed information, see "Managing Wound Care," Chapter 75. | |

Patient Problem/Analyze Cues/Prioritize Hypotheses

# Risk for Infection

*due to* loss of skin barrier/denuded skin, increased metabolic demands, altered nutritional status, invasive procedures/lines, and the hospital environment

***Desired Outcome/Generate Solutions:*** The child exhibits wound healing without signs of burn wound infection (e.g., odor, drainage, increased erythema or edema, increased pain) or systemic infection (e.g., pneumonia or septicemia).

> **Note:** *See assessment/interventions and rationales for* **Injury (Skin/Tissue)** *plus the following.*

| ASSESSMENT—RECOGNIZE CUES/ INTERVENTIONS—TAKE ACTION | RATIONALES |
|---|---|
| Assess the VS every 4 hours and notify the health care provider of findings indicative of infection (e.g., temperature 36° C [96.8° F] or less or 38.5° C [101.3° F] or greater, HR 100 bpm or greater, or RR 30 breaths/minute or more, but will vary depending on age of the child). | Early signs of infection/sepsis include tachycardia, tachypnea, and fever or hypothermia. Early recognition of any abnormality enables prompt treatment and less serious infection. |
| Monitor the LOC every 4 hours. | Disorientation is one of the first signs of overwhelming sepsis/septic shock in patients with burn injury. Knowing the patient's baseline LOC is vital to make an accurate assessment. |
| Monitor for signs of pneumonia every 4 hours (varies depending on the age of the child). | Early recognition facilitates prompt treatment and a less-severe infection.<br><br>• Infant: fever, restlessness, anxiety, grunting, nasal flaring, retractions, tachypnea, and head bobbing.<br><br>• Child and adolescent: fever, chills, cough, chest pain, restlessness, anxiety, and tachypnea. |
| Assess the IV sites (peripheral hourly or central access every 4 hours) for signs of infection (e.g., erythema, warmth, edema). | There is potential for an increased rate of infection because of the child's altered immune response and because the IV site is another entry site for bacteria. |
| Wash your hands before and after working with a child with open wounds or if contact with blood or body fluids is possible. | Hand hygiene is the best method of preventing nosocomial infection. Hand hygiene with an alcohol-based hand sanitizer may be used before and after contact with intact skin. |
| Use gloves as indicated, following standard precautions. | Gloves provide an additional level of protection for the patient by reducing the risk for contamination of open wounds by the bare hands of caregivers. (Wearing gloves also protects the caregiver from contact with the patient's open wounds.) |
| • Depending on developmental age, ensure that the child turns, coughs, and deep breathes or uses incentive spirometer every 2 hours while awake. Younger children can blow bubbles or blow on a pinwheel. | Deep breathing expands alveoli and aids in mobilizing secretions to the airways, and coughing further mobilizes and clears the secretions to help prevent pneumonia. |
| Position the child with the head elevated 15–30 degrees for 1–2 hours after meals. | This position decreases the incidence of aspiration of gastric contents, which could lead to aspiration pneumonia. |
| Screen visitors for colds or other infectious illnesses before they enter the child's room. | The child has an altered immune response and is at greater risk for infection because of the following:<br><br>• Open wounds or denuded skin have lost the protective skin barrier and are potential entry sites for infection.<br><br>• Decreased circulation to the burned area compromises the body's ability to fight infection at the tissue level because fewer leukocytes (white blood cells, which act as scavengers and fight infection) are able to reach damaged tissue.<br><br>• Mature neutrophils, the body's first line of defense against bacterial infection and severe stress, are decreased as immature neutrophils (bands) increase to digest products of the burn injury. |

## Patient Problem/Analyze Cues/Prioritize Hypotheses

# Body Weight Problem (Weight Loss)

*due to* hypermetabolic state and decreased appetite

***Desired Outcome/Generate Solutions:*** Within 1 week of intervention/treatment, the child exhibits adequate nutrition as evidenced by maintenance of or gaining weight without fluid retention.

| ASSESSMENT—RECOGNIZE CUES/ INTERVENTIONS—TAKE ACTION | RATIONALES |
|---|---|
| Assess the weight on the same scale at the same time of day with the same amount of clothing. Frequency depends on the unit policy and/ or prescription of the health care provider. | Consistency with weight measurements helps ensure more accurate results. Weight is a reliable indicator of nutritional status (as long as the child is not edematous). |
| Monitor for hypoglycemia. | Hypoglycemia can result from the stress of injury as glycogen stores in the liver are rapidly depleted. |
| Monitor for hyperglycemia. | Hyperglycemia can occur because of mobilization of glucagon and decreased insulin production. |
| Provide high-calorie, high-protein meals and snacks as well as foods high in vitamin C content. | Because of smaller muscle mass and less body fat than adults, children are at increased risk for protein and calorie deficiency. This diet provides positive nitrogen balance and nutrients needed for wound healing. Energy requirements increase according to size of the burn; caloric requirements may be 2–3 times normal because of the increased metabolic rate. High-protein meals replace protein lost by exudation. |
| Provide foods the child likes and encourage the child to feed self as much as possible. | These measures stimulate appetite and promote cooperation, thereby improving the likelihood of increased intake. |
| Ensure that the child is receiving adequate nutrients. Discuss the child's needs with the health care provider. | If this cannot be accomplished orally, enteral feedings may be necessary. Burns will not heal well without adequate nutrients. Usually parenteral nutrition is used only if the child cannot tolerate enteral feedings. |
| Try to minimize anorexia in the following ways: | Anorexia occurs in many children with burn injury. |
| • Offer small, frequent meals. | • The child may eat better with 4–5 small meals/day rather than three large meals. |
| • Add calories to small meals/fluids (e.g., add ice cream to milk for milkshake or protein powder to pudding) after consultation with health care provider/dietician. | • Enables child to receive increased nutrients with less volume and less energy expenditure. |
| • Make mealtimes pleasant with attractive meals, companionship, and no treatments or unpleasant interruptions. | • Eating is more likely to occur in a more home-like environment. |
| Maintain a neutral thermal environment. | Caloric expenditure is minimized when the child does not need to use energy to cool or heat the body. |
| Ensure that the child is having a normal stooling pattern. Assess for constipation or diarrhea and notify the health care provider if either occurs. | Constipation caused by decreased activity and intake as well as pain medications could further affect the intake because of discomfort and thus interfere with weight gain. Diarrhea would decrease weight as well. |

Patient Problem/Analyze Cues/Prioritize Hypotheses
# Low Self-Esteem

*due to* the child's perception of altered appearance and mobility/skills

***Desired Outcomes/Generate Solutions:*** The child receives emotional support from the onset of injury and discusses feelings related to the change in appearance and mobility/skills after wound healing begins. Within 48–72 hours of this diagnosis, the child relates at least one positive example of his or her appearance/abilities and expresses realistic expectations for the future, if developmentally and medically able to do this.

| ASSESSMENT—RECOGNIZE CUES/ INTERVENTIONS—TAKE ACTION | RATIONALES |
|---|---|
| Assess the support systems and coping mechanisms used in previously stressful situations.  Utilize Child Life Specialists if available. | Optimally, this assessment will mobilize previous effective strategies to assist the child in dealing with the current altered appearance and mobility/skills.  Child Life Specialists work with children to help them cope with their medical experience and can help teach or reinforce effective coping skills. |
| Ensure a positive attitude when caring for the child. | This shows acceptance and encourages the expectation that the child will get better. |
| Point out positive aspects of the child's appearance/abilities. Ask the child during subsequent care to give examples of positive aspects. | Positive reinforcement encourages a child to focus on positive aspects rather than on deficits. |
| Point out evidence of healing. | This promotes a sense of hope. |
| Encourage the child to provide for developmentally appropriate self-care as much as his or her condition allows. | Encouragement enables a child to focus on tasks that he or she can do and promotes a positive self-image in the process. |
| Give honest answers to the child and family regarding care and appearance. | Honesty facilitates building of a trusting nurse–patient/family relationship and assists in developing realistic expectations. |
| Arrange for continued schooling, depending on the age of the child. For younger children, encourage play. | This decreases isolation and provides normalization, which may help self-image. |
| Promote peer contact if possible and prepare peers for the child's appearance. | These measures facilitate acceptance and support. |
| Help the child devise a plan to address and cope with the reactions of others. | This will increase a sense of control. Role-playing may help the child perfect this plan. |
| Support appropriate adaptive behaviors. | This measure builds on strengths. |
| Encourage verbalization about feelings regarding appearance and changes in lifestyle. | This will help identify the child's concerns and anxieties, enabling you to provide more realistic feedback about the child's appearance if appropriate and aid in working on coping strategies. |
| Discuss ways the child can "cover up" disfigurement, dressings, and pressure garments. | This facilitates coping. Examples include clothing (e.g., turtleneck sweaters and larger shirt than normal), wigs, and makeup. |
| Facilitate transition back to group child care, school, and the home environment. Encourage communication of the family and medical staff with other care providers, including school nurse and teachers. | These measures prepare other children and caregivers for the change in the child's appearance and encourage them to make the transition a positive experience. |

## ADDITIONAL PROBLEMS:

## ✔ PATIENT–FAMILY TEACHING AND DISCHARGE PLANNING

When providing child/family teaching, focus on sensory information, avoid giving excessive information, and initiate visiting nurse referral for necessary follow-up teaching and assessment as needed. Utilize a variety of teaching methods (e.g., videos, tablets, and webinars as well as verbal and written) depending on learning style and resources of child/family. Stress the importance of family-centered care (viewing the family as a unit that is the "constant" in the child's life and maintaining or improving the health of the family and its members in a holistic manner). Include information about the following (ensure that written information is at a level the reader can understand):

✔ Type of burn and expected healing time.

✔ Wound care as appropriate:
  • Administering oral pain medication about 1 hour before wound care if needed
  • Cleaning the wound
  • Applying ointment
  • Applying dressing

✔ Treatment of pain (e.g., administering medication on a regular basis, which gives better control and assists the healing process; use of nonpharmaceutical adjuncts such as distraction).

✔ Signs and symptoms of burn wound, graft site, or donor site infection:
  • Purulent drainage or odor
  • Increased redness or swelling
  • Temperature 38.6° C (101.5° F) or greater or per discharge instructions

✔ Ways to prevent infection:
  • Good hand hygiene before and after caring for the wound
  • Dressing changes performed in a clean area with good light
  • Making sure the dressing stays clean and dry

✔ Methods of preventing scars and contractures:
  • Wearing pressure garments as prescribed (usually 23 hours/day)
  • Wearing splints as prescribed (over top of the pressure garment)
  • ROM exercises as prescribed and demonstrated by physical therapist (PT) and/or occupational therapist
  • Child performing as many activities of daily living as possible (e.g., feeding self, combing hair, dressing self)

✔ Care of healing skin:
  • May be dry: Apply lotion (cocoa butter is most often recommended) but avoid those containing alcohol, lanolin, or perfume.
  • May be itchy: Use lotion, prescribed medication (e.g., Benadryl), and distraction.
  • Bathing: Use lukewarm water and be gentle! Pat skin dry rather than rub.
  • Protect new skin over the burned area.
  • Wear comfortable clothing, not constrictive.
  • Try to avoid hitting or bumping the area.
  • Protect from the sun with clothing and sunscreen (Sun Protection Factor [SPF] 15 or higher), per health care provider's recommendation.
  • Do not stay out in cold weather; the burned area is sensitive to cold.

✔ If the child is on any medications: discuss the drug name; route; purpose; type; dosage; precautions; drug–drug, food–drug, and herb–drug interactions; and potential side effects.

✔ Demonstrate drawing up and administering medication and having family member perform return demonstration.

✔ Nutritional needs (the child needs increased calories and protein to heal well):
  • Make pudding with Ensure instead of milk (increases calories).
  • Eat small, frequent meals or three meals with nutritious snacks between meals.
  • Make mealtime a social, shared time. Turn off TV.
  • Feed child when he or she is well rested.
  • If receiving tube feeding: follow procedure for checking placement and administering feeding, checking residual, and recognizing and reporting problems.
  • Vitamins that help skin heal: A and C (found in oranges, grapefruit, tomatoes, broccoli, and carrots).
  • Protein, which promotes skin healing: meat, fish, eggs, peanut butter, chicken, cheese, and milk.

✔ Importance of adequate fluid intake to promote healing (the child should receive at least maintenance fluids or more per the health care provider). How much should the child drink per day? Give parents information they can understand, such as an infant that weighs 9 kg needs 900 mL/day for maintenance fluids, which is 30 oz. If the infant drinks from 4-oz bottles, he or she needs to take eight 4-oz bottles of fluid/day to get maintenance fluids. An older child weighing 40 kg would need 1900 mL/day for maintenance fluids. If this child drinks from 12-oz glasses, he or she would need at least five and a half 12-oz glasses/day. These examples are only for maintenance fluids; the child may need 1½–2 times maintenance fluids to stay well hydrated, depending on the size and stage of healing of the burn injury.

✓ Importance of checking hydration status at least several times a day while the child is still healing from the burn. The less the child weighs and the younger he or she is, the greater the percentage of body weight that is water. Therefore dehydration occurs much more quickly than it would in an older child or adult. The child may still be losing fluid from the burn and using more energy to heal, therefore using more fluid.
  - Is the child alert and interactive? The child would not be as alert and interactive as normal if dehydrated.
  - Check soft spot on top of the head (in children younger than 2 years). If it is sunken in, the child may be dehydrated.
  - Check inside the mouth, not the lips. If dry or sticky and the child is not a mouth breather, the child may be dehydrated.
  - Pinch skin on the abdomen. The child may be dehydrated if the skin sits up like a tent instead of falling down right away. How many wet diapers does the child normally have a day or how many times does he or she normally void? If the number of diapers decreases, they are not as wet as usual, or the child is voiding less often, he or she may be dehydrated.

✓ Adjustment after burn injury, which is often prolonged and painful. Family and individual psychosocial support is important. Reinforce the importance of helping siblings cope/adjust to having a sibling with a potentially long-term injury.

✓ Growth and development (realistic expectations of what the child should be doing at different ages and encouragement of activities that promote normal growth and development).

✓ Feelings the child may experience with reentry to school/society, which vary depending on developmental age and severity of the burn: fear, anger, guilt, depression, withdrawal, altered body image, and anticipating peer response.

✓ Potential for regression. This is normal after a stressful event and/or hospitalization.

✓ Developmentally related risks for burn injuries (see the "Overview/Pathophysiology" section).

✓ Tips for childproofing the home:
  - Set water heater thermostat at 120°F (48.9°C) or less or install antiscald devices in faucets and showerheads in buildings where one does not have access to the water tank (e.g., apartment buildings). In children younger than 5 years with free-flowing water: Water temperature of 120°F (48.9°C) takes 5 minutes for partial or full-thickness burn (second or third degree).

Water temperature of 130°F (54.4°C) takes 30 seconds for partial or full-thickness burn.
Water temperature of 140°F (60°C) takes 5 seconds for partial or full-thickness burn.
  - The younger the child, the thinner the skin, and the quicker the burn occurs and more deeply it penetrates.
  - Never leave a young child alone, especially in the kitchen or bathroom, even to answer the telephone for a minute. Take the child with you.
  - Turn pot handles toward back of the stove and use back burners when cooking.
  - Cover stovetop knobs.
  - Keep appliance cords out of the child's vision and reach (e.g., coffee pot), especially if the appliance contains hot food or liquid.
  - Cover unused electrical outlets with appropriate outlet covers (not the ones that just plug in).
  - Keep hot foods and liquids away from table and counter edges.
  - Do not leave hot foods or liquids on a table with a tablecloth the child can reach.
  - Never carry or hold the child and hot food and/or beverage at the same time.
  - Stress the dangers of open flames; explain what "hot" means.
  - Place a protective cover in front of the radiator, fireplace, or other heating elements.
  - Keep matches, gasoline, lighters, and all other flammable materials locked away and out of the child's reach.
  - Instruct children how to *"stop, drop, and roll"* if their clothes catch fire and how to crawl to safety if a fire occurs in the building they are in.
  - Over 6 months old, apply sunscreen for children and/or sensitive skin with SPF 15 or higher when the child is exposed to sunlight.

✓ Additional tips for preventing fire-related injuries:
  - Install smoke detectors in every bedroom and on each level. Test them monthly and change batteries at least yearly. Having smoke detectors cuts the risk for dying in a fire by 50%.
  - Have at least two multipurpose dry chemical fire extinguishers: one in the kitchen and one in a workshop or area where potential sources of fire exist (e.g., water heater or furnace). Check monthly for signs of damage, corrosion, tampering, and leaks. Always call the fire department before using the fire extinguisher. Use the PASS method (*p*oint, *a*im at the base of the fire, *s*queeze the handle, and *s*weep from side to side).
  - Set up a home emergency fire escape plan and have practice drills using the escape plan at least quarterly. Include a meeting place outside the home in your plan.

✓ First-aid emergency care for a burn injury: Put the burned area under cool running water immediately, remove clothing, cover the burned area loosely with a bandage or clean cloth, and seek medical assistance.

✓ Importance of follow-up care with the health care provider, PT, and any other specialists involved.

✓ Telephone numbers to call for the health care provider, home health nurse, and PT in case any questions or concerns about treatment or injury arise after discharge.

✓ When to call the health care provider:
  • If the child is not eating well or showing signs of dehydration
  • If there is unmanageable behavior at home or school
  • If there are any signs of infection (e.g., healing burn area or donor site looks, feels, or smells different—red, warm, swollen, and very tender to the touch or there is foul-smelling drainage)
  • If there is itching that is not controlled with lotion or medication
  • If the healing/healed area cracks open or splits
  • If contracture occurs
  • If the child's temperature is higher than 38.6°C (101.5°F)
  • If the dressing change is painful despite giving pain medication as prescribed

✓ Referral to community resources, such as National SAFE KIDS Campaign, public health nurse, home health agencies, community support groups, camps for children with burns, psychologists, and financial counseling as appropriate. Additional general information can be obtained by contacting the following organizations:
  • SAFE KIDS Safety Tips: https://www.safekids.org/safetytips.
  • SAFE KIDS The Start Safe: Fire Resources for Kids with an aminated video with Rover the Hound and Freddy the Flashlight, games, and other materials for children 3–6 years old: https://www.safekids.org/start-safe-fire-resources-parents.

• Shriners Hospitals Burn Awareness (for videos, stories, safety tips, and burn prevention materials including Shriners Scald Safety Handout): https://www.shrinerschildrens.org/en/patient-information/patient-services-and-resources/burn-awareness.

• National Fire Protection Association (how to make a home fire escape plan with a video, escape grid that includes Sparky the fire dog, and safety tip sheet) https://nfpa.org/Public-Education/Staying-Safe/Preparedness/Escape-planning.

• American Academy of Pediatrics website for parents with burn treatment and prevention tips: https://www.healthychildren.org (search for "burns"). Or https://www.aap.org/en/search/?context=Healthy%20Children&source=Healthychildren.org&lang=English&k=burns&s=.

• Phoenix Society for Burn Survivors with programs and tools to support young burn victims, siblings, and family members affected by burn injury: https://www.phoenix-society.org/what-we-do/supporting-kids-teens.

• Most burn camps are supported by local/state organizations. Search under "burn camps" for children for individual states. Also look at https://www.kid-scamps.com/special_needs/burn.html and click on your state or the state closest to you because these camps are not located in all states.

• USFA (United States Fire Administration): Keeping kids safe from fire—videos, safety tips, and activities for children: https://www.usfa.fema.gov/prevention/outreach/children.html.

• USFA resources parents/caregivers: Sesame Street Fire Safety Program Family Guide: https://www.usfa.fema.gov/downloads/pdf/publications/ss_family_guide.pdf.

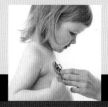

# Child Abuse and Neglect 81

## OVERVIEW/PATHOPHYSIOLOGY

The problem of child abuse and neglect or child maltreatment, formerly called "battered child syndrome," is recognized as a significant but preventable public health issue in the United States. The Centers for Disease Control and Prevention (CDC) (2022) also includes child abuse and neglect as adverse childhood experiences. Survivors often are left permanently disabled, and thousands of victims are overwhelmed by this trauma for the rest of their lives. Fatalities from child abuse and neglect have increased approximately 1.2% over the past 5 years with an estimated 1750 children dying in 2020. Many cases are believed to go unreported/underestimated (Keeshin et al., 2020; United States Department of Health & Human Services [USDHSS], 2022). The total lifetime economic burden of child abuse and neglect was estimated at $529 billion in 2018 (CDC, 2022).

Younger children are more vulnerable to child maltreatment, with the highest rate of victimization occurring in children from birth to 1 year of age. The rate declines as children get older, except for sexual abuse. For all types of child maltreatment the perpetrators most often are one or both of the parents (USDHSS, 2022). With sexual abuse, about 90% of the perpetrators are someone the child or family knows and is experienced by 25% of girls and about 8% of boys at some point in their childhood. This abuse can result in short- and long-term physical (e.g., unwanted pregnancy and physical injuries), mental/emotional (e.g., depression and PTSD), and/or behavioral (e.g., substance abuse including opioid use and risky sexual behavior) health consequences (CDC, n.d.a). The National Center for Missing and Exploited Children (NCMEC, n.d.) received more than 19,000 reports of possible child sex trafficking (CST) in 2022. The data show that when children run away for long periods of time or frequently, they may be running from one unsafe situation to another. One in six of more than 2500 cases of children reported missing to NCMEC (who had run away) were likely victims of CST. About 11% of sex trafficking cases reported in the Child Maltreatment 2020 data were boys (USDHSS, 2022). Child abuse and neglect occur in all cultural, ethnic, occupational, and socioeconomic groups. It is not usually a single event but rather a pattern of behavior that occurs over time. The following factors increase the likelihood of abuse or neglect occurring in families:

- **Parental characteristics:** Predisposition to maltreatment (perhaps having been victims themselves), substance abuse, lack of parenting skills, poor impulse control, emotional immaturity, or any caregiver disability.
- **Child characteristics:** Temperament, physical or cognitive disability that predisposes the child to injury, chronic illness or disability, being born to unmarried parents, or hyperactivity.
- **Environmental characteristics:** Divorce, marital problems, financial strain, inadequate housing, and isolation from support of families or friends.
- **Societal factors:** Increased violence, children viewed as property and not valued, physical methods of punishment, and lack of willingness in community to become involved in family violence issues.

**Note:** *Child Maltreatment 2020 (USDHSS) addresses child abuse and neglect data during the pandemic—noting that the largest group of reporters of suspected maltreatment are education personnel and the lockdowns in 2020 limited their ability to interact and observe their students. Hotlines transitioned to virtual call centers and were open throughout the lockdown.*

Terms include the following:
- **Child maltreatment:** A broad term that includes intentional physical abuse or neglect, emotional abuse or neglect, and sexual abuse (younger than 18 years) usually by an adult caregiver, most often the parent. Some children suffer more than one type of maltreatment, some can be determined to be a victim of up to four types of maltreatment. Neglect is consistently the major type of child maltreatment, 76% of cases in 2020 (USDHSS, 2022).

- **Physical abuse:** The deliberate infliction of physical injury or pain. It may result from punching, beating, kicking, biting, bruising, shaking, burning, or otherwise harming a child and can occur from overdiscipline or physical punishment. About 16.5% suffered physical abuse in 2020 (USDHSS, 2022).
- **Physical neglect:** Failure to provide basic necessities such as food, clothing, shelter, and a safe environment in which the child can grow and develop normally. Infant prenatal

substance exposure is now required to be reported and followed up with a plan of safe care and appropriate referral (USDHSS, 2022).

- **Emotional abuse:** Deliberate attempt to destroy or significantly impair self-esteem or competence by rejecting, ignoring, criticizing, isolating, or terrorizing the child. The most common form is verbal abuse or "belittling."
- **Emotional neglect:** Failure to meet the child's needs for affection, attention, and emotional support. The most common feature is the absence of the normal parent–child attachment and interaction.
- **Sexual abuse:** Contacts or interactions between a child and an adult for the adult's sexual gratification, with or without physical contact, and involves pressuring or forcing a child to engage in sexual acts. It includes pedophilia and all forms of incest and rape. It also includes fondling, oral-genital contact, all forms of intercourse, exhibitionism, voyeurism, and involvement of children in the production of pornography. It is thought to be one of the most common but underreported crimes against children with about 9.6% of reported cases in 2020 that included this form of maltreatment (USDHSS, 2022).
- **Sex trafficking of minors:** Added as a new maltreatment type and refers to recruitment, harboring, transportation, provision, or obtaining a person for the purpose of a sexual act (USDHSS, 2022). The National Center for Missing & Exploited Children (n.d.) notes that this includes sexual acts for items of value (e.g., food, shelter, money, and drugs). It usually is induced by force, fraud, or coercion. About 75% of victims of sex trafficking are 14–17 years old and 19% are 9–13 years old (USDHSS, 2022).
- **Medical care neglect:** Failure to provide needed treatment to infants or children who generally have life-threatening or serious medical conditions. About one-third of these children are younger than 3 years.
- **Medical child abuse (factitious disorder by proxy, Munchausen syndrome by proxy):** Abuse inflicted on a child in which a parent (usually the mother) fabricates symptoms and falsifies medical history or actually causes an illness that results in evaluation and treatment.
- **Abusive head trauma (AHT) (includes shaken baby syndrome):** This inflicted head injury is due to a variety of biomechanical forces including violent shaking of an infant or young child (most often younger than 1 year, with infants 1–3 months at greatest risk), resulting in severe injury. There are high mortality rates in infant victims. Mortality for infants experiencing AHT is at least 25%. Nearly all of these children have serious, long-term health consequences from their injuries, such as vision problems (including cortical blindness), developmental delays, physical disabilities, and hearing loss. AHT is the leading cause of child deaths in the United States due to physical abuse in children under 5 years and accounts for about one-third of all child maltreatment deaths (CDC, n.d.b). About 70% of children surviving AHT have neurologic impairments that include static encephalopathy, cerebral palsy, seizure disorders, cortical blindness, behavioral problems, and learning disabilities. In addition, endocrine dysfunction occurs in many survivors and may not manifest until many years after injury (Narang et al., 2020).

## HEALTH CARE SETTING

Primary care or emergency department with possible hospitalization resulting from complications. Abuse/neglect also may be found during hospitalization for other reasons.

## ASSESSMENT

> **Note:** *History is critical in making a diagnosis. Frequently in child abuse/neglect cases, the history is inconsistent with injury severity, or it changes during evaluation. It is essential that the nurse taking the history be nonjudgmental and report factual information. The nurse needs to identify their own feelings and biases to facilitate this process. This is difficult to do at times, and collegial support is beneficial. History and physical examination will determine needed diagnostic tests.*

***Physical abuse.*** Acts out violently against others; frightened of parents or caregivers; avoids changing clothes (e.g., in gym class); old, new, and multiple injuries; burn or restraint injuries; questionable bruises and welts; questionable burns (e.g., imprint or immersion); questionable fractures (e.g., spiral fracture); questionable lacerations or abrasions (e.g., human bite marks); skull fractures; or internal abdominal injuries.

***Physical neglect.*** Consistently hungry; poor hygiene (e.g., diaper rash or lice) or inappropriate dress for weather; consistently left without supervision; abandoned; begging for or stealing food; constant fatigue and listlessness; frequently absent or tardy for school; failure to gain weight or failure to thrive (FTT); developmentally delayed; assumes adult responsibility; given inappropriate food, drink, or medication; reportedly ingests harmful substances.

***Emotional abuse or neglect.*** Antisocial or destructive behavior; sleep disorders; self-stimulating behaviors such as biting, head banging, rocking, or thumb sucking (in an older child); demanding behaviors; self-destructive, suicide attempt; overly adaptive behavior; emotional or intellectual developmental delays; speech disorders.

***Sexual abuse.*** Recurrent abdominal pain; genital, urethral, or anal trauma; bruises, bleeding, lacerations, or irritation of mouth or throat; torn, stained, or bloody underclothing; sexually transmitted diseases; recurrent urinary tract infections; enuresis (involuntary discharge of urine) or encopresis (incontinence of stool not caused by organic defect or illness); pregnancy; sleep disturbances (e.g., nightmares and night terrors); appetite disturbances (e.g., anorexia or bulimia); neurotic or conductive disorders; withdrawal, guilt, or depression; temper tantrums (in older children); aggressive behaviors; suicidal or runaway threats or behaviors; hysterical or conversion reactions; excessive masturbation; sexualized play in developmentally immature children; school problems; promiscuity;

reluctance to change clothes; substance abuse. Many children have normal genital examinations.

***Medical child abuse (factitious disorder by proxy, Munchausen syndrome by proxy).*** Signs and symptoms occur only when the perpetrator (usually the mother) is present. Common presenting indicators include poisoning, seizures, apnea, bleeding, vomiting, diarrhea, fever, and even cardiopulmonary arrest.

***Abusive head trauma.*** Often there are no external signs of injury other than a change in level of consciousness. The child may have a history of poor feeding, vomiting, lethargy, and irritability occurring for several days or weeks. More severe trauma/shaking may cause brain damage, seizures, blindness, paralysis, and death. On ophthalmologic examination, retinal hemorrhages are seen. The anterior fontanel may be tense or full when the infant is quiet.

## DIAGNOSTIC TESTS

***Radiographs of injured area or skeletal survey.*** Certain findings on radiographic examination are strong indicators of physical abuse. These include metaphyseal "corner" or "bucket handle" fractures of long bones in infants, spiral fractures of long bones in nonambulatory infants, and multiple fractures of the ribs or long bones in varying stages of healing. These findings may help distinguish abuse from osteogenesis imperfecta (an inherited condition marked by abnormally brittle bones that are subject to fracture). A skeletal survey needs to be repeated about 2 weeks after the initial survey. Acute fractures may be missed initially but can be seen when periosteal new bone formation or callus formation occurs.

***Computed tomography or magnetic resonance imaging.*** May reveal subdural hematoma and subarachnoid hemorrhage, hallmark signs of AHT. Computed tomography and magnetic resonance imaging may also diagnose abdominal injuries from abuse.

***Ophthalmology examinations.*** May reveal retinal hemorrhage (usually bilateral), the hallmark sign of AHT.

***Bone scans.*** Detect soft tissue and bone trauma, especially in locating unseen fractures or bone injuries. For example, they can define rib fractures, which are difficult to assess because of overlying structures such as the heart, lungs, and liver.

***Coagulation studies.*** Used in children with many bruises in different stages to differentiate abuse from a medical condition such as leukemia or bleeding or clotting disorders. These studies are also used if intracranial hemorrhage is present. Use topical analgesia with blood draws to decrease anxiety and pain (atraumatic care).

***Complete blood count.*** Helps rule out active bleeding or bleeding disorder. Provide atraumatic care.

***Forensic evaluation.*** In sexually abused children, it may be done to identify evidence such as semen or detect sexually transmitted disease.

## Patient Problem/Analyze Cues/Prioritize Hypotheses

# Injury

*due to* neglect or physical, emotional, or sexual abuse

***Desired Outcome/Generate Solutions:*** After intervention/treatment, the child exhibits no further evidence of abuse or neglect.

| ASSESSMENT—RECOGNIZE CUES/ INTERVENTIONS—TAKE ACTION | RATIONALES |
|---|---|
| Assess the child's physical and mental status as follows:<br>• Note bruises, scars, or other signs of abuse.<br>• Note unusual interactions or responses of the child. | A thorough evaluation must be done on all children in all health care settings. Abuse occurs in all cultural and socioeconomic groups and may not be the admitting diagnosis. |
| Observe interactions between the child and family. | Signs of abuse or neglect may be detected in the way the child interacts with parents and other adults. For example, a child who is emotionally neglected may not want to be held or have eye contact with the parent or other adult. |
| Obtain a detailed history. | This may detect a pattern of trauma or neglect or lack of correlation between the history and severity of the trauma; or the history may change as the examination progresses. |

## ASSESSMENT—RECOGNIZE CUES/ INTERVENTIONS—TAKE ACTION

## RATIONALES

| ASSESSMENT—RECOGNIZE CUES/ INTERVENTIONS—TAKE ACTION | RATIONALES |
| --- | --- |
| Keep factual, detailed, and objective records for documentation. | Medical records may be subpoenaed as evidence in court proceedings and therefore need to be as detailed and objective as possible. Being factual (i.e., no opinions, impressions, or interpretations) is imperative. Records need to include the following:<br><br>• Physical condition (e.g., "Three small, well-delineated, circular lesions, approximately 3–5 mm in diameter and 1 mm in depth, dark purple-red, noted on sole of left foot").<br><br>• Pictures, which are most beneficial in documenting injuries, need to be dated and kept in the patient's chart.<br><br>• The child's behavioral response to parents, others, and environment (e.g., a child with FTT often does not verbally or physically interact with anyone).<br><br>• Specific comments of the child, parents, or other family members and developmental age of the child. Use quotes when appropriate. |
| Use a nonjudgmental, nonthreatening manner when interacting with the child's parents. | Frequently, it is unclear who actually abused the child. The child is more likely to be helped if the parents trust the staff. If the parents feel alienated by the staff, they may deny the child access to care. Parents will be more receptive to teaching in a trusting environment. |
| ⚠ Report all cases of suspected child abuse or neglect. | All 50 states consider health care workers mandatory reporters of child abuse/neglect. |
| ⚠ Keep the child in a safe environment in the hospital (e.g., near the nurses' station). | The suspected abuser may be restricted from visiting, or only certain individuals may be approved to visit. Follow local Child Protective Services (CPS) court documents for visitor information as well as agency policy. |
| ⚠ Assist in removing the child from an unsafe situation (whether verbal or physical neglect or abuse is suspected). Report any suspicious behavior to Social Services in the hospital and CPS in the community. | Nurses are mandated reporters of suspected neglect or abuse in all 50 states. |
| Refer families to social agencies for assistance with finances, food, clothing, and health care. | These measures help ameliorate the causes of neglect. |
| Collaborate with the multidisciplinary health care team involved with the case. | This provides continual evaluation of progress/status of the child in the hospital, foster care, or on return to the home. |
| Help parents identify events that precipitate an abusive act (i.e., crying is a major trigger) and alternative ways to deal with the release of anger (e.g., role-playing). | This may prevent further abuse for this child or siblings. |

## Parent/Caregiver Problem/Analyze Cues/Prioritize Hypotheses

# Impaired Parenting

*due to* the child's, caregiver's, or situational characteristics/temperament that precipitated child abuse or neglect

***Desired Outcome/Generate Solutions:*** Within 1 week after interventions the parents/caregivers begin demonstrating more positive interactions with the child and more appropriate parenting activities and verbalize a more realistic understanding of normal expectations for the child.

| ASSESSMENT—RECOGNIZE CUES/ INTERVENTIONS—TAKE ACTION | RATIONALES |
|---|---|
| Assess/identify the families at risk for further abuse/neglect. | Identifying at-risk families is the first step in helping prevent further abuse or neglect. Such families tend to have immature, single parents; parents who were abused as children; a premature infant; a child younger than 3 years or with a chronic illness or disability; parental substance abuse; poverty; poor housing; and limited social network/support. |
| Assess/observe the parents' interactions with the child. | This is the best way to get a realistic view of the relationship. For example, when feeding the child, the parent may avoid making eye contact or touching the child unless absolutely necessary. |
| Assess the parents' strengths and weaknesses, normal coping behaviors, any cultural practices that may impact the current situation, presence or absence of support systems, and willingness to accept help. | This assessment provides the basis for developing an appropriate plan of care, building trust, and making necessary referrals. |
| Demonstrate age-/developmentally appropriate child-rearing practices, especially communication and discipline. | Parents may care for their child in the way their parents cared for them and may not know age-/developmentally appropriate child-rearing practices. |
| Instruct parents about alternative methods of discipline, such as rewards, time-out, consequences, and verbal disapproval. | Parents may not know any nonviolent methods of discipline. |
| Provide care for the child until the parent is ready to provide care. | This allows parents time to "relax" and observe age-appropriate care. |
| Encourage the parents to participate in care of the child. Reinforce positive behaviors. | This helps build self-esteem and confidence in parents to improve interactions. |
| Focus on positive aspects of the child (e.g., "What beautiful eyes your child has" or "Tell me something your child is good at"). | Parents may have a negative view of the child, and this gives them another perspective. |
| Instruct the family what to expect in terms of growth and development for their child (physical, psychosocial, and cognitive) through role-modeling and having the parents return demonstrations. | Parents will incorporate information better if not "instructed" and feeling as though they are being criticized. This increases their knowledge and reinforces accurate expectations of what is normal for their child, especially if the child has any developmental issues. |
| Also provide education about nutrition, care related to activities of daily living (ADLs), routine well-child care, manifestations of illness, and the importance of caring/loving attitude in dealing with children. | This information increases realistic expectations and chance of positive parenting. |
| Convey a nonjudgmental attitude of genuine concern. | Such an attitude facilitates developing trust and respect and enables parents to observe and develop better methods of caring for their child. |
| Refer the family to appropriate social agencies to assist with financial support, adequate housing, employment, and so on. | This helps to ameliorate risk factors of abuse/neglect. |
| Help identify support systems for the parents such as extended family, neighbors, or support groups. | Support systems decrease family stress and hence decrease the risk for abuse/neglect. |

## Patient Problem/Analyze Cues/Prioritize Hypotheses

# Anxiety

*due to* maltreatment, powerlessness, hospitalization, and potential loss of parents

**Desired Outcomes/Generate Solutions:** Within 72 hours following interventions the child verbalizes source(s) of anxiety and exhibits more interactivity and sociability and less withdrawal. Alternatively, if the child is too young to verbalize, he or she demonstrates more interactivity and sociability and less withdrawal.

| ASSESSMENT—RECOGNIZE CUES/ INTERVENTIONS—TAKE ACTION | RATIONALES |
|---|---|
| Assess the child for signs or verbalization of anxiety. | This enables support and reassurances that are appropriate and beneficial to the child. |
| Provide consistent caregivers and an age-appropriate safe environment. | These measures help relieve the child's anxiety and provide a positive role model for the family. |
| Reassure the child about his or her personal safety. | Verbal reassurance increases a sense of security. |
| Demonstrate acceptance of the child but do not reinforce inappropriate behaviors. | Children need acceptance as well as guidance regarding appropriate behaviors. |
| Support the child in talking about his or her family or stressful events. | Verbalization of anxieties decreases their impact on children. |
| Do not ask too many questions. | This may upset the child and interfere with other professionals' interrogations. |
| Encourage play, especially with the family or appropriate toys such as dollhouse activity. | Play is the "work of the child" and may help reveal the types of relationships perceived by the child. This could include, for example, playing with dolls that represent father, mother, and siblings or drawing pictures of events. The child may tell the story of events with dolls. Drawings often depict fears and reactions to experiences. |
| Incorporate therapeutic play (for children 3 years or older) into care activities if possible. | This helps children cope with new, frightening experiences in a nonthreatening way. For example, have the child check blood pressure on a doll before checking it on the child. |
| Treat the child as you would other children, not as an "abused" victim. | This encourages the child to interact with others rather than promoting isolation. |
| Offer choices whenever possible regarding clothing, diet, and other ADLs; recreation time; and socialization time. | Being allowed to make choices provides a sense of control and decreases a sense of powerlessness and hence anxiety. |

## ✔ PATIENT–FAMILY TEACHING AND DISCHARGE PLANNING

When providing patient–family/foster–family teaching, focus on sensory information, avoid giving excessive information, and initiate a visiting nurse referral for necessary follow-up teaching and assessment as needed. Utilize a variety of teaching methods (e.g., videos, tablets, and webinars as well as verbal and written) depending on learning styles and resources of child/family. Stress family-centered care, which is viewing the family as a unit that is the "constant" in the child's life and maintaining or improving the health of the family and its members in a holistic manner. Include information about the following, ensuring that it is written at a level understandable to the child/family:

✓ Care related to any specific injury.
✓ Realistic expectations for the individual child related to:
  • Growth and development (e.g., regression is normal after a child has been hospitalized and/or severely stressed)
  • Nutrition (e.g., toddler's food jags—may only want one food for every meal for several days)
✓ Guidelines based on developmental level:
  • Safety (e.g., preschooler does not understand the danger of chasing a ball across the street)
  • Need for love and attention
✓ Methods of handling normal developmental problems that increase a parent's stress level (e.g., toddler's negativism, temper tantrums, toilet training, and need for rituals and routines).

✓ Demonstration of care related to ADLs; observe return demonstration by the parents.

✓ Importance of regular well-child visits and provision of routine well-child care.

✓ Suggestions for nonviolent, age/developmentally appropriate methods of disciplining the child (e.g., reward, time-out, consequences, and verbal disapproval).

✓ Identification of stressful situations for the parents and ways to deal with them. For example, if an infant cries for prolonged periods, make sure that infant is clean and dry and is not uncomfortable, hungry, or ill; put the infant in a crib on his or her back and go out of the room but check on the infant about every 10 minutes. DO NOT SHAKE THE BABY. This can cause severe damage.

✓ Review of situations/circumstances that precipitate abuse/violence and of methods to deal with anger constructively.

✓ Importance of providing the child with positive reinforcement of appropriate behavior to build self-esteem.

✓ Teaching the child the difference between "good touch" and "bad touch."

✓ Name of a place a child can go to if being abused (e.g., neighborhood "safe house").

✓ Suggestions for local support systems (e.g., extended family members, church members, and neighbors).

✓ Referrals to community resources, such as parenting classes, support groups, public health nurse, social worker, and financial counseling if appropriate. Additional general information/support can be obtained by contacting the following organizations:

- Parents Anonymous, Inc., at https://www.raisingfuture.org/. This group provides support and resources for overwhelmed families/parents and caregivers and is based in California.
- National Parent Hotline at https://www.nationalparenthelpline.org/find-support or 1-855-4APARENT/1-855-427-2736, launched by Parents Anonymous that provides emotional support and resources for parents and caregivers across America.

- National Child Abuse Hotline at (800) 4-A-CHILD (1-800-422-4453) (call or text) or online https://childhelphotline.org/ with counselors available 24/7.
- Child Help at https://www.childhelp.org with resources for kids, parents, & teachers. Several of the children's resources are *My Yucky Feeling* by Anne Malver (teaching children to trust their gut) and *Cate's Magic Garden* by Betsy Coffeen (reminding young children to use the magic of friendship like Cate does to bring the garden back to life) at https://www.childhelp.org/childrens-resources/reading-resources-for-kids/.
- Prevent Child Abuse America at https://preventchildabuse.org includes a state network site in addition to many other resources. National Center on Shaken Baby Syndrome at https://dontshake.org. This website provides family resources and support. It sponsors the Period of Purple Crying Program: "A New Way to Understand Your Baby's Crying."
- American Academy of Pediatrics Healthy Children—Information and guidance for parents Child Abuse and Neglect: What Parents Should Know https://healthychildren.org/English/safety-prevention/at-home/Pages/What-to-Know-about-Child-Abuse.aspx (updated 3/16/2022).
- Shaken Baby Syndrome: Protect Your Infant From AHT. Provides parents with information and resources for dealing with crying babies to help prevent AHT. https://healthychildren.org/English/safety-prevention/at-home/Pages/Abusive-Head-Trauma-Shaken-Baby-Syndrome.aspx (updated 3/16/2022).
- National Center for Missing & Exploited Children: Child Sex Trafficking in America: A Guide for Parents and Guardians (2022) at https://www.missingkids.org/content/dam/missingkids/pdfs/CSTinAmerica_ParentsGuardians.pdf. This is one of many resources available including 24-hour hotline 1–800-THE-LOST (1-800-843-5678) to be used after reporting your child missing to law enforcement.

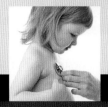

# Cystic Fibrosis 82

## OVERVIEW/PATHOPHYSIOLOGY

Cystic fibrosis (CF) is a chronic, progressive multisystem disease in which there is dysfunction of the exocrine (mucus-producing) glands and abnormal transport of sodium and chloride across the epithelium. This results in abnormally thick secretions, causing obstruction of the small passageways of many organs. Mutation of the CF transmembrane conductance regulator (CFTR) causes the CFTR protein to become dysfunctional, and this leads to the abnormal transport mentioned above. CF is an autosomal recessive hereditary disease with more than 2000 known gene mutations (Cystic Fibrosis Foundation [CFF], 2022; Reed & Shores, 2020). This is why there is such a wide variation in clinical manifestations and why gene therapy remains so challenging.

CF is the most common lethal genetic illness in Caucasian children, adolescents, and young adults (Hockenberry et al., 2019). About 91% of CF cases were identified as Caucasian in 2021, down from about 94% in 2006 (CFF, 2022). The median life expectancy had improved dramatically from about 6 or 7 years in the 1950s to a median age of 53 for children born between 2017 and 2021 (CFF, 2022). The median life expectancy has increased because of specialized care, particularly through the national network of Cystic Fibrosis Foundation (CFF)–accredited centers and new CF therapies that can begin with infants detected through newborn screening (NBS). Research shows that receiving CF care early in life helps children have better nutrition and better overall health than those who are diagnosed later in life. Patients older than 12 years with severe CF are living longer after receiving a lung transplantation (1645 patients reported ever having a lung transplant with a significantly lower number reported in 2020 and 2021), and the median survival rate for children was 5.4 years after lung transplantation between 1999 and 2016 (CFF, 2022, n.d.a). Highlights from the CFF Patient Registry Overview 2021 note that improved trends in infection rates, lung function, pulmonary exacerbations, and survival were observed in 2020 and 2021 and indicated that increased use of elexacaftor/tezacaftor/ivacaftor (a CFTR modulator) seems to be contributing to these better outcomes (in 2022). Also, clinical trials are ongoing to treat key symptoms of CF and improve quality of life.

About 32,000 people in the United States and more than 70,000 worldwide have CF, and around 58% are 18 years or older, with the number of adults continuing to increase.

Historically, about 1000 new cases were diagnosed each year, with some yearly fluctuation from 2019 to 2021, all less than 900. Some of the decrease may be due to reporting during the COVID-19 pandemic, but about 95% were diagnosed by 6 months in 2021 (CFF, 2022). More than 10 million Americans are asymptomatic carriers of one mutation of the *CFTR* gene (CFF, n.d.b). CF is most often seen in Caucasians, but it affects all races and has been increasing steadily in Hispanics (any race) over the past 15 years, from about 6.5% in 2006 to almost 10% in 2021. The percentage of individuals identified as Black or African American has remained steady at about 3.5%, and 1.9% identified as two or more races in 2021 (CFF, 2022).

The health burden of CF includes increased medical costs, reduced quality of life (i.e., time-consuming treatments like chest physiotherapy and medication administration), missed workdays, and premature death (Hermann & Davis, 2019). Parents that have children with complex chronic conditions like CF may face challenges both physically and emotionally in coping with the care of their child (Hockenberry et al., 2019).

## HEALTH CARE SETTING

Primary care, with possible hospitalization for CF exacerbation or other complications.

## ASSESSMENT

Initially involves overall appraisal, including monitoring general activity, physical findings, nutritional status, and chest radiographic examination.

*Signs and symptoms.* Vary widely, as does the severity of involvement of specific organ systems depending on which genetic mutation of CF is present. Patients tend to have periods without acute symptoms and then periods with acute exacerbation of symptoms. The first clinical manifestation may be meconium ileus (obstruction of the small intestine caused by impaction of thick, dry, tenacious meconium—the first stool a newborn passes), or the patient may not have symptoms for months or years.

*Most of the usual symptoms are caused by the following:*
- **Progressive chronic obstructive lung disease:** Initially wheezing and dry cough, progressing to paroxysmal cough that frequently causes posttussive emesis. Other signs include increased dyspnea, barrel chest, mild to severe clubbing of nail beds, cyanosis, and repeated pulmonary infections that cause scarring and bronchiectasis (irreversible dilation and

destruction of the bronchial walls). Numerous complications, such as pneumothorax and hemoptysis, often occur, and about 25% of children also have asthma (CFF, 2022).

- **Pancreatic enzyme deficiency** resulting from duct blockage (present in most children with CF): Stools that are frothy (bulky and large), foul smelling, fat containing (steatorrhea), and float (four *F*s of CF); voracious appetite initially, progressing to loss of appetite late in the disease; weight loss, marked tissue wasting, protuberant abdomen with thin extremities, failure to thrive (FTT), anemia; and evidence of deficiency of fat-soluble vitamins (A, D, E, and K). Complications include pancreatic fibrosis leading to glucose intolerance, diabetes mellitus (DM), and pancreatitis. CF-related DM (CFRD) is very common in people with CF, especially as they get older. In the 2021 CFF Patient Registry Annual Data Summary, about 5% of children under age 18 had CFRD, with an impaired glucose tolerance more prevalent in adolescents. The report also found that 29% of adults had CFRD. The report noted that individuals that had received lung transplants are no longer included in the percentage of patients with CFRD and thus there is a lower prevalence of this complication (2022).
- **Sweat gland dysfunction** resulting in increased sodium and chloride concentrations. Infants "taste" salty and are more susceptible to dehydration (Hockenberry et al., 2019).

*Other gastrointestinal complications.* Include small bowel obstruction in infants, distal intestinal obstruction syndrome in adolescents and adults, and chronic constipation that can lead to rectal prolapse, which occurs in children with CF usually younger than 6 years. Most children experience transient or chronic gastroesophageal reflux (GER) (Reed & Shores, 2020).

*Liver complications.* Biliary cirrhosis and gallbladder dysfunction.

*Other.* Nasal polyps and sinusitis also occur frequently in children with CF.

## DIAGNOSTIC TESTS

CF has been called the "great imitator" because signs of chronic respiratory infection and FTT are symptoms of many other childhood conditions.

*Newborn screening panel.* CF had been added to the NBS panel in all 50 states as of January 1, 2010, and screening is done at the same time as phenylketonuria and other screening tests. The two-tiered process follows:

- *Immunoreactive trypsinogen (IRT) test*: Enables early detection of CF and is done several days after birth (NBS). The IRT can be elevated because of prematurity or a stressful delivery or for other reasons. An elevated IRT requires a repeat test, and there are two methods for following up.
  a. Some states repeat an IRT which is followed by a sweat test if elevated.

  b. The more commonly used method requires CFTR mutation testing to be done after one IRT test is elevated. If one or two variants are identified, then a sweat test is done. If the second test is elevated/positive, make a referral to a CF-accredited care center for further evaluation (CFF, n.d.b; Rosenstein, 2021). It is confirmed by a "sweat test" or mutation analysis (i.e., genetic testing). The combination of these two tests is sensitive 90%–95% of the time.

- *Pilocarpine iontophoresis (quantitative sweat chloride test or "sweat test")*: Production of sweat is stimulated with a special device, and the sweat is collected and measured. Diagnosis is made when the chloride level is equal to or greater than 60 mmol/L along with the presence of clinical symptoms or a family history of CF. Chloride levels of 30–59 mmol/L is considered suggestive and should be repeated. The sweat test is typically done between 2 and 4 weeks of age for infants who have had a positive NBS as full-term infants. Full-term infants usually produce enough sweat by age 2 weeks. This test is considered the gold standard for diagnosing CF and should be done at the CF care center closest to the family (CFF, n.d.b).

- *CFTR (mutation of the gene that codes this regulator) genetic analysis (genetic testing)*: Helps determine whether the child is a carrier or has CF when the NBS cannot be done or has unclear results. Not all mutations cause CF. This information is also helpful in determining which CFTR modulator therapy is tailored to their individual mutation (Dickinson & Paranjape, 2020).

*Chest radiographic examination.* Shows characteristic patchy atelectasis and chronic obstructive emphysema, depending on the severity of pulmonary involvement.

*Pulmonary function tests (usually performed after 5–6 years of age, but new guidelines suggest attempting this as young as 3 years).* Assess the degree of pulmonary disease and response to therapy. In the presence of CF, the test will show decreased forced vital capacity (FVC) and tidal volume, increased airway resistance, increased residual volume, and decreased forced expiratory volume in 1 second ($FEV_1$) and $FEV_1$/FVC ratio (Rosenstein, 2022).

*Pulse oximetry.* Noninvasive, atraumatic method to reveal decreased oxygen saturation (less than 95% or as directed by health care provider).

*Complete blood count.* Increased white blood cells with increased neutrophils on differential count will be present with infection.

*Sputum culture.* For identification of infective organisms and sensitivity of these organisms. Many resistant organisms develop because of the frequency of respiratory infections.

*DNA analysis of chorionic villi or amniotic fluid.* Can establish prenatal diagnosis.

## Patient Problem/Analyze Cues/Prioritize Hypotheses

# Risk for Impaired Airway Clearance

*due to* thick, tenacious mucus in the airways

***Desired Outcome/Generate Solutions:*** Immediately after treatment/interventions, the child expectorates mucus and exhibits improved airway clearance as evidenced by improved breath sounds and heart rate (HR) and respiratory rate (RR) within the child's baseline limits.

| ASSESSMENT—RECOGNIZE CUES/ INTERVENTIONS—TAKE ACTION | RATIONALES |
|---|---|
| Assess the HR, RR, and breath sounds. | This assessment establishes baseline data from which to compare later findings. With ineffective airway clearance, the child will have increased HR and RR. Breath sounds may be decreased with little air movement because of the blocked airway, or adventitious sounds may be increased because of mucus in the airway. |
| Assist the child with sputum expectoration (may be done by respiratory therapist): | Many children swallow sputum and cannot expectorate without assistance/encouragement. |
| • Assess the HR, RR, breath sounds, and O$_2$ saturation before nebulization and after chest physiotherapy. | Assessment before and after treatment monitors the effectiveness of treatment, that is, improved breath sounds and increased O$_2$ saturation. If HR is consistently increased or increasing after chest physiotherapy, the provider should be notified. |
| • Position the child in an upright sitting position, ensuring that he or she does not slouch. | This position facilitates the maximum inhalation of medication and improves the effectiveness of the cough to clear secretions out of the airways. |
| • Administer the nebulization (albuterol) as prescribed 1 hour before or 2 hours after meals. | This treatment opens bronchi to facilitate the removal of secretions after chest physiotherapy. Correlating treatment before or several hours after meals decreases the chance of emesis after chest physiotherapy. |
| • Perform chest physiotherapy after nebulizer treatment. Examples follow. | This helps to loosen secretions and usually causes considerable coughing followed by expectoration of mucus and sometimes vomiting from excessive coughing. Scheduling in relation to meals is essential to provide the maximum benefit of treatment and prevent interference with nutrient ingestion. Treatment before breakfast helps loosen secretions that built up overnight. Treatment before bedtime helps clear secretions that would otherwise provide a medium for bacterial growth. This treatment is performed at least 2–4 times/day for maintenance or routine daily care. The method used depends on age of the child, effectiveness of the technique, the child's/parent's ability to perform/tolerate the technique, and preference of the child/parent. |
| • Chest percussion and postural drainage for 20–40 minutes | Chest percussion loosens secretions, and postural drainage facilitates drainage of secretions so that they can be expectorated. |
| • Oscillating positive expiratory pressure or mucus clearance device (e.g., Flutter, Acapella, Aerobika, and RC-Cornet) typically used for sessions lasting about 20 minutes | These handheld devices have a plastic mouthpiece on one end that the child breathes into. Exhaling into the device vibrates the airways, thereby loosening mucus from the airway walls and accelerating airflow, which facilitates upward movement of mucus so that it can be more readily cleared. These devices are very effective and give children control because they can be used without the assistance of others. |

Continued

| ASSESSMENT—RECOGNIZE CUES/ INTERVENTIONS—TAKE ACTION | RATIONALES |
|---|---|
| • Airway clearance system with high-frequency chest wall oscillation (HFCWO) device (e.g., the vest) used for 20–30 minutes | This inflatable vest fits like a life jacket and is connected by tubes to a generator. The vest inflates and deflates rapidly, applying gentle pressure to the chest. It provides HFCWO to help loosen secretions and increase mucus expectoration. These devices are very effective and give children control because they can be used without the assistance of others. |
| • Suction as necessary.<br><br>Encourage the child to assist with suctioning, if possible (e.g., directing where the suction catheter needs to be used) | For infants/young children or if there is a large volume of mucus, assistance may be needed to clear secretions from the airway. However, children usually cough sufficiently after nebulizer treatment and chest physiotherapy to clear secretions independently.<br><br>Involving children in their care gives them some control over this treatment and their care. |
| Ensure that the child is receiving at least maintenance fluids. | Hydration thins and loosens secretions for easier expectoration. |
| Administer dornase alfa (Pulmozyme) as prescribed. | This medication thins mucus, which will facilitate expectoration. |

## Patient Problem/Analyze Cues/Prioritize Hypotheses

# Impaired Gas Exchange

*due to* airway obstruction occurring with air trapping in the alveoli and airways narrowed by tenacious mucus

***Desired Outcome/Generate Solutions:*** Within 2 hours after treatment/intervention, the child has adequate gas exchange as evidenced by $O_2$ saturation greater than 92% (or consistent with the child's baseline).

| ASSESSMENT—RECOGNIZE CUES/ INTERVENTIONS—TAKE ACTION | RATIONALES |
|---|---|
| ⚠ Along with vital signs, assess respiratory status every 2–4 hours, or more frequently as indicated by the child's condition. | Increased HR and RR would occur with impaired gas exchange, as would chest retractions, increased work of breathing (WOB), nasal flaring, and use of accessory muscles of respiration. These are signs of respiratory distress necessitating prompt intervention/treatment. |
| Ensure continuous monitoring of pulse oximetry readings; report low value (usually 92% or lower). | Decreased $O_2$ saturation can indicate the need for initiation of or increased $O_2$. |
| ⚠ Monitor for behavioral indicators of hypoxia. | Restlessness, mood changes, and/or change in the level of consciousness are early signs of $O_2$ deficiency. Knowing the child's normal behaviors is necessary in order to note changes early. |
| ⚠ Be alert to changes in the child's skin color, such as cyanosis | Cyanosis of the lips and nail beds is a late indicator of hypoxia and a signal of the need for prompt treatment/intervention. Knowing the child's baseline skin color/tone is necessary in order to note changes. |
| Position the child in high-Fowler position and/or leaning forward. | These positions promote comfort and optimal gas exchange by enabling maximal chest expansion. |

Continued

| ASSESSMENT—RECOGNIZE CUES/ INTERVENTIONS—TAKE ACTION | RATIONALES |
|---|---|
| Administer $O_2$ along with humidity through the most appropriate delivery system and at the rate prescribed. | The child's developmental age helps determine the most effective delivery system and flow rate (e.g., nasal cannula for infants with liter flow rate less than 4). Humidity use replaces convective losses of moisture. |
| • Monitor the child on $O_2$ delivery closely.<br><br>  • Ensure the system is functioning properly and not dislodged (e.g., nasal cannula is not in nostrils)<br><br>  • Assess for safety hazards, for example, an active toddler with nasal cannula tubing twisted/occluded and potentially strangling the child. | $O_2$-induced $CO_2$ narcosis is a hazard of $O_2$ therapy in the child with chronic hypercapnia (increased $CO_2$ in the blood). If $O_2$ saturation is consistently greater than 96%, for example, it is likely that the flow rate can be decreased slowly by small increments.<br><br>It is important to assess the entire delivery system—children may be hypoxic because they are not receiving the $O_2$ due to a displaced or disconnected tubing.<br><br>Provide a developmentally appropriate safe environment for the child at all times, "child proof" the area for a toddler. |
| Encourage games or physical exercise appropriate to the child's developmental status and condition (e.g., blowing bubbles, teaching pursed lip breathing, or walking), but avoid overexertion. | Breathing more deeply facilitates clearing of mucus and improves oxygenation. |
| Provide a neutral thermal environment for the child. | This is a room temperature in which the body does not have to use as much energy to stay warm or cool off, thereby enabling the child to use energy to grow or heal. With decreased energy demands, more $O_2$ is available to ensure these needs are met. |
| Coordinate/consolidate care activities with the multidisciplinary team as much as possible and try to have the same staff caring of the child. | Children, especially younger children, become agitated easily in the hospital, especially with frequent encounters with health care team. This increases their respiratory effort and rate as well their energy/oxygen demands. Decreased encounters and familiar staff caring for the children help decrease their respiratory effort and agitation, promote rest, and increase comfort, thus decreasing their oxygen demand. |

## Patient Problem/Analyze Cues/Prioritize Hypotheses

# Body Weight Problem (Weight Loss)

*due to* decreased appetite (advanced disease) or increased metabolic requirements because of increased work of breathing, infection, fatigue, sleep disruptions, and/or malabsorption

***Desired Outcome/Generate Solutions:*** By hospital discharge or within 7 days after treatment/intervention, the child/patient maintains or gains weight and does not have more than two or three stools per day.

| ASSESSMENT—RECOGNIZE CUES/INTERVENTIONS—TAKE ACTION | RATIONALES |
|---|---|
| Assess the daily weight measurements in the hospital and teach the importance of weekly weight measurements at home. | This assesses the effectiveness of nutritional interventions. If the child is losing weight, he or she may not be receiving adequate nutrients or may not be absorbing nutrients properly. |
| Administer the pancreatic enzymes with meals and snacks per the health care provider's prescription if the child has pancreatic insufficiency (most children with CF experience this). | Replacement of enzymes is necessary for proper digestion and absorption of nutrients. Failure to replace pancreatic enzymes would affect the child's growth and ability to fight infection. |
| For young children unable to swallow a capsule, mix powder, granules, or contents of the capsule with a small amount of soft acidic food like applesauce. Follow the administration of enzymes in a small amount of food quickly with infant formula or breast milk. | Protein foods break down this enzyme and can burn the mouth of infants and young children. Using the smallest amount of food possible (e.g., 1–2 tsp of applesauce) helps ensure that the child receives all the medication and following administration with infant formula or breast milk helps ensure digestion. |
| Do not administer enzymes with formula/milk in a bottle or cup. | Pancreatic enzymes curdle milk and formula. In addition, the child may not receive all the medication and may not take the milk/formula in the future if he or she associates it with medication. |
| Monitor and document the frequency and appearance of stools. | Pancreatic enzymes are adjusted to provide normal stooling (i.e., decreased enzymes given with constipation; increased enzymes given with frequent, bulky, foul-smelling stools that float). Normal stooling indicates increased absorption of nutrients. |
| Provide a well-balanced, high-calorie, high-protein, medium- to high-fat diet (require 110%–200% of normal caloric intake/recommended daily allowance). | The severity of lung disease and the degree of impaired intestinal absorption determine each child's needs. |
| Provide adequate salt, especially with fever, hot weather, or exercise. | The child/patient is at risk for electrolyte imbalance (hyponatremia) because sodium concentration in the sweat of a child with CF is 2–5 times greater than that of a child without CF. |
| Administer the supplemental tube feedings (nasogastric tube [NGT] or gastric tube [GT]) or parenteral nutrition (PN) as prescribed. | Measures described in previous interventions alone are not always effective in the child exhibiting FTT. Supplemental feedings through NGT, GT, or PN provide increased calories to treat malnutrition. |
| If prescribed, administer GER medications in a timely manner. | Some reflux medications need to be given before meals or with meals to be most effective. |
| Position/encourage the child to maintain an upright position during and for 1 or 2 hours after eating/receiving enteral feeding and encourage decreased activity. | Lying down during or right after eating increases the risk for reflux, which can increase the risk for respiratory infections. Decreasing activity/energy demands can reduce energy expenditure and decrease the likelihood of emesis after enteral feeding. |

## Patient/Parent Problem/Analyze Cues/Prioritize Hypotheses

# Deficient Knowledge

*due to* unfamiliarity with the purpose, precautions, and potential side effects of prescribed medications

***Desired Outcome/Generate Solutions:*** Within 1 week of diagnosis or change in medication, the patient/parent verbalizes accurate information about the prescribed medications.

| ASSESSMENT—RECOGNIZE CUES/ INTERVENTIONS—TAKE ACTION | RATIONALES |
|---|---|
| **Teach the Following to the Patient/Parent for the Prescribed Medications:** | |
| **Aerosolized Bronchodilators: Albuterol** | This medication helps open the bronchi for easier expectoration of mucus. The route is by nebulizer or metered-dose inhalers (MDIs). |
| • Be alert for and report excitement, nervousness, pharyngitis, bronchospasm, shakiness, palpitations, increased HR, tremors, nausea, and headache. | These are side effects that may indicate the need for dosage adjustment. These are potential side effects and vary with different age groups, e.g., tremor frequency increases with age, excitement occurs in children 2–14 years, and shakiness in children 6–14 years. Side effects also vary with dosage and route of administration (American Pharmacists Association [APhA], 2021). |
| • Be alert for and report nervousness, central nervous system (CNS) stimulation, hyperactivity, and insomnia. | These are side effects that occur more often in younger children than in adults. |
| • Use with caution in patients with cardiovascular disease. | Side effects from these medications are more significant in patients with cardiovascular disease, high blood pressure, or heart failure (APhA, 2021). |
| • All of the previous symptoms may occur with the MDI or nebulization. Notify the prescriber if they persist. | All of these side effects may indicate the need for dosage adjustment or the need for a change in the medication prescribed. |
| • If using an MDI, use with a spacer or holding chamber. Children younger than 4 years need a face mask along with the spacer or holding chamber. | These devices increase drug delivery and efficiency. |
| • Limit caffeinated beverages. | Caffeine may increase side effects such as CNS stimulation and insomnia. |
| • Do not take with beta-adrenergic blocking agents (e.g., propranolol), monoamine oxidase inhibitors (MAOIs), or tricyclic antidepressants. | Propranolol antagonizes the action of albuterol. MAOIs potentiate sympathomimetic effects. Tricyclic antidepressants increase cardiovascular effects. |
| • Do not take with other sympathomimetics. | Albuterol increases cardiovascular effects. |
| • Rinse mouth with water after each inhalation of the MDI. | Rinsing helps moisten a dry mouth and throat |
| **Aerosolized Mucolytic Enzymes: Dornase Alfa (Pulmozyme)** | This medication thins secretions and optimally decreases the number of pulmonary infections. APhA (2021) lists dosages for children 2 to less than 5 years in select patients. Other references specify ranges for infants and children under 2 (Altaf & Parmar, 2022). |
| • Use with an appropriate nebulizer system with a compressor. | A nebulizer unit is available that is made specifically to administer this medication. Patients unable to inhale and exhale for the duration of the whole treatment can use a specialized baby nebulizer. |
| • Be alert to and report pharyngitis, rhinitis, chest pain, voice alteration, rash, hoarseness, and conjunctivitis. | Typically the most common side effects, mild and subside within a few weeks. |
| | **Warning**: Use with caution in infants and children less than 5 years. Safety studies included infants down to 3 months old with some adverse side effects. Some side effects occur more often in younger children than in children 5–10 years of age: cough and rhinitis (APhA, 2021). |

Continued

| ASSESSMENT—RECOGNIZE CUES/ INTERVENTIONS—TAKE ACTION | RATIONALES |
|---|---|
| • Do not dilute or mix with other medications in the nebulizer. | These actions may deactivate the enzyme. |
| • Store ampules in the refrigerator in the foil packet, protected from light and discard if unopened vials are subjected to room temperature for more than 60 hours. | Room temperature may deactivate the medication. |
| • Protect from strong light. Discard the solution if it is cloudy or discolored. | These are signs that the medication may be deactivated. |
| • Use before doing airway clearance techniques | This enhances the effectiveness of the medication. |
| **Oral Inhalation Antibiotics: Tobramycin (e.g., TOBI or TOBI Podhaler)** | These medications help fight *Pseudomonas aeruginosa* infections, which would cause an increase in symptoms. They are FDA approved for adults and children 6 years and older. |
| • Be alert to and report hoarseness, rhinitis, CF exacerbations, shortness of breath, increased and/or productive cough, nosebleed or coughing up blood, sore throat, fever, headache, and pharyngitis. | These are the most common potential side effects of tobramycin by oral inhalation. <br> **Note**: Cough more frequent with powder/Podhaler. |
| • Be alert and report immediately hearing loss or ringing in the ears, increased kidney problems in patients with known or suspected renal issues, worsening muscle weakness in patients with neuromuscular disorders, or severe breathing problems (bronchospasm or wheezing). | These serious side effects are listed under **Warnings/Precautions**, and the health care provider may need to see the patient or adjust the medication. <br> **Warning**: When using TOBI Podhaler (oral capsule powder for inhalation), taste disturbance was reported 2 ½ times more often in children 6 or older than in adults (APhA, 2021). |
| • Store TOBI in the refrigerator. Date and time the drug when removing it from the refrigerator. | TOBI can be used for only 28 days when stored at room temperature (no more than 77°F [25°C]). |
| • Do not use TOBI if the medication is cloudy or contains particles. | These are signs the medication may not work as effectively. |
| • Protect TOBI from intense light. | Light adversely affects TOBI. |
| • Do not take with dornase alfa (Pulmozyme). | When tobramycin and Pulmozyme are mixed, a precipitate may form. |
| • Administer TOBI with the appropriate nebulizer system. | Medication may not be nebulized properly if it is not administered with the appropriate delivery system. |
| • Take the bronchodilator first, then mucolytics (hypertonic saline first, then dornase alfa), then chest physiotherapy, and inhaled tobramycin last. <br> Both forms of this medication need to be taken 12 hours apart and are given in cycles for 28 days and then off for 28 days. | This is the most effective method of administration because when airways are clear, absorption of TOBI is enhanced. <br> Taking this inhaled antibiotic every 12 hours provides maximum benefit. The cycle of 28 days on and 28 days off is the current standard of care for CF patients infected with *P. aeruginosa* (APhA, 2021). |
| • Administer TOBI Podhaler capsules by oral inhalation using Podhaler device, adhering to manufacturer's guidelines for use and handling. | Medication may not be inhaled properly if it is administered without the appropriate delivery system. |
| • Remove the capsule from blister packaging immediately before use. | Medication may not be as effective if not prepared properly. |
| • Inhale the entire contents of the capsule. | Medication may not be as effective if any is left in the capsule. |
| • Administer the TOBI Podhaler within 15–90 minutes after a bronchodilator and administer it last. | This is the most effective method of administration because when airways are clear, absorption of TOBI Podhaler is enhanced. |
| • Ensure that the serum aminoglycoside level is monitored for patients on high-dose aerosolized tobramycin. | This identifies patients who are significant absorbers and may be at risk for ototoxicity and nephrotoxicity. |
| **Pancreatic Enzymes** | These enzymes increase food and nutrient digestion and absorption. |
| • As prescribed, take with meals and snacks within 30 minutes of eating. | Taking enzymes in this manner promotes degradation and absorption of the nutrients just consumed. |

| ASSESSMENT—RECOGNIZE CUES/ INTERVENTIONS—TAKE ACTION | RATIONALES |
| --- | --- |
| • If the patient is an infant or young child, open the capsule and give it in a small amount of nonfat, nonprotein, acidic food (e.g., 1–2 tsp applesauce) at room temperature. | Protein/alkaline foods break down this enzyme and can burn the mouth in an infant/young child. |
| • Administer immediately after mixing or within 15 minutes. | The enzymes may be inactivated in the mixture if not administered quickly and thus, not provide maximum benefit. |
| Follow with breast milk or infant formula to ensure infant or young child received all the enzyme | This ensures complete ingestion and no enzymes remain in the mouth to cause irritation and burning. |
| • Do not mix with milk or formula. | Pancreatic enzymes curdle milk or formula. |
| • Do not chew microspheres or microtabs; swallow capsules or tablets whole. | Chewing or mouth retention before swallowing may cause mucosal irritation and stomatitis. |
| • Monitor stools for frequency and appearance. | Constipation or increased stooling (usually more than 3 stools/day) indicates need to adjust dosage. |
| • Be alert for and report headache, abdominal pain, hyperglycemia, diarrhea, gas, neck pain, nasal congestion, indigestion, and cough. | These are some of the most common side effects and may indicate the need to change the type of enzyme taken or dosage adjustment. Side effects may vary depending on the brand of enzyme taken. |
| • Notify the prescriber if the patient is taking histamine-2 antagonists or gastric acid pump inhibitors (e.g., ranitidine, cimetidine, and omeprazole). | These agents increase the effectiveness of pancreatic enzymes; dosage adjustment may be needed. |
| • Enzymes should not be refrigerated and kept away from heat. | Storing the enzymes properly will improve their effectiveness. Heat will destroy the activity of the enzymes. |
| • They have an expiration date and that should be checked regularly. | The medication may not be as effective after the expiration date. |
| Protect from moisture. Be sure to keep the lid on the bottle tightly sealed after it is opened. | Storing the enzymes properly will improve their effectiveness. |
| **Cystic Fibrosis Transmembrane Conductance Regulator Potentiator/ Modulator: Ivacaftor (Kalydeco)** | There are four CFTR modulators currently. Ivacaftor was the first modulator approved in 2012 by the FDA to treat the underlying cause of CF. It is now approved for 97 specified mutations for use in children 4 months and older (weighing 5 kg or more). The route is oral (APhA, 2021; CFF, n.d.c). |
| • Be alert for and report upper respiratory tract infections (e.g., common cold), oropharyngeal pain, headache, nasopharyngitis or nasal congestion, stomachache, rash, nausea, diarrhea, or dizziness. | These are the most common side effects. |
| • Monitor the liver function tests initially, then every 3 months for the first year, and yearly thereafter. | **Warning/Precautions**: This medication may increase hepatic transaminases. Use with caution with patients with moderate to severe hepatic impairment (APhA, 2021). |
| • Monitor for and immediately report to the health care provider abdominal pain in the right upper abdomen; yellowing of the skin or whites of the eyes; loss of appetite; nausea or vomiting; or dark, amber-colored urine. | These are signs of serious adverse effects involving liver impairment. |
| • Baseline and follow-up eye examinations are recommended in pediatric patients. | **Warnings/Precautions**: Noncongenital cataracts have been reported in pediatric patients taking this medication (APhA, 2021). |
| • This medication interacts with numerous medications. | See a drug book for more detailed information. |
| • Do not take with grapefruit or Seville oranges. | These foods/juices increase the serum concentration of this medication. |
| • For oral granules: Administer before or after high fat–containing foods (e.g., butter, eggs, cheese pizza, and whole milk products). Mix the entire packet with a teaspoon for soft food (e.g., pureed fruits or vegetables, yogurt, applesauce), or 5 mL of liquid (e.g., water, low-fat milk, breast milk, infant formula, or juice). Food or liquid must be at or below room temperature and consumed within 1 hour of mixing with granules. | Medication may not be as effective if not administered properly. |
| • For oral tablets: Administer with high fat–containing foods (e.g., butter, cheese pizza, eggs, peanut butter, and avocado). | |
| Administer medication doses 12 hours apart. | |

Continued

## ASSESSMENT—RECOGNIZE CUES/ INTERVENTIONS—TAKE ACTION

## RATIONALES

- **For Ivacaftor (Kalydeco):** Observe for healthy weight gain.

Improved lung function and decreased sweat chloride levels help patients gain weight and are indicators of the effectiveness of this medication.

### Lumacaftor/Ivacaftor (Orkambi)

Currently approved for treatment of CF patients who are homozygous for the F508del mutation in the CFTR gene. About 44% of people with CF are homozygous for this mutation. (CFF, 2022; Stewart, 2022).

- Be alert for and report chest discomfort, upper abdominal pain, nausea, diarrhea, shortness of breath, upper respiratory infection, increased bronchial secretions, nasal congestion, fatigue, headache, skin rash, or menstrual problems.

These are the most common side effects.

- Monitor ALST, AST, and bilirubin initially, then every 3 months for the first year, and yearly thereafter.

**Warning/Precautions**: This medication may increase hepatic transaminases with or without elevation in total bilirubin. Use with caution with patients with moderate to severe hepatic impairment. (APhA, 2021).

- All other assessments/interventions the same as for Ivacaftor.

Combining two medications may change some of the side effects, while some remain the same.

### Tezacaftor/Ivacaftor (Symdeko®)

Improved FDA-approved combination therapy for individuals 6 years old or older who are homozygous for F508del mutation or individuals with 1 of 154 specified mutations. (CFF, n.d.c; APhA, 2021).

- Be alert for any report of headache, nausea, dizziness, and paranasal sinus congestion.

Most common side effects.

Also see Ivacaftor side effect per APhA, 2021.

- Monitor ALST, AST, and bilirubin initially, then every 3 months for the first year, and yearly thereafter.

**Warning/Precautions**: This medication may increase hepatic transaminases with or without elevation in total bilirubin. Use with caution with patients with moderate to severe hepatic impairment. (APhA, 2021).

- All other assessments/interventions are the same as for Ivacaftor, still interacts with numerous medications but fewer than Ivacaftor, and only comes in tablet form.

Improved combination of two medications changed some of the side effects but additional assessments/interventions unchanged.

- Swallow tablet whole.

Ensure maximum benefit of medication.

Crushing or chewing the tablet may cause increased side effects.

### Elexacaftor/tezacaftor/Ivacaftor (Trikafta®)

First triple combination therapy approved by FDA in October 2019, now approved for ages 6 and older with at least one copy of the F508del mutation or at least one copy of 177 specified mutations. The F508del mutation affects about 85% of individuals with CF (CFF, n.d.c.; CFF, 2022).

- Monitor for and report headache, upper respiratory tract infection, abdominal pain, diarrhea, rashes, nasal congestion, watery nasal drainage, nasal congestion, influenza, sinus congestion, and increased indirect serum bilirubin.

Most common side effects.

- All other assessments/interventions are the same as for Ivacaftor, except it comes in tablet form.

The combination of three medications changed some of the side effects and, thus, some interventions.

- Swallow tablet whole.

Ensure maximum benefit of the medications.

Crushing or chewing the tablet may cause increased side effects.

### Vitamins/Minerals

They supplement the overall diet.

- Take fat-soluble vitamins in water-miscible form (i.e., mixed in a suspension that will not separate) as prescribed.

This action counteracts the malabsorption of fat-soluble vitamins (A, D, E, and K). Examples of water-miscible forms of vitamins include Aquasol A and ADEK.

- Use iron preparations as prescribed.

Malabsorption can cause iron deficiency. Review a drug handbook for more detailed information.

### Antibiotics—Usually Intravenous (IV) (e.g., Ticarcillin and Tobramycin)

These medications are used to treat infections.

| ASSESSMENT—RECOGNIZE CUES/ INTERVENTIONS—TAKE ACTION | RATIONALES |
|---|---|
| • Take as prescribed, usually for at least 10 days and often for several weeks. | Children with CF have frequent respiratory infections and often develop drug resistance. Antibiotics may need to be given for an extended period of time. |
| • Monitor for side effects specific to each individual antibiotic. | Side effects vary, depending on the specific antibiotic. |
| • Monitor the IV site for signs and symptoms of infection (e.g., redness, tenderness, or drainage) and ensure that the dressing is dry and clean at least before and after administration of the antibiotic and/or twice a day. | Home IV antibiotics are usually given through a PICC line or an implanted port. They are less likely to be pulled out than a peripheral IV but can become infected. Both require special care that will be detailed by health care provider. |
| **Azithromycin (oral antibiotic)** | Studies have shown an improvement in lung function and reduction pulmonary exacerbations, in children 6 years or older (APhA, 2021). It is used for its antiinflammatory effects. Consult a drug handbook for more detailed information. |
| **Nonsteroidal Antiinflammatory Drugs (e.g., Ibuprofen)** | Studies have shown a slowed rate of pulmonary decline when taking Ibuprofen in children 6–17 years with mild disease (APhA, 2021). High doses are needed for several years and reduce inflammation in the lungs but not prescribed often due to side effects associated with high doses like kidney problems and ulcers (CFF, n.d.d). Consult a drug handbook for more detailed information. Also see "Osteoarthritis," Chapter 71 for side effects and precautions with these medications. |

## ADDITIONAL PROBLEMS:

| | |
|---|---|
| "Psychosocial Support for the Patient" for relevant clinical problems that pertain to the patient's psychologic status in dealing with a chronic and potentially fatal illness, such as *Fatigue, Anxiety, Difficulty Coping, Anticipatory Grief,* and *Risk for Social Isolation.* | Chapter 8 |
| "Psychosocial Support for the Patient's Family and Significant Other" for relevant clinical problems for family members dealing with a chronic and potentially fatal illness in their loved one, such as *Anxiety, Difficulty Coping,* and *Grief.* **Note**: Parents are also fatigued and at risk for social isolation from care demands. | Chapter 9 |
| "Diabetes Mellitus" for *Risk for Infection* due to chronic disease process. | Chapter 47 |
| "Asthma" for *Anxiety.* | Chapter 77 |
| "Burns" for *Low Self-Esteem* for patients with CF. This could entail delayed puberty, copious sputum and chronic cough, inability to maintain weight, and/or possible presence of a GT and/or long-term central access IV. | Chapter 80 |

## ✔ PATIENT–FAMILY TEACHING AND DISCHARGE PLANNING

When providing child/family teaching, focus on sensory data, avoid excessive information, and initiate a visiting nurse referral for necessary follow-up assessment and teaching as needed. Utilize a variety of teaching methods (e.g., videos, iPad/tablets, and webinars as well as verbal and written) depending on learning style and resources of child/family. Stress family-centered care (viewing the family as a unit that is the "constant" in the child's life and maintaining or improving the health of the family and its members in a holistic manner). Include information about the following and ensure that written information is at a level the reader can understand:

✓ Basic information about the disease process with emphasis on respiratory and gastrointestinal (GI) components.
✓ Maintenance and exacerbation aspects of this chronic disease process.
✓ Diet, including rationale for increased calories, protein, and fat (usually two to three snacks/day).
✓ Administration of pancreatic enzymes such as Creon with meals and snacks (usually a fractional dose given with snacks).
  • If the patient is an infant or young child, may mix contents of capsule, granules, or powder with a small amount of applesauce or other acidic soft food or per specific guidelines for that form of enzyme.

Follow the administration of enzymes in a small amount of food quickly with infant formula or breast milk
  • Do not chew or bite capsule or enteric-coated microspheres.
  • Do not administer in a bottle or cup with fluid.
✓ Need for salt replacement and free access for the child to salt, especially during hot weather, fever, diarrhea, or vomiting.
✓ GI symptoms that signal malabsorption and inadequate enzyme replacement (e.g., bloating, abdominal cramping and distention, and diarrhea).
✓ Need to monitor stools (constipation indicates too much enzyme; frequent fatty loose stools indicate insufficient enzyme).

✓ Administration of nebulizer treatment and chest physiotherapy (i.e., chest percussion and postural drainage, mucus clearance device [e.g., Flutter, Acapella] or a vest airway clearance system [e.g., the vest]). Albuterol nebulizer treatment is done first (1 hour before or 2 hours after meals), then take mucolytic–hypertonic saline and then nebulized Pulmozyme. Chest physiotherapy and suctioning or coughing are administered next and followed by the nebulized antibiotic. Make sure to use the appropriate nebulizer unit with each of the previous medications (they all need different nebulizer units). Stress the importance of routine pulmonary toilet, because thickened mucus is an ideal medium for bacterial growth, which causes pulmonary infections. Also emphasize oral hygiene to prevent oral ulcers and sore throat.

✓ Cleaning and care of equipment (e.g., spacers, nebulizer attachments for albuterol, Pulmozyme, hypertonic saline, and TOBI).

✓ Medications, including drug name; route; purpose; dosage; precautions; drug–drug, food–drug, and herb–drug interactions; and potential adverse effects.

✓ Importance of taking medications at home and at school as directed. Medication in the original container (with prescribing label) and written prescription from the health care provider are needed for the child to be able to take medications at school.

✓ Importance of regular medical follow-up care:
   • Routine immunizations plus pneumococcal polysaccharide vaccination and yearly influenza vaccination
   • Prompt attention to infection (fever, increased coughing, and green sputum)
   • Regular visits with the health care provider

✓ Team care approach, including pediatrician, school nurse and teachers, pulmonologist, or infectious disease physician. Ensure that a genetic referral is made.

✓ Realistic expectations for the child, especially concerning growth and development, participation in school activities and sports, and the child's participation/responsibility for self-care.

✓ Child's legal rights: Section 504 of Rehabilitation Act of 1973. Each student with a disability (physical or mental impairment) is entitled to accommodation in order to attend school and participate as fully as possible in school activities. A child with significant pulmonary involvement may need to be excused from class for 15–30 minutes after receiving a nebulizer treatment and chest physiotherapy because of excessive coughing and expectoration of mucus, or the class schedule might need to be rearranged to accommodate the required treatment (https://www.cff.org/individualized-education-programs-ieps-and-504-plans).

✓ Importance of avoiding environmental exposure to tobacco smoke.

✓ Importance of having yearly screening examinations for depression and anxiety in children 12 years and older as well as their caregivers (Castellani et al., 2018; CFF, 2022).

✓ Telephone numbers to call in case questions or concerns arise about therapy or disease after discharge.

✓ When to call the health care provider:
   • Increased respiratory effort (e.g., increased RR, nasal flaring, and retractions).
   • Excessive coughing and/or coughing up blood.
   • Color change: pallor or cyanosis (blue mucous membranes/lips/tongue or around the eyes). Stress that this is a late sign of a problem.
   • Temperature increase to greater than 101.5°F (38.6°C) lasting more than a few days or a low-grade fever lasting for a week or more or per health care provider's guidelines.
   • Weight loss
   • Abdominal pain or distention, with or without constipation

✓ Referral to community resources such as support groups, specialists working with children affected by CF, CF care center if available, and genetic counselors.

✓ Additional information can be obtained by contacting:
   • Cystic Fibrosis Foundation: https://www.cff.org.
   • Information for the Airway Clearance Therapy using HFCWO
      – Vest Airway Clearance System: https://www.hillrom.com/en/products/the-vest-system-105/# or (800)426-4224
      – Mobile mechanical oscillation therapy: https://www.afflovest.com or call 800-575-1900
   • Compass: https://www.cff.org/support/get-help-cf-foundation-compass or 844-COMPASS (844-266-7277). This program provides personalized service to assist with insurance, financial, legal, and other issues facing families.
   • Managing Cystic Fibrosis-Related Diabetes (CFRD): An Instruction Guide for Parents and Families, 6th (ed.) (2015) and other information per CFRD: https://www.cff.org/managing-cf/cystic-fibrosis-related-diabetes.
   • Stay CF Smart: Eugene the Gene educational series—Animated videos and/or comic book stories to get children familiar with CF from an early age: https://www.cfsource.com/videos-resources#CF-Behind-the-scenes-with-Eugene.

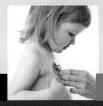

# Diabetes Mellitus in Children 83

## OVERVIEW/PATHOPHYSIOLOGY

Diabetes mellitus (DM) is the most common childhood endocrine disorder and one of the costliest chronic diseases of childhood. It is a disorder of carbohydrate metabolism marked by hyperglycemia and glycosuria, and it results from inadequate production or use of insulin. The major classifications seen in children are as follows:

- **Type 1 DM:** There is an absolute deficiency of insulin secretion resulting from the destruction of beta cells, causing hyperglycemia and ketosis. This destruction is often an immune-mediated or related response. Previously, it was called *insulin-dependent DM (IDDM)* or *juvenile-onset diabetes*. Historically, this was the primary type of diabetes seen in children and one of the most common chronic disorders of childhood. According to the Centers for Disease Control and Prevention (CDC) National Diabetes Statistics Report: Prevalence of Diagnosed Diabetes (2022a), in 2019, approximately 283,000 people younger than 20 years had diabetes (types 1 and 2) in the United States, and about 86% of them had type 1 diabetes. There was a significant increase in this age group between 2002 and 2015 except for those under 5 years and American Indians, mainly from one southwestern tribe. The highest incidence was in Asians/Pacific Islanders, Hispanics, and non-Hispanic Blacks (CDC, 2022b). These children and adolescents are dependent on insulin for survival and to prevent diabetic ketoacidosis (DKA). Individuals diagnosed with type 1 DM in childhood have a high risk for early cardiovascular disease (CVD), and the American Heart Association ranks children with type 1 DM in the highest tier of risk for CVD.
- **Type 2 DM:** There is an insulin resistance with this type, so there is a relative, not absolute, and insulin deficiency. Previously, this was called *non-IDDM* or *adult-onset DM*. Since the 1990s there has been an alarming epidemic of children developing type 2 DM. The SEARCH for Diabetes in

Youth study from 2000 to 2020 notes that racial and ethnic minorities have the highest incidence of youth-onset type 2 diabetes and that the incidence increases with age. The study also noted a significantly increased incidence in all races except White non-Hispanic, with the most prominent in non-Hispanic Blacks, followed by American Indian youth, youth of Hispanic origin, and Asian/Pacific Islander youth in 2017. The study projects a fourfold increase in the prevalence of youth-based type 2 diabetes in the United States by 2050 after accounting for anticipated changes in demography (Perng et al., 2023). Being overweight is a strong risk factor for type 2 DM. In the past, less than 5% of children were diagnosed with type 2 DM. Now, largely because of the obesity epidemic, the number of children and adolescents with type 2 DM have been steadily increasing. The prevalence of obesity in youth 2–19 years in 2017–2020 was greatest in Hispanic children, about 26%, and lowest in non-Hispanic Asian children, about 9%, with the highest percentage in adolescents 12–19 years (CDC, 2022c). Sedentary lifestyle, nonideal diet, and exposure to tobacco are other significant risk factors. Additional risk factors include genetics (e.g., family members with type 2 DM and female gender) and environmental/socioeconomic factors (health insurance, poverty/low socioeconomic status, and stress). The American Diabetes Association (ADA) 2023 Standards of Medical Care notes the importance of assessing the patient/family's financial barriers to care, individualizing treatment of patients with type 2 DM, and the use of diabetes technology. Studies show that some children with type 1 DM, those from low-income, using public insurance, and certain patient groups, including non-Hispanic Black children, are not benefiting from the advances in technology and that diabetes control in type 1 DM in youth is no better than in 2001 (Endocrinology Network Staff, 2022; Lipman and Hawkes, 2021).

> **Note:** *It can be difficult to distinguish between types 1 and 2 DM due to the current obesity epidemic. Diabetes-associated autoantibodies and ketosis may be present in pediatric children and adolescents with clinical features of type 2 DM (including acanthosis nigricans and obesity). Neither type 1 nor 2 DM in children are the same as type 1 or type 2 DM in adults (American Diabetes Association [ADA], 2023).*

- **Neonatal diabetes:** Most often occurs before 6 months of age and is called "neonatal" or "congenital." It rarely occurs after 6 months, and type 1 diabetes rarely occurs before 6 months. It may be transient or permanent, and each is caused by a different gene mutation.
- **Mature-onset diabetes of youth:** This type involves impaired insulin secretion with minimal or no defects in insulin action (in the absence of obesity), usually occurring in individuals younger than 25 years. Symptoms vary depending on the specific gene mutation. It is inherited by an autosomal dominant pattern.
- **Cystic fibrosis–related diabetes (CFRD):** This is one of the most common comorbidities in people with CF. According to the 2021 CFF Patient Registry Annual Data Summary, about 5% of children under age 18 had CFRD with an impaired glucose tolerance more prevalent in adolescents. The report also found that 29% of adults had CFRD but noted that patients that have received lung transplants are no longer included in the % of patients with CFRD. Thus this report shows a lower incidence of CFRD. CFRD shares features with type 1 and type 2 DM, with the primary cause being insulin insufficiency, but insulin resistance also can occur (2022).
- For information on other types, see the adult "Diabetes Mellitus" care plan, Chapter 47, and "Diabetes in Pregnancy," Chapter 90.

## HEALTH CARE SETTING

Primary care, with possible hospital admission because of complications.

## ASSESSMENT

*Signs and symptoms.* These are the same as in the adult DM care plan, except children with type 2 DM usually have hypertension, dyslipidemia, acanthosis nigricans (hypertrophy or thickening of skin with gray, brown, or black pigmentation chiefly in the axilla, other body folds, and sometimes on hands, elbows, and knees), and polycystic ovary syndrome. Females may have vaginitis because of long-standing glycosuria. DKA also may occur in children and adolescents.

## COMPLICATIONS

*Potential for acute crisis.* This is the same as in the adult DM care plan with the addition of cerebral edema in DKA, which occurs more often in children than in adults. Cerebral edema is an uncommon but dangerous consequence of DKA with a mortality rate of 20%–25%. Significant cerebral edema occurs in less than 1% of pediatric DKA cases. The children most at risk for developing cerebral edema are younger and recently diagnosed with diabetes (Glaser, 2022). The 2023 Children and Adolescents: Standards of Care in Diabetes also mentions the possible adverse neurocognitive effects of DKA.

*Long-term complications.* These are the same as in adults, but the micro and macro complications are very aggressive in children with type 2 DM. They occur over a much shorter time frame and the following complications refer to type 2 DM unless noted otherwise. Some children are showing signs of long-term complications when diagnosed. Diabetic retinopathy, the most common complication, may be found during diagnosis and increases over time, with higher incidence with type 2 DM versus type 1 DM. Incidence of nephropathy increases with time with the earliest symptom being microalbuminuria. Diabetic neuropathy rarely occurs in youth but the risk increases with longer duration. Many children have hypertension when diagnosed and this increases the incidence of CVD, retinopathy, and albuminuria (Gonzalez & Freysteinson, 2019; Perng et al., 2023). The progression of vascular abnormalities seems to be higher in type 2 DM than in type 1 of similar duration (e.g., ischemic heart disease and stroke). With type 1 DM, screening for nephropathy, retinopathy, and neuropathy should start after 10–11 years of age or puberty, whichever is earlier, and after 3–5 years of diabetes duration. Children with type 2 DM should have screening for nephropathy, neuropathy, and retinopathy at diagnosis and yearly afterward (ADA, 2023).

> **Note:** *Celiac disease occurs with increased frequency in patients with type 1 DM (1.6%–16.4% of individuals compared with 0.3%–1% in the general population) per the ADA (2023).*

The ADA position paper on the evaluation of Youth-Onset Type 2 Diabetes notes that youth with type 1 diabetes have high rates of diabetes distress, psychiatric symptoms, and diagnoses (e.g., depression and disordered eating behaviors). Symptoms of depression and disordered eating habits are common in youth with type 2 diabetes and are associated with poor glycemic control (Arslanian et al., 2018).

Studies show note that symptoms of depression are present more than twice as much in adolescents with type 2 diabetes than in the general population of adolescents or adults with diabetes. Another study documented that twice as many youths with type 2 diabetes showed symptoms of depression as those with type 1 diabetes (Gonzalez and Freysteinson, 2019).

## DIAGNOSTIC TESTS

The ADA published the most recent *Standards of Medical Care in Diabetes* in 2023. It incorporates the 2018 ADA position statements "Type 1 Diabetes in Children and Adolescents" and "Evaluation and Management of Youth-Onset Type 2 Diabetes."

*Hemoglobin A₁c (HbA₁c):* Value of 6.5% or higher (test must be performed in an appropriately certified laboratory). *OR*

*Fasting plasma glucose.* Will reveal a value of 126 mg/dL or higher. Fasting is defined as no caloric intake for at least 8 hours. *OR*

*Two-hour postprandial plasma glucose.* Will reveal a value of 200 mg/dL or greater during oral glucose tolerance test. *OR*

*Random/casual plasma glucose.* Symptoms of diabetes (polyuria, polydipsia, polyphagia, unexplained weight loss, or hyperglycemic crisis) and a random/casual plasma glucose of 200 mg/dL or greater are diagnostic of diabetes.

Risk-based screening recommendations (ADA, 2023) for type 2 DM or prediabetes in asymptomatic children and adolescents in a clinical setting:

- Overweight with body mass index (BMI) greater than 85th percentile or obese with a body mass and greater than 95% percentile.
- PLUS at least one or more of the following risk factors depending on the degree of their association with diabetes:
  - Maternal history of diabetes or GDM during the child's gestation
  - Family history of type 2 DM in first- or second-degree relatives
  - Belonging to certain race/ethnic groups (Native American, African American, Latino, Asian American, and Pacific Islander)
  - Signs of insulin resistance or conditions associated with insulin resistance such as acanthosis nigricans, hypertension, dyslipidemia, polycystic ovarian syndrome, or small-for-gestational birth weight

Additional risk factors include female gender and low socioeconomic status.

- Begin screening: Age 10 years or at puberty (if puberty begins at an earlier age).
- If the initial test is normal, testing should be done at least every 3 years or more often if BMI is increasing or risk factors increase.

*Fasting lipid panel if type 2 DM suspected.* Dyslipidemia is frequently seen in children with type 2 DM and also needs to be treated. Values vary depending on the age of the child and on whether the reference range is in conventional units or international units.

*Basic metabolic panel (electrolytes, glucose, blood urea nitrogen, and creatinine).* Serum glucose will be elevated, usually greater than 250 mg/dL. Sodium and potassium may be lost because of osmotic diuresis. The higher the glucose level, the greater the dehydration and loss of electrolytes. Serum potassium may be normal on admission, but after fluid and insulin administration, rapid return of potassium to the cells decreases serum potassium, which necessitates monitoring

for cardiac dysrhythmias. Blood urea nitrogen and creatinine likely will be elevated because of dehydration. Also, renal dysfunction occurs when the serum glucose level rises to greater than 600 mg/dL.

*Thyroid-stimulating hormone and thyroxine.* Thyroid hormone increases gluconeogenesis (synthesis of glucose from noncarbohydrate sources such as amino acids and glycerol) and peripheral use of glucose. An elevated or decreased value would affect carbohydrate metabolism and, therefore, plasma glucose. Normal range varies for children depending on their age and the type of reference units reported. Thyroid autoantibodies occur in about 25% of children with type 1 DM at the time of diagnosis. The presence of these autoantibodies is predictive of thyroid dysfunction (ADA, 2023).

*Ketones.* Elevated when insulin is not available and when the body starts to break down stored fats for energy. Ketone bodies are by-products of this fat breakdown, and they accumulate in the blood and urine. Normal range for children is 0 with the qualitative test and 0.5–3 mg/dL (conventional units) or 5–30 mg/L (international units) with the quantitative test.

*Additional data.* *Normal plasma glucose:* A value less than 100 mg/dL.

*Impaired fasting glucose:* 100–125 mg/dL or impaired glucose tolerance if 2-hour postprandial plasma glucose is 140–199 mg/dL. Impaired fasting plasma glucose or impaired glucose tolerance should be monitored on a regular basis, but losing weight and increasing activity can prevent or delay the onset of DM.

*Hemoglobin$_{1c}$ A.* $_{1c}$Assesses control of blood glucose over the preceding 3 months. Normal range for Hemoglobin A$_{1c}$ (HbA$_{1c}$) is 4%–5.6%. The range in children in the past varied depending on age, with higher glucose levels allowed in younger children. The ADA (2023) recommends an A$_{1c}$ goal ranging from less than 7% to less than 8% in children with type 1 diabetes based on a benefit-risk assessment. The target would be highest (less than 8%) in children with a history of severe hypoglycemia, limited life expectancy, or where the harms of treatment are greater than the benefits. An appropriate target range for most children with type 2 diabetes is less than 7% with the less stringent goal of less than 7.5% if there is an increased risk of hypoglycemia. Some selected individual patients may have more stringent A$_{1c}$ goals of less than 6.5% for both types of diabetes. Current guidelines stress that the HbA$_{1c}$ target should be individualized to achieve the best control possible and reassessed over time while decreasing the risk for hypoglycemia (e.g., children younger than 6 years may experience "hypoglycemic unawareness") as well as maintaining normal growth and development.

## Patient/Parent Problem/Analyze Cues/Prioritize Hypotheses

# Deficient Knowledge

*due to* unfamiliarity with blood glucose monitoring

***Desired Outcome/Generate Hypotheses:*** Within 48 hours of this diagnosis, the child/parent demonstrates and verbalizes an accurate understanding of proper blood glucose monitoring and when to monitor for ketones.

| ASSESSMENT—RECOGNIZE CUES/ INTERVENTIONS—TAKE ACTION | RATIONALES |
|---|---|
| Assess the child's/parents' knowledge base about blood glucose monitoring. | Teaching can be more effective when the receiver's knowledge/ understanding has been established. |
| Discuss the reasons for blood glucose testing. | Understanding the purpose of performing tests facilitates adherence. Reasons for blood glucose testing include:<br>• Allows child to relate "how I feel at this time" with the actual blood glucose level.<br>• Gives the child/family some control.<br>• Enables understanding of the effects of food, exercise, insulin, and/ or stress.<br>• Enables adjustments in insulin or diet. |
| Demonstrate the correct use of a glucometer the child will use at home and the proper technique for fingerstick. | There are many different models and strips available commercially. Each system functions a little differently, and it could be overwhelming having to learn a new system at home without assistance or guidance. General guidelines include:<br>• Use side of finger, not the tip, for fingersticks. Sides of the fingers have fewer nerve endings and hurt less. In addition, using the sides decreases loss of sense of touch in fingertips.<br>• Clean hands with soap and warm water. Cleansing helps reduce the risk for infection. Warm water facilitates circulation and hence blood flow.<br>• Avoid the regular use of alcohol-based products to cleanse the skin. Any trace of alcohol left on the skin will interfere with the chemical reaction involved in checking blood glucose. It is okay to use occasionally (e.g., at a picnic), but the finger must be dried carefully and the first drop of blood discarded. Repeated use of alcohol also can lead to thickening of the skin, making fingerstick more difficult and painful.<br>• Hold the hand down, not up, to facilitate blood flow. Placing the hand on a tabletop before a fingerstick may help avoid the natural reflex to withdraw the finger and not get an adequate stick. |
| If the child is using an insulin pump and/or a continuous glucose monitoring (CGM) system, assess user/family understanding and use. | Reassessing child/family's understanding and use of diabetes technology facilitates appropriate application and utilization. A diabetes nurse educator or certified pump trainer is the best resource to assess and reinforce appropriate understanding and use. |
| Discuss when blood glucose testing should be done. | Knowledge and understanding facilitate adherence.<br>• Testing normally should be done at least before each meal and bedtime snack. Checking blood glucose on a regular basis and documenting findings help determine whether adjustments need to be made in insulin/diet/exercise/medication by assessing the pattern of blood glucose levels. The ADA (2023) recommends checking blood glucose up to 6–10 times a day with type 1 diabetes by glucose meter or CGM. |

| ASSESSMENT—RECOGNIZE CUES/ INTERVENTIONS—TAKE ACTION | RATIONALES |
|---|---|
| | • If the child is sick, blood glucose is checked every 2–4 hours. The risk for hyperglycemia is increased when the child is ill (e.g., with headache, fever, and sore throat) or has an infection owing to stress on the body and increased energy demands. Stress causes the adrenal glands to produce more epinephrine, norepinephrine, and cortisol. These stress hormones are "antiinsulin" in their actions, so blood glucose increases and ketones are formed by the liver, breaking down fat stores for energy. As blood glucose increases, the three *P*s (polydipsia, polyuria, and polyphagia) occur, causing dehydration as well as nausea and vomiting owing to ketosis. Blood glucose testing will determine whether changes need to be made in insulin dosage and whether the health care provider should be contacted. |
| | Blood glucose is checked with hypoglycemic or hyperglycemic symptoms to identify which event is occurring and therefore facilitate proper treatment. |
| Explain that if blood glucose is greater than 250–300 mg/dL depending on health care provider's guidelines or if the child is ill, urine should be checked for ketones with every void. | The body starts breaking down stored fats for energy because it cannot use blood glucose for energy. Ketone bodies are by-products of this fat breakdown and can lead to DKA if not controlled/treated. |
| Demonstrate the use of a diary or log to record blood glucose levels, ketones, insulin dose, diet, exercise, and any comments. | Information in this log provides a good overview of how the child is doing and assists the health care provider in making adjustments based on the pattern seen in the log/diary. Be sure to include the date and time of each entry. |
| Instruct the child/parent when to call the health care provider per blood glucose levels or ketones.<br><br>On sick days, instruct child/parent when to call the health care provider. | Understanding when to call improves adherence and decreases complications such as DKA:<br><br>• Blood glucose greater than 250 mg/dL three times in a row or per health care provider's guidelines. At least half of blood glucose values are not in desired range.<br><br>• Blood glucose less than 70 mg/dL twice in 1 week.<br><br>• Ketones moderate or large.<br><br>Understanding when to call improves adherence and decreases the risk of dehydration and DKA.<br><br>• All the above items per blood glucose levels and ketones<br><br>• Vomiting<br><br>• Frequent diarrhea (e.g., five or more times in 6 hours)<br><br>• Change in mental status<br><br>• Any questions or concerns |

## Patient/Parent/Family Problem/Analyze Cues/Prioritize Hypotheses

# Deficient Knowledge

*due to* unfamiliarity with causes, signs and symptoms, and treatment of hypoglycemia and hyperglycemia

***Desired Outcome/Generate Solutions:*** Immediately after instruction, the child/parent/family verbalizes an accurate understanding of possible causes, signs and symptoms, and treatment of hypoglycemia and hyperglycemia.

| ASSESSMENT—RECOGNIZE CUES/ INTERVENTIONS—TAKE ACTION | RATIONALES |
|---|---|
| Assess the child's/parents'/family's understanding about hypoglycemia and hyperglycemia. | Teaching can be more effective when the receiver's baseline knowledge/understanding is determined. |
| Define hypoglycemia. | Knowledge facilitates early recognition of the problem, enabling prompt treatment. Hypoglycemia is defined as a low blood glucose level (less than 60–70 mg/dL or as instructed by health care provider) that occurs rapidly with signs and symptoms noted within minutes to an hour. Hypoglycemia is a potential emergency and needs to be treated promptly. |
| Instruct about the causes of hypoglycemia. | Understanding the causes of hypoglycemia optimally will help decrease occurrences. Causes include<br><br>• too little food or not eating on time,<br>• increased exercise/activity with no increased intake, and<br>• too much insulin. |
| Instruct how to recognize early and late signs and symptoms of hypoglycemia. | Signs and symptoms of hypoglycemia should prompt them to check the blood glucose level.<br><br>• Early signs occurring secondary to adrenaline release are trembling, tachycardia, sweating, headache, anxiety, and hunger.<br>• Later signs and symptoms occurring secondary to cerebral glucose deficit are dizziness, personality/mood changes, slurred speech, loss of coordination, and decreased LOC. Some children may not show early symptoms of adrenaline release or, if younger than 6 years, may not recognize early symptoms. |
| Instruct about the best method for assessing and treating hypoglycemia. | Some signs and symptoms of hypoglycemia and hyperglycemia are difficult to distinguish from one another, but the treatments are different. It is essential to know which reaction a child is experiencing to treat it effectively. Measures include:<br><br>• Checking blood glucose to determine whether the child is hypoglycemic.<br>• In the presence of hypoglycemia, giving 15 g (range 10–20 g, depending on the child's age) of readily absorbed carbohydrates such as 2–8 oz orange juice, 6 oz regular soda, 2–4 glucose tablets, sugar packet, or clear cake gel from grocery store. Candy is not recommended, as it is sometimes too tempting and may be taken by other children (Frohnert and Chase, 2022). If blood glucose is not increased or the child is still having signs and symptoms of hypoglycemia in 15 minutes, treatment is repeated. Easy to remember with "Rule of 15." Keep repeating until blood glucose is back up. This will elevate the plasma glucose level and relieve symptoms of hypoglycemia. Understanding the appropriate initial treatment improves the ability to treat hypoglycemia successfully.<br>• In addition, if it is not time for a meal or snack within 1 hour, giving complex carbohydrates and protein such as bread or crackers with peanut butter or cheese sustains the glucose level inasmuch as readily absorbed carbohydrates (fast-acting or simple sugars) will be out of the system in 45–60 minutes. Complex carbohydrates (e.g., crackers) take 2–3 hours and proteins (e.g., cheese or peanut butter) 3–4 hours to be metabolized. Knowledge of the appropriate follow-up treatment and understanding of the necessity of this treatment improves the ability to resolve the situation successfully. |
| Explain the strategies to prevent hypoglycemia by identifying the pattern of activity or time of day that precedes reactions. | Knowledge of these patterns enables the child/family to prevent or decrease the incidence of hypoglycemia. For example, the patient/parent should record in a log/diary all unusual events or changes in activity or diet to help identify patterns. |

Continued

| ASSESSMENT—RECOGNIZE CUES/ INTERVENTIONS—TAKE ACTION | RATIONALES |
|---|---|
| Instruct about interventions to use if the child is unable to eat, drink, or swallow or is unconscious. | Knowing appropriate treatment improves outcomes. <br>• Glucagon (subcutaneous or intramuscular [IM]) is administered if available to raise the blood glucose level when the child is unable to drink or eat fast-acting carbohydrates. <br>• If glucagon is not available, the child should be positioned on his or her side and honey, corn syrup, or clear cake gel (e.g., Cake Mate gel) rubbed inside the cheek. This position prevents aspiration, especially if giving glucagon, because vomiting may occur. Fast-acting/simple sugars are absorbed through the oral mucosa without danger of aspiration. |
| Define hyperglycemia. | This helps differentiate between hyperglycemia and hypoglycemia. Knowledge enables recognition and discernment of which reaction the child is experiencing. Hyperglycemia is defined as blood glucose levels higher than the target range. Signs and symptoms appear within hours to several days (see signs and symptoms, later). |
| Instruct about the causes of hyperglycemia. | Understanding situations that can result in hyperglycemia (e.g., increased food intake, too little insulin, decreased exercise, infection or illness, and emotional stress) can help the child/family avoid such events. |
| Instruct about the signs and symptoms of hyperglycemia. | Recognition of hyperglycemia enables earlier and more effective treatment and prevents the development of DKA. Signs and symptoms include the three *P*s (polydipsia, polyuria, and polyphagia), fatigue, fruity-smelling breath, and weight loss. |
| Instruct about the treatment for hyperglycemia. | Interventions prevent DKA through early treatment, which include the following: <br>• If blood glucose level is greater than 250 mg/dL or level specific for patient, urine should be checked for ketones. <br>• If ketone results are trace to small, the child should drink extra water and be rechecked for ketones in 2 hours. <br>• If ketone results are medium to large, the health care provider should be contacted. |
| Explain the importance of calling the health care provider if blood glucose is greater than 250 mg/dL or level specific for patient three times in a row. | The provider may need to adjust insulin dosage. |

## Patient/Parent/Family Problem/Analyze Cues/Prioritize Hypotheses

# Deficient Knowledge

*due to* unfamiliarity with meal planning and its relationship to blood glucose

***Desired Outcome/Generate Solutions:*** Within 48 hours after instruction, the child/parent demonstrates the ability to perform meal planning based on blood glucose levels.

| ASSESSMENT—RECOGNIZE CUES/ INTERVENTIONS—TAKE ACTION | RATIONALES |
|---|---|
| Assess the knowledge/understanding of the child/parent/family regarding diet and its relationship to blood glucose. | Teaching can be more effective when the receiver's baseline knowledge/ understanding is determined. |
| Assess the child's weight on admission and daily thereafter (same time of day, same scales, same amount of clothing). | Whether the child is maintaining, losing, or gaining weight may be an indicator of the effectiveness of the diet and treatment and/or adherence to both. |
| Explain the action that different foods (carbohydrates, fats, and proteins) have on blood glucose level. | This information facilitates understanding of the need for adhering to the prescribed diet. For example, carbohydrates raise blood glucose, and simple sugars raise blood glucose more rapidly. Fats and proteins have a less immediate effect on blood glucose level. |

Continued

## ASSESSMENT—RECOGNIZE CUES/ INTERVENTIONS—TAKE ACTION

## RATIONALES

| ASSESSMENT—RECOGNIZE CUES/ INTERVENTIONS—TAKE ACTION | RATIONALES |
|---|---|
| Involve the dietitian in developing and teaching the prescribed meal plan. Medical nutrition therapy is essential. | Dietitians have expertise in designing a plan appropriate for children based on age, cultural background, preferences, and caloric needs. Including these variables in the meal plan increases knowledge, understanding, and hence likelihood of adherence. |
| Use handouts from the dietitian and guidelines in the diabetes book used by your facility for diabetes education (see resources at the end of this care plan) to review the prescribed diet. | Written and verbal explanations increase understanding and promote adherence. |
| As indicated, explain carbohydrate counting. | Understanding the diet plan increases the ability to continue this regimen at home and improves adherence as well. Counting grams of carbohydrates and matching them with the amount of insulin is the diet used most often in children. A no-concentrated-sweets diet and a consistent/constant carb meal plan are other plans used in some facilities. |
| | Recommending resources such as calorieking.com to assist with carbohydrate counting may facilitate compliance, especially if eating out. |
| Review the child's normal schedule and set up a schedule that includes time for blood glucose tests, medication, meals, and snacks. | Having a written schedule facilitates adjustment to new routines. The meal plan is tailored to the child and his or her activity level. Ongoing assessments enable changes as necessary and/or a follow-up dietary consultation. |
| Identify the ideal blood glucose levels for the child. | Diet and activity levels vary more in the younger child. Generally, at younger than 6 years, a child is more likely to have hypoglycemia and less likely to recognize early signs and symptoms, so more frequent blood glucose monitoring is recommended for all children to help maintain appropriate HbA$_{1c}$ for them, usually less than 7%–8%, depending on the type of diabetes and age of child. It is strongly recommended that the HbA$_{1c}$ is individualized for each child to achieve the best possible goal, minimize hypoglycemia or hyperglycemia, and maintain normal growth and development (ADA, 2023). |
| Instruct the parents and family to write meal plans for several days, implementing the use of prescribed foods. | This is one method of assessing and promoting the family's understanding of diet instruction. |
| Provide scenarios for when blood glucose is outside the normal range and have child/family identify ways of adjusting diet, insulin, and/or exercise to get closer to the blood glucose goal. Include how to adjust the insulin and meal plan if ill and cannot eat. | This information facilitates the development of problem-solving skills within the family and assesses their understanding of the interaction among blood glucose, insulin, diet, and exercise. |

## ADDITIONAL PROBLEMS:

## ✔ PATIENT–FAMILY TEACHING AND DISCHARGE PLANNING

Children with DM may have different classifications of DM with varying symptoms and complications. When providing child–family teaching, focus on sensory information, avoid giving excessive information, and initiate a visiting nurse referral for necessary follow-up assessment and teaching as needed. Utilize a variety of teaching methods (e.g., videos, tablets/iPads, and webinars, as well as written and verbal) depending on learning style and resources of child/family. A part of the initial assessment should include asking about existing knowledge of the disease, ability for self-care by child and/or family, and psychologic acceptance. Stress family-centered care, which is viewing the family as a unit that is the "constant" in the child's life and maintaining or improving the health of the family and its members. Include information (ensuring that written material is at a level the reader can understand) about the following:

- ✓ DM: definition, type the child has, brief pathophysiology, and characteristics of specific type.
- ✓ Major influences on blood glucose control: diet, exercise/ activity, insulin/oral medication, and stress/infection.
- ✓ Diet prescribed for the child (most often carbohydrate-counting or no-concentrated-sweets diet). The diet is also low in fat and high in fiber to prevent or decrease problems with blood fats, especially cholesterol and triglycerides. Provide the rationale for three meals and two to three snacks on a consistent schedule as appropriate for the child.
- ✓ Exercise/activity: lowers blood glucose, helps maintain normal cholesterol levels, increases circulation, and is an essential part of a child's life. If exercise is increased or has a different time frame than usual, it may be necessary to adjust the diet (add 15–30 g carbohydrates for each 45–60 minutes of exercise), insulin, or oral medications.
- ✓ Stress or illness/infection: increases blood glucose level; therefore adjustments may be necessary in diet and/or insulin dosage.
- ✓ Insulin: type of insulin; characteristics of particular insulin, including onset, peak, and duration; dose prescribed; and dosing schedule.
  - Have the child/parent demonstrate drawing up each prescribed dose (e.g., Humalog and NPH before breakfast, Humalog, and NPH before supper).
- ✓ Rotation of insulin injection sites:
  - Insulin absorption varies by site (most rapidly in the abdomen, then in the arms, in the hips, and slowest in the thighs).
  - Insulin absorption is affected by the injection site. Massage after injection, exercise of the injected limb, and body temperature increase the rate of absorption.
  - Use all spots in one site before you move on to another site or use the same site for every morning injection and the same site for every evening injection until all spots have been used (gives the same absorption of insulin).
  - Have the child/parent administer insulin using proper technique.
  - At least two people (one could be the child) need to know how to draw up and administer insulin.
- ✓ Other medications, including drug name; purpose; dosage; frequency; precautions; drug–drug, food–drug, and herb–drug interactions; and potential side effects.
- ✓ Honeymoon phase or period with type 1: may occur a short time after diagnosis, usually within 2–8 weeks, and usually lasts 1–3 months, but may last up to a year. Insulin requirement decreases. The child is *not* cured. The insulin requirement will increase again.
- ✓ Acute complications of DM: hypoglycemia and hyperglycemia:
  - Possible causes

- Signs and symptoms
- Treatment
- ✓ Long-term complications (avoid addressing for now if the child has just been diagnosed): microvascular, macrovascular, and joint contractures.
- ✓ Blood glucose monitoring: See details in *Deficient Knowledge* regarding blood glucose monitoring.
- ✓ Sick-day plan of care:
  - Always give insulin if the child is receiving insulin.
  - Check blood glucose at least every 2–4 hours and urine ketones with each void or per health care provider's guidelines. Document in log/diary.
  - If a small amount of ketones is present, increase the fluid intake.
  - If child does not feel like eating, give fluids with sugar such as fruit juice, regular soda, regular Jell-O, and broth-type soups (provide some electrolytes and extra fluid) unless blood glucose is greater than 200 mg/dL. Then give diet fluids.
  - Call the health care provider or nurse educator for the following:
    Nausea and vomiting frequent diarrhea (e.g., five or more times in 6 hours)
    Fruity odor to breath
    Deep, rapid respirations or difficulty breathing
    Decreasing LOC or change in mental status/behavior
    Moderate or high ketones in urine
    Persistent hyperglycemia greater than 250 mg/dL three times in a row or per health care provider's guidelines
- ✓ Prevention of infection:
  - Have good body hygiene with special attention to feet.
  - Report any breaks in skin and treat promptly.
  - Wear only properly fitting shoes and do not go barefooted.
  - Get regular dental checkups.
  - Need for pneumococcal, meningococcal, and yearly influenza vaccines as well as all recommended childhood immunizations.
- ✓ Importance of the child wearing a medical alert necklace or bracelet (depending on age) and carrying a card that states the child has diabetes; the type of diabetes; the child's name, address, and phone number; and the health care provider's name and number.
- ✓ Psychosocial adjustment, initial and ongoing:
  - Reactions of the child: shock, denial, and sadness
  - Reaction of parents: grief reaction
  - Potential ongoing issues for the child: Anxiety and/or depression, eating disorders, and "diabetes distress" (significant negative psychologic reaction related to emotional burdens and worries specific to an individual's experience in having to manage a severe, complicated, and demanding chronic disease such as diabetes—can be seen in children as young as 7–8 years).

✓ Delegation of tasks to the child, based on age and child's abilities (with supervision):

- Older toddler/preschooler: Only offer choices that are acceptable. Assists with choosing and cleaning finger for puncture; tries to identify word or phrase to describe feeling of hypoglycemia. Help choose food; give child a choice of appropriate options.
- School-aged child: Performs finger puncture and blood glucose test. Pushes plunger down on insulin syringe after needle is inserted by parent or gives own injection. Performs ketone test on urine. Recognizes the need to eat on time to avoid hypoglycemia. Verbalizes the treatment for hypoglycemia.
- Older school-aged child: Records blood glucose values in the log/diary. May draw up and inject insulin. Knows meal plan. Can choose the correct foods for snacks.
- Adolescent: Looks for patterns in blood glucose values. Recognizes when to test for ketones. Initiates treatment for ketones (increased fluids). Can plan meals and snacks based on the dietary plan. Can choose appropriate food at a party.

✓ Coordination of care: Need to talk with school nurse and/or other adults who are in close contact with the child (e.g., teachers, scout leaders, all child care providers including grandparents). All caregivers need to have guidelines per diabetes medical management and emergency care plan for hypoglycemia and hyperglycemia.

✓ Legal rights of the child on ADA website: https://diabetes.org/tools-support/know-your-rights/safe-at-school-state-laws/written-care-plans.

- Individuals With Disabilities Education Act: Mandates the federal government to provide funding to education agencies, state and local, to facilitate free and appropriate education to qualifying students with disabilities. This includes children with diabetes because diabetes can, at times, adversely affect school performance in some students. If this can be proved, the school is then required to develop an Individualized Education Program (IEP).
- IEP: Designed by a multidisciplinary team to facilitate special education and therapeutic strategies and goals for each child. The child does not have to be in special education classes. Parents need to be involved in this process.
- Section 504 of Rehabilitation Act of 1973: Each student with a disability is entitled to accommodation to attend school and participate as fully as possible in school activities. This accommodation may be related to a medical condition or an educational issue. For example, the child may need to have extra snacks during the school day and will not be penalized for excessive absences from school that are caused by the diabetes. The 504 Plan may include as many accommodations as necessary for the child to function well at school. Composition of the 504 team may include teachers, school nurses, therapists (physical, occupational, or speech therapists), psychologists, and parents and child as appropriate for the child's needs. Input from the health care provider is vital.

✓ Necessity of having the health care provider's signed prescription form or individualized Diabetes Medical Management Plan (DMMP) detailing guidelines for when to check blood glucose and administer medication or treatment for diabetes-related problems, as well as medications in the original container with prescribing label intact.

✓ Goals of care for a child with diabetes:

- Focus is on a child with diabetes, *not* on the diabetic child.
- Child will have appropriate growth (height and weight).
- Child will have age-appropriate lifestyle (development).
- Child will have near-normal $HbA_{1c}$.
- Child will not have acute complications (hypoglycemia or hyperglycemia).
- Child will have minimal serious complications associated with long-term diabetes.
- Child will be able to perform age-appropriate self-care tasks.

✓ Importance of follow-up care and regular visits to the health care provider and any other specialists working with the child, such as dietitian, physical therapist, or endocrinologist.

✓ Telephone numbers for the family to call if any questions arise about the therapy or disease after discharge.

✓ When to call the health care provider:

- Increased blood glucose greater than 250 mg/dL/level three times in a row or specified by health care provider.
- At least half of blood glucose values are not in the designated range.
- More than two episodes of hypoglycemia per week.
- Moderate-to-large amounts of ketones in urine.

✓ Diabetes camps, which are a fun way for children to learn more about their diabetes and feel less isolated. Listings are available at https://childrenwithdiabetes.com/diabetes-camps.

✓ Referrals to community resources, such as local and national chapters of the ADA https://diabetes.org/ and Juvenile Diabetes Research Foundation (JDRF) https://www.jdrf.org/, public health nurses or home health nurse, diabetes nurse educator or endocrinologist, community teaching programs or support groups for children, diabetes camps, or other resources as necessary.

✓ See "Diabetes Mellitus," Chapter 47, for additional family teaching and discharge planning suggestions and resources.

- Additional resources include the following:
- American Association of Diabetes Educators: https://www.diabeteseducator.org/.

- ADA for Parents: Helping them meet the challenge of having a child with diabetes. Information for parents helping them meet the challenges of having a child with diabetes (e.g., at school/daycare, camp, and importance of talking about everyone's fears) at https://www.diabetes.org/healthy-living/loved-ones. ADA camps https://diabetes.org/get-involved/community/camp/find-a-camp. Blood glucose diary/logbook usually comes with the new meters and can be obtained from the meter manufacturer, from a local pharmacy, or from health care facility caring for child.

- Smartphone Apps for Diabetes Management: Best Diabetes App, updated Aug 2022 at https://www.healthline.com/health/diabetes/top-iphone-an-droid-apps#A-quick-look-at-the-best-diabetes-apps. Some recommended by Diabetes Educators include mySugr at mysugr.com (gives free overview progress report along with many other features) and Calorie King app at calorieking.com (provides carb counting that can be used at home or when eating out).

- Special Considerations for Students at https://diabetes.org/tools-support/know-your-rights/safe-at-school-state-laws/special-considerations include school, child care, camps, and college as well as DMMP, 504 Plan, and IEP under Written Care Plans.

- Frohnert BI, Chase HP. *Understanding Diabetes: A Handbook for People Who Are Living With Diabetes*, 15th ed. 2022 ($25.00); *A First Book for Understanding Diabetes* (synopsis of 15th edition with quick summary of each chapter, $18.00, also available in Spanish for same price); and Chase HP, Messer L. *Understanding Insulin Pumps, Continuous Glucose Monitors and the Artificial Pancreas*, 3rd (ed.), 2017 ($18.00). There is a shipping charge per book. Available at https://www.childrensdiabetes-foundation.org/books/ or call (303) 863-1200.

- Type One Nation (JDRF)—Virtual social network for children older than 13 years and adults with specific groups for teens and parents of children with type 1 DM, also Snail Mail Club for kids and teens with type 1 diabetes around the world (under Virtual Resources—From our Friends and Peers): https://www.jdrf.org/community/typeonenation/.

- JDRF Bag of Hope for children, under 16 years, newly diagnosed with diabetes to help adjust to life with type 1 DM. A few items included are Rufus, the Bear With Diabetes; a book about him, Rufus Come Home; and "*I'm the tougher Than You Can Imagine Type resource folder, with fun and educational*" JDRF No Limits Teen care kit is for teens age 12–17 newly diagnosed with type 1 diabetes. Some items included are Begin with Hope, introductory guide to type 1 diabetes; Bullseye, young adult fiction book about teens journey after diagnosis; and "I'm the Tougher Than You Can Imagine Type" resource folder—with similar material as in child's Bag of Hope. Both are available at https://www.jdrf.org/t1d-resources/newly-diagnosed/.

- Type 1 Diabetes Comics—The online trilogy of comics helps explain type 1 DM to all ages using superheroes. Issues include a young girl admitted with DKA, a teenage boy recently diagnosed with type 1 DM and the stigma associated with DM as well as delving into hypoglycemia. Available at https://revolvecomics.com/read-diabetes-type-1-comics/.

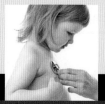

## OVERVIEW/PATHOPHYSIOLOGY

Fractures are common childhood injuries and usually are the result of trauma (falls, motor vehicle or all-terrain vehicle collisions, sports injuries, and child abuse) or bone disease with abnormally fragile bones (osteogenesis imperfecta). They usually result from increased mobility and an immature understanding of potentially dangerous situations. Fractures in infancy are most often caused by trauma or child abuse.

Fractures are a frequent cause of emergency department visits and are an important public health problem. The highest incidence occurs in children between 5 and 9 years of age, and most can be treated on an outpatient basis. The National Health Statistics Reports (Rui et al., 2019) estimate that there are 2.7 million sports- and recreation-related injuries annually in patients 5–24 years, with the highest injury rates in boys aged 10–19 years. The top two sports activities causing ED visits are football and basketball, with an increasing incidence of injuries due to gymnastics or cheerleading and skateboarding. Approximately 20% of these injuries are fractures. In addition, an overview of obesity in children and adolescents notes an increased risk for fracture in obese children (Bradwisch et al., 2020). The percentage of obese children has almost quadrupled in the United States since the 1970s with an increased incidence in non-Hispanic Black, Mexican American, and Hispanic youth (Fryar et al., 2021). Several studies reported that children who take proton pump inhibitors (PPIs) are also at increased risk for fractures compared to those that have not taken PPIs (Freedman et al., 2020; Worchester, 2020).

*Important variables that affect the care of fractures in children compared with adults.*

- Children's bones heal faster than adults'; the younger the child, the faster the bone heals.
- Children's bones are softer and more porous than adults'; rather than a complete break, they may bend, buckle, or partially break in a "greenstick" manner.
- Children's bones have a thicker periosteum and an increased amount of immature bone.
- Children's bones have an open growth plate, or epiphysis. Damage to the growth plate can interrupt and alter growth.
- Children usually only complain when something is wrong. Restlessness, extended periods of crying, and calling for the parent more than usual, as well as disuse of the affected extremity or increased use of the unaffected extremity after a fall or injury are signals that more investigation of the event is needed.

*Most frequent types of fractures in children.*

- **Bends or plastic deformation:** A child's flexible bone can be bent 45 degrees or more before breaking and remains bent when the force is removed. Once bent, it will straighten slowly but not completely. The ossification of bones begins at birth and continues until the child is 18–21 years old. The less ossified the bone, the more easily it bends. Thus this type of injury occurs only in children, most often in the ulna and fibula.
- **Buckle or torus fracture:** Compression of the porous bone as a result of minimal angular trauma. It causes a bulge at the fracture site and occurs most often in young children, usually in the distal radius or ulna.
- **Greenstick fracture:** Break occurs through the periosteum on one side of the bone but only bows or buckles the other side. It occurs most often in the forearm and is the type seen most often in children.
- **Complete fracture:** Break divides the bony fragments. It is classified by the form of the fracture line, such as spiral (from rotational force, often associated with child abuse, especially in infants), oblique, and transverse.
- **Epiphyseal growth plate fracture:** The cartilage growth plate is the weakest part of the long bones. A fracture here can be serious because it can cause growth disruption, arrest, or uneven growth. This fracture is usually classified by the Salter–Harris system (I–V).

*Most common fracture sites in children.* The distal forearm (radius, ulna, or both) is the most common site overall, but this varies with the child's developmental age and size and the type of trauma endured.

## TREATMENT

Most fractures are treated with closed reduction and immobilization of the affected area and heal without complications.

## HEALTH CARE SETTING

Emergency department, with possible hospitalization.

## ASSESSMENT

The child's symptoms, trauma history (should match physical examination), and physical examination are all part of the assessment profile. The history may be difficult to obtain especially with younger children that cannot describe what happened.

**Signs and symptoms.** Vary with the location, severity, and type of injury. Pain or tenderness at the site, decreased range of motion (ROM) or immobility, deformity at the fracture site, crepitus (grating sound heard on movement of the end of the broken bone), gross motion at the injured site, edema, erythema, ecchymosis, muscle spasm, and inability to bear weight may be present.

**Physical assessment.** Involves assessment of the location of the deformity, swelling, ecchymosis, and pain. Vital signs are checked, and neurovascular assessment is performed. ROM should be assessed carefully to prevent more injury to the site.

## DIAGNOSTIC TESTS

**Radiographic examination.** Most effective tool for determining type and location of a fracture. Much of the skeleton of infants and young children is composed of radiolucent growth cartilage that does not appear on radiographs. Observation of gross deformity and point tenderness may be more reliable in diagnosing extremity fractures than a radiograph. Radiographs of the unaffected limb may be obtained for comparison. Radiography of the suspected limb fractures needs to include the joint above and below with a minimum of two views. Radiographs are also taken after fracture reduction and often during the healing process to assess progress.

**Computed tomography, magnetic resonance imaging, and ultrasound.** May be needed to evaluate the fracture in certain circumstances.

## Patient Problem/Analyze Cues/Prioritize Hypotheses

# Acute Pain

*due to* the fracture and other injuries

**Desired Outcome/Generate Solutions:** Within 1 hour following treatment/intervention the child's report of pain/pain level is less than 4 on a 10-point scale (e.g., Wong–Baker Faces scale or numeric scale), or the child exhibits behavior consistent with pain less than 4 on a 10-point scale (e.g., FLACC [*f*ace, *l*egs, *a*ctivity, *c*ry, and *c*onsolability] scale).

| ASSESSMENT—RECOGNIZE CUES/ INTERVENTIONS—TAKE ACTION | RATIONALES |
|---|---|
| Assess the pain before and after analgesia administration and at least every 4 hours using an appropriate pain scale for the child (FLACC, Wong–Baker Faces, Oucher, Poker Chip, and numeric). | This assessment helps determine the degree of pain and effectiveness of the pain medication. |
| Administer the pain medication around the clock for the first 24–48 hours or depending on the severity of the injury. | This decreases or prevents pain more effectively than when given as needed. Prolonged stimulation of pain receptors results in increased sensitivity to painful stimuli and will increase the amount of medication required to relieve pain. |
| Administer analgesia through intravenous (IV) or by mouth (PO) route. Intramuscular (IM) route is rarely used, but if it is the only route possible, use topical anesthetic first. | These measures facilitate atraumatic care and encourage the child to give accurate pain ratings. The child may fear a "shot" and deny pain or refuse pain medication. |
| Assess for muscle spasticity every 4–6 hours by observation or report of the child. | Spasms increase pain, and pain medication alone may not ensure relief. |
| Position, align, and support the affected body part. | Appropriate positioning decreases tension on the affected area, thereby decreasing pain. |
| Use nonpharmacologic pain control measures as appropriate for the child depending on developmental age. | These are adjuncts to pain medication and include rocking, play, toys, music, distraction, relaxation techniques, humor, and massage. |
| Ice and elevate the extremity, especially for the first 24–72 hours. | These measures decrease edema, thereby decreasing pain. |
| Notify the health care provider if relief from pain is not obtained 15 minutes after IV pain medication, 30 minutes after IM pain medication (route rarely used), or 1 hour after PO pain medication was given and after using all the previous measures. | Medication may need to be adjusted for optimal pain control. Prolonged or increasing pain also may signify a fracture complication. See the next patient problem. |

Patient Problem/Analyze Cues/Prioritize Hypotheses

# Risk for Injury (Compartment Syndrome)

*due to* edema following the fracture

***Desired Outcome/Generate Solutions:*** The child's neurovascular checks are within normal limits within 24 hours of the fracture as evidenced by digits that are warm and sensitive to touch, brisk capillary refill (2 seconds or less), peripheral pulse amplitude greater than 2+ on a 0–4+ scale, and minimal or decreased swelling in the affected limb.

| ASSESSMENT—RECOGNIZE CUES/ INTERVENTIONS—TAKE ACTION | RATIONALES |
|---|---|
| Assess the neurovascular status (color, sensation, pulses, warmth, swelling) hourly for the first 24 hours and then every 2–4 hours. Use a measuring tape in millimeter increments to compare circumference of the area distal to the injury to that of the noninjured limb. Or, depending on the size of the child, you should be able to insert one or two fingers into the cast opening. | These checks help determine the presence of peripheral neurovascular dysfunction in the injured limb, which would be evidenced by darker or lighter color than the opposite extremity, decreased sensation, decreased or absent pulse, skin cool to the touch, and increased swelling distal to the injury. |
| Assess the subjective and behavioral indicators of peripheral neurovascular dysfunction. | Complaints of constant or increasing pain (especially on passive movement of the digits) and numbness or tingling in the digits of the injured extremity are subjective indicators of peripheral neurovascular dysfunction. Constant crying or increasing irritability may be seen in young children. |
| Elevate the extremity. | Elevation helps prevent/decrease edema, thereby promoting tissue perfusion. |
| Apply ice during the first 24–72 hours, usually for 20 minutes, as often as possible or per health care providers' order. | Most swelling occurs during the first 24–72 hours. Ice helps decrease edema, thereby promoting tissue perfusion. |
| Notify the health care provider immediately if tissue perfusion deteriorates quickly from baseline. | The child may be developing or experiencing compartment syndrome, **an emergency situation**. For details, see "Fractures," Chapter 69, in the adult care plans for *Risk for Injury (Compartment Syndrome)* due to the interruption of capillary blood flow occurring with increased pressure within the myofascial compartment. |
| Encourage the child to move the involved digits. | Moving toes or fingers in the affected limb improves circulation, thereby decreasing edema and increasing tissue perfusion. **Note:** Inability to move the digits is another sign of compartment syndrome. |

Patient Problem/Analyze Cues/Prioritize Hypotheses

# Risk for Impaired Skin Integrity

*due to* the presence of the immobilization device (bandages, splint, and cast)

***Desired Outcome/Generate Solutions:*** The child's skin remains intact while wearing the immobilization device.

| ASSESSMENT—RECOGNIZE CUES/ INTERVENTIONS—TAKE ACTION | RATIONALES |
|---|---|
| Assess for erythema or irritation caused by the immobilization device every 4 hours. <br> • Check the edges of the immobilization device above and below the fracture site. <br> • If the edges are rough, use petal moleskin to smooth the edges. | Ongoing assessment results in early detection and treatment, thereby decreasing the risk for a break in skin integrity. |

Continued

## ASSESSMENT—RECOGNIZE CUES/ INTERVENTIONS—TAKE ACTION

| ASSESSMENT—RECOGNIZE CUES/ INTERVENTIONS—TAKE ACTION | RATIONALES |
|---|---|
| Assess the immobilization device by running your hand over it to feel for indentations or "hot" spots every 4 hours. | Indentations can cause skin breakdown/pressure. Hot spots (after the cast has dried) may indicate an infection that might occur as a result of a break in skin integrity. |
| Feel around the edges of the immobilization device for tightness/ looseness every 4 hours. | This determines whether the cast/immobilization device fits appropriately and is not too tight or loose. You should be able to insert your fingers between the cast and the child's skin after it dries. If the cast is too tight, it will cause pressure, which can result in decreased tissue perfusion and skin breakdown. If the cast is too loose, it can rub on the skin and cause skin breakdown. |
| Instruct the child or family not to put powder or cornstarch under the cast. | These products may cake and cause skin irritation and breakdown. |
| Caution the child or family not to put anything inside the cast to scratch the skin. | This can cause skin breakdown or become lodged inside the cast. |
| Suggest that the family use cool air blown from a fan or hair dryer to relieve itching or rub the unaffected extremity. | These distraction techniques may keep the child from itching or putting things inside the cast to scratch and cause skin breakdown. |
| Encourage the position changes every 2–4 hours as appropriate. | This improves circulation by preventing prolonged pressure at the same area. |

## ADDITIONAL PROBLEMS:

## ✓ PATIENT–FAMILY TEACHING AND DISCHARGE PLANNING

When providing child–family teaching, focus on sensory data, avoid giving excessive information, and initiate a visiting nurse referral for necessary follow-up assessment and/or teaching as needed. Utilize a variety of teaching methods (e.g., videos, tablets, and webinars as well as written and verbal) depending on learning styles and resources of child/family. All information needs to emphasize that which is developmentally appropriate for the child. Stress family-centered care, which is viewing the family as a unit that is the "constant" in the child's life and maintaining or improving the health of the family and its members in a holistic manner. Include written and verbal information about the following (ensuring that information is at a level the reader can understand):

✓ Proper care of the immobilization device. See *Risk for Impaired Skin Integrity* earlier.

✓ Positioning
  - Elevate injured limb for the first 24–72 hours or per the provider's instructions.
  - Apply ice for 24-72 hours, usually intermittently (on for 20 minute intervals) for as often as possible or per the provider's instructions.

✓ Medications, including drug name; purpose; dosage; frequency; precautions; drug–drug, food–drug; and herb–drug interactions; and potential adverse effects.

✓ Importance of taking medications at home and at school as directed. Medication in the original bottle (with prescribing label) and written prescription from the health care provider are needed for the child to be able to take medication at school.

✓ Legal rights of the child—Section 504 of Rehabilitation Act of 1973: Each student with a disability (whether temporary or permanent) is entitled to accommodation needed to attend school and participate as fully as possible in school activities. This accommodation may be related to a medical or an education issue. The 504 team for this child includes teachers, school nurse, possibly therapists, and parents and child, with input from the health care provider. For example, a child with a long leg cast who has to go up and down steps to change classes would need accommodation—either staying in the same room all day, leaving one class early enough to be able to get to the next class, having someone else carry his or her books, or possibly having a teacher provide lessons at home. As many accommodations can be made as necessary for the child to be able to be successful in school. More details are found at https://www.verywellfamily.com/what-is-a-504-plan-3104706.

✓ Adjustments needed for activities of daily living.

✓ Age-appropriate (developmental age, not just chronologic age) safety measures to help prevent further injuries:
- Childproof the home and play area (include what is appropriate for *all* children in the home).
- Avoid the use of baby walkers, which are responsible for many injuries in infants.
- Proper use of protective equipment (e.g., car safety seats and bicycle helmets).
- Adaptation of a child safety restraint system to accommodate cast/immobilization device.
- Importance of supervising young children while playing.
- Not leaving a child sitting in a shopping cart, because many fall out or manage to tip the cart over. Be sure the shopping cart has a safety belt and that it is secured.
- Realistic expectations for the child.

✓ When to call the health care provider:
- Child complains of pain consistently in the same spot or pain seems to be getting worse.
- Child has tingling or numbness of toes or fingers.
- Child cannot feel something touching fingers or toes.
- Red or sore areas appear around the cast edges.
- Child's fingers or toes are cold when in a warm environment.
- Child's nails stay pale when pressing on them and releasing pressure.
- Child's nails look blue even after elevating limb.
- Child's fingers or toes become very swollen several days after injury. Most swelling should occur in the first 48–72 hours.

- A foul smell comes from the cast.
- A "hot" spot is felt on the cast.
- Staining appears on the cast that was not there when child first came home. This could be an infected area or pressure sore.
- Child complains of constant itching that nothing helps.
- Cast is too tight or too loose.
- The cast starts to break down or fall apart or has indented areas. The cast may need to be reinforced or replaced to provide appropriate support for the injured area.
- Swelling after the first few days, pain, numbness, tingling, red marks or sores, and foul smell are serious signs of a problem. Talk with the child's health care provider immediately. If the health care provider is unavailable, go to the nearest emergency care facility.

✓ Importance of follow-up care.

✓ Referral to community resources for assistance as needed (e.g., in providing a safe home environment and transport to accommodate cast/immobilization device). Additional information can be obtained by contacting the local children's hospital, Social Services, and the following organizations:
- National SAFE KIDS Campaign: http://www.safekids.org
- Pediatric Orthopedic Society of North America/Ortho Kids: https://orthokids.org, with many resources per orthopedic conditions/injuries (e.g., casts and splints)
- Car safety for child with a cast: https://preventinjury.pediatrics.iu.edu/special-needs/child-restraint-options/

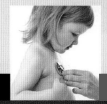

# Gastroenteritis 85

## OVERVIEW/PATHOPHYSIOLOGY

Gastroenteritis, one of the most common infectious diseases seen in children, is an inflammation of the stomach and intestines that accompanies numerous gastrointestinal (GI) disorders. It is one of the leading causes of dehydration and can cause life-threatening complications. Acute infectious gastroenteritis is caused by a variety of bacterial, viral, and parasitic pathogens, with viruses accounting for most of the cases of acute gastroenteritis (AGE) (Gotfried, 2022). Rotavirus infection is still the most common cause of *severe diarrhea* requiring hospitalization in infants and young children worldwide (Bellandi, 2022). Since the introduction of the rotavirus vaccines in 2006 and 2008 and the routine administration of those vaccines, the incidence of rotavirus gastroenteritis has decreased by 58%–90% in the United States from the prevaccine era (Cochran, 2022).

Currently, noroviruses are the leading cause of *severe AGE* in all age groups in the United States and account for nearly 1 million pediatric medical care visits annually. Each year, norovirus is estimated to be responsible for 465,000 ED visits, mainly in young children; 109,000 hospitalizations; and 900 deaths, mostly in adults 65 and older. Norovirus occurs year-round but peaks in the winter, with most outbreaks from November to April. There is also 50% more norovirus illness in years when a new strain of the virus emerges (Centers for Disease Control and Prevention [CDC], n.d.). Norovirus outbreaks occur mainly when infected people spread the virus to others (fecal-oral route), but it is also spread by contaminated food or water or by contact with a surface the virus is on. The foods that primarily are involved in outbreaks include leafy green vegetables (e.g., lettuce), fresh fruits, and shellfish (e.g., oysters).

*Clostridioides difficile* is probably the most common bacterial cause in the United States, with many cases now being community acquired. In the past, it occurred primarily in the hospital in patients receiving antibiotics. Other common causes of infectious bacterial gastroenteritis include *Campylobacter*, *Escherichia coli*, *Salmonella*, and *Shigella* (Gotfried, 2022).

## HEALTH CARE SETTING

Primary care, with possible hospitalization depending on the severity of the illness.

## ASSESSMENT

History is very important, as is physical examination. Signs and symptoms vary widely depending on illness severity. Age,

general health, and environment are factors that predispose children to gastroenteritis.

***Signs and symptoms.*** Children usually present with some degree of the following:

- Diarrhea: Wide range of frequency, volume, and character (e.g., watery and bloody).
- Vomiting: Note onset, frequency, if blood is present, bilious or nonbilious.
- Tenesmus: Painfully urgent but ineffectual attempt to defecate.
- Abdominal pain: Note onset, location, duration, any change, continuous, or intermittent.
- Dehydration: Symptoms vary depending on the degree of dehydration/water deficit.
  - Mild (3%–5%): Normal except for slight thirst, capillary refill less than 2 seconds, decreased urine output (UO). Decreased or low UO varies with age, for example, less than 1 mL/kg/hour for infants, less than 0.5 mL/kg/hour for children, or per the unit's guidelines.
  - Moderate (6%–9%): May be restless, irritable, or lethargic; moderate thirst, eager to drink; slightly increased heart rate (HR); increased respiratory rate (RR); normal to decreased pulses; slightly sunken eyes and anterior fontanelle; decreased tears; dry mucous membranes; prolonged capillary refill time; decreased skin turgor, warm extremities; decreased UO.
  - Severe (greater than or equal to 10%): Lethargic or unconscious; minimal intake, may be unable to drink; tachycardia; weak, thready, or impalpable pulses; increased RR and deep breathing; deeply sunken eyes; absent tears; parched mucous membranes; prolonged or minimal capillary refill and tenting; cold, mottled, cyanotic extremities; minimal or no UO.
- Infants and young children are at increased risk for dehydration due to many factors:
  - A higher percentage of their body weight is water when compared with adults. A newborn's body weight is 75%–80% water, with 40% being extracellular. A preschooler's body weight is 60%–65% water, with 30% being extracellular.
  - Extracellular fluid is lost first with gastroenteritis.
  - The younger the child, the more quickly dehydration occurs.
  - Insensible water loss is also greater in infants and young children through the skin and GI tract because of a proportionally greater body surface area in relation to body

mass. Increased RR also increases insensible water loss, as does a higher metabolic rate.

- Other risk factors for developing AGE include the following:
  - Group child care attendance or exposure to sick contacts.
  - Recent travel in a foreign country.
  - Immunocompromised condition.
  Low socioeconomic status.

The most serious consequences of gastroenteritis are dehydration, electrolyte imbalance, and malnutrition.

## DIAGNOSTIC TESTS

History is very important in determining the source of gastroenteritis and whether there is a need for any tests. In general, laboratory tests are not performed unless the child exhibits severe dehydration, appears toxic (cyanotic, lethargic or irritable, tachypnea, tachycardic, etc.), and has abdominal pain or bloody stools.

**Serum electrolytes.** Determine the severity of electrolyte imbalance and the type of fluid replacement necessary.

**Blood urea nitrogen and creatinine.** Determine hydration and acid–base status in patients but should return to baseline with rehydration.

**Complete blood count.** Hematocrit is often elevated in dehydration. The differential will determine whether viral or bacterial infection is present. In a bacterial infection, the white blood cell (WBC) count is elevated with increased polymorphonuclear leukocytes, especially neutrophils. In a viral infection the WBC count is slightly elevated with increased lymphocytes.

**Blood culture.** Obtained if the child is acutely ill to help determine the cause of illness.

**Stool specimen.** Examined if diarrhea lasts more than a few days based on patient's condition/clinical finds to help determine the cause.

**RT-PCR.** Rapid test to see if rotavirus or norovirus is present in stool specimen. A positive test negates the need for a stool culture.

**Stool culture.** Obtained if blood or mucus is present in stool, when symptoms are severe, or if there is history of travel to a developing country.

**Stool for ova and parasites.** May be used instead of a culture because it is less expensive and often more reliable. A specimen is obtained 3 days in a row.

## Patient Problem/Analyze Cues/Prioritize Hypotheses

# Dehydration

*due to* fluid loss occurring with fever, vomiting, and diarrhea

*Desired Outcome/Generate Solutions:* Within 4 hours after intervention/treatment (for mild-to-moderate dehydration) the infant/child exhibits adequate hydration as evidenced by alertness and responsiveness, anterior fontanel soft and not sunken (in children younger than 2 years), moist oral mucous membranes, elastic abdominal skin turgor, capillary refill less than or equal to 2 seconds, and age-appropriate UO (e.g., infant 2–3 mL/kg/hour, toddler and preschooler 2 mL/kg/hour, school-aged child 1–2 mL/kg/hour, and adolescent 0.5–1 mL/kg/hour).

| ASSESSMENT—RECOGNIZE CUES/ INTERVENTIONS—TAKE ACTION | RATIONALES |
| --- | --- |
| Assess the weight of the child on admission and daily on the same scale, at the same time of day, and wearing the same amount of clothing (infants are weighed without any clothing). Notify the health care provider if the child is losing weight. | Consistency with weight measurements helps ensure more accurate results. Weight is a useful indicator of fluid balance. Weight loss may indicate that the child is not receiving adequate fluid replacement and adjustments need to be made. |
| Assess the vital signs every 4 hours or more often if they are outside baseline parameters. Report abnormalities to the health care provider. | HR is elevated and blood pressure (BP) is normal in compensated shock and low in uncompensated shock. Dehydration can quickly lead to shock in infants and young children in whom a falling BP is a *late* sign of shock. |
| Do not measure temperatures rectally. | Rectal temperature measurements stimulate stooling, which can lead to dehydration. Also, if the child has diarrhea, they cause further irritation to impaired skin. |

## ASSESSMENT—RECOGNIZE CUES/INTERVENTIONS—TAKE ACTION

### RATIONALES

| ASSESSMENT—RECOGNIZE CUES/INTERVENTIONS—TAKE ACTION | RATIONALES |
|---|---|
| Administer oral rehydration solution (ORS), for example, Pedialyte, Enfalyte, Naturalyte, and Ceralyte. | ORS replaces fluid volume in children with minimal-to-moderate dehydration.<br><br>• To make it more palatable for the child, you may add 1 tsp presweetened sugar-free Kool-Aid to chilled 1-L bottle of ORS or try flavored brands of these solutions.<br><br>• Small amounts are given frequently, especially if the child is vomiting, for example, 2–5 mL of ORS via oral syringe or small medication cup every 5 minutes increasing the amount given/consumed as vomiting resolves. The mainstays of treatment of mild-to-moderate dehydration are to improve health outcomes by replacing fluid deficits and to prevent ongoing fluid losses by replacing fluid and electrolytes, as well as glucose, with oral rehydration therapy (ORT). ORT includes rehydration with ORS. The maintenance phase includes fluid and adequate dietary intake. |
| Do not give clear liquids such as apple juice, soda, gelatin, or regular sports drinks. | Liquids with a large amount of simple sugars can exacerbate osmotic effects (stimulating the intestines to excrete more electrolytes and water) associated with diarrhea and vomiting. |
| Do not give tea or soda with caffeine. | Caffeine is a mild diuretic and can increase dehydration as a result of loss of fluid and electrolytes. |
| Do not give chicken or beef broth. | Broths are high in salt and low in carbohydrates. |
| Administer and monitor the nasogastric tube (NGT) fluid replacement (for mild-to-moderate dehydration and vomiting) or intravenous (IV) fluids as prescribed for moderate-to-severe dehydration and vomiting. | If the child is unable to take sufficient ORS orally, the use of NGT with ORS might help initial rehydration and speed up tolerance to refeeding. IV fluid and electrolyte replacement likely will be necessary if this is not successful or if the child is severely dehydrated. |
| Assess the hydration status every 4 hours. | Although the child may be receiving maintenance fluids, he or she may still be dehydrated because of diarrhea, vomiting, and/or insensible water loss. A dehydrated child is likely to exhibit decreasing level of consciousness, sunken anterior fontanel (if younger than 2 years), dry or sticky oral mucous membrane, tented abdominal skin, capillary refill greater than 2 seconds, and decreasing UO. |
| Assess the intake and output every 2–4 hours or per unit policy to ensure that the child has at least minimal UO but that output is not more than intake. | Frequent monitoring is essential to obtain accurate information. The earlier a problem is detected, the sooner appropriate interventions can be made to ensure adequate hydration. |
| After the child is rehydrated, calculate maintenance fluids based on the child's current weight. | The smaller the child, the greater the percentage of body weight is water. To meet minimal fluid requirements, the necessary volume is calculated in the following way (except for neonates whose fluid requirement is different):<br><br>Up to 10 kg: 100 mL/kg/24 hours=_____<br><br>10–20 kg: 50 mL/kg/24 hours=_____<br><br>Greater than 20 kg: 20 mL/kg/24 hours=_____<br><br>total amount=maintenance fluid requirement<br><br>*For example, if child weighs 43 kg:*<br><br>10 kg×100 mL/kg/24 hours=1000 mL/24 hours<br><br>10 kg×50 mL/kg/24 hours=500 mL/24 hours<br><br>23 kg×20 mL/kg/24 hours=460 mL/24 hours<br><br>43 kg=1960 mL/24 hours<br><br>Maintenance fluid requirement is 1960 mL/24 hours or 82 mL/hour. |

Continued

| ASSESSMENT—RECOGNIZE CUES/ INTERVENTIONS—TAKE ACTION | RATIONALES |
|---|---|
| Advocate with health care provider to ensure that the child is receiving at least maintenance fluids. | This is the minimum amount of fluid needed daily to be well hydrated if there are no unusual fluid losses (e.g., fever, diarrhea, and vomiting). |
| Administer the medications as prescribed. | For example, antibiotics are only given to treat the bacterial pathogen causing the diarrhea, ondansetron (Zofran) for vomiting, and probiotics such as *Lactobacillus* GG to decrease the duration of diarrhea. |
| After the child is rehydrated, begin a regular diet as tolerated. | Enteral nutrition stimulates the renewal of intestinal cells, whereas fasting increases gut atrophy and permeability, which can contribute to dehydration. A regular diet is likely to include the following factors: low in fat, avoids high concentrations of simple sugars, and encourages complex carbohydrates such as starches. Examples of an appropriate diet include cereals, lean meats, yogurt, and cooked vegetables. |
| Instruct family members in providing ORS, monitoring intake and output, and assessing for signs of dehydration. | These instructions should improve adherence and promote optimal results. |

## Patient Problem/Analyze Cues/Prioritize Hypotheses

# Risk for Excoriation (Perineal/Perianal Skin)

*due to* irritation caused by frequent stooling

***Desired Outcome/Generate Solutions:*** The child's skin in perineal and perianal areas remains intact.

| ASSESSMENT—RECOGNIZE CUES/ INTERVENTIONS—TAKE ACTION | RATIONALES |
|---|---|
| Assess the perineal and perianal areas for signs of irritation or excoriation with every diaper change. | The earlier the problem is detected, the sooner appropriate interventions can be made to ensure the skin remains intact. |
| Change diapers as soon as they become wet or soiled. | This helps keep skin clean and dry. |
| Cleanse the buttocks gently (pat, do not rub) with water or immerse in tepid water to cleanse. Avoid using soap if possible. | Diarrheal stools are very irritating to the skin. Rubbing the skin every time the diaper is changed would irritate it further. Soap dries skin by removing normal moisturizing skin oils, thereby increasing the potential for irritation and skin breakdown. |
| Do not use commercial baby wipes with alcohol or perfume or baby powder on irritated or excoriated skin. | These products are painful to irritated skin. Baby powder cakes and is difficult to remove. |
| If not contraindicated, apply protective ointments such as petroleum jelly (Vaseline), A&D, or zinc oxide when the child is wearing a diaper. | This measure protects skin from irritation. |
| Leave the diaper area open to air if possible (but not in the presence of explosive diarrhea). Reapply protective ointment before putting the diaper on. | This practice facilitates drying and healing. |
| Instruct the family members in appropriate skin care methods. | This increases the likelihood of the family using these techniques at home. |

## Family Problem/Analyze Cues/Prioritize Hypotheses

# Risk for Disease (Gastroenteritis)

*due to* the transmissible nature of gastroenteritis

**Desired Outcome/Generate Solutions:** After intervention, family members and other children are free of indicators of gastroenteritis.

| ASSESSMENT—RECOGNIZE CUES/ INTERVENTIONS—TAKE ACTION | RATIONALES |
|---|---|
| Implement Standard Precautions as well as appropriate Transmission-Based Precautions. | Standard Precautions reduce the risk for spreading infection, which include the following:<br>• Good hand hygiene: Wash hands before and after working with the child, even with appropriate gloving.<br>• Wear gloves when changing or weighing the diaper.<br>• Wear other personal protective equipment as designated by isolation guidelines. |
| Dispose of linen and other soiled items per hospital protocol. | This will prevent the spread of infection. |
| Apply the diaper securely. | This prevents fecal spread. |
| Try to keep infants and small children from placing hands or objects in contaminated areas. | Gastroenteritis is mostly spread by the fecal–oral route. Infants and young children tend to put their hands in their mouths, and if their hands get into their diaper or stool, fecal–oral spread occurs. |
| Teach children, as appropriate, protective measures such as washing their hands after using the toilet. | This teaching helps prevent the spread of infection. |
| Instruct the family members and visitors in protective measures, especially hand washing and not visiting other patients. | This instruction reduces the risk for spreading infection. |

## Patient Problem

# Body Weight Problem (Weight Loss)

*due to* the inadequate intake and fluid loss occurring with vomiting, diarrhea, and fever

**Desired Outcome/Generate Solutions:** Within 24–48 hours after intervention/treatment, the child maintains or gains weight and exhibits no further vomiting or diarrhea.

| ASSESSMENT—RECOGNIZE CUES/ INTERVENTIONS—TAKE ACTION | RATIONALES |
|---|---|
| Assess the weight on admission and daily (on the same scale, at the same time, with the same clothing—no diaper on infants). | These assessments measure the child's progress in attaining adequate nutrition. Consistency with weight measurements helps ensure more accurate results. |
| If the mother is breastfeeding, encourage her to continue along with giving ORS (if the child has mild-to-moderate dehydration) as described in *Dehydration*, earlier. | This practice tends to reduce the severity and duration of illness by maintaining normal intake so that the child has adequate nutrition. |
| Avoid the BRAT(bananas, rice, apples, and toast) diet. | These foods do not provide complete caloric and protein requirements. They provide excessive carbohydrates and, overall, are also low in electrolytes. Therefore the child does not get needed nutrients. |

Continued

| ASSESSMENT—RECOGNIZE CUES/ INTERVENTIONS—TAKE ACTION | RATIONALES |
|---|---|
| Resume a regular diet when the child is rehydrated as described in *Dehydration*, earlier. | Enteral nutrition stimulates the renewal of intestinal cells and decreases illness duration, whereas fasting increases gut atrophy and permeability. |
| Instruct the family on the appropriate diet as described in *Dehydration*, earlier. | This gains adherence to the treatment plan. |
| Monitor the child's response to feedings. | Monitoring helps assess feeding tolerance.<br><br>• Some children have increased stooling with lactose-containing milk products.<br><br>• Most children do well with lactose-containing milk products, especially if they are eating foods at the same time. |
| Give liquids at room temperature. | Cold liquids stimulate peristalsis and hence diarrhea. |
| Keep the room as odor free as possible. | Minimizing unpleasant or strong (perfume/aftershave) odors increases interest in eating and feelings of well-being. |
| Provide oral hygiene. | This enhances a sense of well-being and improves the chances the child will eat and drink more. |

## ADDITIONAL PROBLEMS:

| | |
|---|---|
| "Psychosocial Support for the Patient's Family and Significant Others" for *Anxiety, Difficulty Coping* (due to situational crisis), and *Deficient Knowledge* (patient's current health status and therapies) | Chapter 9 |
| "Asthma" for *Anxiety* due to illness, loss of control, and medical/nursing interventions | Chapter 77 |

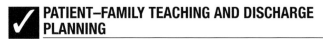

## ✓ PATIENT–FAMILY TEACHING AND DISCHARGE PLANNING

When providing child–family teaching, focus on sensory information, avoid giving excessive information, and arrange for a visiting nurse for follow-up teaching and assessment as needed. Utilize a variety of teaching methods (e.g., videos, tablets, and webinars as well as verbal and written) depending on learning styles and resources of child/family. Stress family-centered care, which is viewing the family as a unit that is the "constant" in the child's life and maintaining or improving the health of the family and its members in a holistic manner. Include information about the following (ensure that written material is at a level the reader can understand):

✓ Pathophysiology of gastroenteritis.

✓ Causes of gastroenteritis: If caused by improper food storage—address proper hygiene, formula or food preparation, handling, and storage.

✓ Contagious aspect of gastroenteritis. It is important to use good hand-washing technique, especially after changing a diaper. Teach children who are old enough to wash their hands after they use the toilet.

✓ Why gastroenteritis can be such a serious problem, especially for infants and young children:

• The younger the child, the greater the percentage of body weight that is water.
  – Premature infant: 85%–90% of body weight is water.
  – Full-term infant: 75%–80% of body weight is water.
  – Preschooler: 60%–65% of body weight is water.
  – Adolescent: 50%–55% of body weight is water.

• Therefore the younger the child, the quicker dehydration can occur (the child loses more fluid than is taken in).

• Problems that cause or increase the severity of dehydration: fever, vomiting, diarrhea, not eating or drinking enough.

✓ Importance of checking hydration status every 2–4 hours when the child is ill with any of the previous problems (the younger the child, the more often status is reassessed):

• Is the child alert and interactive? The child would not be as alert and interactive as normal if dehydrated.

• Check the soft spot on top of the head in children younger than 2 years: if it is sunken, the child may be dehydrated.

• No tears when crying in a child older than 6 months.

• Check inside the mouth, not the lips: if dry or sticky and the child is not a mouth breather, the child is dehydrated.

• Pinch skin on the abdomen: if the skin sits up like a tent instead of falling down right away, the child is dehydrated.

• How many wet diapers does the child normally have per day? If the number is decreased or they are not as wet as normal, the child may be dehydrated.

✓ Feeding of child who has diarrhea:
- If the child is breastfeeding, continue breastfeeding and supplement with ORS (e.g., Pedialyte, Enfalyte, or Ceralyte).
- If the child is taking only formula or milk, it may not be necessary to stop that fluid as long as the child is also taking ORS.
- 1 tsp presweetened sugar-free Kool-Aid can be added to a chilled 1-L bottle of ORS to improve taste or use flavored ORS.

✓ Change diapers frequently:
- Clean after stool with warm water. Pat skin; do not rub.
- Do not use soap if possible. If that is not possible, use mild, nonantiseptic soap.
- Do not use baby wipes containing alcohol or fragrances.
- Avoid powders and corn starch, which trap fluid and get caked.
- Leave skin open to air if irritated, when possible (but not in the presence of explosive diarrhea).
- Put protective ointment such as petroleum jelly (Vaseline), A&D, or zinc oxide on the skin.

✓ Feeding a child who is vomiting: Give small amounts of ORS frequently—the amount varies depending on the age and weight of the child.

✓ After the child is rehydrated, begin a regular diet as tolerated.
- Do not give BRAT (bananas, rice, apples, and toast). This combination does not provide enough calories or protein.
- Use low-fat foods (no peanut butter, potato chips, or hot dogs).
- Give starchy foods such as cooked baby cereal, oatmeal, cream of wheat, rice, nonsugared cereals, noodles, potatoes, bread, and yogurt.
- Give fruits (not packed in syrup), vegetables without butter, and well-cooked chicken, fish, or lean meat.
- Avoid concentrated sweets such as candy or ice cream.
- Most children have no problems drinking formula or milk.

✓ Call the health care provider when:
- There are signs of dehydration.
- There is blood or pus in the stool.
- Child has a fever. Follow temperature-range guidelines per the health care provider.
- The vomiting or diarrhea lasts longer than 8–24 hours (the younger the child, the earlier the health care provider needs to be called).
- Child is not drinking fluids or is less alert than usual.
- Child has abdominal pain for 2 hours or more.
- Child is younger than 6 months and is vomiting or has diarrhea.
- Diaper area is very red or irritated and getting worse.

✓ Reinforce that the child must never receive aspirin with viral illness; acetaminophen or ibuprofen needs to be used for fever or discomfort.

✓ Telephone numbers to call if questions or concerns about the treatment or disease arise after discharge.

✓ Importance of follow-up care.

✓ Importance of getting one of the rotavirus vaccine series (two forms are now available: one has two doses and the other has three doses) for infants less than 6 months unless it is contraindicated. Both vaccines are given orally.

✓ Referral to community resources as necessary.
　Additional online resource for parents:
　Healthychildren.org from American Academy of Pediatrics: (1) Diarrhea https://www.healthychildren.org/English/health-issues/conditions/abdominal/Pages/Diarrhea.aspx and (2) Vomiting with Diarrhea https://www.healthychildren.org/English/tips-tools/symptom-checker/Pages/symptomviewer.aspx?symptom=Vomiting+With+Diarrhea. Note: Both also discuss dehydration.

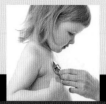

# Otitis Media 86

## OVERVIEW/PATHOPHYSIOLOGY

Otitis media (OM) is the most common reason for visits to the pediatrician or other primary health care provider in the first 3 years of life, the leading cause of antibiotic use, and the most common cause of hearing loss in children. The number of clinician visits for OM has decreased over the years; however, the percentage of children in visits for OM getting antibiotics has remained relatively stable. Factors that may have contributed to the decrease in visits for OM include use of pneumococcal vaccines, increased use of influenza vaccines, and public education campaigns stressing the overuse of antibiotics. Financial issues, for example, missing work to take the child to health care practitioner; child care needs to be increased during illness; and/or lack of health care insurance, probably heightened during the COVID-19 pandemic. Workplace closures and layoffs, impacting families and health care facilities, also contributed to decreased visits for OM. Many factors contribute to OM development, including host (e.g., immune system or anatomic abnormality), infectious (e.g., bacterial or viral pathogen), allergic (e.g., second hand smoke or history of eczema or rhinitis), and environmental (e.g., feeding methods and group child care) factors.

About 25% of infants developed acute OM (AOM) by 1 year of age, an approximate 25% decrease in AOM over the past 20 years, with children experiencing the same contributing factors. This decrease is associated with the introduction of pneumococcal conjugate vaccines and the use of the flu shot. The most common bacterial pathogens for AOM are *Haemophilus influenzae*, *Streptococcus pneumoniae*, and *Moraxella catarrhalis*. There is also an increased incidence of antibiotic-resistant strains of all three pathogens, especially in children frequently treated with antibiotics (Hester, 2019; Levin, 2022). The American Academy of Pediatrics (AAP) updated the Clinical Practice Guidelines for AOM (Lieberthal et al., 2013), which is currently in use. Recommendations included the following:

- Observation/watchful waiting for 48–72 hours without antibiotic treatment for select, otherwise healthy children 6 months to 12 years of age with nonsevere AOM and stressed the importance of follow-up with those children in that time frame.
- It was also stressed that if children treated with antibiotics did not improve or became more ill within 48–72 hours, they needed to be reevaluated.
- Pain assessment and management were stressed in the guidelines also. In addition to pain management, the treatment plan with observation or antibiotics varies depending on the patient's age, severity of symptoms, and whether the AOM is unilateral or bilateral. Oral pain medications such as acetaminophen and ibuprofen are very effective; topical pain may be treated with pain relief drops like benzocaine drops (Hockenberry et al., 2019).

OM includes several conditions ranging from acute to chronic with or without symptoms:

- **OM:** inflammation of the middle ear.
- **AOM:** middle ear inflammation with symptoms of acute illness (fever, pain, irritability) and moderate to severe bulging tympanic membrane (TM) under positive pressure. The TM may be erythematous or opaque with indistinct landmarks.
- **OM with effusion (OME)** or **serous OM:** inflammation of the middle ear without signs and symptoms of acute infection (other than reduced hearing), TM retracted or in neutral position under negative pressure or no pressure, and yellow/amber-colored fluid in the middle ear space. The American Academy of Otolaryngology–Head and Neck Surgery Foundation (AAO-HNSF) noted that 90% of children have OME by 5 years of age. OME is the most common cause of hearing impairment and is very prevalent in children with developmental difficulties. The updated 2016 guidelines emphasizes the importance of proper assessment and treatment. Antibiotics are still frequently prescribed but are not an appropriate treatment for OME (Miyamoto, 2022; Rosenfeld et al., 2016).
- **Chronic OM with effusion:** middle ear effusion lasting more than 3 months.

## HEALTH CARE SETTING

Primary care; possible hospitalization if OM exacerbates a chronic condition or if surgical intervention is required.

## ASSESSMENT

***Signs and symptoms.*** Vary depending on the type of OM, severity, and age of the child.

*Acute otitis media.*

- Infant or young child: fever; possible ear drainage; crying; irritable and fussy; may tug, rub, or hold the affected ear; sleep disturbances; decreased appetite; rolling head side to side; difficult to comfort; possible difficulty hearing.
- Older child: fever, possible ear drainage, complaints of ear hurting, crying, irritable, lethargic, decreased appetite (chewing causes increased ear pain), possible difficulty hearing.

*Otitis media with effusion.* Difficulty hearing, feeling of fullness/pressure in the ear, tinnitus or popping sounds, mild balance disturbances.

### Physical assessment.

*Acute otitis media.* Pneumatic otoscopy reveals bulging, red, opaque, immobile TM (or decreased mobility of TM). Normally, the TM is translucent, light pearly pink or gray, concave, and the malleolus is vertical. Crying, removal of cerumen that thereby irritates the auditory canal, and fever are factors that can cause redness of the TM without infection being present. Postauricular and cervical lymph nodes may be enlarged.

*Otitis media with effusion.* Pneumatic otoscopy may show a slightly injected, dull-gray membrane; obscured landmarks; and fluid visible behind the TM. There is also decreased mobility of the TM.

## DIAGNOSTIC TESTS

**Pneumatic otoscopy.** A pneumatic attachment to the otoscope enables the health care provider to introduce puffs of air into the ear. The TM does not move as well with fluid behind it. This device improves diagnostic accuracy by assessing the mobility of the TM as well as visualizing it.

**Tympanometry.** Method of providing information about the possible presence of a middle ear effusion, including the actual pressures in the middle ear space. This is a quick and simple method of assessing TM mobility.

**Acoustic reflectometry.** Rapid and easy way to measure reflected sound waves from TM; the louder the sound, the greater the likelihood of middle ear effusion. Advantages over tympanometry include that it is unaffected by crying or the presence of cerumen. It is not widely used, however, because there are no specific standards established to determine results.

**Tympanocentesis.** Gold standard for diagnosis of AOM, although it is not routinely used because of cost, effort, and lack of availability. It involves the removal of fluid from the middle ear to identify the bacteria causing the infection. It improves diagnostic accuracy, guides treatment by finding the causative pathogen, and avoids unnecessary medical or surgical intervention. It is especially useful in AOM unresponsive to antibiotics or recurrent AOM.

**Culture and sensitivity.** Not routinely done, but if drainage is present or tympanocentesis is performed, it helps guide treatment in finding the causative pathogen and antibiotics to which it is sensitive.

## Patient Problem/Analyze Cues/Prioritize Hypotheses

# Acute Pain

*due to* increased pressure in the middle ear occurring with fluid and/or infection

***Desired Outcome/Generate Solutions:*** The child is free from pain or has significantly decreased pain (e.g., less than 4 on a 0–10 scale: FLACC [*f*ace, *l*egs, *a*ctivity, *c*ry, and *c*onsolability], Wong–Baker Faces, or a numeric scale [0–10]) within 1 hour after intervention/treatment.

| ASSESSMENT—RECOGNIZE CUES/ INTERVENTIONS—TAKE ACTION | RATIONALES |
|---|---|
| Assess the pain level at least every 4 hours using a developmentally appropriate pain scale for the child (FLACC, Faces, or numeric scale). | A pain scale developmentally appropriate for a child will enable an accurate assessment of the pain level and help evaluate the relief obtained. |
| Administer the antipyretics/analgesics on a regular basis, for example, acetaminophen every 4–6 hours or ibuprofen every 6–8 hours. Both medications are weight-based. | This protocol provides better control of fever and pain than on an as-needed basis. Ibuprofen must not be used on an infant less than 6 months old. |
| Avoid the overdosage of acetaminophen. | Hepatic necrosis can occur. The child must not receive more than 4000 mg/day (American Pharmacists Association, 2021). |
| Reassess the pain level and/or temperature 1 hour after administering medication. | This evaluates the effectiveness of pain relief/fever control measure. |
| Administer the antibiotics, if prescribed. Instruct parents to: | Many cases of mild-to-moderate AOM resolve in 2–3 days without antibiotics. This correlates with the 2013 Clinical Practice Guidelines from the AAP, which are the current guidelines. |
| • Administer the correct dose of medication at the correct time. | This ensures optimal effectiveness of the medication. |
| • Administer all doses (correct number/day and total number of doses prescribed). | The child may feel better after several days, and the parents may stop giving the medication. This may cause OM to reoccur and/or enable antibiotic-resistant bacteria to develop and infect the child. |

| ASSESSMENT—RECOGNIZE CUES/ INTERVENTIONS—TAKE ACTION | RATIONALES |
|---|---|
| • Store medications appropriately. | Many antibiotics have to be refrigerated. |
| Use localized comfort measures based on developmental age that provide maximal comfort for the child.<br><br>• Apply warm compresses to the affected ear or have the child lie on the affected ear on a heating pad on a low setting, covered with a towel to protect the child from potential burns.<br><br>• Apply a wrapped ice bag over the affected ear to decrease edema and pressure. | What is comforting to an infant usually is not comforting to an adolescent. Every child has specific measures that are comforting to him or her. Parents are generally the best source for this information, especially with younger children. |
| Administer analgesic otic drops if prescribed. | These drops may relieve pain but there is not enough evidence to recommend it for routine use (Gaddey et al., 2019). |
| Position for comfort according to the type of OM.<br><br>• AOM: Position with the affected ear in the dependent position.<br><br>• OME: Elevate the head. | Positioning decreases pressure on the TM. |
| Instruct older children to open their eustachian tube by yawning or performing Valsalva maneuver (close your mouth, pinch your nose, and blow air out like trying to blow up a balloon). | This facilitates the drainage of fluid from the middle ear into the pharynx and decreases pressure on the TM. |

## Patient Problem/Analyze Cues/Prioritize Hypotheses

# Dehydration

*due to* losses associated with fever and decreased intake

*Desired Outcome/Generate Solutions:* Within 24 hours of interventions, the child is alert and responsive, the anterior fontanel is soft and not sunken (in a child younger than 2 years), the oral mucous membranes are moist, abdominal skin turgor is good, the child has age-/weight-appropriate urine output (e.g., infant 2–3 mL/kg/hour, toddler and preschool-aged child 2 mL/kg/hour, school-aged child 1–2 mL/kg/hour, and adolescent 0.5–1 mL/kg/hour), and the child receives at least maintenance-level fluids.

| ASSESSMENT—RECOGNIZE CUES/ INTERVENTIONS—TAKE ACTION | RATIONALES |
|---|---|
| Assess the hydration status every 4 hours. Instruct the parents on how to do this and explain its importance. | The younger the child is and the less he or she weighs, the greater the percentage of body weight that is water. The child can become dehydrated easily. Routinely assessing for dehydration in a child who is running a fever and/or has decreased intake facilitates rapid treatment to resolve dehydration. A child who is dehydrated may have a decreasing level of consciousness, sunken anterior fontanel (if younger than 2 years), dry or sticky oral mucous membranes, tenting abdominal skin, and decreasing urine output. |
| Instruct parents when to call the health care provider regarding dehydration. | This facilitates their ability to detect a problem early, thereby ensuring quicker problem resolution. Parents should call under the following conditions:<br><br>• The child is not as alert as usual.<br><br>• The anterior fontanel is sunken.<br><br>• Inside of the mouth is dry or sticky if the child is not a mouth breather.<br><br>• Skin on the abdomen stays up like a tent when pinched.<br><br>• Fewer wet diapers than usual/voiding is less often than usual. |

| ASSESSMENT—RECOGNIZE CUES/ INTERVENTIONS—TAKE ACTION | RATIONALES |
| --- | --- |
| Calculate the maintenance fluids for the child and instruct the family to provide this in terms they can understand. | Specific information enables parents to ensure that their child receives the correct fluid volume. For example, if the child weighs 15 kg, maintenance fluids are 1250 mL/day (42 oz), and if the child drinks from a 6-oz "sippy" cup (180 mL), that child needs to drink at least seven sippy cupfuls (1260 mL) of fluid a day. |
| | Calculation for minimum daily maintenance fluids: |
| | For the child weighing 15 kg: |
| | Up to 10 kg: 100 mL/kg/24 hours = 10 kg $\times$ 100 mL/kg/24 hours = 1000 mL/24 hours |
| | 10–20 kg: 50 mL/kg/24 hours = 5 kg $\times$ 50 mL/kg/24 hours = 250 mL/24 hours 15 kg = 1250 mL/24 hours |
| Offer the child small amounts of fluid at a time and encourage soft food. | Sucking on a nipple or straw or chewing can increase ear pain. |

## Parent Problem/Analyze Cues/Prioritize Hypotheses

# Deficient Knowledge

*due to* unfamiliarity with the disease process and prevention

***Desired Outcome/Generate Solutions:*** Immediately after instruction, the parents verbalize an accurate understanding of the disease process and ways to decrease/prevent future incidents of OM.

| ASSESSMENT—RECOGNIZE CUES/ INTERVENTIONS—TAKE ACTION | RATIONALES |
| --- | --- |
| Assess the parents' knowledge base/understanding of OM, its treatment, and prevention. | Identifying their knowledge/understanding facilitates more effective teaching and helps in correcting misconceptions. |
| Describe the different types of OM and symptoms of each. | Knowledge and understanding improve adherence to the treatment plan. |
| | • AOM: infection of the middle ear; fever and pain may be treated with antibiotics and pain medications. |
| | • OME: inflammation of the middle ear with fluid behind the TM without signs of acute infection; feeling of fullness in the ear; difficulty hearing; and is not treated with antibiotics. |
| Explain that treatment of pain is important, especially in the first few days of OM. | The child is likely to eat and drink more if comfortable, and this facilitates healing. |
| Instruct parents about the importance of giving the full course of antibiotics if they are prescribed and having the ear rechecked when the medication regimen is finished, following the prescriber's guidance. | Adequate treatment of AOM requires the full course of antibiotics; otherwise, OM can reoccur and/or allow an antibiotic-resistant bacteria to infect the child. Ear rechecks assess the effectiveness of treatment. |
| Discuss the preventive feeding practices for an infant. | Feeding practices that prevent OM in infants include the following: |
| | • Feeding the infant in an upright position: facilitates drainage of the middle ear. |
| | • Not putting the infant in bed with a bottle: this increases the incidence of ear infections. |
| | • Decreasing or eliminating the use of a pacifier after 6 months old: sucking on a pacifier causes bacteria to reflux back up into the ear. |
| Explain the importance of avoiding smoking around the child. | Passive smoking increases the incidence of OM. |

# ASSESSMENT—RECOGNIZE CUES/INTERVENTIONS—TAKE ACTION

# RATIONALES

| ASSESSMENT—RECOGNIZE CUES/INTERVENTIONS—TAKE ACTION | RATIONALES |
|---|---|
| Explain the importance of gentle blowing of the nose during upper respiratory infection (URI) rather than forceful nose blowing. | This decreases the risk for transferring organisms from the eustachian tube to the middle ear. |
| Encourage blowing activities (e.g., bubbles, pinwheels) or chewing sugarless gum during a URI. | These activities help promote equalization of pressure in the middle ear. |
| Explain the prevention of ear pain during airplane travel. | Increased atmospheric pressure increases ear pain.<br>• The health care provider may prescribe nasal mucosal shrinking spray if the child has URI or chronic OME to decrease pressure on the TM from edema.<br>• The parent should offer a bottle or pacifier to the infant or give an older child gum during descent to help equalize TM pressure. |
| Describe the potential complications of OM. | Inadequate adherence or nonadherence to treatment may result in the following:<br>• Hearing loss<br>• Perforated, scarred eardrum<br>• Mastoiditis<br>• Cholesteatoma (a cystic mass composed of epithelial cells and cholesterol that occurs as a result of chronic OM). It may occlude the middle ear, or enzymes produced by the cyst may destroy adjacent bones, including the ossicles.<br>• Intracranial infections such as meningitis |

## ADDITIONAL PROBLEMS:

| | |
|---|---|
| "Psychosocial Support for the Patient's Family and Significant Others" for relevant psychosocial problems | Chapter 9 |
| "Asthma" for *Anxiety* | Chapter 77 |

## PATIENT–FAMILY TEACHING AND DISCHARGE PLANNING

When providing child–family teaching, focus on sensory information and avoid giving excessive information. Utilize a variety of teaching methods (e.g., videos, iPads/tablets, and webinars as well as verbal and written) depending on learning style and resources. Stress family-centered care, which is viewing the family as a unit that is the "constant" in the child's life and maintaining or improving the health of the family and its members in a holistic manner. Include information about the following, ensuring that written information is at a level the reader can understand:

✓ Types of ear infections, signs and symptoms, and treatment of each type.

✓ Importance of administering antibiotics as prescribed (can develop resistant strains of bacteria otherwise).

  • Return demonstration of drawing up the correct dose of medication and administering it to the child correctly.

  • Use of a syringe or other calibrated device for administering medication to children.

  • Administering doses at the correct time each day and for the total number of days prescribed.

  • Teach the seven rights of medication administration:
    1. Right child
    2. Right medication
    3. Right dose (i.e., right concentration and right amount/volume of medication)
    4. Right preparation
    5. Right route (e.g., ear drops or oral medication)
    6. Right time
    7. Right documentation—to help keep track of when the child received doses

  • Correct storage of medication (e.g., some need to be refrigerated)

✓ Method of assessing pain in the child and importance of administering analgesic for pain on a regular basis.

✓ Treating fevers correctly:

  • Discuss at what temperature an antipyretic is needed.

  • Explain that fever increases ear pain.

✓ If receiving otic drops, how to administer based on the child's age:

  • Child younger than 3 years, pull the earlobe/pinna down and back.

  • Child older than 3 years, pull the pinna up and back.

✓ Prevention:

  • Never give an infant a bottle to drink while lying down.

- Keep an infant upright during feeding.
- Breastfeed as long as possible.
- Decrease the time a pacifier is used or stop using after 6 months (exception is when flying to prevent ear pain from atmospheric pressure changes).
- Do not smoke around the child or take him or her where smoking occurs.
- If the child will attend group child care, try to place with the least number of children possible.
- Vaccinate the child against pneumococcal and influenza infections.

✓ Signs and symptoms of dehydration:
- The child is not as alert and responsive as usual.
- Soft spot on top of the head may look sunken (for children younger than 2 years).
- Inside of the mouth (not lips) is dry or sticky rather than moist (if the child is not a mouth breather).
- Skin on the abdomen sits up like a tent when gently pinched.
  - Decreased number of wet diapers or same number but not as wet as normal for an infant or young child or decreased number of voids/day in an older child.

✓ Telephone number to call in case any questions arise about therapy or disease after office/emergency department visit.

✓ Importance of follow-up (e.g., many health care providers will do an ear recheck after the child finishes medication).

✓ When to call the health care provider:
- Fever or pain has not decreased after 48–72 hours while on antibiotics.
- Child is showing signs of dehydration.
- Child develops a stiff neck.
- Drainage present from the child's ear canal.

✓ The child needs to have hearing evaluated if the child has had OME for more than 3 months.

✓ Referral to pediatric ear, nose, and throat specialist if OM or OME is chronic.

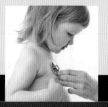

# Poisoning 87

## OVERVIEW/PATHOPHYSIOLOGY

Poisoning can result in death and is a leading cause of hospital visits for children. Safe Kids Worldwide noted that every day in the United States in 2018, 171 children from birth to 14 years were treated in emergency departments (EDs) and about 23 children needed to be hospitalized due to poisoning. The rate of deaths from poisoning decreased by 28% from 2004 to 2018 with one death per week in 2018. Twice as many deaths occurred in Black children as in White and more in boys than girls (Safe Kids Worldwide, 2020a). The 2021 Annual Report of the National Poison Data System (NPDS) reported that poisoning occurred most often through ingestion in about 83% of all cases reported, followed by inhalation/nasal, dermal, and ocular routes, and is seen most often in children younger than 6 years, with the greatest incidence in children younger than 2 years (Gummin et al., 2022). Curiosity and a natural desire to put things in their mouth place younger children at greater risk for accidental poisoning, but poisoning in teenagers is usually more serious. The 2021 Annual Report also showed that children younger than 5 years were involved in 41% of the human poison exposures, whereas about 56% of human exposures were in children 19 years or younger (Gummin et al., 2022). Most of these exposures (about 99%) were unintentional in children less than 6, about 99%, with a smaller percentage (30%) of exposures unintentional in teens. Adolescents (13–19 years) were the only age group in the 2021 Report in which intentional exposures outnumbered unintentional exposures. Despite the high percentage of exposures, only 1.6% of the fatalities in 2021 were in children 5 years or younger, with the primary cause of death related to analgesics. The most common poisons in children 5 years or younger include cosmetics/personal care items such as perfume or soap (10.8%), household cleaning agents such as laundry detergent or floor cleaners (10.7%), analgesics (8.2%), dietary supplements/herbal/homeopathic (7%), and foreign bodies/toys/miscellaneous items such as the silica gel packages that remove moisture from packages, and glow products (6.5%) (Gummin et al., 2022). Hospitalizations in children under 6 years with unsupervised medication exposure/ingestions decreased about 40% from 2009/10 to 2017/18 but still resulted in 130 ED visits and 23 hospitalizations each day. More than 90% of ED visits for accidental medication exposure occurred in children less than 5 when an unsupervised child got into medication on their own and many occurred due to more medications in the home, improperly stored medications,

and/or the medications belonging to grandparents (Safe Kids Worldwide, 2020b).

Adult opioid overdoses have been well publicized, but there has also been a growing concern for children. The Safe Kids Worldwide: Keeping Kids Safe Around Medicine report published in 2020 showed that analgesics caused over twice as many accidental unsupervised medication ingestions and ED visits for one substance ingested in 2017/18 in children less than 6. The 2021 Annual Report of the NPDS noted that pain medication/analgesics are the single most frequent cause of pediatric fatalities reported to Poison Control. About 80% of the deaths in teens 13–19 years were intentional, and analgesics were associated with almost twice as many deaths as any other category even though teens comprised only 8% of the exposures (Gummin et al., 2022). The opioid crisis in the United States is a significant public health issue among children and adolescents. A recent article in JAMA Health Forum noted that the use of prescription and illicit opioids resulted in the deaths of almost 9000 children and adolescents in the United States from 1999 to 2016 with more than a twofold increase in the death rate from opioid poisoning. The article also noted that a recent study by Chua et al. found that 46% of opioid prescriptions for children and young adults in 2019 would have been considered high risk even for adults (Stone et al., 2022). The 2021 National Survey on Drug Use and Health noted that marijuana was the most commonly used illicit drug overall with adolescents 12–17 years having the third highest rate of use, one-third that of adults 18–25 years (Substance Abuse and Mental Health Services Administration, 2022). The 2021 Annual Report of the NPDS listed cannabinoid as an emerging trend with exposures increasing since 2016. Again, the majority were in adults (about 53%), followed by adolescents 13–19 years (about 27%), children 5 years or less (about 14%) and children 6–12 years (about 4.6%), and 1% with unknown ages. For children less than 13 years old, edible marijuana products were the most common exposure (about 41%) followed by plant-based marijuana (about 30%). Children 5 years or younger were the largest age group in exposures with marijuana edibles (Gummin et al., 2022).

Adolescents also have an increased incidence of hospitalization resulting from poisoning, but it is most often intentional and frequently involves inhaling substances. The FDA and Surgeon General declared youth e-cigarette usage an epidemic in 2018. Numerous studies cite the growing incidence of smoking and now e-cigarettes. Although originally advertised as a healthy alternative to cigarette smoking, there is a growing concern with the increased incidence of e-cigarette use or vaping. The 2022 National Youth Tobacco Survey showed high rates of e-cigarette usage in middle- and high-school students. The current study notes that it is difficult to compare these results with previous years, as the survey was solely conducted in schools before 2021 and the 2022 survey utilized an online survey with fewer responses than in past surveys. Increased use of tobacco products was noted in certain populations, for example, students reporting severe psychological distress and students identifying as transgender. Over 70% of the tobacco products used by middle school and high students were e-cigarettes (Park-Lee et al., 2022). There is also an increased teen use of e-cigarettes to inhale cannabis oil (Patterson et al., 2020). The 2019 Annual Report of the AAPCC discussed emerging trends of e-cigarette-associated lung injury that was first noted in July 2019 (Gummin et al., 2020) but is not addressed specifically in the 2021 Annual Report (Gummin et al., 2022). Nicotine toxicity from exposure to e-cigarette devices and nicotine products is also an issue for children 5 and younger, leading to more than 60% of nicotine-related calls to poison control centers (PCCs) (Quail, 2020).

About 93% of all poisoning incidents occur in the home per the 2021 Annual Report of the NPDS data. Inhalation of carbon monoxide is most common in fall and wintertime, and because it is an odorless, colorless, and tasteless gas, it is not easily detected. Most homes have more than 500 toxic substances in them, and one-third of these are in the kitchen. The garage is also particularly dangerous for children, with gasoline and pesticides among the toxic substances housed there. Improper storage of toxic substances and medications, as well as caregiver distractions, are major factors of poisoning in children. Risk factors other than developmental age:

- Boys 12 years or younger are more likely than girls to be poisoned, but this is reversed in adolescents and adults (Gummin et al., 2022)
- Children are more likely to suffer from elevated blood lead levels if they are younger than 5 years and live in homes built before 1978, are non-Hispanic Black children, and have a low income, immigrants or refugee status, or live in large metropolitan areas. Lead service line pipes or poor anticorrosion control have also been found to cause lead poisoning. Any detectable level of lead in the body is abnormal and can cause harm to a child's developing brain. The CDC now recommends screening of all Medicaid-enrolled or -eligible children at 12 and 24 months or at age 24–72 months if they were not previously screened and all children that are identified as high risk for lead poisoning based on the age of housing and socioeconomic risk factors. The blood lead reference value (BLRV) was changed from 5 mg/dL or greater to between 3.5 and 5 mg/dL in 2021. This policy update notes that the BLRV should be used to decide if medical or environmental follow-up actions should be initiated for an individual child (Ruckart et al., 2021).

## HEALTH CARE SETTING

Emergency department with possible hospitalization.

## ASSESSMENT

Varies depending on the source of the poisoning.

**Gastrointestinal system.** Nausea, vomiting, diarrhea, abdominal pain, and anorexia.

**Respiratory system.** Depressed or labored respirations and unexplained cyanosis.

**Circulatory system.** Signs of shock including increased, weak pulse; decreased blood pressure; increased, shallow respirations; pallor; and cool, clammy skin.

**Central nervous system.** Dizziness, overstimulation, pupillary changes, sudden loss of consciousness, behavioral changes, seizures, stupor/lethargy, and coma.

**Integumentary system.** Skin rashes; burns to mouth, esophagus, and stomach; eye inflammation; skin irritations; stains around the mouth; and oral mucous membrane lesions.

### Signs, symptoms, and basic treatment specific to various poisons

**Acetaminophen ingestion.** Included in many over-the-counter medications, acetaminophen is the most common drug ingestion in children. Symptoms occur in stages and are dose dependent (e.g., child may not progress through all stages):

- Stage 1 (first 24 hours): malaise, nausea, vomiting, sweating, pallor, and weakness, or the child may not have symptoms.
- Stage 2 (next 24–72 hours): decrease or disappearance of symptoms in stage 1 and right upper quadrant pain caused by liver damage and increase in liver enzymes.
- Stage 3 (72–96 hours): jaundice, liver necrosis, and possible death from hepatic failure.
- Stage 4: More than 5 days if the child does not die during the hepatic stage (stage 3) and involves gradual recovery.
- Treatment is with the antidote acetylcysteine (Mucomyst).

**Corrosive ingestion.** Toilet and drain cleaners, bleach, ammonia, liquid dishwasher detergent, and denture cleaner. Complaints of severe burning pain in the mouth, throat, and stomach; whitish burns of the mouth and pharynx with edema of the lips, tongue, and pharynx; difficulty swallowing, which leads to drooling; respiratory distress; anxiety and agitation; and shock. Treatment involves diluting the corrosive substance and avoiding emesis, which would increase damage.

**Hydrocarbon ingestion.** Gasoline, kerosene, paint thinner, lamp oil, turpentine, lighter fluid, and some furniture polishes. Gagging, choking, and coughing; nausea, vomiting; characteristic petroleum breath odor; and central nervous system (CNS) depression. Respiratory symptoms of pulmonary involvement include tachypnea, cyanosis, retractions, and grunting. Treatment is symptomatic, but inducing vomiting is generally contraindicated.

**Lead ingestion.** Paint chips from lead-based paint, lead-contaminated dust in the home, soil contaminated with lead, lead solder used in plumbing and artwork, vinyl miniblinds, improperly glazed pottery, and traditional/folk remedies.

Symptoms may be vague with insidious onset. Asymptomatic lead poisoning in children is becoming more common, and even low blood levels (3.5–5 mcg/dL) are linked with irreversible neurocognitive and behavioral impairments (Mayans, 2019; Ruckart et al., 2021). If symptomatic, symptoms may be vague with insidious onset. Children absorb 50% of the lead they ingest and deposit it in their growing bones. Adults absorb only 10% of lead ingested.

- Gastrointestinal: anorexia, nausea, vomiting, and constipation.
- CNS:
  - *Low-dose exposure*—distractibility, impulsivity, hyperactivity, hearing impairment, aggression, mild intellectual deficits, loss of recently acquired developmental skills, and loss of coordination.
  - *High-dose exposure*—lead encephalopathy, mental retardation, severe ataxia, altered level of consciousness (LOC), paralysis, blindness, seizures, coma, and death all can occur.
- Cardiovascular: hypertension, bradycardia.
- Hematologic: anemia.
- Renal: glycosuria, proteinuria, possible acute or chronic renal failure, and impaired calcium function.
- Treatment depends on lead blood level.

**Iron ingestion.** Vitamin supplements with iron are one of the most commonly ingested poisonous substances in children. Iron poisoning occurs in stages ranging from the initial stage (within 6 hours after ingestion) with vomiting, hematemesis, bloody stools, and abdominal pain to the hepatic injury stage (48–96 hours after the ingestion) with seizures, coma, and liver failure. If the child survives, pyloric or duodenal stenosis or hepatic cirrhosis may develop 2–4 weeks after ingestion. Treatment may include lavage or chelation therapy.

**Carbon monoxide inhalation.** Improperly ventilated heaters, wood stoves, and charcoal grills; poorly ventilated automobile. Younger children may present symptoms before older children and adults due to increased respiratory rate and oxygen use.

- *Mild manifestations:* headache, irritability, stomach upset/nausea, and tiredness (similar to early "flu" symptoms).
- *Severe intoxication*, altered LOC, extreme dizziness, hallucinations, and coma. Cherry-red skin has been considered a late sign of most of CO poisoning but occurs rarely. Pallor and cyanosis are more common.

Treatment includes the administration of oxygen and symptomatic treatment.

## DIAGNOSTIC TESTS

History and physical examination help determine necessary tests.

**Arterial blood gases.** May be done if the child is hypoventilating.

**Serum levels.** Blood levels of acetaminophen, salicylate, lead, iron, and alcohol help determine whether treatment with an antidote is necessary.

**Serum carboxyhemoglobin level.** To determine the degree of carbon monoxide poisoning.

## Parent Problem/Analyze Cues/Prioritize Hypotheses

# Risk for Poisoning

*due to* inadequate knowledge about poison prevention

**Desired Outcome/Generate Solutions:** Immediately after teaching, the parents verbalize an accurate understanding of how to childproof all areas (home, babysitter's home, and grandparents' home) in which the child lives or plays.

| ASSESSMENT—RECOGNIZE CUES/ INTERVENTIONS—TAKE ACTION | RATIONALES |
|---|---|
| Assess the parental knowledge level/understanding of potential sources of poisoning. | Teaching can be more effective with a good baseline per the parents' knowledge/understanding. |
| Based on the child's developmental age, discuss the ways in which the child might be exposed to poisons. | Understanding developmentally appropriate behavior enables parents to childproof the home more effectively. For example, a 1-year-old puts everything in the mouth but is not climbing yet, so any potential poison the child could reach while crawling or standing needs to be secured out of his or her reach. |
| Going room by room, discuss the areas that need to be childproofed, with a special emphasis on the kitchen, storage areas, and bathroom. | Many poisonings involve household cleaners or medications. Knowledge of childproofing each area decreases the risk for exposure to potentially toxic substances. |

Continued

| ASSESSMENT—RECOGNIZE CUES/ INTERVENTIONS—TAKE ACTION | RATIONALES |
|---|---|
| Review all materials in the home environment that could be poisonous. | Parents may not be aware of all the potentially poisonous substances in their home. Increased awareness likely will decrease the child's exposure to poisonous substances, including the following:<br>• Household cleaners, disinfectants<br>• Cosmetics<br>• Insecticides<br>• Mouthwash with alcohol in it<br>• Alcohol (beverages or rubbing alcohol)<br>• Liquid dishwasher detergent<br>• Foreign bodies and toys, such as bubble-blowing solution and batteries<br>• Arts, crafts, and office supplies, such as pen and ink<br>• Toxic plants<br>• Hydrocarbons<br>• Prescription and nonprescription medications |
| Describe the ways to childproof the home to prevent poisoning. | Guidelines enhance the parents' ability to effectively and efficiently childproof the home against poisoning. Examples include the following:<br>• Put childproof locks on all kitchen, bathroom, and storage room cabinets.<br>• Make sure all poisonous products are out of reach in locked cabinets.<br>• Do not leave purse/briefcase sitting out that contains medication, cosmetics, or pens.<br>• Buy medications with child-resistant caps but still store in a locked cabinet.<br>• Do not store poisonous substances in food containers or water bottles; store them in the original containers.<br>• Properly dispose of all old medications and other potential poisons that are no longer being used. Dispose of poisons out of the child's reach (i.e., if poison is discarded in the kitchen trashcan and the child can reach the trashcan, it was not disposed "out of the child's reach"). Guidelines for disposing of hazardous household waste are available from the United States Environmental Protection Agency at https://www.epa.gov/hw/household-hazardous-waste-hhw.<br>• Hang or install a carbon monoxide detector on each level of the home on which bedrooms are located.<br>• If the home was built before 1978, have it tested for lead-based paint. |
| Discuss these general guidelines to prevent poisoning:<br>• Stay alert when using poisonous household products. | Poisoning by ingestion or inhalation can occur in a matter of seconds. |
| • Never refer to medicine or vitamins as "candy." | The child may think it is harmless or tastes good. |
| • Do not take medicine in front of young children. | Toddlers and preschoolers often imitate adult behavior. |
| Reinforce the importance of informing family/friends of the previous guidelines. | Even with the home childproofed by the parents, visitors may bring potentially poisonous substances into the home (e.g., grandmother may visit and leave her purse containing a medicine bottle on the floor). |
| Encourage parents to childproof all residences/facilities visited by the child. | The child may be safe at home but not at group childcare or the grandparents' home. |

## Parent Problem/Analyze Cues/Prioritize Hypotheses

# Deficient Knowledge

*due to* unfamiliarity with first aid for toxic ingestion/inhalation/exposure in accidental poisoning

***Desired Outcome/Generate Solutions:*** Immediately after teaching, the parents verbalize an accurate knowledge of steps to take if accidental poisoning occurs.

| ASSESSMENT—RECOGNIZE CUES/ INTERVENTIONS—TAKE ACTION | RATIONALES |
|---|---|
| **Teach Parents the Following:** | |
| Post PCC number on all phones. Also have emergency medical services (EMS) and pediatrician's number readily available. | It is vital to call PCC for a possible ingestion of a toxic substance before administering any antidote to ensure the correct treatment is implemented. Some home treatments may interfere with effective gastric decontamination. |
| If syrup of ipecac is in the child's home, babysitter's home, or any other facility in which the child is cared for, it must be disposed of safely. | The current recommendation is that routine administration of ipecac is avoided in all settings per the American Academy of Pediatrics and PCC. |
| Review the following immediate action response if a child is poisoned:<br>• If swallowed, remove any remaining poison from the child's mouth. Call PCC immediately.<br>• If poison is on the skin, remove contaminated clothing right away without touching the poison and rinse the child's skin with running water. Wash the skin with soap and water and rinse well. Call PCC immediately.<br>• If poison is in the eye, flush the eye with lukewarm to cool water for a full 15 minutes. Call PCC immediately.<br>• If poison is inhaled, move the child to fresh air right away. Call PCC. | Having this knowledge base enables parents to decrease absorption and provide appropriate treatment in the event of poisoning. |
| Discuss the following specific information parents need to give to PCC:<br>• Child's weight and age.<br>• Time the poisoning occurred.<br>• Amount ingested.<br>• Name of poison, if possible. If the medicine bottle or container is available, have it on hand when speaking with PCC. | Specific information enables PCC to direct treatment more appropriately. |

| ADDITIONAL PROBLEMS: | |
|---|---|
| "Psychosocial Support for the Patient's Family and Significant Others" for nursing problems such as *Anxiety* and *Difficulty Coping* for the family whose child is being seen in the emergency department or is hospitalized for a life-threatening condition. | Chapter 9 |
| "Bronchiolitis" for *Dehydration.* The child may be dehydrated because of the effects of ingested substances, treatment for poisoning, or decreased fluid intake. | Chapter 79 |

## ✓ PATIENT–FAMILY TEACHING AND DISCHARGE PLANNING

When providing child–family teaching, focus on sensory information, avoid giving excessive information, and initiate a visiting nurse referral for necessary follow-up teaching and/or to assess safety of the home. Utilize a variety of teaching methods (e.g., videos, iPads/tablets, and webinars as well as verbal and written) depending on the learning style of child/family. Stress family-centered care, which is viewing the family as a unit that is the "constant" in the child's life and maintaining or improving the health of the family and its members. Include information about the following (ensure that written information is at a level the reader can understand):

✓ Contributing factors to the potential for poisoning for each child in the household:
  • Developmental age of the child (e.g., cognitive, physical, and psychosocial)
  • Environmental factors
  • Behavioral problems
  • Level of supervision
✓ Poison prevention tips:
  • Keep all poisonous products out of reach in cabinets locked with safety locks.
  • Know what household products are poisonous or potentially poisonous.
  • Be careful and alert when using poisonous household products.
  • Regularly discard old medications and other potential poisons in a safe manner.
  • Keep all products in their original containers.
  • Remember that many cosmetics and personal products may be poisonous (e.g., aftershave, cologne, hair spray, and fingernail polish remover). Be sure to store them out of the child's reach and where the child cannot climb to get them.
  • Buy products with child-resistant tops.
  • Make sure that poisonous plants are not in the house or yard where the child plays.
  • Put a carbon monoxide detector on each level of the home where bedrooms are located.
  • Keep all medications (prescription and nonprescription) in labeled containers and locked in a cabinet (none in a purse or briefcase or on a counter or dresser).
  • Double-check administering correct dose of medication to the child and using the correct delivery device (i.e., a medication syringe rather than a spoon to administer liquid medication).
  • If the child has to take a prescribed medication on his or her own, leave only one or two doses accessible to the child at a time.
  • If the home was built before 1978, have it tested for lead-based paint.
  • Review the sources of lead poisoning besides paint.
  • Keep alcoholic beverages out of the child's reach and locked up.

✓ Importance of having PCC, EMS, and the health care provider's phone number posted by all phones. Also have the home address and nearest intersection available in case the babysitter or other family member needs to call EMS.
✓ Necessity of close supervision of infants and young children.
✓ Anticipatory guidance for the next milestones the child will achieve and childproofing for each age, including for all children in the family (i.e., what is safe for a 6-month-old is not safe for a 2-year-old). Childproof all residences in which the child stays. Reassess the safety/childproofing frequently.
✓ Referrals to community resources, such as local and National Safe Kids Organization, safety experts, stores with a variety of materials to help childproof a home. Additional information can be obtained by contacting the following organizations:
  • Safe Kids Worldwide: https://www.safekids.org/poisonsafety and Medication Safety Checklist: Tips for parents: https://www.safekids.org/sites/default/files/documents/2020_medicine_safety_checklist-eng.pdf.
  • Nationwide Poison Control Center (PCC): (800) 222-1222, https://aapcc.org, or interactive online help at https://www.poisonhelp.org/help/.
  • Mr. Yuk stickers and related material: https://www.chp.edu/injury-prevention/teachers-and-parents/poison-center/Mr-yuk.
  • CDC's *Up and Away* brochure: https://www.upandaway.org. It provides information and advice on protecting children from an accidental medication overdose.
  • Healthy Children (parenting website backed by pediatricians and the American Academy of Pediatrics providing several references on poisoning as well as other safety and childcare issues): https://healthychildren.org/English/Pages/default.aspx.
✓ Resources for safe management & reduction of hazardous household waste in home:
  • EPA: https://www.epa.gov/hw/household-hazardous-waste-hhw

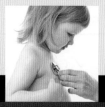

## OVERVIEW/PATHOPHYSIOLOGY

Sickle cell disease (SCD) comprises a group of hereditary blood disorders in which hemoglobin S (HbS) is the dominant hemoglobin. HbS (sickle hemoglobin) replaces normal adult hemoglobin. In HbS, valine, an amino acid, is substituted for glutamine/glutamic acid. Under conditions of dehydration, acidosis, hypoxia, and temperature elevations, HbS changes its molecular structure and forms a crescent or sickle-shaped red blood cell (RBC). This causes the cardinal clinical features of chronic hemolytic anemia and vaso-occlusion, which result from obstruction caused by the sickled RBCs and increased RBC destruction. In most instances, the sickling response is reversible with adequate hydration and oxygenation. After repeated cycles of sickling and unsickling, the RBC remains in the sickled form. The most common and severe form of SCD is hemoglobin SS disease, also called *sickle cell anemia* or *homozygous SCD*, in which the individual inherits a sickle cell gene from each parent.

The inheritance pattern is autosomal recessive (both parents must at least have the sickle cell trait). If both parents have the sickle cell trait, there is a 25% chance that each child will have SCD, a 25% chance that each child will have neither the trait nor the disease, and a 50% chance that each child will have the trait. Therefore a child may not have symptoms (except under rare circumstances) with the trait or have varying degrees of symptoms with the disease. SCD is among the most prevalent genetic diseases in the United States and is common in individuals whose ancestors came from sub-Saharan Africa; Spanish-speaking regions in the Western Hemisphere (South America, Caribbean, and Central America); Saudi Arabia; India; and Mediterranean countries such as Turkey, Greece, and Italy. It is estimated that SCD affects 100,000 Americans and occurs in approximately 1 in every 365 African American births and about 1 in every 16,300 Hispanic American births. About 1 in every 13 African American babies is born with this trait, and all newborns in the United States have been screened for SCD since 2006 (Centers for Disease Control and Prevention [CDC], 2019, 2022). Historically, children with SCD did not survive until adulthood. The life expectancy has increased dramatically from a median age at death of 28 years in 1979 to 43 years in 2017. The SCD-related death rate among Black children younger than 5 years of age has decreased 158% over that same time frame (Payne et al., 2020). Both the increased life expectancy and the decreased death rate of children less than 5 years from SCD are from earlier diagnosis (newborn

screening for SCD), improved preventive measures, ongoing education, and better treatments (Phillips, 2021).

Pain is the leading cause of emergency department visits and hospitalizations. It can occur as early as age 4–6 months and unpredictably throughout a lifetime. There is considerable variation in the severity, frequency, and types of pain among and within affected individuals.

## HEALTH CARE SETTING

Primary care with possible hospitalization for infections or pain crisis.

## ASSESSMENT

***Signs and symptoms:*** Generally do not appear in infants before 4–6 months of age because of high levels of fetal hemoglobin (HbF). Pain is the hallmark manifestation and is caused by vaso-occlusion and the resulting ischemia distal to the occlusion. Pain can range from mild and transient to severe, and it can be localized or generalized, lasting from minutes to days or weeks. The acute painful episode or vaso-occlusive crisis (VOC) is reversible and can occur in the extremities, back, chest, and abdomen. Examples include acute hand–foot syndrome (dactylitis—usually seen in children between 6 months and 2 years old), acute joint inflammation, acute chest syndrome (ACS; a common cause of mortality manifesting as chest pain, decreased oxygen saturation, fever, pneumonia-like cough and shortness of breath), anemia, abdominal pain or gallstones, and priapism. Stroke is another form of vaso-occlusive event and has a high rate of recurrence. In the past, children with SCD were at a much higher risk for having a stroke than children without SCD.

The STOP (Stroke Prevention Trial in Sickle Cell Anemia) protocol has been the endorsed standard of care for children with SCD in the United States. Transcranial Doppler (TCD) ultrasound screening is done on a yearly basis for children with SCD from 2 to 16 years. If an abnormal TCD reading occurs, the child receives regular blood transfusions, which have been shown to decrease the risk for stroke significantly. New guidelines from the American Society of Hematology in 2020 state that after 1 year of regular transfusions, individuals interested in stopping the transfusions need to be evaluated per switching to hydroxyurea therapy (Phillips, 2021). Children with SCD often have nonfunctional spleens owing to "clogging" from the sickled RBCs, and this puts them at increased risk for sepsis. Overwhelming infection/sepsis was the leading cause of death in young children with SCD in the past, but studies show this changing with declining deaths in young children since the advent of universal newborn screening for SCD, daily penicillin prophylaxis for children starting at 2 months and continued until at least 5 years, and routine pneumococcal, *Haemophilus influenzae* type b, and meningococcal vaccines for infants/children (Hockenberry et al., 2017; Kamat, 2020).

*Physical assessment:* History and physical examination, including character, location, severity, and duration of pain, as well as at-home treatment. Information should be obtained about methods used in the past to treat pain crises effectively. An initial pain assessment needs to be done and repeated before and after analgesia.

## DIAGNOSTIC TESTS

> **Note:** *Newborn screening for sickle cell anemia is mandated in all states. Results are sent to the infant's primary care physician. If there is any HbS, a second test is done to confirm the diagnosis (CDC, 2019).*

*Hemoglobin electrophoresis, isoelectric focusing, and high-performance liquid chromatography:* Enable definitive diagnosis of SCD.

*Oximetry:* Noninvasive method that will reveal decreased $O_2$ saturation if it is present.

*Chest radiographic examination:* Helps differentiate between ACS and pneumonia.

*Complete blood count with reticulocytes:* May show increased white blood cells with infection. Hb and hematocrit (Hct) levels usually are much lower than normally seen with anemia. The life span of the normal RBC is decreased from 120 days to 10–14 days, so bone marrow compensates with increased production. Reticulocyte count gives an indication of RBC production by the bone marrow (reticulocytes are immature RBCs).

*Blood culture:* Infection may have triggered a crisis. Sepsis is a leading cause of death in children younger than 5 years.

*Basic metabolic panel:* If signs and symptoms of dehydration are present, it helps assess the degree of dehydration and the need for electrolyte replacement.

## Patient Problem/Analyze Cues/Prioritize Hypotheses

# Acute Pain

*due to* tissue anoxia occurring with vaso-occlusion

*Desired Outcomes/Generate Solutions:* For mild to moderate pain, the child states or demonstrates that pain has decreased within 1 hour of receiving oral medication. For severe pain, the child states or demonstrates that pain has decreased within 24 hours of intervention/treatment. Pain is less than 4 on a 0- to 10-point scale such as FLACC (*face, legs, activity, cry,* and *consolability*), FACES, and numeric.

| ASSESSMENT—RECOGNIZE CUES/ INTERVENTIONS—TAKE ACTION | RATIONALES |
|---|---|
| After establishing a pain scale appropriate for the child (FLACC, Faces, Oucher, Poker Chip, or numeric), assess pain before and after analgesic is administered (within 10–30 minutes after IV medication administration and within 1 hour after oral medication administration). Assess the pain level every 2–4 hours unless on continuous infusion of pain medication, in which case assess hourly. | A developmentally appropriate pain scale helps monitor the degree of pain and effectiveness of the pain medication. |
| Assess the hydration status every 4 hours: level of consciousness (LOC), anterior fontanel if the child is younger than 2 years, oral mucous membranes, abdominal skin turgor, and urine output. | This assessment helps detect and prevent/treat dehydration, which causes vaso-occlusion/pain. A child who is dehydrated may exhibit decreased LOC, sunken anterior fontanel (if younger than 2 years), dry or sticky oral mucous membranes if not a mouth breather, tented abdominal skin, and decreased urine output. |
| Plan a schedule of pain medication around the clock, not as needed. (Usually, patients have a continuous infusion as well as patient-controlled analgesia [PCA].) | Consistent use lowers the total amount of medication with better control. Prolonged stimulation of pain receptors results in increased sensitivity to painful stimuli and will increase the amount of analgesia required to relieve pain. |

| ASSESSMENT—RECOGNIZE CUES/ INTERVENTIONS—TAKE ACTION | RATIONALES |
|---|---|
| Explain how PCA works and that the child cannot give self too much medication. Encourage the child/parent to use PCA when it is needed. | Most experts believe that when a child is capable of pushing the button on the pump, usually by 5–6 years of age, he or she can self-administer pain medication. Some facilities allow PCA by proxy: the parent or the nurse can administer the medication if the child is too ill or cannot understand the concept of pushing the button to relieve the pain. |
| Reassure the child/parent that addiction rarely occurs when medication is used to relieve pain. | Fear of addiction may decrease the use of the PCA/request for pain medication. |
| Do *not* administer meperidine (Demerol). | Demerol increases the risk for normeperidine-induced seizures, *especially* in a child with SCD. |
| Carefully apply warmth to the affected area. | Warmth may be soothing to the child, but it must be applied judiciously because ischemic tissue is fragile. |
| Do *not* apply cold compresses. | Cold promotes sickling and vasoconstriction. |
| Use nonpharmacologic pain control measures as appropriate for the child. | Optimally, comfort measures will distract the child from the pain and augment the effects of pharmacologic measures, but they must not be used to replace them. Examples include distraction (watching TV or playing games), deep breathing, relaxation exercises, music, touch, guided imagery, and massage. |

## Patient Problem/Analyze Cues/Prioritize Hypotheses

# Ineffective Tissue Perfusion (Multisystem)

*due to* vaso-occlusion and anemia

***Desired Outcomes/Generate Solutions:*** Within 2 hours after treatment/intervention, the child's oxygen saturation is maintained at greater than 95% or at a level prescribed by the health care provider. There is no evidence of long-term complications from hypoxia.

| ASSESSMENT—RECOGNIZE CUES/ INTERVENTIONS—TAKE ACTION | RATIONALES |
|---|---|
| Assess the respiratory status and mental status every 2–4 hours and as needed. | Frequent assessment ensures early detection of changes in respiratory status. Tachypnea and increased work of breathing (WOB) are early signs of hypoxia. LOC is a good indicator of oxygen perfusion to the brain. |
| Monitor the pulse oximetry continuously. | This is a noninvasive method of assessing oxygen saturation and noting changes promptly. Results may be less accurate in patients with highly pigmented skin, hypotension, and elevated levels of HbF (Hockenberry et al., 2019; Wood 2022). Thus this must be correlated with other respiratory assessment data. |
| Administer the oxygen as prescribed to keep oxygen saturation levels at greater than 95% or at level appropriate for each individual child. | Delivering oxygen when a child is hypoxic eases WOB. However, it does not reverse the sickling process, and long-term use can depress bone marrow activity and increase the anemia. |
| Elevate the head of bed to a comfortable level for the child. | This facilitates chest expansion by decreasing pressure on the diaphragm. |
| Ensure the incentive spirometry every 1–2 hours while the child is awake as age appropriate. | This treatment facilitates deep breathing and decreases the incidence of acute chest syndrome. Some age-appropriate devices could include pinwheels and bubble wands. |
| Administer the packed RBCs as prescribed. | This treatment improves tissue oxygenation by correcting severe anemia. |

## Patient/Parent/Family Problem/Analyze Cues/Prioritize Hypotheses

# Deficient Knowledge

*due to* unfamiliarity with the disease process of SCD, measures to avoid VOC, home management to prevent severe pain crisis, and the genetics that could result in having other children with this disease

**Desired Outcome/Generate Solutions:** Within 48 hours after instruction, the child/parent/family verbalizes an accurate understanding of the disease process, especially a pain crisis, appropriate treatment, and the genetics of disease transmission.

| ASSESSMENT—RECOGNIZE CUES/ INTERVENTIONS—TAKE ACTION | RATIONALES |
|---|---|
| Assess the knowledge/understanding of SCD and its treatment. | Identifying the child's/parents' knowledge facilitates more effective teaching and helps in correcting misconceptions. |
| Provide the basic information about SCD and measures to minimize sickling. | Knowledge of the disease process promotes adherence to the plan of care, for example, taking prescribed medications such as penicillin and folic acid on a regular basis, staying up to date on immunizations, and avoiding precipitating factors (e.g., dehydration, exposure to individuals who are ill with infections, extreme temperatures, high elevations, and excessive physical activity). |
| Encourage obtaining a medical alert bracelet/necklace and informing significant health professionals/school personnel of the diagnosis. | These actions will help ensure prompt and appropriate treatment. |
| Explain the signs of a developing pain crisis, its significance, and the importance of prompt treatment. Assist parents in identifying methods of assessing pain in their child. | Knowledge about the signs of pain crisis and their significance optimally will result in prompt reporting and treatment, which may avoid a severe VOC. For example, in an infant or toddler, a combination of unusual behaviors such as inconsolability, decreased appetite, unexplained crying, and rapid breathing may indicate discomfort or pain. Older children may complain of mild discomfort or aching. |
| Discuss the home treatment for mild/early symptoms of pain crisis. | The severity of pain crisis may be decreased by early/prompt treatment (e.g., resting, increasing fluid intake to 1–1.5 times the maintenance fluids, and administering pain medication). |
| Discuss the transmission of the disease and refer for genetic counseling as indicated. | This information enables the family to make informed reproductive decisions. See the discussion in the introductory section. |
| Encourage parents/family members to be advocates for the child in the hospital, during appointments with the health care provider, and in group child care or the school setting (e.g., individualized education program [IEP] and/or 504 plan at school). Reinforce that they know the child best and understand what is normal or abnormal in relationship to the child. | Family members may be hesitant to ask questions or advocate for the child; however, they are the best resource. Encouraging advocacy increases the likelihood that the child will receive the best care and facilitates optimal development. |
| Encourage the inclusion of siblings with planning and providing care for the chronically ill child as appropriate. | Including siblings may help them cope with/adapt to having a brother/sister with a chronic illness. |
| Supply the family with information about support groups, local/national sickle cell organizations, and resources for additional information. | Support systems likely will improve their knowledge base about the disease process and therapeutics involved as well as let them know they are not "alone." |
| Encourage the family to have the child receive follow-up visits at a sickle cell clinic on a regular basis. | Follow-up in a sickle cell clinic promotes continuity and quality of care. |

## Patient/Parent Problem/Analyze Cues/Prioritize Hypotheses

# Deficient Knowledge

*due to* unfamiliarity with precautions and side effects of prescribed medications

**Desired Outcome/Generate Solutions:** Within 48 hours after instruction, the child/parent verbalizes accurate information about the prescribed medications, including precautions and side effects.

| ASSESSMENT—RECOGNIZE CUES/ INTERVENTIONS—TAKE ACTION | RATIONALES |
|---|---|
| Provide instructions about the following medications: *Morphine Sulfate* | This medication is an example of an opioid analgesic (administered by intravenous [IV] route in the hospital). |
| Instruct the following: | |
| • Assess the child for the level of sedation, pain relief obtained, $O_2$ saturation, and respiratory and cardiac status. | This assessment helps to evaluate the effectiveness of the medication and the possible need to adjust dosage. Morphine can cause respiratory depression, and if it occurs, $O_2$ saturation will decrease along with the respiratory rate. Many hospitals have a sickle cell weaning score to facilitate adjusting the dosage appropriately (United States Boxed Warning): Serious life-threatening, or fatal respiratory depression may occur, especially during initiation or dose escalation. |
| • Assess for dizziness, drowsiness, itching, nausea, vomiting, constipation, urinary retention, and low blood pressure. Explain that the parent/child should notify the staff or health care provider if any of these symptoms occur. | These side effects may indicate the need to change dosage or the medication itself or to provide additional medication, such as diphenhydramine or naloxone, through continuous IV infusion for itching or an antiemetic for nausea. |
| • Reassure them that analgesics, including opioids, are medically indicated and that high doses may be needed to relieve pain. | There is confusion about the issues of pain control and drug dependence. Children rarely become addicted, and needless suffering may occur as a result of unnecessary fears. |
| *Acetaminophen with oxycodone* | This medication is an example of an oral central analgesic/antipyretic with an added opioid. |
| Instruct the parents/child the following: | |
| • Assess for and report dizziness, drowsiness, itching, gastric distress, nausea, vomiting, abdominal pain, low blood pressure, and constipation, as well as excessive sedation and respiratory depression. | These side effects may indicate the need to adjust or change the medication. |
| • Assess whether pain has decreased within 30 minutes to 1 hour of oral administration. If the child has no relief after several doses of pain medication, the parent's need notifies the health care provider. | This assessment evaluates the effectiveness of the medication because this is the time of peak action. If there is no relief after several doses, the health care provider may increase the dosage. |
| • Explain that there are numerous interactions with other medications. | Administration with certain other medications may increase or decrease the effectiveness of this medication. See a drug book for more specific information. |
| • Ensure that the child does not receive more than 4000 mg/day of acetaminophen. This includes all sources of acetaminophen. For example, it may be used for fever in addition to its use as an analgesic. | As the dose is based on the oxycodone content, the acetaminophen dose may not be monitored as closely. Acetaminophen may cause hepatotoxicity. Most commonly occurs in patients receiving supratherapeutic dosing, more frequent than recommended, and/ or use of multiple acetaminophen-containing products. Hepatoxicity has rarely been reported using recommended dosages (American Pharmacists Association [APA], 2021). |
| *Ibuprofen (nonsteroidal antiinflammatory drug [NSAID])* | This medication augments pain control when administered with morphine or acetaminophen with oxycodone/other analgesic. |

Continued

| ASSESSMENT—RECOGNIZE CUES/ INTERVENTIONS—TAKE ACTION | RATIONALES |
|---|---|
| Instruct the following: | |
| Assess for and report dizziness, drowsiness, and heartburn. | These side effects may indicate the need for the health care provider to adjust the dosage or change medication. |
| Administer with food or milk. | This decreases gastrointestinal (GI) upset. |
| For a discussion of safety issues with NSAIDs, see *Pain* in "Osteoarthritis," Chapter 71. | |
| *Folic acid* | This oral medication enhances the bone marrow's ability to produce new blood cells. |
| *Penicillin* | This is a prophylactic antibiotic. Overwhelming infection/sepsis has been the leading cause of death in young children with SCD. Administered orally. |
| Instruct the following: | |
| • Assess for and report rash, nausea, vomiting, diarrhea, black and hairy tongue, and hypersensitivity reactions. Call 911 promptly if anaphylaxis occurs. | These side effects may indicate the need for the health care provider to adjust the dosage or change the medication. |
| • Stress the importance of daily administration as prescribed at least until the child is 5–6 years old. | This reduces morbidity risks associated with pneumococcal septicemia. It may need to be continued for a longer period if the child has experienced invasive pneumococcal infection, has not received pneumococcal immunizations, is on a hypertransfusion program, or is anatomically asplenic. |
| Administer/take with water on an empty stomach 1 hour before meals or 2 hours after meals; may give with food to decrease GI upset. | Food or milk may decrease absorption. |
| *Docusate* | This oral medication is a stool softener. |
| Instruct the following: | |
| • Assess for and report rash, diarrhea, abdominal cramping, or throat irritation. | These are side effects; the health care provider may need to adjust dosage or change medication. |
| • Administer when the child is taking analgesics. | Analgesics may cause constipation. |
| • Monitor the stool pattern while the child is taking this medication. | It may be necessary to consider adding other medications to facilitate stool passage if docusate is not effective. |
| • If using in liquid form, mix with a small amount (5 mL or less) of sweet-tasting substance (e.g., flavored syrup, jam, or applesauce) | These liquids or foods mask the bitter taste and are not essential food items that the child might refuse later. |
| • Ensure that the child is receiving maintenance fluids unless pulmonary symptoms exist. For calculation of maintenance fluids, see *Dehydration* in "Bronchiolitis," Chapter 79. | This facilitates the effectiveness of the docusate and provides needed hydration for the child with sickle cell pain crisis. Increased fluids may be needed if the child is dehydrated or has insensible losses, for example, with fever. |
| *Acetaminophen* | This oral medication is an analgesic/antipyretic. |
| Instruct the following: | |
| • Administer immediately for mild complaints of pain or discomfort. | This may prevent a pain crisis. |
| • Assess for and report rash. | This side effect may indicate the need for the health care provider to adjust the dosage or change medication. |
| • Ensure that child is receiving the therapeutic dose of acetaminophen. | This helps to provide effective pain relief while avoiding hepatic necrosis. |
| • Ensure that the child does not receive more than 4000 mg/day. This includes all sources of acetaminophen. For example, it may be used for fever in addition to its use as an analgesic. | Acetaminophen may cause hepatotoxicity. Most commonly occurs in patients receiving supratherapeutic dosing, more frequent than recommended, and/or use of multiple acetaminophen-containing products (APhA, 2021). |

## ASSESSMENT—RECOGNIZE CUES/ INTERVENTIONS—TAKE ACTION

## RATIONALES

*Hydroxyurea*

*L-Glutamine (Endari)*

*Crizanlizumab (Adakveo)*

*Voxelotor (Oxbryta)*

This oral medication increases the production of HbF, which prevents the sickling of RBCs, thereby decreasing the incidence of VOCs. Consult a drug handbook for more detailed information.

Oral powder which is an amino acid approved by the FDA in 2017 to help reduce the number and length of hospitalizations for VOC and reduce rates of ACS in children 5 years and older (Phillips, 2021).

IV medication, approved in 2019, reduces the frequency of VOCs, for administration to children greater than or equal to 16 years. Administered monthly (APhA, 2021). Consult a drug handbook for more detailed information.

Oral medication approved in 2019 for the treatment of SCD in children 12 years and older and in 2021 for children 4–11 years. Decreases RBC sickling and hemolysis, increases Hgb, and decreases anemia (FDA, 2021; Phillips, 2021). Consult a drug book for more detailed information.

## ADDITIONAL PROBLEMS:

| | |
|---|---|
| Constipation can occur as a result of narcotic analgesics and decreased mobility. See "Immobility" for *Constipation*. | Chapter 1 |
| "Psychosocial Support for the Patient" for *Anticipatory Grief* | Chapter 8 |
| "Psychosocial Support for the Patient's Family and Significant Others" | Chapter 9 |
| "Asthma" for *Anxiety* due to illness, loss of control, and medical/nursing interventions. | Chapter 77 |
| "Asthma" for *Difficulty Coping* due to having a child with a chronic illness. | Chapter 77 |
| "Bronchiolitis" for *Dehydration* (however, a child with sickle cell pain crisis needs 1–1½ times the maintenance, unless pulmonary symptoms are present, in which case, then only maintenance fluids are needed). Increased fluids may be needed if the child is dehydrated and/or has increased insensible losses (e.g., persistent fever). | Chapter 79 |
| "Diabetes Mellitus" (adult care plan) for *Risk for Infection*. Overwhelming infection/sepsis has been the leading cause of death in young children with SCD, and infection risk is an ongoing concern. | Chapter 47 |

## ✓ PATIENT–FAMILY TEACHING AND DISCHARGE PLANNING

When providing child–family teaching, focus on sensory information, avoid giving excessive instructions, and institute a visiting nurse referral as necessary for follow-up assessment and teaching as needed. Utilize a variety of teaching methods (e.g., videos, iPads/tablets, and webinars, as well as written and verbal) depending on the learning style and resources of child/family. A part of initial assessment should include asking about existing knowledge of the disease, ability for self-care by the child and/or family, and psychologic acceptance. Stress family-centered care (viewing the family as a unit that is the "constant" in the child's life and maintaining or improving the health of the family and its members). Include information about the following (ensure written information is at a level the reader can understand):

✓ Basic pathophysiology about sickle disease and pain crisis.

✓ Cause of the pain, including precipitating factors (e.g., dehydration, infection, fever, hot or cold temperatures, high elevations, excessive physical activity, and stress) and the importance of avoiding same.

✓ For boys, priapism (prolonged erection) is possible with SCD. They need to seek medical attention if erections last more than 3 hours or occur frequently.

✓ Avoiding exposure to individuals who are ill with infections (e.g., do not go in crowded areas during flu season). Overwhelming infection/sepsis is the leading cause of death in young children with SCD.

✓ Importance of maintaining adequate oral intake to prevent dehydration and thereby prevent clumping of HbS.

✓ Signs and symptoms of early pain crisis and treatment (i.e., rest, increase fluids to 1–1½ times the maintenance with specific examples [e.g., a 12-kg child who drinks from a 6-oz cup needs at least 6½ cups of fluid/day], and administer acetaminophen or ibuprofen first; if no relief, try the prescription pain medication from the health care provider).

✓ Maintaining a pain diary, which may be beneficial in finding precipitating factors and effective pain control measures. The most effective treatment in an emergency department also needs to be included in the event the child is seen in another hospital.

✓ Medications, including drug name; route; purpose; dosage; precautions; drug–drug, food–drug, and herb–drug interactions; and potential side effects.

✓ Importance of taking medications at home and school as directed. Medication in the original bottle (with prescribing label) and written prescription from the health care provider are needed for the child to be able to take any medication at school.

✓ Nonpharmacologic methods to relieve pain (Stress that they are used in addition to the pain medication not in place of it):

- Psychological strategies: distraction, guided imagery, virtual reality, education/teaching, and hypnotherapy
- Behavioral strategies: deep breathing, relaxation exercises, self-hypnosis, biofeedback, and behavior modification
- Physical strategies: careful application of heat to painful area, transcutaneous electrical stimulation (TENS), massage, acupuncture/acupressure, and mild exercise, if tolerated

✓ Frequent urination, which is normal with increased fluids; enuresis may occur as a result.

✓ When to contact the health care provider:

- Temperature 38.3°C (101°F) or higher per health care provider's guidelines.
- Pain not relieved by prescribed pain medication (e.g., acetaminophen with hydrocodone).
- The child is pale, lethargic, irritable, or dehydrated.
- Vomiting and/or diarrhea lasting more than a day (time frame varies, shorter time frame for a younger child).
- Shortness of breath or other acute pulmonary symptoms.

✓ Weakness (with or without pain, tingling, loss of speech, or any neurological changes).

✓ Coordination of care. Parents need to discuss the child's illness and need with the school nurse and other adults who are in close contact with the child (e.g., teachers, scout leaders, and group child care providers).

✓ Importance of helping siblings cope with/adapt to having a brother/sister with a chronic illness and including them in planning and/or caring for the chronically ill child depending on their age and interest.

✓ Legal rights of the child:

- Individuals With Disabilities Education Act: Mandates federal government to provide funding to education agencies for free and appropriate education to qualifying students with disabilities, including children with SCD if the disease adversely affects school performance. The school is then required to develop an IEP.
- IEP: A multidisciplinary team designs this plan to facilitate special education and therapeutic strategies and goals for each child. The child does not have to be in special education classes. Parents need to be involved in this process.
- Section 504 of Rehabilitation Act of 1973: Each student with a disability (physical or mental impairment) is entitled to accommodation to attend school and participate as fully as possible in school

activities. This accommodation may be related to a medical condition or an educational issue. For example, the child may leave the classroom to use bathroom facilities without raising his or her hand and will not be penalized for excessive absences from school that are caused by SCD. The 504 Plan may include as many accommodations as necessary for the child to function well. More details can be found at https://www.verywellfamily.com and search for 504 Plan.

✓ Importance of ongoing health care management with the health care provider experienced in dealing with SCD to identify and manage chronic complications:

- Receiving childhood immunizations at the appropriate age, especially pneumococcal, *Haemophilus influenzae* type b, meningococcal, and yearly flu vaccine.
- Prompt attention to symptoms of infection (e.g., fever, sore throat).
- Regular visits with the health care provider, not just when ill.

✓ Telephone numbers to call in case questions or concerns arise about the therapy or disease after discharge.

✓ Additional general information can be obtained by contacting the following organizations:

- The Sickle Cell Information Center: https://scinfo.org (variety of resources for parents, children, and teens, including a list of camps for children with SCD). For example: Education Coloring book for Children: The Bear Necessities of Sickle Cell: https://scinfo.org, then click on resources for patients & families and then click on children and adolescents.
- Sickle Cell Disease Association of America, Inc.: https://www.sicklecelldisease.org.
- St. Jude Children's Research Hospital: https://www. stjude.org./treatment/disease/sickle-cell-disease/educational-resources.html. This website has numerous downloadable handouts about SCD, such as Strokes in Children With Sickle Cell Disease and Your Young Child and Sickle Cell Disease.
- Sickle Cell Speaks: https://sicklecellspeaks.com/ Parents/adolescents/young adults sharing their stories as well info per understanding SCD, managing sickle cell, events, etc.
- Starlight Children's Foundation: https://www.starlight.org. This website provides comfort for hospitalized children and their families. WHY IS PART OF URL HIGHLIGHTED?
- Sickle Cell Summer Camp—Children can experience a variety of enjoyable activities under the direction of health care professionals knowledgeable about SCD and its treatment. It also gives children a chance to develop relationships, talk about their experiences, ask questions, and learn more about their condition. More details can be found at https://cdc.gov, then enter "sickle cell summer camp" in the search box.

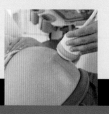

# Bleeding in Pregnancy 89

## OVERVIEW/PATHOPHYSIOLOGY

Hemorrhage during pregnancy continues to be a leading cause of morbidity and mortality. Bleeding can be life threatening when profuse hemorrhage leads to maternal hypovolemia, anemia, and complications such as infection. Major causes of hemorrhage during early pregnancy include *ectopic pregnancy* (implantation outside of the uterus), *threatened spontaneous abortion* (SAB) (confirmed pregnancy with vaginal bleeding), *inevitable SAB* (ruptured membranes with progressive cervical dilation before 20 weeks gestation), *complete SAB* (bleeding and cramping until the passage of the whole conceptus before 20 weeks gestation), *incomplete abortion* (bleeding and cramping with retention of some of the conceptus), *missed abortion* (fetus has died but is retained with the placenta in the uterus), *septic abortion* (from infection) and *gestational trophoblastic disease* (GTD; and includes hydatidiform mole [molar pregnancy]). Hemorrhage later in pregnancy can be due to *cervical insufficiency* (painless dilation of the cervix in the absence of contractions), *placenta previa* (abnormally implanted placenta that partially or completely covers the cervix), *placental abruption* (premature separation from the uterine wall of a normally implanted placenta), *uterine rupture*, or *errors of cord insertion or placental implantation issues*.

## HEALTH CARE SETTING

Primary care or acute care when bleeding persists or surgical intervention is necessary.

## ASSESSMENT

*In early pregnancy*, assessments begin with confirmation of pregnancy, determination of gestational age, and correlation of gestational age with fundal height. The amount and characteristics of bleeding as well as its origin, the severity of pain, and other accompanying signs determine priorities in physical assessment. *In late pregnancy*, medical and nursing assessments are often simultaneous. Bleeding can range from light-pink to dark-brown (old blood) spotting. It may be like heavy menses (up to 1000 mL of blood flows through the placenta). Bleeding can progress rapidly to massive hemorrhage with significant morbidity or mortality for the mother and fetus. When bleeding is associated with a complication of pregnancy, the priorities focus on continuous and ongoing assessment of the following:

*Amount of and characteristics of the bleeding:* Vaginal bleeding can occur at any time during pregnancy. Is the blood viscous, thin, and watery; does it contain clots; is it light pink or bright red or deep red or brown? Is there other tissue, odor, or continuous or recurrent bleeding? A pad count is conducted to maintain an accurate measurement of blood loss.

*Pain:* Was the onset sudden or gradual? Is it localized or generalized, intermittent or continuous, sharp, dull, aching, radiating, or changing? What is its relationship to the uterus or to activities? Pain may be the only sign of an ectopic pregnancy if bleeding is concealed within the abdomen. The abdomen may be tender and exceptionally hard (board-like) as occurs with abruption, and bleeding may be concealed or apparent as the uterine cavity fills with blood.

*Cardiovascular and respiratory status:* Assess for hypertension or hypotension, tachycardia, tachypnea, shortness of breath, postural hypotension, dizziness, lightheadedness, hypoxemia, or syncope.

*Uterine contractions:* Assess for frequency, duration and intensity, resting tone, rupture of membranes, and uterine irritability.

*Condition of the fetus:* Assess for decreased or absent fetal activity relative to gestational age. After 24 weeks gestation, monitor fetal heart rate (FHR) and assess variability, FHR accelerations, FHR decelerations, and FHR changes associated with uterine contractions. Note changes in status from the previous fetal monitor tracings and report to the provider. FHR is assessed as follows: Category 1 is normal, well oxygenated. Category 2 is indeterminate and needs further observation. Category 3 is abnormal and requires action.

*Accompanying signs:* Assess for additional signs of shock with massive blood loss, including cool, pale skin and mucous membranes; oliguria; and altered consciousness. Vaginal discharge before a bleeding episode may range from thin to thick and may be white, yellow, or green. Fever and malodorous vaginal discharge are indications of infection. Assess the woman's anxiety state, as well as her family's emotional response to the bleeding episode.

*Obstetric history:* A thorough history includes the total number of pregnancies (gravidity), the number of live births at more than 20 weeks gestation (parity), and previous abortions or preterm births. Obtain any history of previous bleeding in this pregnancy and any prior pregnancy complications or testing.

## DIAGNOSTIC TESTS

**Obstetric ultrasound:** Transabdominal, transvaginal, or translabial ultrasound locates the gestational sac as intrauterine or ectopic. Real-time ultrasound confirms cardiac activity and a viable fetus. Ultrasound identifies multiple gestation, placental position, number of umbilical vessels, presence of subchorionic hemorrhage (bleeding beneath the outer membrane), and abruption. Ultrasound allows differential diagnosis between the two types of GTD.

**Speculum examination:** A careful speculum vaginal examination safely visualizes the cervix during and after vaginal bleeding, when a sterile-gloved vaginal examination is contraindicated. The examiner can observe dilation and effacement, presence of tissue in the cervix or vaginal vault, polyps, cervical friability, lacerations, or other lesions. Cultures may be obtained. Rupture of membranes can be evaluated using Nitrazine paper or a specimen for microscopic evaluation of ferning (the fern leaf pattern seen with a microscope when amniotic fluid dries).

**Qualitative and quantitative pregnancy tests:** Urine or serum pregnancy tests measure the presence of human chorionic gonadotropin (hCG). The presence of hCG in serum or urine can confirm a pregnancy. Positive results are possible after implantation is complete, 8–10 days after conception, which may occur before or after a missed period. Because the serum concentration of hCG doubles every 1–2 days, serial testing can indicate gestational age. Declining numbers generally indicate SAB or ectopic pregnancy.

**Complete blood count:** Reflects the amount of blood lost, especially by falling levels of hemoglobin (Hgb) and hematocrit (Hct). One pint of blood loss equals approximately 1½-g drop in Hgb and 1%–3% decrease in Hct. Likewise, these factors will rise with each unit of blood replaced. A rising white blood cell count may signal infection. Falling platelets indicate an increasing risk for disseminated intravascular coagulation (DIC). (See "Disseminated Intravascular Coagulation," Chapter 65.)

**Blood Rh factor and antibody screen:** Maternal blood group (ABO) and Rh factor (positive or negative) are determined when medical prenatal care is initiated. An antibody screen (indirect Coombs test) is done to determine whether the Rh-negative woman is sensitized to the Rh antigen. Rh immune globulin (RhoGAM or HypRho-D) is administered within 72 hours after a spontaneous or induced abortion, ectopic pregnancy, or GTD pregnancy; after an external version attempt; after birth with or without a placenta previa or abruptio placenta; at any gestational age; and after maternal abdominal trauma.

**Kleihauer–Betke test:** Checks for the presence of fetal erythrocytes in maternal blood. Fetal–maternal bleeding occurs three to five times more often in pregnancy when the mother experiences abdominal trauma.

**Uterine and fetal heart rate monitoring:** Before gestational viability, uterine activity monitoring alone may be done to demonstrate contraction presence and pattern. In the second and third trimesters, FHR monitoring reveals fetal well-being or fetal response to blood loss, labor, or induction procedures.

Continuous FHR monitoring is used to identify signs of a compromised fetus. Fetal oxygenation may be compromised with a disrupted placental surface area for gas exchange, maternal hypotension, and uterine irritability. The category 2 or category 3 FHR pattern seen with bleeding may include loss of baseline variability, tachycardia or bradycardia, late decelerations, prolonged decelerations, progressively severe variable decelerations, and a sinusoidal pattern. With acute abruptio placenta, there is rapid FHR deceleration indicating imminent fetal demise.

**Nonstress test:** Beginning at 27–32 weeks gestation, this test can demonstrate reactive FHR activity, which indicates adequate fetal oxygenation and an intact central nervous system. Measurement standards differ for the fetus between 32 weeks gestation and term and the fetus less than 32 weeks gestation because the latter's central nervous system is less mature.

PART III: Maternity Nursing Care Plans

## Patient Problems/Analyze Cues/Prioritize Hypotheses

# Risk for Complications Related to Childbirth (Hemorrhage)

*due to* pregnancy-related conditions (SAB [threatened, inevitable, incomplete, complete, or missed], ectopic pregnancy, placenta previa, or abruptio placenta)

# Risk for Complications Related to Childbirth (Shock)

*due to* hypovolemia

**Desired Outcome/Generate Solutions:** Within 2–3 hours of appropriate interventions, the patient returns to a functional level of blood volume/body fluids as measured by return to urinary output greater than 30 mL/hour with urine specific gravity less than 1.030, normotensive blood pressure (90–130/60–80 mm Hg), heart rate (HR) of 60–100 bpm, respiratory rate of 12–20 unlabored breaths/minute, capillary refill time of 2 seconds or less, absence of signs of shock (e.g., alert without anxiety, skin warm and pink, bowel sounds active × 4), and a reactive FHR.

| ASSESSMENT—RECOGNIZE CUES/ INTERVENTIONS—TAKE ACTION | RATIONALES |
|---|---|
| Assess the amount and begin measurement of continuing blood loss, including characteristics and the source/site of blood. As indicated, weigh the saturated linen or peripads and keep a pad count. | Hemorrhage from SAB, placenta previa, or abruptio placenta has different characteristics (see Assessment data, earlier). One gram of weight per scale represents 1 mL blood lost. |
| Assess the accompanying signs and symptoms with blood loss (i.e., pain, fever, and malodorous vaginal discharge) and their duration and association with behaviors (intercourse and activity). | Uterine cramping with hemorrhage may indicate one of the SABs. Deep abdominal pain may signal ectopic pregnancy (with or without bleeding). Painless vaginal bleeding in the third trimester may indicate placenta previa. A board-like, painful abdomen may indicate abruption (with or without dark-red bleeding). Malodorous vaginal discharge may indicate chorioamnionitis (bacteria-caused inflammation of placental membranes). |
| Assess the maternal vital signs (VS) for the signs of shock (hypotension, decreased pulse pressure, tachycardia, delayed capillary refill, cool clammy or mottled skin, and change in mentation and functional ability). Begin assessments every 5–15 minutes and decrease in frequency as her condition improves per agency protocol/health care provider directive. | In a pregnant woman, signs of shock manifest after 25%–30% blood loss. Assessment findings reveal cardiovascular status, degree of hemorrhage, and the results of continuous therapeutic adjustments related to fluid replacement needs. |
| Start and maintain an intravenous (IV) site as soon as possible if one is not in place. Consider the initiation of a second IV site. Use a large-bore needle. | Veins collapse with advancing hemorrhage. Venous access is necessary for the administration of IV fluids. A large needle and a second IV site may be necessary for blood transfusions. |
| Collect a blood specimen for blood type, Rh and antibody screen, complete blood count (CBC), and type and crossmatch per agency protocol and health care provider directives. | This action anticipates the need for fluid replacement therapy as soon as it is available. |
| Administer and carefully monitor the fluid replacement by crystalloid solutions in conjunction with plasma expanders or blood products (e.g., cryoprecipitate, plasma, and packed red blood cells). Monitor for signs of fluid overload (e.g., dyspnea, lung crackles, or cough). | Regardless of the protocol followed, constant adjustments in fluid resuscitation and replacement are necessary during the first 24 hours. Too rapid correction of fluid deficit causes fluid overload, edema, and pulmonary congestion. |
| Insert indwelling catheter and measure urine output hourly. | Urine output returns with recovery from hemorrhagic shock. Its measurement determines replacement adequacy and the patient's changing needs. |
| Monitor laboratory reports: CBC, clotting factors, blood group and Rh, activated partial thromboplastin time (APTT), prothrombin time (PT), and hCG levels. | Hgb and Hct will be lower in the pregnant patient because of hemodilution, and their values will guide fluid replacement. Replacement with packed RBCs raises Hgb 1 g/dL and Hct by approximately 3%. Platelet transfusions increase platelets by 5000/mm$^3$. Fresh frozen plasma raises each clotting factor by 2%–3%. Maintenance of Hct at 30% or greater supports oxygenation and nutrient transport. Platelet levels identify whether thrombocytopenia is present. Platelet values, APTT, PT, and clotting factor values may signal complications (e.g., DIC); hCG levels reveal gestational age/complications (GTD, ectopic pregnancy). |
| Administer the O$_2$ by snug face mask at 8–10 L/minute. | Administering oxygen increases oxygen tension in the circulating blood volume and oxygen delivery to the end organs and fetus. A snug face mask more effectively delivers a higher L/minute flow rate. |
| Position the patient for optimal perfusion (e.g., avoid supine position or use a hip wedge). Use the side-lying position when possible. Change positions every 30 minutes while the patient is awake. Include semi-Fowler position as well, but avoid Trendelenburg position. | These positions ensure adequate circulation to the mother and fetus. When in the supine position a hip wedge prevents compression to the descending aorta or inferior vena cava by the gravid uterus. Semi-Fowler position may enable the fetus to act as a tampon in the third trimester, thereby minimizing bleeding. Trendelenburg position could interfere with adequate maternal respirations. |
| Avoid vaginal or rectal examinations. | These examinations may increase hemorrhage, especially with partial or complete placenta previa. |

Continued

| ASSESSMENT—RECOGNIZE CUES/ INTERVENTIONS—TAKE ACTION | RATIONALES |
|---|---|
| Save expelled conceptus (placenta, membranes, embryo, or fetus). | Anything remaining in the uterus contributes to continued bleeding. The health care provider will evaluate whether the complete or only partial conceptus was passed. Histology studies may be necessary to determine the cause. |
| Ensure meticulous reporting and documentation. | Detailed and accurate communication ensures coordination of diagnosis, changing condition, and therapeutic interventions and maximizes the effectiveness of the entire health care team. |
| Also see "Perioperative Care," Chapter 4. | Dilation and curettage are necessary for a missed or incomplete abortion; laparotomy may be necessary with ectopic pregnancy; cesarean delivery may be necessary for third-trimester bleeding. |

## Fetus Problem/Analyze Cues/Prioritize Hypotheses

# Risk for Impaired Respiratory System Function (Fetal Hypoxia)

*due to* diminished maternal circulation to the uteroplacental unit

**Desired Outcomes/Generate Solutions:** Adequate oxygenation/perfusion to the fetus is demonstrated by fetal activity and FHR variability. After the age of viability, FHR maintains reassuring (category 1) characteristic patterns (i.e., moderate variability, FHR at 110–160 bpm, accelerations may be present or not present, and no late or variable decelerations).

| ASSESSMENT—RECOGNIZE CUES/ INTERVENTIONS—TAKE ACTION | RATIONALES |
|---|---|
| Monitor for fetal distress by repeated nonstress test (NST) as indicated or maintain continuous FHR monitoring at or after 20 weeks gestation. | In the first half of pregnancy, no FHR determination is made. Thereafter FHR and fetal activity reflect fetal oxygenation status. A reactive FHR tracing (an increase of 15 bpm lasting 15 seconds occurring twice in the 20-minute tracing) indicates fetal well-being. Nonreactive FHR indicates hypoxia. Initially, fetal response to hypoxia is increased movements and tachycardia. Bradycardia and decreased movements occur with continued/deepening hypoxia. |
|  | Consideration of preterm behavior and response during the NST is crucial. Before 32 weeks some practitioners consider the NST reactive with an increase in HR of 10 bpm that lasts 10 seconds, occurring twice in the 20-minute period. |
| Administer the $O_2$ by snug face mask at 8–10 L/minute. | Oxygen administration increases oxygen tension in the circulating blood volume and oxygen delivery to the fetus. A snug face mask enhances oxygen delivery to the fetus as well as to the mother. |
| Position the patient for optimal perfusion. For example, if unable to avoid the supine position, use a hip wedge. Encourage a side-lying position. Include semi-Fowler position as well, but avoid Trendelenburg position. Ensure position changes every 30 minutes while the patient is awake. | These positions ensure adequate circulation to the mother and fetus. In the supine position, a hip wedge prevents compression to the descending aorta or inferior vena cava by the gravid uterus. Semi-Fowler position may enable the fetus to act as a tampon in the third trimester, thereby minimizing bleeding. The Trendelenburg position may interfere with adequate maternal respirations. |
| At or after 20 weeks' gestation, assist with amniocentesis and interventions to delay delivery, or facilitate vaginal delivery or cesarean delivery as determined by the health care provider. | Hemorrhage may stop after the placenta (or total conceptus) is removed. The health care provider will assess the fetal lung maturity and then determine the path to take for the best outcome. |
| When the fetus is at 20 weeks' or later gestation, call the neonatal resuscitation team before delivery. | This helps to prepare the team for the delivery of a compromised newborn. Before 20 weeks, the fetus is unable to sustain life after delivery. Twenty weeks or 500 g is used, because dating can be off by a few weeks unless the date of conception is medically confirmed. To err on the side of caution, a resuscitation team would be called until weight and age can be determined. |

## Patient Problem/Analyze Cues/Prioritize Hypotheses

# Acute Pain

*due to* uterine contractions, distention of the lower uterine segment, cervical changes, pressure on adjacent tissues, or tissue trauma (ectopic pregnancy or abruptio placenta)

*Desired Outcomes/Generate Solutions:* Within 1 hour of intervention the patient's subjective perception of pain is at an acceptable level, as evidenced by a report of no more than 2–3 on a 0–10 scale; objective measures such as grimacing are diminished or absent. The patient verbalizes an accurate understanding of her medications and the nonpharmacologic interventions used.

| ASSESSMENT—RECOGNIZE CUES/ INTERVENTIONS—TAKE ACTION | RATIONALES |
|---|---|
| Assess the duration and type of pain, characteristics (intensity, quality, onset, alleviating or aggravating factors), severity by a standard pain scale, and location. | Characteristics and location of pain indicate the cause. Uterine contractions and cramping pain occur with SAB or GTD. Ectopic pregnancy may yield dull aching or severe pain (with ruptured fallopian tube). Abruptio placenta (concealed) may cause severe abdominal pain. |
| Assess and systematically monitor the patient for a verbal report and behavioral signs of pain every 2 hours. | Changes in pain indicate improvement in the patient's condition or development of complications. Behavioral and physiologic responses clarify the presence of pain when the patient is unable to self-report pain. |
| Position for comfort and physiologic response; promote the position changes every 30 minutes while the patient is awake. | Positioning in labor affects anatomic and physiologic responses (i.e., alters the cardiac output, enhances or reduces the effectiveness of uterine contractions, synchronizes abdominal muscle work, and reduces the pressure on the preterm fetal head). Frequent position changes increase comfort and circulation and relieve fatigue. |
| Instruct and assist with appropriate nonpharmacologic methods of pain relief (e.g., breathing and relaxation techniques, application of heat or cold, hydrotherapy, acupressure, effleurage to the abdomen or continuous and firm sacral pressure during each contraction, relaxation conditioned in response to the partner's touch, massage, and music). | Nonpharmacologic methods reduce stress, relieve body tension by promoting relaxation, often increase endorphin levels, and have fewer side effects than medications. Sacral pressure relieves strain put on the sacroiliac joint from the fetal head in the occiput posterior position. |
| Medicate with analgesics or anesthetics as prescribed by the health care provider or anesthetist using the seven rights of medication administration. | The goal of medication administration is to adequately relieve pain without causing maternal or fetal risk. "Seven rights of administration" means right drug, right dose, right preparation, right route, right time, right patient, and right documentation. |

For other assessments, interventions, and rationales, see "Pain," Chapter 5.

## Patient, Partner, and Family Problem/Analyze Cues/Prioritize Hypotheses

# Anxiety

*due to* threat of change in health or death (perceived or actual) to the unborn child or self and/or unknown invasive treatment and its outcome

*Desired Outcome/Generate Solutions:* After interventions, the patient, her partner, and family state that their anxieties and concerns have lessened or resolved.

| ASSESSMENT—RECOGNIZE CUES/ INTERVENTIONS—TAKE ACTION | RATIONALES |
|---|---|
| Assess and acknowledge the concerns and anxieties. | This will help identify the causes of anxiety and focus on what the potential loss of this pregnancy means to the patient and her family. |
| Encourage the verbalization of concerns. | Discussion of concerns makes them more concrete and strengthens coping ability. |
| Provide support with attentive and active listening. | Restating what you have heard them say empowers the patient and family with self-understanding and a sense of control and fosters decision-making. |
| Provide verbal and written sources of information throughout care. | Honest and individualized information develops a knowledge base and helps eliminate anxieties. However, the amount of information and their anxieties may interfere with assimilation. Written information enables later review of information. |
| Discuss the meaning of symptoms and medical interventions ahead of time (if possible). | Knowledge reduces anxiety and body tension and fosters participation in decision-making when possible. |
| For other assessments, interventions, and rationales see the patient problems, in "Psychosocial Support for the Patient," Chapter 8, and "Psychosocial Support for the Patient's Family and Significant Others," Chapter 9. | |

## Patient, Partner, and Family Problem/Analyze Cues/Prioritize Hypotheses

# Grief

*due to* anticipated or actual loss of the unborn child

***Desired Outcome/Generate Solutions:*** Within 24 hours after guidance and support are given by the health care team, the patient, her partner, and family begin expressing their grief or anger, acknowledge that grieving takes a long time with no specific time frames, and begin working with other support persons in or out of the family.

| ASSESSMENT—RECOGNIZE CUES/ INTERVENTIONS—TAKE ACTION | RATIONALES |
|---|---|
| Assess the patient's, partner's, and family's coping methods, strengths, and support systems. | Early, individualized, and continued support helps prevent delayed or complicated grief reactions. |
| Encourage the verbalizing feelings and concerns regarding the potential or actual loss of the unborn child. | The grief and feelings of pregnancy loss are complex and unique for each individual. The ability to communicate fears and express feelings are important elements of sharing grief. |
| Per agency protocol, refer to a social worker, chaplain, and/or grief counselor as needed. | The multidisciplinary team supports the needs of both intuitive and instrumental styles of coping. They assist with decisions and provide support related to pregnancy loss, both in hospital and after discharge. |
| Encourage the continuation with support systems after hospital discharge. | Grief and recovery after losing the pregnancy or child continue for a long time—through as much as a year of bereavement or more and with shadow grief episodes appearing later. |
| Explain that everyone grieves differently. Provide space for and communicate support. | Coping styles vary with individuals and can differ between women and men. |
| Grieve with the patient, partner, and family if this is helpful. | People with intuitive styles of coping (i.e., insightful without consciously reasoning) prefer care that emphasizes emotional and psychological support. |
| For other assessments, interventions, and rationales, see "Psychosocial Support for the Patient," Chapter 8, for *Anticipatory Grief.* | |

## Patient, Partner, and Family Problem/Analyze Cues/Prioritize Hypotheses

# Deficient Knowledge

*due to* unfamiliarity with the effects of bleeding on the pregnancy, fetus, and self; the treatment regimen; and medications

**Desired Outcome/Generate Solutions:**  After instruction, the patient, her partner, and her family members begin to verbalize an accurate understanding of the patient's changing condition, diagnostic and therapeutic procedures, signs and symptoms of developing complications, and plans for follow-up care; and they return demonstrations of the prescribed procedures.

| ASSESSMENT—RECOGNIZE CUES/ INTERVENTIONS—TAKE ACTION | RATIONALES |
|---|---|
| Assess the understanding of the hemorrhagic condition, treatments, and possible outcomes. | This assessment enables the clarification of information and correction of misunderstanding. |
| Ascertain religious practices or preferences. | For example, religious faith may prohibit the use of blood products and indicate the need for alternative treatment. |
| Explain the diagnosis to the patient, her partner, and family; reinforce information provided by other health care providers. Explain the changing maternal and fetal condition, treatment regimen, tests, and medications. | These explanations not only provide accurate information but also reduce stress by eliminating confusion. |
| Speak calmly and clearly in words appropriate to the patient's understanding. | In an already emotionally charged situation the nurse's voice can either increase or reduce anxiety. |
| Anticipate concerns, encourage questions, and include the patient, partner, and family in decision-making as much as possible during hospitalization and follow-up care after discharge. | Evidence-based nursing practice stresses the importance of patient and family preferences in decision-making. For example, with ectopic pregnancy, fertility may be reduced; with GTD, hCG levels need to be monitored; if the client has experienced a repeated SAB, a cervical cerclage may be helpful. |
| For other assessments, interventions, and rationales, see this patient problem in "Psychosocial Support for the Patient," Chapter 8. | |

### ADDITIONAL PROBLEMS:

| | |
|---|---|
| "Immobility" for *Activity (Exercise) Intolerance* | Chapter 1 |
| "Psychosocial Support for the Patient" for *Difficulty Coping* | Chapter 8 |
| "Psychosocial Support for the Patient's Family and Significant Others" for *Difficulty Coping* | Chapter 9 |

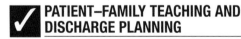

### PATIENT–FAMILY TEACHING AND DISCHARGE PLANNING

Include verbal and written information about the following:
- ✓ Importance of reporting vaginal bleeding to the health care provider in a timely manner.
- ✓ Importance of reporting signs of a complication or worsening condition.
- ✓ Necessity of adhering to prescribed medications, treatment regimen, and scheduled appointments.
- ✓ Medications, including purpose; name; dose; frequency; precautions; and potential side effects or interactions with drugs, foods, and herbs.
- ✓ Measures that help constipation (resulting from bedrest, medications, and pregnancy).
- ✓ How to evaluate fetal movements and contractions (when appropriate)?
- ✓ Balanced diet high in iron; hydration with 8–10 (8-oz) glasses of fluid daily (water is best; avoid caffeinated and sugary drinks).
- ✓ Adherence to restrictions on pelvic rest (e.g., no sexual intercourse and/or tampons, nothing in the vagina).
- ✓ Referral to the American Congress of Obstetricians and Gynecologists, which has an extensive collection of patient education materials available at https://www.acog.org/womens-health/pregnancy.
- ✓ Referral to local or national support organizations:
- ✓ Sidelines is a national organization providing support for women and families experiencing a complicated pregnancy: http://www.sidelines.org
- ✓ March of Dimes: http://www.marchofdimes.com
- ✓ Caring Bridge: http://www.caringbridge.orgPostpartum; Support International: https://www.postpartum.net/

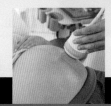

# Diabetes in Pregnancy 90

## OVERVIEW/PATHOPHYSIOLOGY

Diabetes is classified into the following categories: type 1 diabetes mellitus (DM), called *insulin-dependent diabetes;* type 2 DM, called *insulin-resistant diabetes; diabetes dependent* on other specific conditions such as infection or drug induced; and *gestational DM (GDM)*. GDM is defined as carbohydrate intolerance that is first recognized during pregnancy (American College of Obstetrics and Gynecology [ACOG], 2018a). There is a 50% risk for GDM turning to type 2 DM later in life if lifestyle changes are not made. Diabetes poses significant risks to maternal and fetal morbidity and mortality. The incidence of diabetes in pregnancy has increased because more women are delaying pregnancy until relatively late into their reproductive years. Currently, the incidence of gestational diabetes is 2%–10% (Centers for Disease Control and Prevention [CDC], 2022).

## HEALTH CARE SETTING

Primary care (outpatient obstetric clinic, high-risk perinatal clinic) or acute care (inpatient). Patients may be hospitalized for the following: when starting or adjusting insulin, if an infection develops, during the third trimester when diabetes has been poorly controlled and closer maternal and fetal surveillance is indicated.

## ASSESSMENT

At the first prenatal visit all women are screened for clinical risk factors when obtaining a history. If risk factors are identified, such as previous history of GDM, known impaired glucose metabolism, previous macrosomic baby (greater than 4000 g), and obesity (body mass index [BMI] greater than 30), early screening is recommended. An early screen that is negative is repeated for these high-risk women at 24–28 weeks. Between 24 and 28 weeks' gestation, it is recommended that *all pregnant women* be screened for GDM. A two-step screening process is supported by the ACOG. Testing begins with the administration of 50 g of oral glucose solution and requires a 1-hour serum glucose measurement as the initial screening. Screening is recommended even for patients with low risk factors (age younger than 25 years, not a member of an ethnic group at risk for developing type 2 DM, BMI less than 25, no previous history of abnormal glucose tolerance, no previous history of adverse obstetric outcomes that

are usually associated with GDM, and no known diabetes in a first-degree relative [mother, father, siblings]). A one-step approach using a 75-g oral glucose solution followed by a 2-hour serum measurement also may be used.

*Type 1 diabetes mellitus:* Increased risk for abnormal embry-ogenesis (growth, differentiation, and organization of fetal cellular components), spontaneous abortion, sacral agenesis or caudal regression syndrome (absence or deformity of the sacrum), pyelonephritis, preterm labor/birth, polyhydramnios (abnormally high level of amniotic fluid), preeclampsia, ketoacidosis, cesarean delivery, fetal hypoxia, stillbirth, fetal macrosomia (birth weight 4000 g or more) or intrauterine growth restriction (IUGR), birth trauma (e.g., shoulder dystocia because of macrosomia), congenital anomalies (ventral septal defect, transposition of the great vessels), anencephaly (absence of neural tissue in the cranium), open spina bifida (a defect in the closure of the neural tube), holoprosencephaly (absence of midline cerebral structures because of the incomplete division of the forebrain), respiratory distress syndrome (RDS), and neonatal hypoglycemia.

*Type 2 diabetes mellitus/gestational diabetes mellitus:* Increased risk for macrosomia or IUGR (depending on the extent of the maternal illness and glycemic control), pregnancy-induced hypertension (preeclampsia), ketoacidosis, cesarean delivery, hypoxia, RDS, stillbirth, birth trauma, and neonatal hypoglycemia.

> **Note:** *During pregnancy the classic symptoms of diabetes (polydipsia, polyphagia, and polyuria) cannot be used as diagnostic tools because they are normal changes of pregnancy.*

*Renal urinary:* Glucosuria is not a reliable sign of diabetes during pregnancy because of a lowered renal threshold that occurs at that time. If glucose (+1 or higher) appears consistently (two times or more) in the urine, however, the patient needs to be evaluated for GDM.

*Neurologic:* Frequent headaches, fatigue, and drowsiness may be present as a result of maternal insulin resistance. Retinopathy is commonly seen in women with type 1 DM (preexisting disease) caused by abnormal vasculature, capillary rupture, or hemorrhage within the retina. An ophthalmic examination during pregnancy is recommended.

*Cardiovascular:* In patients with long-term diabetes, deterioration of glomerular function can lead to hypertension and superimposed preeclampsia. These women can also develop arteriosclerosis.

*Other symptoms:* Pregnant women with diabetes are at an increased risk for developing preeclampsia. See additional symptoms in "Preeclampsia," Chapter 94.

### Complications—fetal:
- Miscarriage/fetal death
- Embryonic growth delay
- Congenital malformations, especially cardiac and skeletal
- Hypertrophic and congestive cardiomyopathy
- Fetal macrosomia (gigantism)
- Hypoglycemia
- RDS
- Hyperbilirubinemia
- Hypocalcemia IUGR

*Risk factors:* BMI more than $30 \text{ kg/m}^2$, family history of DM, previous history of GDM, previous macrosomic infant, previous unexplained stillbirth, polyhydramnios (past or present), excessive weight gain, history of congenital anomalies in offspring, chronic hypertension, recurrent infections including vaginal monilial, recurrent glucosuria, age older than 30 years, and family origin with a high prevalence of diabetes (African American, Hispanic, Native American, South Asian [India, Pakistan, and Bangladesh], Black Caribbean, Middle Eastern, and South Pacific Islanders).

## DIAGNOSTIC TESTS

*1-hour glucose screening:* Performed between weeks 24 and 28 of the pregnancy or earlier if the patient is identified as high risk. If results are negative in an earlier test, the test is repeated between 24 and 28 weeks in the pregnancy if the patient meets the risk factors (discussed earlier). This test requires the patient to drink a 50-g glucose load, followed in 1 hour by venous plasma measurement. Traditionally, a value of 140 mg/dL or greater was considered abnormal and indicated the need for the 3-hour 100-g oral glucose tolerance test (OGTT). There is evidence that a 130 mg/dL cutoff level identifies 10% more women at risk for GDM. A single set of cutoff criteria is suggested. When a 1-hour value is 190 mg/dL or greater, a fasting glucose should be done before proceeding to the 3-hour test. If the fasting value is 95 mg/dL or greater, the patient is diagnosed as having GDM (Eastern Virginia Medical School [EVMS], 2023).

*3-hour glucose tolerance test:* After fasting for 8–12 hours and abstaining from smoking, a fasting blood sugar (FBS) is drawn, after which the patient drinks a 100-g glucose load followed by serum venous plasma measurements at 1, 2, and 3 hours. Two of the four values need to be abnormal to make the diagnosis of GDM (EVMS, 2023).

> **Note:** *Screening guidelines differ for diagnosing GDM, depending on medical facility preference. The ACOG recommends the 3-hour OGTT for women who test positive with a 1-hour, 50-g OGTT. If two or more blood glucose levels are elevated, the diagnosis is established for GDM.*

> *Fasting: greater than 95 mg/dL*
> *1-hour test: greater than 180 mg/dL*
> *2-hour test: greater than 155 mg/dL*
> *3-hour test: greater than 140 mg/dL*

> **Note:** *The International Association of Diabetes and Pregnancy Study Group recommends using a single 2-hour, 75-g OGTT to screen for gestational diabetes. The American Diabetes Association has endorsed this criterion.*
> *Fasting: 92 mg/dL or higher*
> *2-hour test: 153 mg/dL or higher*

*Glycosylated hemoglobin (HbA$_{1c}$):* Reflects the average blood sugar levels for the 2- to 3-month period before the test. Values may be increased in iron deficiency anemia and decreased in pregnancy. Levels less than 6% are desired in pregnancy. Recent studies have raised questions about the reliability of HbA$_{1c}$ results in the second and third trimesters of pregnancy; therefore it is no longer recommended as a routine assessment of glycemic control in those trimesters (Massachusetts General Hospital, 2020).

*Home glucose monitoring:* The patient at home performs glucose monitoring (obtaining whole blood from a fingerstick) at given intervals prescribed by the health care provider. Taking into account the risk for hypoglycemia, target values during pregnancy are FBS less than 95 mg/dL and 2-hour postprandial (pp) of 120 mg/dL or less. Patients with poor glucose control will have FBS well above 90–95 mg/dL and 2-hour pp well above 120 mg/dL. Careful regulation of maternal glucose levels during pregnancy leads to decreased maternal–fetal compromise and better outcomes.

*Renal function studies:* Normally during pregnancy creatinine clearance is increased, but it is decreased in GDM because of deterioration in glomerular function. A 24-hour urinalysis for protein is recommended early in the pregnancy that can be used as a comparison later if renal function worsens.

*Obstetric ultrasound:* May be done at 2- to 4-week intervals to monitor fetal growth, placental function, amniotic fluid levels, and fetal position and check for the presence of polyhydramnios (excess amniotic fluid). If the primary HbA$_{1c}$ is elevated, a fetal echocardiogram may be done between 20 and 22 weeks gestation. Ultrasounds also assess fetal anomalies for women with pregestational diabetes (Danyao et al., 2020).

*Antepartum fetal monitoring:* Patients with GDM whose blood glucose levels are well controlled by diet are at low risk for fetal complications. Antepartum fetal heart rate testing is limited unless they have hypertension, history of prior stillbirth, or current fetal macrosomia. Any of these conditions would necessitate weekly to twice-weekly testing starting at 32 weeks (or sooner if necessary) to monitor fetal well-being. Ultrasound monitoring of fetal growth is recommended in the last few weeks of pregnancy because of the risk for macrosomia.

## Patient Problem/Analyze Cues/Prioritize Hypotheses

# Risk for Altered Blood Glucose

*due to* fluctuations occurring during pregnancy

**Desired Outcome/Generate Solutions:**  Euglycemia is maintained as evidenced by daily maternal records and prenatal testing results.

| ASSESSMENT—RECOGNIZE CUES/ INTERVENTIONS—TAKE ACTION | RATIONALES |
|---|---|
| **Prenatal:** Assess the patient's HbA$_{1c}$ and blood glucose by the method and timing prescribed by the health care provider. | HbA$_{1c}$ testing is recommended for patients with pregestational DM. HbA$_{1c}$ levels are lower in normal pregnancy because of increased red blood cell turnover. HbA$_{1c}$ less than 6% is associated with a lower risk for congenital anomalies or large-for-gestational-age infants (American Diabetes Association [ADA], 2022). Target blood glucose levels are stricter in pregnancy and are performed by frequent fingersticks. FBS of 95 mg/dL or less, 1-hour pp level of 140 mg/dL or less, and 2-hour pp levels of 120 mg/dL or less are desired target blood glucose levels for pregnant women |
| Assess the patient's urine by dipstick for glucose and ketones and review the maternal monitoring charts as prescribed by the health care provider. | The renal threshold for glycosuria is lower in pregnancy. The pregnant patient is at risk for ketoacidosis at a lower blood sugar rate than the nonpregnant patient. Glycosuria predisposes the patient to urinary tract infections. |
| Assess the daily diet compliance according to the ADA diet prescribed by the dietitian. | GDM may be controlled by diet alone. |
| Explain to the patient with GDM and her family that insulin administration may be necessary as pregnancy progresses. | The body's insulin requirements will increase 2–4 times by the third trimester. If diet repeatedly fails to keep fasting glucose at 95 mg/dL or less, insulin therapy is recommended. |
| Assess the patient's self-administration of human insulin according to the regimen prescribed by the health care provider. | Many pregnant women with diabetes want to administer their own insulin dose. Professional assessment identifies whether the patient's technique is safe or needs refinement by education. |
| Assess the fundal height and compare it to the previous level and gestational week as prescribed by the health care provider. | If euglycemia is not maintained throughout the pregnancy, the fetus is at risk for macrosomia or IUGR. |
| Coordinate referrals after hospital discharge as prescribed, for example, to a perinatologist, endocrinologist, diabetic nurse, dietitian, and medical social worker. | Coordination of referrals fosters continuity of care and timely communication among many health care providers. A team approach benefits the patient and family. |
| **Intrapartum:** Assess and document the blood glucose levels hourly by fingerstick and as prescribed after insulin administration. | Maintenance of euglycemia (75–126 mg/dL [4–7 mmol/L]) in labor reduces the risk for neonatal hypoglycemia, which is especially critical during the first hour after birth when the newborn is no longer experiencing the same glucose level as the mother. |
| If blood glucose rises to 126 mg/dL (7 mmol/L) or higher, begin insulin infusion by a secondary intravenous (IV) line at 2 units/hour in 0.9% normal saline as prescribed by the health care provider. | Blood glucose requirements vary in labor (e.g., food intake is reduced and energy is expended), and oxytocin acts like insulin and drives glucose into the body cells. National Institute for Health and Care Excellence (NICE) guidelines for labor (2020) recommends that blood glucose remains between 75 and 126 mg/dL (4–7 mmol/L) by glucometer. |
| **Postpartum:** Assess the fasting blood glucose levels as prescribed. Encourage the patient to maintain a balanced diet and to have a snack available during breastfeeding | After the placenta is expelled, human placental lactogen (hPL) decreases and the insulin resistance during pregnancy resolves quickly. Insulin needs in the pregestational patient with diabetes are markedly reduced, often below prepregnant needs for 24 hours. The patient with GDM returns to nonpregnant carbohydrate metabolism. |
| Encourage breastfeeding. | Breastfeeding decreases blood glucose levels, and insulin needs are considerably decreased postpartum. Monitoring of blood glucose levels will continue because levels may fluctuate. Because hypoglycemia can occur, regular snacks are encouraged. |

## Patient Problem/Analyze Cues/Prioritize Hypotheses

# Deficient Knowledge

*due to* unfamiliarity with the effects of diabetes on self, the pregnancy, and the fetus

***Desired Outcome/Generate Solutions:*** Immediately after teaching, the patient verbalizes an accurate knowledge about the effects of diabetes on self, the pregnancy, and fetus and adheres to the treatment accordingly.

| ASSESSMENT—RECOGNIZE CUES/ INTERVENTIONS—TAKE ACTION | RATIONALES |
|---|---|
| Explain to the patient and significant others how diabetes affects pregnancy and pregnancy affects diabetes for the mother, fetus, and newborn. | An informed patient is more likely to adhere to the therapeutic plan, which will change frequently as pregnancy advances (e.g., frequent blood sugar checks, frequent clinic visits, insulin injections, dietary monitoring, and fetal surveillance tests), and understand possible problems encountered with pregestational DM and GDM. |
| Encourage adherence to prenatal appointments, daily glucose testing, dietary regimen, and exercise program. | Frequent prenatal visits enable timely modification in the therapeutic regimen to promote optimal pregnancy outcomes (e.g., vaginal delivery without complications, newborn's growth average for gestational age without hypoglycemia, stable DM in postpartum patients with pregestational diabetes, and return to normal FBS for patients with GDM). |
| Encourage patients with pregestational diabetes to develop an individualized plan with their health care provider to maintain good glycemic control before becoming pregnant. | For the woman with pregestational diabetes, euglycemia at conception is associated with fewer congenital malformations in the newborn. Any reduction in HbA$_{1c}$ levels toward the nonpregnant value of 6.1 reduces the risk for congenital malformations. |
| Inform all patients with diabetes about a probable increased need for insulin to maintain euglycemia during pregnancy. | Insulin is the preferred agent for managing both type 1 and type 2 DM in pregnancy and may be necessary for GDM. The body's insulin requirements increase as the pregnancy advances. For the patient with pregestational diabetes taking oral glycemic agents or the patient with GDM, insulin therapy should be considered when nutritional therapy fails to keep fasting blood glucose at or less than 95 mg/dL. |
| For patients with GDM, arrange for one-on-one teaching with a diabetes educator for the following: how to check blood sugars with a glucometer, how to document blood sugars, and the importance of exercise during pregnancy. | A one-on-one session with a diabetes educator experienced with GDM provides an opportunity for questions/interactions and greater patient comprehension. |
| Instruct the patient and her significant others on the signs and symptoms of hypoglycemia, hyperglycemia, diabetic ketoacidosis, and insulin shock. For more information, see "Diabetes Mellitus," Chapter 47, and "Diabetic Ketoacidosis," Chapter 48. | A knowledgeable patient likely will report these symptoms promptly. Although the hormone hPL causes tissue resistance (prolonging hyperglycemia after meals), during periods of fasting, blood glucose levels fall precipitously. Targeted blood sugar levels during pregnancy are lower to protect the fetus. Therefore the patient is more likely to experience swings between hyperglycemia and hypoglycemia. |
| Develop a sick-day plan with the patient. | This information will help the patient maintain adequate glycemic control. For example, the patient should do the following:<br><br>• Check blood sugar and urine for ketones every 2–4 hours during illness.<br><br>• Maintain a normal insulin schedule.<br><br>• Maintain usual meals when possible. Drink plenty of water and/or calorie-free liquids if unable to maintain solid foods. Consume a minimum of 150 g of carbohydrates per day, taken in small amounts over 24 hours.<br><br>• Call the provider if the temperature is 101°F (38.3°C) or greater, ketone level is moderate to high, or the patient is vomiting and unable to keep anything down.<br><br>• The patient may need to be hospitalized for IV fluids and regulation of blood sugar.<br><br>• In diabetes associated with pregnancy, early detection of ketones is critical to fetal mortality because ketoacidosis is a significant factor that contributes to intrauterine death. |

| ASSESSMENT—RECOGNIZE CUES/ INTERVENTIONS—TAKE ACTION | RATIONALES |
|---|---|
| Encourage the patient to maintain or initiate an exercise program. | Exercise improves both cardiopulmonary fitness and glucose metabolism. |
| Suggest that she have hard candy on hand when exercising. | Because moderate exercise increases glucose utilization, hypoglycemia can develop while exercising. |
| Instruct the patient about daily fetal movement counts. | Fetal movement counts are a good first-line indicator of fetal well-being and are performed as follows, beginning at 28 weeks' gestation: The patient lies on her side and counts "distinct fetal movements" (hiccups do not count) daily; 10 movements within a 2-hour period is reassuring. After 10 movements are noted, the count is discontinued. Fewer than 10 movements indicate the need for fetal nonstress testing. |

## Patient Problem/Analyze Cues/Prioritize Hypotheses

# Nonadherence

*due to* cultural habits and lack of knowledge resulting in failure to follow the prescribed dietary regimen for effective glycemic control

***Desired Outcome/Generate Solutions:*** The patient follows the prescribed dietary regimen.

| ASSESSMENT—RECOGNIZE CUES/ INTERVENTIONS—TAKE ACTION | RATIONALES |
|---|---|
| Assess the patient's cultural habits surrounding diet (foods she can and cannot eat, who shops, and who cooks) and exercise patterns. | Working within cultural habits aids in dietary adherence. For example, there may be high carbohydrate consumption, depending on her cultural group: rice for Asian women; tortillas and rice for Hispanic women; and breads and pasta for non-Hispanic Caucasian women. |
| Arrange for a meeting with a dietitian who specializes in diabetes in pregnancy. | A dietitian is trained to answer questions regarding specific foods and meal plans that are appropriate for glycemic control and can act as a resource person for the patient. Nutritional interventions should achieve normal glucose levels and avoid ketosis while maintaining appropriate nutrition and weight gain in pregnancy. |
| Encourage the patient to keep a daily dietary and exercise log. | A log provides a quick reference to compare blood sugars and foods eaten as well as the amount of exercise achieved on a given day. Exercise increases glucose utilization. |
| Praise the patient when blood sugars are within prescribed limits. | Good glycemic control reduces the incidence of maternal and fetal morbidity and mortality. |
| Inform the patient of the risks to self and fetus associated with poor glycemic control related to dietary nonadherence. | Knowledge aids in adherence to the treatment plan. Dietary nonadherence can result in miscarriage, fetal anomalies, fetal macrosomia and increased risk for shoulder dystocia with a vaginal delivery, and increased potential for cesarean delivery. |
| Instruct the patient with insulin-dependent diabetes that she may need to test blood glucose levels at bedtime and during the night. | During periods of fasting, hypoglycemia can develop more quickly when the woman is pregnant. Maternal blood glucose crosses the placental membrane and is taken into fetal circulation. |
| Instruct the patient with type 1 DM to monitor urine with ketone testing strips and to test for ketonuria or ketonemia if becoming hyperglycemic or unwell. | Ketones are weak acids produced when blood sugar is poorly controlled and the body burns fat instead of sugar for energy. Moderate to large (2–4+) ketones may signal ketoacidosis, which necessitates immediate evaluation. If untreated, prolonged ketoacidosis can result in fetal brain damage. |
| Develop a "sick-day plan" with the patient. | See discussion in *Deficient Knowledge*, earlier. |

<u>Patient Problem/Analyze Cues/Prioritize Hypotheses</u>

# Anxiety

*due to* actual or perceived threat to self or fetus because of the effects diabetes may have on the pregnancy

***Desired Outcome/Generate Solutions:*** Within 1–2 hours of intervention, the patient states that her anxiety has lessened or resolved, and she describes appropriate coping mechanisms in managing the anxiety.

| ASSESSMENT—RECOGNIZE CUES/ INTERVENTIONS—TAKE ACTION | RATIONALES |
|---|---|
| Engage in honest communication with the patient; provide empathetic understanding. Listen closely. | This establishes an atmosphere that enables free expression. |
| Assess for verbal and nonverbal cues about the patient's anxiety level. | These cues aid in providing appropriate assistance and support. Levels of anxiety include: <br><br> • *Mild:* restlessness, irritability, increased questions, and focusing on the environment. <br><br> • *Moderate:* inattentiveness, expressions of concern, narrowed perceptions, insomnia, and increased heart rate. <br><br> • *Severe:* expression of feelings of doom, rapid speech, tremors, and poor eye contact. Patients may be preoccupied with the past or unable to understand the present and may have tachycardia, nausea, and hyperventilation. <br><br> • *Panic:* inability to concentrate or communicate, distortion of reality, increased motor activity, vomiting, and tachypnea. |
| Explain that patients with poor glycemic control or who need to initiate first-time insulin use usually are admitted to the hospital for teaching and monitoring. | This offers the potential of a supportive environment that decreases anxiety and increases patient confidence. |
| Encourage the patient to communicate the cause of anxiety, for example, dietary changes, failure to maintain adequate glycemic control, checking blood sugars, and insulin injections. | This information helps determine the patient's knowledge of diabetes in pregnancy and ways in which patient teaching can alleviate anxiety. |
| Provide reassurance and a safe, quiet environment for relaxation. | An anxious person has difficulty learning. |
| Assess at each appointment if the patient has enough supplies to maintain self-care. | Having adequate supplies (e.g., glucometer, test strips, lancets, record book, insulin, syringes, alcohol wipes, and sharps disposal box) on hand may increase adherence to therapy and decrease anxiety. |
| Encourage the patient to attend diabetes classes and support groups for patients with diabetes. | Talking with others who had or are experiencing diabetes in pregnancy aids in establishing outside support resources. Some support groups are listed at the end of this care plan. |
| Inform the patient with GDM that although she has diabetes associated with the pregnancy, her efforts to return to an appropriate weight for height and body build (with a healthy diet and physical activity) can delay or prevent lifelong diabetes. | Having this information may alleviate anxiety and increase adherence to the therapeutic plan. Obesity is strongly associated with the development of type 2 DM. |
| Advise her that if she has other risk factors such as a first-line relative with a history of type 1 or type 2 DM, obesity, and a diet high in carbohydrates and fats, these factors can increase the risk for developing chronic DM during the next 10–15 years. | This information identifies some factors over which she has control, which optimally will decrease anxiety and encourage weight loss, dietary control, and exercise postpartum to prevent the future development of chronic DM. |

## Patient, Partner, and Family Problem

# Deficient Knowledge

*due to* unfamiliarity with the benefits and potential side effects of prescribed medications used to treat GDM

*Desired Outcome/Generate Solutions:* Immediately after teaching, the patient, her partner, and her family (as appropriate) verbalize an accurate understanding of the risks and benefits of medications used during the pregnancy to treat diabetes.

| ASSESSMENT—RECOGNIZE CUES/ INTERVENTIONS—TAKE ACTION | RATIONALES |
|---|---|
| Instruct the patient about prescribed medications: | A knowledgeable patient is more likely to adhere to the therapy, identify and report side effects, and recognize and report precautions that might preclude the use of the prescribed drug. |
| **Sulfonylureas: Second-Generation** | These agents lower blood glucose by stimulating the release of insulin from the pancreas. |
| **Glucophage (Metformin)** **Glyburide (Micronase, DiaBeta, Euglucon)** | Metformin is currently the preferred oral glycemic agent. Patients on all other glycemic agents are encouraged to switch, although glyburide has been shown to be safe and effective in GDM. There is a concern for teratogenicity with other oral agents. Most patients with type 2 DM who have been managed on oral agents are changed to insulin during pregnancy. Administration: by mouth (PO). |
| Instruct the patient to be alert for and report shakiness, sweating, nervousness, headache, and blood sugar level less than 60 mg/dL. | These are signs and symptoms of hypoglycemia. |
| Instruct the patient to be alert for and report blurred vision. | This is a side effect caused by fluctuation in blood glucose levels. |
| Stress the importance of monitoring blood glucose levels as directed. | This helps detect hypoglycemia or hyperglycemia promptly. Preexisting diabetic patients will most likely need to increase their testing frequency during pregnancy. The usual routine in pregnancy is to monitor blood glucose fasting (first thing in the morning before breakfast or taking medications), 2 hours after eating, at bedtime, and when glucose levels have been low or high. Poor glycemic control when taking the oral agent necessitates the initiation of insulin. |
| Instruct the patient to be alert for and report nausea, epigastric fullness, and heartburn. | These are adverse reactions. If these reactions occur consistently, the patient may require dose adjustment or be started on insulin—whichever maintains glycemic control. |
| Caution patients taking nonsteroidal antiinflammatory drugs (NSAIDs) and beta-adrenergic blocking agents to notify the health care provider before taking sulfonylureas. | The hypoglycemic reaction may be potentiated by these medications. |
| **Insulin** | Insulin is the gold standard for glycemic control. It is more protective for perinatal mortality than the oral hypoglycemic agents. |

Continued

| ASSESSMENT—RECOGNIZE CUES/ INTERVENTIONS—TAKE ACTION | RATIONALES |
|---|---|
| **Regular Humalog and Lispro (Rapid Acting), NPH (Intermediate Acting)** | These are parenteral blood glucose–lowering agents that regulate glucose metabolism. Lispro has a more rapid onset of action than regular insulin and does not cross the placenta. |
| | *Administration:* subcutaneous or by insulin pump. Some patients may be started on subcutaneous insulin as an outpatient. This choice is individualized based on patient adherence and comprehension of insulin therapy (drawing up insulin, injecting accurately, and timing doses). Inpatient setting is required for initial teaching of how to use the pump, including monitoring of glucose levels and making necessary insulin dose adjustments. |
| Instruct the patient to be alert for and report shakiness, sweating, nervousness, headache, and low blood sugar levels. | These are signs and symptoms of hypoglycemia, a potential side effect. Some patients may develop symptoms between 60 and 70 mg/dL and others not until 50–60 mg/dL (or lower). |
| Instruct the patient to be alert for and report blurred vision. | This is a side effect secondary to fluctuations in blood glucose levels. |
| Stress the importance of monitoring blood glucose levels as directed. | This aids in the prompt identification of hypoglycemic reactions. |
| Caution patients taking NSAIDs, salicylates, and beta-adrenergic blocking agents to notify their health care provider. | Insulin requirements may be decreased when also taking drugs with hypoglycemic activity. Beta-blockers may mask the symptoms of hypoglycemia and alter glucose metabolism. |
| Caution patients taking terbutaline to notify their health care provider. | Terbutaline is used to decrease uterine myometrial activity (contractions). Beta-sympathomimetics, such as terbutaline, can cause hyperglycemia, and their use is not usually recommended for patients with diabetes. |

## ADDITIONAL PROBLEMS:

| | |
|---|---|
| "Psychosocial Support for the Patient" for relevant problems such as *Difficulty Coping* | Chapter 8 |
| "Psychosocial Support for the Patient's Family and Significant Others" for such problems as *Difficulty Coping* | Chapter 9 |
| "Diabetes Mellitus" | Chapter 47 |
| "Diabetic Ketoacidosis" | Chapter 48 |

## ✔ PATIENT–FAMILY TEACHING AND DISCHARGE PLANNING

Patients with GDM require close monitoring for maternal and fetal well-being. Education is the key to making the pregnancy a success. When providing patient–family teaching, avoid giving excessive information. Part of the initial assessment needs to include asking about existing knowledge of the disease, ability for self-management, and psychologic acceptance. Include written and verbal information about the following:

✓ Recommended glucose levels in pregnancy: Fasting, 60–90 mg/dL; before lunch, dinner, or bedtime snack, 60–105 mg/dL; 2-hour pp, 120 mg/dL or less.

✓ Reminder that stress from illness or infection can increase insulin requirements.

✓ Recognizing warning signs of both hyperglycemia and simple and advanced hypoglycemia and insulin shock, treatment, and factors that contribute to both conditions.

- *Hyperglycemia:* Possible causes include not enough insulin or increased insulin resistance (as seen with advancing gestational age), too much food, stress of illness, emotional stress, and decreased exercise. Patients need to call the health care provider for treatment, which may include increasing insulin dose and/or self-administering an insulin bolus.

- *Hypoglycemia:* Possible causes are too much insulin, too little food, not eating on time, vomiting, and too much exercise. (See the next two items for treatment options.) Review "Diabetes Mellitus," Chapter 47, for further information.

- Foods to treat hypoglycemia such as 4-oz orange juice, 4-oz milk, 4-oz cola drink (not diet cola), 3–4 pieces of hard candy, 3–4 sugar cubes, 2–3 glucose tablets.

- How and when to take glucose tablets. Instruct the patient to keep glucose tablets with her when away from home and food sources. Instruct the patient to use glucose tablets if becoming shaky, nauseated, nervous, headachy, drowsy, and diaphoretic and blood sugar is 60 mg/dL or less.

✓ When to call for emergency services. With advanced hypoglycemia (blood sugar 20–50 mg/dL) the patient may not be the person calling in an emergency situation; this information needs to be communicated to the significant other and family members as well.

✓ Importance of carrying an identification card or wearing a bracelet or necklace that identifies the patient as having diabetes in case of emergency. For patients with GDM, the necklace or bracelet may be obtained at a local pharmacy. If the patient has preexisting diabetes, the previous information may be obtained by contacting the following organization: MedicAlert Foundation, https://www.medicalert.org/.

✓ Importance of adherence to the prescribed health care plan and ready access to hospital and family/social support.

✓ Parameters and guidelines for blood sugar levels as recommended by the health care provider.

✓ Nutritional regimen as recommended by the health care provider. Adequate nutrition and controlled calories are essential to maintaining normoglycemia and appropriate fetal growth.

✓ Medications, including drug name, purpose, dosage, frequency, precautions, administration, and potential side effects. Also discuss potential drug–drug, food–drug, and herb–drug interactions.

✓ How to monitor urine for ketones.

✓ Fetal movement counts (gestational age appropriate).

✓ Referrals to local and national support organizations, including:

- American Diabetes Association (ADA): http://www.diabetes.org
- Sidelines, a national support organization for women and their families experiencing complicated pregnancies: http://www.sidelines.org
- Joslin Diabetes Center: https://www.joslin.org/

# Hyperemesis Gravidarum 91

## OVERVIEW/PATHOPHYSIOLOGY

Nausea and vomiting commonly affect 50%–80% of pregnant women, especially in the first trimester. Although mildly or moderately distressing, nausea and vomiting do not cause metabolic imbalance. Hyperemesis gravidarum (HG), however, is a condition of excessive vomiting in pregnancy affecting 2% of pregnant women in the United States (Jennings, & Mahdy, 2022). HG causes weight loss of 5% or more from prepregnancy weight, dehydration, electrolyte imbalance, acidosis from starvation, and alkalosis from loss of hydrochloric acid. This condition usually begins during the first trimester, after which vomiting becomes intractable and may last throughout the entire pregnancy. The cause is unknown, but theories include rising estrogen and human chorionic gonadotropin levels, displacement of the gastrointestinal (GI) tract, decreased motility caused by an increase in progesterone, decrease in motilin levels, *Helicobacter pylori* infection, and psychogenic factors. Affected women may face multiple disruptions of work, family, and social responsibilities because of the debilitating nature of the condition and repeated hospitalization. The goals of treatment include control of nausea and vomiting, correction of dehydration, restoration of electrolyte balance, and maintenance of adequate nutrition to optimize maternal and fetal/newborn outcomes.

## HEALTH CARE SETTING

Patients are often treated on an outpatient basis with oral medications, home intravenous (IV) infusion therapy to replace fluids and electrolytes, or total parenteral nutrition. Approximately 1%–5% of women who develop HG require hospitalization (Dean, 2014).

## ASSESSMENT

The first priority of care is to determine the severity of the nausea and vomiting problem in patients who can no longer retain solids or liquids as well as the degree of dehydration and weight loss. An early and thorough assessment of previous HG is important because there is an 80% chance of recurrence in subsequent pregnancies. Laboratory studies are prescribed to identify electrolyte imbalances. Patients may exhibit a low-grade fever, increased pulse rate, decreased blood pressure (BP), weakness, dry skin, cracked lips, and poor skin turgor. Patients may look extremely fatigued and listless with a possible loss of 5%–10% of total body weight, be constipated as a result of dehydration, and have a markedly decreased urinary output with ketonemia (presence of ketones in the blood). Women with diabetes who have hyperemesis need to be monitored closely to maintain glycemic control and avoid ketoacidosis. See "Diabetes in Pregnancy," Chapter 90.

**Gastrointestinal:** GI motility is reduced because of increased progesterone and decreased motilin levels. The "expected" nausea and vomiting of pregnancy usually has an onset between 4 and 9 weeks, peaks at about the 12th week, and resolves between 16 and 20 weeks. HG usually begins in the first trimester but may extend throughout the entire pregnancy.

**Fluid and electrolyte imbalance:** With the inability to maintain adequate fluids for hydration and solids for fuel and nutrients, the body experiences an imbalance of the elements necessary for health maintenance, which can lead to maternal ketosis.

**Cardiopulmonary:** The patient may experience one or all of the following: tachycardia, hypotension, postural BP changes, and tachypnea.

**Renal:** Possible presence of oliguria and ketonuria.

**Complications—fetal:** With prolonged dehydration and maternal weight loss, fetal intrauterine growth restriction (IUGR), prematurity, low birth weight, and lower Apgar scores may be seen.

**Physical assessment:** The pregnant patient with hyperemesis looks debilitated and is ill. She is extremely fatigued and pale. A thorough systems assessment is needed to rule out other causes of severe nausea and vomiting, such as gastroenteritis, cholecystitis, pyelonephritis, GI ulcers, or a molar pregnancy (intrauterine benign or neoplastic mass of grape-like vesicles of trophoblastic cells—the embryonic cells that form the chorion).

**Risk factors:** Previous history of hyperemesis, molar pregnancy, multiple gestation, emotional/psychologic stress, gastroesophageal reflux, primigravida, uncontrolled thyroid disease, and increased body weight/obesity.

## DIAGNOSTIC TESTS

**Urine chemistry:** The most important initial laboratory test is urine dipstick measurement of ketonuria (or a specimen may be sent for microscopic urinalysis). Ketones are present with cellular starvation and dehydration from prolonged vomiting.

**Complete blood count:** With dehydration, there likely will be evidence of hemoconcentration (i.e., elevated red blood cell and hematocrit levels).

**Serum chemistry:** Azotemia (increased blood urea nitrogen [BUN]) is seen with salt and water depletion. Serum creatinine will be elevated because of changes in renal function caused by dehydration. Hyponatremia and hypokalemia also may be present because of fluid loss.

**Liver enzymes:** Slight elevations of aspartate aminotransferase and alanine aminotransferase reverse with IV fluid hydration, adequate nutrition, and cessation of vomiting.

**Obstetric ultrasound:** Ultrasound is used to evaluate a normal intrauterine pregnancy versus a molar pregnancy, presence of multiple gestation, fetal growth for IUGR, and amniotic fluid volume/amniotic fluid index.

**Results for complete blood count, electrolyte panel, laboratory tests for liver enzymes and bilirubin levels, and kidney function:** Help to rule out the presence of underlying diseases previously listed.

## Patient Problem/Analyze Cues/Prioritize Hypotheses

# Dehydration

*due to* excessive gastric losses and reduced intravascular and intercellular fluid occurring with nausea and vomiting

**Desired Outcome/Generate Solutions:** Within 24 hours after initiation of treatment, the patient begins to show signs of adequate hydration, as evidenced by decreased emesis, balanced intake and output, and improvement in acid–base balance and electrolyte status.

| ASSESSMENT—RECOGNIZE CUES/ INTERVENTIONS—TAKE ACTION | RATIONALES |
|---|---|
| Assess the characteristics of the patient's nausea/vomiting: frequency, duration, and severity; amount and color of vomitus; accompanying symptoms (abdominal pain, diarrhea, dyspepsia [a vague feeling of discomfort or bloating after eating]); and precipitating factors. Reassess every 8 hours or as indicated. | This comprehensive initial assessment provides a basis for nursing interventions/teaching and a subsequent comparison for changes. |
| Assess for signs of dehydration: dry mucous membranes, poor skin turgor, decreased BP, increased pulse, possible low-grade fever, and increases in urine specific gravity, BUN, and hematocrit. | With fluid losses, blood and urine become concentrated, circulating blood volume decreases, BP may decrease, and the heart rate increases to compensate. |
| Assess for signs of electrolyte imbalance every 8 hours (muscle weakness, cramps, irritability, and irregular heartbeats) and monitor the results of the prescribed laboratory studies. | Potassium and magnesium are lost with prolonged vomiting. Muscles, including the myocardium, are weakened by the loss of these electrolytes. Severe potassium loss affects the kidneys' ability to concentrate urine. |
| Initiate and monitor the IV hydration, including electrolyte replacement, while keeping the patient nothing by mouth for 48 hours, as prescribed by the health care provider. | This approach aids in resting GI motility, resolving dehydration, and improving electrolyte balance caused by intractable vomiting. |
| Administer parenteral nutrition as prescribed by the health care provider. Secure the assistance of the clinical pharmacist and/or dietitian to manage the patient's nutrition. | Total nutritional needs can be met with parenteral nutrition, thereby helping to ensure adequate fetal growth and preventing maternal malnutrition. |
| Encourage the patient to take approximately 100 mL (e.g., in 1-oz portions hourly), preferably of electrolyte-containing liquid, between each meal and to avoid fluids with meals. | This measure prevents dehydration between meals and overdistention of the stomach during meals, allowing more space for caloric foods, and may prevent nausea. |

## Patient Problem/Analyze Cues/Prioritize Hypotheses

# Body Weight Problem (Weight Loss)

*due to* the inability to ingest, digest, and absorb sufficient nutrients and calories because of prolonged vomiting

**Desired Outcome/Generate Solutions:** Within 1 week of interventions/treatment, the patient increases her nutritional intake and demonstrates improvement in her acid–base balance, electrolytes, and nutritional status.

| ASSESSMENT—RECOGNIZE CUES/ INTERVENTIONS—TAKE ACTION | RATIONALES |
|---|---|
| Assess the weight at admission (or initial encounter) and document the daily morning weight on the same scale. Compare with prepregnant weight and monitor the continued weight loss or gain. | Weight changes indicate progress with treatment and resolution of the condition or severity of losses and risk for maternal and fetal malnutrition. |
| Assess for signs of starvation every 8 hours (e.g., jaundice, bleeding from mucous membranes, and ketonuria). | Insufficient nutrition may cause hypothrombinemia, depleted vitamin C and B complexes, and ketosis. |
| Initiate and titrate the enteral (nasogastric) feeding or parenteral nutrition (by intravascular therapy) as prescribed by the health care provider and agency protocols. | These are effective methods with which to administer nutrients and hydration when oral ingestion of food and fluids is not possible. |
| Start the patient on oral intake when acute nausea resolves, beginning as prescribed with clear liquids (broth and bland juices) and advancing to solid foods as tolerated. | Because an individual tolerates liquids and foods differently, it is important to gradually test that foods and pattern of eating are better tolerated. |
| Suggest alternative dietary patterns (e.g., frequent small and dry meals, six or more per day, and followed by clear liquids). | Small, frequent, and dry meals may reduce nausea and vomiting from a distended stomach. |
| Suggest eating meals with the highest protein-calorie intake when the nausea is the least problematic, possibly within 30 minutes to 1 hour after taking medication for nausea and vomiting. | When the meal providing the most nutrition is consumed at the time the patient is most likely to retain it, the patient may be able to absorb higher protein and nutrient levels necessary for pregnancy. |
| Suggest high-protein supplemental beverages. | Liquids may be easier to tolerate than solid foods. |
| As indicated, suggest that the patient avoid food odors and foods that are greasy, highly spiced, rich, or overly sweet. | These measures prevent stimulating the gag reflex or increasing acid reflux. However, because some individuals prefer salty and spicy foods, the patient should try anything that is appealing and that she believes she will be able to keep down. |
| Encourage the patient to stay upright for 2 hours after eating. | This prevents esophageal spasms that can be caused by the reflux of acid and food into the esophagus. Gravity aids in facilitating the movement of food through the esophagus to the stomach and into the small intestine. |
| Administer the prescribed therapies for nausea: antiemetic medications such as pyridoxine (vitamin $B_6$), metoclopramide (Reglan), or promethazine (Phenergan). | These therapies are known to decrease nausea and may enable the patient to ingest and retain fluid and food nutrients, vitamins, proteins, carbohydrates, and fats from oral intake. |
| Refer for acupuncture as prescribed by the health care provider or encourage the patient to wear an acupressure wristband. | Many women report less nausea and vomiting with acupuncture treatment or with the wristband. |

## Patient Problem/Analyze Cues/Prioritize Hypotheses

# Anxiety

*due to* actual or perceived threat to self and fetus because of inadequate nutritional status and increasing debilitation from prolonged vomiting

**Desired Outcome/Generate Solutions:**  Within 1–2 hours of intervention, the patient verbalizes her anxieties, assesses her support systems, and uses appropriate coping mechanisms for the management of self and family needs.

| ASSESSMENT—RECOGNIZE CUES/ INTERVENTIONS—TAKE ACTION | RATIONALES |
|---|---|
| Establish a therapeutic relationship with honest nurse–patient communication, unconditional positive regard, active listening, and empathetic understanding. | Fostering a trusting relationship promotes the patient's ability to assess her feelings, discuss her situation, and freely express her needs and concerns. |

Continued

| ASSESSMENT—RECOGNIZE CUES/ INTERVENTIONS—TAKE ACTION | RATIONALES |
|---|---|
| Encourage the patient to develop self-awareness and communicate the causes of her anxiety. | Self-awareness and the ability to communicate anxiety and characteristics of her situation aid in developing a care plan specific to her needs, such as whether home or hospital treatment will be more helpful. Examples of causes that may be contributing to the patient's anxiety include weight loss, frustration with constant nausea and vomiting, ambivalence about the pregnancy, fear for the well-being of the preborn baby, lack of support from significant other and family, inability to care for self or others, and loss of income if unable to work. |
| Assist with making arrangements for admittance to the hospital, if prescribed by the health care provider, or arrange for assistance of the medical social worker (MSW) as soon as possible after admission, per hospital protocol. | Patients with severe nausea and vomiting who demonstrate changes in laboratory values and weight loss need to be admitted to the hospital for hydration, nutritional supplementation, medications, and monitoring of weight loss or gain. This assistance will provide a supportive environment that decreases anxiety and increases the patient's comfort. |
| Be alert for verbal and nonverbal cues about the patient's anxiety level. | These cues aid in providing appropriate assistance and support. Levels of anxiety include the following: <br><br>• *Mild:* restlessness, irritability, increased questions, focusing on the environment. <br><br>• *Moderate:* inattentiveness, expressions of concern, narrowed perceptions, insomnia, and increased heart rate. <br><br>• *Severe:* expression of feelings of doom, rapid speech, tremors, and poor eye contact. The patient may be preoccupied with the past or unable to understand the present and may have tachycardia, increased nausea and vomiting, and hyperventilation. <br><br>• *Panic:* inability to concentrate or communicate, distortion of reality, increased motor activity, and increased vomiting and tachypnea. |
| Refer to Social Services when available to assist with psychosocial needs and discharge planning. | Social Services provides counseling, support, and resources for written material. Other options include Internet chat groups, which enable communication with others who are experiencing similar circumstances, as well as other resources within the community. |
| In collaboration with the health care provider, refer to a mental health professional as needed. | A mental health professional (i.e., psychiatric nurse practitioner, counselor, and psychologist) enables evaluation for possible psychologic factors that may be contributing to the anxiety and hyperemesis. Supportive counseling or intervention may be beneficial in identifying the cause. |
| Involve assistance from the hospital chaplain or the patient's personal spiritual/religious advisor if the patient desires. | Pastoral care and sharing of concerns with a trusted spiritual advisor may decrease anxiety and provide continuity of support after hospital discharge. |
| Assist the patient to have undisturbed sleep, and provide a quiet, restful environment free of odors that cause discomfort. | Rest enhances coping mechanisms by decreasing physical and psychologic stress. The nurse can coordinate treatment interventions and visitation around the patient's need for rest. |

## Patient Problem/Analyze Cues/Prioritize Hypotheses

# Difficulty Coping

*due to* loss of control over changing health status, changing role with her family's needs, and maintenance of adequate nutritional intake

***Desired Outcome/Generate Solutions:*** Within the 24-hour period after interventions, the patient verbalizes her concerns, fears, strengths, and weaknesses and identifies personal coping mechanisms and support systems.

| ASSESSMENT—RECOGNIZE CUES/ INTERVENTIONS—TAKE ACTION | RATIONALES |
|---|---|
| Establish honest and empathetic communication with the patient. | Empathy and honesty promote effective communication. For example, "Please tell me what I can do to help you through this stressful time in your pregnancy." |
| Assess the patient's stressors and perceptions and the ability to understand her current health status. | Evaluation of the factors that stress the patient as well as her perceptions and comprehension level enable the mutual development of an individualized care plan. |
| Identify the patient's support systems. If possible, assess their interactions with the patient and assist with the development of a family plan to adapt to daily living changes. | Involvement of the family unit enables the identification of strengths and weaknesses and aids in planning the patient's care, thereby reducing stress and promoting effective coping. |
| Discuss the patient's cultural beliefs that affect her present situation, decision-making abilities, and previous methods of coping with life problems. | Cultural beliefs positively or negatively affect her ability to handle her condition. Maximizing her participation in planning and home management increases successful planning. Previous styles and successes with problems in the past may empower the patient and be reliable predictors of how she will cope with current problems. |
| Enlist assistance from MSW, dietitian, and spiritual support individuals as indicated. | The MSW can follow the patient after hospital discharge, knows community resources, and is trained to assist with financial and psychosocial needs. The dietitian develops parenteral and oral diet plans to enhance the patient's ability to ingest, digest, and absorb fuels and nutrients. Spiritual support, related to the patient's spiritual/religious preferences, assists with finding meaning and hopefulness in a debilitating situation. |
| Instruct the patient on how to effectively use her time when she feels well (e.g., performing activities of daily living or doing errands). | This information will give some sense of control over her situation while also promoting involvement with her larger life and family. |

## Patient, Partner, and Family Problem

# Deficient Knowledge

*due to* unfamiliarity with the effects HG has on self, the pregnancy, fetus, and family; the treatment; and expected outcomes of care

**Desired Outcome/Generate Solutions:** Immediately after teaching, the patient, her partner, and her family verbalize accurate knowledge about HG, its treatment, and the expected outcome.

| ASSESSMENT—RECOGNIZE CUES/ INTERVENTIONS—TAKE ACTION | RATIONALES |
|---|---|
| Assess the patient's, her partner's, and family's knowledge and past experiences with HG. As indicated, explain the effect it has on the patient and the fetus. | Hyperemesis causes decreased maternal–fetal placental transfer of nutrients and IUGR. Information motivates adherence to treatments and enables the understanding of possible consequences from nonadherence. |
| Explain the various treatment options, as described in earlier patient problems. | Treatments may include IV hydration, medications (IV, intramuscular [IM], by mouth [PO]), total parenteral nutrition, home care, and hospitalization. Explanation of treatment options helps the patient and health care provider decide on a care plan that is most beneficial to the patient and fetus. |
| Instruct the patient about signs and symptoms that may indicate worsening HG and dehydration (e.g., inability to keep solids or liquids down for the previous 12 hours, dizziness, extreme fatigue, poor skin turgor, decreased and/or caramel-colored urine, and weight loss). | A knowledgeable patient likely will report symptoms promptly. Early evaluation and treatment may decrease the severity of the condition. |
| Explain the expected outcomes that adequate fluid and nutritional intake will have on fetal development (i.e., it will increase maternal–fetal placental transfer of nutrients and optimize intrauterine fetal growth). | This information reinforces the need for the patient's adherence to possible hospitalization or home infusion, IV fluids, or parenteral nutrition. |

Continued

| ASSESSMENT—RECOGNIZE CUES/ INTERVENTIONS—TAKE ACTION | RATIONALES |
|---|---|
| Encourage the patient to avoid brushing her teeth within 1–2 hours after meals or on arising in the morning. | This action may stimulate the gag reflex and aggravate vomiting in women who are pregnant. |
| Encourage good daily oral hygiene after vomiting episodes. | This prevents dental decay that may accompany contact with the acids present in emesis and for some may help decrease nausea. For example, the patient may use mouthwash and brush and floss teeth when she feels the least nauseated. |

## Patient Problem/Analyze Cues/Prioritize Hypotheses

# Deficient Knowledge (regarding medications)

*due to* unfamiliarity with the purpose, potential side effects, nonprescribed devices, and safety of prescribed medications used during HG

*Desired Outcome/Generate Solutions:* Immediately after teaching, the patient verbalizes an accurate understanding of the risks, benefits, and precautions of medications used during pregnancy in the treatment of HG.

| ASSESSMENT—RECOGNIZE CUES/ INTERVENTIONS—TAKE ACTION | RATIONALES |
|---|---|
| Instruct the patient about prescribed medications: | A knowledgeable patient is more likely to adhere to the therapy, identify and report significant side effects, and recognize and report precautions that might preclude the use of the prescribed medication. |
| • **Metoclopramide Hydrochloride (Reglan)** | This is an antiemetic that works on the chemoreceptor trigger zone in the brain to decrease nausea and vomiting. It helps move food through the GI tract, counteracting the effects of progesterone produced at higher levels in pregnancy. Reglan may be given inpatient or outpatient. *Administration:* PO/IM/IV. |
| Caution the patient to be alert for and report twitching of the eyelids or muscles surrounding the eyes, hands, or legs. | These extrapyramidal reactions may be seen with high IV doses. |
| Caution the patient to be alert for and report involuntary repetitious movements of the muscles of the face, limbs, and trunk. | This is a sign of tardive dyskinesia (a syndrome of potentially irreversible involuntary repetitious movements) and a serious side effect seen with long-term use. |
| Instruct the patient to be alert for and report drowsiness, restlessness, lethargy, fatigue, seizures, lactation, and constipation. | These are common side effects. |
| Explain that caution is necessary in patients with seizure disorders. | This medication may lower the seizure threshold. |
| **Pantoprazole (Protonix)** | Antiulcer/proton pump inhibitor. *Administration:* PO/IV. |
| Instruct the patient to be alert for and report diarrhea, abdominal pain, headache, heartburn, skin rash, and dizziness. | These are possible side effects. Patients must avoid activities that require alertness until the medication's effect on the central nervous system (CNS) is known. |
| **Promethazine (Phenergan)** | Antiemetic/antihistamine/tranquilizer. *Administration:* PO/IV/IM/rectal. |
| Instruct the patient to be alert for and report dizziness, drowsiness, dry mouth, blurred vision, fatigue, and urinary retention. | These are common side effects. Patients must avoid activities that require alertness until the medication's effect on the CNS is known. |
| Explain that precautions are needed for patients taking other CNS depressants such as opioids. | Medication interactions can occur, necessitating a lower dose of opioids. |

| ASSESSMENT—RECOGNIZE CUES/ INTERVENTIONS—TAKE ACTION | RATIONALES |
|---|---|
| • Administer IV doses through a large-bore vein, not in the hand or wrist, and in a running IV line. Stop the infusion immediately if burning or pain occurs with IV administration | IV administration can cause severe pain at the infusion site. |
| **Prochlorperazine (Compazine)** | Antiemetic. *Administration:* PO/IM/IV/rectal. |
| Instruct the patient to be alert for and report drowsiness, dizziness, blurred vision, and fatigue. | These are common CNS side effects. Patients must avoid activities that require alertness until the medication's effect on the CNS is known. |
| Caution the patient to be alert for and report involuntary movements and decreased BP. | Extrapyramidal reactions and hypotension are seen with IV administration. |
| Instruct the patient to be alert for and report seizures, dry mouth, constipation, and urinary retention. | These are less common side effects. |
| **Ondansetron (Zofran)** | Antiemetic. *Administration:* PO/IM/IV. |
| Instruct the patient to be alert for and report pain, redness, and burning at the site of injection. | These signs can occur as a local reaction with IM injection or IV infiltration. |
| Instruct the patient to be alert for and report anxiety, dizziness, drowsiness, headache, constipation, and diarrhea. | These are common side effects. |
| Caution the patient to be alert for and report involuntary movements. | Extrapyramidal reactions are rare CNS side effects. |
| Explain that caution is necessary in patients with liver disease. | Liver clearance of this medication is reduced in patients with hepatic impairment. |
| **Diphenhydramine (Benadryl)** | This antihistamine can be used as an antiemetic, reducing nausea and vomiting in mild cases. *Administration:* PO/IV. |
| Instruct the patient of the potential for mild drowsiness and dry mouth. | These are common side effects. |
| **Motion Sickness Band** | This motion sickness device is worn on both wrists, applying gentle pressure to acupressure points on the wrists. It is available without a prescription and comes in various brands; some are battery operated. |

## ADDITIONAL PROBLEMS:

| | |
|---|---|
| "Immobility" for relevant patient problems (The patient may be on self-imposed bedrest for comfort reasons.) | Chapter 1 |
| "Psychosocial Support for the Patient" for relevant patient problems such as: *Anxiety* and *Fatigue* (due to interrupted sleep) | Chapter 8 |
| "Psychosocial Support for the Patient's Family and Significant Others" for relevant problems such as *Difficulty Coping* | Chapter 9 |

## ✔ PATIENT–FAMILY TEACHING AND DISCHARGE PLANNING

Include verbal and written information about the following:
✓ Possible causes and effects HG has on the pregnancy and fetus.
✓ Signs and symptoms the patient need to report to her health care provider.
✓ Treatment interventions and medications for HG.
✓ Importance of attaining as much rest as possible.
✓ Nutritional options that would be most beneficial to the patient.
✓ Importance of eating small, frequent meals during the day.
✓ Importance and timing of oral hydration.
✓ Importance of avoiding lying down or reclining for 2 hours after eating.
✓ If parenteral nutrition is needed, the importance of maintaining insertion site and reporting any signs of site infection and pump malfunction.
✓ Importance of frequent clinic visits if being monitored on an outpatient basis and the date and time of the next clinic visit.
✓ Importance of informing the health care provider of any physical and emotional changes that may exacerbate the hyperemesis.

✓ Medications, including drug name, purpose, dosage, frequency, precautions, and potential side effects. Also explain relevant drug–drug, food–drug, and herb–drug interactions.

✓ Importance of monitoring fetal well-being with ultrasound and nonstress test.

✓ Referral to local and national support organizations, including Sidelines, a national support organization for women and their families experiencing complicated pregnancies, at http://www.sidelines.org.

✓ Patient education materials may be found at:
- American College of Obstetricians and Gynecologists has an extensive collection of patient education materials available at https://www.acog.org/womens-health/pregnancy
- Pregnancy Sickness Support: http://www.pregnancysicknesssupport.org.uk

## OVERVIEW/PATHOPHYSIOLOGY

Labor and birth are natural human processes, and for most women, minimal interventions are required. The philosophy that birth is a normal, natural process works best in an environment of continuous labor support, shared information, and decision-making and where interventions are viewed and practiced on a continuum from noninvasive to least invasive based on the wishes of the laboring woman and at the discretion of the health care provider. Nurses working in the intrapartum setting have a broad knowledge of the physiologic and psychologic stressors faced by the laboring woman. The nurse provides family-centered care, supporting the natural labor and birthing process and the woman's wishes regarding her care. Uncomplicated labor occurs at term (completion of 38 weeks gestation), with a single fetus in a vertex presentation with labor initiated by spontaneous and effective contractions, and with birth completed within 24 hours.

Initiation of labor is a complex process involving a combination of factors that work in conjunction to stimulate myometrial activity and, in turn, initiate the onset of labor. These factors may include oxytocin release from the posterior pituitary, uterine distention or stretching, increasing uterine pressure due to the term fetus, increased maternal prostaglandin and fetal cortisol levels, placental aging, and changes in estrogen and progesterone ratios. The exact mechanisms that initiate spontaneous labor have been researched but are not completely understood.

Premonitory signs of labor such as weight loss of 1–3 lb (0.45–1.36 kg) before the start of labor, lightening, urinary frequency, a change in vaginal discharge including bloody show, the loss of the mucus plug, and irregular contractions are often reported before true labor begins. True labor is distinguished from false labor by contractions that become progressively more frequent and regular and by discomfort beginning in the back and radiating toward the abdomen causing cervical dilation, cervical effacement, and fetal descent. Duration of labor depends on fetal presentation, fetal size, position of the fetus, and a multitude of factors, including pelvic structure, the woman's body mass, and birthing position. Whether the woman is a primipara (first-time pregnancy past the 20th-week gestation) or multiparous (this pregnancy is past the 20th week and the woman has already delivered an infant weighing more than 500 g) can influence how rapidly labor progresses.

Labor is divided into four stages. The first stage of labor, which is cervical dilation to 10 cm, is divided into latent (0–3 cm dilation), active (4–7 cm dilation), and transitional (8–10 cm dilation) phases. Stage two is measured from compete cervical dilation to the birth of the baby. Stage two may have a latent or passive phase of descent and/or an active phase facilitating open glottis pushing with contractions. Stage three is from the birth of the baby to the expulsion of the placenta. Stage four is the immediate postpartum recovery phase occurring from the delivery of the placenta and encompassing the first 2 hours postdelivery.

## HEALTH CARE SETTING

Primary care and acute care in an inpatient hospital setting or free-standing birth center. Home births occur in some geographic areas.

## ASSESSMENT

On the mother's arrival to the perinatal unit, the nurse obtains a thorough admission assessment. Assessment is focused on current and prior obstetric history, the patient's medical history, known allergies, and presenting labor symptoms. A review of the prenatal record is optimal and easily done with the increasing use of electronic medical records. After about 36 week's gestation in areas without electronic medical records, most health care providers provide copies of the woman's prenatal records to the delivering hospital or birthing center so that they are readily available if the woman comes in to be assessed. A review of laboratory data and prenatal testing allows for a more comprehensive assessment. Risk factors for the pregnancy will be assessed and documented along with maternal preferences for childbirth, including pain control options. If the patient has had no prenatal care or no records are available, the admission assessment will include appropriate laboratory or diagnostic testing.

### Signs and symptoms:

*Rule out labor:* Women may come to the hospital to "rule out" labor, unsure if the signs and symptoms they are experiencing indicate they are in labor. The pregnant woman is evaluated and, if found to be in labor, is admitted. If the woman is found not to be in labor, she is sent home with verbal and written instructions regarding the signs of true labor, when to see the health care provider, and follow-up phone numbers.

*Uterine contractions:* Characteristics of true labor include contractions that increase in frequency, duration, and strength over time and cause cervical dilation, effacement, and fetal descent. Typically with true labor the woman's contractions will increase with walking because this increases myometrial irritability. Uterine contractions (UCs) will continue even when the woman tries to sleep or rest. In early labor the patient will be able to walk and talk through the contraction. Often the woman in early labor is encouraged to ambulate and change positions frequently rather than labor in bed, allowing gravity to facilitate labor progress.

*Low back pain:* Back pain that begins in the low back and radiates to the front is indicative of true labor. The woman may also report a "tightening" across the abdomen that begins in the back or back pain that does not completely go away because the fetal head is applying pressure to the maternal structures.

*Bloody show:* Pink or reddish-brown vaginal discharge likely will be present, resulting from cervical softening and changes due to effacement.

*Mucus plug:* Loss of the mucus plug will have occurred.

*Rupture of membranes:* Rupture of membranes occurs when the amniotic sac breaks and the patient begins to leak amniotic fluid. The amniotic fluid surrounds and protects the baby within the uterus. When the patients' membranes rupture or "water breaks," it will be assessed for color (normal color is clear; if the fluid appears greenish or meconium stained, it is an indication that the baby has had their first bowel movement while in-utero), amount, odor (the fluid should not have a foul or malodorous smell), and the time the patient started leaking.

## THE DIAGNOSTIC TESTS

*Admission vital signs:* Temperature, pulse, respirations, and blood pressure measurements are obtained. These are compared with prepregnant and prenatal records. Pain level is assessed using a valid pain tool. The woman's acceptable pain level is documented. The woman is placed in semi-Fowler position, usually in a left tilt using a wedge or pillow under the right hip, to optimize uterine perfusion. A baseline electronic fetal heart rate (FHR) monitoring strip with uterine activity of at least 20-minute duration is obtained on admission. The frequency and duration of contractions, along with the category of the FHR tracing, should be obtained.

*Cervical evaluation:* A sterile vaginal examination is performed by the registered nurse (RN) or health care provider to assess cervical dilation, effacement, and station of the fetal presenting part.

*Sterile speculum examination:* A sterile speculum is inserted into the vagina to visualize amniotic fluid leaking from the cervical os or pooling of amniotic fluid in the vagina. This fluid is tested with Nitrazine paper. If positive for amniotic fluid, the paper will turn from yellow to dark blue or green-blue, and the pH will be greater than 6. False-positive results may be seen in the presence of semen, blood, vaginal infections, or alkaline antiseptics. Using a cotton swab, a sample of vaginal fluid is taken from the posterior vaginal fornix (the posterior space below the cervix) and examined under the microscope for the presence of a ferning pattern that amniotic fluid makes when it dries on a slide.

*PAMG-1 (AmniSure):* The test detects trace amounts of a protein, PAMG-1, expressed by the cells of the decidua and is found in amniotic fluid. The test is performed by swabbing a sterile polyester swab into the vaginal secretions. The swab is then rinsed with a vial of solvent for 1 minute and thrown away. A test strip is dipped into the vial for 5–10 minutes and then read. One line indicates no rupture of membranes. Two lines indicate a rupture of membranes. No lines indicate an invalid test. The test has a 99% accuracy rate.

*External uterine and fetal monitoring:* Before placing the electronic fetal monitor (EFM), the RN or provider may perform Leopold maneuvers, a systemic assessment in which the external maternal abdomen is palpated. This is intended to determine fetal presentation before placing the external fetal monitors onto the maternal abdomen. External uterine monitoring is done to evaluate FHR, variability, and periodic and episodic changes for fetal well-being. UC presence, frequency, and duration are also monitored using a toco transducer. The RN or practitioner may also palpate the strength of UC as mild (tense fundus but easily indents to fingertip touch), moderate (firm fundus, difficult to indent with fingertip pressure), or strong (hard, firm fundus that does not indent to fingertips) and will ensure that the uterus is relaxing between contractions. The EFM provides a permanent record of the FHR and UCs. In the United States, the EFM may be used continuously or intermittently, or FHR may be intermittently auscultated (IA) if the patient is considered low risk. FHR will be determined, evaluated, and documented every 30 minutes during the first stage of labor and every 15 minutes during the active phase of pushing during stage two. If there are risk factors, FHR is identified, evaluated, and documented every 15 minutes during the first stage of labor and every 5 minutes during the active pushing phase of stage two (Perry et al., 2018).

## Patient Problem/Analyze Cues/Prioritize Hypotheses

# Anxiety

*due to* unfamiliar surroundings, processes, and procedures

*Desired Outcome/Generate Solutions:* Within 1 hour of intervention, the patient states that her anxiety has lessened or resolved, and she describes effective coping mechanisms.

| ASSESSMENT—RECOGNIZE CUES/ INTERVENTIONS—TAKE ACTION | RATIONALES |
|---|---|
| On admission, provide a brief tour of the unit, familiarize the patient and family with the room and where food and supplies may be found, provide contact phone numbers and rules regarding visitation, and discuss parking and the use of electronics. | Familiarity with the layout of the room and unit and knowledge of where to find important items or locations such as dietary supplies, linens, pay phones, and bathrooms will increase independence and decrease anxiety. Knowing the rules for visiting, cell phone use, and taking pictures/videos, among other concerns, will help decrease anxiety. |
| Assess which prenatal classes, reading materials, and hospital tours the patient may have attended or participated in. | Assessment of classes the patient attended and the educational needs of the patient and her family enables the nurse to teach the patient's specific needs, thereby helping to reduce anxiety. Identifying educational gaps enables the nurse to provide materials and teach specific educational topics to women in early labor and provides distraction as well. |
| Engage the patient and family in discussions regarding their previous experiences being hospitalized and their expectations and methods for successful coping during stressful events in the past. | Birth is often the first time a woman is hospitalized. Assessing previous experiences and acknowledging concerns show respect and provide the nurse with helpful information. Reflecting on successful methods used to cope with anxiety in the past during stressful situations enables the patient to call on her own strengths. |
| Assess for verbal and nonverbal cues regarding the patient's anxiety level. | Verbal as well as nonverbal cues can provide the nurse with insights into how the patient is coping with the hospitalization and the labor process. Examples of nonverbal cues that might indicate anxiety are not making eye contact, fidgeting, being distracted, or ignoring teaching. Anxiety decreases the patient's ability to focus and relax. Relaxation is important in labor to provide adequate oxygenation and promote optimal labor progress. |
| Explain the purpose of any equipment or procedure (monitoring fetal status, IV, and sterile vaginal examination) to the patient along with rationales and options for care. | Explanation or demonstration of procedures or equipment and their use or purpose will provide information and decrease anxiety. Patients often are fearful or concerned that a procedure will hurt or ask, "Why is this being done?" Informed consent and explanations of treatment options are necessary to provide the opportunity for shared decision-making and facilitate the cooperation and trust of the patient. |
| | For example, to assess fetal well-being and contraction status, the nurse will use EFM or IA. Explanation of these methods, when and how often they will occur, and the information they provide should be shared with the patient to gain acceptance and cooperation and ease anxiety. Explanation of findings and progress is part of family-centered care and part of the shared decision-making process. |
| Review the stages of labor as they occur, reassuring the woman and family of normal expectations and behaviors, while providing coaching and support. | The patient may become fearful if she does not understand what is happening to her body during labor or feels something is abnormal. Explaining, in lay terms, the labor process, expected progress, and what to expect while providing encouragement and support enhances the patient's and family's coping skills and well-being and decrease anxiety. |
| Encourage doula (professional or lay-support person) support of the laboring woman when available. | Continuous support by the doula in labor has been shown to reduce medical interventions and provide the woman with additional support that reassures her as labor progresses. Women report a greater satisfaction with their labors when they have continuous labor support (Perry et al., 2018). |
| Offer praise and encouragement to family members or other support person and offer breaks. Acknowledge that labor support can be difficult. | Instructing and supporting family members to provide relaxation techniques through demonstration and return demonstration allows the family to support the woman in labor as part of family-centered nursing care. |

## Patient, Partner, and Family Problem

# Deficient Knowledge

*due to* misinformation, late or no prenatal care, or lack of prenatal class attendance

***Desired Outcome/Generate Solutions:*** Immediately after instruction, the patient, partner, and family verbalize accurate knowledge of the admission procedure and expectant labor and delivery care.

| ASSESSMENT—RECOGNIZE CUES/ INTERVENTIONS—TAKE ACTION | RATIONALES |
|---|---|
| Assess the patient's, her partner's, and family's understanding of the birth process and whether they attended prenatal classes. | Assessing the knowledge base and expectations initiates a relationship based on trust. Educational assessment facilitates the nurse's teaching and helps meet individual educational needs regarding labor and birth. |
| Engage the patient in an open discussion about her birth plan if she has one, including who will attend the delivery and any wishes she may have regarding the delivery. Share the birth plan with other members of the health care team so that collaboration occurs and the patient and family feel valued and heard. | Acknowledging and assisting the woman to meet her birthing goals based on her birthing plan necessitates clear communication. Having and meeting birth plans increases the woman's sense of control and decreases anxiety. Communicating that the health and well-being of the mother and baby may necessitate adjustment of the birthing plans is important to gain trust and cooperation. |
| Assess which plans or questions the woman has regarding pain management in labor. | Acknowledging the woman's wishes for pain management is a vital part of family-centered care. Active listening to the woman shows respect. If the patient has not taken childbirth classes that discussed pain and anesthesia or analgesia, the nurse needs to explain options for pain management, ideally in early labor when the woman is able to focus on the information and ask questions so that she can make an informed decision. Some women will want to know their options regarding pain management and will choose to wait and see how labor progresses before selecting a specific method of analgesia or anesthesia. The nurse works with the patient and family to support their goals for pain management. |
| Provide culturally sensitive care to the patient, her partner, and the family, adapting care to their individual needs. | Culturally sensitive nursing care shows respect and acknowledges people as individuals and the influence that culture may have on their individual coping styles. Different cultures approach labor and birth differently. For example, in some cultures the woman may labor very quietly and in others the woman may be very demonstrative. Some cultures insist on many people being present at the delivery, and other cultures may not wish any men in attendance. The nurse works with the woman and family to provide safe, culturally appropriate family-centered care in an atmosphere of shared decision-making. |

## Patient Problem/Analyze Cues/Prioritize Hypotheses

# Dehydration

*due to* decreased oral intake in labor, mouth breathing, and diaphoresis

***Desired Outcome/Generate Solutions:*** The patient becomes adequately hydrated throughout labor as evidenced by normal elastic skin turgor, moist mucous membranes, and urinary output measured at a minimum of 30 mL/hour.

| ASSESSMENT—RECOGNIZE CUES/ INTERVENTIONS—TAKE ACTION | RATIONALES |
|---|---|
| Monitor the hydration status (see the desired outcome) and measure urine specific gravity as needed. | The expected urine specific gravity range is 1.005–1.030. An excess of 1.030 indicates dehydration. |
| Assess her temperature every 2–4 hours per agency policy. | An elevated temperature is associated with dehydration. |
| Monitor the pulse and blood pressure per agency policy. | Increased pulse and decreased blood pressure indicate dehydration. |
| Encourage steady, modest amounts of fluids and light snacks in early labor (e.g., fruit juice, Jell-O, broth, clear soups, Popsicles, tea, sports drink, and clear carbonated beverages). Provide ice chips if the patient does not wish to drink fluids. | There is slowed gastric emptying in labor, so if large volumes of food or liquids are consumed, vomiting may occur, although few women choose to eat or drink large quantities after active labor begins. |
| Instruct the patient to take solid food with caution while in labor. | Solids are avoided after active labor begins because of the risk for aspiration of gastric contents if emergency anesthesia is required. Although the risk is low, solid food in labor is only provided at the discretion of the anesthesiologist and per agency policy. |
| Discuss IV fluids with the patient in early labor or on admission if possible to assess her preference. (An IV line may or may not be part of admission protocols, depending on unit policy.) | This provides the patient with information and rationales regarding IV administration of fluids. |
| | Administration of IV fluids for hydration, commonly normal saline or lactated Ringer solution, is an option in labor, especially for the patient who is nauseated or not taking adequate fluids by mouth. IV hydration in labor may have the added benefit of shortening labor and is necessary for some forms of analgesia or anesthesia. Some facilities strongly suggest or require IV access in case of emergency. |
| Provide comfort care for the diaphoretic patient. Maintain the room at a comfortable temperature for her. Remove excess clothing or linens as needed and change her gown to keep her dry and comfortable. Provide cool washcloths or ice packs to help maintain comfort as well as hand-held or electric fans. | Labor is strenuous work and elevates the body's temperature. The woman may perspire in an attempt to cool her body. |

## Patient Problem/Analyze Cues/Prioritize Hypotheses

# Acute Pain

*due to* cervical dilation, muscle hypoxia from uterine contractions, a full bladder, or stretching of maternal tissues

***Desired Outcomes/Generate Solutions:*** Using a pain scale, the patient states that she is coping with pain to her satisfaction using pharmacologic or nonpharmacologic pain relief methods based on her preference and birth plan. Nonverbal cues, such as grimacing, are absent or declining in frequency.

| ASSESSMENT—RECOGNIZE CUES/ INTERVENTIONS—TAKE ACTION | RATIONALES |
|---|---|
| Encourage the patient to verbalize her level of acceptable pain using a valid pain scale. | Documentation and understanding of the patient's individual acceptable pain level enable the nurse to work with the patient in providing adequate pain relief. The nurse recognizes that pain is unique for each person. |
| Assess for behavioral or physiologic indicators of pain at frequent intervals (e.g., every 1–2 hours or during scheduled vital sign assessments). | Pain in labor occurs from stretching, lactic acid buildup, muscle hypoxia, and pressure on the pelvic structure and from the fetal head. Increased heart rate, respirations, and blood pressure occur in response to increased pain. |
| Assess for verbal and nonverbal cues indicating pain. | Examples of nonverbal cues include facial grimacing, moaning, and muscle tension in the extremities along with increased anxiety. The patient may not be aware of these cues; encourage her to use relaxation techniques such as breathing and visualization to decrease muscle tension and decrease the pain–fear–tension cycle. |

Continued

## ASSESSMENT—RECOGNIZE CUES/INTERVENTIONS—TAKE ACTION

## RATIONALES

| ASSESSMENT—RECOGNIZE CUES/INTERVENTIONS—TAKE ACTION | RATIONALES |
|---|---|
| Instruct and encourage the relaxation and breathing techniques. | Relaxation and breathing techniques promote adequate oxygenation to the tissues and decrease physiologic responses to pain. |
| Encourage emptying of the bladder every 2 hours or more frequently as needed. | A full bladder can cause discomfort and impede fetal descent. Use of a bedpan or bedside commode may be necessary if the woman does not wish to ambulate or has received medications. Catheterization may be necessary with some regional anesthetics because of motor blockade. |
| Keep the laboring woman's environment as quiet as possible. | A quiet environment free of noise and distraction promotes rest and conserves energy. |
| Instruct and assist with nonpharmacologic comfort measures (e.g., breathing techniques, effleurage [gliding stroke] to the abdomen, application of heat and cold, acupressure or acupuncture, continuous and firm counterpressure to the sacral area during each contraction, pelvic rocking, relaxation conditioned in response to the partner's touch, massage, music, hydrotherapy, and transcutaneous electrical nerve stimulation). | Nonpharmacologic methods may promote relaxation, decrease muscle tension, and provide distraction from pain and give the woman a sense of control. The support person may need to vary the method, depending on the stage of labor and position of the fetus (e.g., counterpressure to the sacrum reduces pain from back labor and occiput-posterior presentations). Cutaneous methods such as therapeutic touch, massage, counterpressure, application of heat or cold, and acupressure rely on interrupting the transmission of sensation. Location, technique, and depth of massage may vary but can decrease perceptions of pain. |
| Use other comfort measures that incorporate the senses. | Nonpharmacologic comfort measures that incorporate the senses include stimulation of visual, olfactory, and auditory stimuli to block pain impulses. These comfort measures include the use of focal points, guided imagery, music, hypnosis, aromatherapy, and keeping the patient dry and clean. |
| Change the woman's position frequently, at least every 30 minutes, and encourage ambulation or an upright position in labor. Explain to her that labor progresses more quickly if she remains relaxed and upright. | Frequent position changes assist in comfort and needs to be based on the patient's comfort level, preference, safety, and privacy. The nurse can suggest and demonstrate appropriate laboring positions that increase comfort. |
| Advise the laboring woman to avoid the supine position. | This position causes decreased uteroplacental blood flow and cardiac return. If the woman wishes to lie down, a side-lying or a left or right tilt to the pelvis is recommended to increase blood flow to the heart and to the uterus.<br><br>**Note:** Administration of regional anesthetics may negate the use of ambulation and some positions, especially if there is motor blockade. |
| Suggest the following actions/positions. | Hands-and-knees position may be effective in the rotation of the fetus from occiput posterior to occiput anterior and may reduce back labor. The use of this position and the upright position shortens labor for both the first and second stages of labor and is associated with a decreased use of pain medication.<br><br>Use of a birthing ball, peanut labor ball, lunging, squatting at the side of the bed, and the various positioning capabilities of the birthing bed facilitate patient comfort and should be encouraged as long as the well-being of the mother and fetus is established.<br><br>Laboring on the toilet or squatting decreases the pressure of presenting parts and allows gravity to assist with dilation and descent for some women and is encouraged as long as fetal well-being is assessed. |
| Medicate with analgesic or anesthetics as prescribed by the health care provider or anesthetist. | The types of medications used for pain management in labor may include those that cause a sedative effect to the woman so that she may doze or sleep between contractions; or a numbing of the lower abdomen so that she has reduced or no pain during labor. |

## ASSESSMENT—RECOGNIZE CUES/ INTERVENTIONS—TAKE ACTION

## RATIONALES

As indicated, keep the side rails up and advise the patient she will need assistance with ambulation if she is being treated with opioid-type medications. Advise not to attempt to ambulate with regional anesthesia such as epidural.

Common medications used for pain management in labor include opioids, synthetic opioids, opioid agonist-antagonists, and regional anesthesia. These medications have different side effects but offer some blunting or dulling of pain. The safety of the patient who has received these medications is paramount.

**Note:** Medications may cause a change in the labor progress and a decrease in contractions; thus they are usually not given until labor is well established. Respiratory depression in the newborn may occur if given too close to delivery. Naloxone (Narcan) is an opioid agonist and may be given to reverse the respiratory depressive effect to the newborn if opioids are given to the patient within 4 hours of delivery.

### ✔ PATIENT–FAMILY TEACHING AND DISCHARGE PLANNING

Labor and birth are a part of the normal human process. Education and teaching regarding the signs of true labor, the stages of labor, normal expectations, and labor support and pain management ideally should occur in prenatal classes or in early labor when the woman and her family are ready for this information. (For problems that can occur before or after delivery, see the subsequent chapters.) Include written and verbal information about the following:

✓ Signs and symptoms of true labor.
✓ When to call the health care provider or come to the hospital.
✓ Danger signs that require prompt reporting to the health care provider.
✓ Availability and choice of pain management methods.
✓ Availability of labor support/doula services.

# Postpartum Wound Infection 93

## OVERVIEW/PATHOPHYSIOLOGY

Wound infection is one of the postpartum (puerperal) infections that can develop after childbirth. Puerperal infection is a leading cause of maternal death worldwide. In the United States the infection rate for patients with a cesarean delivery is approximately 10%–15%, whereas it is approximately 2% for patients who give birth vaginally. Prophylactic broad-spectrum antibiotic therapy has been shown to be beneficial for women undergoing cesarean delivery or having a vaginal delivery who experience a third- or fourth-degree laceration. Wound infections after childbirth can develop anywhere there is a break in the skin or mucous membranes, which provides a portal of entry for bacteria. Wound infections are classified as early onset (within 48 hours) or late onset (after the first 48 hours) and develop from endogenous or exogenous bacteria. When identified early, most postpartum wound infections can be successfully treated with antibiotic therapy. Late-onset wounds may require incision and drainage, wound débridement, and multiple antibiotic therapy. Wound cultures may be necessary to identify the causative organism. When there is little to no improvement in wound site infection with first-choice antibiotics, methicillin-resistant *Staphylococcus aureus* (MRSA) infection must be considered and treated appropriately and aggressively.

The definition for puerperal infection centers on fever. A diagnosis is established with a fever of 100.4°F (38°C) or higher occurring in 2 or more days in the first 10 days postpartum, not including the first 24 hours (when dehydration and the exertion of labor can contribute to a low-grade fever).

The following are other types of postpartum infections:

*Endometritis:* An infection of the endometrium is the most common postpartum infection. It usually starts at the open site of placental attachment. It can spread easily through the interconnected genital tract or to a wound.

*Urinary tract infection ([UTI] or cystitis):* Bladder infections readily respond to antibiotics when identified early. Postpartum women with diabetes, women who have been catheterized, and women with lacerations extending into the urethral meatus are most at risk for UTI.

*Mastitis:* Infections of the breast usually involve one breast, manifest about 2 weeks after delivery, and are usually preventable with good hand hygiene, frequent feedings with an adequate transfer of milk, and daily variation of the newborn's feeding positions at the breast. If left untreated, mastitis may become an abscess.

*Septic pelvic thrombophlebitis:* Patients generally do not appear ill and may have minimal to no pain. A patient who persistently has a fever and does not respond to multiple antibiotic therapies may have this condition. Treatment includes both anticoagulant and antibiotic therapy.

## HEALTH CARE SETTING

Primary care (outpatient clinic), acute care (hospital), or home care; rehospitalization is common.

## ASSESSMENT

Assessments of the wound and other systemic signs of infection are necessary for all postpartum patients. Assess the postcesarean patient and those with other risk factors more frequently to monitor and report early signs of infection. The defining characteristics of wound infection are fever, pain or tenderness, edema, redness (erythema) surrounding the wound, induration (hardened tissue under the skin), purulent drainage, and separation of wound edges or wound dehiscence.

**Cardiopulmonary:** Tachycardia, hypotension, tachypnea, or syncope may be seen in the acutely ill patient when sepsis is present.

**Fever:** The temperature pattern may vary with the type of infection. It may be 101°F (38.3°C) or higher, with or without spiking episodes. With mild infection the patient may remain afebrile. Headache and overall "body aches" may accompany fever.

**Chills:** The patient may feel she cannot get warm even in the presence of an elevated temperature. Body shakes may accompany the chills. An overall flu-like feeling may be present.

**Malaise:** A feeling of generalized uneasiness, discomfort, and fatigue may be present.

**Pain:** Pain may be present with light or deep external palpation of the abdomen or wound site, or with bimanual palpation of the uterus. Cervical motion tenderness on bimanual examination may be present with a uterine infection. With an episiotomy infection, pain may be localized (throbbing, aching, or sharp) and deep tissue in nature. The patient may describe a sensation of vaginal pressure or "fullness."

**Vaginal discharge:** With an episiotomy infection, discharge may be purulent. It may be foul smelling if endometritis coexists with the infected episiotomy.

**Abdominal surgical incision:** The area around the incision is often erythematous and warm to the touch, and it may become edematous. If the tissue is very congested (indurated), it may have a "woody" appearance and feel hard to palpation. If the wound is not already open and draining bloody, serosanguineous, or purulent discharge, it may be probed with a cotton-tipped applicator to promote drainage. Dehiscence may or may not occur.

**Episiotomy or perineal laceration:** A thorough wound assessment may be guided by the acronym REEDA to monitor localized *r*edness (erythema), *e*dema, *e*cchymosis (bruising), *d*rainage (exudates), and *a*pproximation of skin edges. Dehiscence of the episiotomy may or may not occur. Any episiotomy or laceration, whether or not infected, interrupts tissue integrity and can lead to stress incontinence, pelvic floor prolapse, anal incontinence, and pelvic floor muscle dysfunction.

**Complications—neonatal:** If the maternal infection is caused by an antepartum uterine infection (chorioamnionitis), the neonate is at increased risk for infection or sepsis and generally would be admitted to the intensive care nursery for close and careful monitoring. Group B streptococcus (GBS) is the leading cause of newborn sepsis. When an infection occurs in the newborn, it usually manifests as pneumonia and/or meningitis within the first 24 hours of life. The presentation is fulminant, and the neonate deteriorates rapidly. Untreated, the infant mortality rate is high. A late-onset GBS infection typically presents as meningitis after 7–10 days. The mortality rate is low; however, survivors have significant neurologic sequelae.

**Physical assessment:** Patients presenting with wound infections may not appear or report feeling acutely ill. Some mild infections, such as cellulitis, respond well to early oral antibiotic therapy. More serious wound infections will require double or triple intravenous (IV) antibiotic therapy administration, wound débridement, or daily wound packing that allows the open incision to heal from the inside out by secondary intention (tissue granulation). In some instances, as in the case when there is a large blood clot behind the incision, reopening the complete incision may be necessary. This condition requires the use of a wound vacuum device or secondary surgical closure using retention sutures and extended hospitalization.

Early assessment and treatment are critical in reducing maternal morbidity/mortality. Sepsis is rare but can occur.

**Risk factors:** Risk factors associated with postpartum infections include obesity, hemorrhage, anemia, history of chorioamnionitis, prolonged rupture of membranes, multiple vaginal examinations, invasive procedures, corticosteroid therapy, advanced age, malnutrition, immunosuppression, type 1 diabetes, low socioeconomic status, malnutrition, positive GBS culture, prolonged preoperative hospitalization, long labor, hemorrhage (loss of leukocytes), duration of the surgery (cesarean delivery or postpartum tubal ligation), razor shaving of the operative site, use of electrosurgical knife, use of open drains (e.g., Jackson Pratt, Penrose), closure technique (suture vs staples), and emergency surgery (e.g., for fetal distress).

## DIAGNOSTIC TESTS

**Complete blood count with differential:** Leukocytes (white blood cells) will be elevated in the presence of infection. The differential lists the five types of leukocytes, which all perform a special function. The type of leukocyte elevation will depend on the type of infection present.

**Blood cultures:** During acute febrile illness, blood cultures may identify the source of bacteria causing the infection, and sensitivity analysis determines the most effective antibiotic therapy.

**Gram stain and culture of foul-smelling lochia:** Helps to identify *Clostridia*, anaerobes, and *Chlamydia* and indicates sensitivity analysis for the most effective antibiotic to use.

**Urinalysis for microscopy:** Detects the presence of UTI, which may be seen postoperatively after removal of an indwelling urinary catheter or if the patient experienced catheterization during labor.

**Pelvic ultrasound:** Detects and locates possible abscesses and hematomas.

**Computed tomography and magnetic resonance imaging:** In patients who do not respond to antibiotic therapy and have a negative ultrasound examination, these studies can detect obscure pelvic abscesses and pelvic thrombi.

## Patient Problem/Analyze Cues/Prioritize Hypotheses

# Impaired Skin and Tissue Integrity

*due to* wound infection and/or dehiscence

**Desired Outcome/Generate Solutions:** After initiation of therapy, the patient describes sensations and characteristics of the infected wound that necessitate nursing intervention and measures she can take to improve wound condition, and she begins to regain integrity in skin and underlying tissue without evidence of complications.

## ASSESSMENT—RECOGNIZE CUES/ INTERVENTIONS—TAKE ACTION

## RATIONALES

| ASSESSMENT—RECOGNIZE CUES/ INTERVENTIONS—TAKE ACTION | RATIONALES |
|---|---|
| Assess the pain every 2 hours after vaginal and cesarean childbirth and provide pain relief with analgesics, warm compresses, or sitz baths for episiotomy incisions, as prescribed by the health care provider. | Pain relief encourages patient movement. Both increased movement and heat increase circulation to promote wound healing. |
| Assess the cesarean surgical site, episiotomy, or other wounds every 4 hours for REEDA (see the description under "Assessment"). | Early identification of infection and prompt reporting of the need for medical intervention reduce maternal morbidity, the possibility of rehospitalization, and the length of treatment.<br><br>• *Cesarean surgical site:* redness surrounding incision, abdomen warm to touch, drainage from incision, wound dehiscence (incision partially or fully open), and evisceration (protrusion of an organ, usually bowel, through open surgical wound).<br><br>• *Episiotomy:* extreme pain in any position but especially sitting, foul-smelling vaginal odor in the absence of abdominal tenderness, drainage of pus, or dehiscence of sutures. The patient may use a mirror for self-examination or ask a family member to examine her perineum. |
| Assess the temperature, pulse, respirations, and pain characteristics every 2–4 hours. | This assessment aids in the early identification of a developing postpartum infection. A temperature increase to 100.4°F (38°C) or higher in 2 of the first 10 days postpartum indicates infection. Pulse rises with fever and increases more with sepsis. Tachypnea may develop with sepsis. |
| Demonstrate and have the patient, family, or significant other return demonstrations of the ability to practice scrupulous hand hygiene, cleansing of the wound area, and aseptic techniques to care for the wound, such as wearing gloves (nonsterile acceptable) after thorough hand washing, disposing of soiled dressings in plastic bags, maintaining a clean field for irrigation and packing, using alternatives to tapes for holding dressings in place, applying a new dressing as prescribed, and maintaining a clean and dry wound environment after discharge to home with outpatient care. | Hand hygiene and regular changes of dressings, including frequent changing of peripads, remove bacteria and thereby reduce the incidence of contamination. Tape can cause skin reactions and break down sensitive tissue. Maintaining a clean and dry wound provides an optimal environment to assist the body's natural healing processes. |
| As prescribed by the health care provider at hospital discharge, provide a referral to community health nursing for supervision of progressive wound changes, monitoring the patient's care, or providing daily dressing changes if wound care is complex. | Professional referral decreases stress on the patient and family, reinforces newly learned skills, improves knowledge, and assists with unforeseen problems during the transition to home care (e.g., adaptation to the home environment, conflict with work commitments, or uneasiness in self-management of a surgical wound). Home care also enables the patient to be home, which decreases medical costs. |
| Encourage the patient to eat a well-balanced diet that includes protein, carbohydrates, fruits, vegetables, and adequate fluid intake. | An adequate diet provides nutrients, especially vitamin C, and a positive nitrogen state, which promote wound healing. Adequate hydration also promotes wound healing. |
| Encourage the patient to report changes that indicate complications and to keep all medical appointments. | Good communication likely will promote early identification of complications. Adherence to appointments enables timely evaluation of the wound's healing process and initiation of care in response to complications. |
| Provide abdominal support or a binder after a cesarean delivery or bilateral tubal ligation. | A binder provides support and decreases stretching/tension on muscles or the surrounding tissue of the wound to promote healing. This is especially important with patients who are obese. |

## Patient, Partner, and Family Problem/Analyze Cues/Prioritize Hypotheses

# Deficient Knowledge (Medications)

*due to* unfamiliarity with the therapeutic medication regimen and potential side effects of the prescribed medications used for treating wound infections

***Desired Outcome/Generate Solutions:*** Immediately after instruction, the patient, her partner, and family (as indicated) verbalize an accurate understanding of the risks and benefits of medications used in treating postpartum wound infections.

| ASSESSMENT—RECOGNIZE CUES/ INTERVENTIONS—TAKE ACTION | RATIONALES |
|---|---|
| Instruct the patient about prescribed medications: | A knowledgeable patient is more likely to adhere to the therapy, identify and report side effects, and recognize and report precautions that might preclude the use of the prescribed medication. |
| **Antimicrobials** | These agents may be used as a perioperative prophylaxis, treating potential wound cellulitis/infection. |
| ⚠ **Cephalosporins** | |
| Cefazolin (Ancef, Kefzol), cefoxitin (Mefoxin), cefotetan (Cefotan), cefoperazone (Cefobid), cephalexin (Keflex) | *Administration:* IV, by mouth (PO), intramuscular (IM). |
| Instruct patients who are breastfeeding that cephalosporins will be present in low concentrations in breast milk. | Patients can breastfeed without it causing a problem to the infant. |
| Caution is necessary for patients with sensitivity to penicillins. Consult the provider before administering if a penicillin allergy is present. | Cross-sensitivity with penicillins is possible. Serious and possible fatal reactions can occur. |
| Explain the importance of following the complete course for all prescribed medications and taking them on time. | These measures reduce the risk for reinfection, prevent the development of antibiotic resistance, and maintain a constant level of medication in the bloodstream. |
| Instruct the patient to be alert for and report diarrhea, nausea, vomiting, stomach cramps, and anorexia. | These are possible side effects. |
| Caution the patient to be alert for and report excessive and explosive diarrhea. | *Clostridiodes difficile* infection is a potentially serious side effect in which the normal flora of the bowel is reduced by antibiotic therapy, and the anaerobic organism *C. difficile* multiplies and produces its toxins, causing severe diarrhea. This problem necessitates discontinuation of the antibiotic and laboratory evaluation of a stool sample. |
| Caution the patient to be alert for a rash and pruritus. | These may be signs of an allergic reaction. |
| ⚠ **Penicillins** | |
| Penicillin, amoxicillin, amoxicillin/clavulanate potassium (Augmentin), and ampicillin-sulbactam (Unasyn) | *Administration:* IV/IM/PO. *Breastfeeding:* Okay with amoxicillin. |
| Caution is necessary for patients with sensitivity to cephalosporins. Consult the provider before administering if a cephalosporin allergy is present. | Cross-sensitivity with cephalosporins is possible. Serious and possible fatal reactions can occur. |
| Advise the patient to follow the complete course for all prescribed medications and take them on time. | These measures reduce the risk for reinfection, prevent the development of antibiotic resistance, and maintain a constant level of medication in the bloodstream. |
| Instruct the patient to be alert for and report nausea, indigestion, and vomiting. | These are possible side effects. |
| Instruct the patient to monitor for and report itching, rash, and shortness of breath. | These indicators may signal an allergic reaction. |
| Caution the patient to be alert for and report excessive and explosive diarrhea. | See discussion of *C. difficile*, earlier. |
| ⚠ **Aminoglycosides** | |
| Gentamicin (Garamycin) | *Administration:* IM/IV. *Breastfeeding:* May continue. |

| ASSESSMENT—RECOGNIZE CUES/ INTERVENTIONS—TAKE ACTION | RATIONALES |
|---|---|
| Instruct the patient to be alert for and report lethargy, confusion, respiratory depression, visual disturbances, depression, weight loss, hypotension or hypertension, decreased appetite, rash, itching, headache, nausea, vomiting, and hearing loss. | These are potential adverse and allergic reactions. |
| Caution the patient to be alert for and report excessive and explosive diarrhea. | See discussion of *C. difficile*, earlier. |
| Caution use in patients with neuromuscular disorders and in patients with impaired renal function. | This medication may lead to neurotoxicity and nephrotoxicity. |

### Other Antibiotics

### Clindamycin (Cleocin)

| | |
|---|---|
| | *Administration:* IV/IM/PO. |
| | *Breastfeeding:* May continue. |
| Instruct the patient to monitor for and report itching and rash. | These signs can occur with allergic reactions. |
| Instruct the patient to be alert for and report diarrhea, nausea, vomiting, stomach cramps, and anorexia. | These are possible adverse reactions. |
| Advise the patient to follow the complete course for all prescribed medications and take them on time. | These measures reduce the risk for reinfection, prevent the development of antibiotic resistance, and maintain a constant level of medication in the bloodstream. |
| Caution the patient to be alert for and report excessive and explosive diarrhea. | See discussion of *C. difficile*, earlier. |
| Caution use in patients with a history of colitis. | This drug may exacerbate the colitis. |
| Instruct the patient to be alert for and report redness, swelling, and pain at IV insertion site. | Thrombophlebitis can occur after IV infusion of clindamycin. |
| Caution use in patients with renal disease. | The injectable drug is potentially nephrotoxic. |

### Linezolid (Zyvox)

| | |
|---|---|
| | This antibiotic is used to treat complicated skin and skin structure infections caused by MRSA. |
| | *Administration:* IV/PO. |
| Caution use in patients with hypertension. | This drug may increase preexisting hypertension. |
| Instruct the patient to ensure that the provider is aware of breastfeeding status and discuss the risks and benefits of breastfeeding | There is very little information that exists regarding the use of linezolid in breastfeeding mothers. Research has shown that linezolid is excreted into breast milk (Rowe et al., 2014). Therefore infants exposed to linezolid should be monitored for signs of diarrhea. |
| Instruct the patient to be alert for and report diarrhea, headache, nausea, vomiting, insomnia, constipation, rash, dizziness, and fever. | These are possible side effects. |
| Caution patients taking selective serotonin reuptake inhibitors (SSRIs) to be alert for and report cognitive dysfunction, hyperpyrexia, hyperreflexia, and incoordination. | Serotonin syndrome can be associated with the coadministration of Zyvox and SSRIs. |
| Instruct the patient to be alert for and immediately report visual blurring, changes in color vision, or loss of vision. | Peripheral and optic neuropathy may be associated with the drug when it is used beyond the recommended treatment (more than 28 days). |
| Instruct the patient to be alert for and immediately report repeated episodes of nausea and vomiting. | Lactic acidosis is a possible side effect. |

Continued

| ASSESSMENT—RECOGNIZE CUES/ INTERVENTIONS—TAKE ACTION | RATIONALES |
|---|---|
| Instruct the patient to be alert for and report excessive and explosive diarrhea. | See discussion of *C. difficile*, earlier. |
| Instruct the patient to avoid ingesting excessive amounts of foods or beverages with high tyramine content while taking this drug. | Foods with greater than 100 mg of tyramine (e.g., red wine, aged cheese) may enhance the pressor response of this drug and increase blood pressure (BP). |
| Instruct the patient to avoid medications containing pseudoephedrine HCl or phenylpropanolamine HCl. | Zyvox enhances the increases in systolic BP caused by pseudoephedrine HCl or phenylpropanolamine HCl. |

**Analgesics**

**Morphine Sulfate**

| | This opiate analgesic (opioid) is used in the treatment of moderate-to-severe pain.<br>*Administration:* IV/IM/PO. |
|---|---|
| Encourage breastfeeding before taking the analgesic. | Breastfeeding generally is accepted as safe. Taking the medication after breastfeeding reduces the possibility of medication influence on the infant. |
| Instruct the patient to be alert for and report itching and rash. | Itching is a potential side effect, but itching and rash are possible allergic reactions. |
| Instruct the patient to be alert for and report weakness, headache, restlessness, agitation, hallucinations, and disorientation. | These are possible adverse reactions. |
| Caution the patient to arise slowly from a supine position or have assistance with ambulating after receiving this medication. | Morphine is a central nervous system (CNS) depressant. It may impair mental and/or physical abilities and cause hypotension. |
| Caution the patient to avoid activities that require alertness until the drug's effect on the CNS is known. | Drowsiness is a common side effect. |
| Caution use with other CNS depressants. | Morphine can potentiate CNS effects of these drugs. |
| Caution use in patients with seizure disorder. | Seizures may result from high doses. |
| Caution use in patients with renal/hepatic insufficiency. | Morphine's active metabolite may accumulate and potentiate the sedative effects. |

**Oxycodone With Acetaminophen (Percocet) and Hydrocodone With Acetaminophen (Vicodin)**

| | These are opioid analgesics used to treat moderate to moderately severe pain.<br>*Administration:* PO. |
|---|---|
| Encourage the patient to breastfeed before taking the medication and to follow carefully the prescribed dose regimen. | Both analgesics are commonly used in postpartum women. Breastfeeding just before taking the medication and adhering to the prescribed therapy reduce any threat to the newborn. |
| Instruct the patient to be alert for and report nausea, vomiting, itching, dizziness, and headache. | These are common adverse reactions. |
| Instruct the patient to be alert for and report itching with a rash. | These are signs of a possible allergic reaction. |
| Instruct the patient to be alert for and report shortness of breath. | This adverse reaction may indicate an overdose. |
| Caution the patient to arise slowly from a supine position or have assistance with ambulating after taking this medication. | These drugs are CNS depressants. They may impair mental and/or physical abilities and cause hypotension. |
| Caution the patient to avoid activities that require alertness until the drug's effect on the CNS is known. | Drowsiness is a common side effect. |

## Patient, Partner, and Family Problem/Analyze Cues/Prioritize Hypotheses
# Deficient Knowledge

*due to* unfamiliarity with the effects of postpartum wound infection on the self and neonate and the importance of following the treatment course

***Desired Outcome/Generate Solutions:*** Immediately after instruction, the patient, her partner, and family (as indicated) verbalize accurate knowledge about the effects of postpartum wound infections and the associated treatment on the patient and neonate.

| ASSESSMENT—RECOGNIZE CUES/ INTERVENTIONS—TAKE ACTION | RATIONALES |
|---|---|
| Instruct the patient, her partner, and family about the effects postpartum wound infection may have on the mother and newborn and the likely treatments for the infection. | Information helps patients adhere to treatments, report symptoms in a timely manner, and understand the consequences of nonadherence. Effects an infection may have on the mother include pain, fever, chills, wound dehiscence, sepsis, and increased morbidity/mortality. For the neonate, effects include fever, possible rapid deterioration, and increased morbidity/mortality. Rehospitalization or illness may interrupt breastfeeding and infant bonding. Likely treatments include IV antibiotics and fluids, wound packing, secondary wound closure, and possible lengthy hospitalization or home treatments. |
| Instruct the patient about signs and symptoms of worsening wound infection and its complications that need to be reported after hospital discharge. | This teaching intervention enables the patient, her partner, and family to recognize and report such signs as increasing fever; foul-smelling vaginal discharge; failure of lochia to progress from rubra to serosa to alba and its timely completion; spreading abdominal cellulites; severe pain; vaginal bleeding; wound drainage; seroma; hematoma; dehiscence; necrotizing fasciitis; and signs of disseminated intravascular coagulation (see "Disseminated Intravascular Coagulation," Chapter 65). Early evaluation and treatment result in decreased maternal morbidity. |
| Explain treatment options such as daily wound packing or secondary wound closure and IV or PO antibiotics used to treat the infection and decrease the risk for further infection. | After hospital treatment of acute infection with IV antibiotics, treating the patient at home is preferred. If a secondary wound closure is done, it requires readmittance to the hospital (or an extended stay if the infection occurs before hospital discharge). Daily wound care consists of inspection, irrigation, débridement, packing, and dressing applications. (See "Managing Wound Care," Chapter 75, for more information.) |
| Explain to the patient and her partner that intercourse is not recommended during the process of wound healing, especially in the presence of wound dehiscence. | Usually, intercourse is not recommended until 6 weeks postpartum. This time frame allows the placental attachment site to heal, cervical closure, lochia (vaginal discharge) to stop, and incisions to heal without the risk for introducing bacteria. |

## Patient, Partner, and Family Problem/Analyze Cues/Prioritize Hypotheses
# Difficulty Coping

*due to* a shift in health status of the family member, the need to provide an optimal environment for wound healing while providing for newborn care and feeding, or family roles shift

***Desired Outcome/Generate Solutions:*** Within 2–4 hours after interventions, the patient, her partner, and family (as indicated) begin to express their feelings and identify ways to modify their daily living patterns to meet physical, psychosocial, and spiritual needs of the patient and newborn.

| ASSESSMENT—RECOGNIZE CUES/ INTERVENTIONS—TAKE ACTION | RATIONALES |
|---|---|
| Assess the patient's, her partner's, and family's acceptance and confidence in caring for the wound on an outpatient basis, clarifying their perceptions about the patient's current health status and daily needs. | This assessment evaluates their comfort level with providing home wound care and enables the mutual development of an individualized plan for the patient to take control of her own care. |
| Review attachment documentation immediately after birth and observe variations in the patient's/family's attitudes and behaviors with their newborn over the course of the hospital stay. Provide family-centered care (FCC) in the hospital. | Appropriate support and interventions depend on an accurate assessment of attitudes and behaviors to distinguish what is related to the complication versus psychologic causes, cultural practices, or interrupted attachment. FCC prevents needless separation of the mother and newborn. |
| Assess for signs of complications with parenting (e.g., being unable to take on the role of daily infant care and feeding; lack of interest in caring for and feeding the newborn; lack of consistent and ongoing support from family members, friends, church group support, and neighbors; reference to self or newborn as ugly or problematic; difficulty with sleep; and loss of appetite). | Parents usually attach without ambivalence to their newborn, want to parent their newborn, and have the energy and motivation to do so, but they also may need to develop infant care and decision-making skills as new parents and learn to balance individual needs with infant needs on a daily basis. A maternal infection complicates this process. |
| Establish empathetic communication and encourage open expression of feelings and thoughts by the patient, her partner, family, and others involved with the patient, newborn, and family after hospital discharge. | Honesty and empathy promote effective therapeutic communication and support. For example, "I know this is difficult to deal with while also caring for a newborn. Let's talk about it. I want to be of support to you in this unexpected transition." |
| Help the patient, her partner, and family identify and develop a daily pattern to meet individual needs, incorporate the newborn into the family, continue with lactation preferences (pumping, breastfeeding, or bottle feeding), promote wound healing, support maternal rest, and have an effective support system. | The healthy family pulls together in a crisis. Adaptation is most effective when the support system is consistent, flexible, and related to individual needs. The patient may need assistance with personal care, newborn care/feeding, parenting her other children, and homemaking tasks to modify her daily living so that wound healing can occur. |
| Arrange community referrals (e.g., visiting nurse service, lactation consultant, or postpartum doula support as appropriate). | Support in the home environment is likely to promote healthier adaptation and strengthen the family system. |
| Affirm that lifestyle adjustments are for a limited time (e.g., increased rest, dressing changes, frequent clinic visits, taking medications, and interrupted maternal role fulfillment). | This information may promote family decision-making, facilitate acceptance of outside support and assistance, and reinforce patience with the healing process of an infected wound. |
| Explain diagnostic tests and medical interventions (e.g., blood work to monitor for further infection, ultrasound to check for abscess) and procedures (e.g., wound packing, secondary wound closure). | Anticipating the needs of the patient, her partner, and family and explaining what to expect will strengthen their coping mechanisms. |

## ADDITIONAL PROBLEMS:

| | |
|---|---|
| "Immobility" for relevant patient problems such as *Risk for Deep Vein Thrombosis* and *Activity Intolerance*. | Chapter 1 |
| "Psychosocial Support for the Patient" for problems such as *Anxiety* | Chapter 8 |
| "Psychosocial Support for the Patient's Family and Significant Others" for such problems as *Difficulty Coping* | Chapter 9 |
| "Managing Wound Care" | Chapter 75 |
| "Preeclampsia" for *Risk for Caregiver Role Strain* | Chapter 94 |
| "Preterm Labor" for *Risk for Difficulty Performing Breastfeeding* | Chapter 95 |

 **PATIENT–FAMILY TEACHING AND DISCHARGE PLANNING**

Wound infections place a great deal of strain on the patient and family dynamics. A proactive approach to anticipating patient and family needs for education and support will decrease their level of anxiety and optimize outcomes. Referral to a wound care specialist may be necessary at any time during the assessment/healing process. Include verbal and written information about the following:

✓ Signs and symptoms of wound infection.

✓ Wound care (cleansing, packing, and dressing); instructions will vary depending on the facility and provider preference. Check with the health care provider for specific instructions. Also see care plans in "Managing Wound Care," Chapter 75.

✓ Importance and timing of good hand hygiene.

✓ Where to obtain dressing materials for home care (prescriptions for supplies that may be acquired through a pharmacy or medical supply store).

✓ Importance of adequate rest, nutrition, and oral hydration for effective wound healing.

✓ Importance of compliance with the prescribed health care regimen and ready access to hospital and family/social support.

✓ Medications, including drug name, purpose, dosage, frequency, precautions, potential drug reactions, and side effects. Also discuss potential drug–drug, food–drug, and herb–drug interactions.

✓ Referral to local and national support organizations, including lactation consultants and Sidelines, a national support organization for women and their families experiencing complicated pregnancies, at http://www.sidelines.org.

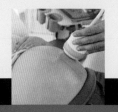

# Preeclampsia 94

## OVERVIEW/PATHOPHYSIOLOGY

Hypertensive disorders of pregnancy are among the most frequently reported medical complications of pregnancy and are steadily increasing in incidence. The American College of Obstetrics and Gynecology (ACOG) categorizes hypertensive disorders of pregnancy as follows: gestational hypertension, preeclampsia, preeclampsia with severe features, eclampsia, HELLP ("H" stands for hemolysis of red blood cells [RBCs]; "EL" stands for elevated liver enzymes; and "LP" stands for low platelets) syndrome, chronic (preexisting) hypertension, chronic hypertension with superimposed preeclampsia, and chronic hypertension with superimposed preeclampsia with severe features (ACOG, 2020a).

**Preeclampsia/eclampsia:** Preeclampsia is a pregnancy-specific syndrome affecting approximately 3%–5% of pregnant women. Diagnosis is based on new-onset hypertension occurring after 20-week gestation in a previously normotensive patient. Blood pressure (BP) is elevated (more than 140 mm Hg systolic, more than 90 mm Hg diastolic) on two separate readings, taken at least 4 hours apart and accompanied by significant proteinuria (greater than 300 mg in 24 hours or protein/creatinine ratio more than 0.3 mg/dL). Preeclampsia is no longer classified as mild or moderate but may present with severe features (see Preeclampsia Assessments, later in this section) and can progress to eclampsia or HELLP syndrome.

- *HELLP syndrome* is a laboratory diagnosis for a severe variant of preeclampsia associated with high maternal and fetal morbidity.
- *Eclampsia:* When severe preeclampsia has progressed to generalized seizures, it is called eclampsia. Seizures may occur during the antepartum, intrapartum, or postpartum period. Coma often follows a seizure.

**Gestational hypertension:** BP elevation after 20-week gestation occurs without proteinuria. It may be transient or chronic and often resolves before 12-week postpartum. Despite hypertension, good pregnancy outcomes are expected.

**Chronic hypertension:** BP elevation occurring before pregnancy or before 20-week gestation. Chronic hypertension is defined by ACOG as systolic BP of 140 mm Hg or greater, diastolic BP of 90 mm Hg or greater, or both, documented on two occasions more than 4–6 hours apart. Chronic hypertension is more prevalent with increasing late childbearing and rising rates of obesity.

**Chronic hypertension with superimposed preeclampsia:** A common complication for a chronic hypertensive woman, superimposed preeclampsia occurs in 25% of these pregnancies. Preconception screening and lifestyle changes are encouraged to attain a prepregnancy normotensive state.

Although the cause of preeclampsia remains unknown, the pathology is believed to begin shortly after conception with placental abnormalities and eventually presents with the resulting generalized vasoconstriction, vasospasms, and endothelial cell damage causing decreased circulation and oxygenation for all organ systems, including the gravid uterus and fetus, and redistribution of intravascular fluid (edema). Serious and lifelong complications can develop in any affected organ system, including the brain, kidney, liver, and uteroplacental unit. Often the presenting signs are the classic signs of hypertension accompanied by proteinuria. As this multisystem disorder progresses, varied clinical manifestations may demonstrate the more severe effects on each organ system. The only known cure is the delivery of the newborn and removal of the placenta.

## HEALTH CARE SETTING

Primary care and acute care antepartum and intrapartum hospital units. Outpatient and home care are possible for preeclampsia without severe features.

## ASSESSMENT

**Preeclampsia Assessments: Signs and Symptoms**

| Preeclampsia | Preeclampsia With Severe Features |
|---|---|
| • BP elevated × 2, 4–6 hours apart on bedrest: systolic BP (SBP) 140–160 mm Hg or 30 mm Hg over baseline; diastolic BP (DBP) 90–110 mm Hg or 15 mm Hg over baseline (DBP 90 mm Hg or higher in the second trimester). | • BP elevated × 2, 4–6 hours apart on bedrest: SBP greater than 160 mm Hg; DBP greater than 110 mm Hg |

Continued

## Preeclampsia Assessments: Signs and Symptoms

| Preeclampsia | Preeclampsia With Severe Features |
|---|---|
| • Mean arterial pressure (MAP) 105 mm Hg or higher or increased by 20 mm Hg from baseline. | • MAP higher than 105 mm Hg |
| • Proteinuria: Greater than 0.3 g in 24-hour collection; 2+ or 3+ on random dipstick (without urinary tract infection), or protein/creatinine ratio greater than or equal to 0.3 mg/dL. | • Proteinuria: Greater than 3 g/L in a 24-hour collection; protein/creatinine ratio greater than or equal to 0.3 mg/dL, or 2+, 3+, or more on dipstick |
| | • Increased sodium retention |
| • Reflexia: 2+ or less (normal response). | • Hyperreflexia: 3+ or more; clonus |
| • Headache: Absent or transient. | • Headache: Continuous or severe, affective changes, and nausea/vomiting |
| • No vision changes. | • Vision: Blurred, scotoma, diplopia, photophobia, and retinal detachment (spontaneously reattaches later) |
| • No epigastric pain. | • Epigastric pain: Present (impending convulsion) |
| • Normal urine output. | • Oliguria: Urine output less than 30 mL/hour. |
| • Laboratory studies: Platelets normal, hematocrit (Hct) normal or decreased, liver enzymes begin to rise, serum creatinine greater than 1.1 mg/dL or doubling (in the absence of renal disease). | • Laboratory studies: Liver enzymes (alanine aminotransferase [ALT], aspartate aminotransferase [AST], and lactate dehydrogenase [LDH]) will be elevated. |
| | • Increased Hct indicates hemoconcentration. |
| | • Elevated serum creatinine signals renal compromise. When these values are accompanied by thrombocytopenia, it is crucial to monitor for HELLP syndrome. |
| | • Thrombocytopenia: Less than 100,000/μL. |
| • Weight gain: More than 1.5 kg (3.3 lb)/month or more than 0.5 kg (1.1 lb/week) in the third trimester. Edema is not considered diagnostic but should not remain after 8–12 hours bedrest. | • Edema: Generalized, dyspnea, rales/crackles (pulmonary edema) |
| • Placenta: Decreased placental perfusion. | • Placenta: Markedly reduced perfusion results in intrauterine growth restriction (IUGR). |
| • Risk for oligohydramnios. | • Risk for abruptio placenta. |
| | • Labor: Late decelerations. |
| • Early placental aging not apparent yet. | • Placental evaluation after birth: Intervillous thrombosis, ischemic necrosis (white spots), infant smaller than expected for gestational age. |

Additional reportable signs include decreased fetal movement (fetal compromise), spontaneous bruising, prolonged bleeding, and epistaxis (thrombocytopenia).

**Risk factors:** A thorough medical history is important in the early identification of risk factors. This needs to include nulliparity (status of a woman who has not carried the pregnancy and given birth after 20-week gestation), African American race, history of preeclampsia, renal disease, diabetes mellitus, hypothyroidism, age younger than 20 years or older than 40 years, family history of preeclampsia (mother/sister), chronic hypertension, thrombophilias (antiphospholipid syndrome, proteins C and S, antithrombin deficiency, and factor V Leiden), multifetal pregnancy, oocyte donation or donor insemination, autoimmune disorders including systemic lupus erythematosus or antiphospholipid syndrome, urinary tract infections, obesity, and gestational trophoblastic disease (molar pregnancy).

## DIAGNOSTIC TESTS

**Complete blood count:** May be within accepted ranges. Changes reflect hemodynamic changes. Hct rises with hemoconcentration. Platelets drop (thrombocytopenia) with hemoconcentration and with HELLP syndrome. Hemoglobin (Hgb) falls with hemolysis.

**Renal function studies:** Proteinuria 0.3 g or more in a 24-hour urine specimen is diagnostic of preeclampsia. With kidney involvement, blood tests may show rising serum creatinine, uric acid, and blood urea nitrogen. Elevated creatinine clearance in a 24-hour urine collection indicates reduced renal function.

**Liver function tests:** ALT, AST, and LDH rise with severe preeclampsia and rise even further with HELLP syndrome.

**Coagulation studies:** Platelet count decreases in severe preeclampsia and HELLP syndrome. Intrinsic or extrinsic factors may induce clot formation and deplete clotting factors, leading to hemorrhage.

**Obstetric ultrasound:** Serial ultrasound examinations are commonly used to estimate fetal growth and amniotic fluid index (AFI).

**Daily fetal activity monitoring, nonstress testing, and biophysical profile:** These tests assess uteroplacental perfusion.

## Patient Problem/Analyze Cues/Prioritize Hypotheses

# Altered Blood Pressure

*due to* biochemical changes that cause vasoconstriction and vasospasm

***Desired Outcome/Generate Solutions:*** Within 24 hours after interventions, the patient begins to return to normotensive BP and pulse for the pregnancy and participates in her health care regimen.

| ASSESSMENT—RECOGNIZE CUES/ INTERVENTIONS—TAKE ACTION | RATIONALES |
|---|---|
| Assess and document the BP and pulse every 1–4 hours as indicated. | Hypertension results from biochemical changes that cause vasoconstriction and vasospasm. Rising BP values indicate the progression of preeclampsia. |
| Measure urine volume and proteinuria hourly or per protocol. Maintain a strict intake and output (I&O). | As preeclampsia becomes severe, glomerular endothelial damage allows protein molecules to pass into the urine. Hypovolemia and damage to blood vessel walls decrease circulation to the kidneys. |
| For patients with worsening preeclampsia, explain the importance of bedrest with bathroom privileges and frequent use of lateral position. | Bedrest and lateral positioning facilitate venous return to the heart, which lowers BP and increases perfusion of the kidneys and uteroplacental unit. |
| Administer the prescribed antihypertensive medication (i.e., hydralazine [Apresoline], labetalol HCl [Normodyne], or Nifedipine [Procardia]) | Antihypertensives lower BP by vasodilation and decreasing systemic vascular resistance. |
| Prepare for cesarean delivery if indicated by the severity of preeclampsia and as determined by the health care provider. | Delivery (of placenta) is the definitive way to halt the progression of preeclampsia. Cesarean delivery is selected when induction and vaginal delivery are ruled out. |

## Patient Problem/Analyze Cues/Prioritize Hypotheses

# Fluid Imbalance (Fluid Overload)

*due to* vasoconstriction, vasospasms, and endothelial cell damage resulting in the redistribution of intravascular fluid (edema)

***Desired Outcome/Generate Solutions:*** Fluid volume normalizes within 8–12 hours, as evidenced by decreased BP, normal rate and quality of pulse, unlabored respirations, urine output greater than 30 mL/hour without proteinuria, usual pregnancy weight gain, absence of pitting edema, and Hct within normal limits (WNL).

| ASSESSMENT—RECOGNIZE CUES/ INTERVENTIONS—TAKE ACTION | RATIONALES |
|---|---|
| [!] Assess the BP; heart rate, rhythm, and quality; respiratory rate (RR); and lung sounds every 1–4 hours. | Increasing hypertension occurs with worsening vasoconstriction and increasing peripheral vascular resistance. Pulse increases and quality changes occur to compensate for hypovolemia. Pulmonary edema causes dyspnea. |
| Assess the presence, degree, and location of edema every 1–8 hours. Weigh the patient daily. Report significant findings. | Edema develops as fluid shifts from the vascular to the extravascular spaces. Weight gain can be an indicator of fluid retention. |
| [!] Assess deep tendon reflexes (DTRs) and for the presence of clonus every 1–4 hours. | Increasing hyperreflexia signals a worsening condition. DTRs correspond to the peripheral neurologic condition. Clonus relates to central neurologic irritability. For more details about DTRs and clonus, see *Risk for Disease*, later. |
| [!] Assess for headaches: presence, location, and severity every 1–4 hours. | Headaches increase in intensity and frequency with advancing brain edema. |

| ASSESSMENT—RECOGNIZE CUES/ INTERVENTIONS—TAKE ACTION | RATIONALES |
|---|---|
| ⚠ Assess for mental changes, irritability, and level of consciousness every 1–4 hours. | Changes in mentation indicate a worsening condition with increased central nervous system (CNS) edema. |
| ⚠ Monitor the fluid intake and urine output every 1–4 hours. If indicated, limit fluid intake to 2000–3000 mL/day (PO and intravenous [IV]). | Fluid retention could lead to pulmonary edema when severe. Oliguria (urine output less than 30 mL/hour) signals renal system compromise. |
| ⚠ Collect a 24-hour urine specimen to measure proteinuria and creatinine if prescribed by the health care provider. Measure proteinuria with a dipstick every void. | As preeclampsia becomes severe, glomerular endothelial damage allows protein molecules and creatinine to pass into the urine. |
| ⚠ Monitor for hemodynamic changes by the following laboratory values: | Hemodynamic changes result from increasingly severe preeclampsia. |
| • Hct | Hct rises with hemoconcentration. |
| • Hgb | Hgb falls as RBCs are damaged in turbulent blood flow (vasospasms). |
| • Platelets | Platelet decrease indicates HELLP syndrome. |
| • Liver enzymes | Liver function enzymes rise with increased liver compromise. |
| • Serum creatinine and uric acid | Serum creatinine and uric acid increase with reduced glomerular filtration and indicate nephron function. |

## Fetus Problem/Analyze Cues/Prioritize Hypotheses

# Impaired Gas Exchange (Fetal Hypoxia)

*due to* progressive vasospasms of the uterine spiral arteries and reduced blood flow to the placenta

***Desired Outcome/Generate Solutions:*** Within 8–12 hours of interventions, fetal status stabilizes and improves as evidenced by improved fetal activity, reassuring nonstress testing (NST), and fetus tolerating labor and vaginal delivery.

| ASSESSMENT—RECOGNIZE CUES/ INTERVENTIONS—TAKE ACTION | RATIONALES |
|---|---|
| Measure the fundal height. | Monitoring progressive fetal growth identifies the potential development of IUGR, which results from maternal vasospasm, vasoconstriction, and hypovolemia and will affect uteroplacental blood flow and oxygenation. |
| Monitor the ultrasound and AFI results after 28-week gestation. | Serial ultrasound examinations monitor for the potential development of IUGR. AFI measurement identifies oligohydramnios. Maternal vasospasms and vasoconstriction decrease uteroplacental perfusion, causing fetal hypoxia, and can result in IUGR and oligohydramnios. |
| Instruct the mother on how to assess the fetal activity by performing and recording daily fetal movement counts per agency/hospital protocol. | Decreased fetal movements may indicate fetal hypoxia. |
| Assess the fetal heart rate (FHR) patterns by continuous FHR monitoring or NST per agency protocol. | These procedures monitor for uteroplacental insufficiency and fetal hypoxia. Reactive NST: two FHR accelerations in a 20-minute period are indicative of adequate oxygenation and an intact fetal CNS. |
| ⚠ Assess for signs of abruptio placenta: uterine hypertonus; dark, nonclotting vaginal bleeding; abdominal pain; uterine tenderness; and fetal distress signs. | Abruptio placenta may occur spontaneously with hypertension. |
| ⚠ Assess the fetal response to medication: misoprostol (Cytotec), dinoprostone (Cervidil insert or Prepidil Gel), oxytocin induction, and magnesium sulfate. | Some cervical ripening agents (misoprostol) or oxytocin may cause uterine hyperstimulation or tachysystole, resulting in fetal hypoxia with nonreassuring (categories 2 and 3) FHR pattern. Magnesium sulfate may cause hypermagnesemia in the newborn (depression of respiratory and neurologic systems). |

## Patient Problem/Analyze Cues/Prioritize Hypotheses

# Risk for Disease

*due to* abnormal blood profile; effects of vasoconstriction, vasospasm, endo-thelial cell damage, and tissue hypoxia in every organ system; and/or develop-ment of disseminated intravascular coagulation (DIC)

**Desired Outcomes/Generate Solutions:** The patient remains free of complications caused by preeclampsia on the maternal cardiovascular, hematologic, renal, neurologic, respiratory, and hepatic systems as evidenced by a return to normotensive BP, MAP below 105 mm Hg, nega-tive or trace proteinuria, normal urine output, reflexes of 2+, and clear vision. The patient has normal hematology values within 12–24 hours after expulsion of an intact placenta.

| ASSESSMENT—RECOGNIZE CUES/ INTERVENTIONS—TAKE ACTION | RATIONALES |
|---|---|
| Assess the symptoms along with maternal reports of worsening disease: changes in CNS signs, visual changes, pain (degree, type, and location), urinary output and proteinuria, and weight gain. In addition, assess the FHR pattern, maternal vital signs, and the effects of medications every 1–4 hours. Document and communicate the results as indicated. | Symptoms from organ system damage with progressive vasoconstriction, vasospasms, and endothelial cell damage reflect the severity of preeclampsia. Epigastric pain is considered a late sign and is associated with impending convulsion. Twitching of facial muscles often precedes a grand mal seizure. Confusion, combative behavior, or coma often follows a seizure. |
| Maintain a therapeutic environment: quiet, darkened room; limited visitors; and left lateral positioning. Initiate seizure precautions. | A therapeutic environment reduces stimuli that may heighten seizure activity. |
| Explain to the patient the importance of eating a balanced pregnancy diet at least three times/day with adequate protein, calcium, zinc, magnesium, sodium, folate, vitamins C and E, and roughage. Explain that her food should contain no added salt, and she needs to drink 8–10 (8-oz) glasses of water/day. | Diet influences disease progression. Protein replaces protein lost in the urine. Adequate dietary antioxidants may facilitate prostacyclin/ thromboxane balance, leading to vasodilation and lower BP. Roughage and fluids may prevent constipation. |
| Administer the IV magnesium sulfate as prescribed with before and after assessments of DTRs/clonus, BP, respirations, urine output, FHR, medication effects, and signs of magnesium toxicity. | Magnesium sulfate depresses the CNS (seizure prophylaxis) and relaxes smooth muscle, thereby decreasing BP and slowing respirations. If respirations fall to less than 12/minute, this is a sign of too much magnesium. In fact, the cascade into respiratory arrest followed by cardiac arrest can be quite rapid (1 hour to a few hours), whereas DTRs become hyperreactive along with signs of clonus (rapidly alternating contractions and relaxations of a skeletal muscle) before a seizure, and depressed DTRs can occur with too much medication (see the next rationale). Because magnesium sulfate is excreted through the kidneys, urinary output of at least 30 mL/hour is a sign that the kidneys are functioning adequately. A reactive (category 1) FHR is reassuring of fetal well-being. |
| As prescribed, administer the IV magnesium sulfate as an IV piggyback (IVPB) by infusion pump. | The IV route most accurately controls dosage and intervention responses if toxicity develops. |
| Follow agency protocols to ensure safe medication administration. | Overdose and overhydration are best prevented with an infusion pump. |
| Assess the therapeutic blood levels of magnesium periodically per the health care provider directive during pregnancy, labor, and postpartum. | A loading dose of 4–6 g over 20 minutes, followed by 2 g/hour as a maintenance dose provides a therapeutic plasma level of 4–8 mg/dL (4–7 mEq/L) without toxicity. At 8–12 mg/dL (8–10 mEq/L) DTRs become absent, at 14 mg/dL (13–15 mEq/L) respiratory arrest occurs, at 30 mg/dL (more than 20–25 mEq/L) cardiac arrest occurs. |
| Keep an ampule of calcium gluconate at the bedside. If symptoms indicate and as prescribed, administer 1 g (10 mL of a 10% solution) over a period of 3 minutes. | Calcium gluconate is the antidote administered to counteract adverse toxic effects from magnesium. |
| Assess the renal function every 2 hours or as often as prescribed by the health care provider: strict hourly I&O, proteinuria assessment, and periodic serum magnesium assessments. | Magnesium is excreted through the kidneys. Oliguria indicates renal compromise (if fluid intake is adequate). Serum toxic levels develop quickly with renal failure. |

Continued

| ASSESSMENT—RECOGNIZE CUES/ INTERVENTIONS—TAKE ACTION | RATIONALES |
|---|---|
| **!** Obtain baseline parameters (FHR pattern, maternal VS, uterine activity) before administration of oxytocin or cervical ripening agent. | Baseline findings WNL rule out maternal or fetal contraindications. Infusion pump and IVPB administration of oxytocin decrease the risk for fluid overload and allow rapid response to complications. Follow agency protocols for the safe administration of these medications. |
| **!** Administer the following cautiously and as prescribed: cervical ripening agents, for example, misoprostol (Cytotec) or dinoprostone (Cervidil insert or Prepidil Gel), and oxytocin for labor induction. | Hyperstimulation of the uterus from ripening agents or oxytocin can cause a rupture of the uterus. |
| **!** Perform invasive procedures as minimally as possible. | Invasive procedures (e.g., vaginal examination, internal maternal or fetal monitoring, IV therapy, catheterization, anesthesia [epidural or spinal], or cesarean delivery) may cause infection as external microscopic organisms are moved internally. |
| **!** Maintain a safe environment with padded bedside rails, oxygen by face mask, connected and working suctioning equipment, and maternal and fetal assessment equipment. | Preparation before a seizure occurs enables immediate response by the health care team. |
| **!** Assess for other complications: blood oozing at the IV site, epistaxis, and petechiae. | These are early signs of DIC. Vascular endothelial damage from preeclampsia can activate the intrinsic coagulation pathway and result in DIC. For more information, see "Disseminated Intravascular Coagulation," Chapter 65. |

## Fetus Problem/Analyze Cues/Prioritize Hypotheses

# Risk for Perinatal Problems (Intrauterine Growth Restriction)

*due to* the progressively severe effects of vasospasm and decreased circulation to the uteroplacental unit (may require preterm delivery of the newborn and the placenta)

***Desired Outcome/Generate Solutions:*** Daily and timely interventions limit the progression of preeclampsia (see previous patient problems for optimal signs) and promote the delivery of a healthy newborn as close as possible to term.

| ASSESSMENT—RECOGNIZE CUES/ INTERVENTIONS—TAKE ACTION | RATIONALES |
|---|---|
| Assess carefully for side effects when administering the following medications to prevent eclampsia in pregnancy and labor: magnesium sulfate, labetalol HCl (Normodyne), hydralazine (Apresoline), or nifedipine (Procardia) | Newborn hypermagnesemia (depression of the neurologic and respiratory systems) may follow maternal magnesium sulfate therapy (see discussion, earlier). Good maternal renal functioning is needed for the elimination of magnesium. Do not give nifedipine with magnesium sulfate because the combination may significantly drop the BP. Care must be taken not to decrease the BP too rapidly because this may affect uterine perfusion and oxygenation to the fetus. Hydralazine overdose can lead to abruptio placenta. |
| **!** Administer prescribed oxytocin carefully by IVPB with infusion pump and following the agency/health care provider protocol for increasing and decreasing the dosage. | Uterine hyperstimulation with oxytocin causes fetal hypoxia, rapid labor and delivery, and possible CNS injury in the preterm newborn. Higher oxytocin dosages are often needed for a woman on magnesium sulfate during labor. Follow agency protocols for the safe administration of this medication. |
| Confer with the health care provider regarding the results of the test for fetal lung maturity if a preterm birth is planned. | Respiratory distress syndrome (RDS) develops in the preterm infant born before lung surfactant is mature (evidenced by two parts lecithin per one part sphingomyelin [L/S ratio]). RDS is a leading cause of infant mortality. |
| Administer maternal corticosteroid therapy (betamethasone 12 mg intramuscular [IM]×2 doses 24 hours apart or dexamethasone 6 mg IM×4 doses 12 hours apart). | Corticosteroids stimulate fetal lung maturity by inducing the release of lung surfactants. |

| ASSESSMENT—RECOGNIZE CUES/ INTERVENTIONS—TAKE ACTION | RATIONALES |
|---|---|
| Administer NST every 4 hours or as prescribed in pregnancy and perform FHR and uterine monitoring in labor, with documentation every ½–1 hour or per agency protocol. | Adverse effects of severe preeclampsia, magnesium, cervical ripening agents, and oxytocin may cause fetal distress as reflected by nonreassuring (category 2 or 3) FHR patterns. |
| Arrange for neonatologist and resuscitation team to be present at the delivery for newborn care with delivery of an infant of a preeclamptic mother, whether preterm or term delivery. | Their presence is vital during preeclampsia and after an eclamptic seizure. Disease progression, gestational age limitations, and medications may lead to asphyxia and other severe complications in the newborn. |

## Patient, Partner, and Family Problem/Analyze Cues/Prioritize Hypotheses

# Deficient Knowledge

*due to* unfamiliarity with the effects of preeclampsia on the mother, fetus, and delivery; effects of treatments and medications; and the potential impact of medications and treatment regimen on daily family life

***Desired Outcome/Generate Solutions:*** Immediately after instruction, the patient, her partner, family, and others (as indicated) begin to participate in her therapeutic regimen by accurately monitoring and reporting weight, BP, urine protein, edema, fetal activity, signs of improving or worsening preeclampsia, and side effects or effectiveness of medications.

| ASSESSMENT—RECOGNIZE CUES/ INTERVENTIONS—TAKE ACTION | RATIONALES |
|---|---|
| Assess the woman's ability to assume self-care responsibilities, report symptoms, the impact of language on communication, her support systems, her culture and beliefs about illness, and the home environment. | Physical, psychosocial, and environmental factors determine whether home care is a viable option in mild preeclampsia. Some individuals need more educational and medical intervention than others. |
| Develop an educational plan that uses several modes of instruction tailored to the patient's and family's information needs and cognitive ability. | Comprehension improves when education is given at an individual's level of understanding. Using verbal, auditory, and kinesthetic modes enhances learning and retention. |
| Inform the patient and her family about the effects of preeclampsia on pregnancy, delivery, and maternal and fetal well-being. | An informed patient and family are more likely to adhere to the prescribed therapy and participate in the therapeutic regimen. |
| As indicated, instruct on self-assessment and reporting of clinical signs and symptoms: how to take and record her own BP, measure urine protein, maintain a daily weight record, assess edema, count and report fetal activity, and report signs of worsening preeclampsia. | Self-care instruction provides closer surveillance of changing preeclampsia, improves responses by health care providers, and may prevent the worsening of preeclampsia. |
| Explain self-care with a balanced pregnancy diet (adequate protein, calcium, zinc, magnesium, sodium, folate, vitamins C and E, and roughage); adequate fluids as prescribed; preference for left side-lying positions; sufficient rest and relaxation; understanding treatments and medications; and the impact of these on maternal and fetal well-being. | A nutritious diet and adequate fluids influence disease progression. Rest and relaxation promote diuresis. Antihypertensive medications (hydralazine [Apresoline] and labetalol HCl [Normodyne]) are preferred in a hypertensive crisis. Patients with chronic hypertension before preeclampsia may be on labetalol HCl (beta-blocker), or nifedipine (Procardia). |
| Instruct the patient to distinguish between magnesium sulfate side effects and toxicity. | The most common side effects of magnesium sulfate therapy include lethargy, weakness, sweating and flushing, nausea and vomiting, headaches, and slurred speech. Signs of developing toxicity include loss of DTRs, oliguria, respiratory depression (RR less than 12/minute), respiratory arrest, and cardiac arrest. |
| Support the family and other caregivers in assisting with the patient's responsibilities, helping manage the preeclampsia regimen, and providing emotional support. | Family involvement promotes the patient's self-efficacy with participation in the regimen and her sense of control, enhances her coping skills, and reduces anxiety and fears. |

## Caregiver Problem/Analyze Cues/Prioritize Hypotheses

# Risk for Caregiver Role Strain

*due to* the care that the partner, family member, or support person needs to provide not only to the patient but also possibly to other children to ensure the patient adheres to therapeutic rest and thereby prolongs the gestational period

***Desired Outcome/Generate Solutions:*** Within 24 hours of this diagnosis, the caregiver verbalizes concerns/frustrations about caregiving responsibilities, identifies at least one other support person, and recognizes at least one change that would make his or her job easier.

| ASSESSMENT—RECOGNIZE CUES/ INTERVENTIONS—TAKE ACTION | RATIONALES |
|---|---|
| Assess and encourage the caregiver to relate feelings and concerns regarding added responsibilities. Help the caregiver clarify responsibilities with the patient and other family members. | This validates the caregiver's concerns and helps him or her understand whether expectations are realistic. |
| Encourage the caregiver to identify activities that would benefit from outside assistance. | This confirms the caregiver's need to seek help and facilitates that help. |
| Involve social services in support of the caregiver establishing a plan for time-outs or for referrals to community support groups. | This also confirms the need to seek help and provides the caregiver with coping mechanisms. During times of stress, caregivers may know they need help but may not know where to find it. |

## Patient and Partner Problem/Analyze Cues/Prioritize Hypotheses

# Risk for Impaired Parent–Child Attachment (Interrupted Bonding)

*due to* separation from the preterm or compromised newborn

***Desired Outcome/Generate Solutions:*** Within 24 hours of receiving encouragement, information, and support from the health care team, the parents verbalize concerns and begin the parenting of their newborn.

| ASSESSMENT—RECOGNIZE CUES/ INTERVENTIONS—TAKE ACTION | RATIONALES |
|---|---|
| Assess the parental perception of their situation, individual concerns, and strengths. | Identifying perceptions, verbalizing concerns, and identifying strengths (sensitivity to newborn cues, understanding of preterm abilities, and provision of reciprocal relationship) enable effective and realistic planning. |
| Establish a trusting and nurturing nurse, patient, and family relationship. | The quality of the nurse–patient relationship is key to successful transitioning and parenting a preterm or compromised newborn. Nurturing the parents promotes the development of the parent–infant relationships. |
| Encourage the parents and family to verbalize fears and concerns. | Parents and family are already grieving real and potential losses (e.g., possible newborn death, inability to deliver at term or deliver a healthy newborn, idealized dreams of parenting the newborn, and seeing the newborn attached to tubes and ventilators). Verbalizing fears and concerns provide validation of their concerns and enables reassessment. |
| Before labor, provide anticipatory guidance for the realities of a possible preterm birth, a preterm infant, and separation from the newborn in the newborn intensive care unit (NICU). | Time to process, rehearse, and develop understanding empowers parents and fosters self-efficacy. |

| ASSESSMENT—RECOGNIZE CUES/ INTERVENTIONS—TAKE ACTION | RATIONALES |
|---|---|
| Encourage and assist the parents to attach and interact with their newborn in the NICU. | Parents may have to resolve the realities of the NICU, along with the newborn's preterm appearance and capacity, and learn new ways to interact in the NICU setting. The newborn could have tubes inserted, be attached to a heart rate monitor and pulse oximeter, and be in an Isolette. Over time parents can learn to do some daily care (e.g., take axillary temperatures, change diapers, bathe very delicate skin, and learn preterm cues that signal fatigue and other issues). |
| Encourage the mother to breastfeed or provide breast milk for her baby. | Breastfeeding enhances maternal sensitivity to her newborn. Support and assistance by the hospital staff significantly influence success with breastfeeding and the development of maternal role attainment. Establishing an early pumping regimen can be beneficial in creating an adequate milk supply for the baby in NICU or who is premature and unable to latch. |
| Support and praise the parents' behaviors that foster secure rather than avoidant or ambivalent attachment. | The parents' support, consistency, warmth, and sensitivity in responding to their baby facilitate secure attachment. |
| If the mother is too ill to be with her newborn, arrange for the father, family, and others to visit, keep her informed of the baby's condition, and bring her photos or other mementos. | These actions encourage the development of mother–infant attachment. They may decrease her fears as well. |
| Refer the parents to a perinatal social worker and offer referrals to ongoing support groups as appropriate. | Professional support may facilitate parental adaptation and foster self-efficacy. |

## ADDITIONAL PROBLEMS:

## ✓ PATIENT–FAMILY TEACHING AND DISCHARGE PLANNING

Preeclampsia is a progressive disease in which monitoring for maternal and fetal changes is of critical importance. Include verbal and written information about the following:

✓ Signs and symptoms of worsening preeclampsia (headache, increased edema, oliguria, right upper quadrant pain, decreased fetal movement, nausea, and vomiting) and importance of contacting the health care provider promptly if they occur.

✓ Seizure precautions.

✓ Medications, including drug name, purpose, dosage, frequency, precautions, potential drug reactions, and side effects. Also discuss potential drug–drug, food–drug, and herb–drug interactions.

✓ Importance of adherence to the prescribed health care regimen and ready access to hospital and family/social support.

✓ Parameters and guidelines for home bedrest.

✓ Measures that help with side effects of prolonged bedrest such as constipation, muscle pain, back pain, and muscle weakness.

✓ Fetal movement counts.

✓ The American Congress of Obstetricians and Gynecologists has an extensive collection of patient education materials available at https://www.acog.org/womens-health/pregnancy.

✓ Referrals to national and local support agencies, including:

• Sidelines, a national support organization for women and their families experiencing complicated pregnancies: http://www.sidelines.org

• March of Dimes: http://www.marchofdimes.com

# Preterm Labor 95

## OVERVIEW/PATHOPHYSIOLOGY

Preterm labor (PTL) is the onset of contractions that affect cervical change, either dilation or effacement, after 20 weeks' gestation and before the 37th week of gestation. Birth before completion of the 37th week is considered preterm. Most preterm births (PTBs) occur between 34 and 36 weeks. *Late-preterm infant birth* is the term given to infants born between 34 weeks and 0 days and 36 weeks and 6 days. All pregnant women are considered at risk for PTL, although approximately 12% of all pregnancies end in PTL (American College of Obstetrics and Gynecology [ACOG], 2016).

It is not known what causes PTL; however, it is associated with infections such as chorioamnionitis, periodontitis, and vaginal bacteriosis. Because the mechanisms that initiate term labor are multifactorial and not completely understood, exactly what causes PTL continues to be researched. Some risk factors for PTL have been identified. See the following table for details. The end results of PTL are increased uterine irritability, decreased placental functioning, increased prostaglandin synthesis, cervical changes, and the risk for PTB. Prematurity is a leading cause of infant mortality in the United States. The risk for serious health problems, including physical or neurologic impairment, is greatest in preterm infants born before 34 weeks, but PTL infants are at an increased risk compared with infants born at term.

## HEALTH CARE SETTING

Some patients may be managed by primary care on an outpatient basis with frequent clinic evaluation or in a high-risk perinatal clinic. Others may receive acute care in an inpatient antepartum setting.

## ASSESSMENT

Symptoms of PTL may range from subtle to obvious. Many symptoms do not cause pain. PTL does not present in the same way as labor at term. All pregnant women need to be taught the symptoms of PTL during early prenatal visits and then be reassessed at each prenatal visit. The mother may feel that the baby is "balling up" in her abdomen and describe a "heavy" feeling in the perineum or pelvic pressure, or she may note a change or increase in vaginal discharge.

***Contractions/uterine tightening:*** As the pregnancy progresses, so does the frequency of uterine activity. Uterine tightening/contractions begin in the second trimester as the uterus enlarges and continue throughout the pregnancy. These contractions are called *Braxton Hicks*. They occur at irregular intervals, usually are painless, and do not change the cervix. PTL may feel like light menstrual-like cramping or strong, palpable contractions. PTL is diagnosed when uterine contractions are persistent and accompanied by cervical change, either dilation or effacement.

***Backache:*** This is a very common complaint in pregnancy. Any woman with a history of PTL/preterm delivery who complains of new-onset backache needs to be evaluated for cervical changes, especially if she describes the backache as low and lumbar/sacral in location, deep tissue in nature, or a dull aching sensation that radiates around the hips to the lower abdomen/pelvic area and down the thighs.

***Pelvic pressure:*** The woman may state that she feels the "baby has dropped." Pelvic pressure may be described as a constant or intermittent "heaviness" or a sensation of "fullness in the pelvis."

***Abdominal cramping:*** Gastrointestinal symptoms such as increased flatus or diarrhea may be present. The abdomen may be tender to palpate, as is seen with chorioamnionitis (inflammatory reaction in the amniotic membranes caused by bacteria or virus).

***Vaginal discharge:*** An increase in vaginal discharge is expected during pregnancy because of hormonal changes. Discharge may be thick or thin in consistency, and clear, "milky white," or light yellow. It may become watery, as with preterm premature rupture of membranes (PPROMs), or bloody, as with placental abruption or when the cervix dilates and its surface vessels break. Vaginal itching or burning or a foul odor may indicate an infection. Vaginal bleeding may range from light-pink spotting to bright-red bleeding.

***Fever:*** The temperature may range from 98.6°F (37°C) to 101°F (38.3°C) or higher if an infection is present.

***General complaints:*** Other symptoms may include a feeling of unease and body aches. The woman may state, "I just feel different."

***Physical assessment:*** Even with vague symptoms, cervical changes may be taking place. Therefore it is important not to underestimate reported symptoms. Early evaluation and treatment are critical in attempting to stop PTL and preventing fetal morbidity and mortality.

### Risks for Preterm Labor

#### Medical Risks

The following three groups of women are at the greatest risk for preterm labor (PTL) and preterm birth (PTB):

- women who have had a previous PTB;
- women who are pregnant with twins, triplets, or more; and
- women with certain uterine or cervical abnormalities or who have had prior cervical or uterine surgeries.

If a woman has any of these three risk factors, it is especially important for her to know the signs and symptoms of PTL and what to do if they occur.

Certain medical conditions during pregnancy may increase the likelihood that a woman will have PTL. These conditions include

- urinary tract infections (UTIs), vaginal infections, sexually transmitted infections, and possibly other infections;
- diabetes;
- high blood pressure (BP);
- clotting disorders (thrombophilia);
- bleeding from the vagina;
- certain birth defects in the baby;
- being pregnant with a single fetus after in vitro fertilization;
- being underweight before pregnancy;
- obesity;
- one or more midtrimester pregnancy losses;
- polyhydramnios;
- placenta abruption; placenta previa; and
- having a short cervix.

#### Lifestyle and Environmental Risks

Some studies have found that certain lifestyle factors may put a woman at greater risk for PTL. These factors include

- late or no prenatal care;
- grand multiparity;
- smoking;
- drinking alcohol;
- using illegal drugs;
- exposure to the medication diethylstilbestrol;
- domestic violence, including physical, sexual, or emotional abuse;
- lack of social support;
- stress;
- working the night shift; and
- long working hours with long periods of standing.

- Short time period between pregnancies (less than 6–9 months between birth and the beginning of the next pregnancy) (see March of Dimes, http://www.marchofdimes.org).

#### Complications—fetal:

- Preterm delivery
- Respiratory distress syndrome (RDS)
- Patent ductus arteriosus (PDA—an abnormal opening between the pulmonary artery and aorta)
- Intraventricular hemorrhage (IVH)
- Sepsis
- Necrotizing enterocolitis (ischemic, inflammatory bowel disorder that can lead to perforation and peritonitis)
- Hyperbilirubinemia
- Hypoglycemia
- Impaired/immature immunologic system
- Neonatal death

## DIAGNOSTIC TESTS

There are several biochemical markers and assessments that assist in the diagnosis of PTL.

**Cervical evaluation:** Sterile speculum cervical examinations provide information about cervical effacement, cervical dilation, and whether amniotic fluid is leaking or abnormal secretions are present in the vagina. Cervical or vaginal secretions can be collected for a ferning test (rupture of membranes) or fetal fibronectin (fFN) test, or cultures may be obtained to diagnose an infection.

**Transvaginal ultrasonography:** May be used to measure cervical length when cervical effacement is less than 80% and to evaluate funneling of the internal cervical os as well as effacement and dilation of the cervix. The shorter the cervix, the greater the risk for PTL. The shortest acceptable length is 30 mm. Less than 25 mm is considered a shortened cervix and is associated with PTL (Son et al., 2016). Vaginal progesterone, 17-alpha-hydroxyprogesterone caproate (17P), may be used as a treatment for PTL in women with an asymptomatic shortened cervix or previous spontaneous PTB (Shapiro-Mendoza et al., 2016).

**Fetal fibronectin:** fFNs are glycoproteins present in the cervical and vaginal secretions early in pregnancy. After 22 weeks' gestation, they are not detectable in vaginal secretions. Their presence returns within 2 weeks of delivery, whether it is preterm or term. Therefore negative fFN results between 24 and 35 weeks' gestation are strongly associated with not going into labor for the next 1–2 weeks. The negative predictive power of fFN is used to avoid further and unnecessary interventions for the woman at risk for PTL. A positive fFN finding is less predictive of labor because false-positive results occur with recent sexual intercourse, vaginal bleeding, amniotic fluid, or recent cervical examinations. The health care provider gathers the sample for testing before doing a vaginal examination for cervical changes because the lubricant used for manual vaginal examinations may interfere with test results.

**Uterine contraction evaluation:** A diagnosis of PTL is made when the cervix is more than 2 cm dilated and the patient presents with regular contractions. Other criteria include a cervical examination showing more than or equal to 80% effaced or a change in cervical dilation with regular contractions. The focus of care is on stopping PTL if the intervention can begin before the woman has reached 3-cm cervical dilation. If PTL cannot be stopped, management is focused on maternal safety and reduction of the preterm infant's risk for RDS.

**Preterm premature rupture of membrane:** PPROM precedes PTL in 25% of PTBs. See discussion in "Preterm Premature Rupture of Membranes," Chapter 96.

**Urinalysis for microscopy:** UTIs are associated with PTL. A clean-catch urine specimen needs to be obtained when attempting to rule out PTL, even when the patient does not have symptoms. When a UTI is present, antibiotic therapy will be initiated.

## Patient Problem/Analyze Cues/Prioritize Hypotheses

# Anxiety

*due to* perceived or actual threats to self and well-being of the fetus and inadequate time to prepare for labor/delivery

**Desired Outcomes/Generate Solutions:** Immediately after intervention, the patient describes the symptoms of anxiety she is feeling. Within 1–2 hours of intervention, the patient reports that the detrimental anxiety reactions are lessened.

| ASSESSMENT—RECOGNIZE CUES/ INTERVENTIONS—TAKE ACTION | RATIONALES |
|---|---|
| Assess the maternal level of understanding, language, and ability to communicate her feelings and concerns, culture-bound anxiety, and the impact of fatigue. | Assessment provides information about the woman's and family's emotional needs, communication needs, and cognitive level. When interventions are provided at the appropriate level and understood, behavioral changes take place. Anxiety can be culture related and is manifested differently from culture to culture. |
| Assess the maternal vital signs (VS) and fetal heart rate (FHR) patterns per agency protocol. | Maternal temperature and pulse rise if an infection is present. Physiologic stress reaction also increases pulse and respirations. Muscle tension and vasoconstriction may cause uteroplacental insufficiency and reduce oxygenation to the fetus as evidenced by nonreassuring (category 2 or 3) FHR patterns. |
| Help the patient anticipate and problem-solve her needs related to procedures, procedural side effects, how they affect her and her unborn baby, her changing labor status, the fetal condition, and hoped-for outcomes. | Anxiety is reduced with clarification of needs, medical interventions, procedures, and anticipated medications. |
| Encourage questions and verbalization of concerns. Answer honestly, while maintaining an optimistic attitude. | When concerns are verbalized and clarified, the nurse can give realistic feedback and provide appropriate emotional support. |

Continued

| ASSESSMENT—RECOGNIZE CUES/ INTERVENTIONS—TAKE ACTION | RATIONALES |
|---|---|
| Assess and guide the patient to develop a personal support system and use community resources while in the hospital in anticipation of her return home to self-care and outpatient monitoring. | Refer to interventions and rationales for support under *Difficulty Coping*, later. |
| Encourage self-nurturing with rest, assistance with relaxation techniques, prayer or meditation as related to the woman's faith, and administration of sedatives if prescribed when other measures are insufficient. | When the usual quiescence of the uterus is interrupted by the threat of preterm delivery, the mother and family can become severely stressed. Rest, meditation, prayer, and focused relaxation improve physiologic, psychologic, and spiritual well-being. |

## Patient Problem/Analyze Cues/Prioritize Hypotheses

# Impaired Mobility

*due to* prescribed rest to prevent the effects of activity on advancing preterm labor.

***Desired Outcome/Generate Solutions:*** Within 1–2 hours after interventions, the patient describes her at-home situation, mobilizes appropriate support for home care (or family while in the hospital), and verbalizes plans to reduce her activity level as prescribed.

| ASSESSMENT—RECOGNIZE CUES/ INTERVENTIONS—TAKE ACTION | RATIONALES |
|---|---|
| Assess the readiness of the patient, her partner, and family to learn from within their cultural context. Assess the ability of the family unit to assume care responsibilities in preparation for the patient's discharge to home care. | Changes in family functioning and behavior occur when education is given at the appropriate level of understanding. Barriers to effective functioning may include familial conflicts and uncontrollable outside stressors. |
| Explain ways to maintain muscle strength with prescribed activity reduction or possible bed rest, the reasons for bed rest or activity reduction, and the frequent use of left lateral positioning. | Physical deconditioning develops quickly with bed rest and may take weeks to reverse (muscle atrophy, cardiovascular changes, and maternal weight loss). Understanding the value of reducing fetal pressure on the cervix and increasing uterine perfusion promotes adherence to lateral positioning. There is no current evidence that supports *strict* bed rest as beneficial or identifies the level of reduced activity that is beneficial for the mother or baby. A thorough explanation of activity limits and positioning encourages adherence through improved understanding. |
| Provide comfort measures (back rubs, frequent position changes while awake, and reduced noise and stimuli in the room) and uninterrupted periods of rest/sleep. | These interventions decrease muscle tension and fatigue while promoting relaxation and a sense of well-being. |
| Assist with the development of plans for adjustments in family functioning and mobilizing a support team, which may include personal and community resources. | Being able to rely on a team of support for the care of other children and accomplishing family needs reduces physical tension and mental anxiety. |
| Assist with diversional activity plans (e.g., at home get dressed daily and rest on the couch; learn sedentary hobbies [e.g., knitting]; read; watch television; use a laptop computer, smartphone, or other methods to communicate with friends and access support and information; listen to books on tape; and plan appropriate friend/ family visits [at home or in hospital]). | Making plans for acceptable diversional activities decreases anxiety and a sense of isolation. |

## Patient and Fetus Problem/Analyze Cues/Prioritize Hypotheses

# Risk for Perinatal Problems (Side Effects of Tocolytics and Other Drugs)

*due to* the need to decrease uterine contractions

**Desired Outcome/Generate Solutions:** After 1–4 hours of tocolytic therapy, uterine contractions begin to decrease without manifestation of toxic side effects in the mother or the fetus.

| ASSESSMENT—RECOGNIZE CUES/ INTERVENTIONS—TAKE ACTION | RATIONALES |
|---|---|
| Assess the VS (especially BP, heart rate [HR], and respiratory rate [RR]) and cardiac rhythm. Auscultate lung sounds. Note reports of dyspnea or chest tightness. | Many adverse side effects of tocolytic medications alter these physiologic parameters. |
| Before beginning tocolytic therapy, hydrate with a bolus if intravenous (IV) fluids are prescribed. | Hydration reduces the risk for hypotension and promotes renal clearance. It also may decrease uterine contractions. |
| **!** Administer tocolytic medications (magnesium sulfate, terbutaline, nifedipine, and indomethacin) per agency policy. Use an infusion pump if IV magnesium sulfate is being administered. | IV administration by infusion pump takes effect quickly and can be discontinued quickly if adverse reactions occur. Commonly used in the United States as tocolytics, magnesium sulfate and terbutaline are not approved by the US Food and Drug Administration for this purpose and are used off label to inhibit the contractions of PTL. However, they should not be used for more than 24–48 hours. |
| Assess for side effects of tocolytics. | |
| • Terbutaline: Monitor serum potassium level before administration and periodically afterward, along with glucose level. Instruct the patient to report and assess for tachycardia (maternal or fetal), heart palpitations, chest pain, shortness of breath, headache, weakness, and nausea. | As a beta-adrenergic agonist (beta-sympathomimetic), terbutaline relaxes smooth muscles, thus inhibiting uterine contractions while causing bronchial dilation and accelerating the HR. HR greater than 120 bpm is associated with decreased cardiac output and may necessitate discontinuance of the medication. An overdose may cause cardiac arrest. Common adverse metabolic side effects with this medication are hyperglycemia and hypokalemia. Terbutaline is recommended for use for 24 hours and only in an inpatient setting. The neonate needs to be closely monitored for hypoglycemia after birth until feeding is well established. |
| • Magnesium sulfate: Assess the serum magnesium levels as prescribed during therapy. Assess for and report depressed deep tendon reflexes, significant changes in VS from baseline, including decreased BP, reduced respirations (less than 14/minute), drowsiness, oxygen saturation less than 95%, changes in the level of consciousness, hot flashes, blurred vision, slurred speech, reduced FHR variability, and serum hypocalcemia. | As a central nervous system (CNS) depressant, magnesium sulfate relaxes smooth muscles, thereby decreasing uterine contraction frequency/intensity and relaxing blood vessel walls. An overdose may cause respiratory paralysis and cardiac arrest. |
| Keep calcium gluconate on hand. | Normal magnesium levels are 1.5–2.5 mEq/L or 1.7–2.4 mg/dL. *Therapeutic* levels are 4–7.5 mEq/L or 5–8 mg/dL. |
| | Magnesium sulfate affects the actions/concentrations of $K^+$ and $Ca^{2+}$, and therefore calcium gluconate is used as an antidote to reverse magnesium sulfate toxicity. |
| **!** Administer nifedipine as prescribed. Assess for hypotension, dizziness, facial flushing, headache, nausea, and peripheral edema (fluid retention). Dose is given orally, not sublingually. | As a calcium channel blocker, nifedipine relaxes smooth muscles, thereby decreasing the amplitude and frequency of uterine activity and contractility of the cardiac muscle and dilating blood vessel walls. An overdose may cause heart failure. There is a risk of severe hypotension and skeletal muscle blockade if given with magnesium sulfate. |

Continued

| ASSESSMENT—RECOGNIZE CUES/ INTERVENTIONS—TAKE ACTION | RATIONALES |
|---|---|
| Administer indomethacin as prescribed. Assess for side effects (e.g., heartburn, nausea, and vomiting). | As a prostaglandin inhibitor, indomethacin plays a role in decreasing uterine contractions of labor. When given after 32 weeks' gestation, it has been associated with premature closure of PDA in the fetus and persistent pulmonary hypertension in newborns. After 48 hours, amniotic fluid index measured by ultrasound, perinatology consult, and weekly fetal echocardiography may be prescribed. |
| Administer betamethasone or dexamethasone as prescribed by the health care provider. | These corticosteroids reduce the effects of RDS, IVH, and necrotizing enterocolitis in the preterm neonate when delivery is anticipated to be less than 34 weeks and after the gestation of viability. They also accelerate the maturation of the CNS and fetal organs, including cardiovascular. |
| Assess the intake and output (I&O) every 1–8 hours as prescribed. | Hydration is often the first treatment for PTL. Assessing I&O promotes interventions for adequate hydration while reducing the risk for fluid overload. Pulmonary edema is a risk with tocolytic medications. Magnesium sulfate is excreted through the kidneys, and therefore urinary output of at least 30 mL/hour is a sign the kidneys are functioning properly. |

## Patient Problem/Analyze Cues/Prioritize Hypotheses

# Constipation

*due to* decreased peristalsis occurring with immobility, stress, lack of exercise, and prolonged bed rest

***Desired Outcome/Generate Solutions:*** The patient has regular bowel movements and minimal discomfort from gas and hard stooling within 2–3 days of interventions, thereby reducing the risk for preterm contractions.

| ASSESSMENT—RECOGNIZE CUES/ INTERVENTIONS—TAKE ACTION | RATIONALES |
|---|---|
| Assess the patient's usual bowel status and whether she requires laxatives or stool softeners on a routine basis. | This assessment identifies whether constipation is playing a role in PTL. Constipation often occurs with pregnancy because the descending colon vies for space with the uterus as it enlarges and because progesterone, one of the hormones produced in pregnancy, decreases gastric motility. However, in a patient prone to PTL who is on bed rest, constipation can be exacerbated because of the decrease in peristalsis associated with inactivity. |
| Explain the effects of constipation in a patient prone to PTL. | Constipation or gastric irritability can increase uterine irritability in the form of contractions. This would increase the risk for PTL. |
| Encourage the intake of at least 8–10 glasses of water/day and increasing dietary fiber or adding a fiber laxative or stool softener to her daily regimen. | These measures provide bulk and aid in keeping the stool soft to promote evacuation. |

## Patient, Partner, and Family Problem/Analyze Cues/Prioritize Hypotheses

# Deficient Knowledge

*due to* unfamiliarity with the effects of preterm labor on self and the fetus

***Desired Outcome/Generate Solutions:*** The patient, her partner, and her family verbalize an accurate knowledge about the effects of PTL on the patient, her pregnancy, and her fetus.

| ASSESSMENT—RECOGNIZE CUES/ INTERVENTIONS—TAKE ACTION | RATIONALES |
|---|---|
| Assess the patient, her partner, and her family regarding attitudes about the patient's care (allowed self-care and care contributed by the family). Encourage self-efficacy for learning about her condition and the necessary care for herself and the fetus. | Encourages the patient and her family to be proactive in her care and reporting of problems. |
| Discuss with the patient and her family the signs of PTL, its treatment, and its effects on delivery and on the newborn. Develop an assessment and reporting plan with her. | Adequate information helps to identify problems early and promote adherence to the therapeutic regimen. The effects PTL and delivery have on the newborn can be life threatening (i.e., RDS, hypoglycemia, IVH, sepsis, and necrotizing enterocolitis), and can lead to neonatal death. |
| Actively use written material in the discussion. | Written materials reinforce learning and retention. |
| Explain the importance of access to a specialized facility and the possible need to transport the pregnant woman (if she lives in a rural area) to a distant hospital. | Delivering a preterm infant at a tertiary or secondary hospital facility with perinatal and neonatal specialists and a neonatal intensive care unit (NICU) provides the greatest opportunity for infant survival. |
| Instruct *all* pregnant women about the signs and symptoms of PTL. | An informed patient likely will report these symptoms promptly. See introductory information for detailed signs and symptoms of PTL. Barring the presence of chorioamnionitis, the earlier PTL is diagnosed, the better the chance for prolonging the pregnancy and decreasing fetal morbidity and mortality. |
| Question the patient at each prenatal visit, starting at the beginning of the second trimester, if she is experiencing any signs or symptoms of PTL/contractions. | Early recognition of PTL (see signs and symptoms in the assessment data) may lead to prolonging the gestational period and decreasing fetal morbidity and mortality. |
| Encourage the patient to report even vague or subtle symptoms no matter the time of day or night. Provide written instructions and telephone numbers to call if concerns or changes arise. | Uterine contractions may be painless. Fewer than 50% of patients in PTL are aware of their contractions, and many do not realize that PTL can be serious. Women who present with PTL account for approximately 12% of PTB (ACOG, 2016), and PTB accounts for almost 70% of all neonatal mortality not caused by congenital anomalies (ACOG, 2016). |
| Instruct the patient on how to do daily fetal movement (kick) counts. | Fetal movement (kick) counts done twice a day are a good first-line indicator of fetal well-being and are performed as follows, beginning at 28 weeks' gestation: The patient lies on her side and counts "distinct fetal movements" (hiccups do not count); 10 movements within a 2-hour period are considered reassuring. After 10 movements are discerned, the count is discontinued. Fewer than 10 movements in a 2-hour period signal the need for fetal nonstress testing. |
| Instruct the patient on how to palpate contractions. To palpate contractions, the patient lies comfortably on her side. She spreads her fingers apart and places one hand on the left side and the other on the right side of her abdomen. She will palpate the abdomen using her fingertips. When the uterus is relaxed, the abdomen should feel soft. She should palpate contractions for 1 hour. In the presence of a contraction the uterus should feel hard, tight, or firm under her fingertips. She then times the duration of the contraction from the beginning of one contraction to the end of that contraction. The frequency of contractions is measured from the beginning of one contraction to the beginning of the next contraction. Contractions will vary in frequency and duration. The patient needs to record whether contractions are palpated only or also experienced as a specific sensation. If the patient experiences more than 4 contractions/hour, she needs to call her primary provider. Contractions may be mild to severe in intensity and difficult for a gravida I (first pregnancy) mother to discern as PTL. | Timely reporting of preterm contractions to her health care provider can play a significant role in affecting outcome. Palpation and awareness of contractions enable the patient to be an active participant in her health care. |

Continued

| ASSESSMENT—RECOGNIZE CUES/ INTERVENTIONS—TAKE ACTION | RATIONALES |
|---|---|
| Instruct the patient to drink at least 10 8-oz glasses of water per day, tapering her intake during the last few hours before sleep. | The uterus is a muscle and will respond to dehydration by cramping/contracting. Adequate oral hydration is a preventive measure for PTL. |
| Explain to the patient and her partner the effect that sexual foreplay or intercourse may have on PTL. Advise the patient to avoid all forms of sexual stimulation. | This information promotes patient/partner understanding and adherence. Sexual intercourse may increase uterine contractions and promote cervical change. Increased uterine activity also may be caused by breast stimulation, female orgasm, and prostaglandin in male ejaculate. |

## Patient Problem/Analyze Cues/Prioritize Hypotheses

# Difficulty Coping

*due to* adjustment in lifestyle to provide an optimal environment for the fetus or lack of support from family, friends, and community

***Desired Outcome/Generate Solutions:*** Within the 24-hour period after intervention, the patient verbalizes feelings and identifies strengths and coping behaviors that provide the best pregnancy outcome for herself and her fetus.

| ASSESSMENT—RECOGNIZE CUES/ INTERVENTIONS—TAKE ACTION | RATIONALES |
|---|---|
| Assess the patient's perceptions and ability to understand her current health status regarding PTL. | Evaluation of the patient's perceptions and comprehension enables the development of an individualized care plan. |
| Provide referral sources for support groups, written material, Internet chat groups, or home help if the patient is on home bed rest or hospitalization. Involve social services as needed. | Communicating with or learning about others who have experienced similar circumstances may aid in the development of positive coping mechanisms. |
| Help the patient identify or develop a support system. | Having a support system will aid in the patient's overall care and reduction of stress to promote positive coping behaviors. |
| Arrange community referrals as appropriate or at the request of the patient. | Support in the home environment promotes healthier adaptations and may avert crises. |
| Offer realistic hope for continuing the pregnancy to a safe gestation. Help the patient and family develop realistic expectations for the future if a preterm delivery occurs and to identify support persons or systems that will help them plan for the future. | These measures foster realistic expectations about a preterm neonate's health status (in the absence of congenital anomalies) and promote adaptation to possible changes in family dynamics. |
| Advise the patient and family that hospitalization and medical interventions in preventing a PTB may not always be effective or wise. | Medications, bed rest, and hydration are not always successful in stopping PTL. In some instances, an early delivery may be in the best interest of the mother, fetus, or both, as would be the case in the presence of infection, nonreassuring (categories 2 and 3) FHR tracings, severe oligohydramnios (abnormally low amount of amniotic fluid), anhydramnios (no amniotic fluid), and congenital anomalies. |
| Affirm that lifestyle adjustment (e.g., no work, bed rest, and no intercourse) is for a limited time. | This information facilitates acceptance of outside support and assistance and reinforces the knowledge that routine or increased activity with PTL may increase the risk for cervical change and possible preterm delivery. |

## Caregiver Problem/Analyze Cues/Prioritize Hypotheses

# Risk for Caregiver Role Strain

*due to* the care the patient's partner, family member, or support person needs to provide not only to the patient but also possibly to other family members in order for the patient to remain compliant and prolong the gestational period

*Desired Outcome/Generate Solutions:* Within 24 hours after interventions, the caregiver verbalizes concerns/frustrations about caregiving responsibilities, identifies at least one other support person, and recognizes at least one change that would make his or her job easier.

| ASSESSMENT—RECOGNIZE CUES/ INTERVENTIONS—TAKE ACTION | RATIONALES |
|---|---|
| Encourage the caregiver and the patient to relate their feelings and concerns regarding their roles and to problem-solve together. | This validates concerns and helps them understand if expectations are realistic. Mutual participation in planning fosters self-efficacy for both. |
| Acknowledge the caregiver's role in the patient's care; identify and praise strengths. | This reinforces positive ways of dealing with the current health crisis and promotes a sense of involvement and appreciation. |
| Involve social services in support of the caregiver in helping establish a plan for time-outs. | Social services can provide the caregiver with a weekly viable goal and coping mechanisms and identify resources available to the caregiver and family. |
| Provide the patient and caregiver with status reports on the effectiveness of the patient's bed rest, decreased activity, stopping work, or inability to participate in routine household activities. | Reassuring the patient and caregiver that the support and assistance are positively affecting the patient's health likely will promote more of the same. |
| Affirm that this situation is for a limited time. | This information facilitates the patient's and caregiver's acceptance in receiving and giving support and assistance. |
| Encourage diversional activities (e.g., time alone away from home or hospital and other children) and interactions with support persons or systems outside the family. | Promoting respite enhances coping and helps family members remain focused and supportive of the patient. For example, "I know this must be a difficult time and you want to stay with her, but I will call you if any changes occur." |

## Patient Problem/Analyze Cues/Prioritize Hypotheses

# Risk for Difficulty Performing Breastfeeding

*due to* a break in the continuity of the normal breastfeeding process resulting from a premature and/or ill infant

*Desired Outcome/Generate Solutions:* The patient produces breast milk using a breast pump or makes an informed decision regarding which method of feeding most benefits the infant's needs and her own emotional/physical state of well-being.

| ASSESSMENT—RECOGNIZE CUES/ INTERVENTIONS—TAKE ACTION | RATIONALES |
|---|---|
| When possible, encourage the mother to visit the baby in NICU as soon as possible after the delivery. Provide the mother with written information on care, including breastfeeding support provided in the NICU. | These measures promote the bonding process, encourage communication with the baby's care providers, and provide an opportunity to have questions answered. Breastfeeding support enables the new mother to reach her goals to provide milk for her baby. |
| Encourage the mother to breastfeed or express milk for later feeding of the infant. | In the preterm infant, it is not always possible or recommended to feed at the breast. However, supporting the mother's efforts to provide breast milk by teaching manual hand expression and pumping facilitates lactogenesis and promotes psychologic benefits for the mother by involving her in the infant's daily care and reinforcing the importance her breast milk has to the health of her infant. |
| Explain the benefits of breast milk for the preterm infant. | For the preterm infant, breast milk decreases the incidence of infectious complications and metabolic disturbances. Maternal antibodies in breast milk also promote immunologic health because the preterm infant's immune system is immature. Breast milk also helps establish nonpathogenic bacterial flora in the newborn intestinal tract and stimulates the passage of stool. |

Continued

| ASSESSMENT—RECOGNIZE CUES/ INTERVENTIONS—TAKE ACTION | RATIONALES |
|---|---|
| If the mother chooses to breastfeed by expressing milk for later infant feeding, assist her with breast pump operation and arrange for the acquisition of an electric breast pump for home use as needed. | A breast pump aids in producing/sustaining breast milk for later infant feeding. |
| As indicated, instruct about manual expression, storage, and transport of milk. | These measures aid in the success of producing milk and the safety of its storage. |
| Encourage the mother to verbalize her feelings and concerns and to clarify her questions. | Verbalizing feelings and concerns makes them more concrete and manageable. Clarification of questions enables the development of self-efficacy. Tension can interfere with establishing an adequate milk supply. |
| Reassure the patient that breastfeeding can be successful even with initial separation after birth. Explain her the physical process of how lactation occurs after birth. | This information helps decrease her anxiety about "not having enough milk" and helps her understand the importance of breast stimulation through actual breastfeeding or pumping. Delivery of the placenta causes a decrease in progesterone and an increase in prolactin, the hormone that stimulates lactogenesis (milk production). Prolactin is released from the anterior pituitary gland during breastfeeding or with nipple stimulation as with breast pumping and manual hand expression. Prolactin levels increase with each breastfeeding session and, in turn, stimulate milk production. Oxytocin is released from the posterior pituitary gland at the same time and causes the milk ejection reflex, or milk "letdown." During the course of breastfeeding, these hormones are released and regulated on a supply-and-demand basis. Encouragement of a regular pumping and manual hand-expression regimen (eight times in 24 hours) promotes the best milk supply. |
| Provide support to the mother through referral to a lactation consultant (a certified lactation consultant is known as IBCLC) available within the hospital or as an outside consultant. | Lactation consultants teach the mother how to use a breast pump or, in actual infant breastfeeding, how to position the infant for comfort and ease of nursing, how to use nipple shields and other lactation support as needed, and how to manage engorgement, inverted or flat nipples, milk supply problems, plugged ducts, sore nipples, and infant sucking problems. |
| Explain the importance of adequate oral hydration (10–12 glasses of fluids per day), nutrition (a balanced diet with about 300–500 calories more than a nonpregnant diet), and rest. | Adequate maternal caloric intake, oral hydration, and rest help meet the periods of increased demand for breast milk during the infant's growth spurts and maintain a consistent supply of breast milk. |

## ADDITIONAL PROBLEMS:

## ✓ PATIENT–FAMILY TEACHING AND DISCHARGE PLANNING

PTL and PTB can have lifelong effects on the child and family. Early diagnosis and treatment are imperative. Education about the signs and symptoms of PTL needs to be a part of every woman's prenatal care. Include verbal and written information about the following:

- ✓ Potential risk factors for PTL that may be present early in prenatal care.
- ✓ Signs and symptoms of PTL.
- ✓ Palpation of contractions.
- ✓ Promptly reporting any signs of UTI.
- ✓ Importance of adequate oral hydration during the pregnancy.
- ✓ Importance of compliance with routine prenatal care.
- ✓ Medications, including drug name, purpose, dosage, frequency, precautions, potential drug reactions, and potential side effects. Also discuss potential drug–drug, food–drug, and herb–drug interactions.
- ✓ Measures that help with constipation, which occurs frequently in pregnancy and can be exacerbated with bed rest.
- ✓ Measures for coping with muscle pain, back pain, and muscle weakness that can be present with prolonged bed rest.

✓ Fetal movement counts.
✓ Referral to local and national support organizations, including:
  - Sidelines, a national support organization for women and their families experiencing complicated pregnancies: http://www.sidelines.org
  - March of Dimes: http://www.marchofdimes.com

- La Leche League: http://www.lalecheleague.org
- American Congress of Obstetricians and Gynecologists has an extensive collection of patient education materials available at http://www.acog.org/Resources_And_Publications/Patient_Education_FAQs_List

## OVERVIEW/PATHOPHYSIOLOGY

When membranes rupture before the onset of labor, it is called *premature rupture of membranes (PROMs)*. PROM occurs in approximately 10% of pregnancies (ACOG, 2020b). *Preterm premature rupture of membrane (PPROM)* is the leakage of amniotic fluid occurring before 37 weeks gestation. From early in pregnancy, the slightly alkaline (pH 7.0–7.5) amniotic fluid is produced within the amniotic sac. As pregnancy advances, fetal urine significantly contributes to the volume. Fetal breathing and swallowing reabsorb the amniotic fluid, which is formed, absorbed, and replaced within a 4-hour period. Amniotic fluid volume at term is approximately 500–1000 mL. Amniotic fluid provides an environment that protects the fetus from trauma and injury, provides even distribution of temperature, contains an antibacterial substance, and enables the fetus to move and develop without pressure. Amniotic fluid levels are a good indicator of fetal kidney function and lung maturity. Although the exact cause of PPROM is unknown, infection is identified as a risk factor that often precedes PPROM. PPROM may occur without an obvious cause. Risk for a preterm birth is high when PPROM occurs. Despite medical management, approximately half of patients with PPROM deliver within 1–2 weeks of onset.

## HEALTH CARE SETTING

The woman may be evaluated in the health care provider's office or clinic. She is managed by obstetricians or perinatologists as an outpatient or inpatient, depending on the week of gestation. Hospital sites may vary depending on gestational age and level of care needed for a high-risk pregnancy and neonate. Previability PPROM (gestation 14–24 weeks) occurs in less than 1% of pregnancies, and management is planned around the risks for infection and maternal complications. Parents are included in decision-making.

## ASSESSMENT

Patients may have difficulty determining the presence of ruptured membranes because symptoms are not always obvious and leaking amniotic fluid can be confused with leaking urine. Consider carefully any complaint of watery vaginal discharge or sudden gush of fluid. Assess the timing and occurrence of the initial loss of fluid. On some occasions, leakage of amniotic fluid may stop, or it may resume without signs of infection.

**Vaginal discharge:** Patients may experience a "sudden gush" or sensation that something "popped," followed by a slow leakage of clear, watery fluid from the vagina, and may state that the amount being leaked requires the use of a sanitary pad. The fluid may be blood tinged or meconium stained. The amount, color, and odor of the fluid need to be evaluated. Vaginal bleeding may accompany PPROM and range from light-pink spotting to bleeding as with a heavy menses.

**Backache:** May or may not be present with PPROM. In the presence of infection, there may be low lumbar/sacral pain that is deep tissue in nature or a dull, aching sensation that may radiate around the hips to the lower abdomen/pelvic area. If abruptio placenta is present with PPROM, the back pain may be mild or severe.

**Abdominal pain/cramping or uterine cramping contractions:** There may be a feeling of pelvic pressure or fullness, menstrual-like cramping, or contractions. Aching thighs may accompany uterine cramping. In the presence of infection, the patient may complain of abdominal/uterine tenderness or pain. If abruptio placenta accompanies PPROM, the pain may be mild to severe.

**Fever:** May occur in the presence of an infection, and the temperature may be 101°F (38.3°C) or higher.

**Complications—fetal:** Risks to the fetus depend on gestational age at the time of PPROM, the severity of PPROM (the amount of amniotic fluid remaining), and the presence of infection.

- Prematurity
- Fetal infections/sepsis
- Hypoxia and asphyxia caused by umbilical cord compression/prolapse
- Fetal deformities with PPROM at an early gestational age (i.e., pulmonary hypoplasia, facial anomalies, and limb position defects) due to prolonged oligohydramnios (deficiency of amniotic fluid)
- Abruptio placenta
- Fetal death

**Physical assessment:** In many cases, the cause of PPROM is unknown and there is no forewarning. Therefore it is important to evaluate changes in vaginal discharge. A timely diagnosis of PPROM is critical to optimize outcomes.

**Risk factors:** Maternal infections precede PPROM 30%–40% of the time. Urinary tract infection (UTI); genital tract infections such as *Chlamydia trachomatis*, gonorrhea, bacterial vaginosis, or trichomoniasis; chorioamnionitis (intraamniotic infection); and group B streptococcus are contributing factors to PPROM. Other risk factors include low socioeconomic status, smoking, multiple gestation, incompetent cervix (painless cervical dilation before term without contractions), previous history of PPROM, diethylstilbestrol exposure, amniocentesis, chorionic villi sampling, coitus, poor nutrition, bleeding in pregnancy, polyhydramnios (excess of amniotic fluid), cervical cerclage (a suture used for holding the cervix closed during a pregnancy), previous cervical laceration or surgery, placental abruption (abnormal separation of the placenta from the wall of the uterus before delivery), history of midtrimester pregnancy loss, cocaine use, hypertension, diabetes, and Ehlers–Danlos syndrome (a group of inherited connective tissue diseases).

## DIAGNOSTIC TESTS

***Sterile speculum examination:*** A sterile speculum is inserted into the vagina to visualize amniotic fluid leaking from the cervical os or pooling of amniotic fluid in the vagina. If visual examination of pooling of fluid is inconclusive, the fluid is tested with Nitrazine paper. If positive for amniotic fluid, the paper will turn from yellow to dark blue or green-blue, and the pH will be greater than 6. False-positive results may be seen in the presence of semen, blood, vaginal infections, or alkaline antiseptics. Using a cotton swab, a sample of vaginal fluid is taken from the posterior vaginal fornix (the posterior space below the cervix) and examined under the microscope for the presence of a ferning pattern that amniotic fluid makes when it dries on a slide. A digital examination of the cervix is not recommended in a patient with suspected PPROM who is not in labor. Some agencies use an immunoassay test PAMG-1 (AmniSure) to confirm the rupture of membranes. The test detects trace amounts of a protein, PAMG-1, expressed by the cells of the decidua and found in amniotic fluid. The test is performed by swabbing a sterile polyester swab into the vaginal secretions. The swab is then rinsed with a vial of solvent for

1 minute and thrown away. A test strip is dipped into the vial for 5–10 minutes and then read. One line indicates no rupture of membranes. Two lines indicate a positive test for rupture of membranes. No lines indicate an invalid test. The test has a 99% accuracy rate. Because a digital cervical examination can increase the risk for infection, the cervix is visually inspected for dilation and effacement.

***External uterine and fetal monitoring:*** External uterine monitoring is done to evaluate fetal well-being and uterine contraction presence, frequency, and duration. Category 1 fetal heart rate (FHR) pattern is a sign that the fetus is well oxygenated. Category 2 is indeterminate and needs further observation, and category 3 is abnormal and requires action. Category 2 or 3 FHR patterns (decreased variability, moderate-to-severe variable decelerations, and late decelerations) suggest fetal compromise, which can be caused by umbilical cord compression, cord prolapse, or infection that may accompany PPROM.

***Obstetric ultrasound:*** Abdominal ultrasound is used to confirm gestational age, calculate amniotic fluid index (AFI) and biophysical profile (BPP), rule out multiple gestation, and determine placental location and fetal presentation. AFI is calculated by dividing the uterus into four quadrants and measuring the fluid "pockets" during the ultrasound. Normal value for the AFI is between 10 and 20 mL of amniotic fluid. A normal rating on the BPP is 6–8 out of 10.

***Amniocentesis:*** Transabdominal aspiration of amniotic fluid to test for fetal lung maturity and the presence of chorioamnionitis.

***Blood Rh factor and antibody screen:*** This test needs to be a part of the routine prenatal screening. In patients with no prenatal care who have PPROM, this laboratory test is performed on admittance to determine the need for administration of Rh immune globulin to a Rh-negative mother if her newborn is Rh positive.

## Patient and Fetus Problem/Analyze Cues/Prioritize Hypotheses

# Risk for Infection (Amniotic Fluid Infection)

*due to* bacterial spread (often from ascending movement of vaginal bacteria)

***Desired Outcome/Generate Solutions:*** The amniotic fluid is clear without offensive odor; maternal temperature remains less than 99.5°F (37.5°C).

| ASSESSMENT—RECOGNIZE CUES/ INTERVENTIONS—TAKE ACTION | RATIONALES |
|---|---|
| Assist the health care provider with sterile speculum examination, collection of amniotic fluid, Nitrazine paper test, PAMG-1 immunoassay test, and observation of ferning by microscope. | These assessments can confirm the diagnosis of PPROM. |
| Assist with collecting specimens from amniocentesis. Collect a catheterized urine specimen and vaginal secretions for culture. | UTI, group B streptococcus, *C. trachomatis*, gonorrhea, bacterial vaginosis, and trichomoniasis organisms are common causes of maternal vaginal tract infections and chorioamnionitis. |
| After PPROM has been confirmed, begin maternal assessments: monitor the maternal vital signs every 4 hours; palpate the uterus for tenderness; and monitor vaginal secretions for color, amount, and odor every 8 hours. | Fever, uterine tenderness, and changes in vaginal discharge characteristics are signs of infection. Prompt notification of these signs to the health care provider may decrease the risk for further compromise to the fetus or mother. |

| ASSESSMENT—RECOGNIZE CUES/ INTERVENTIONS—TAKE ACTION | RATIONALES |
|---|---|
| Apply an FHR monitor and perform a nonstress test (NST) every 8 hours. | A reactive NST reflects adequate fetal oxygenation status. Category 2 or 3 FHR patterns (decreased variability, variable decelerations, or late decelerations) are associated with fetal compromise and indicate a need for further testing or action. Fetal tachycardia is a sign of infection, as is decreased variability. |
| Arrange for other tests of fetal well-being (e.g., BPP, amniocentesis for lecithin-to-sphingomyelin [L/S] ratio, and phosphatidyl glycerol [PG] and ultrasound for AFI). | BPP is a noninvasive test that assesses fetal breathing movement, gross body movement, fetal tone, AFI, and FHR to determine fetal oxygenation status. |
| | L/S ratio and PG identify lung maturity/readiness for neonatal breathing. AFI measurement, a part of the BPP, identifies oligohydramnios by measuring amniotic fluid volumes and helps the health care provider make decisions for the optimal time of delivery. |
| Collect serial maternal specimens of blood for complete blood count and urine for urinalysis as prescribed by the health care provider (e.g., daily). | White blood cell differential rises with infection. Bacteria are present in the urine if a UTI develops. |
| Administer antibiotics as prescribed by the health care provider. | Prophylactic antibiotics prevent or reduce the effects of maternal–fetal infections and may reduce morbidity and prolong the pregnancy. |
| Instruct and assist the patient with good hygiene: frequent hand hygiene, daily showering, wiping the perineum from front to back, and changing the peripad every 2 hours (if a pad is worn). | These practices prevent the spread of microorganisms from the environment to the genital area. A moist, warm peripad fosters bacterial growth. |

## Patient and Partner Problem/Analyze Cues/Prioritize Hypotheses

# Deficient Knowledge

*due to* unfamiliarity with the signs and symptoms of PPROM, its effects on the pregnancy and fetus, and guidelines to follow for an optimal outcome

*Desired Outcome/Generate Solutions:* Immediately after teaching, the patient and her partner verbalize an accurate knowledge about the effects of PPROM on the patient and fetus, as well as its signs and symptoms, prescribed medications, and treatment guidelines for an optimal outcome.

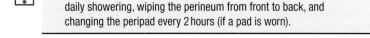

| ASSESSMENT—RECOGNIZE CUES/ INTERVENTIONS—TAKE ACTION | RATIONALES |
|---|---|
| Instruct the patient and family or significant about other signs and symptoms of PPROM and chorioamnionitis (intraamniotic infection), which may be present after PPROM. | A knowledgeable patient likely will report symptoms promptly and understand the consequences of nonadherence. PPROM plays a major factor in the morbidity and mortality of the neonate, depending on gestational age. See the introductory information for signs and symptoms of PPROM. Indicators of chorioamnionitis include abdominal pain, uterine tenderness, fever, chills, foul vaginal odor, and contractions. |
| Inform the patient and significant other about the effects PPROM can have on the patient and fetus. | Information facilitates adherence to the treatment regimen. Amniotic fluid is critical to fetal development. See the "Assessment" section, for fetal and newborn risks. PPROM also increases maternal risks: chorioamnionitis (see previous symptoms), abruptio placenta (premature separation of the placenta), and a postpartum risk for endometritis (inflammation of the endometrial lining of the uterus). Maternal death from sepsis is rare, but it can occur. |
| Discuss the risks/benefits of conservative management (delaying delivery and monitoring the pregnant woman for signs of infection and the fetus for signs of distress) versus active delivery with anticipated extrauterine support for a preterm infant, despite the risk for respiratory distress syndrome (RDS), infection, and neonatal death. | When there are no signs of maternal infection or cervical change and the intrauterine environment is safe for both the mother and fetus, conservative management may buy time for fetal lung maturation. In the presence of a uterine infection, however, delivery is advised. Treating the mother postpartum and the fetus in an extrauterine environment improves maternal–fetal well-being. |

| ASSESSMENT—RECOGNIZE CUES/ INTERVENTIONS—TAKE ACTION | RATIONALES |
|---|---|
| Instruct the patient on how to do daily fetal movement counts. | Beginning at 28 weeks' gestation, fetal movement is assessed as an indicator of fetal well-being. One of several methods is performed as follows: The patient lies on her side and counts "distinct fetal movement" (hiccups do not count) daily; 10 movements within a 2-hour period are reassuring. After 10 movements, the count is discontinued. Fewer than 10 movements indicate the need for fetal NST. There are cell phone applications to assist patients with record keeping of fetal movement count (kick counts). |
| Instruct about palpation of contractions, which may accompany PPROM (gestation appropriate). The patient lies comfortably on her side. She will spread her fingers apart and place one hand on the left side and the other on the right side of the abdomen. Palpation is done with the fingertips of both hands. When the uterus is relaxed, the abdomen should feel soft. When a contraction occurs, the uterus will feel hard, tight, or firm under the fingertips. She will time the duration from the beginning of the contraction to the end of the contraction. Duration of the contraction is not an indicator of contraction intensity. The woman also will be asked to note the frequency of contractions—the time from the beginning of one contraction to the beginning of the next contraction. | A knowledgeable patient likely will report an increase in contractions promptly: for a singleton pregnancy, four contractions/hour or more; for a multiple pregnancy, six contractions/hour or more. Palpation and awareness of contractions enable the patient to be an active participant in her health care. Timely reporting of contractions can play a significant role in optimal maternal–fetal outcome. Although contraction frequency alone is insufficient in diagnosing preterm labor, it can serve as a helpful guideline. |
| Instruct the patient to report signs and symptoms of infection (elevated fever, chills, body aches), decrease or changes in fetal movement (gestation appropriate), and elevated maternal blood glucose levels in patients with diabetes. | After prolonged rupture of membranes, an intraamniotic infection often develops. These are common signs of an intraamniotic infection. |
| For patients on antibiotic therapy, caution about the importance of following the complete course and taking them on time. | These measures prevent the development of antibiotic resistance and maintain a constant level of medication in the bloodstream. |
| Instruct the patient on antibiotic therapy to be alert for and report excessive and explosive diarrhea. | *Clostridioides difficile* is a potentially serious side effect in which the normal flora of the bowel is reduced by antibiotic therapy and the anaerobic organism *C. difficile* multiplies and produces its toxins, causing severe diarrhea. This problem necessitates discontinuation of the antibiotic and laboratory evaluation of a stool sample. |
| Explain the purpose of the antenatal glucocorticoids betamethasone and dexamethasone if these medications are prescribed. | Antenatal glucocorticoids accelerate the development of fetal lungs and help reduce the effects of RDS, intraventricular hemorrhage, and necrotizing enterocolitis in the neonate when delivery is anticipated to be preterm and after 24 weeks gestation. They also accelerate the maturation of other organs (e.g., the central nervous system [CNS] and the cardiovascular system).<br>• Betamethasone: two doses of 12 mg given by intramuscular (IM) injection 24 hours apart.<br>• Dexamethasone: four doses of 6 mg given by IM injection 12 hours apart.<br>• Maximum benefit is 48 hours after administration. |
| Instruct the patient to observe for side effects of corticosteroid therapy and to promptly report her observations. | Possible side effects of corticosteroid medication include reduced maternal–fetal resistance to infection, impaired glucose tolerance (people with borderline gestational diabetes may develop true gestational diabetes), and suppression of maternal or neonatal adrenal function. Usually, a rise in blood glucose is seen for approximately 48–96 hours after administration, and it may necessitate intravenous insulin. |

Continued

| ASSESSMENT—RECOGNIZE CUES/ INTERVENTIONS—TAKE ACTION | RATIONALES |
|---|---|
| Explain the purpose of Rh immune globulin (human) RhoGAM if it is prescribed. | This agent prevents the formation of antibodies to the Rh-positive antigen in the mother's blood and prevents hemolytic disease in a future Rh-positive fetus/newborn if the mother has not already been sensitized by the presence of Rh-positive blood. *Administration:* IM only to nonsensitized Rh-negative women after bleeding any time during the pregnancy, after spontaneous abortion, or after delivery. Recommended administration is within 72 hours after the bleeding episode or delivery. |
| Advise the patient that she may note discomfort at the site of injection. | This is a common side effect. |

### Patient Problem/Analyze Cues/Prioritize Hypotheses

# Difficulty Coping

*due to* health crisis, sense of vulnerability, inadequate support systems, and needed adjustment in lifestyle to provide an optimal environment for the fetus and prolong the gestational period

*Desired Outcome/Generate Solutions:*  Within 24 hours of interventions, the patient verbalizes feelings, identifies strengths, exhibits positive coping behaviors, and modifies her lifestyle to provide the best pregnancy outcome for her fetus.

| ASSESSMENT—RECOGNIZE CUES/ INTERVENTIONS—TAKE ACTION | RATIONALES |
|---|---|
| Assess the patient's perceptions and ability to understand the current health status of herself and fetus. | Evaluation of the patient's comprehension enables the development of an individualized care plan. |
| Help the patient identify previous stressors and methods of coping with stressful situations in life. | Recalling previous situations when she was able to handle the problem may strengthen effective coping now with current problems. |
| Provide the patient with resources for support groups, written information, Internet chat groups, or home helpers. | Talking with others who have experienced similar circumstances may aid in the development of coping mechanisms. A home helper, for example, likely will decrease pressure on the patient and thereby promote coping abilities. |
| Assist and affirm the patient's efforts to set realistic goals for lifestyle adjustments and for her support systems. | Participation in decision-making, use of realistic personal and professional resources, and evaluation of potential effects or problems enable a more successful adaptation and facilitate effective coping. |
| Assess and acknowledge the influence of the patient's cultural beliefs, norms, and values regarding coping during pregnancy. | This shows respect for the patient's coping style and a willingness to integrate her beliefs and practices into health care prescriptions. You might ask, "Could you tell me how you and your family are coping with this pregnancy?" Be mindful that different cultures perceive pregnancy in various ways. For example, some patients come from countries in which maternal and fetal mortality rate is high and daily survival is the major focus. Their method of coping may be emotional detachment from the fetus. The current pregnancy may not seem as important as the children and family that are already at home and need care. |
| Involve assistance of social services when available. | Social services provide counseling and make recommendations for referrals. Both home management and hospital management may require outside assistance to care for family members or pets at home. |

| ASSESSMENT—RECOGNIZE CUES/ INTERVENTIONS—TAKE ACTION | RATIONALES |
|---|---|
| Provide the patient and family with information regarding the effectiveness of hospitalization bed rest versus home bed rest. | This information helps the patient and her health care provider decide the best method of management. Patients on bed rest at home must be able to remain lying down in alternating side-lying positions (occasionally sitting up propped with pillows) and avoid doing housework, laundry, cooking, or shopping. The side-lying position improves uteroplacental blood flow and oxygenation, which, in turn, improve the chance of reaccumulation of amniotic fluid. Hospitalization is often recommended to monitor signs of infection or fetal compromise. Providers inform, educate, and involve parents in the decision-making process after increasing their knowledge level. |
| Encourage the patient and family to verbalize their concerns in a supportive environment. | This will help alleviate stress, anxiety, and misconceptions. See *Anxiety* in "Preterm Labor," Chapter 95. |

## Patient Problem/Analyze Cues/Prioritize Hypotheses

# Deficient Knowledge

*due to* unfamiliarity with deconditioning, muscle weakness, back pain, and decreased circulation that can occur with prescribed bed rest

**Desired Outcome/Generate Solutions:** Within 24 hours of this diagnosis, the patient verbalizes an understanding of and demonstrates measures to reduce or relieve back pain and improve circulation.

| ASSESSMENT—RECOGNIZE CUES/ INTERVENTIONS—TAKE ACTION | RATIONALES |
|---|---|
| Instruct the patient to recognize signs and symptoms of back pain related to bed rest versus back pain associated with contraction activity. | A knowledgeable patient optimally will discern the different causes of back pain and report these symptoms accordingly. Back pain related to bed rest is usually thoracic to lumbar and superficial and will be improved by position change or massage to promote circulation. Back pain related to contraction activity is usually lumbar/sacral and deep tissue, and it may radiate to the hips and low abdominal/pelvic area. Position change and massage may decrease intensity. |
| Inform the patient about the probable causes of muscle pain, weakness, and back pain. | This information aids in patient understanding and optimally in adherence to therapeutic management. For example, probable causes include lack of use of certain muscles, delay in change of positioning, increasing weight of the uterus, and dehydration, which can lead to the buildup of lactic acid in the muscles and cause pain. |
| Instruct the patient leg exercises to perform for the period in which she is on bed rest. | Leg exercises promote peripheral tissue perfusion and decrease the risk for deep vein thrombosis (DVT) and muscle wasting. Calf-pumping (ankle dorsiflexion–plantar flexion) and ankle-circling exercises are examples of leg exercises. The patient needs to repeat each movement 10 times, performing each exercise hourly during extended periods of immobility, provided the patient is free of symptoms of DVT. Passive and active range of motion exercises are often instructed by the physical therapist to promote circulation and maintain strength in the patient with activity restriction. |
| Encourage the patient to change positions frequently in bed, from alternating side-lying positions to sitting propped up with pillows. Explain how to use pillows between the knees to prevent pressure on the back. | Changing position at frequent intervals (e.g., every 2 hours) promotes circulation and decreases pressure and hence discomfort on tissues, joints, and muscles. Pillows provide support and decrease strain on muscles and promote comfort. |

Continued

| ASSESSMENT—RECOGNIZE CUES/ INTERVENTIONS—TAKE ACTION | RATIONALES |
|---|---|
| Caution the patient to *avoid* the supine position. | The supine position places pressure on the aorta by the enlarging fetus. This could result in a vasovagal response, which would decrease maternal blood pressure and cause diaphoresis, nausea, dizziness, and decreased uteroplacental perfusion. |
| Provide the patient with a referral for physical or massage therapy for back pain related to prolonged bed rest. | Professional interventions likely will aid in promoting circulation and patient comfort. |

## Patient, Partner, and Family Problem/Analyze Cues/Prioritize Hypotheses

# Grief

*due to* the potential or actual fetal loss that could occur with PPROM

**Desired Outcome/Generate Solutions:**  The patient, her partner, and family verbalize their feelings and identify and use support systems to aid them in the grief process within 24 hours of interventions.

| ASSESSMENT—RECOGNIZE CUES/ INTERVENTIONS—TAKE ACTION | RATIONALES |
|---|---|
| Encourage the patient and significant others to verbalize their feelings and concerns regarding the potential for the loss of their baby. | This measure validates concerns and conveys the message that grief is a normal and expected reaction to the potential loss of a baby. |
| Assess and accept behavioral responses. | Disbelief, denial, guilt, anger, and depression are normal reactions to grief. |
| Explain the stages of grief and that there is no specific time frame in which to go through the process. | This information enables the patient to understand where she or her family members may be in the grief process. Stages include (1) shock and numbness; (2) denial and searching-yearning; (3) anger, guilt, and sense of failure; (4) depression and disorganization; and (5) resolution. |
| Clarify misconceptions about the potential risk for fetal loss with PPROM. | This allows the patient and significant others to process the information regarding PPROM appropriately while not providing false hope. The gestational age at which PPROM occurs plays a significant role in treatment options and outcome. The earlier the gestational age at delivery, the higher the risk for fetal loss. A gestational age of 24 weeks is considered viable, but with each passing day and week, there is a better opportunity for fetal survival and decreased morbidity barring preexisting fetal complications such as cardiac, respiratory, and CNS problems. |
| If available, involve social services when a loss is perceived or present. | Social services provide resources and referrals for individual counseling and support groups for bereaved parents and grandparents, which may help the participants feel less isolated. Social Services also can guide the family through the disposition of the infant if deaths occur. |
| If a loss occurs, provide the patient and her significant others with support if they decide to see and hold the baby and place appropriate items in a memory/keepsake box. | These measures assist with the grieving process by enabling parents/grandparents to spend time with and affirm their baby. Such items as footprints and a lock of hair may be tucked away and not looked at right away, but it may help to know they are there. |

## ADDITIONAL PROBLEMS:

| | |
|---|---|
| "Immobility" for such patient problems as *Constipation* | Chapter 1 |
| Palliative and End-of-Life Care for *Risk for Spiritual Distress* | Chapter 7 |
| "Psychosocial Support for the Patient" for patient problems such as *Fatigue, Anxiety, Difficulty Coping,* and *Anticipatory Grief* | Chapter 8 |
| "Psychosocial Support for the Patient's Family and Significant Others" for *Difficulty Coping* | Chapter 9 |

## ✓ PATIENT–FAMILY TEACHING AND DISCHARGE PLANNING

PPROM is potentially life threatening to the fetus, depending on gestational age at the time of occurrence. When reviewing the symptoms of PPROM and the importance of the patient adhering to the therapeutic regimen with the hope of decreasing fetal morbidity and mortality, include verbal and written information about the following:

- ✓ Signs and symptoms of ruptured membranes, a developing infection, and the importance of contacting the health care provider in a timely manner.
- ✓ Signs and symptoms of preterm labor (see discussion in Chapter 95) because it may precede or follow PPROM.
- ✓ Palpation of contractions and uterine tenderness.
- ✓ Importance of adherence to prenatal care.
- ✓ Importance of a well-balanced prenatal diet.
- ✓ Potential risk factors for PPROM that may be present early in the pregnancy.
- ✓ Measures for muscle pain, back pain, and muscle weakness that can be present with prolonged bed rest with bathroom privileges. See *Deficient Knowledge,* earlier.
- ✓ Measures that help with constipation, which occurs frequently in pregnancy and can be exacerbated with bed rest.
- ✓ How to read a thermometer accurately.
- ✓ How to avoid intercourse but maintain intimacy with her husband or partner.
- ✓ Availability of social services and spiritual care.
- ✓ Medications, including drug name, purpose, dosage, frequency, precautions, and potential side effects. Also discuss potential drug–drug, food–drug, and herb–drug interactions.
- ✓ Fetal movement counts.
- ✓ The American Congress of Obstetricians and Gynecologists has an extensive collection of patient education materials available at https://www.acog.org/womens-health/pregnancy Referral to local and national support organizations, including:
  - Sidelines, a national support organization for women and their families experiencing complicated pregnancies: http://www.sidelines.org
  - March of Dimes: http://www.marchofdimes.com

# Breastfeeding 97

## OVERVIEW/PATHOPHYSIOLOGY

Worldwide, breastfeeding is recognized as the preferred method and gold standard of infant feeding and nutrition. It has been shown to result in improved infant and maternal health in both developing and industrialized worlds. Many organizations such as the American Academy of Pediatrics and the World Health Organization recommend that new mothers exclusively breastfeed for at least 6 months and/or longer.

### Benefits of breastfeeding

Breastfeeding has many health benefits for both mother and baby. A mother's breast milk is custom-made just for her baby. It contains many antibodies that help protect the infant from illness, which is particularly important in those early months when the infant's immune system is very immature. When either the mother or her baby is exposed to a virus or bacteria, the mother's immune system triggers the production of antibodies that enters into the breast milk. Breastfed infants have also been shown to have a reduced risk for many illnesses and diseases, such as asthma, ear infections, diabetes, necrotizing enterocolitis, childhood obesity, eczema, and sudden infant death syndrome.

Mothers may also experience an array of health benefits from breastfeeding. Studies have shown that breastfeeding can help reduce the mother's risk for developing type 2 diabetes, certain types of breast cancer, postpartum depression, and ovarian cancer. As a result of the release of the hormone oxytocin during breastfeeding, mothers can also have reduced blood loss after birth. Mothers who breastfeed may also experience an increase in weight loss. Breastfeeding burns about 500 extra calories per day for producing milk, which, in turn, can lead to faster weight loss after pregnancy. In addition, mothers who exclusively breastfeed experience the financial benefits of breastfeeding because they do not have to buy formula. According to the Office of Women's Health and US Department of Health and Human Services (2019), formula and feeding supplies may cost over $1500 per year.

### Contraindications to breastfeeding

For some mothers, breastfeeding may not be an option. There are a limited number of medical conditions in which breastfeeding is contraindicated. One example is infants diagnosed with galactosemia. Galactosemia is a metabolic disorder in which the body cannot break down or metabolize galactose, a simple sugar found in milk. Without proper diagnosis and interventions, galactosemia can be life-threatening in newborns. Infants with this disorder require a lactose-free formula. It is also recommended that mothers diagnosed with the following problems refrain from breastfeeding: human immunodeficiency virus, active herpes simplex virus infection with lesion on the breast, human T-cell lymphotropic virus type I or type II, active varicella, and those suspected or confirmed with having Ebola virus, because these infections may be transmitted through breast milk or from direct contact with the infected area. Certain medications can also be contraindicated in breastfeeding. It is important that the mother consults with her health care provider about the safety of prescribed medications and breastfeeding.

### Breast milk

Breast milk production begins during pregnancy. It is composed of different nutrients that the baby needs to help it grow. Over time, the composition of the breast milk will change to meet the needs of the growing baby. The first few days after the birth of the newborn, the breasts will produce a thick, sticky yellowish milk called colostrum. Colostrum, which is also referred to as "liquid gold," is very rich in nutrients and antibodies that will help protect the baby from infections. It also helps the infant's digestive system to grow and work. As the breast milk begins to mature, it will shift to transitional milk. The mother can expect to make transitional milk from 2–5 days after delivery and up to 2 weeks after delivery. With the production of transitional milk, the mother can expect her breasts to become fuller and firmer. She may also notice that the milk is more of a bluish-white color. Around 10–15 days after birth, the milk changes over to mature breast milk. The mature milk is lower in protein but has a higher fat and carbohydrate content.

### Techniques and signs of effective breastfeeding

Breastfeeding, although a natural process, does not always come without its challenges and is not always easy for every mother or baby. It is important that health care providers provide patients with the proper tools and support needed to make breastfeeding successful. When educating the patient about breastfeeding, providers need to start with the basics.

**Positioning:** Mothers must be shown and taught the different breastfeeding positions, so that they can choose the one that works best for them. Some of the most common positions include cradle, side lying, clutch/football hold, and cross-cradle. Regardless of the position that is chosen, the patient needs to make sure that she and the baby are positioned comfortably. She must not be in a straining or "curled-up" posture, her nipples need to be free from pain, and the infant should be relaxed and supported.

**Latching:** It is important to instruct the mother on how to obtain an effective latch (how the baby's mouth attaches to the nipple and areola). When latching, the mother should place the baby facing toward the breast. She should compress her breast with her free hand in the shape of a C, to help the baby take more of the breast tissue into its mouth. The baby should not be attached to just the nipple, as this will cause pain and can lead to nipple injury. Using her free hand to support the head, the mother will bring the baby to the breast, chin-first. The nipple needs to be aimed upward toward the roof of the infant's mouth. When latched properly, the baby's chin should be pressed close to the breast, their lips should be flared out, and their nose is free. To assess if the infant is effectively latched, encourage the mother to observe the sucking and swallowing pattern of the infant. Typically, the infant starts a feeding with rapid, shallow suckling, which triggers the release of the milk or letdown. Once the milk is released, the baby's suck will become deeper and longer. When the infant is latched correctly, the mother should not experience any nipple pain. Nipple pain during a feeding is a sign of a poor latch, and adjustment is needed to prevent injury.

**Hunger cues:** It is also imperative that the parents understand when their baby is hungry. Parents often associate a baby crying with hunger; however, babies normally exhibit other signs that they need to be fed, before they began to cry. Crying is usually a late sign of hunger for infants. The parent needs to watch for feeding cues or signs of hunger and offer the breast in response. Some early hunger signs that the baby may demonstrate are: being more awake and active, opening and closing their mouth, turning their head toward the breast or chest, making sucking motions with their mouth, smacking their lips or sticking out their tongue, sucking on their finger, hands or clothing, and clenching their hands into fists. Infants that are fed based on hunger cues, rather than a feeding schedule, have been associated with increased breastfeeding duration, increased milk intake, and faster regain of birth weight. When the newborn is adequately fed or finished eating, they will relax their hands and body. They may also release or push away from the breast and are overall more content.

**Assessing milk intake:** A common concern of parents is knowing whether their baby is getting enough breast milk. Encourage mothers to monitor the infant's output. They need to keep a written record of the number of wet and dirty diapers per day; give them a guide as to what is expected. The baby's voids and stool will increase as they consume more breast milk. For example, on the second to third day of life, the newborn should have at least two wet and dirty diapers, but by the

fourth to fifth day, they should have at least five wet diapers per day. Fewer than the recommended amount of wet and dirty diapers or dark yellow or orange urine are signs of inadequate intake and must be reported to the child's health care. Newborn weight gain can also be used as a sign of adequate milk intake. It is normal for babies to lose weight after birth, with an average weight loss of 4–5 oz within the first few days after birth. This weight loss can continue up to 5 days. The baby should start to regain their birth weight by 2 weeks of age. Those infants who do not gain weight and continue to lose weight are at risk for becoming dehydrated and/or developing jaundice. If the cause of weight loss cannot be determined, the infant may require supplementation with formula.

## Common breastfeeding complications

**Breast and nipple pain:** One of the most common problems that breastfeeding mothers report is breast and nipple pain. It is also the second most common reason mothers stop breastfeeding. There are many causes to breast and nipple pain, including, but not limited to, use of poor feeding techniques (bad positioning and/or latch), nipple injury, engorgement, plugged milk ducts, nipple and breast infections, newborn with ankyloglossia (tongue tie), and improper nipple care. To help determine the possible cause of the pain, the health care provider needs to examine the mother and the newborn and perform a visual assessment of the mother while breastfeeding. Most cases of breast and nipple pain are a result of improper breastfeeding techniques; that is why it is important to watch the mother as she is breastfeeding, to make corrections as needed. If not fixed, poor positioning and latching can lead to nipple injury and can result in ineffective emptying of the breast, which, in turn, can lead to engorgement, plugged ducts, and breast infections.

**Engorgement:** Breast engorgement happens when the breasts are overfilled with milk. It can make the breast feel full or swollen and can cause pain and tenderness. Mothers often experience engorgement as they began to produce milk, typically the first few days after birth. Other causes include missing feedings, producing more milk than the baby can consume, and the use of poor breastfeeding techniques, which results in the ineffective emptying of the breast. Management of engorgement focuses on the removal of the milk from breast. Thus encourage mothers to breastfeed more often, at least every 2 hours and at least twice at night. The use of warm compresses or a warm shower before feeding will also help with letdown (release of the milk). After or between feedings, the mother may apply a cold compress to the breast to decrease swelling and pain. If the mother is having trouble with properly breastfeeding her baby, she needs to seek support from her health care provider or a lactation consultant.

**Clogged milk duct:** Milk ducts are small tubes in the breast that carry milk from the glandular tissue to the nipples. Sometimes, these ducts get blocked with milk, which prevents the flow of breast milk. Signs and symptoms of a clogged milk duct include a tender or painful lump in one area of the breast and pain during letdown. The mother may also have complaints of swelling and engorgement at the affected site. Clogged milk ducts can occur when mothers skip or miss feedings, if she is wearing tight clothing or bras, and due to poor latch-on and positing. To help open the blocked milk duct and relieve symptoms, mothers should continue breastfeeding their baby, making sure to start feeds on the affected breast; this will help empty the breast. They can also apply warm compresses or take a warm shower and massage the clog. Lastly, the mother needs to refer to her health care provider or lactation consultant for assistance with improving feeding techniques. If the clogged milk duct is not diagnosed and properly treated, it can progress to a more serious condition called mastitis.

**Mastitis:** Mastitis is a localized inflammation of the breast that can be infectious (most common) or noninfectious. Symptoms typically include fever, swelling, breast pain, redness,

and muscle pain. Noninfectious mastitis is usually caused by milk stasis, which is the buildup of milk within the breast tissue. Oftentimes noninfectious mastitis will progress to a mastitis with infection because of the bacteria growth in the stagnant milk. Mastitis tends to occur as a result of prolonged engorgement or poor drainage caused by blocked milk ducts, inefficient milk removal or infrequent feedings, oversupply of milk, and nipple trauma and pressure on the breast from tight-fitting clothing or bras. Mothers who suspect that they may have mastitis must seek treatment from a medical provider. Treatment will depend upon the severity of the infection and may include antibiotic therapy, use of fever reducers, and pain relievers such as ibuprofen and acetaminophen. In severe cases of mastitis the patient may require minor surgery to help drain any abscesses that may have formed due to the infection.

## Patient Problem/Analyze Cues/Prioritize Hypotheses

# Risk for Impaired Skin Integrity

*due to* the use of improper breastfeeding technique (often from poor newborn latch-on and/or positioning).

*Desired Outcome/Generate Solutions:* Within 24 hours of this diagnosis, the patient will demonstrate how to properly latch and position her newborn to the breast, and the skin around the nipple will remain intact.

| ASSESSMENT—RECOGNIZE CUES/ INTERVENTIONS—TAKE ACTION | RATIONALES |
|---|---|
| Observe and assess the patient while breastfeeding. | The assessment can confirm the diagnosis. The use of poor breastfeeding techniques is a common cause for nipple injury. |
| Assist the patient with breastfeeding. | The clinician will be able to help the patient correct any poor breastfeeding techniques. |
| Consult with a lactation consultant in the patient's care. | Lactation consultants are experts in breastfeeding. They can provide additional support and education to the patient. |
| Provide patient with resources for outpatient breastfeeding support. | The patient may require additional breastfeeding help after leaving the hospital. |
| Educate patient on how to properly care for her nipples while breastfeeding: <br>• She needs to use only water to wash breast and nipples; encourage the patient to avoid using soaps or detergents. <br>• Avoid harsh washing and/or drying of her breast and nipples. <br>• Nursing pads are to be changed often when they become moist. <br>• Encourage patients to apply a little breast milk on nipples after feedings to help protect them from injury. | Soaps and aggressive washing and/or drying of the breast and nipples can cause them to be dry and crack. <br><br>The patient needs to avoid excessive moisture of the nipples and breast because it can increase her risk for obtaining an infection. <br><br>Breast milk contains natural antibodies, which can help prevent and treat breast and nipple injury. |

## Patient Problem/Analyze Cues/Prioritize Hypotheses

# Breast Engorgement

*due to* the excess accumulation of milk in the breast or the increased blood flow to the breast as a result of the onset of lactation.

*Desired Outcome/Generate Solutions:* Within 48 hours after interventions, the patient will verbalize a decrease in engorgement symptoms.

| ASSESSMENT—RECOGNIZE CUES/ INTERVENTIONS—TAKE ACTION | RATIONALES |
|---|---|
| Assess for and instruct the patient about the signs and symptoms of engorgement. Common symptoms include<br><br>• breast that feels full and firm/hard,<br><br>• breast tenderness or pain,<br><br>• swollen breast, and<br><br>• breast that are warm to the touch. | The assessment can confirm the diagnosis.<br><br>When the patient understands the symptoms associated with engorgement, she can differentiate it from other breastfeeding complications. |
| Assess patient's breastfeeding history (including, but not limited to, when breastfeeding was initiated, frequency of breastfeeding; and any problems she is having with breastfeeding or have had with breastfeeding in the past). | It is important to have an understanding of the patient's current and past breastfeeding routine because it can provide insight into the possible cause of the engorgement. |
| Observe and assist the patient with breastfeeding. | The clinician will have the opportunity to ensure the patient is using good feeding techniques, and help the patient make corrections as needed. Improper positioning and latching can cause the inadequate removal of milk and result in engorgement. |
| Encourage the patient to breastfeed or express milk at least every 2 hours and at least twice during the night. If patient has problems latching baby due to swelling, have patient express milk manually or with breast pump. | To effectively manage engorgement, the patient needs to remove the milk from her breast. By regularly nursing, the patient can prevent excess milk accumulation.<br><br>Swollen and hardened nipples can make it difficult for the baby to nurse. Patients may find that expressing small amounts of milk before breastfeeding may soften and decrease swelling around nipples, therefore making it easier for the baby to latch. However, the use of a breast pump should be limited to immediately prior to nursing because the overuse can stimulate the production of more milk, thus increasing the engorgement. |
| Provide the patient with cold compresses. Instruct the patient to apply the cold compresses to her breast after or between feeding. | Applying something cold to the breast can help relieve pain and swelling. Patient needs to avoid the cold compress before feedings because it can decrease milk flow. |
| Encourage the patient to apply a warm compress or take a warm shower before nursing. | Applying heat can help enhance and encourage letdown and aid with the removal of milk. |
| Administer a mild pain reliever (acetaminophen or ibuprofen) for pain, as prescribed. | Some patients may experience pain with engorgement, pain medication can help decrease this discomfort. |
| Educate patient on to how to prevent engorgement; which can include the following:<br><br>• Breastfeeding or expressing milk at least every 2 hours and at least twice during the night.<br><br>• Avoiding missing feedings.<br><br>• Massaging the breast while nursing.<br><br>• Alternating breasts with each feeding.<br><br>• Asking for help if experiencing problems with breastfeeding. | To prevent engorgement, encourage the patient to perform interventions that result in the emptying of the breast. Missing or skipping feedings and poor latch and positioning can cause the overfilling of milk in the breast, which results in engorgement. It is important that patients seek help if they are having problems with breastfeeding to help prevent engorgement and further complications. |
| Consult with a lactation consultant in the patient's care. | Lactation consultants are experts in breastfeeding. They can provide additional support and education to the patient. |
| Provide patient with resources for outpatient breastfeeding support. | The patient may require additional breastfeeding help after leaving the hospital. |

Patient Problem/Analyze Cues/Prioritize Hypotheses

# Deficient Knowledge

*due* to unfamiliarity with how to breastfeed and/or ineffective breastfeeding

***Desired Outcome/Generate Solutions:*** Patient will verbalize and demonstrate proper breastfeeding techniques. The patient will also accurately verbalize the signs of effective breastfeeding (infant will gain weight appropriately and will have an adequate output for age, and the fontanelles are flat and soft).

| ASSESSMENT—RECOGNIZE CUES/ INTERVENTIONS—TAKE ACTION | RATIONALES |
|---|---|
| Assess the patient's health, prenatal, medication, and breastfeeding (if she has breastfed before) history. | It is important to identify those patients that may be at risk for having breastfeeding complications, in an effort to provide the patient with the proper support and education. |
| Assess the patient's knowledge on breastfeeding and any concerns that she may have. | Getting an understanding of the patient's past and current knowledge and concerns about breastfeeding helps the clinician tailor their education to meet the specific needs of the patient. |
| Instruct about four of the most commonly used breastfeeding positions (cradle, side lying, clutch/football, cross-cradle) and assist with performing each position. | There are several different positions that the patient can use to breastfeed. Allowing the patient to try different positions provides her with the opportunity to find the one that is most comfortable for her. |
| Assist with properly latching newborn. Educate on the signs of an effective latch. | An improper latch can lead to nipple injury and pain. If a poor latch is not corrected, it can result in complications like plugged milk ducts, engorgement, and more severe problems like mastitis. |
| Instruct the patient on how to properly care for nipples while breastfeeding:<br><br>• Use only water to wash breast and nipples; encourage the patient to avoid using soaps or detergents.<br>• Avoid harsh washing and/or drying of her breast and nipples.<br>• Change nursing pads often when they become moist.<br>• Encourage the patient to apply a little breast milk on nipples after feedings to help protect them from injury. | Good breast and nipple care can help prevent injury and pain. |
| Explain the signs of effective breastfeeding. | This intervention enables the patient to recognize if breastfeeding is being done correctly or if changes need to be made. |
| Educate patient on when to seek out help from a health care provider. | This intervention enables the patient to recognize and report signs of breast infections; like mastitis (redness, hardness, pain, swelling in breast; fever; and flu like symptoms) and thrush (flaky, itchy, or shiny skin on nipples or areola; cracked and/or red nipples; shooting or stabbing pain in breast during or after feeding). |
| Encourage the patient to maintain a healthy diet and take prenatal vitamins. Instruct them about alcohol consumption, caffeine, and foods to avoid while breastfeeding. | Breastfeeding mothers need to eat a well-balanced diet and take their prenatal vitamins to help them meet the nutritional and energy needs required to produce breast milk.<br><br>Although not drinking alcohol is the safest option for breastfeeding mothers, consuming a moderate amount of alcohol (up to one standard drink) has not shown to be harmful. If drinking, the patient must wait at least 2 hours before nursing.<br><br>Caffeine passes from mother to infant through breast milk. However, most breastfeeding women can drink about two to three cups of a caffeinated beverage a day without significant effects to the baby. Nonetheless, if the infant shows signs of sensitivity (irritability or difficulty sleeping) to caffeine, the mother may need to lessen that amount.<br><br>Although there are not many foods that the patient cannot eat, they must avoid eating fish with high concentrations of mercury. Mercury can be harmful to the brain and nervous system if exposed to too much of it over time. |

| ASSESSMENT—RECOGNIZE CUES/ INTERVENTIONS—TAKE ACTION | RATIONALES |
|---|---|
| Involve the lactation consultant in the patient's care. Educate patient on when to seek out help from a lactation consultant. | Lactation consultants are experts in breastfeeding. They can provide additional support and education to the patient. |
| Prior to discharging mother and newborn, ensure that an infant follow-up appointment has been made. | It is important that a health care provider assesses the newborn to ensure that they are healthy and are growing appropriately. |

## ADDITIONAL PROBLEM:

| "Psychosocial Support for the Patient" for relevant problems such as *Fatigue* (interrupted sleep) and *Anxiety* | Chapter 8 |
|---|---|

## ✓ PATIENT–FAMILY TEACHING AND DISCHARGE PLANNING

Breastfeeding is considered the best source of nutrition for most babies. It provides many health benefits for both the mother and the baby. Include written and verbal information about the following:

✓ Different breastfeeding positions and how to obtain a good latch.

✓ Signs and symptoms of breastfeeding complications and when to call the health care provider; and the importance of contacting them in a timely manner.

✓ Signs of effective breastfeeding.

✓ Proper breast and nipple care.

✓ Nutrition while breastfeeding.

✓ When to follow up with health care provider for scheduled appointments.

✓ Contact information for lactation support if needed. Many birthing centers have community support groups for breastfeeding mothers.

✓ Online resources:

- Office on Women's Health: https://www.womenshealth.gov/breastfeeding/breastfeeding-resources
- La Leche League U.S.A.: https://lllusa.org/; WIC Breastfeeding Support: https://wicbreastfeeding.fns.usda.gov/

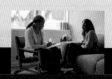

# Delirium 98

## OVERVIEW/PATHOPHYSIOLOGY

Delirium is a reversible disturbance of attention, consciousness, cognition, and perception that occurs in varying degrees. It develops over a short period of time (hours or a few days) and generally lasts less than 3 months. By comparison, dementia is not reversible and is a chronic syndrome (see *Dementia—Alzheimer's Type*, Chapter 101). However, dementia is often the diagnosis assigned to someone who may actually have delirium. Delirium can be caused by several factors, such as medications, substance use disorder, fluid, electrolyte or metabolic imbalances, sleep deprivation, hypoxia, fever, and infection. It is often one of the first symptoms of life-threatening conditions such as sepsis or pneumonia. If the underlying condition is treated promptly, delirium is usually reversible.

## HEALTH CARE SETTING

Acute care, long-term care

## ASSESSMENT

A variety of manifestations may occur, such as agitation, altered personality, decreased or altered level of consciousness (LOC), altered cognitive functioning, impaired memory, hallucinations, lack of self-awareness, restlessness, wandering, and incoherent or rambling speech.

## DIAGNOSTIC STUDIES

Blood tests such as complete blood count (CBC) are done to check for infection; blood chemistries are done to rule out fluid, electrolyte and metabolic imbalances, and to check renal function. A urinalysis should be completed as well because a urinary tract infection is the number one cause of delirium in older adults, including those with dementia. Pulse oximetry or arterial blood gases (ABGs) are done to check for hypoxia and metabolic disorders. A chest x-ray may be done to assess for pneumonia; an electrocardiogram may indicate a cardiac dysrhythmia (which may be the cause for reduced cardiac output). In some cases, magnetic resonance imaging and computed tomography (CT scan) may be done if a brain lesion is suspected.

## Patient Problem/Analyze Cues/Prioritize Hypotheses

# Confusion

*due to* decreased renal or cardiac function; altered sensory/perceptual reception occurring with poor vision or hearing; short-term memory loss occurring with decreased brain oxygenation or fluid/electrolyte imbalance

***Desired Outcome/Generate Outcomes:*** Optimally, acute confusion diminishes following interventions.

| ASSESSMENT—RECOGNIZE CUES/ INTERVENTIONS—TAKE ACTION | RATIONALES |
|---|---|
| Assess the patient's baseline LOC and mental status on admission. Obtain preconfusion functional and mental status abilities from significant other or clinical caregiver. | It is important to obtain a baseline for subsequent assessments of a patient's confusion. |
| Administer a quick tool that tests cognitive function, such as the Mini-Cog (https://mini-cog.com/). This test has two components: a three-item recall test for memory and a clock-drawing test. The scores for both actions are combined for a final score. | The Mini-Cog is a screening tool that assesses cognitive function and can be used to indicate whether further diagnostic testing is needed. |

| ASSESSMENT—RECOGNIZE CUES/ INTERVENTIONS—TAKE ACTION | RATIONALES |
|---|---|
| Test short-term memory by showing the patient how to use the call light, having the patient return the demonstration, and then waiting at least 5 minutes before having the patient demonstrate the use of the call light again. Document the patient's actions in behavioral terms; describe the "confused" behavior specifically. | Inability to remember beyond 5 minutes indicates poor short-term memory. |
| Identify the cause of acute confusion (delirium). | Acute confusion is caused by physical and psychosocial conditions and not by age alone. For example, oximetry or ABG values may reveal low oxygenation levels, serum glucose or fingerstick glucose may reveal high or low glucose level, and electrolytes and CBC will ascertain imbalances and/or the presence of elevated white blood cell count as a determinant of infection. Hydration status may be determined by pinching skin over the sternum or forehead for turgor (tenting may occur with dehydration) and checking for dry mucous membranes and a furrowed tongue. |
| Obtain a complete history, including all medications (prescribed, over-the-counter [OTC], herbal products, and recreational substances). | The use of medications and other substances may be a cause of cognitive impairment. |
| Assess for pain using a rating scale of 0–10. If the patient is unable to use a scale, assess for behavioral cues such as grimacing, clenched fists, frowning, and hitting. The FLACC pain scale includes these behaviors and is done to assess pain in nonverbal patients or patients who are unable to self-report.<br><br>Ask the family or significant other to assist in identifying pain behaviors. (See "Pain," Chapter 5, for more interventions.) | Acute confusion can be a sign of pain. |
| Treat the patient for pain, as prescribed, and monitor behaviors. | If pain is the cause of the confusion, the patient's behavior should change accordingly. |
| Review the cardiac status. Assess the apical pulse and notify the health care provider of an irregular pulse or decreased pulse rate that is new to the patient. If the patient is on a cardiac monitor or telemetry, watch for dysrhythmias; notify the health care provider accordingly. | Dysrhythmias and other cardiac dysfunctions may result in decreased oxygenation, which can lead to confusion. |
| Review the current medications, including OTC drugs. | Toxic levels of certain medications, such as digoxin, cause acute confusion. Medications that are anticholinergic also can cause confusion, as can drug interactions. |
| Use the 3-minute confusion assessment method (3D-CAM) to help identify the presence or absence of delirium, and for ongoing monitoring. | The 3D-CAM tool (Marcantonio et al., 2014) can be administered in a short period of time. It is a simple, standardized tool that can be used by bedside clinicians to identify and monitor the presence or absence of delirium. |
| Monitor the intake and output at least every 8 hours. | Optimally, output should match intake. Dehydration can result in acute confusion. |
| Review the patient's creatinine clearance test to assess renal function. | Renal function plays an important role in fluid balance and is the main mechanism of drug clearance. Blood urea nitrogen and serum creatinine are affected by hydration status and in older patients reveal only part of the picture. Therefore, to fully understand and assess renal function in older patients, creatinine clearance must be tested. |
| When first meeting the patient, introduce yourself, address the patient by name, and speak slowly and clearly. | The patient may be anxious and not understand why strangers are in the room. |
| Have the patient wear glasses and hearing aids or keep them close to the bedside and within easy reach for patient use. | Glasses and hearing aids are likely to help decrease sensory confusion. |
| Keep the patient's urinal and other routinely used items within easy reach of the patient. | A confused patient may wait until it is too late to seek assistance with toileting. |

Continued

| ASSESSMENT—RECOGNIZE CUES/ INTERVENTIONS—TAKE ACTION | RATIONALES |
|---|---|
| If the patient has short-term memory problems, take them to the toilet or offer the urinal or bedpan every 2 hours while awake and every 4 hours during the night. Establish a toileting schedule and post it on the patient care plan and, inconspicuously, at the bedside. | A patient with a short-term memory problem cannot be expected to use the call light. Establishing a toileting schedule can help to prevent episodes of incontinence. |
| ⚠ Check on the patient at least every 30 minutes and every time you pass the room. Place the patient close to the nurses' station if possible. Provide an environment that is nonstimulating and safe. | A confused patient requires extra safety precautions. Excessive stimulation may cause anxiety and/or agitation. |
| Provide television, radio, or music based on the patient's preference. | These measures may provide distraction and stimulation. A favorite TV show, for example, may be comforting. |
| Attempt to reorient the patient to his or her surroundings as needed. Keep a clock with large numerals and a large print calendar at the bedside; verbally remind the patient of the date and day as needed. Use a whiteboard if available to write the date and update daily. | Reorientation may decrease confusion. |
| Tell the patient in simple terms what is occurring. For example, "It's time to eat breakfast," "This medicine is for your heart," "I'm going to help you get out of bed." | Sentences that are more complex may not be understood. |
| Encourage the patient's significant other to bring items familiar to the patient, including blanket, bedspread, and pictures of family and pets. | Familiar items may promote orientation while also providing comfort. |
| If the patient becomes belligerent, angry, or argumentative while you are attempting to reorient, **stop this approach**. Do not argue with the patient or the patient's interpretation of the environment. State, "I can understand why you may [hear, think, see] that." | This approach prevents the escalation of anger in a confused person. |
| ⚠ If the patient displays hostile behavior or misperceives your role (e.g., nurse becomes thief, jailer), leave the room. Return in 15 minutes. Introduce yourself to the patient as though you had never met. Begin dialogue anew. | Patients who are acutely confused have poor short-term memory and may not remember the previous encounter or that you were involved in that encounter. |
| If the patient attempts to leave the hospital, walk with them and attempt distraction. Ask the patient to tell you about the destination. For example, "That sounds like a wonderful place! Tell me about it." Keep your tone pleasant and conversational. Continue walking with the patient away from exits and doors around the unit. After a few minutes, attempt to guide the patient back to the room. Offer refreshments and a rest. For example, "We've been walking for a while and I'm a little tired. Why don't we sit and have some juice while we talk?" | Distraction is an effective means of reversing a behavior in a patient who is confused. |
| If the patient has a permanent or severe cognitive impairment, check on her or him at least every 30 minutes and reorient to baseline mental status as indicated; however, do not argue with the patient about his or her perception of reality. | Arguing can cause a cognitively impaired person to become aggressive and combative. **Note:** Individuals with severe cognitive impairment (e.g., Alzheimer's disease or dementia) also can experience acute confusional states (i.e., delirium) and can be returned to their baseline mental state. |
| If the patient tries to climb out of bed, offer a urinal or bedpan or assist to the commode. | The patient may need to use the toilet. |
| ⚠ Alternatively, if the patient is not on bedrest, place the patient in a chair or wheelchair at the nurses' station. | This action provides added supervision to promote a patient's safety while also promoting stimulation and preventing isolation. |
| ⚠ If the patient continues to try to climb out of bed, obtain a sitter or electronic camera or telemetry device to monitor the patient continuously. | Some facilities offer electronic camera/telemetry monitoring where a caregiver can speak to the patient to remind him or her not to get out of bed or notify the nurses if the patient continues to try to leave the bed. An in-room sitter will help the patient as needed and prevent injuries from falling. |

| ASSESSMENT—RECOGNIZE CUES/ INTERVENTIONS—TAKE ACTION | RATIONALES |
|---|---|
| Bargain with the patient. Try to establish an agreement to stay for a defined period, such as until the health care provider, meal, or significant other arrives. | This is a delaying strategy to defuse anger. Because of poor memory and attention span, the patient may forget he or she wanted to leave. |
| Have the patient's significant other talk with the patient by phone or come in and sit with the patient if the patient's behavior requires checking more often than every 30 minutes. | These actions by the significant other may help promote the patient's safety. |
| If the patient is attempting to pull out tubes, hide them (e.g., under blankets). Put a stockinette mesh dressing over intravenous (IV) lines. Tape feeding tubes to the side of the patient's face using paper tape and drape the tube behind the patient's ear. | Keeping these items out of the patient's sight may reduce the chance of interference with them. |
| Evaluate the continued need for certain therapies. For example, if the patient is now drinking, contact the provider to discontinue the IV line; if the patient is eating, contact the provider to discontinue the feeding tube; if the patient has an indwelling urethral catheter, obtain an order to discontinue the catheter and begin a toileting routine. | Such therapies may become irritating stimuli. |
| Use restraints with caution and according to agency policy. Restraints should only be done as a last resort, after all measures have failed and when the patient is a safety risk to self and others. | Patients can become more agitated when wrist and arm restraints are used. |
| See also "Dementia—Alzheimer's Type," Chapter 101, as appropriate. | |

## Patient Problem/Analyze Cues/Prioritize Hypotheses

# Risk for Injury

*due to* impaired cognition

***Desired Outcomes/Generate Outcomes:*** The patient sustains no evidence of injury or harm as a result of mental status or sensory losses.

For "Assessment—Recognize Cues/Interventions—Take Action" and "Rationales," refer to "General Care of Patients with Neurologic Disorders," Chapter 36, for *Risk for Falls*.

### ADDITIONAL PROBLEMS:

| | |
|---|---|
| "Older Adult Care" for *Confusion, Risk for Aspiration, Risk for Dehydration* | Chapter 3 |
| "Psychosocial Support for the Patient" for *Anxiety* | Chapter 8 |
| "Psychosocial Support for the Patient's Family and Significant Others" for two separate *Difficulty Coping* problems. | Chapter 9 |

### ✓ PATIENT–FAMILY TEACHING AND DISCHARGE PLANNING

- ✓ Medications, including drug name; purpose; dosage; frequency; precautions; drug–drug, food–drug, and herb–drug interactions; and potential side effects.
- ✓ Importance of following up with medical care as well as psychiatric care as needed.
- ✓ Importance of maintaining a healthy lifestyle—balanced diet, exercise, and regular adequate sleep patterns.
- ✓ Emphasize to the family that the delirium may be short-lived and diminish once the underlying condition is resolved.
- ✓ Emphasize safety measures to the patient and family. Assist the patient as needed with activities of daily living and ambulation.
- ✓ Provide teaching to the patient (as appropriate) and family about the cause of the delirium, if known, and measures being done to treat it.
- ✓ Assess the home environment and resources needed. Assess whether the patient will be able to return to the previous living environment or whether in-home assistance is needed or consideration of another arrangement.
- ✓ Refer to community resources (Meals on Wheels, adult day care services) as appropriate.

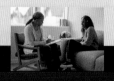

## OVERVIEW/PATHOPHYSIOLOGY

*Anxiety* is a neurochemical reaction involving the hypothalamus–pituitary–adrenal axis. It is a response to a real or perceived threat and often precedes significant changes, for example, beginning new employment. When it is prolonged or excessive, crippling physical and psychologic symptoms may develop. The anxiety disorders are characterized by anxiety symptoms and behavioral efforts to avoid these symptoms. They are the most common psychiatric disorders in the United States. Comorbidity with depression is common. Acute anxiety creates physical sensations of arousal (fight or flight), an emotional state of panic, decreased cognitive problem-solving ability, and altered spiritual state with hopelessness and/or helplessness. Anxiety is considered abnormal when reasons for it are not evident or when manifestations are excessive in intensity and duration. Psychologic *stress* refers to the response of an individual appraising the environment and concluding that it exceeds his or her resources and jeopardizes well-being. Some stressors are universal, whereas others are person specific because of highly individual interpretations of events.

Anxiety is always part of the stress response and has four levels, ranging from mild to panic. Normally, a person experiencing mild-to-moderate anxiety uses voluntary behaviors called *coping skills*, that is, distraction, deliberate avoidance, and information seeking. The use of coping skills is a positive adaptation to stress and anxiety. Another common response is the use of unconscious defense mechanisms, including repression, suppression, projection, introjection, reaction formation, undoing, displacement, denial, and regression. Unconscious defense mechanisms are negative and maladaptive. Depending on the level of anxiety, work, personal, and/or social functions may be disrupted. If stress continues at an unbearable level or if the individual lacks sufficient biologic mechanisms for coping, an anxiety disorder may develop. There are six major categories.

***Generalized anxiety disorder.*** Characterized by excessive, uncontrollable worrying that out of proportion to the impact of events. This lasts over a period of at least 6 months. Symptoms include motor tension (trembling; shakiness; muscle tension, aches, soreness; easy fatigue), autonomic hyperactivity (shortness of breath, palpitations, sweating, dry mouth, dizziness, nausea, diarrhea, frequent urination), and scanning behavior (feeling on edge, having an exaggerated startle response, difficulty concentrating, sleep disturbance, irritability).

***Panic disorder.*** Characterized by a sudden onset of intense fear or discomfort with at least four of the following symptoms: palpitations or pounding heart, sweating, trembling or shaking, sensations of smothering or difficulty breathing, feeling of choking, chest pain, nausea, feeling dizzy or faint, feeling of unreality or losing control, numbness, and chills or flushes. Normal function is impeded, there is a severely altered perceptual field, and the person may have a misinterpretation of reality.

***Phobias.*** Characterized by a persistent and severe fear of a clearly identifiable object or situation despite awareness that the fear is unreasonable. There are two types: specific and social. Specific phobias are subdivided into five types: animals, natural environment (e.g., lightning), blood-injection-injury type, situational (e.g., flying, tunnels or bridges), and other (situations that could lead to choking or contracting an illness). *Social phobia* relates to profound fear of social or performance situations in which embarrassment could occur.

*Agoraphobia* is characterized by feelings of intense fear of being alone in open or public places where escape might be difficult. Individuals with agoraphobia become immobilized with anxiety and may find it impossible to leave their homes.

***Acute stress disorder.*** Like posttraumatic stress disorder (PTSD), the problem begins with exposure to an identifiable traumatic event, with a response of intense fear, helplessness, or horror. The person's usual coping skills are ineffective. In addition, the person shows dissociative symptoms, that is, subjective sense of numbing, feeling "in a daze," depersonalization, or amnesia, and clearly tries to avoid stimuli that arouse recollection of the trauma. But just like PTSD, the victim reexperiences the trauma and shows functional impairment in social, occupational, and problem-solving skills. The key difference is that this syndrome occurs within 4 weeks of the traumatic event and only lasts 2 days to 4 weeks. The degree of response generally depends on the person's prior experience.

***Anxiety disorder caused by a general medical condition.*** May be characterized by severe anxiety, panic attacks, or obsessions or compulsions. The cause is clearly related to a medical problem, excluding delirium. History, physical examination, and laboratory findings support a specific diagnosis, for example, hypoglycemia, pheochromocytoma, or thyroid disease.

***Anxiety disorder not otherwise specified.*** Describes an individual with significant anxiety or phobic avoidance but not enough symptoms to meet the criteria for other anxiety or adjustment disorder diagnoses. The patient may show a mixed anxiety-depressive picture or demonstrate social phobic symptoms related to having another medical problem (such as Parkinson disease), or present with insufficient data to rule out a general medical condition or substance abuse.

## HEALTH CARE SETTING

Depends on the type of anxiety disorder. Primary (outpatient) care is likely for most categories, and possibly emergency department care for panic disorders. If the patient has developed agoraphobia, psychiatric home care may be the best care option. Some patients may be hospitalized for physiologic problems or to treat psychiatric needs.

## ASSESSMENT

*Physical indicators.* Dry mouth, elevated heart rate, blood pressure or respiratory rate, diarrhea, increased urination, nausea, diaphoresis, hyperventilation, fatigue, insomnia, sexual dysfunction, irritability, and being tense.

*Emotional indicators.* From slight discomfort and restlessness to fear, sense of impending doom, helplessness, insecurity, low self-confidence, anger, and/or guilt.

*Cognitive indicators.* Mild anxiety produces increased awareness and problem-solving skills. Higher levels produce narrowed or distorted perceptual field; missed details; diminished problem-solving skills; and catastrophic, dichotomous thoughts resulting in deteriorated logical thinking.

*Social indicators.* Occupational, social, and familial role, for example, marital and parental functioning may be adversely affected by anxiety and therefore needs to be assessed. High levels of anxiety may result in social withdrawal.

*Spiritual indicators.* Hopelessness/helplessness, feeling of being cut off from God, and anger at God may be experienced.

*Suicidality.* Suicide assessment is critical with anxious patients, especially those with panic disorder. For patients suffering dual diagnoses of depression and substance abuse or other anxiety disorders, risk for self-injury is even greater. Suicidal assessment includes questions to determine the presence of suicidal ideation, intent, presence, and lethality of any plan. Essential questions to ask include the following:

- Have you thought of hurting yourself?
- Are you presently thinking about hurting yourself?
- If you have been thinking about suicide, do you have a plan?
- What is the plan?
- Have you thought about what life would be like for others if you were no longer a part of it?

A previous history of suicide attempts combined with depression places the patient at higher risk in the present. A patient whose depression is lifting is at higher risk for suicide than a severely depressed individual. The improvement may result in an increase in energy. This increased energy is not enough to make the patient feel well or hopeful, but it is enough to carry out a suicidal plan.

## DIAGNOSTIC TESTS

There is no specific diagnostic test for anxiety disorders. The diagnosis of anxiety is made through history, interview of the patient and family, and observation of verbal and nonverbal behaviors. There are a few reliable and effective scales to assess anxiety that include the Severity Measure for Generalized Anxiety Disorder, the Anxiety Symptoms Questionnaire, Patient Health Questionnaire Anxiety and Depression Scale, Hamilton Anxiety Rating Scale, and Beck Anxiety Inventory.

## Patient and Significant Other Problems/Analyze Cues/Prioritize Hypotheses

# Deficient Knowledge

*due to* unfamiliarity with the causes, signs and symptoms, and treatment of anxiety or specific anxiety disorders

*Desired Outcome/Generate Solutions:* By discharge (if inpatient) or after 2 weeks of outpatient treatment, the patient and significant other verbalize accurate information about at least two of the possible causes of anxiety, four of the signs and symptoms of the specific anxiety disorder, and the available treatment options.

| ASSESSMENT—RECOGNIZE CUES/ INTERVENTIONS—TAKE ACTION | RATIONALES |
|---|---|
| Assess the patient's understanding of anxiety, its signs and symptoms, and its treatment. | This assessment helps the nurse reinforce, as needed, information about anxiety and correct any misunderstanding. Many people lack understanding about the physiologic basis for anxiety and that feeling a little worry is different from the overwhelming anxiety experienced by those who have an anxiety disorder. |
| Inform the patient and significant other that anxiety disorders are physiologic disorders caused by the interplay of many factors, such as stress, imbalance in brain chemistry, psychodynamic factors, faulty learning, and genetics. | Many people with anxiety disorders lack the knowledge that anxiety disorders represent a complex interplay of treatable biologic, genetic, and environmental factors. |

Continued

| ASSESSMENT—RECOGNIZE CUES/ INTERVENTIONS—TAKE ACTION | RATIONALES |
|---|---|
| Inform the patient and significant other about the holistic nature of anxiety, which produces physical, emotional, cognitive, social, and spiritual symptoms. | Often, people believe that anxiety equates with nervousness and are not aware of other signs and symptoms that make this a holistic disorder. |
| Inform the patient and significant other that anxiety disorders are treatable. | Receiving information about potential treatments may help to alleviate the feelings of hopelessness and anxiety the patient may be experiencing. |
| Medications are usually indicated for the treatment of these disorders and may include antidepressants and anxiolytics or a combination of medications. In addition, other interventions are useful, including dietary interventions (e.g., elimination of caffeinated products), and behavioral therapy, which may include breathing control, exercise, relaxation techniques, and psychological interventions (i.e., distraction, positive self-talk, psychoeducation, exposure therapy, systematic desensitization, implosive therapy, social interventions, cognitive behavioral therapy, and stress and time management interventions). For more information about medications, See *Deficient Knowledge* (regarding prescribed medications), later. | |

## Patient Problem/Analyze Cues/Prioritize Hypotheses

# Anxiety (Recurring Panic Attacks)

*due to* the lack of knowledge regarding the cause and treatment

**Desired Outcomes/Generate Solutions:** Within 48 hours of treatment/intervention, the patient verbalizes methods for dealing with panic attacks and the understanding that panic attacks are not life threatening and that they are time limited and demonstrates this knowledge accordingly. Within 2 weeks, the patient will express having reduced anxiety and fewer panic attacks.

| ASSESSMENT—RECOGNIZE CUES/ INTERVENTIONS—TAKE ACTION | RATIONALES |
|---|---|
| Assess the patient's current understanding of the nature and cause of and treatments for panic disorders as well as current coping strategies employed by the patient. | Most patients who experience panic attacks have experienced several attacks before obtaining an accurate diagnosis. Panic attacks have an unexpected, abrupt onset and peak within 10 minutes. Patients with panic attacks fear they are losing control or "going crazy." Some believe they are having a heart attack or are dying. |
| | Patients sometimes adopt unhealthy coping strategies, such as restricting their movement (i.e., avoiding bridges if they have experienced a panic attack on a bridge or avoiding shopping in stores if this is where a panic attack occurred). It is important to provide information that the patient can understand and use to make appropriate lifestyle changes. |
| Administer the medication as prescribed for panic attacks. | Panic attacks are neurobiologic events that respond to medications. See *Deficient Knowledge* (regarding prescribed medications), later. |
| Provide instruction on reducing or eliminating dietary substances that may promote anxiety and panic, such as caffeine, food coloring, artificial sweeteners, and monosodium glutamate (MSG). | Caffeine increases feelings of anxiety. However, caffeine withdrawal symptoms also can stimulate panic. Therefore the plan needs to include a focus on reducing consumption first, followed by elimination from the diet. Some individuals are sensitive to food colorings, artificial sweeteners, and MSG. This sensitivity is experienced as increased anxiety. |
| Provide instruction about relaxation techniques; assist with practicing imagery, deep breathing, progressive relaxation, and use of relaxation tapes. | Relaxation is effective in reducing anxiety. The patient's ability to master relaxation techniques provides a sense of control and enhances self-care ability. |

| ASSESSMENT—RECOGNIZE CUES/ INTERVENTIONS—TAKE ACTION | RATIONALES |
|---|---|
| Stay with the patient during panic attacks. Use short, simple directions. Encourage the patient to use relaxation, remind the patient that the attack is time limited. Ask the patients to identify their feelings. | During a panic attack, the ability to refocus is limited. The patient needs reassurance that he or she is not dying and that this will pass. |
| Encourage patients to describe and discuss their feelings. | This helps patients to recognize what is happening to them. |
| Move the patient to a calm, quiet, less stimulating environment. | Expressing feelings help the patients increase their awareness of the correlation between feelings and actions. |
| **Remain calm**. | A calm quiet environment will help to identify and reduce stimulation including interactions with other patients that provoke anxiety |
|  | If the nurse meets the patient's anxiety with their own anxiety, it will likely increase the patient's negative behavior. |
| Instruct the patient to self-administer anxiolytic medication when the first signs and symptoms of a panic attack start and initiate coping strategies to ward off the most severe symptoms. | This information empowers the patient by providing a strategy to deal with panic attacks. As patients become aware of early signs of oncoming panic, taking the prescribed anxiolytics and initiating relaxation and cognitive strategies to reduce the magnitude of the event will increase a sense of mastery over panic anxiety. |

## Patient Problem/Analyze Cues/Prioritize Hypotheses

# Impaired Psychologic Function (Agoraphobia)

*due to* anxiety disorder

**Desired Outcome/Generate Solutions:** By discharge (if inpatient) or after 4 weeks of outpatient treatment, the patient demonstrates behavior consistent with increased social interaction.

| ASSESSMENT—RECOGNIZE CUES/ INTERVENTIONS—TAKE ACTION | RATIONALES |
|---|---|
| Assess the degree of social isolation experienced by the patient in response to agoraphobia. | It is critical to know how isolated the patient has become secondary to agoraphobia. If the patient no longer leaves her or his home and has no contact with anyone except those who either live in the home or those who come to visit, the social phobia is very severe and will require more intense work to overcome it, including home visits. |
| Provide the patient with activities that promote socialization without promoting avoidance of activities yet do not increase anxiety. Assist the patient in a graded exposure plan to gradually increase independent functions and interactions with others. | Gradual exposure is effective in treating agoraphobia. Help patients understand that avoidance behaviors are their mechanism for avoiding anxiety. |
| Assist the patient with practicing relaxation techniques. | Relaxation helps mitigate impending panic attacks. |
| Discuss alternatives for social interaction. Introduce individual therapy before group therapy with a goal of joining group activities and therapy gradually. Involve family in group activities. | Patients may need assistance with developing activity plans. Appropriate alternatives for social interaction may be volunteer work in small groups and taking a friend to a social event to increase comfort. Introduce social interaction as tolerated. |

## Patient Problem/Analyze Cues/Prioritize Solutions

# Difficulty Coping

*due to* a perceived inadequate level of control or support/resources in dealing with situational crises

**Desired Outcome/Generate Outcomes:** Within 24–48 hours of intervention/treatment, the patient begins to identify ineffective coping behaviors and consequences, expresses feelings appropriately, identifies options, uses resources effectively, and uses effective problem-solving techniques.

| ASSESSMENT—RECOGNIZE CUES/ INTERVENTIONS—TAKE ACTION | RATIONALES |
|---|---|
| Assess the patient's previous successful methods of coping with life problems. | How individuals have handled problems in the past is a reliable predictor of how current problems will be handled. Successful methods reinforce effective coping strategies. |
| Determine the use of substances (alcohol, other drugs, smoking, and eating patterns). | The patient may have used substances as coping mechanisms to control anxiety. This pattern can interfere with the ability to deal with the current situation. |
| Provide information regarding different ways to deal with situations that promote anxious feelings, for example, identification and appropriate expression of feelings and problem-solving skills. | This information provides patients with an opportunity to learn new coping skills. |
| Role-play and rehearse new skills. | Role-playing promotes skill acquisition in a nonthreatening environment and increases coping mechanisms |
| Encourage and support patients in evaluating their lifestyle and identifying activities and stresses of family, work, and social situations. | These measures enable patients to examine areas of life that may contribute to anxiety and make decisions about how to engender changes gradually without adding undue anxiety. |
| Assist with identifying some short- and long-term goals focused on making life changes and decreasing anxiety. | Goals help provide direction in making necessary changes. Cognitive behavioral therapy, systematic desensitization, or emotionally focused therapy are effective treatments for making life changes and decreasing anxiety. |
| Assist the patient with breaking responsibilities into manageable units. | Small steps enhance the success and avoid the anxiety that comes from facing a huge task and feeling overwhelmed. |
| Suggest incorporating stress management techniques (e.g., relaxation) into a typical day. | This encourages the patient to take care of self, take control, and decrease stress. These techniques help patients manage their anxiety. |
| Emphasize the importance of balance in life. | A life out of balance adds tremendously to stress and anxiety. Changes such as getting adequate sleep, nutrition, exercise, quiet time, work time, family time, and spiritual time enhance the quality of life, decrease anxiety, and increase a sense of power and control. |
| Refer to outside resources, including support groups, psychotherapy, religious resources, and community recreation resources. | Many people benefit from the support of other people and resources to help keep life in balance and monitor stress level. |

## Family Problem/Analyze Cues/Prioritize Hypotheses

# Difficulty Coping (Family)

*due to* family disorganization and role changes

***Desired Outcomes/Generate Solutions:*** Within 24–48 hours of interventions, family members begin to identify resources within themselves to deal with the situation; interact appropriately with the patient, providing support and assistance as needed; recognize their own needs for support; seek assistance; and use resources effectively.

| ASSESSMENT—RECOGNIZE CUES/ INTERVENTIONS—TAKE·ACTION | RATIONALES |
|---|---|
| Assess the level of information available to and understood by the family. | Lack of understanding about the patient's anxiety disorder can lead to unhealthy interaction patterns and contribute to the anxiety felt by family members. |
| Identify the role of the patient and current family roles and discuss how illness has changed the family organization. | Patients' disabilities (e.g., resulting in inability to go to work or maintain the household) interfere with their usual role in the family structure and can substantially contribute to family stress and disorganization. |

| ASSESSMENT—RECOGNIZE CUES/ INTERVENTIONS—TAKE ACTION | RATIONALES |
|---|---|
| Help the family identify other factors besides the patient's illness that affect their ability to provide support to one another. | This takes the focus off of the patient as "the problem" and helps family members examine each of their individual responsibilities and behaviors. |
| Discuss the psychoneurologic basis of anxiety to reduce stigmatizing the patient with having an anxiety disorder. | This helps the family understand and accept behaviors that may be very difficult and reduces labeling the patient as weak or "crazy," which can aggravate the stigma of having an anxiety disorder. |
| Help the family to be supportive of the patient but to recognize to whom the disorder belongs and who is responsible for the resolution of the disorder. | This recognition promotes self-responsibility. Individuals with the disorder can seek support and ask for help, but it is not the responsibility of the family to seek treatment on their behalf. |
| Provide instruction to the family in constructive problem-solving skills. | These skills help the family learn new ways to deal with conflicts and reduce anxiety-provoking situations. |
| Refer the family to appropriate community resources. | The family may need additional assistance (e.g., from counselors, psychotherapy, Social Services, financial advisors, and spiritual advisor) to work through family issues and remain intact. |

## Patient Problem/Analyze Cues/Prioritize Hypotheses

# Deficient Knowledge

*due to* unfamiliarity with the prescribed medications, their purpose, and their potential side effects

***Desired Outcome/Generate Solutions:*** By discharge (if inpatient) or after 4 weeks of outpatient treatment, the patient verbalizes accurate information about the prescribed medications and their side effects.

| ASSESSMENT—RECOGNIZE CUES/ INTERVENTIONS—TAKE ACTION | RATIONALES |
|---|---|
| Assess the patient's knowledge about the prescribed medications and her or his understanding of the importance of taking medications as prescribed. | This assessment helps the nurse to reinforce, as needed, information about the medications and correct any misunderstanding. |
| Provide instruction about the physiologic action of anxiolytics and/or antidepressants and how they alleviate symptoms of the patient's anxiety disorder. | Anxiety disorders are neurobiologic occurrences that respond to both anxiolytics and antidepressants. Many people who experience anxiety are fearful of taking medications because they fear drug dependence and view taking it as a sign of weakness. |
| Explain the importance of taking antidepressant medications as prescribed. | These medications require certain blood levels to be therapeutic; therefore patients need to take them daily at the dose and time interval prescribed. |
| Inform the patient about the side-effect profile and its management of prescribed medications. | The anxiolytic medications, as well as each class of antidepressants, carry specific side-effect profiles. Knowledge about expected side effects, ways to manage these side effects, and how long potential side effects may last is important for ensuring therapy adherence. |
| **Tricyclic antidepressants (TCAs):** Amitriptyline, desipramine, and imipramine are examples of TCAs. They are not used often but are used when selective serotonin reuptake inhibitors (SSRIs) are not proving to be effective. | TCAs are very effective for anxiety disorders because of their sedating properties to promote sleep restoration. |
| For patients taking TCAs, provide information about the following: | |
| • Drink at least 8 glasses of water a day and add high-fiber foods to the diet. | Water and high-fiber foods combat constipation, a potential anticholinergic effect. |
| • Rise from a sitting position slowly. Discuss the risks of falling related to dizziness associated with orthostatic hypotension. | Orthostatic hypotension is a potential side effect. |

| ASSESSMENT—RECOGNIZE CUES/ INTERVENTIONS—TAKE ACTION | RATIONALES |
|---|---|
| • Suck on sugar-free candy or mints or use sugar-free chewing gum. | These products combat dry mouth, a potential anticholinergic effect. |
| • Establish a sleep routine and regular exercise. | Regular sleep and exercise combat feelings of fatigue associated with these medications. |
| • Limit the intake of refined sugars and carbohydrates. | Weight gain is a common occurrence with these medications and eating sugar and carbohydrates can cause added weight gain and carbohydrate cravings. |
| • Caution is needed for patients with epilepsy or other seizure disorder. | TCAs lower the seizure threshold. |
| • Be alert for and report signs of cardiac toxicity. Explain that patients older than 40 years need an electrocardiogram evaluation before treatment and periodically thereafter. | These medications may decrease the vagal influence on the heart secondary to muscarinic blockade and by acting directly on the bundle of His to slow conduction. Both effects increase the risk for dysrhythmias. |
| • Discuss the possible drug interactions. | The combination of tricyclics with monoamine oxidase (MAO) inhibitors can cause severe hypertension. The combination of tricyclics with central nervous system (CNS) depressants, such as alcohol, antihistamines, opioids, and barbiturates, can cause severe CNS depression. Because of the anticholinergic effects of tricyclics, any other anticholinergic drug, including over-the-counter antihistamines and sleeping aids, needs to be avoided. |
| ⚠ **SSRIs:** Examples include fluoxetine, sertraline, paroxetine, citalopram, and escitalopram | SSRIs are helpful not only for patients with depression and obsessive-compulsive symptoms but also for patients with panic and anxiety disorders. |
| Provide information about SSRIs: | |
| • Inform the patient that the following can occur: nausea, headache, nervousness, insomnia, anxiety, agitation, sexual dysfunction, dizziness, fatigue, rash, diarrhea, excessive sweating, and anorexia with weight loss. | These are reported side effects. Because these medications can increase anxiety, it is recommended that treatment be started at very low doses and increased gradually. |
| • Discuss the possible drug interactions. | Interaction with MAO inhibitors can cause serotonin syndrome, a potentially life-threatening event. Symptoms include anxiety, diaphoresis, rigidity, hyperthermia, autonomic hyperactivity, and coma. Because of this possibility, MAO inhibitors must be withdrawn at least 14 days before starting an SSRI, and when an SSRI is discontinued, at least 5 weeks must elapse before an MAO inhibitor is given. |
| ⚠ **Other antidepressant medications:** Common examples include bupropion, mirtazapine, trazadone, duloxetine, venlafaxine, and desvenlafaxine. | Antidepressants are frequently prescribed for the treatment of anxiety disorders because of their effectiveness and low side-effect profile. |
| Provide information about other antidepressant medications: | |
| • Remind the patient to take the medication as prescribed daily and not to abruptly discontinue the medication. Explain that a gradual tapering is necessary when being taken off the medication. | Venlafaxine, in particular, when abruptly withdrawn, causes an uncomfortable discontinuation syndrome including dizziness, nausea, blurred vision, headache, and general malaise. Patients must be monitored carefully during the tapering period to avoid serious withdrawal symptoms. |
| ⚠ **Benzodiazepines:** diazepam, chlordiazepoxide, lorazepam, alprazolam, and clonazepam | These benzodiazepines are used for generalized anxiety disorder. Alprazolam also can be used for panic disorder. |
| Provide information about benzodiazepines: | |
| • Drowsiness, impairment of intellectual function, impairment of memory, ataxia, and reduced motor coordination can occur. | These are common side effects that subside as tolerance to the drug develops. |
| • For patients who use these medications for sleep, there may be daytime fatigue, drowsiness, and cognitive impairments that can continue while awake. | These are common side effects that subside as tolerance to the medication develops. |

| ASSESSMENT—RECOGNIZE CUES/ INTERVENTIONS—TAKE ACTION | RATIONALES |
|---|---|
| • A gradual tapering is necessary when being taken off the medication. | Abrupt discontinuation of the benzodiazepines can result in a recurrence of target symptoms such as anxiety. Gradual tapering is also necessary to prevent the occurrence of seizures. |
| • Nausea, vomiting, impaired appetite, dry mouth, and constipation may occur. | These are gastrointestinal (GI) symptoms associated with this medication. |
| • Take the medication with food. | Taking the medication with food may ease GI distress. |
| • Report worsening of depression symptoms. | This effect may occur in patients who are both depressed and anxious. |
| • Older adults need to take the smallest possible therapeutic dose. | Older adults taking this drug are at increased risk for incontinence, memory disturbances, dizziness, and falls. |
| • Pregnant women and nursing mothers must avoid using benzodiazepines. | Benzodiazepines are excreted in breast milk of nursing mothers. They also cross the placenta and are associated with an increased risk for certain birth defects. |
| • Decrease or stop smoking altogether. | Nicotine decreases the effectiveness of benzodiazepines. |
| **Nonbenzodiazepine:** buspirone | Buspirone is indicated in the treatment of generalized anxiety disorder. It does not increase depression, so it is a good choice when anxiety and depression coexist. It is not effective in treating other anxiety disorders. |
| Instruct patients taking buspirone the following: | Patients need to know the proper dosage, side effects, expected therapeutic effects, and precautions for their prescribed drugs. |
| • Be alert for dizziness, drowsiness, nausea, excitement, and headache. | These are common side effects. |
| • Take buspirone on a continual dosing schedule two or three times daily. | Buspirone has a short half-life. |
| • This medication can cause liver and kidney toxicity. Patients with kidney or liver impairment must be monitored for this adverse effect. | Buspirone is metabolized in the liver and excreted predominantly by the kidneys. |
| **Noradrenergic medications:** clonidine, propranolol, gabapentin, and pregabalin | These medications are used for off-label treatment of anxiety. Propranolol is used in the treatment of performance anxiety found in some forms of social phobia and in panic disorder. Clonidine is used to block the physiologic symptoms of opioid withdrawal. Pregabalin and gabapentin, anticonvulsant medications, show positive results in the treatment of anxiety disorders. |

## ADDITIONAL PROBLEMS:

"Major Depression" for     Chapter 102
*Risk for Suicide*
*Risk for Hopelessness*
*Low Self-Esteem*

## ✔ PATIENT–FAMILY TEACHING AND DISCHARGE PLANNING

The patient with an anxiety disorder experiences a wide variety of symptoms that affect the ability to learn and retain information. Instruction must be geared toward a time when the patient is not experiencing anxiety or medication has begun to calm the person and improve abilities to concentrate and learn. Verbal instruction needs to be simple and supplemented with written materials to which the patient and family can refer at a later time. Demonstrate and practice with the patient self-calming strategies, such as relaxation techniques, deep breathing, and "five senses" exercise, and instruct the patient to practice daily even when not anxious. Ensure that follow-up treatment is scheduled and that the patient and family understand the need to take medication as prescribed. Psychiatric home care might be a valuable part of the discharge planning to facilitate compliance with the discharge plan. In addition, provide verbal and written information about the following ssues:

✓ Medications, including drug name; purpose; dosage; frequency; precautions; drug–drug, food–drug, and herb–drug interactions; and potential side effects.

✓ Thought-stopping techniques to deal with negativism.

✓ Reducing catastrophic, dichotomous thinking to promote realistic appraisal of anxiety-provoking event.

✓ Importance of maintaining a healthy lifestyle—balanced diet, minimal to no caffeine, decrease or stop smoking, exercise, and regular adequate sleep patterns—for remaining in remission.

✓ Importance of continuing medication use long after symptoms have gone.

✓ Importance of social support and strategies to obtain it.

✓ Importance of using constructive coping skills to deal with stress.

✓ Importance of using relaxation techniques to minimize stress.

✓ Importance of maintaining or achieving spiritual well-being.

✓ Importance of follow-up care, including day treatment programs, appointments with psychiatrists and therapists, home care psychiatric nurses, and a vocational rehabilitation program if indicated.

✓ Referrals to community resources for support and education. Additional information can be obtained by contacting the following organizations:

- Anxiety Disorders Association of America: www. adaa.org
- National Alliance for the Mentally Ill for information on all of the anxiety disorders: https://nami.org/Home
- National Institute of Mental Health for information on anxiety disorders: www.nimh.nih.gov

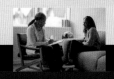

# Bipolar Disorder (Manic Component) 100

## OVERVIEW/PATHOPHYSIOLOGY

Bipolar disorder is a mood disorder characterized by episodes of major depression and mania or hypomania. (In this chapter, we will focus on the assessment and treatment of mania; see the care plan for "Major Depression," Chapter 102, for specifics regarding depression.) Bipolar disorder affects 46 million people or 0.6% worldwide and is associated with high rates of relapse and suicide.

*Mania* is characterized by a period in which there is a dramatic change in mood; the individual is either elated and expansive or irritable. For the diagnosis to be made, this change in mood must last 1 week (or most of the day, almost daily, if hospitalization is required). At least three other symptoms from the following list must be present: inflated self-esteem or grandiosity; decreased need for sleep; pressured speech; flight of ideas; distractibility; increased involvement in goal-directed activities or psychomotor agitation; and overinvolvement in pleasurable activities with potentially damaging consequences. Examples of this behavior include hypersexuality, impulsive spending, and other reckless and dangerous behaviors.

*Hypomania* is characterized by at least 4 days of abnormally and persistently elevated, expansive, or irritable mood accompanied by at least three additional symptoms seen in a manic episode.

The median age of onset is 25 years. In women, hormonal factors may account for a greater rate of rapid cycling (having at least four episodes of extremely high or low moods within 1 year), but in general, women and men are equally affected with this disorder. There is no difference in prevalence rates by race or ethnicity. Twenty-five percent of those diagnosed with bipolar disorder are elderly (65 years or older). Bipolar disorder is a chronic, relapsing, and episodic disease. In individuals 40 years or older who experience a first episode of mania, it is most likely related to medical conditions such as substance abuse or a cerebrovascular disorder. About 50% of bipolar patients have concurrent substance abuse disorders. Cigarette smoking is significantly more prevalent among individuals with bipolar disorder than among those without the disorder. Theories that explain the causation of bipolar disorder include disorders in brain function or structure and genetic factors. Sleep deprivation may trigger manic/hypomanic episodes.

## HEALTH CARE SETTING

Most patients may be treated as outpatients except those who are at high risk for suicide, represent a danger to others, or are experiencing a psychotic mania. Acute care (inpatient

psychiatric unit) stays are brief and focus on restabilization. Patients with bipolar disorder require long-term medication management; intensive psychosocial support to function within the community; and possibly individual, group, and family therapy.

## ASSESSMENT

Like depression, the assessment of mania involves much more than an assessment of mood. This is a holistic disorder that results in changes in self-attitude (feelings of self-worth) as well as vital sense (sense of physical well-being) and spiritual sense. Depression diminishes self-worth, self-attitude, and vital sense, whereas mania may increase these perceptions.

***Feelings, attitudes, and knowledge.*** During manic episodes, patients express inflated views of themselves. Many manic patients state that they enjoyed the euphoric feeling and, because of this, refused medications. After the mania has subsided, the patient is confronted with the consequences of behaviors and actions engaged in while manic. Being faced with the reality of those behaviors and their consequences produces negative feelings expressed as shame, humiliation, denial, anger, fear of experiencing a relapse, fear of passing the disorder onto children, and fear of cycling into an episode of depression.

***Elevated mood or irritability.*** Patients may be excessively cheerful and unusually elated or display irritability over the smallest matters. This irritability increases when others attempt to reason with them. A manic person may display a haughty or superior attitude toward others. They may display overt anger, particularly if their requests or behaviors are challenged.

***Increased self-attitude.*** Patients may express and act in unusually optimistic fashion, engaging in behaviors that reflect poor judgment, and may act in inappropriate, dangerous, or indiscreet ways. For example, a normally conservative person may engage in sexual indiscretions or speak in overly critical or judgmental terms, often at inappropriate times and about sensitive subjects.

***Increased vital sense.*** The person with mania has increased energy and may appear tireless in the face of physical and mental efforts that would greatly tax unaffected individuals. He or she may feel completely refreshed after only a few minutes or hours of sleep.

***Spiritual issues.*** Bipolar disorder mania carries with it many negative experiences—such as marital and family problems, divorce, legal difficulties, financial ruin, and unemployment—that contribute to the downward spiral of self-appraisals. Spirituality is an important, though often a neglected, aspect of assessment, especially during the acute episode. Bipolar disorder can lead to a crisis in faith in self, others, life, and ultimately God. This loss of faith and hope contributes significantly to the risk for suicide.

**Additional signs.** Manic individuals may experience a voracious appetite or may be too busy to eat.

**Suicidality.** Suicide assessment is critical with manic patients. Individuals with bipolar disorder account for 25% of completed suicide. The presence of psychotic thinking, hyperactivity, impulsiveness, and possible substance abuse increases suicide risk significantly. It is important to ask questions to determine the presence of suicidal ideation and the lethality of any plan. Essential questions to ask include the following:

- Have you thought of hurting yourself?
- Are you presently thinking about hurting yourself?
- If you have been thinking about suicide, do you have a plan? What is the plan?
- Have you thought about what life would be like for others if you were no longer a part of it?

A previous history of suicide attempts places the patient at high risk for attempting suicide. (See *Risk for Suicide* in "Major Depression," Chapter 102.)

## DIAGNOSTIC TESTS

There are no diagnostic tests to diagnose bipolar disorder mania. Diagnosis is made through history, interview of the patient and family, and observation of verbal and nonverbal behaviors. To be diagnosed with bipolar disorder, the individual must meet the criteria spelled out in the *Diagnostic and Statistical Manual of Mental Disorders*, fifth edition (American Psychiatric Association, 2013). The Young Mania Rating Scale is an effective instrument to quantify the degree of mania. Some are misdiagnosed as schizophrenia when bipolar would be more appropriate.

### Patient Problem/Analyze Cues/Prioritize Hypotheses

# Risk for Injury (to Self and Others)

*due to* impulsivity/agitation occurring with manic excitement

**Desired Outcome/Generate Outcomes:** By the time of discharge from an inpatient psychiatric unit, the patient demonstrates increased self-control and decreased hyperactivity.

| ASSESSMENT—RECOGNIZE CUES/ INTERVENTIONS—TAKE ACTION | RATIONALES |
|---|---|
| Continually assess the patient's response to frustrations or difficult situations. | This enables early intervention and helps patients manage situations independently, if possible. |
| Continually assess to ensure that the patient's environment is safe. Remove objects that could be dangerous and rearrange the room to decrease environmental risks to prevent accidental/purposeful injury to self or others. | Hyperactive behavior and grandiose thinking can lead to destructive actions with possible harm to self or others. Physical safety of the patient and others is a priority. |
| Decrease environmental stimuli, assign a private room (if possible), avoid exposure to situations of predictable high stimulation, and remove the patient from the area if he or she becomes agitated. | Patients may be unable to focus attention on relevant stimuli and will be reacting/responding to all environmental stimuli. |
| When necessary, limit contact between the patient and other patients or restrict visitation during manic or agitated states. | The patient may need to regain self-control before interacting with others. |
| Intervene at the earliest signs of agitation. Use direct verbal interventions prompting appropriate behavior, redirect or remove the patient from the difficult situation, establish voluntary time-out or move to a quiet room, use physical control (e.g., hold the patient) if absolutely necessary. Offer and administer as-needed medications, preferably before the patient's behavior escalates and becomes destructive. | Early intervention assists patients in regaining control, defuses a difficult situation, prevents violence, and enables treatment to continue in the least-restrictive manner. **Note:** Physical hold/restraints are used only as a last resort. |
| Until the patient is calm, avoid analyzing or problem-solving regarding the prevention of violence or collecting information about precipitating events or provoking stimuli. | Questioning the patient will only add to agitation. Analyze and problem-solve when the patient is calm. |
| Communicate the rationale for taking action using a concrete, direct, and simple approach. | People are unable to process complicated communication when they are agitated or upset. |
| When the patient is ready to leave the quiet area or time-out location, allow gradual reentry to the area of greater stimulation. | The patient has diminished tolerance for environmental stimuli; gradual reentry fosters coping skills. |

| ASSESSMENT—RECOGNIZE CUES/ INTERVENTIONS—TAKE ACTION | RATIONALES |
|---|---|
| Do not argue with the patient if they verbalize put-downs or unrealistic or grandiose ideas. | Challenging the patient only increases agitation and reinforces undesirable behavior. |
| Ignore or minimize attention given to bizarre dress or use of profanity, while placing clear limits on destructive behavior. Set and maintain limits regarding inappropriate behaviors. | This avoids reinforcing negative behavior while providing controls for potentially dangerous behavior. Limit setting is necessary to help the patient learn appropriate behaviors. |
| Avoid unnecessary delay of gratification when the patient makes a request. If refusal is necessary, make sure the rationale is given in nonjudgmental and concrete manner. | Patients in a hyperactive state do not tolerate waiting or delays, which add to frustration or agitation level. Any unnecessary delays could trigger aggressive behavior. |
| Offer alternatives when available. | This uses the patient's distractibility to decrease the frustration of having a request refused. For example, "I don't have any soda. Would you like a glass of juice?" |
| When the patient is less agitated and labile, provide information about alternative problem-solving strategies. | When calm, patients are able to hear and retain information. |
| When the patient is calm, help to examine the antecedents/precipitants to agitation. | This promotes early recognition of the developing problem, enabling patients to plan for alternative responses and intervene in a timely fashion. |
| Collaborate with the patient to identify alternative behaviors that are acceptable to both the patient and staff. Role-play how to use these behaviors if appropriate. | Patients are more apt to follow through if the alternatives are mutually agreed on. This practice enables patients to "try on" new behaviors while calm and ready to learn. |
| Give positive reinforcement when the patient attempts to deal with difficult situations without violence. | Praise increases patients' sense of success and increases the likelihood that desired behaviors will be repeated. |
| Administer the following medications as prescribed: | |
| **Antimanic medications:** lithium carbonate, divalproex sodium, valproic acid, valproate, carbamazepine, topiramate, oxcarbazepine, tiagabine, and lamotrigine | Lithium is the drug of choice for mania and is indicated for the alleviation of hyperactive symptoms. Some patients do not respond to or are intolerant of lithium and may need alternative medications, which may include divalproex, carbamazepine, topiramate, valproic acid, valproate, tiagabine, or lamotrigine. |
| **Atypical antipsychotics with mood-stabilizing effects:** olanzapine, quetiapine, haloperidol, aripiprazole, clozapine, paliperidone, risperidone, ziprasidone | Atypical antipsychotics have been found to be helpful as adjuncts to mood stabilizers. Olanzapine is well tolerated and is also helpful in treating the anxiety symptoms in bipolar depression. For the treatment of acute mania, haloperidol, risperidone, and olanzapine have shown the best efficacy. |
| Provide restraint or seclusion per agency policy. | These measures may be necessary for brief periods to protect the patient, staff, and others. Use cautiously and as a last resort. |
| Prepare the patient for electroconvulsive therapy (ECT) if indicated. | In a severely manic episode, ECT may be recommended. ECT is one of the most effective treatment options and is especially useful for individuals who need a rapid treatment response, cannot take or are refusing medications, or do not respond to other treatment modalities. |

### Patient and Significant Other Problems/Analyze Cues/Prioritize Hypotheses

# Deficient Knowledge

*due to* unfamiliarity with the causes, signs and symptoms, and treatment of bipolar disorder mania

***Desired Outcome/Generate Solutions:*** Within 24 hours of instruction, the patient and/or significant others verbalize accurate information about at least two possible causes of bipolar disorder, four signs and symptoms of the disorder, and available treatment options.

| ASSESSMENT—RECOGNIZE CUES/ INTERVENTIONS—TAKE ACTION | RATIONALES |
|---|---|
| Assess the level of knowledge of the patient and significant others regarding the causes of bipolar disorder, signs and symptoms of the disorder, and the available treatment options. | Initially, it is difficult to diagnose bipolar disorder and is sometimes misdiagnosed as schizophrenia. Patients and their significant others may have faulty perceptions about it. Unless corrected, these faulty perceptions may interfere with treatment adherence on the part of the patient and weaken support for treatment adherence from the significant others. |
| Provide information to the patient and significant others about bipolar disorder and mania. | Providing education about the physical basis for the disorder increases understanding and acceptance and decreases blaming behavior. |
| Provide information to the patient and significant others about relapse, decreased nutrition, and poor hygiene. | If the patient and significant others can recognize possible relapse or decompensation, the patient can seek early interventions. |
| Inform the patient and significant others that there are treatments available for bipolar disorder. Stress the importance of taking medications and adhering to the prescribed treatment plan. | Medications are essential to stabilize and maintain mood. However, they are not enough. Comprehensive treatment involves intensive outpatient programs, frequent office visits, crisis telephone calls, family involvement, and psychosocial interventions including psychoeducation, suicide prevention, psychotherapy for depression, and limit setting in mania and hypomania. Management of bipolar disorder is a lifelong commitment. Knowledge and acceptance of the diagnosis often increase the adherence to treatment. |

## Patient Problem/Analyze Cues/Prioritize Hypotheses

# Body Weight Problem (Weight Loss)

*due to* inadequate intake in relation to metabolic expenditures

***Desired Outcome/Generate Solutions:*** Immediately after interventions, the patient displays increased attention to eating behaviors.

| ASSESSMENT—RECOGNIZE CUES/ INTERVENTIONS—TAKE ACTION | RATIONALES |
|---|---|
| Establish a baseline regarding nutritional and fluid intake as well as activity level. | This assessment is necessary to quantify deficits, needs, and progress toward goals. |
| Weigh the patient daily. | This is another form of quantification that provides information about therapeutic needs and effectiveness of interventions. |
| Serve meals in a setting with minimal distractions. | This encourages patients to focus on eating and prevents other distractions from interfering with food intake. |
| Stay with the patient during mealtime, even if this means walking with the patient. | This provides support and encouragement for patients to take in adequate nutrition and does not set the unrealistic expectation that patients must sit during mealtime. |
| Provide finger foods, snacks, and juices. Provide high protein, high caloric food/beverages that can be consumed while walking (i.e., protein bars, protein shakes, nutritional supplements) | Patients will most likely eat small frequent meals on the move, and this allows a reasonable accommodation for this behavior. |
| Enable the patient to choose food when he or she is able to make choices. | Encouraging choices before patients are ready may add to confusion. However, if patients can handle choices, this increases a sense of control. |
| Refer to a dietitian as indicated. | It may be useful to involve an expert in determining patients' nutritional needs and the most appropriate options for meeting these needs. |
| Administer the vitamins and mineral supplements as prescribed. | Supplements help correct dietary deficiencies and improve nutritional status. |

## Patient Problem/Analyze Cues/Prioritize Hypotheses

# Risk for Self-Care Deficit

*due to* impulsivity and lack of concern

***Desired Outcome/Generate Solutions:*** Immediately after interventions, the patient performs self-care activities within his or her level of ability.

| ASSESSMENT—RECOGNIZE CUES/ INTERVENTIONS—TAKE ACTION | RATIONALES |
|---|---|
| Assess the patient's current level of functioning; reevaluate daily. | Patients' abilities for self-care may change daily. This information is needed to plan or modify care. |
| Provide physical assistance, supervision, simple directions, reminders, encouragement, and support as needed. | This helps patients focus on the task. Providing only required assistance fosters independence. |
| If possible, use the patient's clothing and toiletries. Have family, friends, or support system bring patient's personal items to the hospital. | Patients may have been disorganized entering the hospital or hospitalized as an emergency measure, so their own belongings were left at home. Having personal clothing and supplies supports autonomy and self-esteem. |
| As appropriate, limit the choices regarding clothing. | During periods of extreme hyperactivity and distractibility, patients may be unable to make appropriate choices or to care for personal belongings. |
| As the patient's condition improves, set goals to establish minimum standards for self-care (e.g., taking a bath every other day). | Setting goals promotes the idea that patients are responsible for themselves and enhances a sense of self-worth. |

## Patient Problem/Analyze Cues/Prioritize Hypotheses

# Deficient Knowledge

*due to* unfamiliarity with medication use, including the purpose and potential side effects of prescribed medications

***Desired Outcome/Generate Solutions:*** Immediately after teaching interventions, the patient verbalizes accurate information about the prescribed medications.

| ASSESSMENT—RECOGNIZE CUES/ INTERVENTIONS—TAKE ACTION | RATIONALES |
|---|---|
| Assess the patient's level of knowledge regarding the prescribed medications. | Education needs to be directed to assess deficits in knowledge regarding the expected benefits of taking the prescribed drug, potential side effects, and how to deal with them. Knowledge increases adherence to taking the prescribed medications. |
| In simple terms, explain the physiologic action of mood stabilizers. | Patients may have little or no understating regarding the purpose and actions of these medications. |
| Emphasize the importance of taking the medication as prescribed and the need for follow-up blood tests to monitor medication serum level. | The medication requires certain blood levels to be therapeutic, and therefore patients need to take it at the dose and time interval prescribed. The scheduled serum evaluations ensure that the medication level remains within therapeutic range. |
| **Antimanic medications for adults:** lithium carbonate or lithium citrate | Lithium provides mood stability and prevents dangerous highs and despairing lows experienced in bipolar disorder. |
| Provide instructions about the following: | |
| • How to monitor for swelling of feet or hands, fine hand tremor, mild diarrhea, muscle weakness, fatigue, memory and concentration difficulties, metallic taste, nausea or abdominal discomfort, polydipsia, polyuria. | These are common side effects. |

Continued

| ASSESSMENT—RECOGNIZE CUES/ INTERVENTIONS—TAKE ACTION | RATIONALES |
|---|---|
| • The importance of monitoring intake and output, sodium intake, and weight and how to elevate legs when sitting or lying down. | These are interventions for the prevention of edema of the feet and hands. |
| • The importance of notifying the health care provider if urinary output decreases. | This may be a sign of increasing serum level of lithium. |
| • When to notify the prescriber if tremors interfere with work. | A medication that interferes with work may result in adherence issues. Smaller, more frequent doses may help. In addition, tremors worsen when patients are anxious. |
| • The need to take lithium with meals, replace fluids lost secondary to diarrhea, and notify the prescriber if diarrhea becomes severe. | Some people can have nausea from lithium. At higher doses, loose stools or even diarrhea are frequently noted. The prescriber may need to change the medication. |
| Caution the patient that if any of the following symptoms occur while taking lithium—muscle weakness, fatigue, memory problems, or concentration difficulties—he or she must avoid driving or operating hazardous equipment during this period, use reminders and cues for memory deficits, and notify the prescriber if these symptoms become severe. | These are interventions to prevent harm to self and others. The prescriber may change to another medication. |
| Encourage the patient to use sugarless candies, mints, or throat lozenges and engage in frequent oral hygiene. | These are interventions for metallic taste and the dry mouth that can be associated with some medications. |
| Caution that large amounts of sugar-free candies may cause excessive gas and diarrhea. | Diarrhea from the sugar substitutes in candies may be confused with side effects of the medications. |
| Explain that drinking large amounts of fluids is a normal mechanism for coping with the side effect of increased urine. | This information provides reassurance for polydipsia. |
| Explain in simple terms the importance of having laboratory work done as prescribed as well as being alert to signs and symptoms of lithium toxicity. | This helps ensure that the serum lithium level is maintained between 0.6 and 1.2 mEq/L. Mild toxic lithium effects, including impaired concentration, lethargy, tremor, slurred speech, and nausea, may be seen at plasma levels of 1–1.5 mEq/L. Moderate toxic lithium effects, including confusion, disorientation, drowsiness, unsteady gait, dysarthria, and muscle fasciculations, may be seen at plasma levels of 1.6–2.5 mEq/L. Severe toxic lithium effects, including impaired consciousness with progression to coma, delirium, ataxia, impaired renal function, and convulsions, may be seen at plasma levels greater than 2.5 mEq/L. Laboratories have established critically high lithium values that are used for clinician notification. Usually, these concentrations are greater than 2 mEq/L, although some facilities may consider lithium concentrations greater than 1.5 mEq/L as their critically high lithium level (Souza et al., 2013). Usually, after stabilization is achieved, laboratory work is done every 1–2 weeks during the first 2 months and every 3–6 months during long-term maintenance. |
| Caution the patient to avoid alcohol or other central nervous system depressant medications. | These substances may increase serum lithium level. Risk for injury may increase with the combination because of sedation and/or dizziness. |
| Advise the patient to notify the prescriber if pregnant or planning to become pregnant and to avoid breastfeeding while taking this medication. | Safe use during pregnancy and breastfeeding has not been established. |
| Advise the patient to notify the prescriber before taking any other prescription or over-the-counter medication. Consult with pharmacist for possible drug interactions. | Many other medications interact with lithium to either increase or decrease the serum level. For example, when combined with lithium, nonsteroidal antiinflammatory drugs can increase lithium levels in the blood, resulting in an increased risk for serious adverse effects. |
| Caution the patient not to discontinue this medication abruptly. | This could lead to exacerbation of manic symptoms. |

| ASSESSMENT—RECOGNIZE CUES/INTERVENTIONS—TAKE ACTION | RATIONALES |
|---|---|
| **Antiseizure medications with mood-stabilizing effects:** divalproex sodium or valproic acid, carbamazepine, topiramate, lamotrigine, oxcarbazepine | These medications generally are used when lithium does not work or when side effects from lithium are intolerable to the patient. |
| **Atypical antipsychotics with mood-stabilizing effects:** olanzapine, quetiapine, aripiprazole, clozapine, paliperidone, risperidone, ziprasidone | Each of the atypical antipsychotics is effective in managing mania. Olanzapine often is better tolerated than lithium. Quetiapine is also effective in treating the anxiety symptoms in bipolar depression. |
| Instruct the patient to be alert for anorexia, nausea, vomiting, drowsiness (most common), and tremor. | These are common side effects. |

## ADDITIONAL PROBLEMS:

| "Major Depression" for | Chapter 102 |
|---|---|
| *Risk for Suicide* | |
| *Risk for Hopelessness* | |
| *Low Self-Esteem* | |

## PATIENT–FAMILY TEACHING AND DISCHARGE PLANNING

The patient with a bipolar disorder mania experiences a wide variety of symptoms that affect the ability to learn and retain information. Patient teaching must be geared toward a time when medication has begun to decrease hyperactive symptoms and improve abilities to concentrate and learn. Verbal instructions need to be simple and supplemented with reading materials the patient and/or significant other and family can refer to later. Ensure that follow-up treatment is scheduled and that the patient and/or significant other and family understand the need to get prescriptions filled and the importance of taking the medication as prescribed. Consider whether the patient has transportation available to get to follow-up treatment. Psychiatric home care might be a valuable part of the discharge planning to facilitate adherence to the discharge plan. In addition, provide the patient and/or significant other/family with verbal and written information about the following issues:

- ✓ Medications, including drug name; purpose; dosage; frequency; precautions; drug–drug, food–drug, and herb–drug interactions; and potential side effects.

- ✓ Importance of laboratory follow-up tests for serum lithium levels.
- ✓ Importance of maintaining a healthy lifestyle—balanced diet, minimal to no caffeine or alcohol, exercise, and regular adequate sleep patterns—to ensure remaining in remission.
- ✓ Importance of continuing medication use for life.
- ✓ Importance of social support and strategies for obtaining it.
- ✓ Importance of using community follow-up resources; for example, psychiatrist, psychiatric nurse, intensive outpatient, support groups, family counseling.
- ✓ Importance of maintaining or achieving spiritual well-being.
- ✓ Referrals to community resources for support and education. Additional information can be obtained by contacting the following organizations:
  - Depression and Bipolar Support Alliance (DBSA): www.dbsalliance.org. The DBSA provides education as well as support to individuals and families affected by depression and bipolar illnesses.
  - National Alliance on Mental Illness (NAMI) is the nation's largest grassroots mental health organization dedicated to building better lives for the millions of Americans affected by mental illness. NAMI advocates for access to services, treatment, support services, and research. They are steadfast in their commitment to raise awareness and building a community of hope for all of those in need (https://www.nami.org/Home).

# Dementia—Alzheimer's Type 101

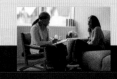

## OVERVIEW/PATHOPHYSIOLOGY

Dementia is a progressively deteriorating cognitive disorder that is part of a category of psychiatric disorders classified as *Neurocognitive Disorders* in the fifth edition of the *Diagnostic and Statistical Manual of Mental Disorders* (American Psychiatric Association, 2013). Delirium is characterized by an acute change in cognition and consciousness that occurs over a short period of time (see "Delirium," Chapter 98). Dementia is characterized by multiple cognitive deficits that include impairment in memory, perception, language, behavior, affect, and motor ability. The dementias are also classified according to etiology: dementia of the Alzheimer's type; vascular dementia; Lewy body disease; frontotemporal degeneration; and neurocognitive disorder due to other general medical conditions, such as human immunodeficiency virus disease, head trauma, Parkinson disease, Huntington disease, Pick disease, and Prion disease (formerly known as Creutzfeldt–Jakob disease); substance-induced persisting dementia; dementia due to multiple etiologies; and dementia not otherwise specified.

The most common form is Alzheimer's disease (AD), a primary dementia accounting for approximately 60%–80% of dementia diagnoses (Alzheimer's Association, 2022; CDC, 2019), and it is the focus of this care plan. Although AD is age related, it does not represent the normal process of aging. It occurs with distinctive brain lesions without any certain physiologic basis. The brain lesions are neurofibrillary tangles and neuritic plaques that take up space in the brain, replacing normal tissue in the cell body of the neuron. There are multiple theories to explain the occurrence of AD, including genetic transmission, a decrease in acetylcholine, beta-amyloid activity, impact of a head injury, mini strokes, lack of estrogen, immunologic factors, effects of a slow-acting virus, and environmental factors.

AD affects an estimated 6.5 million Americans, making it the most common neuropsychiatric illness in older adults (Alzheimer's Association, 2022). Its diagnosis covers deficits in memory, problem-solving, attention, and cognition. The actual course of the disorder follows a predictable pattern of early, middle, and late stages of progression, each displaying characteristic behaviors and requiring a different focus of treatment. The early stage is also referred to as the *mild stage* (the patient has cognitive changes such a memory loss, difficulty with tasks at work or socially); the middle stage or *moderate stage* evidenced by forgetting events or personal history, forgetting their address or phone number; difficulty choosing clothes for the correct weather conditions or seasons, difficulty controlling bowel or bladder, or suspiciousness, delusions or compulsive behaviors; and the late stage or the *severe stage*, when the patient loses the ability to respond to their environment, they need around-the-clock care, lose the ability to walk, sit, and eventually swallow. Seizures and psychotic symptoms are common in late stages. Death inevitably occurs as a result of neurologic complications imposed by the brain lesions.

AD represents the clinical prototype for chronic cognitive disorders. The care required by the Alzheimer's patient, especially in the middle and late stages of the disorder, is essentially the same care required by all dementia patients regardless of type. The cognitive symptoms of dementia involve serious memory impairment as well as significant alterations in language and perceptual acuity and abilities to abstract, problem-solve, and make appropriate judgments. Patients ultimately experience loss of all memory (amnesia), agnosia (inability to recognize objects, people, places), and aphasia (loss of meaningful verbal communication). Noncognitive behavioral symptoms can be just as profound. These include significant personality changes, purposeless movements, agitation and aggression, overreaction to situations, irritable and repetitive behavior, and emotional disinhibition.

## HEALTH CARE SETTING

In the early stage of AD, care takes place in the home and primary care setting. By the end of the early stage of the disease, additional services such as home care and use of adult day care are needed to safely maintain the patient at home. At the end of the early stage and moving into the middle stage, the decision regarding where to place the patient begins. The patient is generally moved into residential care in the middle stage, and during the late stage, care is frequently provided in a skilled nursing facility and sometimes a specialized, locked dementia unit (sometimes called a "memory unit") for safety.

## ASSESSMENT

### Psychiatric assessment

Involves assessment of primary and secondary psychiatric manifestations of AD and differential diagnosis from delirium, psychosis, depression, anxiety, and phobias.

*Family history.* Dementing illness, psychiatric disease, neurologic disease, substance-use disorders.

***Social history.*** Education, past level of functioning per occupational history, close relationships and children, current living situation, and history and present substance use.

***Medical history.*** All past and present medical illnesses, especially cardiovascular; past surgeries; past trauma, especially to the head; allergies; and medications.

***Psychiatric history.*** Psychotic illness; depressive illness; other psychiatric illnesses; psychiatric symptoms, especially mood lability and psychotic symptoms; past and current treatments; hospitalizations; suicidal ideation; and violence or aggression.

***Present illness.*** Length of cognitive loss and degree of memory loss:

- Short-term memory loss so significant that the patient is no longer able to remember and perform activities of daily living (ADLs)
- Other presenting problems, physical symptoms and injuries, functional deficits, psychiatric symptoms
- Personality changes, including low tolerance for normal frustrations, oversensitivity to remarks of others, lack of initiative, decreased attention span, diminished emotional presence, emotional lability, restlessness
- Difficulty with word finding and comprehension; thought blocking

***Mental status examination.*** Appearance, behavior, speech, mood, hallucinations, delusions, paranoid ideation, anxiety, phobias, cognition, insight and judgment, behavioral disturbances such as agitation, combativeness, screaming, and catastrophic reactions.

## Physical assessment

***Psychomotor functioning.*** Difficulty in carrying out new or complex motor tasks is apparent in the early stages; difficulty in carrying out activities such as dressing, eating, and walking becomes apparent in the middle stages. Unsteadiness of gait coupled with confusion poses a significant risk for falls during the middle stages. In addition, marked psychomotor agitation is common. Restlessness, agitation, and aimless pacing replace normal motion.

***Nutrition and elimination.*** Eating difficulties may present in the early stages. The patient may forget that he or she has just eaten, exhibit lax table manners, fail to know it is mealtime without prompting, experience changes in taste and appetite, express denial of hunger or need to eat, and experience weight loss. As the disease progresses, the patient does not respond to the need for elimination, which necessitates the caregiver to plan regular bathroom breaks. Constipation and incontinence of urine and feces become problems. Additionally, as the disease progresses, patients may forget to swallow food, which increases the risk for choking and/or aspiration.

***Activity and rest.*** Fatigue increases the severity of symptoms, especially as evening approaches. Patients may reverse days and nights, with wakefulness and aimless wandering at night indicative of disturbance of sleep rhythms. Patients may be content to sit and watch others. The main activity may be hoarding inanimate objects, hiding articles, wandering, or engaging in repetitive motions.

***Hygiene.*** As the disease progresses, so does dependence on the caregiver to meet basic hygiene needs. Appearance may be disheveled, and patients may have body odor. Clothing may be inappropriate for the situation or weather conditions. Patients may forget to go to the bathroom and the steps involved in toileting.

***Social assessment.*** Patients may ignore rules of social conduct and exhibit inappropriate behavior and disinhibition. Speech may be fragmented; family roles may be altered/reversed as patients become more dependent.

***Spiritual assessment.*** An assessment of the patient's faith tradition, practices, level of commitment, and connection to a faith community is critical. In the early stage of AD, the patient may have full awareness of the journey that lies ahead, and spirituality may offer support and comfort in ways that nothing else can. As the disease progresses and deficits become greater, it is difficult to assess the patient's spiritual needs. However, because long-term memory remains intact long after the short-term memory is gone, patients may still be comforted by spiritual traditions such as worship services, prayers, and hymns that are a vivid part of his or her history. Moreover, care of the Alzheimer's patient is so demanding that spiritual needs of the caregiver must be assessed and support provided. A faith community may provide invaluable assistance in the actual care of the patient, providing the caregiver with respite and help with day-to-day activities.

## DIAGNOSTIC TESTS

Obtaining an accurate differential diagnosis of dementia is essential. AD is basically a rule-out disorder; that is, the diagnosis is made after family history, laboratory tests, and brain imaging eliminate other disorders with similar cognitive deficits. Sources of information needed to make a differential diagnosis of dementia include a full neurologic assessment, laboratory tests to rule out metabolic factors, and family history of the patient's past behavior and symptom progression. Mini-Cog (or other cognitive screening) and functional assessment of ADLs provide the necessary information. Computed tomography (CT) identifies structural deficits. Brain imaging with positron emission tomography (PET) provides the clinician with information about changes in the metabolic activity and neurochemical characteristics associated with dementia. Typically, testing of patients in the early stage of AD reveals a normal electroencephalogram, CT scan, and magnetic resonance imaging study, and generally, laboratory tests are within normal range. A comprehensive psychiatric assessment provides additional information. Use of the Functional Assessment Staging Tool allows for staging the disease, facilitates recognition of cognitive and functional abilities and deficits of each stage of AD, and enables planning for the appropriate adjustments to care.

## Family and Significant Other Problems/Analyze Cues/Prioritize Hypotheses

# Deficient Knowledge

*due to* unfamiliarity with the disease progression and care of the dementia patient

***Desired Outcome/Generate Solutions:*** By the time the diagnosis of AD is confirmed, family/significant others relay accurate information and expectations about the course of the disease and the role they will play in the care of their loved one.

| ASSESSMENT—RECOGNIZE CUES/ INTERVENTIONS—TAKE ACTION | RATIONALES |
|---|---|
| Assess the significant other's/family's understanding about the disease process and expected care that will be needed for their loved one. | This assessment enables the nurse to reinforce, as needed, information about AD and correct any misunderstandings. |
| Provide information about the staging of the disease and changes to expect in their loved one. | The family plays an integral role in the care of their loved one. Initially, they are the informants, providing information that facilitates diagnosis; they move into the role of advocate, then primary caregiver, and finally the patient supporter. Staging is discussed in the overview section. |
| Provide written information regarding educational resources, such as the *36-Hour Day* (Mace & Rabins, 2021) and identification of appropriate support groups. | The cited book presents a compilation of family experiences with the disorder at different stages. Although there are other helpful books, this one remains the definitive resource for family caregivers. Support groups for family members offer an ongoing, practical socioeducational source, even in the early stage. They provide a safe place to explore issues such as whether the patient should stop driving; whether other people should be told about the diagnosis; whether the patient should wear an ID bracelet or carry a card indicating a dementia diagnosis; what the healthy spouse should do to handle the sexual desires of the affected spouse when the unaffected spouse no longer feels as though he or she has an adult relationship. |
| Coach the family to recall past memories in talking with their loved one. | Families feel more comfortable and are more likely to continue to interact with the patient if they know that reduced animation in the patient's face is part of the disease. Conversation may have noticeable pauses with less spontaneous speech; conversations should be short and simple. Reassuring the patient decreases overconcern about minor matters; touch continues to be important; and sharing important memories from the past helps maintain links to the patient even if the response is minimal. |
| Teach about safety issues. | Safety issues become the responsibility of the caregiver early in the disorder. The patient with AD needs room to pace and may fail to notice scatter rugs, spills on the floor, and changes in floor elevations, which increase the risk for falls. Other safety concerns deal with wandering, unsteady gait, forgetting the stove is turned on, and using toxic substances inappropriately. |
| Provide information about legal matters. | Decisions about durability and health care power of attorney need to be decided in the early stage of the disease when the patient is still competent. Legal counsel may be desirable for decisions regarding financial matters. |
| Provide information about health care resources. | The job of the family caregiver is overwhelming. Family members need to consider the use of adult day care centers and varieties of respite care, even in the early stage of the illness. Use of home health services also may be of valuable assistance. |
| Teach strategies to deal with behavioral issues such as wandering, rummaging, incontinence, difficulty following directions, and profound memory loss. | The more knowledge the family has regarding strategies to deal with these various behaviors, the better they will be able to care for the patient. |

## Patient Problem/Analyze Cues/Prioritize Hypotheses
# Deficient Knowledge: Risk for Injury

*due to* impaired judgment and inability to recognize the danger in the environment

***Desired Outcome/Generate Solutions:*** The patient remains free of signs and symptoms of trauma/injury.

| ASSESSMENT—RECOGNIZE CUES/ INTERVENTIONS—TAKE ACTION | RATIONALES |
|---|---|
| Assess the degree of impairment in the patient's abilities. Assist the caregiver to identify risks and potential hazards that may cause harm in the patient's environment and the necessary interventions that must be made to ensure safety. | Patients with impulsive behavior are at increased risk for harm because they are less able to control their own behaviors. Patients may have visual/perceptual deficits that increase the risk for falls. Caregivers need a heightened awareness of potential risks in the environment and need to take appropriate action. |
| Eliminate or minimize identified environmental risks. | Because a person with a cognitive deficit is unable to take responsibility for basic safety needs, the caregiver must eliminate as many risks as possible: take knobs off of or disable the stove, remove scatter rugs, place a safety gate at the top and bottom of stairs, and make sure doors to the outside are locked. |
| Routinely monitor the patient's behavior. Initiate the interventions to prevent negative behaviors from escalating. | Close observation of the patient's behavior allows early identification of problematic behaviors (e.g., increasing agitation) and enables early intervention. |
| Use distraction or redirection of the patient's attention when agitated or dangerous behavior such as climbing out of bed occurs. | Using the patient's distractibility avoids confrontation or behavioral escalation and helps maintain safety. |
| Ensure that the patient wears an ID bracelet providing name, phone number, and diagnosis. Do not allow the patient to have access to stairways or exits. | Because of memory deficits and confusion, these patients may not be able to provide this basic identifying information. The ID bracelet facilitates the patient's safe return. |
| Ensure that doors to the outside are locked. Make sure there is supervision and/or activities if the patient is regularly awake at night. | Taking appropriate preventive measures facilitates safety without constant supervision. Activities keep the patient occupied and limit wandering. |
| Ensure that the patient is dressed appropriately for weather/physical environment and individual needs. | Patients with cognitive disorders many times experience seasonal disorientation. In addition, AD affects the hypothalamus gland, making the person feel cold. The patient is not able to make appropriate choices regarding dress. |
| Inspect the patient's skin during care activities. | Identification of rashes, lacerations, and areas of ecchymosis enables necessary treatment and signals the need for closer monitoring and protective interventions. |
| Attend to nonverbal expressions of physiologic discomfort. | The patient may lack the ability to express needs clearly but may give clues to a problem by grimacing, sweating, doubling over, or panting. |
| Monitor for polypharmacy and drug interactions, medication side effects; signs of overmedication, for example, gastrointestinal (GI) upset; extrapyramidal symptoms; and orthostatic hypotension. | Drugs easily build up to toxic levels in older adults, and the patient may not be able to report any signs or symptoms that would indicate drug toxicity. |

## Patient Problem/Analyze Cues/Prioritize Hypotheses
# Deficient Knowledge: Impaired Memory (Dementia)

*due to* physiologic changes occurring with the progressive course of AD

***Desired Outcome/Generate Solutions:*** The patient remains calm and displays fewer undesirable behaviors.

| ASSESSMENT—RECOGNIZE CUES/ INTERVENTIONS—TAKE ACTION | RATIONALES |
|---|---|
| Assess the degree of confusion experienced by the patient with AD and how much short-term memory the patient still retains. | Loss of short-term memory prevents the AD patient from learning. Being unable to learn presents significant environmental safety issues that must be confronted. For example, a patient could exit the home or facility where he/she resides and may become lost. |
| Provide a predictable environment with orientation cues. | A calm environment with scheduled activities, adequate lighting, low noise level, calendars, clocks, and frequent verbal orientation helps maintain the patient's sense of calm and security. |
| Always address the patient by name. | Patients may respond to their own names long after they no longer recognize their significant others. Names are an integral part of self-identity; using the person's name is a part of reality orientation. |
| Communicate with the patient using a low voice, slow speech, and eye contact. | Deliberate communication techniques such as these increase the patient's attention and the chance for comprehension. Calm begets calm. |
| Simplify directions into a step-by-step process, giving one direction at a time and using simple and clear words. | As the disease progresses, the patient's ability to comprehend complex directions and interactions diminishes greatly. Simplicity is the key to effective communication. |
| Encourage the patient's response, allow pauses in interaction, and use open-ended comments and phrases. | These interventions invite a verbal response. |
| Listen carefully to the content of the patient's speech even if it is incomprehensible. | The patient may be having difficulty processing and decoding messages. However, listeners need to continue to show interest and encouragement to keep the communication going. |
| Offer interpretations regarding the patient's statements, meanings, and words. If the patient struggles to find a word, supply the word if possible. | Assisting patients in processing words promotes continuing communication efforts and decreases frustration. |
| Avoid negative comments, taking argumentative stands, confrontations, and criticism. | These aggressive responses only serve to increase frustration, agitation, and inappropriate behaviors. Cognitively impaired patients have no internal controls over their thinking and communications. |
| Listen carefully to the patient's stories. | As memory continues to fail, patients are unable to reenter the reality of their caregivers. To argue or reason with the patient only causes more anxiety. It is more important to provide an emotional connection with the patient than to correct the details of his or her stories. |
| Monitor for hallucinations. Observe the patient for verbal and nonverbal cues of responding to hallucinations. Validate the presence of the patient's hallucinatory experiences. | Validating that the patient is hearing voices allows some discussion of fears associated with the experience and permits assurance that the experience is part of the illness. |
| Allow the patient to hoard safe objects within reason. | This provides patients with a sense of security. |
| Provide musical stimulation using selections that would have been popular during the patient's adolescent and early adult years. | Music is a powerful intervention. People who no longer can speak can many times sing. Music can calm an agitated mood and encourage socialization and movement. If music is agitating, stop playing the music. Another genre of music may be helpful (i.e. hymns). |
| Provide useful and productive outlets for the patient to engage in repetitive activities, for example, folding and unfolding laundry, collecting junk mail, dusting, and sweeping floors. | This measure acknowledges that repetitive activities are a normal expression of illness but channels these activities in a way that increases the patient's self-esteem and may decrease restlessness. |
| Ensure that the environment is quiet, calm, and visually nondistracting. | These qualities help to avoid visual/auditory overload. |
| Provide touch to the patient in a caring way. | Touch enhances the perception of self and body boundaries and communicates caring. |

| ASSESSMENT—RECOGNIZE CUES/ INTERVENTIONS—TAKE ACTION | RATIONALES |
|---|---|
| Use reminiscence therapy with props such as photo albums, old music, historical events, and mementos. Encourage the patient to talk about memories and feelings attached to these items. | This measure aids in preservation of self by recalling past accomplishments and events, increases the patient's sense of security, and encourages sharing that keeps the patient linked to others socially. |
| Encourage intellectual activity such as word games, discussion of current events, and storytelling. | This provides patients with normalcy and connection to others and the world and stimulates remaining cognitive abilities. |
| Suggest that the caregiver accompany the patient on short outings in the car, taking walks, and going shopping. | This decreases the sense of isolation, increases physical stamina, and provides sensory pleasure. |

## Patient, Family, and Significant Other Problems/Analyze Cues/Prioritize Hypotheses

# Grief

*due to* awareness on the part of the patient and significant others/family that something is seriously wrong because changes in memory and behaviors are increasingly evident

***Desired Outcome/Generate Solutions:*** The patient, family, and significant other discuss loss and participate in planning for the future.

| ASSESSMENT—RECOGNIZE CUES/ INTERVENTIONS—TAKE ACTION | RATIONALES |
|---|---|
| Assess for and encourage the patient and family to discuss feelings associated with anticipated losses. | This conveys the message that grief is a normal and expected reaction to the diagnosis of AD, with which progression and decline are certain. |
| Acknowledge expressions of anger and statements of despair and hopelessness, such as "I and my family would be better off if I were dead." | Feelings of anger may be the patient's way of dealing with underlying feelings of despair. Despairing and hopeless statements may be indicative of suicidal ideation. These should be explored, and appropriate action taken to protect the patient from self-directed harm (see *Risk for Suicide* in "Major Depression," Chapter 102). |
| Provide honest answers and do not give false reassurances or gloomy predictions. | Honesty promotes a trusting relationship and open communication. False reassurances or predictions of gloom are not helpful. |
| Discuss with the patient and significant other/family ways they can plan for the future. Recognize and respect generational and cultural differences. | Participation in problem-solving increases a sense of control. Effective communication, respect, and compassion are strengthening. While the patient is cognitively able, it would be best to plan for the identification of a health care agent to make a decision when the patient is unable. |
| Emphasize that this is a disease in which research is active and ongoing and that it is possible the disease will progress slowly. | Real hope may exist for the future. |
| Assist the patient, significant other, and family to identify strengths they see in themselves, in each other, and in available support systems. | This emphasizes that there are supports and resources to help work through grief. |
| Encourage the family to participate in a support group for caregivers of Alzheimer's patients. | Support groups not only provide valuable information but also communicate to caregivers that they are not alone as they struggle to manage the illness. |

Caregiver Problem/Analyze Cues/Prioritize Hypotheses

# Risk for Caregiver Role Strain

*due to* the severity of the patient's illness, the duration of care required, and the complexity and increasing number of caregiving tasks

***Desired Outcome/Generate Solutions:*** The caregiver exhibits behaviors consistent with a healthy lifestyle.

| ASSESSMENT—RECOGNIZE CUES/ INTERVENTIONS—TAKE ACTION | RATIONALES |
|---|---|
| Assess the caregiver's physical/emotional/spiritual condition and the caregiving demands that are present. | This assessment helps to determine the individual care needs of the caregiver. |
| Determine the caregiver's level of responsibility, involvement in, and anticipated duration of care involved. | This helps the caregiver realistically assess what is involved in a commitment to providing care. |
| Identify the strengths of the caregiver and the patient. | This identifies positive aspects of each so that they may be incorporated into daily activities. |
| Encourage the caregiver to discuss personal perspectives and views about the situation. | This allows venting of concerns and provides opportunities for the validation and acceptance of the caregiver's issues. |
| Explore available supports and resources. Facilitate decision-making regarding the least restrictive, safe living environments. | This enables the evaluation of adequacy of current resources. |
| Encourage and offer to facilitate family conferences to develop a plan for family involvement in care activities. | The more people who are involved in care, the less risk that one person will become overwhelmed. |
| Identify additional resources, including financial, legal, and respite care. | Referral to community resources can decrease the burden of caregiving. |
| Identify equipment needs/resources and other environmental adaptations. Consider occupational therapy (OT) consultation. | Appropriate equipment and environmental modifications promote patient safety and ease the care burden on the primary caregiver. An OT consult may be helpful to provide adaptive tools the AD patient can use. This will enable improved quality of life for the patient and caregivers by extending the patient's independence and ability to participate in self-care activities for a longer period of time. |
| Teach caregiver/family techniques and strategies to deal with acting out and disoriented behaviors, as well as incontinence and other physical challenges. | This increases a sense of control and competency of the caregiver and family. |
| Teach caregivers the importance of continuing to engage in their own self-care activities. | Risk for caregiver burden, burnout, and stress is greatly diminished if the caregiver takes time for self—for example, continuing a hobby, pursuing social activities, and taking care of personal needs. |
| Encourage and help the caregiver/family to plan for changes that may be necessary, such as home care services, use of adult day care, and eventual placement in a long-term facility. | Planning is essential for these eventualities. As the disease progresses, the burden of care outstrips the resources of the caregiver. |

Caregiver and Family Problem/Analyze Cues/Prioritize Hypotheses

# Deficient Knowledge

*due to* unfamiliarity with the rationale, potential side effects, and interventions for side effects of the prescribed medications

***Desired Outcome/Generate Solutions:*** Immediately after teaching, the caregiver and/or family verbalize accurate information about the rationale for use of certain medications, their common side effects, and methods for dealing with those side effects.

| ASSESSMENT—RECOGNIZE CUES/ INTERVENTIONS—TAKE ACTION | RATIONALES |
|---|---|
| In the early stages of AD for the patient, as well as ongoing for the caregivers and/or family, assess their knowledge level regarding the use of cholinesterase inhibitors and/or an N-methyl-D-aspartate (NMDA) antagonists as part of the treatment plan for AD. | As the disease progresses and the patient's memory continues to deteriorate, the caregiver's and/or family's role in administering and monitoring the effects of the prescribed medications becomes increasingly important. |
| Describe the physiologic action of **cholinesterase inhibitors** and how they improve cognition. | There are three cholinesterase inhibitors used to manage AD symptoms. Donepezil is used to manage mild to severe AD. Rivastigmine tartrate is used to manage mild-to-moderate AD. Galantine can be used in any stage of AD. These medications do not cure AD, but they may potentially slow cognitive decline by slowing the breakdown of acetylcholine released by intact cholinergic neurons. |
| Describe the physiologic action of **memantine** and the rationale for including it in the medication regimen along with a cholinesterase inhibitor. | Memantine is an NMDA receptor antagonist that targets glutamate, the main excitatory neurotransmitter, and blocks the glutamate from attaching to nerve cells. Specifically, memantine targets the NMDA receptors, another chemical and structural system involved in memory. Researchers believe that too much stimulation of nerve cells by glutamate may be responsible for the degeneration of nerves that occurs in some neurologic disorders such as AD. It is the first medication to be developed that targets symptoms during the moderate to severe stages of AD. It is taken in conjunction with a cholinesterase inhibitor. |
| Advise the patient, caregiver, and family that these medications ideally will slow the progression of AD, but that these medications do not cure AD. | Slowing the progression of AD may delay nursing home placement by as much as a year. Patients, family members and caregivers need to have realistic expectations about the potential benefits of these medications. |
| Teach the side-effect profile of the specific prescribed medication and methods for dealing with those effects as follows: | Knowledge about expected side effects and adverse effects is important for promoting adherence to the therapeutic regimen. |
| • Be alert for headache, fatigue, dizziness, confusion, nausea, vomiting, diarrhea, upset stomach, poor appetite, abdominal pain, rhinitis, and skin rash. | These are common side effects that, if severe, should be reported to the prescriber for possible decrease in dosage or gradual discontinuation. |
| • Take the medication exactly as prescribed around the clock and ideally, on an empty stomach. However, if GI upset occurs, take with meals. | Absorption is increased when taken on an empty stomach, but a full stomach may decrease gastric upset. |
| • Maintain appointments for regular blood work and medical follow-up while adjusting to the medication. Caution is necessary for patients with renal and hepatic disease, seizures, sick sinus syndrome, and GI bleeding. | This is especially important if the patient has preexisting medical conditions, such as renal, liver, or cardiac disease, because these medications may affect these organs. |
| • Avoid concomitant use of AD medications with nonsteroidal antiinflammatory drugs (NSAIDs) by assessing the patient's medication regimen. Explore any herbs or supplements taken. | Concomitant use of NSAIDs, herbs, or supplements may increase the effects and risk for toxicity associated with AD medications. Potential drug–herb interactions should be examined. |
| Describe the physiologic action of caprylidene and the rationale for including it in the medication regimen for AD. | Caprylidene is a medical food used in mild-to-moderate AD. It is metabolized into ketone bodies the brain uses for energy when its ability to process glucose is impaired. |
| Describe the physiologic action of memantine/donepezil and how it aids in the treatment of moderate to severe AD. | Memantine/donepezil is a fixed-dose combination medication that combines memantine and donepezil to ease medication administration and enhance adherence. |
| See care plans for "Anxiety Disorders," Chapter 99, "Major Depression," Chapter 102, and "Schizophrenia," Chapter 103, for a review of antidepressants, anxiolytics, and antipsychotic medications. | Patients with AD may also suffer from depression, anxiety, and psychosis at a clinically significant severity. If depression or anxiety symptoms are severe, psychotropic medications may be indicated and can significantly decrease distress. |

## ADDITIONAL PROBLEMS:

| | |
|---|---|
| "Psychosocial Support for the Patient's Family and Significant Others" for problems as appropriate | Chapter 9 |
| "Anxiety Disorders" for *Difficulty Coping* problems | Chapter 99 |
| "Bipolar Disorder (Manic Component)" for *Body Weight Problem (Weight Loss)* | Chapter 100 |

 ## PATIENT–FAMILY TEACHING AND DISCHARGE PLANNING

The patient with dementia—Alzheimer's type—progresses through predictable stages, each with characteristic symptoms and behaviors that directly affect the ability to effectively process and use new information. As the disease progresses, the patient requires increasing amounts of physical care, and the caregiver/family requires information and support. Dementia is a family disease.

As soon as the diagnosis is made, education and support of the family begins. They need information on the nature and expected progress of the disease and use of memory triggers; establishment of a schedule for basic activities, such as bathing, toileting, meals, and naps; monitoring for intake and output, weight, and skin status; recognition of nonverbal indications of needs and problems; use of redirection and distraction to reduce difficult behaviors; identification of new symptoms or changes; physical and mental activities; necessary environmental modifications, safety measures, and legal issues; sources of information and support; and community resources for caregiving assistance and respite.

Teaching must be geared toward a time when medication has begun to lift mood and to clear thinking processes; otherwise, it is a wasted effort. Verbal teaching should be simple and supplemented with reading materials the patient and family can refer to at a later time. Ensure that follow-up treatment is scheduled and that the patient and/or significant other and family understand the need to get prescriptions filled and to consistently take medication as prescribed. Consider whether the patient has transportation available to get to follow-up treatment. Psychiatric home care might be a valuable part of the discharge planning to facilitate compliance with the discharge plan and for caregiver support. In addition, provide the patient and/or significant other and family with verbal and written information about the following issues:

- ✓ Nature and expected course of AD.
- ✓ Medications, including drug name; purpose; dosage; frequency; precautions; drug–drug, food–drug, and herb–drug interactions; and potential side effects.
- ✓ Strategies to deal with difficult behaviors.
- ✓ Strategies to maintain patient safety.
- ✓ Importance of self-care for the caregiver.
- ✓ Importance of using all available supports to aid in caregiving.
- ✓ Importance of caregiver and family engaging in honest expression of feelings and confronting negative emotions.
- ✓ Importance of caregiver using relaxation techniques to minimize stress.
- ✓ Importance of maintaining or achieving spiritual well-being for the patient and caregiver.
- ✓ Referrals to community resources for support and education. Additional information can be obtained by contacting the following organizations:
  - Alzheimer's Association (https://alz.org) provides a 24-hour hotline, free publications, and information for local chapters.
  - AARP (www.aarp.org) is an advocacy group for older adults; it also provides (for a reasonable fee) training materials associated with reminiscence therapy.
  - Alzheimer's Disease Education and Reference Center is available through National Institute on Aging (www.nia.nih.gov), which provides electronic newsletters and evidence-based resources.

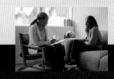

# Major Depression 102

## OVERVIEW/PATHOPHYSIOLOGY

Major depression is one of the most common psychiatric disorders, affecting 16 million adults in the United States. Major depressive disorder is characterized by a persistently depressed mood (profound sadness or apathy, irritability, emptiness or hopelessness) lasting for at least 2 weeks. At least four other symptoms must be present from the following list: lack of interest or pleasure in all or almost all activities, changes in appetite or weight, insomnia or hypersomnia, psychomotor agitation or retardation, loss of energy, feelings of worthlessness and guilt; difficulty concentrating or making decisions; and recurrent thoughts of death or suicidal ideation, plans, or attempts.

Major depression affects emotional, cognitive, behavioral, and spiritual dimensions. Depression may range from mild to moderate states to severe states with or without psychotic features. Major depression can begin at any age, although it usually begins in the mid-20s and 30s. However, there is a significant increase in depression in adolescents. Nearly 3 million adolescents (11%) between the ages of 13 and 18 reported experiencing depression. This is higher than the rate for adults. These adolescents are at risk for periods of depression throughout their life. The primary risk factors for depression include prior history of depression, family history of depression, prior suicide attempts, female gender, age of onset younger than 40 years, postpartum period, medical comorbidity, lack of social support, stressful life events, adverse childhood experiences, and current substance abuse. There are many theories to explain the causation of depression. Research supports the influence of the following factors: sleep disturbance; effects of pharmacologic substances, including many of the antihypertensive, steroidal, cardiovascular, and antipsychotic medications; neuronal factors that involve injury or malfunction of the brain, such as stroke, Parkinson's disease, and deficiencies in neurotransmitters; thyroid dysfunction; genetic factors; and psychodynamic factors.

## HEALTH CARE SETTING

Care of patients with major depression can be managed by primary care providers, psychiatrists, psychologists, or psychiatric nurse practitioners/clinical specialists in either the inpatient or outpatient setting. Some patients may require brief acute care hospitalizations in a psychiatric unit for severe depression, suicidal ideation, and/or homicidal ideation. The patient experiencing major depression also may participate in intensive outpatient programs.

## ASSESSMENT

The assessment of major depression involves much more than an assessment of mood. It is a disorder that results in changes in the following:

*Feelings, attitudes, and knowledge.* Sadness, lack of joy and happiness about anything, shame, humiliation, fear of stigma if others find out about depression, denial, anger, fear of experiencing a relapse, and fear of passing the disorder on to children.

*Signs of low mood.* Withdrawal from activities that once provided pleasure as well as from social interactions; negativism and unhappiness expressed in persistent sadness or frequent crying.

*Signs of lowered self-worth.* Self-deprecating, guilty, hopelessness, or self-blaming comments are common.

*Signs of decreased physical well-being.* A depressed person may neglect personal appearance or let assignments, tasks, and projects slide. Decreased energy is common, with the depressed person complaining of fatigue and inanition (exhaustion; lack of vigor or enthusiasm). A decreased ability to concentrate makes problem solving difficult. Decision-making also may be difficult.

*Spiritual issues.* Depression carries with it many negative experiences, such as marital and family problems, divorce, and unemployment, which contribute to the downward spiral of self-appraisals. Depression can lead to a crisis of faith in self, others, life, and ultimately God. This loss of faith and hope contributes significantly to the risk for suicide.

*Additional signs.* Some depressed individuals experience decreased appetite leading to weight loss. Others experience an increase in appetite and weight gain. A change in sleep pattern is characteristic of depression, with difficulty falling asleep, awakening in the middle of the night, and/or awakening in the early morning hours being common. Others may experience a need for excessive sleep and have difficulty awakening. A decline in sexual interest and activity is a characteristic of depressed individuals.

*Suicidality.* Suicide assessment is critical with depressed patients and includes questions to determine the presence of suicidal ideation and the lethality of any plan. Essential questions to ask include the following:

- When you feel depressed, what thoughts go through your mind?
- Have you thought of hurting yourself?
- Are you presently thinking about hurting yourself?
- If you have been thinking about suicide, do you have a plan?
- What is the plan?
- Have you thought about what life would be like for others if you were no longer a part of it?

A previous history of suicide attempts combined with depression places the patient at higher risk in the present for attempting suicide. A patient whose depression is lifting is at higher risk for suicide than a severely depressed individual because increased energy usually is manifested before improved mood. This increased energy is not enough to make the patient feel good or hopeful, but it is enough to carry out a suicidal plan.

## DIAGNOSTIC TESTS

The diagnosis of depression is made through history, interview of the patient and family, and observation of verbal and nonverbal behaviors. Laboratory tests that can rule out a medical basis for depression symptoms include thyroid and liver function tests. A number of effective scales are available to quantify the degree of depression, such as the Patient Health Questionnaire-9, the Beck Depression Inventory, the Hamilton Depression Scale, and the Geriatric Depression Scale.

## Patient Problem/Analyze Cues/Prioritize Hypotheses

# Risk for Suicide

*due to* depressed mood and feelings of hopelessness

**Desired Outcome/Generate Solutions:** By discharge (if inpatient) or by the end of 4 weeks (if outpatient), the patient expresses and demonstrates that he or she is free of suicidal thinking.

| ASSESSMENT—RECOGNIZE CUES/ INTERVENTIONS—TAKE ACTION | RATIONALES |
|---|---|
| Complete an initial suicide assessment (using the following questions): | The degree of hopelessness expressed by the patient is important in assessing the risk for suicide. The more the patient has thought out the plan, the greater the risk. The risk for suicide is increased if the patient has a history of a previous attempt or there is a family history of suicide and depression. Patients who display impulsive behaviors are more likely to attempt suicide without giving clues. Patients who are experiencing psychotic thinking, especially when there are "voices" that encourage self-harm, are at great risk. Use of alcohol/substance abuse in the presence of any of the above risk factors increases the overall risk for a suicide attempt. A high risk for suicide should prompt hospitalization. |
| Ask the patient if they feel like hurting themselves or others. | |
| Ask if they have a plan. Assess the plan. | |
| Assess the planned method. | |
| The amount of effort to deceive possible rescuer increases the risk of completed suicide. | |
| | The more developed the plan is, the higher the risk for suicide will be. |
| | Methods of suicide are more lethal depending on accessibility to the means to commit suicide. For example, a patient with three bottles of pills is more lethal that the patient that needs to make an appointment to see the care provider for a prescription. If the method is gun shot, the method is more lethal if the patient has the accessibility to a gun. |
| | If a person says they are going to one place to commit the act, but goes to another place, then they make it more difficult for family or friends to rescue. |
| ⚠ Reassess for suicidality, especially during times of change. | Changes such as the patient's mood improving, medication regimen being altered, discharge planning being initiated, and increasing withdrawal are all signals to reassess suicidality. Suicide risk is greatest in the first few weeks after treatment is begun. The patient may be feeling a little better but not well enough to feel hopeful and may have regained enough energy to actually act on suicidal thoughts. |
| Administer the antidepressant medication (selective serotonin reuptake inhibitors [SSRIs] or tricyclic antidepressants [TCAs]) or instruct the patient regarding the importance of taking medication as prescribed. | Suicidal thinking is a symptom of depression, which is can be treated through appropriate medications. |
| | Keep in mind that with antidepressants, the patient may have increased energy and increased energy puts the patient at higher risk for suicide. |

| ASSESSMENT—RECOGNIZE CUES/ INTERVENTIONS—TAKE ACTION | RATIONALES |
| --- | --- |
| If the patient is taking monoamine oxidase inhibitors (MAOIs) the patient needs to be educated on dietary restrictions. | The MAOIs break down monoamine neurotransmitters. Because of this, patients need to avoid certain foods containing tyramines |
| Inform the significant other about safety precautions and to be alert for changes in the patient's behavior and/or verbalization that would indicate an increase in suicidal thinking. | Using available support provides a safety net for the patient and communicates that he or she is not alone but that others are concerned and involved in care. |
| If the patient is hospitalized, implement the following: | |
| • Monitor at least every 15 minutes for moderate risk, preferably staggering monitoring times so that the patient does not take advantage of a guaranteed window of time to engage in suicidal behavior. Provide constant one-on-one observation for serious risk. Place the patient in a room close to the nurses' station. Do not assign to a single room. Accompany the patient to all off-unit activities or restrict him or her to the unit. Ask the patient to remain in view of the staff at all times. | Providing close observation may prevent suicidal attempts. |
| • Remove items such as belts, scarves, razor blades, shoelaces, scissors, phone cords, call bell cords—anything that could be used for self-harm. Check all items brought into the unit by patients. Instruct the family members to avoid bringing into the unit any hazardous items. | This provides environmental safety and removes potential suicide weapons. |
| • Provide supervision when the patient is in the bathroom—the door must remain open with a staff member outside. | It is important to remove all opportunities to engage in self-harmful behaviors. |
| • Perform a mouth check to make sure the patient swallows medications that are administered. | This prevents saving up medications to overdose or discarding and not taking. |
| • Ensure that nursing rounds are made at frequent but irregular intervals, especially at times that are predictably busy for the staff such as a change of shift. | It is important that staff surveillance not be predictable; otherwise, patients would be able to identify a possible suicide window. In addition, it is essential to maintain awareness of the patient's location at all times. |
| • Routinely check the environment for hazards and ensure environmental safety. | Minimizing opportunities for self-harm (e.g., keeping doors, windows, and access to stairways and the roof locked and monitoring cleaning, chemical, and repair supplies) is an ongoing concern requiring constant vigilance. |
| • Initiate a safety plan with the patient. | Involving the patient in creating a safety plan advances trust between the patient and nurse while promoting self-care and monitoring. |
| | The safety plan may include a set of actions the patient agrees to initiate when suicidal feelings increase, for example, approaching the nurse for one-on-one interactions, requesting an as-needed medication to reduce anxiety, and creating a list of friends or support persons the patient can call. |

## Patient and Significant Other Problems/Analyze Cues/Prioritize Hypotheses

# Deficient Knowledge

*due to* unfamiliarity with the causes, signs and symptoms, and treatment of depression

***Desired Outcome/Generate Solutions:*** By discharge (if inpatient) or after 4 weeks of outpatient treatment, the patient and significant others verbalize accurate information about at least two of the possible causes of depression, four of the signs and symptoms of depression, and use of medications, psychotherapy, and/or electroconvulsive therapy as treatment.

| ASSESSMENT—RECOGNIZE CUES/ INTERVENTIONS—TAKE ACTION | RATIONALES |
|---|---|
| Assess the patient's and significant other's knowledge about depression and its causes. | Depression is a physiologic disorder caused by the interplay of many factors such as stress, loss, imbalance in brain chemistry, and genetics. It is one of the most common psychiatric disorder. Many people believe that depression is caused by character weakness. This belief contributes to the stigma experienced by depressed individuals and interferes with seeking treatment. |
| Inform the patient and significant other about the major symptoms of depression. These include sadness and loss of interest in normal activities, plus at least four of the following: changes in appetite or weight, insomnia or hypersomnia almost every day, loss of interest in sex, or psychomotor agitation or retardation almost daily, feelings of worthlessness and guilt, difficulty concentrating or making decisions, recurrent thoughts of death or suicidal ideation with or recurrent thoughts of death or suicidal ideation with or without plans, or suicide attempts. | Many people believe depression equates with sadness and fail to recognize the many other signs and symptoms that make this a holistic disorder. If the depressed individual expresses sadness through irritability, the conclusion that depression is present may be missed and, consequently, necessary treatment may be delayed or avoided entirely. |
| Explain that depression is treatable. | Medications are usually indicated for treatment. They do not solve the stressors or problems that may have precipitated or resulted from the depression, but they provide the energy to deal with these issues. A combination of antidepressants and psychotherapy generally helps to relieve the symptoms of depression in weeks. Psychotherapy alone may be indicated for mild depression related to situational causes. |
| Explain the use of ECT as a treatment modality for major depression, if appropriate. | Because ECT is associated with many false beliefs, patients and families must be educated. ECT may be used to treat patients who do not respond to antidepressant medications after several trials and psychotherapy. It is relatively safe and well tolerated and is given as a series of 6–12 treatments administered 2–3 times a week under brief anesthesia. The patient and significant other/family may fear ECT because of misinformation in media portrayals. If it is recommended, it provides an opportunity for education that presents ECT as a positive treatment alternative. |

## Patient Problem/Analyze Cues/Prioritize Hypotheses

# Deficient Knowledge

*due to* unfamiliarity with medication use in depression, including potential side effects

*Desired Outcome/Generate Solutions:* By discharge (if inpatient) or after 4 weeks of outpatient treatment, the patient verbalizes accurate information about the prescribed medications and their potential side effects.

| ASSESSMENT—RECOGNIZE CUES/ INTERVENTIONS—TAKE ACTION | RATIONALES |
|---|---|
| Assess the patient's knowledge level regarding the use of medication to improve depressive symptoms. | It is essential to ascertain what patients know and do not know about the medications prescribed to treat their depression. Frequently patients hold faulty and inaccurate views about medications. This may interfere with adherence to a prescribed medication regimen. |
| Provide instruction about the physiologic action of the prescribed antidepressant and how it alleviates symptoms of depression. | Many depressed patients resist taking medications because they fear becoming "addicted"; however, antidepressants are not addictive drugs. Providing the patient with information about the medication's physiologic action helps with adherence. |

| ASSESSMENT—RECOGNIZE CUES/ INTERVENTIONS—TAKE ACTION | RATIONALES |
|---|---|
| Caution about the importance of taking the medication at the prescribed dose and time interval. | Some medications require certain blood levels to be therapeutic; therefore, patients need to take them at the dose and time prescribed. |
| Provide information about the side-effect profile of the specific prescribed medication, including interventions to combat these effects, for the following: | Each class of antidepressants carries with it a specific side-effect profile. Knowledge about expected side effects, ways to manage these side effects, and the length of time these side effects last is important in ensuring adherence. |
| **TCAs:** There are several used for major depressive disorder. They act on neurotransmitter pathways. For more information, see this patient problem in "Anxiety Disorders," Chapter 99. | These medications are effective in decreasing signs and symptoms of depression but can produce some troublesome anticholinergic side effects, including urinary hesitancy or retention, dry mouth, blurred vision, fatigue, weight gain, and orthostatic changes, some of which are transient in nature. Additionally, they can cause cardiac QT prolongation (heart block). Electrocardiograms (ECGs) must be monitored intermittently. |
| **SSRIs:** These medications are the most commonly used medications for depression and are generally the first line of prescribed medication for depression. For more information, see this patient problem in "Anxiety Disorders," Chapter 99. | SSRIs are effective, safe, and tolerable. These agents enhance the serotonergic function by inhibiting serotonin uptake, which increases bioavailability, thus promoting an antidepressant effect. |
| **Dual-mechanism agents:** venlafaxine, nefazodone HCl, mirtazapine, duloxetine, levomilnacipran, and desvenlafaxine | These medications inhibit both norepinephrine and serotonin uptake and are used when tricyclics and SSRIs fail to improve symptoms. |
| • Emphasize the importance of frequent blood pressure (BP) measurements for patients taking venlafaxine. For more information, see this patient problem in "Anxiety Disorders," Chapter 99. | At doses greater than 200 mg/day, venlafaxine causes an increase in BP. |
| **Norepinephrine–Dopamine Reuptake Inhibitor:** | This medication blocks the reuptake of both norepinephrine and dopamine. |
| • Inform the patient to be alert for anticholinergic side effects, decreased libido, and the potential for drug interactions. | These are common side effects. |
| • Be aware of the risk for seizures. | Risk increases with bupropion, although seizures have been reported with reboxetine use as well. |
| **Miscellaneous Antidepressants:** | |
| Provide instructions about the following: | |
| • Watch for anticholinergic effects such as urinary hesitancy or retention, dry mouth, blurred vision, sedation, hypotension, and risk for falling related to dizziness associated with hypotension. | These are common side effects and can be managed by encouraging patients to drink sufficient water and avoid exertion in high temperatures and activities that require mental alertness while adjusting to the medication. |
| • Be aware of the risk for seizures. | Risk is moderate with trazodone and increases with amoxapine and maprotiline. |
| • Be aware of the risk for cardiac toxicity. Patients older than 40 years need an ECG evaluation before treatment and periodically thereafter. | There is a significant risk with maprotiline. |
| **MAOIs:** | MAOIs are used when patients have not responded to other antidepressants. When MAO activity is reduced in the central nervous system, there is increased dopamine, serotonin, norepinephrine, and epinephrine at the receptor sites, thereby promoting an antidepressant effect. |
| • Caution the patient to be alert to the potential for mild sedation and hypotension. | These are common side effects. |

Continued

| ASSESSMENT—RECOGNIZE CUES/ INTERVENTIONS—TAKE ACTION | RATIONALES |
|---|---|
| • Provide instruction about MAOI dietary restrictions. | MAOIs combined with dietary tyramine can cause a life-threatening hypertensive crisis. Dietary restrictions include avocados; fermented bean curd; fermented soybean; soybean paste; figs; bananas; fermented, smoked, or aged meats; liver; bologna, pepperoni, and salami; dried, cured, fermented, or smoked fish; practically all cheeses; yeast extract; some imported beers; Chianti wine; protein dietary supplements; soups that contain protein extract; shrimp paste; and soy sauce. Large amounts of chocolate, fava beans, ginseng, and caffeine also may cause a reaction. The transdermal form of the MAOI selegiline does not require dietary restrictions. |
| • Instruct the patient to watch for possible drug interactions and the need to avoid all prescription and over-the-counter drugs unless they have been specifically approved by the provider. | MAOIs can interact with many medications to cause potentially serious results. Use of ephedrine or amphetamines can lead to hypertensive crisis. The interaction of TCAs with MAOIs can cause severe hypertension. Do not use SSRIs with MAOIs because together they can cause serotonin syndrome, a potentially life-threatening event. Symptoms include anxiety, diaphoresis, rigidity, hyperthermia, autonomic hyperactivity, and coma. Because of this possibility, MAOIs must be withdrawn at least 14 days before starting an SSRI, and when an SSRI is discontinued, at least 5 weeks must elapse before an MAOI is given. Antihypertensive drugs combined with MAOIs may result in the excessive lowering of BP. |

## Patient Problem/Analyze Cues/Prioritize Hypotheses

# Risk for Hopelessness

*due to* losses, stressors, and the burdensome symptoms of depression

***Desired Outcome/Generate Solutions:*** By discharge (if inpatient) or by the end of 4 weeks of outpatient treatment, the patient verbalizes feelings and acceptance of life situations over which he or she has no control, demonstrates independent problem-solving techniques to take control over life, and does not demonstrate or verbalize suicidality.

| ASSESSMENT—RECOGNIZE CUES/ INTERVENTIONS—TAKE ACTION | RATIONALES |
|---|---|
| Assess the individual signs of hopelessness. | This helps focus attention on areas of individual need. These signs may include decreased physical activity, social withdrawal, and comments made by patients that indicate hopelessness and despair. |
| Assess the unhealthy behaviors used to cope with feelings. | The patient may have tried to overcome feelings of hopelessness with harmful and ineffective behaviors (e.g., withdrawal, substance abuse, avoidance). Identifying ineffective and harmful behaviors provides an opportunity for change. |
| Encourage the patient to identify and verbalize feelings and perceptions. | The process of identifying feelings that underlie and drive behaviors enables patients to begin taking control of their lives. |
| Express hope to the patient with realistic comments about the patient's strengths and resources. | Patients may feel hopeless, but it is helpful to hear positive expressions from others. |
| Help the patient identify areas of life that are under their control. | A patient's emotional state may interfere with problem solving. Assistance may be required to identify areas that are under his or her control and to have clarity about options for taking control. |

| ASSESSMENT—RECOGNIZE CUES/ INTERVENTIONS—TAKE ACTION | RATIONALES |
|---|---|
| Encourage the patient to assume responsibility for self-care, for example, setting realistic goals, scheduling activities, and making independent decisions. | Helping patients set realistic goals increases feelings of control and provides satisfaction when goals are achieved, thereby decreasing feelings of hopelessness. |
| Help the patient identify areas of life situations that are not within his or her ability to control. Discuss feelings associated with this lack of control. | The patient needs to recognize and resolve feelings associated with the inability to control certain life situations before acceptance can be achieved and hopefulness becomes possible. |
| Encourage the patient to examine spiritual supports that may provide hope. | Many people find that spiritual beliefs and practices are a great source of hope. |
| Conduct a suicide assessment to determine the level of suicide risk (see earlier). | High risk will necessitate hospitalization. |
| Provide information to the patient about crisis intervention services such as suicide hotlines and other resources. | It is vital to provide patients with resources for support and safety when thoughts and feelings about suicide become difficult to manage. |
| Administer the antidepressant medication or emphasize the importance of taking medication as prescribed (see *Deficient Knowledge* regarding medications, earlier). | Suicidal thinking is a symptom of depression that is ameliorated through appropriate medication. |
| For additional interventions, see *Risk for Suicide*, earlier. | |

## Patient Problem/Analyze Cues/Prioritize Hypotheses

# Low Self-Esteem

*due to* the repeated negative reinforcement of self-appraisal, which is symptomatic of depression

***Desired Outcome/Generate Solutions:*** By discharge (if inpatient) or after 4 weeks of outpatient treatment, the patient demonstrates behaviors consistent with increased self-esteem.

| ASSESSMENT—RECOGNIZE CUES/ INTERVENTIONS—TAKE ACTION | RATIONALES |
|---|---|
| Assess the patient's level of self-esteem. | It is essential to identify the manifestations of low self-esteem, including neglect of personal hygiene and dress, withdrawal from social activities, and self-deprecatory comments, any of which signals a negative thought pattern. |
| Encourage the patient to engage in self-care grooming activities. | Attending to grooming is often an initial step in feeling better about oneself. |
| Provide positive reinforcement for all observable accomplishments. | Patients with low self-esteem do not benefit from flattery or insincere praise. Honest, positive feedback enhances self-esteem. |
| Encourage the patient to participate in simple recreational activities or art projects, proceeding to more complex activities in a group setting. | Initially, patients may be too overwhelmed to engage in activities that involve more than one person. |
| If the patient persists in self-deprecation, place a limit on the length of time you will listen to negativity. | Time limits allow patients a safe time and place to vent negative feelings and demonstrate thought stopping, the conscious interruption of negative thoughts. For example, agree to 10 minutes of negativity followed by 10 minutes of positive comments. |
| Provide instructions about thought-stopping techniques and positive reframing. | Many depressed people engage in self-critical thinking and need to be taught to consciously stop that type of thinking and substitute positive thinking in its place. |
| Explore the patient's personal strengths and suggest making a list to use as a reminder when negative thoughts return. | Having a written list to review can help patients during difficult times. |

## Patient Problem/Analyze Cues/Prioritize Hypotheses

# Grief

*due to* actual, perceived, or anticipated loss

***Desired Outcome/Generate Solutions:*** By discharge (if inpatient) or by the end of 4 weeks of outpatient treatment, the patient demonstrates progress in dealing with stages of grief at his or her own pace, participates in work/self-care activities at his or her own pace, and verbalizes a sense of progress toward resolution of grief and hope for the future.

| ASSESSMENT—RECOGNIZE CUES/ INTERVENTIONS—TAKE ACTION | RATIONALES |
| --- | --- |
| Assess the losses that have occurred in the patient's life. Discuss the meaning these losses have had for the patient. | Many people deny the importance/impact of a loss. They fail to recognize, acknowledge, or talk about their pain and act as if everything is fine. This has a cumulative effect on the individual. Denial requires physical and psychological energy. When individuals become clinically depressed, they are often already in a physically and emotionally depleted state. |
| Discuss the cultural practices and religious beliefs and ways in which the patient has dealt with past losses. | Cultural practices and religious beliefs influence how people express and accept the grieving process. |
| Encourage the patient to identify and verbalize feelings and examine the relationship between feelings and the event/stressor. | Verbalizing feelings in a nonthreatening environment can help patients deal with unrecognized/unresolved issues that may be contributing to depression. It also helps patients connect the response (feeling) to the stressor or precipitating event. |
| Discuss the healthy ways to identify and cope with underlying feelings of hurt, rejection, and anger. | This helps expand the patient's repertoire of coping strategies. |
| If indicated, tell stories of how others have coped with similar situations. | Patients often feel alone. They may feel they are the only ones with these feelings. Providing examples provides possible solutions, suggests that the problem is manageable, and informs patients that others have experienced the same feelings. |
| Inform the patient about the expected stages of grief and acknowledge the reality of associated feelings, such as guilt, anger, and powerlessness. | This information helps the patient realize the normalcy of feelings and may alleviate some of the guilt generated by these feelings. |
| Help the patient name the problem, identify the need to address the problem differently, and fully describe all aspects of the problem. | Once patients have clarity about the problem, they can address their individual issues. |
| Help the patient identify and recognize early signs of depression and plan ways to alleviate these signs. Assist with formulating a plan that recognizes the need for outside support if symptoms continue and/or worsen. | This actively involves the patient and conveys the message that the patient is not powerless but rather that options are available. |

| ADDITIONAL PROBLEMS: | |
| --- | --- |
| "Anxiety Disorders" for *Impaired Psychologic Function (Agoraphobia)* | Chapter 99 |
| "Bipolar Disorder (Manic Component)" for *Body Weight Problem (Weight Loss)* | Chapter 100 |
| *Risk for Self-Care Deficit* | |
| "Substance-Related and Addictive Disorders" for *Risk for Impaired Family Functioning* | Chapter 104 |

 **PATIENT–FAMILY TEACHING AND DISCHARGE PLANNING**

Patients with major depression experience a wide variety of symptoms that affect their ability to learn and retain information. Teaching is most effective when medication and therapy have begun to alleviate the depressed symptoms and clear thought processes. Verbal instruction needs to be simple and supplemented with reading materials the patient and/or significant other and family can refer to later. Ensure that follow-up treatment is scheduled and that the patient and/or significant other and family understand the need to get prescriptions filled and the importance of taking medication as prescribed. Consider whether the patient has transportation available to get to follow-up treatment. Also consider whether the patient is financially able to purchase the prescribed medications. Psychiatric home care might be a valuable part of the discharge planning to facilitate adherence to the discharge plan. In addition, provide the patient and/or significant other/family verbal and written information about the following issues:

- ✓ Remission/exacerbation aspects of depression.
- ✓ Medications, including drug name; purpose; dosage; frequency; precautions; drug–drug, food–drug, and herb–drug interactions; and potential side effects.
- ✓ Importance of continuing medication even after depressed symptoms are reduced.
- ✓ Importance of maintaining a healthy lifestyle—balanced diet, exercise, and regular adequate sleep patterns—to facilitate remaining in remission.
- ✓ Importance of social support and strategies for obtaining it.
- ✓ Importance of using constructive coping skills to deal with stress.
- ✓ Importance of honest expression of feelings and confronting of negative emotions.

- ✓ Thought-stopping techniques for dealing with negativism.
- ✓ Importance of using relaxation techniques to minimize stress.
- ✓ Importance of maintaining or achieving spiritual well-being.
- ✓ Importance of follow-up care, including day treatment programs, appointments with psychiatrists and therapists, and vocational rehabilitation program if indicated.
- ✓ Referrals to community resources for support and education. Additional information can be obtained by contacting the following organizations:
  - Depression and Bipolar Support Alliance (DBSA): www.dbsalliance.org. The DBSA provides education as well as support to individuals and families affected by depression and bipolar illnesses.
  - **Samaritans 24-Hour Crisis Hotline (212) 673-3000: Free 24-hour emotional support and crisis response hotline**. https://samaritansnyc.org/24-hour-crisis-hotline/
  - National Alliance on Mental Illness https://www.nami.org/Home
  - Referrals to websites that provide clinical information on the disease process and medications, such as www.WebMD.com.

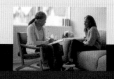

## OVERVIEW/PATHOPHYSIOLOGY

Schizophrenia is a neurobiologic disorder of the brain categorized as a thought disorder with disturbances in thinking, feeling, perceiving, and relating to others and the environment. Schizophrenia is a mixture of both positive and negative symptoms that are present for a significant part of a 1-month period but with continuous signs of disturbances persisting for at least 6 months. It is characterized by delusions, hallucinations, disorganized speech and behavior, and other symptoms that cause social or occupational dysfunction.

Schizophrenia is considered one of the most profoundly disabling of the major mental disorders, with less than 1% of the population suffering (Keltner & Steele, 2019). It can occur at any age, but it tends to first develop (or at least become evident) between adolescence and young adulthood. Men typically develop signs earlier than women, but the incidence for men and women is about the same. Risk factors include maternal starvation and infections during fetal development, complications during childbirth, childbirth that occurs in late winter or early spring, and living in an urban environment. The nature of these factors suggests a neurodevelopmental pathologic process in schizophrenia, but the exact pathophysiologic mechanism associated with these risk factors is unknown. Theories of causation include genetics, autoimmune factors, neuroanatomic changes, the dopamine hypothesis (people with schizophrenia appear to have excessive dopamine levels), and psychologic factors. Schizophrenia is classified as positive (type I) or negative (type II). Positive schizophrenia is when symptoms are exaggerated or embellished. For example, some positive symptoms are agitation, delusions, bizarre behavior, grandiosity, hallucinations, excitement, hostility, insomnia, or suspiciousness. Negative symptoms could include lack of conversation (perhaps communication difficulties) lack of energy, lack of social interactions or withdrawal, blunted effect, poor grooming and hygiene, or attention deficits.

## HEALTH CARE SETTING

Most patients with schizophrenia receive treatment across a variety of settings, including inpatient and partial hospitalization (day treatment), psychiatric home care, and crisis stabilization units. Community services include assertive community treatment, outpatient therapy, case management, and psychosocial rehabilitation.

## ASSESSMENT

Schizophrenia affects many aspects of a person's being. How the individual looks, feels, thinks, interacts with others, and moves in the world are all drastically affected by this disorder. A thorough assessment focuses not only on the bizarre behaviors that are characteristic of the disease, but also on the whole person—his or her physical, cultural, environmental, biological, psychological, emotional, social, and spiritual dimensions.

**Biologic.** A thorough history and physical examination are essential to rule out a medical illness, delirium, or substance use that could cause the psychiatric symptoms. It is essential to screen for comorbid treatable medical illnesses. People with schizophrenia have a higher mortality rate from physical illness and often have smoking-related illnesses such as emphysema and other pulmonary and cardiac disorders. The patient may appear awkward and uncoordinated, with poor motor skills and abnormalities in eye tracking.

**Psychologic.** Many patients report prodromal symptoms of tension and nervousness, lack of interest in eating, difficulty concentrating, difficulty in making choices, disturbed sleep, decreased enjoyment and loss of interest, poor hygiene, restlessness, forgetfulness, depression, social withdrawal from friends, feeling that others are laughing at them, feeling bad for no reason, thinking about religion more, hearing voices or seeing things, and feeling too excited. These symptoms are often ignored and may result in treatment delays.

**Appearance.** Individuals with schizophrenia may neglect hygiene and personal appearance. As the disease advances, they may lose weight and forget to bathe.

**Objective behaviors.** Patients may display stereotypy (idiosyncratic, repetitive, purposeless movements), echopraxia (involuntary imitation of another's movements), and waxy flexibility (posture held in odd or unusual fixed position for extended periods). Patients may display altered mood states ranging from heightened emotional activity to severely limited emotional responses. Affect, the outward expression of mood, may be described as flat, blunted, or full range, or it may be described as inappropriate. Other common emotional symptoms include affective lability, ambivalence, and apathy.

**Delusions.** Delusions are beliefs that are held despite clear contradictory evidence. Sometimes, they are plausible; at other times, the delusions expressed are bizarre, implausible, and not derived from ordinary life experiences. Delusions of persecution are the most common type. Delusions of grandeur are also commonly expressed. Ideas of reference are delusional ideas in which patients believe the actions of others are directed toward them. Two other forms of delusional thinking include thought broadcasting—the belief that one's thoughts can be heard by others—and thought insertion—the belief that thoughts of others can be inserted into one's mind. It is important to assess the content of the delusion; the degree of conviction with which the delusion is held; how extensively other aspects of the patient's life are incorporated into the delusion; the degree of internal consistency, organization, and logic evidenced in the delusion; and the impact exerted on the patient's life by this delusion.

**Hallucinations.** A hallucination is an alteration in sensory perception. Command hallucinations are auditory hallucinations that instruct a person to act in specific ways and can range from innocuous to life threatening. When patients experience auditory hallucinations, it is critical to determine whether these voices are commanding them to harm themselves or others. Although hallucinations can be experienced in all sensory modalities, auditory hallucinations are the most common in schizophrenia. Patients may not spontaneously share their hallucinations, and in order to assess for them, nurses may need to rely on observations of the patient's behavior, including pauses in a conversation during which the patient seems to be preoccupied or seems to be listening to someone other than the interviewer, looking toward the perceived source of a voice, or responding to the voices in some manner. It is important to not argue with the patient about the hallucinations, but rather, in a kind, calm voice indicates that you don't see or hear what they are seeing/hearing. For example: "I don't hear that" or "I don't see that."

**Disorganized communication.** Both speech content and patterns are important to assess. Abrupt shifts in conversational focus are typical of disorganized communication and are referred to as *loose association*. The most severe shifts may occur after only one or two words, referred to as *word salad*—a jumble of unrelated words. A less severe shift may occur after one or two phrases, referred to as *flight of ideas*. The least severe shift in the focus occurs when a new topic is repeatedly suggested and pursued from the current topic, referred to as *tangentiality*. In addition to abrupt shifts from one topic to another, the person with schizophrenia experiences thought blocking, in which thoughts and psychic activity unexpectedly cease. Language may be difficult to understand and may begin to serve as a tool of self-expression rather than a tool of communication. Sometimes, the person creates completely new words, referred to as *neologisms*.

**Cognitive impairments.** Although cognitive impairments vary widely from patient to patient, several problems are consistent across most patients; these include hypervigilance (increased and sustained attention to external stimuli over an extended time), a diminished ability to distinguish relevant from irrelevant stimuli, familiar cues going unrecognized or being improperly interpreted, and diminished information processing leading to inappropriate or illogical conclusions from available observations and information.

- *Memory and orientation:* Individuals with schizophrenia display impairments in memory and abstract thinking. Although orientation to time, place, and person remains relatively intact unless the person is preoccupied with delusions and hallucinations, all aspects of memory are affected in schizophrenia. Patients may experience a diminished ability to recall within seconds newly learned information. Both short- and long-term memories are often affected.
- *Insight and judgment:* Insight and judgment depend on cognitive functions that are frequently impaired in people with schizophrenia.
- *Affective symptoms:* Affective symptoms involve the emotions expressed and experience. The range of emotions and behavior could include a labile, unstable, or erratic mood. Depression is often noted, and it is crucial to assess for this as it could put the patient at an increased risk of suicide (see *Risk for Suicide* in "Major Depression," Chapter 102).

**Social issues.** As the disorder progresses, individuals become increasingly socially isolated. People with schizophrenia have difficulty connecting with others on a one-to-one basis. Emotional blunting, inability to form emotional attachments, problems with face and affect recognition, inability to recall past interactions, problems making decisions or using appropriate judgment in difficult situations, and poverty of speech and language all serve to separate and isolate the individual.

**Spiritual issues.** Persons with schizophrenia may experience delusions and hallucinations with religious content, and some health care providers tend to dismiss religious verbalizations as psychotic expressions. However, the contrary is true. Religion and spirituality can be a source of comfort to patients dealing with a terrible disease. It is important to assess religious commitment, religious practices, and spiritual issues such as the meaning of the illness to the individual, the role of God, and sources of hope and support.

**Suicidality.** An important priority of care is patient safety. Suicide assessment is critical in schizophrenia. The presence of psychotic thinking and command hallucinations, coupled with possible substance abuse, increases the suicide risk significantly. Suicide is also more likely in someone who is

- hopeless,
- male,
- socially isolated,
- in worsening health,
- suffering from a recent loss or rejection,
- lacking support from other people, and
- having family stress or instability.

It is important to ask questions to determine the presence of suicidal ideation and the lethality of any plan. Essential questions to ask include the following:

- Have you thought of hurting/killing yourself?
- Are you presently thinking about hurting/killing yourself?
- If you have been thinking about suicide, do you have a plan? What is the plan?
- Have you thought about what the life of others would be like if you were no longer a part of it?

Consider using the SAD PERSONS suicide assessment tool to quantify the risk for suicide.

## DIAGNOSTIC TESTS

There are no specific tests to diagnose schizophrenia. Diagnosis is made using the criteria put forth in the *Diagnostic and Statistical Manual of Mental Disorders*, fifth edition (American Psychiatric Association, 2013). Diagnosis is made through history, interview of the patient and family, and observation of verbal and nonverbal behaviors. Assessment needs to include the mini mental status exam and review of spiritual and cultural beliefs. Review psychological, biological, social, and environmental factors that may determine the effect on the presentation of the patient.

The Abnormal Involuntary Movement Scale (AIMS) and Simpson-Angus Rating Scale are tools used to evaluate movement abnormalities related to medications. AIMS is a 12-item clinician-rated scale to assess the severity of dyskinesia (specifically, orofacial movements and extremity and truncal movements) in patients taking neuroleptic medications. Items are scored on a 0 (none) to 4 (severe) Likert scale. The scale provides a total score (items 1 through 7), or item 8 can be used in isolation as an indication of the overall severity of symptoms. These tools are beneficial in assessing the severity of extrapyramidal symptoms (EPS) or tardive dyskinesia.

## Patient, Family, and Significant Other Problem/Analyze Cues/Prioritize Hypotheses

# Deficient Knowledge

*due to* unfamiliarity with the causes, signs and symptoms, and treatment of schizophrenia

*Desired Outcome/Generate Solutions:* Before discharge from the care facility or after 4 weeks of outpatient treatment, the patient and/or family/significant others verbalize accurate information about at least two of the possible causes of schizophrenia, four of the signs and symptoms of the disorder, and the available treatment options.

| ASSESSMENT—RECOGNIZE CUES/ INTERVENTIONS—TAKE ACTION | RATIONALES |
|---|---|
| Assess the patient's and significant other's understanding of schizophrenia. | Schizophrenia is a physiologic disorder caused by the interplay of many factors such as stress, genetics, infectious-autoimmune factors, neuroanatomic changes, the dopamine hypothesis, and psychologic factors. Providing education about the physical basis for the disorder increases understanding and acceptance and decreases blaming behavior. |
| Inform the patient about depression, self-destructive behavior, or other psychiatric problems. | The patient may have very limited knowledge of or insight into his or her behavior and emotions. |
| Provide instruction about social skills, such as approaching another person for an interaction, appropriate conversation topics, and active listening. Give the patient feedback regarding social interactions. | The patient may lack skills and confidence in social interactions; this may contribute to the anxiety, depression, or social isolation. |
| Help these patients identify some positive aspects about themselves. You may point out these characteristics, behaviors, or activities as observations, without arguing with the patients about their feelings. | These patients may see only their negative self-evaluations and not recognize positive characteristics. Although their feelings are real to them, your positive comments present a different perspective that they can examine and begin to incorporate into their self-evaluations. |
| Don't be judgmental. Treat with respect. Establish trust and involve the patient in treatment planning | Treating a patient with respect and dignity helps to establish trust. Trust is key to a therapeutic relationship. |
| Explain that there are treatments, including medications, available for schizophrenia. Comprehensive treatment involves short or long-term inpatient and partial hospitalization, day treatment, psychiatric home care, and crisis stabilization. Community services include assertive community treatment, outpatient therapy, case management, and psychosocial rehabilitation. and partial hospitalization, day treatment, psychiatric home | Medications are essential to stabilize and maintain patients with schizophrenia. They decrease psychotic thinking, hallucinations, and delusions. Some drugs target negative symptoms. However, medications are not the only treatment needed for schizophrenia. Patients may not be aware of existing treatment programs in the community and regimens for schizophrenia. |
| Involve patients as much as possible in planning their own treatments. | Participation in planning their care can help to increase a sense of responsibility and control. |

## Patient Problem/Analyze Cues/Prioritize Hypotheses
# Deficient Knowledge

*due to* unfamiliarity with the medications used in schizophrenia, including their purpose and potential side effects

***Desired Outcome/Generate Solutions:*** Before discharge from the care facility or after 4 weeks of outpatient treatment, the patient verbalizes accurate information about the prescribed medications.

| ASSESSMENT—RECOGNIZE CUES/ INTERVENTIONS—TAKE ACTION | RATIONALES |
|---|---|
| Assess the patient's knowledge about the physiologic action of antipsychotic medications. | Direct education to assess deficits in knowledge regarding the expected benefits of taking the prescribed drug, potential side effects, and how to deal with them. Knowledge increases adherence to taking the prescribed medications. |
| Ensure the patient is aware that antipsychotics generally take 2–6 weeks to reach the expected effects. Educate the patient on the importance of reaching the balance between effectiveness and the side effects. | |
| Provide information about the side-effect profiles of the specific prescribed medication as well as interventions to ease the effects. | A knowledgeable patient is likely to report adverse symptoms and know how to intervene properly for others, which optimally will promote adherence. |
| Explain the metabolic changes that may occur while taking antipsychotic medications. | Most atypical antipsychotic medications are associated with weight gain, hyperglycemia, dyslipidemia, and insulin resistance. |
| **Typical (first-generation) antipsychotic agents:** chlorpromazine thioridazine perphenazine, fluphenazine, haloperidol, and cariprazine. | Typical antipsychotics block all dopamine receptors in the central nervous system (CNS) and can produce serious movement disorders, referred to as *EPS*. |
| • Explain that sedation, orthostatic hypotension, and anticholinergic effects can occur. Explain the importance of changing positions slowly. | These are common side effects of first-generation antipsychotic agents. Changing positions (lying to standing or sitting to standing) suddenly causes blood to pool to the legs simply because of gravity. When this happens, the blood pressure drops and the body tries to shunt the blood back upward to provide the brain with oxygen. If this does not happen right away, the patient may be symptomatic due to the blood pressure dropping. Symptoms of orthostatic hypotension can be dizziness, weakness, blurry vision, nausea, or syncope. |
| • Inform the patient to be alert for EPS, including acute dystonia (impaired muscle tone), parkinsonism, akathisia (restlessness, agitation), and tardive dyskinesia (involuntary movements of the face, trunk, and limbs) using the AIMS. AIMS shall be assessed at least once every 6 months or more frequently as necessary by symptom assessment or as determined by the prescribing practitioner. | These are adverse effects of first-generation antipsychotic drugs, with tardive dyskinesia being the most serious. Use of AIMS enables objective quantification of changes in movements and permits early intervention before the appearance of tardive dyskinesia. |
| • Explain the potential for neuroleptic malignant syndrome (NMS). This is an idiosyncratic hypersensitivity to antipsychotics that is believed to affect the body's thermoregulatory mechanism. It is a rare but serious reaction that carries with it a 4% risk for mortality. Symptoms include high fever, sweating, unstable blood pressure, stupor, muscular rigidity, and autonomic dysfunction. | Early identification and treatment of individuals with NMS improve the outcome. |
| • Caution the patient that there is a risk for seizures. | Antipsychotics can reduce the seizure threshold and must be used with caution in patients with epilepsy or other seizure disorder. |
| • Emphasize the importance of avoiding all products with anticholinergic actions, including antihistamines and specific over-the-counter sleeping aids. | Products with anticholinergic properties intensify the anticholinergic responses to antipsychotic drugs, including dry mouth, constipation, blurred vision, urinary hesitancy, and tachycardia. |

Continued

| ASSESSMENT—RECOGNIZE CUES/ INTERVENTIONS—TAKE ACTION | RATIONALES |
|---|---|
| • Explain the importance of avoiding alcohol and other medications with CNS-depressant actions, for example, antihistamines, opioids, and barbiturates. | Antipsychotics can intensify CNS depression caused by alcohol and other medications. |
| • Explain the importance of avoiding smoking while taking clozapine, olanzapine, thiothexine, trifluoperazine. | Smoking decreases the serum level of these medications. |
| • For patients taking chlorpromazine, thioridazine, fluphenazine decanoate, perphenazine, or trifluoperazine, emphasize the importance of avoiding excessive exposure to sunlight, using sunscreen, and wearing protective clothing. | These medications belong to the phenothiazine class, which causes sensitization of the skin to ultraviolet light, thus increasing the chance of severe sunburn. |
| • Provide information that sexual dysfunction is a possible side effect and needs to be reported to the prescriber rather than stopping the medication. | It is important that the patient not discontinue the medication abruptly, but rather report it so that the prescriber can intervene accordingly. |
| **Atypical (second-generation) antipsychotic agents:** clozapine risperidone, olanzapine quetiapine, ziprasidone aripiprazole lurasidone | Atypical antipsychotics are more selective in blocking specific dopamine receptors. Because of this, they are associated with less risk for EPS. |
| • Explain that patients taking clozapine need to be watchful for drowsiness and sedation, hypersalivation, tachycardia, constipation, and postural hypotension. | These are common side effects. |
| • Explain that patients taking clozapine need weekly hematologic monitoring for the first 6 months of treatment, and after 6 months, the monitoring is monthly. Advise the patient that clozapine will not be dispensed if a blood test is not done. | Agranulocytosis (a marked decrease in granulocytes, a type of white blood cell) occurs in 1%–2% of patients, with an overall risk for death of about 1 in 5000. Agranulocytosis usually occurs in the first 6 months. Regular monitoring for agranulocytosis is essential to detect problems early. |
| • Caution that patients taking clozapine, especially those with seizure disorder, are at risk for seizures. | Generalized tonic–clonic seizures occur in 3% of patients, and the risk is dose related, with a higher incidence in patients receiving doses greater than 600 mg. Patients who have experienced a seizure need to be warned not to drive a car or participate in other potentially hazardous activities while on this medication. |
| • Explain that patients taking clozapine need to avoid medications that can suppress bone marrow function, such as carbamazepine and many cancer drugs. Cimetidine and erythromycin increase levels of clozapine, leading to toxicity. Smoking and phenytoin can decrease levels of clozapine, thus diminishing its efficacy. | These are drug-to-drug interactions that can occur when they are combined with clozapine. |
| • Advise patients taking risperidone that there is a risk for insomnia, agitation, anxiety, constipation, nausea, dyspepsia, vomiting, dizziness, and sedation. | These are common side effects. |
| • Advise patients taking risperidone to be watchful for EPS. | This is an adverse effect that is dose related (reported in doses greater than 10 mg/day). |
| • Explain that patients taking olanzapine to watch for headache, insomnia, constipation, weight gain, akathisia, and tremor. | These are common side effects. |
| • Explain that patients taking quetiapine need to watch for headache, somnolence, constipation, and weight gain. | These are common side effects. |
| • Caution patients taking ziprasidone who have a history of cardiac disease, low electrolyte levels, or family history of QT prolongation that they are at risk for electrocardiogram changes, specifically QT prolongation. | This is a common side effect. |
| Stress to the patient and significant others that medications must be taken regularly and continually to be effective; medications must not be discontinued because the patient's mood is stable. | A relatively constant blood level, within the therapeutic range, is necessary for successful maintenance treatment. |

## ADDITIONAL PROBLEMS:

## ✔ PATIENT–FAMILY TEACHING AND DISCHARGE PLANNING

Patients with schizophrenia experience a wide variety of symptoms that affect their ability to learn and retain information. Teaching must be geared toward a time when medication has begun to decrease the psychotic symptoms, thoughts are more organized, and communication is more effective. Verbal instruction needs to be simple and supplemented with reading materials that the patient and/or significant other and family can refer to at a later time.

Most patients with schizophrenia experience memory deficits, so retention of new information does not come easily. Repetition and attention to clarity and simplicity of teaching approaches and materials facilitate learning. Ensure that follow-up treatment is scheduled and that the patient and/or significant other and family understand the need to get prescriptions filled and to take medications as prescribed. Consider whether the patient has transportation available to get to follow-up treatment. Psychiatric home care might be a valuable part of the discharge planning to facilitate adherence to the discharge plan. In addition, provide the patient and/or significant other/family with verbal and written information about the following issues:

- ✔ Medications, including drug name; purpose; dosage; frequency; precautions; drug–drug, food–drug, and herb–drug interactions; and potential side effects.
- ✔ Importance of laboratory follow-up tests if the patient is taking clozapine.
- ✔ Importance of maintaining a healthy lifestyle—balanced diet, minimal to no caffeine or alcohol, exercise, limit the amount of smoking, and regular adequate sleep patterns—to facilitate remaining in remission.
- ✔ Importance of continuing medication use, probably for a lifetime.
- ✔ Importance of social support and strategies to obtain it.
- ✔ Importance of using community resources, for example, psychiatrist, psychiatric nurse, intensive outpatient support groups, family counseling, psychosocial programs including club houses, and other patient-run support groups.
- ✔ Importance of following up with medical care as well as psychiatric care.
- ✔ Importance of maintaining or achieving spiritual well-being.
- ✔ Referrals to community resources for support and education. Additional information can be obtained by contacting the following organizations:
  - Johnson & Johnson Patient Assistance Foundation, Inc. provides access to medicines for uninsured individuals who lack the financial resources to pay for them https://www.jjpaf.org/.
  - Lilly Cares Patient Assistance Program, at Eli Lilly and Company, https://www.lillycares.com/assets/pdf/lilly_cares_application.pdf. This program was designed to assist providers, patients, and the patient caregivers through reimbursement support and temporary provision of olanzapine and other drugs at no charge to eligible patients.
  - National Alliance for the Mentally Ill (NAMI) at https://www.nami.org/Home. Contact NAMI chapter in local state for information and schedule or contact the national office of NAMI. The NAMI Family to Family Education Program is a 12-session comprehensive course for families of people with serious mental illnesses.
  - Mental Illness Education Project, Inc. (www.miepvideos.org) has a videotape for families and mental health professionals titled "Families Coping with Mental Illness."
  - Mental Health America is a community-based nonprofit that helps those with mental illness. They provide education to patients and family (https://www.mhanational.org/).
  - MedicAlert Foundation (www.medicalert.org) provides a simple tool to ensure that people with schizophrenia receive proper care in an emergency department or to help family members find a loved one who has stopped taking medication and is experiencing behavioral problems in public. MedicAlert has a program for people who cannot afford the membership fees.
  - National Institute of Mental Health Public Inquiries (www.nimh.nih.gov) has a booklet prepared by the Schizophrenia Research Branch titled, *Schizophrenia: Questions and Answers* (DHHS Publication No. ADM 90-1457).

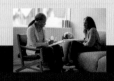

## OVERVIEW/PATHOPHYSIOLOGY

Substance use disorders are a major health issue in the United States. The connection between substance use and social and health problems is well documented and includes such issues as an increase in illegal and violent activities associated with the sale and distribution of illegal drugs, the current national opioid crisis, major health problems including the spread of human immuno-deficiency virus and other communicable diseases among intrave-nous (IV) drug users, developmental issues of "crack babies" born to addicted mothers, fetal alcohol syndrome babies, low-birth-weight babies, domestic violence, and child abuse/neglect. Deaths caused by motor vehicular collisions are often directly linked to alcohol consumption. In addition, there are a full range of med-ical complications that are a direct result of alcohol use disorders (AUDs), including cardiovascular, respiratory, hematologic, ner-vous, digestive, endocrine, metabolic, skin, musculoskeletal, geni-tourinary problems, and nutritional deficiencies.

According to the *Diagnostic and Statistical Manual of Men-tal Disorders*, fifth edition (DSM-5; American Psychiatric Association [APA], 2013), the essential feature of a substance use disorder is a cluster of cognitive, behavioral, social, and physiologic symptoms indicating that the individual contin-ues using a substance despite significant substance-related problems and dangers. There is an underlying change in brain circuits that may persist beyond detoxification. This is evidenced by a patient being sober for many years and remains vulnerable to the effects on exposure at a later time. DSM-5 diagnosis for each substance is based on the number of symptoms on a continuum from mild to severe: mild (two or three symptoms), moderate (four or five symptoms), and severe (six or more symptoms). Each substance the person uses will receive its own diagnosis in relation to its severity on this spectrum, for example, AUD—Severe; Stimulant Use Disorder—Moderate.

Identifying the specific drugs used is essential for individu-alized treatment of toxicity and withdrawal. However, it is the outcome of psychoactive drug use, shared in common by all drug classifications, that is most likely to account for the prob-lems associated with the disorder. These properties include acute and chronic structural and functional changes in the brain associated with drug intake; variable effects on the per-son taking the drugs; tolerance and reinforcing properties that are unique characteristics of most psychoactive substances and are not found in other pharmacologic classifications; and the

treatment concepts of recovery and relapse prevention after cessation of drug use.

## HEALTH CARE SETTING

Treatment of substance use disorders occurs in multiple health care settings. Acute detoxification usually takes place in an acute care/hospital facility. However, long-term care takes place in various community settings: outpatient or par-tial hospitalization therapy, vocational supports, family ther-apy, residential programs, and employee assistance programs. Treatment adjuncts include support group programming such as Alcoholics Anonymous (AA), Narcotics Anonymous (NA), and Celebrate Recovery.

## ASSESSMENT (ALCOHOL USE DISORDER)

Assessment focuses on AUD as a prototype for the category of *Substance Use Disorders* because it constitutes the most frequently used and misused psychoactive substance in the United States.

Screening tools have been developed and are used to aid health care providers in making a diagnosis of an AUD or in identifying those who are at risk for an AUD. The Alcohol Use Disorder Identification Test (AUDIT) is a questionnaire used to identify people with AUD or with risky alcohol use. The pro-vider reviews the questions and explains the significance with the patient. The CAGE assessment is a four-question assess-ment that identifies substance use disorders but does not iden-tify at risk behavior.

The tools help nurses identify the extent of the issues related to the alcohol disorder.

Major symptoms supportive of a diagnosis of AUD:

- Withdrawal symptoms. May use more of the substance to avoid withdrawal.
- Tolerance, as evidenced by needing more alcohol to get the same effect or consuming the same amount with less effect.
- Indiscriminate or regular drinking (or cravings) despite social or medical contraindications.
- Significant interference with psychosocial functioning in family and job relationships.
- Frequent absences, especially after time off.
- Drinking in hazardous situations or arrests for driving while under the influence of alcohol.

***Assessment interview.*** This includes family history, history of alcohol and other drugs used by the patient, and a description of behavior patterns described previously. It is important to ask about preexisting mental disorders (co-occuring disorders), metabolic conditions, cardiac and gas exchange problems, prescribed medications, and head injuries, all of which have symptoms that sometimes mimic acute intoxication or withdrawal symptoms.

***Psychologic symptoms, behavior patterns, and defense mechanisms.*** The patient uses *denial* to insist that they do not have a problem despite concrete evidence to the contrary. *Rationalization* appears in the form of self-imposed rules that explain the person's drinking habits as legitimate. Statements may be made such as "I only drink on weekends" or "I limit myself to beer, none of the hard stuff for me." *Projection* is evidenced in the blaming of external forces for stimulating the need to drink, for example, a nagging spouse or a stressful job. *Blackouts* refers to a period of time when the person functions socially but has no memory of that time. The hippocampus is not able to record short-term memory related to high blood alcohol levels.

### Physical indicators/examination

- Activity/rest: Difficulty sleeping, not feeling well rested.
- Cardiovascular: Peripheral pulses weak, irregular, or rapid; hypertension common in the early withdrawal stage from alcohol but may become labile and progress to hypotension as withdrawal progresses; tachycardia common in early withdrawal; dysrhythmias may be identified; other abnormalities depending on underlying heart disease/concurrent drug use.
- Elimination: Diarrhea, varied bowel sounds resulting from gastric complications such as gastric hemorrhage or distention.
- Nutrition and fluid intake: Nausea, vomiting, and food intolerance; difficulty chewing and swallowing food; muscle wasting; dry, dull hair; swollen salivary glands, inflamed buccal cavity, capillary fragility (malnutrition); possible generalized tissue edema resulting from protein deficiency; gastric distention, ascites, liver enlargement (seen in cirrhosis with long-term use).
- Pain/discomfort: Possible constant upper abdominal pain and tenderness radiating to the back (pancreatic inflammation).
- Respiratory: History of smoking; recurrent/chronic respiratory problems; tachypnea (with hyperactive state of alcohol withdrawal); diminished breath sounds.
- Neurosensory: Internal shakes or tremors, headache, dizziness, blurred vision, blackouts.
- Psychiatric: Possible dual diagnoses of mental illness, for example, schizophrenia, bipolar disorder, major depressive disorder, and anxiety.
- Level of consciousness/orientation: Confusion, stupor, hyperactivity, distorted thought processes, slurred/incoherent speech.
- Affect/mood/behavior: May be fearful, anxious, easily startled, inappropriate, irritable, labile, physically/verbally abusive, depressed, or paranoid.

***Withdrawal assessment.*** Monitor the patient every 4–6 hours with Clinical Institute Withdrawal Assessment—Alcohol, Revised

until the score is less than 10 for 24 hours, when medication for withdrawal is usually no longer necessary. Patients with scores greater than 15 are at a higher risk of delirium tremens (DTs) which can be life threatening.

- Early symptoms (6–12 hours after alcohol use cessation): Temperature, pulse, respirations, and systolic blood pressure (SBP) elevated; palpitations; slight diaphoresis; oriented × 3; mild anxiety and restlessness; restless sleep; tremulousness; decreased appetite; nausea.
- 12–24 hours after alcohol use cessation: Increased diaphoresis; intermittent confusion; transient visual and auditory hallucinations, primarily at night; increased anxiety and motor restlessness; insomnia; nightmares; nausea, vomiting, anorexia.
- 24–48 hours after alcohol use cessation: Additional symptoms may include generalized tonic–clonic seizures.
- Later (48–72 hours after alcohol use cessation): Severe additional symptoms. Pulse 120–140 bpm; increased temperature; increased diastolic blood pressure and SBP; marked diaphoresis; marked disorientation and confusion; frightening visual, auditory, and tactile hallucinations (predominantly visual); illusions (misinterpretation of objects); delusions; DTs; disturbances in consciousness; agitation, panic states; inability to sleep; gross uncontrollable tremors, convulsions; inability to ingest any oral fluids or foods.

***Safety assessment.*** History of recurrent accidents, such as falls, fractures, lacerations, burns, bruises, blackouts, seizures, or automobile accidents.

***Suicidal assessment.*** Alcoholic suicide attempts may be as much as 30% higher than the national average, and impulsivity is increased during intoxication.

***Social assessment.*** Dysfunctional family system; problems in current relationships; frequent sick days off work/school; history of arrests because of fighting with others or driving while intoxicated, disorderly conduct, or automobile collisions.

***Spiritual assessment.*** It is important to assess for spiritual beliefs, practices, faith traditions, and commitment to those traditions. Many alcoholics and others addicted to substances find recovery through the spiritual program models of AA, NA, and Celebrate Recovery. Spiritual beliefs may provide the anchor that prevents an addicted individual from considering suicide.

## DIAGNOSTIC TESTS

Blood alcohol and drug levels can be obtained. However, the diagnosis of *AUD* is generally made through interview history and physical and psychiatric examinations. The diagnosis is made by confirmation of the presence of the four major symptoms of AUD listed previously. Two of the most common assessment screening tools used to establish problem severity are the AUDIT and the CAGE questionnaires.

## Patient Problem/Analyze Cues/Prioritize Hypotheses

# Risk for Injury

*due to* altered cognitive function occurring with alcohol withdrawal

***Desired Outcome/Generate Solutions:*** During the withdrawal period, the patient does not exhibit evidence of physical trauma caused by alcohol withdrawal.

| ASSESSMENT—RECOGNIZE CUES/ INTERVENTIONS—TAKE ACTION | RATIONALES |
|---|---|
| Assess the stage of alcohol withdrawal and severity of symptoms. Monitor the vital signs, gait and motor coordination, presence and severity of tremors, mental status, and electrolyte status. | The greater the severity of symptoms, the more likely the patient will experience increasing disorientation, confusion, and restlessness. As the withdrawal progresses, the risk for a fall or injury increases significantly. |
| When monitoring for withdrawal hallucinations, be mindful not to confuse them with hallucinations from DTs. | Withdrawal hallucinations may occur 12–24 hours after the last alcoholic drink and usually resolve within 48 hours. Patients usually are aware that the unusual sensations are not real but may need support to manage the symptoms until resolution. |
| Monitor for the development of DTs. | DTs usually begin 48–72 hours after the last alcoholic drink. Signs and symptoms include disorientation, confusion, severe anxiety, hallucinations (primarily visual and tactile), profuse sweating, seizures, hypertension, racing/irregular heartbeat, severe tremors, and low-grade fever. |
|  | DTs can be life threatening, require medical attention, and are managed in an acute care setting. |
| Monitor for seizure activity; institute seizure precautions: bed in lowest position with side rails padded. | Withdrawal seizures usually occur within 24–48 hours after the last alcoholic drink. |
| Keep the communication simple. | As withdrawal progresses, the patient's ability to comprehend complex directions and interactions diminishes greatly. Simplicity is the key to effective communication. |
| Continue to orient the patient to surroundings and call light or communication system. | As the blood alcohol level drops, disorientation increases and can last several days. |
| Maintain a calm, quiet environment. | Controlling the amount of external stimulation and keeping it at a minimal level promote calm in the patient. |
| Administer the IV/oral (PO) fluids with caution as indicated. | Careful fluid replacement corrects dehydration and facilitates the renal clearance of toxins. Excessive alcohol use damages the cardiac muscle and/or conduction system. Overhydration poses a significant risk to cardiac functioning. |
| Administer medications as prescribed and be alert for side effects: |  |
| • Benzodiazepines: lorazepam, diazepam, or chlordiazepoxide | These medications are commonly used to control neuronal activity as alcohol is detoxified from the body. Either IV or PO route is preferred. These agents produce muscle relaxation, which is effective in controlling the "shakes," trembling, and ataxic movements, as well as preventing seizures. They are usually initiated at a high dose and tapered and discontinued within 96 hours. They must be used cautiously in patients with hepatic disease because the liver metabolizes them. |
| • Benzodiazepine use with hepatic disease: oxazepam | This may be the medication of choice for patients with liver disease. Although it does not produce quite the dramatic effects of controlling withdrawal symptoms, it has a shorter half-life, so it is safer in the presence of hepatic disease. |

| ASSESSMENT—RECOGNIZE CUES/ INTERVENTIONS—TAKE ACTION | RATIONALES |
|---|---|
| • Anticonvulsants such as phenobarbital or carbamazepine | These medications are highly effective in suppressing withdrawal symptoms and are effective anticonvulsants. Use must be monitored to prevent exacerbation of respiratory depression. |
| • Antipsychotics such as haloperidol or olanzapine | Antipsychotic medications may be used with DTs, specifically for symptoms of psychosis or severe agitation. |

## Patient Problem/Analyze Cues/Prioritize Hypotheses

# Risk for Denial

*due to* the lack of control of alcohol use resulting in the minimization of its symptoms and effects

***Desired Outcome/Generate Solutions:*** Before discharge from the care facility or after 4 weeks, if outpatient, the patient acknowledges that his or her drinking is out of control and that his or her life has become unmanageable.

| ASSESSMENT—RECOGNIZE CUES/ INTERVENTIONS—TAKE ACTION | RATIONALES |
|---|---|
| Assess the patient's level of denial versus acceptance that his/her alcohol use is a major problem and responsible for disruption in every area of their life. | Denial interferes with the patient's ability to participate in treatment. It is important for the patient to take personal responsibility for their recovery. |
| Encourage the patient to self-admit to an alcoholism treatment program. | Self-admittance is preferred because the element of denial has been addressed to a certain degree. Self-admission also may indicate readiness to refrain from alcohol use. |
| Assure the patient that alcoholism is a physiologic, chronic illness and not a moral problem. | This demonstrates a nonjudgmental attitude; it is easier to accept treatment for an illness than for what is perceived as a moral or emotional weakness or flaw. |
| Encourage the patient to compile a written list of the harmful consequences of excessive alcohol use experienced over the time they have been drinking. Ask the patient to show the list to another nurse, peer, or member of AA, NA, or Celebrate Recovery (if the patient is participating in support programming). | These interventions help break through the process of denial. Acknowledging the consequences of excessive alcohol use on one's life can help the patient move past denial and facilitate further progression through the stages of change. |
| Ask the patient to compile a list of situations that influenced excessive drinking and discuss ways to respond that do not involve drinking. | To help avoid relapse, it is important to know which situations triggered excessive drinking in the past and how to avoid those situations. If avoidance is not possible, teach coping skills to use when confronted with situations that have triggered alcohol use in the past. |

## Patient Problem/Analyze Cues/Prioritize Hypotheses

# Body Weight Problem (Weight Loss)

*due to* poor dietary intake

***Desired Outcomes/Generate Solutions:*** Within 1 week of interventions/instruction, the patient verbalizes an accurate understanding of the effects of alcohol and reduced dietary intake on nutritional status and demonstrates nutritional intake adequate for their needs.

| ASSESSMENT—RECOGNIZE CUES/ INTERVENTIONS—TAKE ACTION | RATIONALES |
|---|---|
| Assess for abdominal distention, tenderness, and the presence and quality of bowel sounds. | Excessive alcohol intake may irritate gastric mucosa and result in epigastric pain and hyperactive bowel sounds. Other, more serious gastrointestinal (GI) effects may occur secondary to GI bleed, hepatitis, and cirrhosis. |
| Note the presence of nausea/vomiting and diarrhea. | These signs are frequently among the first indicators of alcohol withdrawal and may interfere with establishing adequate nutritional intake. |
| Assess the patient's ability to feed self. | A number of factors, including tremors, mental status changes, and hallucinations, may interfere with independent feeding and signal the need for assistance. |
| Refer to a dietitian as indicated. | Expert advice may be necessary to coordinate the patient's nutritional regimen. |
| Provide small, easily digested, and frequent feedings/snacks as desired; increase as tolerated. | Small feedings may enhance the intake and toleration of nutrients by limiting gastric distress. As appetite and ability to tolerate food increase, adjustments are made to the diet to ensure that adequate calories and nutrition are supplied for tissue repair and healing and restoration of energy and vitality. |
| Review the liver function tests. | Liver function status influences the choice of diet and the need for/effectiveness of supplemental therapy. |
| Provide a diet high in protein with about 50% of the calories supplied by carbohydrates. | This diet provides for energy needs and tissue healing while stabilizing blood sugar levels. |
| Administer the medications as prescribed: | |
| • Antacids, antiemetics, and antidiarrheals | These medications reduce gastric irritation. |
| • Thiamine and vitamins | Thiamine and supplemental vitamins help to reverse deficiencies caused by chronic alcohol use. |
| Ensure the patient has nothing by mouth, if indicated. | It may be necessary to reduce gastric/pancreatic stimulation in the presence of GI bleeding or excessive vomiting. |

## Patient Problem/Analyze Cues/Prioritize Hypotheses

# Deficient Knowledge

*due to* unfamiliarity with the prescribed medications, rationale for use, and potential side effects

***Desired Outcome/Generate Solutions:*** Immediately after instruction, the patient verbalizes accurate information about the prescribed medication, including rationale for use and common side effects.

| ASSESSMENT—RECOGNIZE CUES/ INTERVENTIONS—TAKE ACTION | RATIONALES |
|---|---|
| Assess the patient's level of knowledge of the medications used in treatment. | Knowledge increases adherence to a prescribed medication regimen. In addition, because some of the medications used to treat AUD carry significant and dangerous risks, the patient must be informed regarding these risks. |
| Provide instruction about the medications that are sometimes used as adjuncts to AUDs treatment: | |

| ASSESSMENT—RECOGNIZE CUES/ INTERVENTIONS—TAKE ACTION | RATIONALES |
|---|---|
| **Disulfiram (Antabuse)** | |
| | This agonist medication is used as a deterrent to impulsive drinking. |
| Explain the risks of consuming ethanol (ETOH) or ETOH-containing substances while taking disulfiram. | Possible outcomes of using alcohol or substances that contain ETOH while on Disulfiram include the following: severe nausea, vomiting, hypotension, headache, cardiovascular collapse, heart palpitations, seizures, or death. Education on potential adverse reactions may increase adherence and decrease the potential for negative outcomes. |
| Inform the patient both verbally and in writing of the serious side effects that occur while taking disulfiram when ingesting alcohol or other substances containing alcohol such as cough syrups or cold remedies. | Potential side effects are so serious that informed consent is essential to document patient understanding, willingness to comply with the treatment regimen, and accepting the potential risks associated with disulfiram administration. |
| Reinforce the following: | |
| • Do not ingest any form of alcohol (beer, wine, liquor, vinegars, cough medicines, sauces, aftershave lotions, liniments, mouthwash, or cologne). | Doing so may cause a severe, even life-threatening reaction. Knowledge of substances to avoid may increase adherence to the treatment regimen and decrease the potential risks associated with disulfiram administration. |
| • Take the medication daily (at bedtime if it produces fatigue or dizziness). Crush or mix the tablet with liquid if necessary. | Taking medications as directed increases efficacy and ensures positive patient outcomes. |
| • Wear or carry medical identification with you at all times. | This alerts any medical emergency personnel that the patient is taking disulfiram, thereby preventing the administration of ETOH-containing substances if the patient becomes unresponsive. |
| • Keep appointments for follow-up laboratory tests. | Disulfiram may worsen coexisting conditions such as diabetes mellitus, hypothyroidism, chronic and acute nephritis, and hepatic disease. It also increases prothrombin time. When these conditions exist, blood sugar monitoring, kidney and liver function tests, thyroid tests, and prothrombin times need scheduled follow-up evaluations. |
| • The metallic aftertaste is temporary and will disappear after the medication is discontinued.<br>• Avoid consuming ETOH or ETOH-containing substances for 14 days after discontinuing disulfiram. | It takes up to 2 weeks for disulfiram to be totally metabolized by the body. Using ETOH-containing substances before disulfiram is fully metabolized can lead to unpleasant symptoms such as nausea, vomiting, and excessive diaphoresis. |
| • Avoid driving or performing tasks that require alertness while taking disulfiram unless the response to the medication is known. | Drowsiness, fatigue, or blurred vision may occur with disulfiram administration. |
| **Naltrexone (ReVia); Long-Acting Injectable Formulation (Vivitrol)** | |
| | This is an opioid antagonist originally used as a treatment for heroin use but has now been approved for the treatment of AUD. The drug reduces the cravings for alcohol and works best when accompanied by psychosocial treatment. |
| Provide instructions about adverse effects: difficulty sleeping, anxiety, nervousness, headache, low energy, abdominal pain, cramps, nausea, vomiting, delayed ejaculations, decreased potency, skin rash, chills, increased thirst, and joint and muscle pain. | These common adverse effects need to be reported to the prescriber. Adverse side effects may prevent patient adherence to naltrexone administration. |
| Reinforce the following: | |
| • **Naltrexone** decreases cravings and will make it easier not to drink. It also blocks the effects of opioids. | Educating the patient on the mechanism of action of **naltrexone** can increase adherence to the treatment regimen. |
| • Wear a medical identification tag. Notify other health professionals that you are taking this medication. | This alerts emergency medical personnel that the patient is taking **naltrexone**, which helps in choosing appropriate medication regimens if the patient becomes unresponsive. |

Continued

| ASSESSMENT—RECOGNIZE CUES/ INTERVENTIONS—TAKE ACTION | RATIONALES |
|---|---|
| • Avoid the use of heroin or other opiate drugs. | Small doses may have no effect, but large doses can cause death, serious injury, or coma. Patient education may increase adherence to and the proper administration of naltrexone. |
| • Report any signs and symptoms of adverse effects. | This enables the health care provider to adjust dosages or change the treatment plan if necessary. |
| • Keep appointments for follow-up blood tests and treatment program. | Frequent monitoring and adherence to medication management and treatment programs increase the patient's possibility of becoming and remaining ETOH free. |
| **Ondansetron** | |
| Explain that ondansetron is a serotonin receptor antagonist and is useful in reducing alcohol consumption and craving in patients with early-onset AUDs. | Patient education may increase adherence to the treatment regimen. ondansetron use can help to minimize the negative effects of ETOH cessation. |
| **Nalmefene** | |
| Inform the patient that nalmefene is an opioid antagonist that is similar in structure to naltrexone and is used often in emergency department treatment. It is less toxic to the liver and effective in preventing relapse to heavy drinking. It has few side effects. | Patient education may increase adherence to the treatment regimen. Nalmefene can be used as an alternative to naltrexone for patients with liver issues. |
| **Acamprosate** | |
| Inform the patient that acamprosate is a synthetic compound that is associated with increased abstinence through decreased alcohol craving. | Patient education may increase adherence to the treatment regimen. Acamprosate may be an effective tool for the patient to use until coping skills and support systems are in place. |

## Family Problem/Analyze Cues/Prioritize Hypotheses

# Risk for Impaired Family Functioning

*due to* the long-term pattern of the patient's alcohol use

**Desired Outcome/Generate Solutions:**  Before the patient is discharged from the care facility or after 4 weeks if the patient is outpatient, family members verbalize the dysfunctional behavioral dynamics present within the family system, the difference between caring and enabling, and the available services and treatment options that would help the family.

| ASSESSMENT—RECOGNIZE CUES/ INTERVENTIONS—TAKE ACTION | RATIONALES |
|---|---|
| Assess for and provide the family members with an opportunity to discuss their experiences of living with the disabling effects of AUD. | This validates their experience and encourages open discussions of the problem. |
| Educate the family members about the effects of AUD on the family system. | This information enables recognition that the dynamics in their family, although dysfunctional, are a predictable response to having a family member addicted to alcohol. It also encourages engagement in a realistic appraisal of the family's dynamics. |
| Provide family members with a list of services and available treatment options. | This validates that AUD has seriously and negatively affected the family unit. It normalizes seeking the aid and support of professionals to help address maladaptive family patterns. |

## ASSESSMENT—RECOGNIZE CUES/ INTERVENTIONS—TAKE ACTION    RATIONALES

| ASSESSMENT—RECOGNIZE CUES/ INTERVENTIONS—TAKE ACTION | RATIONALES |
|---|---|
| Define the term *enabling* for family members. Encourage each of them to identify at least one time when he or she enabled the patient. Offer family members alternative choices to enabling behaviors. Have them practice what they will do and say when a situation arises. | It is important to reframe helping behavior as enabling behavior for family members to recognize the pattern. It is also important for them to realize that changing these patterns requires practice and feedback. During times of anxiety, it is normal to fall back on previous patterns of behaving. |
| If in a relationship, encourage the couple to consider couples therapy to begin to discuss regrets and resentments that have occurred because of alcohol use. | It is important to begin to talk about unresolved feelings related to alcohol use that have been buried. This process needs to be undertaken with a professional who can act as a mediator and teach the couple how to communicate without blaming, which is a common dynamic in a relationship affected by alcohol use. |
| Explain how the roles have changed within the family because of alcohol use. | AUD produces dramatic role shifts that families are unaware of when they are amid problems such as codependence. Presenting this emotionally charged information in a concrete, didactic manner increases the ability to hear the information. |
| Encourage family members to talk about their needs and identify that caring is different from enabling. Foster understanding that caring behaviors are different from enabling behaviors. | Social and emotional isolation and denial of needs are common in families affected by alcohol use. Enabling behaviors are frequently intended as, and misunderstood to be, caring behaviors. |
| Encourage the family to attend Al-Anon meetings. | Significant change will require long-term commitment and support. |

### ADDITIONAL PROBLEMS:

### ✓ PATIENT–FAMILY TEACHING AND DISCHARGE PLANNING

The patient with a substance use disorder suffers from a problem that will affect every area of their life. To remain free of the use of substances, the patient will likely benefit from lifelong adjunctive treatment support through AA, NA, or Celebrate Recovery. The patient and family need to recognize that substance use disorders are family problems necessitating professional counseling and that alcoholism is a relentlessly progressive disease with profound medical, psychologic, social, and spiritual implications. Provide the patient and family with verbal and written information about the following issues:

- ✓ The nature and expected course of alcoholism/AUD/substance use disorder.
- ✓ Medications, including drug name; purpose; dosage; frequency; precautions; drug–drug, food–drug, and herb–drug interactions; and potential side effects.
- ✓ Withdrawal process—what to expect.
- ✓ Nutritional issues.
- ✓ Emergency measures.
- ✓ Importance of social support and strategies to obtain it; importance of changing social support if that support promotes drug use.
- ✓ Importance of using relaxation techniques to minimize stress.
- ✓ Importance of maintaining or achieving spiritual well-being.
- ✓ Importance of lifestyle issues such as benefits of exercise.
- ✓ Importance of group support for continued adjunctive treatment through AA, NA, or Celebrate Recovery.
- ✓ Additional information can be obtained by contacting the following organizations:
  - Al-Anon Family Groups: https://al-anon.org/
  - AA: https://www.aa.org/
  - Celebrate Recovery: https://www.celebraterecovery.com/
  - Substance Abuse and Mental Health Services Administration: www.samsha.gov
  - National Institute on Alcohol Abuse and Alcoholism: www.niaaa.nih.gov
  - National Institute on Drug Abuse: www.nida.nih.gov
  - Online AA Recovery: www.aaonline.net/index.html

# Bibliography

## Part I: Medical-Surgical Nursing Care Plans
### Section 1: General Care Plans

Abebe, W. (2019). Review of herbal medications with the potential to cause bleeding: Dental implications, and risk prediction and prevention avenues. *EPMA Journal, 10*, 51–64. https://doi.org/10.1007/s13167-018-0158-2.

American Cancer Society. (n.d.a). *Cervical cancer.* Retrieved from: https://www.cancer.org/cancer/cervical-cancer.html.

American Cancer Society. (n.d.b). *Prostate cancer.* Retrieved from: https://www.cancer.org/cancer/prostate-cancer.html.

American Cancer Society. (2018). *Hodgkin lymphoma risk factors.* Retrieved from: https://www.cancer.org/cancer/hodgkin-lymphoma/causes-risks-prevention/risk-factors.html.

American Cancer Society. (2021a). *Cancer treatment & survivorship facts & figures.* Retrieved from: https://www.cancer.org/research/cancer-facts-statistics/survivor-facts-figures.html.

American Cancer Society. (2021b). *The American Cancer Society guidelines for the early detection of cancer.* Retrieved from: https://www.cancer.org/healthy/find-cancer-early/american-cancer-society-guidelines-for-the-early-detection-of-cancer.html.

American Cancer Society. (2021c). *The American Cancer Society guidelines for the prevention and early treatment of cervical cancer.* Retrieved from: https://www.cancer.org/cancer/cervical-cancer/detection-diagnosis-staging/cervical-cancer-screening-guidelines.html.

American Cancer Society. (2021d). *Recommendations for prostate cancer early detection.* Retrieved from: https://www.cancer.org/cancer/prostate-cancer/detection-diagnosis-staging/acs-recommendations.html.

American Cancer Society. (2022a). *Cancer facts & figures 2022.* Retrieved from: https://www.cancer.org/research/cancer-facts-statistics.html.

American Cancer Society. (2022b). *Colorectal facts & figures 2020–2022.* Retrieved from: https://www.cancer.org/research/cancer-facts-statistics.html.

American Cancer Society. (2022c). *Key statistics for breast cancer.* Retrieved from: https://www.cancer.org/cancer/breast-cancer/about/how-common-is-breast-cancer.html.

American Cancer Society. (2022d). *Key statistics for ovarian cancer.* Retrieved from: https://www.cancer.org/cancer/ovarian-cancer/about/key-statistics.html.

American Cancer Society. (2022e). *Lesbian, gay, bisexual, transgender and queer (LGBTQ) people and cancer fact sheet.* Retrieved from: https://www.cancer.org/content/dam/cancer-org/cancer-control/en/booklets-flyers/lgbtq-people-with-cancer-fact-sheet.pdf.

American Psychological Association. (2015a). Guidelines for psychological practice with transgender and gender nonconforming people. *The American Psychologist, 70*(9), 832–864.

American Psychological Association. (2015b). Understanding transgender people, gender identity and gender expression. *The American Psychologist.* Retrieved from: http://www.apa.org/topics/lgbt/transgender.aspx.

Borg, G. A. (1982). Psychophysical bases of perceived exertion. *Medicine and Science in Sports and Exercise, 14*, 377–381.

Centers for Disease Control and Prevention. (2016a). *How infections spread.* Retrieved from: https://www.cdc.gov/infectioncontrol/spread/.

Centers for Disease Control and Prevention. (2016b). *Standard precautions for all patient care.* Retrieved from: https://www.cdc.gov/infectioncontrol/basics/standard-precautions.html.

Centers for Disease Control and Prevention. (2016c). *Transmission-based precautions.* Retrieved from: https://www.cdc.gov/infectioncontrol/basics/transmission-based-precautions.html.

Centers for Disease Control and Prevention. (2020). *Hand hygiene guidance.* Retrieved from: https://www.cdc.gov/handhygiene/providers/guideline.html.

Centers for Disease Control and Prevention. (2021a). *HPV vaccine.* Retrieved from: https://www.cdc.gov/hpv/parents/vaccine-for-hpv.html.

Centers for Disease Control and Prevention. (2021b). *Screening tests.* Retrieved from: https://www.cdc.gov/cancer/dcpc/prevention/screening.htm.

Centers for Disease Control and Prevention. (2022a). *Chronic diseases in America.* Retrieved from: https://www.cdc.gov/chronicdisease/resources/infographic/chronic-diseases.htm.

Centers for Disease Control and Prevention. (2022b). *Colorectal cancer screening tests.* Retrieved from: https://www.cdc.gov/cancer/colorectal/basic_info/screening/tests.htm.

Chou, R., Gordon, D. B., de Leon-Casasola, O. A., Rosenberg, J. M., Bickler, S., Brennan, T., Carter, T., Cassidy, C. L., Chittenden, E. H., Degenhardt, E., Griffith, S., Manworren, R., McCarberg, B., Montgomery, R., Murphy, J., Perkal, M. F., Suresh, S., Sluka, K., Strassels, S., … Wu, C. L. (2016). Guidelines on the management of postoperative pain. *The Journal of Pain, 17*(2), 131–157.

Dickey, L., Karasic, D., & Sharon, N. (2017). *Guidelines for the primary and gender affirming care of transgender and gender non-binary people: Mental health considerations with transgender and gender nonconforming clients.* San Francisco, CA: UCSF. Retrieved from: http://www.transhealth.ucsf.edu/trans?page=guideline-mental-health.

Edmiston, C. E., Leaper, D. J., Barnes, S., Johnson, H. B., Barnden, M., Paulsen, M. H., Wolfe, J. L., & Truitt, K. (2019). Revisiting perioperative hair removal practices. *AORN Journal, 109*(5), 583. https://doi.org/10.1002/aorn.12662.

Faghani, S., & Ghaffari, F. (2016). Effects of sexual rehabilitation using the PLISSIT model on quality of sexual life and sexual functioning in post-mastectomy breast cancer survivors. *Asian Pacific Journal of Cancer Prevention, 17*(11), 4845–4851. https://doi.org/10.22034/APJCP.2016.17.11.4845. PMID: 28030909; PMCID: PMC5454684.

Harding, M. M., Kwong, J., Hagler, D., & Reinisch, C. (2023). *Lewis's medical-surgical nursing* (12th ed.). St. Louis, MO: Elsevier.

Healthy People 2020. (2014). *Lesbian, gay, bisexual, and transgender health.* Retrieved from: http://www.healthypeople.gov/2020/topics-objectives/topic/lesbian-gay-bisexual-and-transgender-health.

Hui, D., & Bruera, E. (2017). The Edmonton symptom assessment 25 years later. *Journal of Pain and Symptom Management, 53*, 630–643.

Institute for Safe Medication Practices (ISMP). (2016). *Medication safety alert: Worth repeating…recent PCA by proxy events suggests reassessment of practices that may have fallen by the wayside. (September 22, 2016).* Retrieved from: http://www.ismp.org.

Kang, Y., & Demiris, G. (2018). Self-report pain assessment tools for cognitively intact older adults: Integrative review. *International Journal of Older People Nursing, 13*(2), e12170. https://doi.org/10.1111/opn.12170.

LeFebvre, K. B., Rogers, B., & Wolles, B. (2020). Cancer constipation: clinical summary of the ONS Guidelines(™) for opioid-induced and non-opioid-related cancer constipation. *Clinical Journal of Oncology Nursing, 24*(6), 685–688. https://doi.org/10.1188/20.CJON.685-688.

Lilley, L. L., Rainforth Collins, S., & Snyder, J. S. (2023). *Pharmacology and the nursing process* (10th ed.). St. Louis, MO: Elsevier.

Marks, A., & Marchand, L. (2022). *Near death awareness. Fast facts and concepts #118*. Palliative Care Network of Wisconsin. https://www.mypcnow.org/fast-fact/near-death-awareness/

National Cancer Institute. (n.d.). *Pack years (definition)*. Retrieved from: https://www.cancer.gov/publications/dictionaries/cancer-terms/def/pack-year.

National Cancer Institute. (2021a). *Cancer stat facts: Cervical cancer*. Retrieved from: https://seer.cancer.gov/statfacts/html/cervix.html.

National Cancer Institute. (2021b). *Cancer stat facts: Hodgkin lymphoma*. Retrieved from: https://seer.cancer.gov/statfacts/html/hodg.html.

National Cancer Institute. (2021c). *Cancer stat facts: Leukemia*. Retrieved from: https://seer.cancer.gov/statfacts/html/leuks.html.

National Cancer Institute. (2021d). *Cancer stat facts: Non-Hodgkin lymphoma*. Retrieved from: https://seer.cancer.gov/statfacts/html/nhl.html.

National Cancer Institute. (2021e). *Cancer stat facts: Ovarian cancer*. Retrieved from: https://seer.cancer.gov/statfacts/html/ovary.html.

National Cancer Institute. (2021f). *Cancer stat facts: Prostate cancer*. Retrieved from: https://seer.cancer.gov/statfacts/html/prost.html.

National Cancer Institute. (2021g). *Cancer stat facts: Testicular cancer*. Retrieved from: https://seer.cancer.gov/statfacts/html/testis.html.

National Cancer Institute. (2021h). *Head and neck cancers*. Retrieved from: https://www.cancer.org/research/cancer-facts-statistics/survivor-facts-figures.html.

National Cancer Institute. (2021i). *Lung cancer screening PDQ®*. Retrieved from: https://www.cancer.gov/types/lung/patient/lung-screening-pdq.

National Cancer Institute. (2021j). *SEER cancer stat facts: Lung and bronchus cancer*. Retrieved from: https://seer.cancer.gov/statfacts/html/lungb.html.

National Cancer Institute. (2022a). *Leukemia—Health professional version*. Retrieved from: https://www.cancer.gov/types/leukemia/hp.

National Cancer Institute. (2022b). *PDQ® adult central nervous system tumors treatment*. Retrieved from: https://www.cancer.gov/types/brain/hp/adult-brain-treatment-pdq.

National Cancer Institute. (2022c). *Survival rates for bladder cancer*. Retrieved from: https://www.cancer.org/cancer/bladder-cancer/detection-diagnosis-staging/survival-rates.html.

Olson, J., Schrager, S. M., Belzer, M., Simons, L. K., & Clark, L. F. (2015). Baseline physiologic and psychologic characteristics of transgender youth seeking care for gender dysmorphia. *Journal of Adolescent Health, 57*(4), 374–380.

Population Reference Bureau. (2022). *Fact sheet: Aging in the U.S.* https://www.prb.org/resources/fact-sheet-aging-in-the-united-states/.

Puchalski, C. (2020). *The FICA spiritual history tool*. The GW Institute for Spirituality and Health (GWish). https://smhs.gwu.edu/spirituality-health/program/transforming-practice-health-settings/clinical-fica-tool.

Qureshi, R. I., Zha, P., Kim, S., Hindin, P., Naqui, Z., Holly, C., Dubbs, W., & Ritch, W. (2017). Health care needs and care utilization among lesbian, gay, bisexual, and transgender populations in New Jersey. *Journal of Homosexuality*, 2–14.

Rafferty, J. (2022). *Gender identity development in children*. American Academy of Pediatrics. Retrieved from: www.aap.org.

The Joint Commission (TJC). (2023). *Hospital national patient safety goals*. Retrieved from: https://www.jointcommission.org/standards/national-patient-safety-goals/hospital-national-patient-safety-goals/.

Williams, N. (2017). The Borg Rating of Perceived Exertion (RPE) scale. *Occupational Medicine, 67*(5), 404–405.

World Professional Association for Transgender Health (WPATH). (2011). *Standards of care for the health of transsexual, transgender, and gender nonconforming people*. 7th ed. Retrieved from: http://www.wpath.org.

World Professional Association for Transgender Health (WPATH). (2017). *Standards of care version 8*. Retrieved from: WPATH.org/publications/SOC.

### Section 2: Respiratory Care Plans

American Lung Association. (2021). *What causes COPD?* Retrieved from: https://www.lung.org/lung-health-diseases/lung-disease-lookup/copd/what-causes-copd.

Centers for Disease Control and Prevention. (2020). *Venous thromboembolism (blood clots)*. Retrieved from: https://www.cdc.gov/ncbddd/dvt/facts.html.

Centers for Disease Control and Prevention (CDC). (2021a). *Leading causes of death*. Retrieved from: https://www.cdc.gov/nchs/nvss/leading-causes-of-death.htm.

Centers for Disease Control and Prevention (CDC). (2021b). *Who needs a flu vaccine?* Retrieved from: https://www.cdc.gov/flu/prevent/vaccinations.htm.

Centers for Disease Control and Prevention (CDC). (2022a). *FastStats: Deaths and mortality*. Retrieved from: https://www.cdc.gov/nchs/fastats/default.htm.

Centers for Disease Control and Prevention (CDC). (2022b). *Pneumococcal vaccine recommendations*. Retrieved from: https://www.cdc.gov/vaccines/vpd/pneumo/hcp/recommendations.html.

Centers for Disease Control and Prevention (CDC). (2022c). *Tuberculosis: Data and statistics*. Retrieved from: https://www.cdc.gov/tb/statistics/

Harding, M. M., Kwong, J., Hagler, D., & Reinisch, C. (2023). *Lewis's medical-surgical nursing* (12th ed.). St. Louis, MO: Elsevier.

Light, R.W. (2017). *Primary spontaneous pneumothorax in adults*. UpToDate. Retrieved from: http://www.uptodate.com/contents/primary-spontaneous-pneumothorax-in-adults.

McDonald, C. F. (2014). Oxygen therapy for COPD. *Journal of Thoracic Disease, 6*(11), 1632–1639. https://doi.org/10.3978/j.issn.2072-1439.2014.10.23.

McKnight, C. L., & Burns, B. (2021). Pneumothorax. In: *StatPearls*. National Library of Medicine. Retrieved from: https://www.ncbi.nlm.nih.gov/books/NBK441885/.

World Health Organization. (2021). *Tuberculosis*. Retrieved from: https://www.who.int/news-room/fact-sheets/detail/tuberculosis.

### Section 3: Cardiovascular Care Plans

Advanced Cardiac Life Support Algorithms. (n.d.). *ACLS medical training*. Retrieved from: https://www.aclsmedicaltraining.com/acls-algorithms/.

Centers for Disease Control and Prevention, National Center for Health Statistics. (2021a). *FastStats: Hypertension*. Retrieved from: https://www.cdc.gov/nchs/fastats/hypertension.htm.

Centers for Disease Control and Prevention, National Center for Health Statistics. (2021b). *Underlying cause of death 1999-2020 on CDC WONDER online database, released in 2021*. Retrieved from: http://wonder.cdc.gov/ucd-icd10.html.

Harding, M. M., Kwong, J., Hagler, D., & Reinisch, C. (2023). *Lewis's medical-surgical nursing* (12th ed.). St. Louis, MO: Elsevier.

National Heart, Lung and Blood Institute. (2022a). *Heart failure*. Retrieved from: https://www.nhlbi.nih.gov/health/heart-failure.

National Heart, Lung and Blood Institute. (2022b). *Venous thromboembolism*. Retrieved from: https://www.nhlbi.nih.gov/health/venous-thromboembolism.

Whelton, P. K., Carey, R. M., Aronow, W. S., Casey Jr., D. E., Collins, K. J., Himmelfarb, C. D., DePalma, S. M., Gidding, S., Jamerson, K. A., Jones, D. W., MacLaughlin, E. J., Munter, P., Ovbiagele, B., Smith Jr., S. C., Spencer, C. C., Stafford, R. S., Taler, S. J., Thomas, R. J., Williams Sr., K. A., … Wright, J. T. (2018). 2017 ACC/AHA/AAPA/ABC/ACPM/AGS/APhA/ASH/ASPC/NMA/PCNA guidelines for the prevention, detection, evaluation, and management of high blood pressure in adults: A report of the American College of Cardiology/American Heart Association Task Force on Clinical Practice Guidelines. *Journal of the American College of Cardiology, 71*, e127.

### Section 4: Renal-Urinary Care Plans

American Nephrology Nurses' Association (ANNA) Specialty Practice Networks. (2021). *Renal transplantation fact sheet*. Retrieved from: https://www.annanurse.org/download/reference/practice/transplantFactSheet.pdf.

Gomez, N. (2017). *ANNA nephrology nursing scope and standards of practice* (8th ed.). Pitman, NJ: American Nephrology Nurses' Association.

Harding, M. M., Kwong, J., Hagler, D., & Reinisch, C. (2023). *Lewis's medical-surgical nursing* (12th ed.). St. Louis, MO: Elsevier.

Kidney International: Kidney Disease Improving Global Outcomes (KDIGO). (2021). *Clinical practice guidelines for the management of blood pressure in chronic kidney disease*. https://www.kidney-international.org/action/showPdf?pii=S0085-2538%2820%2931270-9.

Leslie, S.W., Sajjad, H., & Murphy, P.B. (2022). Renal calculi. In: *StatPearls [Internet]*. Treasure Island, FL: StatPearls Publishing. https://www.ncbi.nlm.nih.gov/books/NBK442014/.

National Kidney Foundation, (2015). KDOQI Clinical practice guideline for Hemodialysis adequacy: 2015 update. *American Journal of Kidney Diseases, 5*, 884–930.

Rabinowitz, R., & Cubillos, J. (2020). Renal anomalies. https://www.merckmanuals.com/professional/pediatrics/congenital-renal-and-genitourinary-anomalies/renal-anomalies.

### Section 5: Neurologic Care Plans

Ahn, S.-N., Lee, J.-W., & Hwang, S. (2016). Tactile perception for stroke induce changes in electroencephalography. *Hong Kong Journal of Occupational Therapy, 28*, 1–6.

American Spinal Injury Association (ASIA). *Impairment scale*. https://www.icf-casestudies.org/introduction/spinal-cord-injury-sci/american-spinal-injury-association-asia-impairment-scale.

Bay, E. H., & Chartier, K. S. (2014). Chronic morbidities after traumatic brain injury. *The Journal of Neuroscience Nursing: Journal of the American Association of Neuroscience Nurses, 46*(3), 142–152.

Bishop, B. S. (2017). Multiple sclerosis. In T. M. Buttaro, J. Trylbuski, & P. Polgar-Bailey (Eds.), *Primary care a collaborative practice* (5th ed., pp. 1044–1050). St. Louis, MO: Elsevier.

Blissett, P. A. (Ed.), (2014). *Cervical spine surgery a guide to preoperative and postoperative patient care: AANN clinical practice guideline series*. Chicago, IL: American Association of Neuroscience Nurses.

Chaudhuri, K. R., Bhidayasiri, R., & Laar, T. V. (2016). Unmet needs in Parkinson's disease: New horizons in a changing landscape. *Parkinsonism and Related Disorders Journal, 33*(1), S2–S8.

Graykoski, J. (2017). Cerebrovascular events. In T. M. Buttaro, J. Trybulski, & P. Polgar-Bailey (Eds.), *Primary care a collaborative practice* (5th ed., pp. 1010–1016). St. Louis, MO: Elsevier.

Green, T. L., McNair, N. D., Hinkle, J. L., Middleton, S., Miller, E. T., Perrin, S., Power, M., Southerland, A. M., Summers, D. V., & American Heart Association Stroke Nursing Committee of the Council on Cardiovascular and Stroke Nursing and the Stroke Council, (2021). Care of the patient with acute ischemic stroke (posthyperacute and prehospital discharge): Update to 2009 comprehensive nursing care scientific statement: A scientific statement from the American Heart Association. *Stroke, 52*(5), e179–e197. https://doi.org/10.1161/STR.0000000000000357.

Harding, M. M., Kwong, J., Hagler, D., & Reinisch, C. (2023). *Lewis's medical-surgical nursing* (12th ed.). St. Louis, MO: Elsevier.

Herpich, F., & Rincon, F. (2020). Management of acute ischemic stroke. *Critical Care Medicine, 48*(11), 1654–1663. Open Access PMC7540624. https://www.ncbi.nlm.nih.gov/pmc/articles/PMC7540624/.

Jordan, B. L. (2017). Parkinson disease. In: *Primary care: A collaborative practice* (5th ed., pp. 1050–1054). St. Louis, MO: Elsevier.

Kolkin, S. (2017). Guillain-Barre syndrome. In: *Primary care: A collaborative practice* (5th ed., pp. 1028–1030). St. Louis, MO: Elsevier.

Le, N. M., & McCube, K. (2017). Movement disorders and essential tremor. In: *Primary care: A collaborative practice* (5th ed., pp. 1040–1043). St. Louis, MO: Elsevier.

Oliveira, D. C. A. M. D. P., Pereira, C. U., & Freitas, Z. M. D. P. (2016). Prognosis of patients with traumatic brain injury after implementation of a nurse assessment protocol. *The Journal of Neuroscience Nursing: Journal of the American Association of Neuroscience Nurses, 48*(5), 278–284.

O'Neill, D. W., & Jennings, R. M. (2017). Infections of the central nervous system. In: *Primary care: A collaborative practice* (pp. 1037–1040) (5th ed.). St. Louis, MO: Elsevier.

Secore, K. L. (2017). Seizure disorder. In: *Primary care: A collaborative practice* (pp. 1054–1063) (5th ed.). St. Louis, MO: Elsevier.

Seizure Assessment in the Emergency Department. (2017). *Overview, pathophysiology, etiology*. Retrieved from: http://emedicine.medscape.com/article/1609294-overview.

Teran, F., Harper-Kirksey, K., & Jagoda, A. (2015). Clinical decision making in seizures and status epilepticus. *Emergency Medicine Practice, 17*(1), 1–24. quiz 24–25. Retrieved from: https://www.ncbi.nlm.nih.gov/pubmed/25902572.

Varghese, R., Chakrabarty, J., & Menon, G. (2017). Nursing management of adults with severe traumatic brain injury: A narrative review. *Indian Journal of Critical Care Medicine, 21*(10), 684–697. https://doi.org/10.4103/ijccm.IJCCM_233_17.

West, T. A. (Ed.). (2016). *Care of adult and children with seizures and epilepsy: AANN clinical practice guideline series*. Chicago, IL: American Association of Neuroscience Nurses.

Winstein, C. J., Stein, J., Arena, R., Bates, B., Cherney, L. L., Cramer, S. C., Deruyter, F., Eng, J. J., Fisher, B., Harvey, R. L., Lang, C. E., MacKay-Lyons, M., Ottenbacher, K. J., Pugh, S., Reeves, M. J., Richards, W. S., & Zorowitz, R. D. (2016). Guidelines for adult stroke rehabilitation and recovery. *Stroke: A Journal of Cerebral Circulation, 47*(6), e98–e169.

### Section 6: Endocrine Care Plans

Alexander, E. K., Pearce, E. N., Brent, G. A., Brown, R. S., Chen, H., Dosiou, C., Grobman, W. A., Laurberg, P., Lazarus, J. H., Mandel, S. J., Peeters, R. P., & Sullivan, S. (2017). 2017 Guidelines of the American Thyroid Association for the diagnosis and management of thyroid disease during pregnancy and the postpartum. *Thyroid, 27*(3), 315–389.

American Diabetes Association. (2023). *Hypoglycemia (low blood sugar)*. https://www.diabetes.org/healthy-living/medication-treatments/blood-glucose-testing-and-control/hypoglycemia.

American Diabetes Association. (2022). *Standards of medical care in diabetes—2022 abridged for primary care providers.* https://diabetesjournals.org/clinical/article/40/1/10/139035/Standards-of-Medical-Care-in-Diabetes-2022.

Centers for Disease Control and Prevention (CDC). (2022). *Gestational diabetes.* Retrieved from: https://www.cdc.gov/diabetes/basics/gestational.html.

Cuesta, M., & Thompson, C. J. (2016). The syndrome of inappropriate antidiuresis (SIAD): Best practice and research. *Clinical Endocrinology and Metabolism, 30*(2), 175–187.

Fayfman, M., Pasquel, F. J., & Umpierrez, G. E. (2017). Management of hyperglycemic crises: Diabetic ketoacidosis and hyperglycemic hyperosmolar state. *The Medical Clinics of North America, 101*(3), 587–606.

Garber, A. J., Handelsman, Y., Grunberger, G., Einhorn, D., Abrahamson, M. J., Barzilay, J. I., Blonde, L., Bush, M. A., DeFronzo, R. A., Garber, J. R., Garvey, W. T., Hirsch, I. B., Jellinger, P. S., McGill, J. B., Mechanick, J. I., Perrault, L., Rosenblit, P. D., Samson, S., & Umpierrez, G. E. (2017). Consensus statement by the American Association of Clinical Endocrinologists and American College of Endocrinology on the comprehensive type 2 diabetes management algorithm – 2017 executive summary. *Endocrine Practice, 23*(2), 207–238.

Harding, M. M., Kwong, J., Hagler, D., & Reinisch, C. (2023). *Lewis's medical-surgical nursing* (12th ed.). St. Louis, MO: Elsevier.

LeFevre, M. L., & U.S. Preventive Services Task Force. (2015). Screening for thyroid dysfunction: U.S. Preventive Services Task Force recommendation statement. *Annals of Internal Medicine, 162*(9), 641–650.

Lilley, L. L., Rainforth Collins, S., & Snyder, J. S. (2023). *Pharmacology and the nursing process* (10th ed.). St. Louis, MO: Elsevier.

Masri-Iraqi, H., Hirsch, D., Herzberg, D., Lifshitz, A., Tsvetov, G., Benbasset, C., & Shimon, I. (2017). Central diabetes insipidus: Clinical characteristics and long-term course in a large cohort of adults. *Endocrine Practice, 23*(5), 600–604.

Merck Professional Manual. (2022). *Symptoms of inappropriate ADH secretion (SIADH).* Retrieved from: https://www.merckmanuals.com/professional/endocrine-and-metabolic-disorders/electrolyte-disorders/syndrome-of-inappropriate-adh-secretion-siadh.

NIH National Institute of Diabetes and Digestive Kidney Diseases. (2017). *Continuous glucose monitoring.* Retrieved from: https://www.niddk.nih.gov/health-information/diabetes/overview/managing-diabetes/continuous-glucose-monitoring.

Umpierrez, G., & Korytkowski, M. (2016). Diabetic emergencies—Ketoacidosis, hyperglycaemic hyperosmolar state and hypoglycaemia. *Nature Reviews. Endocrinology, 12*(4), 222–232.

Verbalis, J. G. (2016). Disorders of water balance. In K. Skorecki, G. M. Chertow, & P. A. Marsden (Eds.), *Brenner & Rector's the kidney* (Vol. 1, 10th ed., pp. 460–510). Philadelphia, PA: Elsevier.

Wang, S., Li, D., Ni, M., Jia, W., Zhang, Q., He, J., & Jia, G. (2017). Clinical predictors of diabetes insipidus after transcranial surgery for pituitary adenoma. *World Neurosurgery, 101*, 1–10.

## Section 7: Gastrointestinal Care Plans

Barnes, E. L., Raffals, L., Long, M. D., Syal, G., Kayal, M., Ananthakrishnan, A., Cohen, B., Pekow, J., Deepak, P., Colombel, J., Herfarth, H. H., & Sandler, R. S. (2020). Disease and treatment patterns among patients with pouch-related conditions in a cohort of large tertiary care inflammatory bowel disease centers in the United States. *Crohn's & Colitis, 360*(2), 3. https://doi.org/10.1093/crocol/otaa039.

Blank-Reid, C. (2017). Abdominal trauma: Dealing with the damage, ED insider. *Nursing, 37*(4), 4–11.

Cadagan, M. (2022). *Appendicitis—The eponymous examination.* Life in the Fastlane. https://litfl.com/appendicitis-eponyms/.

Colwell, J. C., McNichol, L., & Boarini, J. (2017). North America wound, ostomy, and continence and enterostomal therapy nurses current ostomy care practice related to peristomal skin issues. *Journal of Wound, Ostomy, and Continence Nursing, 44*(3), 257–261.

Craig, S. (2017). *Appendicitis.* MedScape. Retrieved from: http://emedicine.medscape.com/article/773895-overview.

Dubinsky, M., & Rosh, J. (March 18 and 19, 2016). *Course directors: Great debates and updates in inflammatory bowel disease conference.* San Francisco, CA: Imedex, LLCC.

Fang, S., Kraft, C S., Dhere, T., Srinivasan, J., Begley, B., Weinstein, D., & Shaffer, V. O. (2016). Successful treatment of chronic pouchitis utilizing fecal microbiota transplantation (FMT): A case report. *International Journal of Colorectal Disease, 31*(5), 1093–1094.

Harding, M. M., Kwong, J., Hagler, D., & Reinisch, C. (2023). *Lewis's medical-surgical nursing* (12th ed.). St. Louis, MO: Elsevier.

Kennedy, P., Wagner, M., Castéra, L., Hong, C. W., Johnson, C. L., Sirlin, C. B., & Taouli, B. (2018). Quantitative elastography methods in liver disease: Current evidence and future directions. *Radiology, 286*(3), 738–763. https://doi.org/10.1148/radiol.2018170601.

Kistangari, G., Lopez, R., & Shen, B. (2017). Frequency and risk factors of *Clostridium difficile* infection in hospitalized patients with pouchitis: A population-based study. *Inflammatory Bowel Diseases, 23*(4), 661–671.

Levine, J. S., & Burakoff, R. (2016). Inflammatory bowel disease: Medical considerations. In N. J. Greenberger, R. S. Blumberg, & R. Burakoff (Eds.), *Current diagnosis & treatment: Gastroenterology, hepatology, & endoscopy* (3rd ed.). New York: McGraw Hill Education.

McPhee, S. J., & Papadakis, M. A. (2016). *Current medical diagnosis & treatment* (55th ed.). Stanford, CT: Appleton & Lange.

Nordqvist, C. (2017, April 25). Appendicitis: Signs, symptoms, and treatment. *Medical News Today.* Retrieved from: http://www.medicalnewstoday.com/articles/158806.php.

Prinz, A., Colwell, J. C., Cross, H. H., Mantel, J., Perkins, J., & Walker, C. A. (2015). Discharge planning for a patient with a new ostomy: Best practice for clinicians. *Journal of Wound, Ostomy, and Continence Nursing, 42*(1), 79–82.

Young, M., & Dhruv, M. (2021). *Percutaneous transhepatic cholangiogram.* Bethesda, MD: NIH National Library of Medicine. https://www.ncbi.nlm.nih.gov/books/NBK493190/.

## Section 8: Hematologic Care Plans

Arepally, G. M. (2017). Heparin-induced thrombocytopenia. *Blood, 129*, 2864–2872.

Cooper, N. (2017). State of the art: How I manage immune thrombocytopenia. *British Journal of Haematology, 177*, 39–54.

Fraenkel, P. G. (2017). Anemia of inflammation a review. *Medical Clinical of North America, 101*, 285–296.

Gerds, A. T., & Dao, K. H. (2017). Polycythemia vera management and challenges in the community health setting. *Oncology, 92*, 179–189.

Harding, M. M., Kwong, J., Hagler, D., & Reinisch, C. (2023). *Lewis's medical-surgical nursing* (12th ed.). St. Louis, MO: Elsevier.

Kaushansky, K., Lichtman, M., Prchal, J., Levi, M., Burns, L., & Linch, D. C. (2022). *Williams manual of hematology* (10th ed.). New York: McGraw-Hill.

Pagana, K. D., & Pagana, T. J. (2018). *Mosby's manual of diagnostic and laboratory tests* (7th ed.). St. Louis, MO: Elsevier Mosby.

Parnes, A., & Ravi, A. (2016). Polycythemia and thrombocytosis. *Primary Care: Clinics in Office Practice, 43*, 589–605.

Squizzato, A., Hunt, B. J., Kinasewitz, G. T., Cate, H. T., Thachil, J., Levi, M., Vicente, V., D'Angelo, A., & Di Nisio, M. (2016). Supportive management strategies for disseminated intravascular coagulation: An international consensus. *Journal of Thrombosis and Haemostasis*, *115*, 896–904.

Wolfe, L. (2016). Ruxolitinib in myelofibrosis and polycythemia vera. *Journal of the Advanced Practitioner in Oncology*, 436–444.

### Section 9: Musculoskeletal Care Plans

Arthritis Foundation. (n.d.). *Arthritis Today drug guide*. Retrieved from: http://www.arthritis.org/living-with-arthritis/treatments/medication/drug-guide/.

Dunkin, M. A. (n.d.). *Lab test guide*. Retrieved from: http://www.arthritis.org/living-with-arthritis/tools-resources/lab-test-guide/index.php.

Harding, M. M., Kwong, J., Hagler, D., & Reinisch, C. (2023). *Lewis's medical-surgical nursing* (12th ed.). St. Louis, MO: Elsevier.

National Osteoporosis Foundation. (n.d). *What is osteoporosis and what causes it?* Retrieved from: www.nof.org/patients/what-is-osteoporosis/.

NIH National Library of Medicine. (n.d.). *Musculoskeletal disorders*. https://www.ncbi.nlm.nih.gov/books/NBK559512/

### Section 10: Special Needs Care Plans

Berríos-Torres, S. I., Umscheid, C. A., Bratzler, D. W., Leas, B., Stone, E. C., Kelz, R. R., Reinke, C. E., Morgan, S., Solomkin, J. S., Mazuski, J. E., Dellinger, P., Itani, K. M. F., Berbari, E. F., Segreti, J., Parvizi, J., Blanchard, J., Allen, G., Kluytmans, J. J. W., Donlan, R., & Schecter, W. P. Healthcare Infection Control Practices Advisory Committee. (2017). Centers for Disease Control and Prevention guideline for the prevention of surgical site infection. *JAMA Surgery*, *152*(8), 784–791. Retrieved from: https://www.scribd.com/document/367755381/CDC-Berrios-Torres-S-Et-Al-Prevention-Guideline-for-the-Prevention-of-Surgical-Site-Infection-2017#.

Braden Scale II: Predicting pressure injuries (n.d.). Retrieved from: http://www.bradenscale.com.

Centers for Disease Control and Prevention. (2017). *About adult BMI*. Retrieved from: https://www.cdc.gov.healthyyweight/assessing/bmi/adult/index.html.

Centers for Disease Control and Prevention. (2021). *HIV in the United States and dependent areas*. Retrieved from: https://www.cdc.gov/hiv/statistics/overview/ataglance.html.

Delmore, B., Cohen, J. M., O'Neill, D., Chu, A., Pham, V., & Chiu, E. (2017). Reducing postsurgical wound complications: A critical review. *Advances in Skin and Wound Care*, *30*(6), 272–286.

McClave, S., Taylor, B. E., Martindale, R. G., Warren, M. M., Johnson, D. R., Braunschweig, C., McCarthy, M. S., Davanos, E., Rice, T. W., Cresci, G. A, Gervasio, J. M., Sacks, G. S., Roberts, P. R., & Compher, C. (2016). Guidelines for the provision and assessment of nutrition support therapy in the adult critically ill patient. Society of Critical Care Medicine (SCCM) and American Society for Parenteral and Enteral Nutrition (A.S.P.E.N.). *Journal of Parenteral and Enteral Nutrition*, *40*(1), 159–211.

National Institute of Health: National Heart, Lung, and Blood Institute. (1998). *Table IV-2, classification of overweight and obesity by BMI, waist circumference and associated disease risk*. Retrieved from: https://www.ncbi.nlm.nih.gov/books/NBK2004/table/A242/.

National Pressure Ulcer Advisory Panel. (2016). *NPUAP pressure injury stages*. Retrieved from: http://www.npuap.org/resources/educational-and-clinical-resources/npuap-pressure-injury-stages/.

Stotts, N. A. (2016). Wound infection: Diagnosis and management. In R. A. Bryant & D. P. Nix (Eds.), *Acute & chronic wounds* (5th ed.). St. Louis, MO: Elsevier. https://musculoskeletalkey.com/wound-infection-diagnosis-and-management/.

Thompson, M. A., Horberg, M. A., Agwu, A. L., Colasanti, J. A., Jain, M. K., Short, W. R., Singh, T., & Aberg, J. A. (2020). Primary care guidance for persons with human immunodeficiency virus: 2020 update by the HIV Medicine Association of the Infectious Diseases Society of America. *Clinical Infectious Diseases*, *73*(11), e3572–e3605. https://doi.org/10.1093/cid/ciaa1391.

US Department of Health and Human Services. (2017). *Taking HIV medicine to stay healthy and prevent transmission*. Retrieved from: https://www.hiv.gov/tasp/.

US Department of Health and Human Services. (2018). *AIDS info: Offering information on HIV/AIDS treatment, prevention, and research*. Retrieved from: https://aidsinfo.nih.gov/guidelines.

US Department of Health and Human Services. *HIV basics*. Retrieved from: https://www.hiv.gov/hiv-basics/overview/about-hiv-and-aids/what-are-hiv-and-aids/.

US Department of Health and Human Services Panel on Antiretroviral Guidelines for Adults and Adolescents. (2018). *Guidelines for the use of antiretroviral agents in adults and adolescents living with HIV*. Retrieved from: https://aidsinfo.nih.gov/contentfiles/lvguidelines/adultandadolescentgl.pdf.

## Part II:  Pediatric Nursing Care Plans
### 77. Asthma

American Pharmacists Association. (2021). *Lexicomp: Pediatric & neonatal dosage handbook* (28th ed.). Riverwoods, IL: Wolters Kluwer.

Centers for Disease Control and Prevention. (2022a). *Most recent asthma data, 2020*. https://www.cdc.gov/asthma/Most_recent_national_asthma_data.htm.

Centers for Disease Control and Prevention. (2022b). *AsthmaStats: Uncontrolled asthma among children with current asthma, 2018-2020*. https://www.cdc.gov/asthma/asthma_stats/uncontrolled-asthma-children-2018-2020.htm.

National Heart, Lung, and Blood Institute. (2020). *2020 Focused updates to the asthma management guidelines: A report from the National Asthma Education and Prevention Program Coordinating Committee Expert Panel Working Group. NIH Publication No. 20-HL-8140, Dec 2020*. https://www.nhlbi.nih.gov/resources/2020-focused-updates-asthma-management-guidelines.

National Institute of Health. (2022). *News Release: Scientists find racial and ethnic disparities in use of pediatric acute asthma care*. https://www.nih.gov/news-events/news-releases/scientists-find-racial-ethnic-disparities-use-pediatric-acute-asthma-care.

### 78. Attention-Deficit Hyperactivity Disorder

American Academy of Pediatrics. (2019). Clinical practice guidelines for diagnosis, evaluation, and treatment of attention-deficit/hyperactivity disorder in children and adolescents. *Pediatrics*, *144*(4), e20192528. https://doi.org/10.1542/peds.2019-2528. or https://pediatrics.aappublications.org/content/144/4/e20192528.

American Psychiatric Association. (2013). *Diagnostic and statistical manual of mental disorders* (5th ed.). Washington, DC: APA.

American Pharmacists Association. (2021). *Lexicomp: Pediatric & neonatal dosage handbook* (28th ed.). Riverwoods, IL: Wolters Kluwer.

Bitsko, R. H., Claussen, A. H., Lichtein, J., Black, L. I., Jones, S. E., Danielson, M. L., Hoenig, J. M., Davis Jack, S. P., Brody, D. J., Gyawali, S., Maenner, M. J., Warner, M., Holland, K. M., Perou, R., Crosby, A. E., Blumberg, S. J., Avenevoli, S., Kaminski, J. W., & Ghandour, R. M. (2022). Mental health surveillance among children – United States, 2013–2019. *MMWR Supplements*, *71*(Suppl. 2), 1–42. https://doi.org/10.15585/mmwr.su7102a1.

CHADD. (n.d.a.). *About ADHD – Overview.* https://chadd.org/about-adhd/overview.

CHADD. (n.d.b.). *Managing medications.* https://chadd.org/for-parents/managing-medication/.

Gephart, H. (2020). The diagnosis of attention-deficit/hyperactivity disorder (ADHDA). *Contemporary Pediatrics, 37*(10), 20–22. https://www.comtemporarypediatrics.com/view/the-dx-of-adhd.

Gray, L., Loring, W., Malow, B., Pryor, E., Turner-Henson, A., & Rice, M. (2020). Do parent ADHD symptoms influence sleep and sleep habits of children with ADHD? A pilot study. *Pediatric Nursing, 46*(1), 18–25. www.pediatricnursing.net/issues/20janfeb/.

Hockenberry, M., Wilson, D., & Rodgers, C. (2019). *Wong's nursing care of infants and children* (11th ed.). St. Louis, MO: Elsevier.

Wesemann, D., & Van Cleve, S. (2018). ADHD: From childhood to adulthood. *The Nurse Practitioner, 43*(3), 8–15. www.tnpj.com.

Zhao, X., Page, T., Altszuler, A., Pelham, 3rd., W., Kipp, H., Gnagy, E., Coxe, S., Schatz, N., & Zimlich, R. (2019). ADHD guideline update: What's new, what's changed. *Contemporary Pediatrics, 37*(2), 20–21. www.Contemporarypediatrics.com.

## 79. Bronchiolitis

American Academy of Pediatrics. (2014). Clinical practice guidelines: The diagnosis, management, & prevention of bronchiolitis. *Pediatrics, 134*(5), e1474–e1502. https://doi.org/10.1542/peds.2014-2742.

American Academy of Pediatrics. (2022). *Updated guidance: Use of Palivizumab prophylaxis to prevent hospitalization from severe respiratory syncytial virus infection during the 2022-2023 RSV season.* https://www.aap.org/en/pages/2019-novel-coronavirus-covid-19-infections/clinical-guidance/interim-guidance-for-use-of-palivizumab-prophylaxis-to-prevent-hospitalization/

Centers for Disease Control and Prevention. (n.d.a). *RSV transmission.* https://www.cdc.gov/rsv/about/transmission.html.

Centers for Disease Control and Prevention. (n.d.b). *RSV: Research and surveillance.* https://www.cdc.gov/rsv/research/index.html?CDC_AA_efVal=https%3A%2F%2Fwww.cdc.gov%2Frsv%2Fresearch%2Fus-surveillance.html.

Centers for Disease Control and Prevention. (2022). RSV in infants and children. https://www.cdc.gov/rsv/downloads/RSV-in-Infants-and-Young-Children.pdf.

Freeman, J., & Bajaj, L. (2022). Is home oxygen therapy an alternative to hospitalization for bronchiolitis? *Pediatrics, 150*(4), e2022058042. https://doi.org/10.1542/peds.2022-058042.

Hockenberry, M., Wilson, D., & Rodgers, C. (2019). *Wong's nursing care of infants and children* (11th ed.). St. Louis, MO: Elsevier.

Justice, N. A., Le, J. K., & Bronchiolitis. (2022). *StatPearls [Internet].* Treasure Island, FL: StatPearls Publishing. Available from: https://www.ncbi.nlm.nih.gov/books/NBK441959/.

## 80. Burns

Consumer Products Safety Commission. (2022). *2021 Fireworks annual report: Firework-related deaths, emergency department-treated injuries, and enforcements activities during 2019.* https://www.cpsc.gov/s3fs-public/2021-Fireworks-Annual-Report.pdf.

Hockenberry, M., Wilson, D., & Rodgers, C. (2019). *Wong's nursing care of infants and children* (11th ed.). St. Louis, MO: Elsevier.

Loos, M., Almekinders, C., Heymans, M., de Vries, A., & Bakx, R. (2020). Incidence and characteristics of non-accidental burns in children: A systemic review. *Burns, 46*(6), 1243–1253. https://doi.org/10.1016/j.burns.2020.01.008.

Merk & Co., Inc. (2023). Figures (A) Rule of nines (for adults) and (B) Lund-Browder chart (for children) for estimating extent of burns. *MSD manual professional version.* https://www.msdmanuals.com/professional/multimedia/figure/a-rule-of-nines-for-adults-and-b-lund-browder-chart-for-children-for-estimating-extent-of-burns.

Safe Kids Worldwide. (2022). *Fast facts: Fire and burn injury among children in 2020 (2022 Update).* https://www.safekids.org/sites/default/files/documents/2022_fire_and_burn_fast_facts.pdf.

## 81. Child Abuse and Neglect

Centers for Disease Control and Prevention. (n.d.a). *Preventing child sexual abuse.* https://www.cdc.gov/violenceprevention/pdf/can/factsheetCSA508.pdf.

Centers for Disease Control and Prevention. (n.d.b). *Preventing abusive head trauma.* https://www.cdc.gov/violenceprevention/childabuseandneglect/Abusive-Head-Trauma.html.

Centers for Disease Control and Prevention. (2022). *Preventing child abuse & neglect.* https://www.cdc.gov/violenceprevention/childabuseandneglect/fastfact.html.

Keeshin, B., Forkey, H. C., Fouras, G., & MacMillan, H. L. (2020). Children exposed to maltreatment: Assessment and the role of psychotropic medication. *Pediatrics, 145*(2). https://publications.aap.org/pediatrics/article/145/2/e20193751/68268/Children-Exposed-to-Maltreatment-Assessment-and.

Narang, S., Fingarson, A., Lukefahr, J., & Council on Child Abuse and Neglect. (2020). Abusive head trauma in infants and children. *Pediatrics, 145*(4), e20200203. https://doi.org/10.1542/peds.2020-0203.

National Center for Missing and Exploited Children (NCMEC). (n.d.). *The issues – Child sex trafficking.* https://www.missingkids.org/theissues/trafficking.

U.S. Department of Health & Human Services, Administration for Children and Families, Administration on Children, Youth and Families, Children's Bureau. (2022). *Child maltreatment 2020.* https://www.acf.hhs.gov/cb/data-research/child-treatment.

## 82. Cystic Fibrosis

American Pharmacists Association (APhA). (2021). *Lexicomp: Pediatric & neonatal dosage handbook* (28th ed.). Riverwoods, IL: Wolters Kluwer.

Altaf, R., & Parmar, M. (2022). Dornase alfa. In: StatPearls [Internet]. Treasure Island, FL: StatPearls Publishing. Available from: https://www.ncbi.nlm.nih.gov/books/NBK556018/.

Castellani, C., Duff. A., Bell, S., Heijerman, H., Munck, A., Ratjen, F., Sermet-Gaudelus, I., Southern, K., Barben, J., Flume, P., Hodkova, P., Kashirskaya, N., Kirszenbaum, M., Madge, S., Oxley, H., Plant, B., Schwarzenberg, S., Smyth, A., Taccetti, G., ... Drevinek, P. (2018). ECFS best practice guidelines: The 2018 revision. *Journal of Cystic Fibrosis, 17*(2), 153–178. https://www.cysticfibrosisjournal.com/article/S1569-1993(18)30029-8/fulltext.

Cystic Fibrosis Foundation. (n.d.a). *Cystic fibrosis-related diabetes.* https://www.cff.org/managing-cf/cystic-fibrosis-related-diabetes.

Cystic Fibrosis Foundation. (n.d.b). *Lung transplant today.* https://www.cff.org/managing-cf/lung-transplant-today.

Cystic Fibrosis Foundation. (n.d.c). *Testing and genetics.* https://www.cff.org/intro-cf#testing-and-genetics.

Cystic Fibrosis Foundation. (n.d.d.). *Medications.* https://www.cff.org/managing-cf/medications.

Cystic Fibrosis Foundation. (n.d.e). *Inflammation.* https://cff.org/research-clinical-trials/research-inflammation.

Cystic Fibrosis Foundation. (2022). *Patient registry, Annual data report 2021.* https://www.cff.org/medical-professionals/patient-registry.

Dickinson, K., & Paranjape, S. (2020). Triple combination therapy for cystic fibrosis is here! *Contemporary Peds Journal, 37*(2), 17–19.

Hermann, E., & Davis, S. (2019). Motivational interviewing for providers managing adolescents with cystic fibrosis. *Pediatric Nursing, 45*(6), 267–272. www.pediatricnursing.net/issues/19novdec/abstr.1.html.

Hockenberry, M., Wilson, D., & Rodgers, C. (2019). *Wong's nursing care of infants and children* (11th ed.). St. Louis, MO: Elsevier.

Reed, A., & Shores, D. (2020). Gastrointestinal manifestations of cystic fibrosis: A primer for pediatricians. *Contemporary PEDS Journal, 37*(2), 12–16. https://www.contemporarypediatrics.com/view/gastrointestinal-manifestations-cystic-fibrosis-primer-pediatricians.

Rosenstein, B. (2022). Cystic fibrosis. *MSD manual.* Retrieved from: https://www.msdmanuals.com/professional/pediatrics/cystic-fibrosis-cf/cystic-fibrosis#

Stewart, J. (2022). *Orkambi FDA approval history.* Retrieved from: https://www.drugs.com/history/orkambi.html.

## 83. Diabetes Mellitus in Children

American Diabetes Association. (2023). Children and adolescents: Standards of medical care in diabetes—2023. *Diabetes Care 2023, 46*(Suppl. 1), S230–S253. https://doi.org/10.2337/dc23-S014.

Arslanian, S., Bacha, F., Grey, M., Marcus, M., White, N., & Zeitler, P. (2018). Evaluation and management of youth-onset type 2 diabetes: A position statement by the American Diabetes Association. *Diabetes Care, 41*(12), 2648–2668. https://doi.org/10.2337/dci18-0052.

Centers for Disease Control and Prevention. (2022a). *National diabetes statistics report: Prevalence of diagnosed diabetes.* https://www.cdc.gov/diabetes/data/statistics-report/diagnosed-diabetes.html.

Centers for Disease Control and Prevention. (2022b). *Rates of new diagnosed cases of type 1 and type 2 diabetes continue to rise among children, teens.*

Centers for Disease Control and Prevention. (2022c). *Childhood obesity facts.* https://www.cdc.gov/obesity/data/childhood.html.

Cystic Fibrosis Foundation. (2022). *Patient registry, annual data report 2021.* https://www.cff.org/medical-professionals/patient-registry.

Endocrinology Network Staff. (2022). *In pediatric type 1 diabetes, race, income, insurance remain barriers to insulin pump use.* https://www.contemporarypediatrics.com/view/pediatric-type1-diabetes-barriers-insulin-pump-use.

Frohnert, B., & Chase, H. P. (2022). *Understanding diabetes: A handbook for people of all ages who are living with diabetes* (15th ed.). Aurora, CO: Children's Diabetes Foundation of America.

Glaser, N. (2022). *Diabetic ketoacidosis in children: Cerebral edema injury (cerebral edema).* Update.com. https://update.com/contents/diabetic-ketoacidosis-in-children-cerebral-injury-cerebral-edema.

Gonzalez, K., & Freysteinson, W. (2019). Youth-onset type 2 diabetes mellitus in primary practice: A review. *Pediatric Nursing, 45*(6), 293–296. 288www.pediatricnursing.net/issues/19novdec/.

Krewson, C. (2023). *Diabetes in youth expected to rise in coming decades.* Retrieved from: https://www.contemporarypediatrics.com/view/diabetes-in-youth-expected-to-rise-in-coming-decades.

Lipman, T., & Hawkes, C. (2021). Racial and socioeconomic disparities in pediatric type 1 diabetes: Time for a paradigm shift in approach. *Diabetes Care, 44*(1), 14–16. https://doi.org/10.2337/dci20-0048 or https://care.diabetesjournals.org/content/diacare/44/1/14.full.pdf.

Perng, W., Conway, R., Mayer-Davis, E., & Dabelea, D. (2023). Youth-onset type 2 diabetes: The epidemiology of an awakening epidemic. *Diabetes Care, 46*(3), 490–499. https://doi.org/10.2337/dci22-0046.

## 84. Fractures in Children

Bradwisch, S., Smith, E., Mooney, C., & Scaccia, D. (2020). Obesity in children and adolescents: an overview. *Nursing, 50*(11), 60–66. https://doi.org/10.1097/01.NURSE.0000718908.20119.01.

Freedman, M., & Farber, J. (2020). *PPI exposure increases risk of fractures.* Contemporary Pediatrics. https://www.contemporarypediatrics.com/view/ppi-exposure-increases-risk-fractures.

Fryar, C., Carroll, M., & Afful, J. (2020). *Prevalence of overweight, obesity, and severe obesity among children and adolescents aged 2-19 years: United States, 1963-1965 through 2017-2018.* Health E-States. https://www.cdc.gov/nchs/data/hestat/obesity-child-17-18/obesity-child.htm.

Rui, P., Ashman, A., & Akinseye, A. (2019). Emergency department visits for injuries sustained during sports and recreational activities by patients aged 5-24 years, 2010-2016. *National Health Statics Report, 133*, 1–14.

U.S. Department of Health and Human Services, Centers for Disease Control and Prevention, National Center for Health Statistics. (2019). *Emergency department visits for injuries sustained during sports and recreational activities by patients aged 5–24 years, 2010–2016.* Retrieved from: https://www.cdc.gov/nchs/data/nhsr/nhsr133-508.pdf.

Worchester, S. (2020). PPI use linked with increased fracture risk in children *JAMA Pediatrics.* Retrieved from: https://www.mdedge.com/pediatrics/article/219097/gastroenterology/ppi-use-linked-increased-fracture-risk-children?sso=truesso.

## 85. Gastroenteritis

Bellandi, D. (2022). Rotavirus leads global diarrhea hospitalizations among young children. *JAMA, 28*(15), 1490. https://jamanetwork.com/journals/jama/article-abstract/2797408.

Centers for Disease Control and Prevention. (n.d.). *Burden of Norovirus illness in the U.S.* https://www.cdc.gov/norovirus/trends-outbreaks/burden-US.html.

Cochran, W. (2022). *Overview of gastrointestinal disorders in neonates and infants. Merck manual professional version.* Retrieved from: https://www.merckmanuals.com/professional/pediatrics/gastrointestinal-disorders-in-neonates-and-infants/overview-of-gastrointestinal-disorders-in-neonates-and-infants?query=gastroteritis%20in%20children.

Gotfried, J. (2022). *Overview of gastroenteritis. Merck manual professional version.* Retrieved from: https://www.merckmanuals.com/professional/gastrointestinal-disorders/gastroenteritis/overview-of-gastroenteritis?query=gastroenteritis.

## 86. Otitis Media

American Pharmacists Association. (2021). *Lexicomp: Pediatric & neonatal dosage handbook* (28th ed.). Riverwoods, IL: Wolters Kluwer.

Gaddey, H., Wright, M., & Nelson, T. (2019). Otitis media: Rapid evidence review. *American Family Physician, 100*(6), 350–356. https://www.aafp.org/afp/2019/0915/p350.html.

Hester, M. (2019). *Latest guidance on diagnosing, treating acute otitis media.* Contemporary Pediatrics. https://www.contemporarypediatrics.com/view/latest-guidance-diagnosing-treating-acute-otitis-media.

Hockenberry, M., Wilson, D., & Rodgers, C. (2019). *Wong's nursing care of infants and children* (11th ed.). St. Louis, MO: Elsevier.

Levin, L. (2022). *Prescribing antibiotics for kids in 2022.* Contemporary Pediatrics. Retrieved from: https://www.contemporarypediatrics.com/view/prescribing-antibiotics-for-kids-in-2022.

Lieberthal, A., Carroll, A., Chonmaitree, T., Ganiats, T., Hoberman, A., Jackson, M., Joffe, M., Miller, D., Rosenfeld, R., Sevilla, X., Schwartz, R., Thomas, P., & Tunkel, D. (2013). Clinical Practice Guideline: The diagnosis and management of acute otitis media. *Pediatrics, 131*(3), e964–e999. https://doi.org/10.1542/peds.2012-3488.https://pediatrics.aappublications.org/content/131/3/e964.full.

Miyamoto, R. (2022). *Otitis media (secretory)*. https://www.merckmanuals.com/professional/ear,-nose,-and-throat-disorders/middle-ear-and-tympanic-membrane-disorders/otitis-media-secretory#top.

Rosenfeld, R. M., Shin, J. J., Schwartz, S. R., Coggins, R., Gagnon, L., Hackell, J. M., Hoelting, D., Hunter, L. L., Kummer, A. W., Payne, S. C., Poe, D. S., Veling, M., Vila, P. M., Walsh, S. A., & Corrigan, M. D. (2016). Clinical practice guideline: Otitis media with effusion executive summary (update). *Otolaryngology – Head and Neck Surgery, 154*(2), 201–214. https://doi.org/10.1177/0194599815624407.

### 87. Poisoning

Gummin, D., Mowry, J., Beuhler, M., Spyker, D., Rivers, L., Feldman, R., Brown, K., Nathaniel, P. T., Bronstein, A., & Weber, J. (2022). 2021 Annual report of the National Poison Data System© (NPDS) from America's Poison Centers: 39th annual report. *Clinical Toxicology, 60*(12), 1381–1643. https://doi.org/10.1080/15563650.2022.2132768.

Mayans, L. (2019). Lead poisoning in children. *American Family Physician, 100*(1), 24–30. https://www.aafp.org/afp/2019/0701/afp20190701p24.pdf.

Park-Lee, E., Ren, C., Cooper, M., Cornelius, M., Jamal, A., & Cullen, K. A. (2022). Tobacco product use among middle and high school students—United States. *Morbidity and Mortality Weekly Report, 71*, 1429–1435. https://doi.org/10.15585/mmwr.mm7145a1. https://www.cdc.gov/mmwr/volumes/71/wr/pdfs/mm7145a1-H.pdf.

Patterson, M., Williams-Jones, P., & Lewis, T. (2020). Consequences of the vaping epidemic on adolescents. *Nursing, 50*(7), 30–37. www.Nursing2020.com.

Quail, M. T. (2020). Nicotine toxicity: Protecting children from e-cigarette exposure. *Nursing, 50*(1), 44–48. www.Nursing2020.com.

Ruckart, P., Jones, R., Courtney, J., LeBlanc, T., Jackson, W., Karwowski, M., Cheng, P., Allwood, P., Svendsen, E., & Breysse, P. (2021). Update of the Blood Lead Reference Value—United States, 2021. *Morbidity and Mortality Weekly Report, 70*(43), 1509–1512. https://doi.org/10.15585/mmwr.mm7043a4.

Safe Kids Worldwide. (2020a). *Fast facts: Poisoning among children ages 0-14 in 2018 (fact sheet)*. https://www.safekids.org/sites/default/files/documents/2020_fast_facts_poisonings_v1.pdf.

Safe Kids Worldwide. (2020b). *Keeping kids safe around medicine: Insights and implications*. https://www.safekids.org/sites/default/files/medicine_safety_study_2020-v14.pdf.

Stone, E., Tormohlen, K., McCourt, A., Schmid, I., Stuart, E., Davis, C., Bicket, M., & McGinty, E. (2022). Association between state opioid prescribing cap laws and receipt of opioid prescriptions among children and adolescents. *JAMA Health Forum, 3*(8), e222461. https://doi.org/10.1001/jamahealthforum.2022.2461.

Substance Abuse and Mental Health Services Administration. (2022). *Key substance use and mental health indicators in the United States: Results from the 2021 National Survey on Drug Use and Health (HHS Publication No. PEP22-07-01-005, NSDUH Series H-57)*. Center for Behavioral Health Statistics and Quality, Substance Abuse and Mental Health Services Administration. https://www.samhsa.gov/data/report/2021-nsduh-annual-national-report.

### 88. Sickle Cell Pain Crisis

American Pharmacists Association. (2021). *Lexicomp: Pediatric & neonatal dosage handbook* (28th ed.). Riverwoods, IL: Wolters Kluwer.

Centers for Disease Control and Prevention. (2019). *Get screened to know your sickle cell status (fact sheet)*. https://www.cdc.gov/ncbddd/sicklecell/documents/Factsheet_scicklecell_status.pdf.

Centers for Disease Control and Prevention. (2022). *Data and statistics on sickle cell disease*. https://www.cdc.gov/ncbddd/sicklecell/data.html.

Federal Drug Administration. (2021). FDA approves drug to treat sickle cell disease in patients 4 up to 11 years. *FDA News Release*. https://www.fda.gov/drugs/news-events-human-drugs/fda-approves-drug-treat-sickle-cell-disease-patients-aged-4-11-years.

Hockenberry, M., Wilson, D., & Rodgers, C. (2019). *Wong's nursing care of infants and children* (11th ed.). St. Louis, MO: Elsevier.

Kamat, D. (2020). *Hemoglobinopathies and sickle cell disease*. American Academy of Pediatrics. Pediatric Care Online. https://doi.org/10.1542/aap.ppcqr.396170.

Payne, A., Mehal, J., Chapman, C., Haberling, D., Richardson, L., Bean, C., & Hooper, W. (2020). Trends in sickle cell disease–related mortality in the United States, 1979 to 2017. *Annals of Emergency Medicine, 76*(3S), S28–36. https://pubmed.ncbi.nlm.nih.gov/32928459/.

Phillips, S. (2021). Caring for an individual with sickle cell disease: Nurses play a pivotal role in ensuring optimal care. *American Nurse, 16*(6), 6–10. https://www.myamericannurse.com/caring-for-sickle-cell-disease/.

Wood, K. (2022). *Measurement of gas exchange*. https://www.merckmanuals.com/professional/pulmonary-disorders/tests-of-pulmonary-function-pft/measurement-of-gas-exchange#.

### Part III:   Maternity Nursing Care Plans

American Academy of Pediatrics. (2022). *Policy statement: Breastfeeding and the use of human milk*. American Academy of Pediatrics. Available from: https://publications.aap.org/pediatrics/article/150/1/e2022057988/188347/Policy-Statement-Breastfeeding-and-the-Use-of?autologincheck=redirected.

American College of Obstetrics and Gynecology. (2016). Management of preterm labor. In: *ACOG practice bulletin, 171*. Washington, DC.

American College of Obstetrics and Gynecology. (2017). Postpartum hemorrhage. In: *ACOG practice bulletin, 183*. Washington, DC.

American College of Obstetrics and Gynecology. (2018a). Gestational diabetes. In: *ACOG practice bulletin, 190*. Washington, DC.

American College of Obstetrics and Gynecology. (2018b). Nausea and vomiting in pregnancy. In: *ACOG practice bulletin, 189*. Washington, DC.

American College of Obstetrics and Gynecology. (2019). Chronic hypertension in pregnancy. In: *ACOG practice bulletin, 203*. Washington, DC.

American College of Obstetrics and Gynecology. (2020a). Gestational hypertension and preeclampsia. In: *ACOG practice bulletin, 222*. Washington, DC.

American College of Obstetrics and Gynecology. (2020b). Premature rupture of membranes. In: *ACOG practice bulletin, 217*. Washington, DC.

American Diabetes Association. (2022). Management of diabetes in pregnancy: Standards of medical care in diabetes. *Diabetes Care, 45*(Suppl. 1), S232–S243. https://doi.org/10.2337/dc22-S015.

Centers for Disease Control and Prevention. (2022). *Gestational diabetes*. Available from: https://www.cdc.gov/diabetes/basics/gestational.html.

Danyao, J., Rich-Edwards, J. W., Chen, C., Huang, Y., Wang, Y., Xu, X., Lu, J. Liu, Z., Gao, Y., Zou, S., Zhou, H., & Wang, H. Gestational diabetes mellitus: Predictive value of fetal growth measurements by ultrasonography at 22–24 weeks: A retrospective cohort study of medical records. *Nutrients, 12*(12), 3645. doi: 10.3390/nu12123645. Available from: https://www.ncbi.nlm.nih.gov/pmc/articles/PMC7760346/.

Dean, C. (2014). Helping women prepare for hyperemesis gravidarum. *British Journal of Midwifery, 22*(12), 847–852.

Eastern Virginia Medical School. (2023). *Screening for diabetes in pregnancy.* Norfolk, VA: Eastern Virginia Medical School (EVMS).

Ehsanipoor, R. M., & Satin, A. J. (2023). *Labor: Overview of normal and abnormal progression.* Waltham, MA: UpToDate. Available at: https://www.uptodate.com/contents/labor-overview-of-normal-and-abnormal-progression.

Jennings, L. K., & Mahdy, H. (2022). Hyperemesis gravidarum. In: *StatPearls [Internet].* Treasure Island, FL: StatPearls Publishing. Retrieved from: https://www.ncbi.nlm.nih.gov/books/NBK532917/.

Massachusetts General Hospital. (2020). *HBAIC can underestimate maternal glycemia during pregnancy.* Available from: https://advances.massgeneral.org/obgyn/journal.aspx?id=1557.

National Institute for Health and Care Excellence (NICE). (2020). *Diabetes in pregnancy: Management from preconception to the postnatal period.* Retrieved from: https://www.nice.org.uk/guidance/ng3.

Office of Women's Health & U.S. Department Health & Human Services. (2019). *Making the decision to breastfeed.* https://www.womenshealth.gov/breastfeeding/making-decision-breastfeed.

Perry, S. E., & Hockenberry, M. J. (2018). *Maternal child nursing care* (6th ed.). St. Louis, MO: Elsevier.

Rowe, H. E., Felkins, K., Cooper, S. D., & Hale, T. W. (2014). Transfer of linezolid into breast milk. *Journal of Human Lactation, 30*(4), 410–412. https://doi.org/10.1177/0890334414546045.

Shapiro-Mendoza, C. K., Barfield, W. D., Henderson, Z., James, A., Howse, J. L., Iskander, J., & Thorpe, P. G. (2016). CDC grand rounds: Public health strategies to prevent preterm birth. *Morbidity and Mortality Weekly Report, 65*(32), 826–830.

Son, M., Grobman, W. A., Ayala, N. K., & Miller, E. S. (2016). A universal mid-trimester transvaginal cervical length screening program and its associated reduced preterm birth rate. *American Journal of Obstetrics and Gynecology, 214*(3), 365.e1–365.e5.

Spencer, J. (2019). *Patient education: Common breastfeeding problems (beyond the basics).* Waltham, MA: UpToDate. Available from: https://www.uptodate.com/contents/common-breastfeeding-problems-beyond-the-basics?topicRef=1196&source=see_link.

## Part IV: Psychiatric–Mental Health Nursing Care Plans

Alzheimer's Association. (2022). *2022 Alzheimer's disease facts and figures.* https://www.alz.org/media/Documents/alzheimers-facts-and-figures.pdf.

American Psychiatric Association. (2013). *Diagnostic and statistical manual of mental disorders* (5th ed.). Washington, DC: APA.

Centers for Disease Control and Prevention (CDC). (2019). *What is dementia?* Retrieved from: https://www.ncbi.nlm.nih.gov/books/NBK538266/.

de Souza, C., Vedana, K. G., Mercedes, B. P., & Miasso A. I. (2013). Bipolar disorder and medication: Adherence, patients' knowledge and serum monitoring of lithium carbonate. *Revista Latino-Americana de Enfermagem, 21*(2), 624–631.

Halter, M. J. (2017). *Varcarolis' foundations of psychiatric-mental health nursing: A clinical approach* (8th ed.). St. Louis, MO: Elsevier.

Keltner, N. L., & Steele, D. (2019). *Psychiatric nursing* (7th ed.). St. Louis, MO: Elsevier.

Mace, N. L., & Rabins, P. V. (2017). *The 36-hour day: A family guide to caring for people who have Alzheimer's disease, related dementias and memory loss* (6th ed.). New York: Warner Books.

Marcantonio, E. R., Ngo, L. H., O'Connor, M., Jones, R. N., Crane, P. K., Metzger, E. D., & Inouye, S. K. (2014). 3-D CAM: Derivation and validation of a 3-minute diagnostic interview for CAM-defined delirium: A cross-sectional diagnostic test study. *Annals of Internal Medicine, 161*(8), 554–561. https://doi.org/10.7326/M14-0865. Available from https://pubmed.ncbi.nlm.nih.gov/25329203/.

# Index